NURSING NOW
Today's Issues, Tomorrow's Trends
9th Edition

NURSING NOW

Today's Issues, Tomorrow's Trends

9th Edition

Joseph T. Catalano, PhD, RN

Program Consultant, Author,
Professor Emeritus
East Central University
Ada, Oklahoma

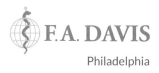

F.A. DAVIS

Philadelphia

F. A. Davis Company
1915 Arch Street
Philadelphia, PA 19103
www.fadavis.com

Printed in the United States of America

Last digit indicates print number: 10 9 8 7 6 5 4 3 2 1

Sponsoring Editor: Haleahy Craven
Manager of Project and eProject Management: Catherine Carroll
Content Project Manager: Amanda Minutola
Design & Illustrations Manager: Carolyn O'Brien

As new scientific information becomes available through basic and clinical research, recommended treatments and drug therapies undergo changes. The author(s) and publisher have done everything possible to make this book accurate, up to date, and in accord with accepted standards at the time of publication. The author(s), editors, and publisher are not responsible for errors or omissions or for consequences from application of the book, and make no warranty, expressed or implied, in regard to the contents of the book. Any practice described in this book should be applied by the reader in accordance with professional standards of care used in regard to the unique circumstances that may apply in each situation. The reader is advised always to check product information (package inserts) for changes and new information regarding dose and contraindications before administering any drug. Caution is especially urged when using new or infrequently ordered drugs.

Library of Congress Control Number: 2023941576

Dedication

To all those dedicated nurses and nursing students who provided heroic care for the severely ill patients during the COVID-19 pandemic, some of whom became infected with the virus yet returned to work after recovering and some of whom gave their lives for others. Jesus said: "There is no greater love than to lay down one's life for a friend" (John 15:13). During the pandemic, nurses laid down their lives for complete strangers. How great is that love?

Preface

Global pandemics. Warming oceans. Rising sea levels. Devastating hurricanes. Empowered autocrats. Mass shootings. Racial inequity. Nursing shortages. No wonder some believe that the apocalypse is near! Yet, through it all, nurses and the profession of nursing have had the courage and strength to survive it with kindness and caring. If you are a nurse or a nursing student, you should be proud to belong to a profession that has been recognized as one of key health-care workers who placed their lives on the line to stop one of the deadliest pandemics in history. It brings to mind Florence Nightingale working during the Crimean War with inadequate supplies, understaffed, and in a potentially lethal environment. Since Nightingale's time, nurses have been the first line of defense; however, in today's health-care system, it is taking place in a much bigger scale.

Despite challenging situations, nurses are ideal for confronting and resolving overwhelming conditions because of their firsthand experience working directly with patients. By tapping into that experience, they face a wide variety of health-care threats head-on. Although nurses were called heroes during the pandemic, most of them really did not like the title. They preferred to say they were just doing their jobs. Because of the pandemic and the fallout it produced, the landscape of health-care has changed. In response to these changes, the profession continues to progress and evolve at a rapid rate, and the ninth edition of *Nursing Now: Today's Issues, Tomorrow's Trends* is keeping up with that progress. This edition includes loads of new information and the latest topics! We believe you will be more than delighted with the new version of this text, as it remains truly unique among issues and trends books. The ninth edition retains the eye-appealing and user-friendly format that made previous editions so popular along with instructor and student resources found online.

The rapid rate of transformations in health care continues to affect the profession of nursing. Demographic shifts have become the new norm as the baby boomer bulge reaches the heart of retirement age and new immigrants gain political savvy and power. The Affordable Care Act (ACA) is back on track with the advent of a new administration, offering even more health-care options for the poor and disadvantaged. Nurses, as always, lead the vanguard in directing and managing the many new evolutions in health care. Quality of care rather than the number of services provided is becoming the outcome measure for the provision of health care at all levels.

We have been listening to our readers and have incorporated a number of their suggestions into the text. One of the chapters that nursing students will find most useful is the chapter on the NCLEX licensure examination, now call the Next Generation NCLEX (NGN). The National Council of State Boards of Nursing (NCSBN), the people who write the examination, have developed a whole new set of questions that are based on the Clinical Judgment Measurement Model (CJMM), which measures how you make valid decisions, incorporate your clinical judgment, and use your decision-making skills. These questions are more complicated than the former types of questions seen on the exam. This chapter gives you a chance to see what these questions look like and how to answer them before you sit down at the NGN computer.

Graduates from today's nursing programs have opportunities for professional practice and advancement that could only be dreamed of a few years ago.

Yes, the demands are many, but the rewards are great. Today's nursing students must learn more, do more, and be more. Students entering nursing schools today come from increasingly diverse cultural, personal, and educational backgrounds. They must master a tremendous amount of information and learn a wide variety of skills so that they can pass the licensure examination and become highly skilled registered nurses.

The ninth edition of *Nursing Now* offers students a starting point to influence the future of health care in the United States. With the tremendous nursing shortage looming around the corner, there will be a need not only for more nurses but for more nurses with knowledge and skills to practice in an increasingly complicated and crowded health-care system. We are very excited about the revised text and believe its quality and content meet the high standards demanded by our readers.

The book's primary purpose remains the same as in past editions. It presents an overview and synthesis of the important issues and trends that are basic to the development of professional nursing and that affect nursing both today and into the future. Our readers tell us that the book can be used both at the beginning of the student's educational process as an introduction to nursing course and toward the end of the process as an issues and trends course. Some instructors even use it throughout their programs, incorporating chapters as the content is reflected in their course presentations. Nursing students remain the primary intended audience for *Nursing Now*. However, practicing nurses have reported there is a sufficiently wide range of current issues and topics covered in enough depth to be useful for their practice.

A dichotomy that nurses face on a daily basis is the ability to hold on to key unchanging principles while working in a constantly changing environment. Simply stated, a nurse's ability to adapt to changes in the health-care system while remaining focused on providing high-quality care is the basis for a successful professional practice. The only way that nurses will be able to effectively practice their profession in a demanding health-care system is to remain firmly rooted in those values and beliefs that have always served as their source of strength. Even more so than in the past, nurses need to look to each other for the inspiration and strength that allow them to succeed. Professional organizations still serve as the single-most powerful force for nurses, and membership in professional organizations is becoming increasingly important.

It is our belief that this book will help future nurses become familiar with the important issues and trends that affect the profession and health care. The nursing profession needs highly skilled nurses who can be civil, teach, do research, solve complicated patient problems, provide highly skilled care, obtain advanced degrees, and influence the political realm that so affects all aspects of health care. The leaders of the profession will come from those students who have a clear understanding of what it means to be a professional nurse and are willing to invest effort in attaining their goals.

Joseph T. Catalano, PhD, RN

Acknowledgments

I would like to acknowledge the many nurse authors who have published informative and enlightening books and articles during the pandemic years. Your works express the commitment and dedication to the pledge we take as RNs to provide the most informed and skilled care possible.

Reviewers

Civita M. Allard, MS, RN
Professor
Utica University
Utica, New York

Mary C. Carrico, MSN, RN
Professor, Nursing
West Kentucky Community and Technical College
Paducah, Kentucky

Tiffany Cox, RN, PhD, MPPA, CNE
Instructor/Course Coordinator
Holmes Community College
Ridgeland, Mississippi

Amy K. Cutler, RN, MSN
Adjunct Professor
Dominican University
Orangeburg, New York

Kimberly A. Davies, DNP, RN, COI
Director of Nursing Programs
State University of New York, College of Technology
  at Canton
Canton, New York

Catherine M. DeChance, PhD, RN
Faculty Program Director
Excelsior College, Utica College, SUNY Empire
Albany, New York

M. Kathleen Dwinnells, PhD, RN, CNS, CNE, NE-BC
Professor
Kent State University at Trumbull
Warren, Ohio

Sabrina Ehmke, DNP, RNC-OB, NPD-BC
Assistant Professor
Minnesota State University, Mankato
Mankato, Minnesota

Janet Lee Harper, BSN, MN, RN
Nursing Instructor
Riverside College of Health Careers
Newport News, Virginia

Anne Hustad, DNP, RN, CNE
Professor, Department Head of Nursing
Olney Central College
Olney, Illinois

Nancy Lada, RN, MScN
Professor, Nursing Studies
Algonquin College
Ottawa, Ontario

Vanessa Ervin Lyons, PhD, RN, CNOR, CNE
Access and Success Coordinator
West Kentucky Community and Technical College
Paducah, Kentucky

Barbara J. Miller, MSN, RN
Professor of Nursing
Community College of Allegheny County
Pittsburgh, Pennsylvania

Elizabeth S. Miller, DNP, RN, CCM, CMSRN
Assistant Dean of Nursing
Arizona College of Nursing - Falls Church, VA
Falls Church, Virginia

Contributors

Mary Abadie, RN, MSN, CPNP
Assistant Professor, Retired
Southern University and A&M College
School of Nursing
Baton Rouge, Louisiana

Tonia Aiken, RN, BSN, JD
President and CEO
Aiken Development Group
New Orleans, Louisiana

Sharon M. Bator, PhD, RN
Associate Professor
Denver College of Nursing
Denver, Colorado

Barbara Bellfield, MS, RNP-C, RN
Family Nurse Practitioner
Oxnard, California

Cynthia Bienemy, RN, PhD
Director, Louisiana Center for Nursing
Louisiana State Board of Nursing
Baton Rouge, Louisiana

Doris Brown, MEd, MS, RN, CNS
Public Health Executive Director
Robert Wood Johnson Nurse Fellow 2006–2009
Baton Rouge, Louisiana

Sandra Brown, RN, DNS, APRN, FNP-BC CNE, ANEF, FAAN
Professor
Director of NP and DNP Program
Woman's Hospital Endowed Professor
Southern University and A&M College
School of Nursing
Baton Rouge, Louisiana

Joseph T. Catalano, PhD, RN
Program Consultant, Author
Professor Emeritus
Ada, Oklahoma

Sarah T. Catalano
Graphic Designer
The Chickasaw Nation
Ada, Oklahoma

Captain Dr. Leah S. Cullins, MSN, APRN, FNP-BC
Assistant Professor
Southern University School of Nursing
Undergraduate & Graduate Programs
Southern University and A&M College
Baton Rouge, Louisiana

Lydia DeSantis, RN, PhD, FAAN
University of Miami
School of Nursing
Miami, Florida

Joan Anny Ellis, RN, PhD
Faculty Development Specialist
Chamberlain University
Baton Rouge, Louisiana

Mary Evans, JD, RN
Colorado Springs, Colorado

Betty L. Fomby-White, RN, PhD
Professor, Retired
Southern University and A&M College
School of Nursing
Baton Rouge, Louisiana

Donna Gentile O'Donnell, RN, MSN
Health Research Advisory Committee
Thomas Jefferson University
Philadelphia, Pennsylvania

Anita H. Hansberry, RN, MS
Assistant Professor, Retired
Southern University and A&M College
School of Nursing
Baton Rouge, Louisiana

Nicole Harder, RN, BN, MPA
Coordinator, Learning Laboratories
Helen Glass Centre for Nursing
Faculty of Nursing
University of Manitoba
Winnipeg, Manitoba, Canada

Jacqueline J. Hill, RN, PhD
Associate Professor
Interim Dean of College of Nursing and
    Allied Health
Southern University A&M College
Baton Rouge, Louisiana

Edna Hull, PhD, RN, CNE
Associate Professor, Retired
Southern University and A&M College,
    Baton Rouge
Associate Editor
Teaching and Learning in Nursing
Senior Contributing Faculty Member
Walden University

Sharon W. Hutchinson, PhD, MN, RN, CNE
Chair and Professor
Dillard University
College of Nursing
New Orleans, Louisiana

Cindy Krentz, DNP, RN
Assistant Professor of Nursing
Assistant Chairperson of the Nursing Department
Metropolitan State College
Denver, Colorado

Joyce Miller, BSN, CPE, CCM
Medical Case Manager
KorVel Corporation
Baton Rouge, Louisiana

Karen Mills, MSN, RN
Nurse Family Partnership State Nurse Consultant, Retired
Louisiana Office of Public Health
Baton Rouge, Louisiana

Roberta Mowdy, PMHNP-BC
Chickasaw Nation Division of Health
Ada, Oklahoma

Joseph Mulinari, PhD, RN
College of Mount Saint Vincent
Department of Nursing
Bronx, New York

Linda Newcomer, RN, MSN
Instructor
East Central University
Department of Nursing
Ada, Oklahoma

Robert Newcomer, PhD
Assistant Professor, Retired
East Central University
Ada, Oklahoma

Janet S. Rami, RN, PhD
Professor Emeritus
Southern University and A&M College
School of Nursing
Baton Rouge, Louisiana

Diane Ream, DNP, RN
Director of Finance and Operations
All for Kids Home Health
Denver, Colorado

Viki Saidleman, MS, RN
Instructor
East Central University
Department of Nursing
Ada, Oklahoma

Nancy C. Sharts-Hopko, RN, PhD, FAAN
Professor
Villanova University
Villanova, Pennsylvania

Enrica K. Singleton, RN, PhD
Professor, Retired
Southern University and A&M College
School of Nursing
Baton Rouge, Louisiana

Wanda Raby Spurlock, DNS, RN, BC, CNS, FNGNA
Associate Professor
Southern University and A&M College
School of Nursing
Baton Rouge, Louisiana

Melissa Stewart DNS, RN, CPE
Assistant Professor
National Consultant, Health Literacy Theorist
Louisiana State University, Eunice
Baton Rouge, Louisiana

Cheryl Taylor, PhD, RN, FAAN
Chairperson, Graduate Nursing Programs (MSN, PhD, & DNP)
Associate Professor of Nursing
Southern University and A&M College
Jewel L. and James Prestage Endowed Professor/ Kellogg
National League for Nursing Consultant to the National Student Nurses' Association
FNINR, National Institute of Nursing Research, Ambassador
Jonas Scholar Mentor
Baton Rouge, Louisiana

Karen Tomajan, MS, RN, NEA-BC
Director of the Nursing Practice/Magnet Program
John Muir Health Center
American Nurses Credentialing Center Magnet Recognition Program
Concord, California

Esperanza Villanueva-Joyce, EdD, CNS, RN
Nurse Consultant

Karen Lynn Webb, MSN, RN, PhDc
Assistant Professor
Appalachian State University
Department of Nursing
Boone, North Carolina

Kathleen Mary Young, RN, C, MA
Instructor
Western Michigan University
Kalamazoo, Michigan

Contents

Available Online Only

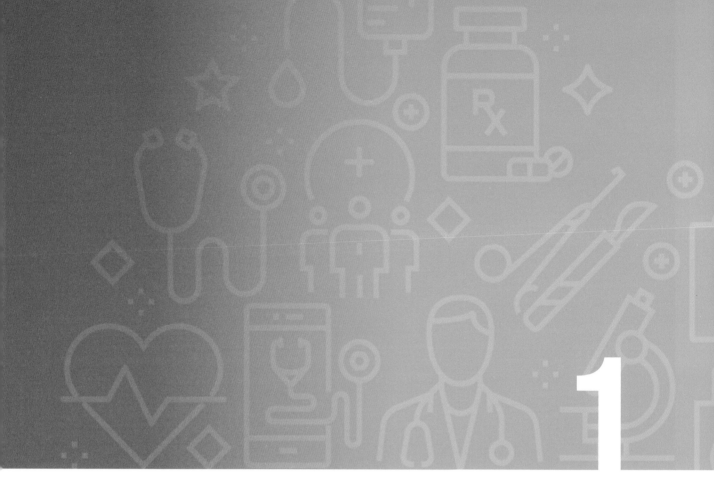

1

The Evolution
of Nursing

The Development of a Profession

Joseph T. Catalano

1

Learning Objectives

After completing this chapter, the reader will be able to:

- Define the terms *position*, *job*, *occupation*, and *profession*
- Compare the three approaches to defining a profession
- Analyze those traits defining a profession that nursing has attained
- Evaluate why nursing has failed to attain some of the traits that define a profession
- Correlate the concept of power with its important characteristics

INTRODUCTION

Since the time of Florence Nightingale, each generation of nurses, in its own way, has fostered the movement to professionalize the image of nurses and nursing. The struggle to change the status of nurses—from that of female domestic servants to one of high-level health-care providers who base their **protocols** on scientific principles—has been a primary goal of nursing leaders for many years.

At some levels in nursing, the question of **professionalism** takes on immense significance.[1] However, to the busy **staff nurse**—who is trying to allocate patient assignments for a shift, distribute the medications at 9 a.m. to patients, and supervise two aides, a **licensed practical nurse (LPN)** or licensed vocational nurse (LVN), and a nursing student—the issue may not seem very significant at all.

Indeed, when nurses were first developing their identity separately from that of physicians, there was no thought about their being part of a **profession**.[2] Over the years, as the scope of practice and responsibilities have expanded, nurses have been recognized as the professionals they are.

This chapter presents some of the current thoughts concerning nursing as a profession.

WHAT IS A PROFESSION?

For almost 100 years, experts in social science have been attempting to develop a foolproof approach to determining what constitutes a profession but with only minimal success.[3]

What Do You Think?

Do you care if nursing is considered a profession? How will it affect the way you practice nursing?

Of the many researchers and theorists who have attempted to identify the traits that define a profession, Abraham Flexner, Elizabeth Bixler, and Eliza Pavalko are most widely accepted as the leaders in the field. These three social scientists have determined that the following common characteristics are important:

- High intellectual level
- High level of individual responsibility and **accountability**
- Specialized body of knowledge
- Knowledge that can be learned in institutions of higher education
- Public service and altruistic activities
- Public service valued over financial gain
- Relatively high degree of **autonomy** and independence of practice
- Well-organized and strong organization representing the members of the profession and controlling the quality of practice
- A **code of ethics** that guides the members of the profession in their practice
- Strong professional identity and commitment to the development of the profession
- Demonstration of professional competency and possession of a legally recognized license[4]

NURSING AS A PROFESSION

How does nursing compare with other professions when measured against these widely accepted professional traits? The profession of nursing meets most of the criteria but falls short in a few areas.

High Intellectual Level

In the early stages of the development of nursing practice, this criterion did not apply. Florence Nightingale raised the bar for education, and graduates of her school were considered to be highly educated compared with other women of that time. However, by today's standards, most of the tasks performed by these early nurses are generally considered to be menial and routine.

As health care has advanced and made great strides in technology, pharmacology, and all branches of the physical sciences, a high level of intellectual functioning is required for even relatively simple nursing tasks, such as taking a patient's temperature or blood pressure using automated equipment. On a daily basis, nurses use **assessment** skills and knowledge, have the ability to reason, and make routine judgments based on patients' conditions. Without a doubt, professional nurses must function at a high intellectual level.

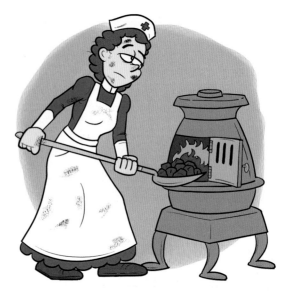

Patient comfort during the Civil War had additional meaning.

High Level of Individual Responsibility and Accountability

Not too long ago, a nurse was rarely, if ever, named as a **defendant** in a malpractice suit. In general, the public did not view nurses as having enough knowledge to be held accountable for errors that were made in patient care. This is not the case in the health-care system today. Nurses are often the primary, and frequently the only, defendants named when errors are made that result in injury to the patient. Nurses must be accountable and demonstrate a high level of individual responsibility for the care and services they provide.[5]

The concept of accountability has legal, ethical, and professional implications that include accepting responsibility for actions taken to provide **patient** care and for the consequences of actions that are not performed. Nurses can no longer state that "the physician told me to do it" as a method of avoiding responsibility for their actions.

Specialized Body of Knowledge

Most early nursing skills were based either on traditional ways of doing things or on the intuitive knowledge of the individual nurse. As nursing developed into an identifiable, separate discipline, a specialized body of knowledge called *nursing science* was compiled through the research efforts of nurses with advanced educational degrees.[3] As the body of specialized nursing knowledge continues to grow, it forms a theoretical basis for the **best practices** movement in nursing today. As more nurses obtain advanced degrees, conduct research, and develop philosophies and theories about nursing, this body of knowledge will increase in scope and quantity.

Evidence-Based Practice

In professional nursing today, there is an increasing emphasis on **evidence-based practice (EBP)**.[6] Almost all of the currently used nursing theories address this issue in some way. Simply stated, EBP is the practice of nursing in which interventions are based on data from research that demonstrates that they are appropriate and successful. It involves a systematic process of uncovering, evaluating, and using information from research as the basis for making decisions about and providing patient care.[7] Many nursing practices and interventions of the past were performed merely because they had always been done that way (accustomed practice) or because of deductions from physiological or pathophysiological information. Patients have become more adept in the use of information technology, and as a result, many now have a higher level of knowledge about their illnesses than in the past. This increase in knowledge levels, use of online health-care information, and demand for higher-quality care constitute one of the driving forces behind the use of EBP.

The development of information technology has made EBP in nursing a reality. In the past, nurses relied primarily on units within their own facilities for information about the success of treatments, decisions about health care, and outcomes for patients. Nursing education now requires nursing students to perform research for papers and projects so that by the time of graduation, they feel comfortable accessing a wide range of the best and most current information through electronic sources. Of course, one of the key limiting factors of EBP is the quality of the information on which the practice is based. Evaluating the quality of information on the Internet can be difficult at times.

> *Evidence-based practice is the practice of nursing in which interventions are based on data from research that demonstrates that they are appropriate and successful.*

The first step in developing an EBP is to identify exactly what the intervention is supposed to accomplish. Once the goal or patient outcome is identified, the nurse needs to evaluate current practices to determine whether they are delivering the desired patient outcomes. If the current practices are unsuccessful or if the nurse feels they can be more efficient with fewer complications, research sources need to be collected. These can be from published journal articles (either electronic or hard copy) and from presentations at research or practice conferences, which often present the most current information. Then a plan should be developed to implement the new findings. This process can be applied to changing policy and procedures or developing training programs for facility staff. The most current research data should always be used when initiating new practices or modifying old ones. For more information on EBP, go to Chapter 24.

Public Service and Altruistic Activities

When defining nursing, almost all major nursing theorists include a statement that refers to a goal of helping patients adapt to illness and achieve their highest level of functioning. The public (variously referred to as consumers, **clients**, patients, individuals, or humans) is the focal point of all nursing models and nursing practice. The public-service function of nursing has always been recognized and acknowledged by society's willingness to continue to educate nurses in public, tax-supported institutions and in private schools. In addition, nursing has been viewed universally as an altruistic profession composed of selfless individuals who place the lives and well-being of their patients above their personal safety. In the earliest days, dedicated nurses provided care for victims of deadly plagues with little regard for their own welfare. Today, nurses are found in remote and often hostile areas, providing care for the sick and dying, working 12-hour shifts, being on call, and working rotating shifts.

Few individuals enter nursing to become rich and famous. It is likely that those who do so for these reasons quickly become disappointed and move on

Issues Now

Web Sites: Friends or Foes?

Have a paper or report to do for class? Need information on pheochromocytoma, Smith-Strang disease, Kawasaki disease? No problem, look it up on the Web, right? Well, yes and no. Without question, there is a tremendous amount of information about almost any subject available just a few mouse clicks away. But the bigger question is, how good is that information? Anyone can post almost anything online these days, and there are no organizations or agencies that oversee or review the information for quality, accuracy, or objectivity. So how are you supposed to know what is credible and what is not? Although there is no foolproof method for determining the quality of any given Web site, some telltale markers can point you in the right direction when you are rating the quality of the information you seek.

Marker 1: Peer Review

All major professional journals have a peer-review process that requires any manuscript submitted to be reviewed by two or three professionals who are considered experts, or at least knowledgeable, in the subject matter. Peer review is one of the key elements in ensuring the accuracy of the information in the manuscript. When considering an Internet source, look for a clear statement of the source of the information and how that information is reviewed. If the information is from an established source, such as a recognized professional journal, it has been peer reviewed and has a higher degree of accuracy. Examine the format and writing style of the document. If it seems to be very choppy, or if the style, tone, or point of view changes throughout the article, it is an indication that it was not well edited and probably was not peer reviewed. Use the information with caution.

Marker 2: Author Credentials

The author's name, titles, and credentials should be listed. Be cautious if no author or publisher is listed. Of course, anyone can use another person's name as the author, but it is relatively easy to cross-check authors' names through other databases, such as those found in libraries. Before accepting the information as gospel, it is probably worth looking up the author to see what other articles or books they have written. Another key to determining author credentials is to establish who owns the Web site. In general, personal Web pages are less likely to contain authoritative information. You can also look at the last three letters in the domain name of the Web address. Domain names ending in *.gov, .org*, or *.edu* tend to have higher-quality information. Also, see whether the information has a copyright. If the information is copyrighted, the person felt strongly enough about the content to make sure that others could not use it as their original information.

Marker 3: Prejudice and Bias

Although there is almost always a small degree of prejudice and *bias* in all written material, most legitimate authors strive to be as objective as possible. Many times, if you read a document with a critical eye, you can discern obvious prejudicial viewpoints. See if the author has a vested interest in the content of the document. For example, an article about the effects of tobacco use on the respiratory system written by a scientist who was hired by a tobacco company would probably have a decidedly different viewpoint than an article written by a scientist who was employed by the National Health Information Center. See if contact information is provided by the author and who the sponsor or publisher of the document is. If these are not provided, be suspicious about the information.

Issues Now (continued)

Marker 4: Timeliness

Of course, all of us want the most recent information we can find and sometimes mistakenly assume that because it is on the Web, it is new. Some information on the Internet has been around since Tim Berners-Lee invented the World Wide Web in 1989, so some of the material can be very outdated. See if you can determine when the site was last updated and how extensively the information was revised. It is also a good practice to look to other sources (e.g., Internet, journals, books) to compare the material for currency. Many Web sites have links to related information. If those links have messages such as "Page not found" or "Link no longer available," be extremely cautious with the information. Good links should connect you to other reliable sites.

Marker 5: Presentation

Although the old saying is that you can't judge a book by its cover, experienced Internet users can often tell a lot about a Web site by its presentation. Some look well developed and professional, and others look very amateurish. There is no guarantee that the slick-looking Web sites are better, but it is one factor to consider in the overall evaluation of the information you are seeking. Take a look at the graphics. They should be balanced with the text and help explain or demonstrate information in the text. If the graphics seem to be just decorative, it should raise a red flag about the content of the site. Some sites use a compressed format that requires special programs such as Adobe Acrobat to view them. If you do not have access to these programs, the information in the site is unusable. Move on to the next site.

In summary, the Internet can be a valuable source of information about a wide variety of subjects. However, each source needs to be evaluated carefully. Following the five markers discussed here will place you on the path to deciding the quality of the information presented in any Web site.

Sources: *McClennan Community College Library Services, December 1, 2022, Searching the Internet: Evaluating Web sources, https://mclennan.libguides .com/searchingInternet/searchInternet/eval; E. Peterson, A guide to using the Internet for research, May 20, 2020, https://elizabethjpeterson.com/2020/05/ using-the-internet-for-research-guide.*

to other career fields. Although the pay scale has increased tremendously since the early 2000s, nursing, at best, provides a middle-class income. Surveys among students entering nursing programs continue to indicate that the primary reason for wishing to become a nurse is to "help others" or "make a difference" in someone's life and to have "job security." Rarely do these beginning students include "to make a lot of money" as their motivation.[7]

The altruistic attitude of nurses was well evidenced during the COVID-19 pandemic. The dedication and selflessness of nurses harkened back to earlier epidemics and even to the time of Florence Nightingale, when nurses were always on the front lines providing lifesaving care and comfort to those who needed it most.

During the COVID-19 pandemic, dedicated nurses continued to go to work day after day and give high-quality care in the war against this deadly virus. Ironically, the first and most deadly year of the pandemic was also the Year of the Nurse, which received little attention in the media. It proved to be a year in which professional nurses were doing what they always do best: facing dangerous conditions to serve the public in all settings and to provide comfort to those who were dying without family nearby.

COVID-19 changed health care in ways that rocked the whole system and all its members, including nurses. We now take for granted social distancing, no personal contact, masks at all times, universal testing, and other workplace safety measures that initially seemed burdensome and unrealistic. The pandemic also forced health-care institutions to take a new look at staffing ratios that not only provide high-quality patient care but also are necessary for the safety of nurses and other staff. In the face of shortages of equipment and staff, innovative nurses used their problem-solving skills to overcome intimidating odds.

As the pandemic begins to resolve into an endemic event, we can begin to calculate its true cost. Although nurses and health care seem to have brought the virus and its variants under control, the cost in dollars and human life was tremendous. Ideally, moving forward, everyone who might be touched by similar outbreaks will be better prepared to identify them early on and muster the forces to defeat them.[8]

Well-Organized and Strong Representation

Professional organizations represent the members of the profession and control the quality of professional practice. The National League for Nursing (NLN) and the American Nurses Association (ANA) are the two major national organizations that represent nursing in today's health-care system. The NLN is primarily responsible for regulating the quality of the educational programs that prepare nurses for the practice of nursing, whereas the ANA is more concerned with the quality of nursing practice in the daily health-care setting. These and other organizations are discussed in more detail in Chapter 5.

Both of these groups are well organized, but neither can be considered powerful when compared with other professional organizations, such as the American Hospital Association (AHA), the American Medical Association (AMA), or the American Bar Association (ABA). One reason for their lack of strength is that fewer than 10 percent of all nurses in the United States are members of any professional organization at the national level. Many nurses do belong to specialty organizations that represent a specific area of practice, but these lack sufficient political power to produce changes in health-care laws and policies at the national level.

Nurses' Code of Ethics

Nursing has several codes of ethics that are used to guide nursing practice. The ANA Code of Ethics for Nurses, the most widely used in the United States, was first published in 1971 and was updated in 1985, 2001, and 2015. The current 2015 ANA Code of Ethics, while maintaining the integrity found in earlier versions, is now more relevant to current health-care and nursing practices.[9] This code of ethics is recognized by other professions as a standard with which others are compared. The nurses' code of ethics and its implications are discussed in greater detail in Chapter 6.

Competency and Professional License

Nurses must pass a national licensure examination to demonstrate that they are qualified to practice nursing. Nurses are allowed to practice only after passing this examination. The granting of a nursing **license** is a legal activity conducted by the individual state under the **regulations** contained in that state's nurse practice act.

WHEN NURSING FALLS SHORT OF THE CRITERIA

Professional Identity and Development

Many new nurses face the issue of whether nursing, to them, is a job or a career. A job is commonly considered to be a group of positions, tasks, or assignments similar in nature and level of skill, that can be carried out by one or more individuals. There is relatively little commitment to a job, and many individuals move from one job to another with little regard to the long-term outcomes. A career, in contrast, is usually viewed as a person's major lifework, which progresses and develops as the person grows older. Careers and professions have many of the same characteristics, including a formal education, full-time employment, requirement for lifelong learning, and a dedication to what is being achieved. Although an increasing number of nurses view nursing as their life's work, many still treat nursing more as a job.

MEMBERS OF THE HEALTH-CARE TEAM

The health-care delivery system employs large numbers of diagnosticians, technicians, direct care **providers**, administrators, and support staff (Table 1.1). It is estimated that more than 300 job titles are used to describe health-care workers. Among these are nurses, nurse practitioners, physicians, physician assistants, social workers, physical therapists, occupational therapists, respiratory therapists, clinical psychologists, and pharmacists. All of these individuals provide services that are essential to daily operation of the health-care delivery system in this country.

Table 1.1   Other Key Health-Care Team Members

Title	Credential	Practice
Physician (MD)	License—medical	Medical—limited only by specialization; some serve as primary care providers.
Physician (DO)	License—osteopath	Medical, with focus on body movement and holistic health—similar to MD. Can serve as primary care providers.
Physician (DC)	License—chiropractor	Limited—focus on spinal column and nervous system. Unable to prescribe medications.
Physician (DPM)	License—podiatry	Limited—foot health. Can prescribe medications, perform foot surgery.
Physician assistant	Certification—no individual license	Practices on physician's license. Practice limited by medical practice act and wishes of supervising physician.
LPN/LVN	License	Nursing—limited; basic nursing practice skills under the direction of a higher-level provider.
Social worker	License	Increasingly important as health care becomes more complex. Resolves financial, housing, psychosocial, and employment problems; does discharge planning and assists patients in transfer between facilities. May serve in case management roles to coordinate services.
Physical therapist	License	Focuses on helping patients maintain or regain the highest level of function possible after strokes, spinal cord injury, arthritis, or residual effects of traumatic accidents. Helps prevent physical decline and regain the ability to groom, eat, and walk through individualized range-of-motion and exercise programs. Therapy occurs in hospitals, clinics, or the community.
Respiratory therapist	License	Strives to restore normal or as near to normal as possible pulmonary functioning by conducting diagnostic tests and administering treatments that have been prescribed by a physician.
Clinical psychologist	License	Helps patients to manage mental health problems. Private practice, clinics.
Pharmacist	License	Distributes prescribed and over-the-counter medications, educates patients, monitors appropriate medication selections, detects interactions and untoward responses in community pharmacies and institutional settings. Valuable resource for nurses.

Of particular importance among this array of health-care workers are various types of nurses: registered nurses, licensed practical (vocational) nurses, nurse practitioners, case managers, and clinical nurse specialists. Each of these requires a different type of educational background, clinical expertise, and, sometimes, professional credentialing. In general, all nurses make valuable contributions within the health-care delivery system. There has been an increased demand for nurses who are educated to deliver care in the community setting and in long-term health-care settings rather than in the hospital. There has also been a need for nurse case managers who are prepared to coordinate care for vulnerable populations requiring costly services over extended periods.[10] Nursing education programs attempt to meet these needs by preparing individuals who can practice independently and autonomously, network, collaborate, and coordinate services. These programs also offer more clinical experiences in rehabilitation, nursing home, and community settings.

What Do You Think?

List and rate several of your recent experiences with the health-care system. In what roles did you observe registered nurses functioning?

Advanced Practice Registered Nurses

For individuals who are unfamiliar with the health-care delivery system, it is sometimes difficult to understand the similarities and differences between nursing titles and roles. This confusion is particularly evident in the case of clinical nurse specialists (CNSs) and nurse practitioners (NPs), who are sometimes collectively referred to as advanced practice registered nurses (APRNs).[11] To become an APRN, a registered nurse must first obtain an advanced degree in nursing. After taking a certification examination, the APRN is then qualified to provide patient care at a higher level, similar to what a family practice physician might perform. They are legally allowed to assess and diagnose patients, independently prescribe medications in most states, order laboratory and other tests, and develop both current and future treatment plans of care. The education of nursing students, other nurses and staff, and patients is an essential element of their roles as APRNs.[12]

The APRN Consensus Model regulates the roles an APRN may choose for their specialization, which often focuses on a specific patient population. These roles are described in the following subsections.

Nurse Practitioner

In general, nurse practitioners (NPs) are prepared to provide direct patient care in primary care settings, focusing on health promotion, illness prevention, early diagnosis, and treatment of common **health** problems. Their educational preparation varies, but in most cases, individuals successfully complete a graduate nurse practitioner program and are certified by the American Nurses Credentialing Center (ANCC) or an appropriate professional nursing organization. Depending on the individual state nurse practice act, NPs have a range of responsibilities for diagnosing diseases and prescribing both treatments and medications.[13] A growing number of states now grant NPs direct third-party reimbursement for their services without a physician.

Certified Nurse Midwife

Certified nurse midwives (CNMs) have similar advanced practice education except that it focuses on the care of pregnant women before, during, and after the birth process. They also have extensive education in the care of newborn infants. Focusing on women's reproductive health, CNMs use a holistic approach to care for the woman's physical and mental health, all aspects of reproduction, the safety and health of both the mother and child, and life-span development.

Certified Nurse Specialist

Certified nurse specialists (CNSs) usually practice in secondary- or tertiary-care settings and focus on care of individuals who are experiencing an acute illness or an exacerbation of a chronic condition. In general, they are prepared at the graduate level and are ANCC certified.[13] These highly skilled practitioners are comfortable working in high-tech environments with seriously ill individuals and their families. Because of the nature of their work, they are excellent health-care educators and physician collaborators. Acting as a mentor, educator, and advocate within their facility, the CNS performs an inimitable function in advanced practice nursing. They encourage and promote the many changes that occur in a facility to improve patient care. They oversee and act as a supervisor for other nurses to ensure that they are using the highest-quality evidence-based care for patients. The CNS may not be providing direct patient care on a unit or throughout the facility, yet their advanced education can help implement and foster changes facility-wide. Attempts have been made to combine the roles of the CNS and NP so that the best qualities of both roles are preserved. The goal of this combination would be to provide high-quality care in a wide array of health-care settings to individuals who have a wide range of health problems. Advocates of this movement include the NLN, the American Association of Colleges of Nursing (AACN), and the ANA. Titling for this new blended role is unconfirmed, and state legislatures may make the final decisions through their licensing laws.[14] As such, titling, educational preparation, and practice privileges will probably vary from one state to another.

Certified Registered Nurse Anesthetist

Unlike the other APRN roles, certified registered nurse anesthetists (CRNAs) have no specific patient population. They administer a wide range of medications that induce sleep and sedation, generally classified as **anesthetics**, to patients in a number of settings but particularly during surgery. Because of the inherent dangers associated with anesthetics and **anesthesia**, CRNAs are responsible for patient safety before, during, and after any procedure in which anesthesia is involved. As with the other APRN roles, CRNAs need to educate families and patients on the aftereffects of medications to make sure the recovery period goes smoothly and the patient receives the best possible care.

Further Specialization for Advanced Practice Nurses

In addition to the patient populations already discussed, APRNs may select from a number of other patient populations as their focus in which to obtain a recognized certification. These specialties include the following:

• Family/individual life span
• Adult–gerontology
• Neonatal
• Pediatrics
• Women's health
• Psychiatric–mental health

APRNs may also choose to remain APRNs without a certified specialty and focus on a patient population or role such as oncology care, orthopedic patients, emergency department, or case management.[14]

Case Managers

One argument for the blended NP–CNS role is the need for case managers who possess the expertise of both levels of preparation. Case managers coordinate services for patients with high-risk or long-term health problems who require access to the full continuum of health-care services. Case managers provide services in various settings, such as acute care facilities, rehabilitation centers, and community agencies. They also work for managed-care companies, insurance companies, and private case-management agencies. Their roles vary according to the circumstances of their employment; however, their overall goal is to coordinate the use of health-care services in the most efficient and cost-effective manner possible.[15]

Case management is the glue that holds health-care services together across practitioners, agencies, funding sources, locations, and time. Titling, educational preparation, and certification of nurse case managers are now available. The ANCC has developed certification eligibility criteria for nurse case managers, and an

examination is available. At this time, case managers can be physicians, social workers, RNs, LPNs, and even well-intentioned laypersons with little health-care education.

EMPOWERMENT IN NURSING

One concern that has plagued nursing, almost from its development as a separate health-care specialty, is the relatively large amount of personal responsibility shouldered by nurses combined with a relatively small amount of control over their practice. This imbalance between authority and responsibility is the source of disempowerment. Even in today's society, with its concerns about equal opportunity, equal pay, and collegial relationships, some nurses still seem uncomfortable with the concepts of power in and control of their practice. Their discomfort may arise from the belief that nursing is a helping and caring profession whose goals are separate from issues of power.

Although power and **empowerment** usually go hand in hand, they are slightly different in concept.[16] While *empowerment* helps the nurse to take action and perform those activities that promote patient care, *power* is associated with control and authority.

> *Depending on the individual state nurse practice act, NPs have a range of responsibilities for diagnosing diseases and prescribing both treatments and medications.*

Historically, nurses were mostly powerless, and previous attempts at gaining power and control over their practice were met with much resistance. Nevertheless, all nurses use an authoritative voice in their daily practice, even if they do not realize it. Nurses can understand the sources of their influence, learn how to increase it, and use it in providing patient care.[17]

The Nature of Power

The term *power* has many meanings. From the standpoint of nursing, power is probably best defined as the ability or capacity to exert influence over another person or group of persons.[16] In other words, power is the ability to get other people to do things even when they do not want to do them. Although power in itself is neither good nor bad, it can be used to produce either good or bad results.

Power is always a two-way street. By its very definition, when power is exerted by one person, another person is affected; that is, the use of power by one person requires that another person give up some of their power. Individuals are always in a state of change, either increasing their power or losing some; the balance of power rarely remains static.

Nurses who are empowered have a strong, positive attitude; are highly motivated; and use that motivation to motivate others on their team. They share their sources of power and raise the satisfaction levels and the quality of care on their unit.[18]

Powerlessness in nurses is almost never a positive attribute. Nurses who lack power are likely to be ineffective in their care and practice. They may lack the ability to respond in crisis situations, may be viewed as lazy, and may create feelings of irritation and frustration in the rest of the team. Internally, they may feel they are failures at their jobs. They are more likely to be unhappy with their profession, to burn out quickly, to feel isolated, and to contribute to poor patient outcomes.[16] To survive, they may use coping mechanisms such as passive-aggressive behavior, negativism, and hostility that can create a toxic work environment for all of the team.[16]

Origins of Power

If power is such an important part of nursing and the practice of nurses, where does it come from? Although there are many sources, some of them would be inappropriate or unacceptable for those in a helping and caring profession. The following list includes some of the more accessible and acceptable sources of power that nurses should consider using in their practice:[16]

- Referent
- Expert
- Reward
- Coercive
- Legitimate
- Collective

Referent Power

The referent source of power depends on establishing and maintaining a close personal relationship with someone. In any close personal relationship, one individual often will do something they would really rather not do because of the relationship. This ability to change the actions of another is an exercise of power.

Nurses often obtain power from this source when they establish and maintain good therapeutic relationships with their patients. Patients take medications, tolerate uncomfortable treatments, and participate in demanding activities that they would likely prefer to avoid because the nurse has good relationships with them. Likewise, nurses who have good collegial relationships with other nurses, departments, and health-care providers are often able to obtain what they want from these individuals or groups in providing care to patients.

Expert Power

The expert source of power derives from the amount of knowledge, skill, or expertise that an individual or group has. This power source is exercised by the individual or group when knowledge, skill, or expertise is either used or withheld in order to influence the behavior of others. Nurses should have at least a minimal amount of this type of power because of their education and experience. It follows logically that increasing the level of nurses' education will, or should, increase this expert power. As nurses attain and remain in positions of power longer, the increased experience also aids the use of expert power. Nurses in advanced practice roles are good examples of those who have expert power. Their additional education and experience provide these nurses with the ability to practice skills at a higher level than nurses prepared at the basic education level.

> *By demonstrating their knowledge of the patient's condition, recent laboratory tests, and other elements that are vital to the patient's recovery, nurses demonstrate their expert power. This knowledge may increase the amount of respect they are given by health-care providers.*

By demonstrating their knowledge of the patient's condition, recent laboratory tests, and other elements that are vital to the patient's recovery, nurses demonstrate their expert power. This knowledge may increase the amount of respect they are given by health-care providers. Nurses access this expert source of power when they use their knowledge to teach, counsel, or motivate patients to follow a plan of care. Nurses can also use expert power when dealing with other health-care providers.

Power of Rewards

The reward source of power depends on the ability of one person to grant another some type of reward for specific behaviors or changes in behavior. The rewards can take on many different forms, including personal favors, promotions, money, expanded privileges, and eradication of punishments. Nurses, in their daily provision of care, can use this source of power to influence patient behavior. For example, a nurse can give a patient extra praise for completing the prescribed range-of-motion exercises. There are many aspects of the daily care of patients over which nurses have a substantial amount of reward power. This reward source of power is also the underlying principle in the process of behavior modification.

Coercive Power

The coercive source of power is the flip side of the reward power source. The ability to reprimand, withhold rewards, and threaten punishment is the key element underlying the coercive source of power. Although nurses do have access to this source of power, it is probably one that they use minimally, if at all. Not only does the use of coercive power destroy therapeutic and personal relationships, but it can also be considered unethical and even illegal in certain situations. Threatening patients with an injection if they do not take their oral medications may motivate

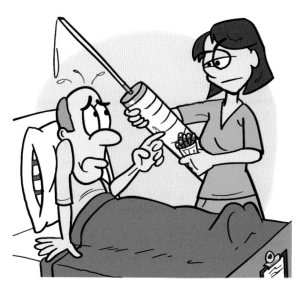

"Take the pill or I'll give you a shot!"

them to take those medications, but it is generally not considered to be a good example of a therapeutic communication technique.

Legitimate Power

The legitimate source of power depends on a legislative or legal act that gives the individual or organization a right to make decisions that they might not otherwise have the authority to make. Most obviously, political figures and **legislators** have this source of power. This power can also be disseminated and delegated to others through legislative acts. In nursing, the state board of nursing has access to the legitimate source of power because of its establishment under the nurse practice act of that state. Similarly, nurses have access to the legitimate source of power when they are licensed by the state under the provisions in the nurse practice act or when they are appointed to positions within a health-care agency. Nursing decisions made about patient care can come only from individuals who have a legitimate source of power to make those decisions—that is, licensed nurses.

Collective Power

The collective source of power is often used in a broader context than individual patient care and is the underlying source for many other sources of power. When a large group of individuals who have similar beliefs, desires, or needs become organized, a collective source of power exists.[17] For individuals who belong to professions, the professional organization is the focal point for this source of power. The main goal of any organization is to influence policies that affect the members of the organization. This influence is usually in the form of political activities carried out by politicians and **lobbyists**.

Professional organizations that can deliver large numbers of votes have a powerful means of influencing politicians. The use of the collective source of power contains elements of reward, coercive, expert, and even referent sources. Each source may come into play at one time or another.

How Do Nurses Become Empowered?

Despite some feelings of powerlessness as a group, nurses really do have access to some important and rather substantial sources of power. Nurses can be empowered from several sources. Empowerment can

Issues in Practice

Kasey is an RN who has worked on the busy surgical unit of a large city hospital for the past 6 years. As one of three RNs on the unit's day shift, she often serves as the charge nurse when the assigned charge nurse has a day off. She is hardworking, caring, and well organized and provides high-quality care for the often very unstable postoperative patients the unit receives on a daily basis.

About 2 weeks ago, Kasey's mother was admitted for a high-risk surgical removal of a brain tumor that was not responding to chemotherapy or radiation therapy. The surgery did not go well, and Kasey's mother was admitted to the surgical unit after the procedure. During the past 2 weeks, she has shown a gradual but steady decline in condition and is no longer able to recognize her family, speak, or do any self-care. It is believed she will probably not live more than another week.

Per hospital policy, Kasey is not assigned to care for her mother; however, during her shifts, Kasey spends more and more time with her mother, sometimes to the detriment of her assigned patients. She is also beginning to make more demands on the unit nursing staff, often overseeing their care and requesting that only certain nurses care for her mother. One of the other nurses on the unit suggested that Kasey's mother be moved to a less specialized unit. When Kasey heard about the suggestion, she became livid and, in the middle of the nurses' station, loudly scolded the nurse for her insensitivity.

Questions for Thought

1. Is the practice of not allowing nurses to provide care for their relatives evidence based or accustomed practice? How would you find out?
2. Identify the steps in making this policy evidence based.
3. Do you think nurses should be allowed to care for relatives? Why? Why not?

---

originate from the social structure of the work setting when nurses work to increase their control over the workplace and feel more satisfied with the care they provide.[16] Relationships are also a very strong source of empowerment by sharing power with others, particularly those who are often viewed as having more power than nurses. Empowerment can result from a group effort, from an environmental change, or from the individual nurse's own efforts at self-growth and actualization. Most commonly, it is gained through a combination of all three factors.

What can nurses, either as individuals or as a group, do to increase their power?

Professional Unity

Probably the first, and certainly the most important, way in which nurses can gain power in all areas is through professional unity. The most powerful groups are those that are best organized and most united. The power that a professional organization has is directly related to the size of its membership. According to the ANA, there were approximately 4.2 million actively practicing nurses and 355,000 Advanced Practice Nurses in the United States in 2022. It is not difficult to imagine the power that the ANA could have to influence legislators and legislation if all of those nurses were members of the organization rather than the approximately 300,000 who actually do belong.[17]

Political Activity

A second way in which nurses can gain power is by becoming involved in **political action**. Although many nurses are uncomfortable taking a politically active role, they must realize that they are affected by politics and political decisions in every phase of their daily nursing activities.

The simple truth is that if nurses do not become involved in politics and participate in important legislation that influences their practice, someone other than nurses will be making those decisions for them. The average legislator knows little about issues such as patients' rights, national health insurance, quality of nursing care, third-party reimbursement for nurses, and expanded practice roles for nurses, yet they make decisions about these issues almost daily. It would seem logical that more informed and better decisions could be made if nurses took an active part in the legislative process.

Accountability and Professionalism

A third method of increasing power is by demonstrating the characteristics of accountability and professionalism. Nursing has made great strides in these two areas in recent years. Nurses, through professional organizations, have been working hard to establish standards for high-quality patient care. More important, nurses are now concerned with demonstrating competence and delivering high-quality patient care through processes such as peer review and evaluation. By accepting responsibility for the care that they provide and by setting the standards to guide that care, nurses are taking the power to govern nursing away from non-nursing groups.

> *Probably the first, and certainly the most important, way in which nurses can gain power in all areas is through professional unity. The most powerful groups are those that are best organized and most united.*

Networking

Finally, nurses can gain power through establishing a nurse-support network. It is common knowledge that the old boy system remains alive and well in many segments of 21st-century society. The old boy system, which is found in most large organizations, ranging from universities to businesses and governmental agencies, provides individuals, usually white men, with the encouragement, support, and nurturing that allow them to move up quickly through the ranks in the organization to achieve high administrative positions. An important element in making this system work involves never criticizing another "old boy" in public, even though there may be major differences of opinion in private. Presenting a united front is extremely important in maintaining power within this system. Nursing and nursing organizations have never had this type of system for the advancement of nurses.

Part of the difficulty in establishing a nurse-support network is that nurses have not been in high-level positions for very long. The framework for a support system for nurses is now in place; with some commitment to the concept and some activity, it can grow into a well-developed network to allow the brightest, best, and most ambitious people in the profession to achieve high-level positions.[18]

Conclusion

Ongoing changes in the health-care system are having a major impact on how and where nursing is practiced and even on who practices it. If nurses utilize their tremendous potential power by banding together as a profession, they can influence decisions about the direction in which health care is going. Subsequently, nurses, in addition to politicians, health-care providers, hospital administrators, and insurance companies, will be shaping the future of the nursing profession and health care itself. Nurses were at the table for the formation of the Affordable Care Act. It is essential that they be involved in any modifications or revisions that are made to it in the future.

Nursing has made great strides in achieving professional status in the health-care system. Currently, many nurses accept that nursing is a profession and therefore are not very concerned about furthering the process. Even as nursing has matured and evolved into a field of study with an identifiable body of knowledge, some of the questions and problems that have plagued this profession persist. In addition, advances in technology, management, and society have raised new questions about the nature and role of nursing in the health-care system. Only by understanding and exploring the issues of professionalism will nurses be prepared to practice effectively in the present and meet the complex challenges of the future.

CRITICAL-THINKING EXERCISES

- Distinguish between an occupation and a profession.
- Is nursing a profession? Defend your position.
- Discuss four ways in which nursing can improve its professional status.

- Name the three sources of power to which nurses have the most access. Discuss how nurses can best use these sources of power to improve nursing, nursing care, and the health-care system.

NCLEX-STYLE QUESTIONS

1. Which qualities are characteristic of a profession? **Select all that apply**.
   1. Specialized body of knowledge
   2. High level of individual responsibility and accountability
   3. Potential for high pay
   4. Relatively high degree of autonomy
   5. A code of ethics
2. An APRN discusses the possible causes of a patient's abnormal laboratory work with the patient's physician. What source of power is the APRN demonstrating?
   1. Referent
   2. Expert
   3. Rewards
   4. Coercive
3. Yolanda is doing research for a nursing paper on lung cancer, and she wonders if the Web site she's looking at is credible. What finding should make her suspicious of the content on the site?
   1. There are no credentials listed after the authors' names.
   2. The domain name of the site's Web address ends in *.edu*.
   3. The articles are from a current peer-reviewed journal.
   4. The study she's reading about was funded by the American Cancer Society.
4. _____ is the ability or capacity to exert influence over another person or group of persons.

5. Whose scope of practice is NOT regulated by the state board of nursing?
   1. Registered nurse
   2. Licensed practical nurse
   3. Case manager
   4. Physician assistant
6. Reggie is doing online research for his nursing fundamentals class. In the article he's reading, several links that he has clicked on returned the message "Page not found." What should Reggie do next?
   1. Stop clicking the links and keep reading.
   2. Find a more up-to-date source for his information.
   3. Write an angry e-mail to the site's administrator.
   4. Click more links to see if they work.
7. Some states require that APRNs practice under the license of a physician. What area of the nursing profession is being limited by these regulations?
   1. Specialized body of knowledge
   2. Public service and altruistic activities
   3. A code of ethics that guides members in their practice
   4. Autonomy and independence of practice
8. Place the steps of developing an evidence-based practice in the order they should occur.
   1. Evaluate effectiveness of current practices.
   2. Identify the goal of the intervention.
   3. Develop a plan to implement new findings.
   4. Train staff to use the new intervention.
   5. Search for practices that are demonstrably more effective.

9. For decades, Homans sign was used to assess for the presence of deep vein thrombosis (DVT) in the lower leg. However, after many studies called into question the risks involved with and the diagnostic value of Homans sign, it has fallen out of favor. What is this an example of?
   1. Accustomed practice
   2. Evidence-based practice
   3. Specialized body of knowledge
   4. A nursing intervention

10. To increase their power, what should nurses do? **Select all that apply**.
    1. Network
    2. Become politically active
    3. Demonstrate professionalism
    4. Join professional organizations
    5. March in demonstrations

References

1. Poorchangizi B, Borhani F, Abbaszadeh A, Mirzaee M, Farokhzadian J. Professional values of nurses and nursing students: A comparative study. *Biomedical Central Medical Education*, 19(1):438, 2019. https://doi.org/10.1186/s12909-019-1878-2

2. Creighton L, Smart A. Professionalism in nursing: Working as part of a team. *Nursing Times*; 118: 5, 2022. https://www.nursingtimes.net/clinical-archive/leadership/professionalism-in-nursing-2-working-as-part-of-a-team-04-04-2022/

3. Williams E. Define professionalism in nursing. *Chron*, March 25, 2022. https://work.chron.com/define-professionalism-nursing-15763.html

4. Institute of Medicine (US) Committee on Enhancing Environmental Health Content in Nursing Practice; Pope AM, Snyder MA, Mood LH, editors. Nursing Health & Environment: Strengthening the Relationship to Improve the Public's Health. Washington (DC): National Academies Press (US); 1995. 4, Nursing Education and Professional Development. Available from: https://www.ncbi.nlm.nih.gov/books/NBK232399/

5. Nurse liability laws. LegalMatch, 2022. https://www.legalmatch.com/law-library/article/nurse-liability-laws.html

6. Wilson B, Austria M. What is evidence-based practice? University of Utah Health, February 26, 2021. http://accelerate.uofuhealth.utah.edu/improvement/what-is-evidence-based-practice

7. Connor L, Dean J, McNett M, Tydings D, et al. Evidence-based practice improves patient outcomes and healthcare system return on investment: Findings from a scoping review. *Sigma Nursing*, 20(1):6–15, 2023. https://sigmapubs.onlinelibrary.wiley.com/doi/10.1111/wvn.12621

8. Treston C. COVID-19 in the year of the nurse. *Journal of the Association of Nurses AIDS Care*, 31(3):359–360, 2020. https://doi.org/10.1097/JNC.0000000000000173

9. American Nurses Association. *Code of Ethics for Nurses with Interpretive Statements*. Silver Spring, MD: American Nurses Association, 2015. https://www.nursingworld.org/practice-policy/nursing-excellence/ethics/code-of-ethics-for-nurses

10. Rupp S. 7 Advantages of a BSN degree. *Electronic Health Reporter*, April 12, 2022. https://electronichealthreporter.com/7-advantages-of-a-bsn-degree/

11. Physician and nurse relationships. Center for Health Ethics, University of Missouri, n.d. https://medicine.missouri.edu/centers-institutes-labs/health-ethics/faq/physician-nurse-relationships

12. No idea with philosophy of nursing? Here're some examples. New Health Advisor, 2023. https://www.newhealthadvisor.org/Nursing-Philosophy-Examples.html

13. Fulton D. What is an advanced practice registered nurse? *Nursing and Health Care*, April 4, 2022. https://www.gcu.edu/blog/nursing-health-care/what-advanced-practice-registered-nurse

14. APRN Consensus Model: The consensus model for APRN regulation, licensure, accreditation, certification and education. National Council of State Boards of Nursing, n.d. https://www.ncsbn.org/aprn-consensus.htm

15. Davis E. Duties and types of case managers. *VeryWell Health*, March 20, 2022. https://www.verywellhealth.com/what-does-a-case-manager-do-1738560

16. Woodend K, Thibeault C, Lemonde M, McCabe J. Power and power dynamics in nursing leadership. *Leadership for Nurses in Clinical Settings* [online course], 2022. https://ecampusontario.pressbooks.pub/nursingleadership/chapter/power-and-power-dynamics-in-nursing-leadership/

17. Business Bliss Consultants FZE. The definition of empowerment in nursing. Nursing Answers.net, February 11, 2020. https://nursinganswers.net/essays/the-definition-of-empowerment-nursing-essay.php

18. Ayele K. What leadership styles use empowerment? Leadership, May 11, 2022. https://www.leadership.contractors/what-leadership-styles-use-empowerment

Historical Perspectives

2

Joseph T. Catalano

Learning Objectives

After completing this chapter, the reader will be able to:

- Explain why studying the history of health care and nursing is important to the nursing profession
- Name three "historical threads" found in the study of nursing history and discuss why they are important
- Discuss Christian influences on health care and nursing
- Discuss the influences of the Renaissance and Reformation on health care and nursing
- Describe the major changes in health care and nursing during and immediately after World War II
- Identify key historical persons who advanced the profession of nursing

UNDERSTANDING OUR HISTORY

Knowledge about the profession's past can help us understand how nursing developed and even suggest solutions to problems that face the profession today. Several threads run throughout the history of nursing, including society's beliefs about the causes of illness, the value placed on individual life, and the role of women in society. The wars of modern history have also had a significant impact on nursing, particularly in influencing the development of technology and guiding the direction of health care. This chapter is not a treatise on the history of health care and nursing but rather an introduction to some key historical milestones and individuals who helped to form the foundations of health care and nursing care.

ORIGINS OF NURSING

According to the American Nurses Association (ANA), nursing is the protection, promotion, and optimization of clients' health and abilities; the prevention of disease and **illness**; and the alleviation of suffering through the **diagnosis** and treatment of human response to disease and injury. This comprehensive and modern definition of nursing was only derived after centuries of development. However, one of the common elements seen throughout the history of nursing is the belief that by providing care to the ill and injured, including individuals, families, and communities, optimal health and quality of life could be restored or maintained.

Before Nursing

Nursing, as it is currently practiced with its emphasis on theory and best practices, is a relatively recent development in the historical timeline. The major concern of most early civilizations was the survival and propagation of the tribe or group. Because illness and injury threatened this survival, many primitive health-care practices grew from processes of trial and error. In prehistoric times, women were the primary care providers for the ill and injured because they were the ones who were at home while the men were off fighting or hunting. Evil spirits were thought to be the cause of many illnesses, and the medicine men and women who practiced witchcraft to ward off or rid the group of spirits were considered religious figures.

Driving Out Demons

In ancient Eastern civilizations, starting from about 3500 BC, health care was intertwined with religion. Taoism emphasized balance and the driving of demons out of the ailing body. Acupuncture developed over the next several thousands of years, and medicinal herbs were used in preventive health care.

In Southeast Asia, Hinduism emphasized the need for good hygiene, and written records would soon chronicle a number of surgical procedures. This was also the first culture to document medical treatment outside the home. The rise of Buddhism around 530 BC caused a surge in interest in health care, leading to the development of public hospitals and the requirement of high standards for doctors and other hospital workers. Buddhists emphasized good hygiene and prevention of disease. The development of medical knowledge was somewhat hindered by the refusal of physicians to come in contact with blood and infectious body secretions and the prohibition against dissection of the human body.

Ancient Sciences

During the same period, the ancient Egyptians' belief that all disease was caused by evil spirits and punishing gods was changing. Health-care providers from that time showed a well-developed understanding of the basis of disease. Writings from 1500 BC refer to surgical procedures, the role of the midwife, bandaging, **preventive care**, and even birth control. Women enjoyed a higher status in Egyptian society and even worked in hospitals.[1] Physicians, however, were still men, who served in multiple roles as surgeons, priests, architects, and politicians.

The Babylonian Empire, united in 2100 BC, was a civilization that focused on astrology and what we now call holistic health practices. Its health-care practices

included special diets, massage therapy, and rest to drive evil spirits from a body. People would go to the marketplace to seek advice on how to treat their ailments. During the height of the empire, strict guidelines governed doctors' fees and responsibilities in medical practice. There is also evidence from this period of child care and treatment of some diseases in special temples, but most care still took place in the home.

By 1900 BC, the Hebrews had formed a nation along the Mediterranean and adopted many of the health practices of the neighboring civilizations. They integrated elements of the Egyptian sanitary laws to form the Mosaic Code of Laws, which, as in many other cultures, mixed religion and medicine. Caring for widows, orphans, the poor, and strangers in need was part of daily life and an essential element of their religious laws. Hebrews had good knowledge of anatomy and physiology, especially the circulatory system. Physician-priests routinely performed operations such as surgical deliveries (named cesarean deliveries later by the Romans), amputations, and circumcisions. They also enforced rules of purification, performed sacrifices, and conducted rituals related to food preparation. They believed strongly in praying to their one god for help in times of plagues and disaster for healing and cure. Women's role in their society was a mixture of being a step lower than men and being held in high esteem. The Old Testament is filled with women of great strength and character, yet in everyday society, they did not have much stature. There were no specific prohibitions against women providing care of the sick and injured, and as in most early societies, this care was given at home.

> *The major concern of most early civilizations was the survival of the group, and because illness and injury threatened this survival, many primitive health-care practices grew from processes of trial and error.*

What Do You Think?

How might the study of nursing history inform your nursing practice? What do you expect to learn?

The Father of Medicine

Ancient Greek culture focused on appeasing the gods, and its medical practice was no exception. The god Apollo was devoted to medicine and good health.

The Greeks performed sacrifices to appease the gods and practiced abortion and infanticide in an attempt to control the population. People took hot baths at spas to improve health, but the sick and injured were cared for at clinics. Although women were held in high esteem, they were not permitted to provide any health care outside the home.

Around 400 BC, the writings of Hippocrates began to change medical practice in Greece. One of a roving group of physician-priests, Hippocrates is today called "the father of medicine." His beliefs focused on harmony with the natural law instead of on appeasing the gods. He emphasized treating the whole client—mind, body, spirit, and environment—and diagnosing on the basis of symptoms rather than on an isolated idea of a disease. He was also concerned with ethical standards for physicians, expressed in the now-famous Hippocratic Oath.

Health Care in the Roman Empire

Ancient Romans clung to superstitions and polytheism as the foundations for medical and religious practices. The dominant Roman Empire ruled from around 290 BC and absorbed useful elements of whatever culture it conquered—including the Greeks and Hebrews. The Romans developed quite an advanced system of medicine and a pharmacology that included more than 600 medications derived from herbs and plants. Roman physicians were eventually able to distinguish among various conditions and to perform many kinds of surgeries. They also did physical therapy for athletes; diagnosed symptoms of infections; identified job-related dangers of lead, mercury, and asbestos; and published medical textbooks.

The Romans' advances in creating an unlimited supply of clean water through aqueducts were critical in maintaining the good health of the citizens, as were central heating, spas and baths, and advanced systems for sewage disposal. Because the great Roman armies were so crucial to the empire, they developed early hospitals to care for sick and injured soldiers. These were mobile and were staffed by female and male attendants who performed duties that would today be thought of as nursing care. Their skill set included cleaning and bandaging wounds, feeding and washing clients, and providing comfort to the wounded and dying. In many ways, women enjoyed an equal status in society. Most care, including the practice of midwifery, was still provided in the home.

Early Efforts at Nursing

Although caring for the ill and injured had become an established element in most early societies, the concept of a special group to provide this care evolved some time later. The concept of nurse grew primarily from the care provided by Christian orders of nuns who were dedicated solely to the care of the sick and dying.

The Sanctity of Life

The rise of Christianity, starting from 30 AD, brought with it a strong belief in the sanctity of all human life. Christians considered practices such as human sacrifice, infanticide, and abortion—which had been common in Roman society—to be murder. Following the teachings of Jesus meant that caring for the sick, poor, and disadvantaged was of primary importance, and groups of believers soon organized to offer care for those in need.

Early writings of the Christian period record women's important role in ministering to the sick and providing food and care for the poor and homeless. Wealthy Roman women who had converted to Christianity established hospital-like institutions and residences for these caregivers in their homes. The term *nurse* is thought to have originated in this period from the Latin word *nutrire*, meaning "to nourish, nurture, or suckle a child." The majority of care was still provided by a family member in the home. Most early Christian hospitals were roadside houses for sick travelers, as well as for the poor and destitute, who were cared for by male and female attendants alike. The attendants learned from a process of trial and error and from observing others.

A Time of Disease

The Dark Ages, from roughly 500 to 1000 AD, were marked by widespread poverty, illness, and death. Plagues and other diseases, such as smallpox, leprosy, and diphtheria, ravaged the known world and killed

> *The term **nurse** is thought to have originated in this period from the Latin word **nutrire**, meaning 'to nourish, nurture, or suckle a child.'*

large segments of populations. Health care at this time was almost nonexistent.

However, the strong beliefs of the Catholic Church, which was based in Rome, produced monasteries and convents that became centers for the care of the poor and the sick. By 500 AD, there were several religious **nursing orders** in what are today England, France, and Italy. Men and women worked there and also traveled to rural areas where they were needed, combining religious rituals and prayers with home remedies and providing treatments such as bandaging, cautery, bloodletting, enemas, and leeching. The biggest contribution to health care in this period may have been the insistence on cleanliness and hygiene, which lessened the spread of infections. Medieval nurses did not have any formal schooling but learned through apprenticeships with older monks or nuns. Eventually, hospitals came to be built outside of monastery grounds. Also established were secular orders, which could provide a wider range of services to the sick because they were not limited by religious restrictions and obligations.

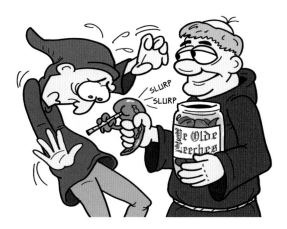

Leeches were cutting-edge medical practice.

Early Military Hospitals

At the end of the Dark Ages, a series of holy wars and invasions, including the Crusades, produced many sick and injured who were far from home. Military nursing orders developed to care for the soldiers, but these were made up exclusively of men who wore suits of armor to protect themselves against attacks. These orders, with the emblem of a Red Cross, were

extremely well organized and dedicated, and they existed well into the Renaissance.

Development of the Modern Nurse

Current society readily accepts technology and scientific breakthroughs; however, earlier religion-based societies had more difficulty moving forward with these developments, which were sometimes seen as works of Satan. The Renaissance developed into a battle between progressive thinkers and a very conservative governance structure that resisted change.

Health Care in the Renaissance

In the intellectual reawakening of the Renaissance in Europe, starting in about 1350, nursing emerged in a form that would be recognizable today and formed the cornerstone of what we now know as a profession. Inventions from this time include the microscope and thermometer, but the use of more modern diagnoses and treatments was viewed with skepticism. Monastic hospitals still regarded the restoration of health as secondary to the salvation of the soul. Major political changes initiated by the Protestant Reformation in 1517 had the greatest effect on the health care of the period. In Catholic nation-states, including Italy, France, and Spain, health care remained generally unchanged from that of the Middle Ages, although the number of male nursing orders gradually decreased. By 1500, the majority of health care was provided by female religious orders.

What Do You Think?

Imagine yourself living in one of the historical periods discussed in this chapter. Given your or your family's health-care problems, how would your lives be different?

A Nursing Hierarchy

In the nation-states that broke away from the Catholic Church, such as England, Germany, and the Netherlands, health care soon degenerated to a state even worse than that of the Middle Ages. The role of women was reduced under Protestant leadership, and the male nurse all but disappeared. Secular nursing orders gradually took over the duties of the many substandard hospitals that had been established in metropolitan areas. The most famous of these was the Sisters of Charity, established in 1600.

These orders were the first to establish a nursing hierarchy. Primary nurses were called *sisters*, and those assisting them were called *helpers* and *watchers*. At this time, people began to recognize the benefits of skilled nursing care. The first nursing textbooks appeared, and the use of midwives became widespread. Although hospitals were gaining importance, most clients still received health care at home.

The Industrial Revolution (1760–1840) caused a flood of people throughout Europe to move from rural areas into cities. Cramped living situations caused very bad health conditions and the spread of disease and plagues. Factory owners supported some forms of health care to keep their workers on the job, and this led to an early form of community health nursing. The Sisters of Charity expanded their care to include home care. Only a few male nursing orders survived the Protestant Reformation and Industrial Revolution. Several non-Catholic nursing orders were founded, including one by the famous Quaker Elizabeth Fry. In London in 1840, Fry established the Society of Protestant Sisters of Charity, which provided training to nurses who cared for the sick and poor, including prisoners and children.

NURSING IN THE UNITED STATES

Five hospitals existed in America before the Revolutionary War; they housed the homeless and the poor and included rudimentary infirmaries. However, there were no identifiable groups of nurses for these infirmaries.[2] Health care in America at this time reflected that of the European countries from which the settlers had come. Infant mortality rates were very high, ranging between 50 and 75 percent.[2] One of the first schools of nursing was established in 1640 by the Sisters of St. Ursula in Quebec, and Spanish and French religious orders would establish hospital-based training schools in the New World over the next 100 years.

In Colonial Times

During the Revolutionary War, there were no organized medical or nursing corps, but small groups of untrained volunteers cared for the wounded and sick in their homes or in churches or barns. In 1751,

Benjamin Franklin founded Pennsylvania Hospital, the first U.S. hospital dedicated to treating the sick.

Between the Revolutionary War and the Civil War, health care in the United States increased markedly with the influx of religious nursing orders from Europe. More early schools of nursing developed at this time. Despite the rapid increase in the number of hospitals, most nursing care was still given at home by family members. Hospitals were considered a last resort where people went to die; consequently, the hospitals had very high mortality rates.

When the States Went to War

The Civil War caused more death and injury than any other war in the history of the United States, and the demand for nurses increased dramatically. Women volunteers (as many as 6,000 for the North and 1,000 for the South) began to follow the armies to the battlefields to provide basic nursing care, although many of these volunteers were untrained. Large numbers of women came out of their homes to work in the hospitals, and a number of African American volunteers in the North paved the way for others to enter the health-care field in the future. During the Civil War (1861–1865), some nurses were on the army payroll, but others were paid by the U.S. Sanitary Commission or by volunteer agencies. During the Spanish-American War (1898), nurses were civilian contract nurses. Dr. Anita Newcomb McGee, the acting assistant surgeon during the war, was responsible for the establishment of the Army Nurse Corps (ANC) after the war in 1901. In 1920, ANC personnel were given "relative rank," or officer-equivalent ranks, but army and navy nurses did not receive actual military ranks until 1944.

> **The Civil War caused more death and injury than any other war in the history of the United States, and the demand for nurses increased dramatically.**

After 1914

Prior to the beginning of World War I, nurses' primary duties were to carry out the orders of physicians, clean, cook, and empty bedpans. Most of the duties carried out by physicians at that time would fall well within today's scope of practice for nurses. However, in the face of the large numbers of injured produced in World War I, nurses' roles rapidly expanded,

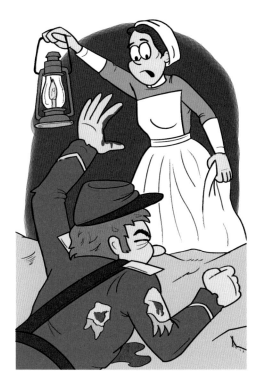

During the Civil War, women volunteers followed the armies and provided basic nursing care.

and they began to be recognized for their skills in providing care and saving lives.

Untrained Nurses

At the beginning of World War I, there were only about 400 nurses in the Army Nurse Corps, but by 1917, that number had swelled to 21,000. Because many hospitals were recruiting uneducated women to provide basic care, a committee on nursing was formed to establish standards, and eventually the Red Cross began a training program for nurse's aides. This was supported by physicians but opposed by many nursing leaders who were concerned that such a program relegated nursing to "women's work," which would be seen as something anyone could do with minimal training. Because nurse's aides were a cheap source of labor, they began to replace more trained nurses in hospitals. Unfortunately, this also resulted in a lower quality of care and started a cost-saving practice that continues today.

Between Wars

After the war, a segment of the nursing profession began to focus on improving the educational standards of nursing care. At the time, 90 percent of nursing care was still given at home, but nurses began to practice in industry and in branches of government outside of the military. The standards of nursing care were low, and external quality controls were nonexistent.

The Great Depression took its toll on health care and nursing, as funds dried up, jobs became scarce, and many nursing schools closed. At this time, the federal government became one of the largest employers of nurses. The newly organized Joint Committee on Nursing recommended that jobs go to more qualified nurses and that the workday be reduced from 12 to 8 hours, although these measures were not widely implemented.[1] During this period, hospitals became the primary source of health care, supported by hospital insurance programs. As the size of hospitals increased, more nursing jobs became available.

Establishing Standards

World War II produced another nursing shortage, and in response, Congress passed the Bolton Act, which shortened hospital-based diploma programs from 36 to 30 months. The new Cadet Nurse Corps established minimum educational standards for nursing programs and forbade discrimination on the basis of race, creed, or sex.[2] Many schools revised and improved their curricula to meet these new standards.

To encourage more nurses to enter the military, the U.S. government granted women full commissioned status and gave them the same pay as men with the same rank. Male nurses who served in the war worked as orderlies rather than RNs. Men did not become part of the ANC until 1955.

Modern Times: Emerging Specialties

The single largest transformation of the practice of nursing occurred during World War II. Navy and army nurses had such a positive image that nursing attracted more women volunteers to the armed services than to any other occupation at the time. Nurses were revered as selfless heroes under fire in several movies produced during the war. Even nurses captured by the Japanese were allowed to keep practicing because their role was so highly respected. On the battlefields and at rear area hospitals, they often worked together with untrained care providers and physicians, thus initiating the concept of a health-care team.

A Team of Nurses

The advancements in health care made during World War II required that nurses receive more highly specialized education to meet clients' unique needs. After the war, many of the highly educated and experienced nurses left the profession to raise families, and their vacancies were filled by graduates of new programs that trained licensed practical nurses (LPNs) and licensed vocational nurses (LVNs) in just 1 year. At this time, the concept of team nursing came to be widely accepted, although it removed the registered nurses (RNs) from direct client care, requiring them to serve as team leaders.

A Growing Need

Technical nursing programs, which granted associate degrees (associate degree nurse [ADN]) at 2-year community colleges, were developed as a quick-fix solution to help with the nursing shortage. With the postwar baby boom, the need for nurses continued to grow, and what was supposed to have been a temporary resolution to a short-term problem became a permanent fixture. By the mid-1960s, ADNs outnumbered nurses with baccalaureate degrees (BSNs) and LPNs. Also, ADNs won the right to take the same licensing examinations as RN graduates from diploma and BSN programs.

> *Medieval nurses did not have any formal schooling but learned through apprenticeships with older monks or nuns.*

After World War II, technology developed during the war began to be transformed for use in civilian life, including health care. This made the health-care system increasingly complicated, and some major nursing leaders questioned whether 1- or 2-year LPN and ADN programs were adequate to meet the needs of a profession on the brink of an explosion of knowledge. Slowly, the number of BSN programs and graduate-level programs began to increase.

Vietnam: Traveling Hospitals

The mobile army surgical hospital (MASH) units that had been developed during the Korean War were replaced during the Vietnam War with medical unit, self-contained transportable (MUST) hospitals, which were staffed by nurses and physicians. Some 5,000 nurses served in this war, and for the first time, graduates of 2-year ADN programs were commissioned into the armed services. (However, the armed services now commission only nurses with a BSN.) Several navy nurses were injured in the line of duty, and one army nurse was killed. The efforts of these and other women who served are recognized at the Vietnam Women's Memorial in Washington, dedicated in 1993.

THE EVOLUTION OF SYMBOLS IN NURSING

All professions have symbols that are easily identified and connected with the work and services they provide. In the past, when most of the population was illiterate, these symbols were helpful in distinguishing one professional from another. In modern society, the symbols connect the professions to their historical roots and provide the philosophical basis for the work they do.

The Lamp

The simple definition of a lamp is a device that provides a continuous source of light for an extended period of time. The first evidence of lamp use, a hollowed-out stone with oil residue in it, can be traced back to 10,000 BC. Early variations on the oil lamp included seashell lamps and coconut lamps. Since then, technology has advanced lamps to clay bowls, pottery, wood, and various types of metals.

Pushing Back Darkness

The significance of the lamp is really the significance of light. Its origins can be traced back to the first attempts of human beings to control fire and use it as a tool of survival. These early humans soon found that fire extended their day, was a source of warmth on cold nights, kept wild animals from attacking, and was useful for cooking.

Light, first in the form of torches and candles and later in the form of the oil lamp, has been used by human beings for thousands of years to push back the darkness of night. It dispelled fear and allowed people to pursue learning long after the sun went down.

The lamp has long been used as a religious symbol. It often represents the eternal flame that dispels darkness and evil. Commonly found in Christian symbolism is the Lady of Light, often depicted as radiant and glowing brightly and filled with goodness, purity, and wisdom. The lamp can also represent the flame of life, eventually extinguished by death.

As schools and universities developed during the Middle Ages, many adopted the lamp as a symbol of learning. The burning of the lamp signifies the continual seeking of knowledge and the pushing back of the darkness of illiteracy. It also symbolizes the enlightenment that accompanies knowledge. The coats of arms or logos used by many universities contain the image of a lamp.

A Sign of Caring

The lamp was first introduced as a symbol for the nursing profession at the time of Florence Nightingale. In addition to her fame as an early health-care reformer and pioneer, she became well known for her role in caring for injured soldiers during the Crimean War. She made history when she took her 38 nurses to Turkey to try to improve the squalid, filthy conditions she found in the primitive British field hospitals. As Nightingale and her nurses made their night rounds, caring for the wounded in unlit wards, they carried lamps to light the way. For the wounded and suffering, these lamps became signs of caring, comfort, and often the difference between life and death.

> **Large numbers of women came out of their homes to work in the hospitals, and a number of African American volunteers in the North paved the way for others to enter the health-care field in the future.**

Nightingale's lamp was not the often-depicted genie or Aladdin's lamp. Rather, Nightingale would have used one of the many lamps in circulation around the wards, picking up whichever was closest at hand. The most common type used was the ordinary camp lamp, or a Turkish candle lantern. She later became immortalized as the "lady with a lamp" in a poem written by Longfellow ("Santa Filomena").

For graduate nurses, the lamp, or candle, retains its significance as a symbol of the ideals and selfless devotion of Florence Nightingale. It also signifies the knowledge and learning that the graduates have attained during their years in the nursing program. Some nursing graduates physically carry a candle during their pinning ceremonies that symbolically represents the brightly burning lamp of their knowledge, skills, care, and devotion as they go forth to minister to the sick and injured in their nursing practice.

The Nursing Pin

Unlikely as it may seem, the modern nursing pin can trace its origins to the heavy protective war shields used by soldiers as far back as the Greek and Roman empires. The primary purpose of these shields was to protect the warriors from the spears, swords, and arrows of the opposing army, but they could also be used as weapons to knock down the enemy. Adorned with the emblems of the soldier's country and his particular unit in the army, these ancient war shields also served as a quick way to distinguish friend from foe.

During the Crusades, the Knights Hospitallers were formed to provide medical care for the wounded and sick. The Knights wore black tunics over their armor, carried no weapons, and wore a white Maltese cross on chains around their necks. Those wearing this cross became known for their skill in treating the injured and healing the wounded. Since that time, the Maltese cross has been recognized as a symbol of those who care for the sick. Although large by today's standards, the Maltese cross is often considered the first true nursing pin.

The shields of some medieval knights were painted with the coats of arms of the kings they were defending. Only the best knights, recognized for their skill in battle, strength, honesty, and dedication to the service of the king, were permitted to use the king's coat of arms on their shields. The coat of arms displayed to the world the characteristics by which the king wished to be known. A classic example is the symbol of the lion, found on the shields of the knights who served King Richard the Lionheart, which indicated the king's fearlessness and power.

Similarly, during the Middle Ages when most of the population was illiterate, tradesmen and craft guilds began adopting symbols as pictorial representations of their services, skills, and crafts. Modern companies use trademarks and brand names in the same way today. Medieval schools and universities also began using symbols to represent their values and goals. The modern practice of branding the university, or adopting an official symbol or logo for the school, can be traced back to these early practices. These symbols were embossed on clothing, buttons, badges, and pins that were worn by members of the group. Also traceable to this time in history are the shields and badges worn by firefighters and law enforcement officers. Although these shields offer little in the way of protection from arrows and spears, they symbolize official authority and identify the wearer as belonging to a unique, specially trained group.

The first modern nursing pin is attributed to Florence Nightingale. After receiving the medal of the Red Cross of St. George from Queen Victoria for her selfless service to the injured and dying in the Crimean War, Nightingale chose to extend the honor she had received to her most outstanding graduate nurses by awarding each of them a badge of excellence. The badge or pin she designed for her school is a deepblue Maltese cross (Fig. 2.1). In the center of the cross is a relief image of Nightingale's head. As the number of nursing schools increased, each program designed a unique pin to represent its own particular values, philosophies, beliefs, and goals.

The pinning ceremony is part of a long tradition that acknowledges nursing graduates as belonging to a unique group and identifies them as new members of the health-care community. The historical origins of the pin remind nursing professionals of what it symbolizes. Like the badge worn by law enforcement officers, it is also a sign of their legal authority as licensed professionals. Nursing graduates wear their pins proudly in the work setting as evidence of their successful completion of the nursing program.

The Cap

It is rare to see a nurse wearing the traditional nursing cap in today's modern hospitals. However, the cap has a long, rich history. Throughout much of history, women were required to keep their heads covered with some type of garment. This practice was prevalent in the early Hebrew, Greek, and Roman cultures that served as the roots for modern Western society and the current profession of nursing. Few women in Western society wear any type of regular hair cover now. A few groups of nuns still wear traditional head

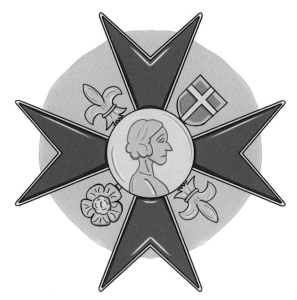

Figure 2.1 Florence Nightingale's nursing excellence pin.

coverings as they were required to do in the past, although most orders have gone to a civilian dress code that does not require the traditional veil.

A Symbol of Service

The origins of what we identify as modern nursing can be traced back to an early Christian era group of women called *deaconesses*. Deaconesses were set apart from other women of the period by their white head coverings, which indicated that their primary service was to care for the sick. During the early centuries of Christianity, groups of deaconesses banded together and formed what later became religious orders that were prevalent in the Holy Roman Empire. The former deaconesses, now recognized as religious order nuns, remained the primary providers of care for the sick throughout the Middle Ages. The traditional garb of nuns, the long-robed habit with the wimple or veil, can be considered the first official nurse's uniform. Each religious order had its own unique style of habit and wimple. The order the nun belonged to could be easily identified from the habit or veil she was wearing.

Religious orders continued to be the primary source of care for the sick well into the 19th century. However, as the Industrial Revolution progressed and the concept of the modern hospital developed, the care of the sick moved away from religious orders to care by laypeople who did not wear the nun's robe and veil.

By the time Florence Nightingale trained at the Institute of Protestant Deaconesses in Germany, the veil had evolved into a white cap that signified "service to others." However, Florence Nightingale lived and practiced nursing during the Victorian era, which required "proper" women to keep their heads covered. The nursing cap Florence Nightingale wore was similar to the head garb worn by cleaning ladies of the day. It was hood shaped with a ruffle around the face and tied under the chin (Fig. 2.2). This early cap served multiple purposes. It met the requirements of the times for women to keep their heads covered; it kept the nurse's long hair, which was fashionable during the Victorian era, up and off her face; and it kept the hair from becoming soiled. An unintended benefit was that it kept contaminants from the hair from infecting wounds.

A Cap for Every School

In the United States, the first standardized nursing cap is generally attributed to Bellevue Training School in New York City around 1874. The cap's primary purpose was to keep the nurse's long hair from getting in the way, but it also identified nurses who had graduated from Bellevue. The Bellevue cap covered

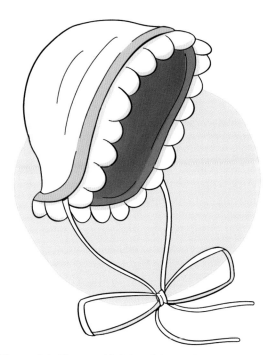

Figure 2.2 Florence Nightingale's nursing cap.

the whole head to just above the ears and resembled a modern knitted ski hat except that it was made of white linen with a rolled fringe at the bottom.

As the number of nursing schools increased, there was a corresponding increase in the need for unique caps. Each nursing school designed its own cap. Nursing caps became very frilly, elaborate, and sometimes large and unwieldy. Some caps adopted the upside-down ice cream cone shape, similar to the cloth cone through which ether was given as an anesthetic. By looking at the cap, a person could still determine the school from which the nurse had graduated.

Traditionally, in the 3-year hospital-based schools of nursing, there were two separate ceremonies—one for capping and one for pinning. The capping ceremony usually took place after the student completed the initial 6 months of classroom education, which was considered the probationary period of the program. Capping indicated that the student was now off probation and that she had earned the right to wear the cap during clinical rotations in the hospital.

During nursing school, the cap was also used as a sign of rank and status. In the 3-year hospital-based nursing schools, first-year students wore plain white caps. Second-year students had a vertical black band added to the edge of the cap, and third-year students were given a second vertical black band. When the student graduated, the vertical black bands were removed, and a horizontal black band was placed across the front of the cap.

Unchanging Values

As shorter hair became an acceptable style for women in the 20th century, the nursing cap lost its function of controlling long hair. However, it continued as a status symbol and a source of pride and identity for the graduates of nursing schools into the 1970s. As technology increased in the health-care work environment, the traditional nursing cap became more of an obstacle for nurses in the practice setting. Also, research demonstrated that the cap, rather than protecting clients from infection by organisms from the nurse's hair, actually helped to colonize organisms. By the 1980s, health-care facilities no longer required nurses to wear caps as part of the uniform, and nursing schools eliminated the cap as a mandatory item of students' uniforms.

Most nursing programs have eliminated the capping ceremony as a throwback to an era that was repressive to women. However, the nursing cap connects graduates to a rich and long history. It retains its significance, from the time of Florence Nightingale, as a sign that the primary goal of nursing is "service to those in need." The nursing cap is a reminder of the unchanging values of wisdom, faith, honesty, trust, and dedication. These values are as important in today's modern, technology-filled hospitals as they were in the era when washing floors was a required basic nursing skill.

What Do You Think?

Does your nursing school have a unique nursing cap that was used in the past? What is the symbolism of the cap's design?

NURSING LEADERS

The nursing profession as it is practiced today owes a great deal to several outstanding nurses who had a vision for the future. The few discussed here are representative of the great drive and dedication of the many individuals who created change and influenced the development of the nursing profession.

Florence Nightingale (1820–1910)

Universally regarded as the founder of modern nursing, Florence Nightingale dedicated her long life to improving health care and nursing standards. Raised in England, Nightingale was considered highly educated for her time. Through travels with her family, she became aware of the substandard health care in many countries in Europe. In 1851, she attended a 3-month nurses' training program at the church-run hospital in Kaiserswerth, Germany. She was impressed with the program but believed this brief training was insufficient. She later ran a private nursing home and realized that the only way to improve health care was to educate women to be reliable, high-quality nurses.[3]

Volunteering Under Fire

Plans to develop a school of nursing in England were interrupted in 1854 by a cholera epidemic. Nightingale volunteered her services and learned a great deal about how to prevent the spread of disease. When the Crimean War broke out that same year, she obtained permission to take a group of 37 volunteer nurses into the battlefield area. British medical officers initially refused the assistance of Nightingale's nurses. As conditions worsened, the medical officers became overwhelmed with the care of large numbers of patients and reluctantly allowed the nurses to care for the wounded in the primitive hospital.

After just 6 months of the nurses cleaning and bandaging wounds, cooking, and cleaning the wards, the mortality rate dropped from 42 percent to 2 percent.[3] Nightingale expanded her reform to include supplies, a military post office, convalescent camps for long-term recovery, and residences for soldiers' families. She also began to help with the care given at the front lines. At the height of her work in the war, Nightingale supervised 125 nurses in several large hospitals. Her accomplishments were recognized by the Queen of England, and she was the first woman ever to be awarded with the medal of the Order of Merit, the highest award given to English civilians Also, in April 1904, Nightingale was awarded this scroll and the title of "Lady of Grace of the Order of St John Royal Order of Chivalry." The scroll is contained within a metal casket and features a large seal attached by a silk cord.

What Do You Think?

What would current nursing practice and nursing education be like without the influences of Florence Nightingale?

A Health-Care Reformer

The war experience strengthened Nightingale's convictions that nursing education required major reform. Believing that nursing schools should be run by nurses and be independent of hospitals and physicians, she advocated a program of at least 1 year that included basic biological science, techniques to improve nursing care, and supervised practice. She regarded nursing as a lifelong career and felt that nurses should be in direct contact with clients rather than cooking and cleaning. She worked tirelessly for the reform of health care and nursing and was appointed to many related committees and commissions. A prolific writer, she wrote extensively about improving hospital conditions, sanitation, nursing education, and health care in general.

Her famous Florence Nightingale School of Nursing and Midwifery opened in 1860 and began to train nurses, who were in great demand throughout Europe and the United States. At this school, Nightingale advocated health maintenance and the concept that nursing was both an art and a science. She taught that each person should be treated as an individual and that nurses should meet the needs of clients, not the demands of physicians.

The school flourished, although it faced strong opposition from physicians who felt that nurses were already overeducated. Many early graduates went on to become important nursing leaders. Nightingale's ideas were somewhat diluted during the first half of the 20th century, but they have since resurfaced and are now evaluated in the light of a rapidly changing health-care system.[3]

Isabel Adams Hampton Robb (1860–1910)

Isabel Adams Hampton Robb started out as a teacher in her home province of Ontario, Canada, but in 1881 she went to New York City to train to be a nurse. After graduation, she moved to Rome and became a superintendent of a hospital there. She had always focused on the academic rather than the clinical side of nursing. In Italy, her conviction grew that nurses needed a solid theoretical education—a belief that was not well accepted by the medical community of the time. From that point on, she dedicated her life to raising the standards of nursing education in the United States, first as director of the Illinois Training School for Nurses, a school that was unique for its time in that it was university based and emphasized academic learning. Some of her unique ideas for the time were to develop and implement a grading policy for nursing students that required nurses to prove their abilities in order to be awarded a diploma. She also advocated for the reduction of the long hours involved in training nurses. She later headed the new Johns Hopkins Training School for Nurses and implemented her ideas there as well.[4]

Hampton Robb brought together leaders from key nursing schools to form the American Society of Superintendents of Training Schools for Nurses, and she served as its chairwoman. The group was the precursor to the National League for Nursing, which was dedicated to improving the standards for nursing

> *The war experience strengthened Nightingale's convictions that nursing education required major reform. Believing that nursing schools should be run by nurses and be independent of hospitals and physicians, she advocated a program of at least 1 year that included basic biological science, techniques to improve nursing care, and supervised practice.*

education. In 1896, Hampton Robb became the first president of a group for staff nurses in active practice called the Nurses Associated Alumnae of the United States and Canada, which would later become the American Nurses Association (ANA), dedicated to the improvement of clinical practice.[4] She later helped develop the *American Journal of Nursing*, the first professional journal dedicated to the improvement of nursing, which is still the official journal of the ANA.

Lillian Wald (1867–1940)

Lillian Wald was raised in Ohio and graduated from the New York Hospital Training School for Nurses in 1901. After working as a hospital nurse, she entered medical school, but encounters with New York's poor and sick caused her to change direction. She instead opened the Henry Street Settlement, a storefront health clinic in one of the poorest sections of the city, which organized nurses to make home visits, focusing on sanitary conditions and children's health.[5] Wald became a dedicated social reformer, an efficient fundraiser, and an eloquent speaker. Although women still did not have the right to vote, her political influence was felt worldwide.

Under Wald's auspices, Columbia University developed courses to prepare nurses for careers in public health. Wald also advocated wellness education, which the medical community did not value at the time. However, the Metropolitan Life Insurance Company saw the value in her beliefs and asked her to organize its nursing branch. She is also credited with founding the American Red Cross's Town and Country Nursing Service and with initiating the concept of school nursing. In 1912, she founded and became the first president of the National Organization for Public Health Nursing. She was the first to place nurses in public schools.[5] Many child health and wellness programs in use today are based on her efforts. Current proposals for health-care reform often include her ideas about public health nursing, independent clinics, and health maintenance.

What Do You Think?

Who is your favorite historical nursing leader? What are some of that person's characteristics that appeal to you? Is there a current nurse or nurse educator who is a role model for you? What are some of that person's characteristics that appeal to you?

Lavinia Lloyd Dock (1858–1956)

Lavinia Lloyd Dock left her home in Pennsylvania in 1885 to attend New York's Hunter-Bellevue School of Nursing. Her contributions as a reformer focused on the professionalization of nursing and the equality of women.[6] She noticed that many of her fellow students struggled to learn about all the medications that were becoming available, and she would later write the first medication textbook for nurses. She worked alongside Lillian Wald at the Henry Street Settlement and Isabel Hampton Robb at Johns Hopkins Hospital.

Like Wald, Dock believed that poverty and squalor contributed to poor health, and she dedicated herself to social reform to address these problems.[6] However, she soon learned that her influence was limited because she was a woman, and she spent most of her career dedicated to the pursuit of equal rights. For 20 years, she lobbied legislators at all levels about women's right to vote, believing that this was the only way to influence social reform and health care. Exemplifying the diverse ways that nurses can help achieve higher-quality health care, Dock is considered one of the most influential leaders in the early 20th century.

Annie W. Goodrich (1866–1954)

Annie Goodrich provided nursing care at Lillian Wald's Henry Street Settlement in New York after receiving her nursing degree. She was known as an outstanding nursing educator and ran a number of nursing schools in New York. In 1910, she was appointed as state inspector of nursing schools, a position that up to that time had been held only by physicians. After the U.S. Army asked her to survey its hospital nursing departments, Goodrich proposed that it organize its own nursing school. The school opened later that year, with her as its dean, and this school served as the model for others established at army hospitals during World War I.

To respond to the need for nurses in the war, Goodrich also established a nursing training program at Vassar College. After the war, other colleges and universities slowly began to develop their own nursing programs. Goodrich had demonstrated that teaching theoretical information in a classroom was just as important as clinical practice in training highly skilled nurses. When the war was over, Goodrich returned to the Henry Street Settlement and then became a nursing educator, eventually serving as dean at the Yale School of Nursing. Her many writings about nursing education and her experiences with military nursing have been a great contribution to the nursing profession.[7]

Loretta C. Ford (1920–)

Credited with founding nurse practitioner (NP) practice, Loretta C. Ford was born in New York City. She received her diploma in nursing from the Robert Wood Johnson University Hospital in New Brunswick, New Jersey. She held a staff nurse position there until she accepted a commission as an officer in the U.S. Army Air Force in 1943. After the war, she was accepted into the bachelor of science (BS) program at the University of Colorado College of Nursing. She earned her BS in 1949 and her master of science in nursing in 1951. Subsequently, she worked as a public health nurse in Boulder, Colorado, and then for the Boulder County Health Department, where she served as director from 1956 to 1958.[8]

Ford began her career in education in 1955, when she was appointed assistant professor at the University of Colorado College of Nursing in Denver. She received her doctorate in education from the University of Colorado in 1961 and became a professor in 1965.

During her time at University of Colorado, she began working with a pediatrician, Dr. Henry K. Silver. Together, they noted that there was a severe regional shortage of family care physicians and pediatricians, particularly in the rural and underserved areas of Colorado. In response, they came up with an innovative approach to the health-care provider shortage. They applied for and received a small grant from the university in 1965, which led to the creation of a demonstration project that focused on extending the role of the nurse in the health-care community.[9] It was so effective that they published their findings, which later became the blueprint for an educational curriculum for NPs.

Soon after the pilot project was completed, the University of Colorado started the first formal NP program in the country. Initially, it was a certificate program for nurses with a baccalaureate in nursing degree. Ford believed that the nurse practitioner philosophy should be to provide a holistic approach to the client's health. Nurse practitioners should focus on health, functionality, and daily living, as well as give the client feedback on how they are progressing.[8]

At first, the NP program prepared nurses in child and family care, educating clients in preventive health. The extremely popular program eventually became a master's degree program. It also expanded its focus to a broader population as it grew, including caring for adults. Ford's program educated NPs to integrate the traditional role of the nurse with advanced medical training and community health, thereby providing clients with high-quality care and education not found in the traditional health-care setting.

Ford became the founding dean of the University of Rochester School of Nursing and director of the Nursing Service at the University Hospital in 1972. The school now has nine specialty NP programs, including child psychiatry, which helps fill a need for mental health services in rural upstate New York.[9] In 2003, she was awarded the Blackwell Award (named for the first female doctor in America) from Hobart and William Smith Colleges, which is given to a woman whose life exemplifies outstanding service to humanity. Among many other

accolades, she was inducted into the National Women's Hall of Fame in 2011 for being recognized as an internationally renowned nursing leader who has transformed the profession of nursing and made health care more accessible to the general public. Ford is now retired and living in Florida; however, she has remained involved with the University of Rochester School of Nursing. She still consults and lectures on the historical development of the nurse practitioner along with issues in advanced nursing practice and health-care policy.

NPs are found in every corner of the health-care system today. More than 150,000 NPs work within the United States, and the number grows daily. In many states, NPs can function independently and provide services such as ordering, performing, and interpreting diagnostic tests. They can diagnose and treat acute and chronic conditions such as diabetes, high blood pressure, infections, and injuries. In some states, they are legally permitted to prescribe medications independently. Although still receiving some resistance from physicians' groups, NPs have transformed both the health-care system and the profession of nursing.[8]

Issues Now

Travel Nursing as a Career

As a nursing student, you may have heard of *travel nursing* or *traveling nurses* but may not really know what travel nursing is or if it might be something you would be interested in as a career. Much like the recruitment posters for the armed services, "See the World" seems to be an attractive slogan for those looking for new experiences and adventure. However, there may be some drawbacks to travel nursing.

In general, travel nurse staffing companies require a BSN or higher degree. This standard allows the nurses to meet any staffing requirements of individual facilities. Research has demonstrated improved client outcomes with the use of BSN staffing, so it is important to health-care organizations. Travel nurses differ from agency nurses in several ways. Travel nurses are usually committed to working for a facility for a predetermined length of time, usually about 3 months. To allow preparation for travel to the facility, they are scheduled for their time about 2 months before their start date. Agency nurses generally work on a per diem (by the day) basis and live near the facility. They work a few days at a time to meet a short-term staffing need. Travel nurses provide more continuity of care and fill in for long-term needs, such as extended illness, maternity leave, or even sabbatical leave.

Travel nurses can select where they want to work and the time period of the work schedule. They usually follow the schedule required by the facility but have scheduled days off like other nurses. Their salaries tend to be higher; and, depending on the company, the benefits may range from "bare bones" to what regular staffers would receive at a large health-care facility. Some staffing agencies also pay for the nurse's license and housing costs. Staffing agencies have a group of employees who support the nurse and act as liaisons with the facilities to resolve any problems that may arise. Salaries are a bit complicated to

(continued)

Issues Now (continued)

calculate, depending on benefits, but usually work out to a range of $40 to $50 or more per hour ($80,000 to $105,000 or more per year). Tax-free benefits can include stipends for incidentals such as laundry, Wi-Fi use, phone, and free, private, quality housing located conveniently near the work facility. Because these stipends do not qualify as income, they are not taxed as part of the salary of a travel nurse. Even better, stipends are not performance or hours based, so nurses keep their stipend no matter what happens; however, stipends are usually calculated as a fixed sum on the initial contract.

A nurse must be careful when selecting a travel nurse staffing company. The nurse should investigate the company carefully, talk to other nurses it employs, and examine the benefits closely. Generally, the larger the firm, the more locations it serves and the better the benefits and support services. Some nurses use travel nurse employment to research locations in which they may be interned and then permanently relocate when they find the ideal location.

Requirements for travel nurses include the following:

- At least 1 year of experience
- For specialty areas (obstetrics, intensive care, emergency, etc.), an additional year in that area
- BSN preferred but not required
- Basic life support (BLS), advanced cardiovascular life support (ACLS), certification in specialty area (e.g., critical care registered nurse [CCRN] for intensive care unit)
- Belong to Nurse Compact Licensure state or obtain nursing license in the state you are going to practice
- Remain current in competency with continuing education units (CEUs) or other requirements

So, if you want to be a travel nurse, the opportunities are out there. Travel nursing certainly provides a high degree of autonomy and control of your schedule and career. One of the key elements reported by nurses for career satisfaction is quality of life. The freedom of choice provided by travel nursing would certainly fulfill that need.

Source: *American Traveler, What is a travel nurse? January 12, 2022, https://www.americantraveler.com/what-is-a-travel-nurse.*

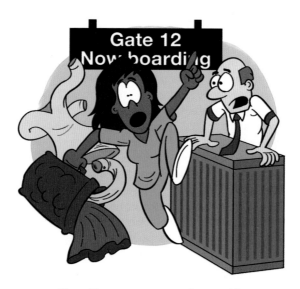

Traveling nurses see the world.

Conclusion

Nursing and the modern health-care system are in a time of transition. How will the various health-care professions address the challenges posed by shrinking health-care budgets, increasing insurance and medical costs, and a large population of aging baby boomers? Nurses at all levels can find creative solutions to meet these challenges with professionalism and empowerment, just as nursing's foremothers did.

Nightingale invaded the hospital run by the British Army with 37 of her best-educated nurses and made massive changes in health outcomes. She singlehandedly reworked the education system for nurses in the face of a physician-run and highly resistant health-care system. Hampton Robb pushed for nursing education at the university level at a time when there were hardly any women in college. Loretta Ford conceived and nurtured the role of advanced practice nurse despite strong objections from her physician colleagues.

Although many of the difficulties with today's health-care system, and those of nursing in particular, can be traced back to the historical development of the profession, they cannot stop creative, strong-willed, and persistent nurses from moving the profession forward. Knowledge of nursing's historical roots can help us understand these current difficulties. That same historical knowledge can point the way to innovative solutions. For example, nurses today still typically have a high level of responsibility but a low level of power; however, when nurses unite, they can sometimes move mountains (sometimes called legislators, physicians, and administrators).

There are untold *opportunities* for today's nurses to be change agents in defining the roles that nurses fill and empowering nurses to have a strong voice in the 21st-century health-care system. Those who belong to the nursing profession have a responsibility not only to learn from the past but also to use those lessons to make nursing the premier profession for the future.

CRITICAL-THINKING EXERCISES

- Trace the history of your nursing school. Who were the leaders in the foundation of the school? Write a short biography for each one, listing their accomplishments.
- If you know any retired nurses, contact them and ask if they would be willing to talk to you about their practice. Develop an oral history of what they experienced and compare it to nursing practice today.
- Start a journal of your own experiences as a nursing student. Maintain this journal throughout your career. Make sure to include interesting instructors and clients with whom you are in contact.

NCLEX-STYLE QUESTIONS

1. Which of these nursing leaders helped develop the *American Journal of Nursing?*
   1. Florence Nightingale
   2. Isabel Adams Hampton Robb
   3. Lillian Wald
   4. Lavinia Lloyd Dock
2. In what way did Hippocrates' beliefs about illness and medicine differ from those of other ancient Greek physician-priests?
   1. Hippocrates believed in treating the whole client, not just in appeasing the gods.
   2. Hippocrates believed in diagnosis through mystical visions.
   3. Hippocrates believed that the physician was never to be questioned.
   4. Hippocrates believed in treating the body, not the spirit.
3. Place the events in the development of nursing in the Christian church in the order in which they occurred.
   1. Monks and nuns, often with little training, cared for the poor and the sick.
   2. After the Protestant Reformation, nursing care in countries that broke away from the Catholic Church fell into disarray.

3. During the Crusades, Knights Hospitallers cared for those who became sick or were wounded in battle.
4. Wealthy Roman women who had converted to Christianity established hospital-like institutions.

4. Which historical thread explains the evolution of health-care providers from shamans and priests to nurses and physicians?
   1. The value placed on individual life
   2. The role of women in society
   3. The beliefs about the causes of illness
   4. The effects of large-scale war on society
5. What effect did World War II have on the development of U.S. nursing? **Select all that apply**.
   1. The U.S. government commissioned nurses and paid them the same as men with the same rank.
   2. Working with physicians and untrained personnel, nurses initiated the concept of the health-care team.
   3. The nursing shortage immediately after World War II led to ADNs outnumbering BSNs by the 1960s.
   4. The number of BSN and graduate nursing programs exploded.
   5. The image of the nursing profession was especially positive, in part because of the heroic portrayal of nurses in movies produced during the war.
6. Which of the following nursing leaders is best known for her work outside the field of nursing?
   1. Annie W. Goodrich
   2. Loretta C. Ford
   3. Lavinia Lloyd Dock
   4. Lillian Wald

7. What effect did the Renaissance have on the role of nursing?
   1. Nursing care fell to female religious orders as the number of male nursing orders decreased.
   2. Nursing became more scientific because of the invention of the microscope and the thermometer.
   3. Nursing became more secular, and faith in the teachings of the Catholic Church waivered.
   4. Nursing in countries that broke away from the Catholic Church advanced swiftly.
8. What does the nursing lamp symbolize? **Select all that apply**.
   1. Life
   2. Learning
   3. Fire
   4. Sacrifice
   5. Caring
9. What was the status of organized medical care in the American colonies before they gained their independence?
   1. People were cared for at home; only five hospitals existed for the homeless and poor before the Revolutionary War.
   2. Nurses trained in religious orders in Europe immigrated to the colonies in large numbers.
   3. Hospitals were well known for their success in treating a variety of serious illnesses.
   4. Benjamin Franklin organized and trained medical volunteers to aid the injured and sick during the Revolutionary War.
10. In addition to their development of central heating, baths, and advanced systems for sewage disposal, the ancient Romans maintained the good health of citizens with _____, which supplied clean water.

References

1. Duffin J. *History of Medicine: A Scandalously Short Introduction* (3rd ed.). Toronto: University of Toronto Press, 2021.
2. Wyatt L. *A History of Nursing.* New York: Amberley Publishing, 2019.
3. Keeling A, Hehman M, Kirchgesener J. *History of Professional Nursing in the United States.* New York: Springer, 2018.
4. Isabel Hampton Robb—Nursing theorist. Retrieved January 8, 2023, from http://nursing-theory.org/nursing-theorists/Isabel-Hampton-Robb.php
5. Henry Street Settlement. Lillian Wald, n.d. https://www.henrystreet.org/about/our-history/lillian-wald
6. Bradford-Burnam MA. Lavinia Lloyd Dock: An activist in nursing and social reform. Dissertation, Ohio State University, 1998.
7. Annie Warburton Goodrich (1866–1954), 1976 inductee. American Nurses Association, n.d. https://www.nursingworld.org/ana/about-ana/history/hall-of-fame/1976-1982-inductees
8. Brennan C. Tracing the history of the nurse practitioner profession in 2020, the Year of the Nurse. *Journal of Pediatric Healthcare*, 34(2):83–84, 2020. https://doi.org/10.1016/j.pedhc.2019.12.005
9. Time Line Stories: Loretta Ford. Women in Exploration, n.d. https://www.womeninexploration.org/timeline/loretta-ford/

Theories and Models of Nursing

3

Joseph T. Catalano

Learning Objectives

After completing this chapter, the reader will be able to:

- Explain why theories and models are important to the profession of nursing
- Analyze the four key concepts found in nursing theories and models
- Interrelate systems theory as an important element in understanding nursing theories and models
- Evaluate how the four parts of all systems interact
- Synthesize three nursing theories, identifying how the different nursing theorists define the key concepts in their theories
- Compare and contrast a middle-range theory with a grand nursing theory

CARING FOR REAL PEOPLE

For many nurses, and for most nursing students, the terms **theory** and **model** evoke images of textbooks filled with abstract, obscure words and convoluted sentences. The visceral response is often, "Why is this important? I want to take care of real people!" The simple answer is that understanding and using practice models, especially the middle-range theories and models, will help you be a better nurse and provide better care to real people. For example, during the height of the COVID-19 pandemic, a number of middle-range nursing theories (discussed later in this chapter) were used to conduct research projects to identify best practices in nursing care of these patients. One such project was conducted by Zahourek using the Griffith model of Intentionality: The Matrix of Healing. The research showed that writing vital signs and care-related messages to nurses, respiratory therapists, and other caregivers on the glass doors of intensive care units during the pandemic actually helped increase nursing retention. The study also showed that positioning patients on their stomachs rather than on their backs helped increase their oxygenation levels. Nurses and institutions that use professional practice models find that the quality of patient care improves with the knowledge and use of practice models, and nurses have more satisfaction with their careers and remain current with trends and changes in technology.[1]

DIFFERENCES BETWEEN THEORIES AND MODELS

What Is a Theory?

Although *theory* and *model* are not synonymous, in nursing practice they are often used interchangeably. Strictly speaking, a theory refers to a speculative statement involving some element of reality that has not been proved. For example, the theory of relativity has never been proved, although the results have often been observed.

The nursing profession tends to use *theory* when attempting to explain apparent relationships between observed behaviors and their effects on a patient's health. In this nursing context, the goal of a theory is to describe and explain a particular nursing action to make a **hypothesis**, which predicts the effect on a patient's outcome, such as improved health or recovery from illness. For example, the action of turning an unresponsive patient from side to side every 2 hours should help to prevent skin breakdown and improve respiratory function.

In the early days of nursing, theories were very simple and reflected the knowledge base of the time. With the rapid growth in health-care knowledge and **technology**, nursing theory also has expanded and evolved to help nurses provide **higher-quality care** in increasingly complex patient conditions. Nursing theories provide a framework to plan for decision making when new patient needs are encountered. They also provide a method for nurses to communicate with each other and with other members of the health-care team. Guiding the development of research and helping to formulate a nurse's values and **goals**, nursing theories are one of the key elements in nursing's development as a profession.

In recent years, nursing has been moving toward using research findings to guide nursing practice. This approach, called *evidence-based practice*, is an important element in improving nursing care and proving many of the long-standing theories that the nursing profession has developed over the years.[1]

> *Mr. X had surgery for intestinal cancer 4 days ago. He has a colostomy and needs to learn how to take care of it at home because he is going to be discharged from the hospital in 2 days. When the nurses attempt to teach him colostomy care, he looks away, makes sarcastic personal comments about the nurses, and generally displays a belligerent and hostile attitude.*

What Is a Model?

A model is a hypothetical representation of something that exists in reality. The purpose of a model is to explain a complex reality in a systematic and organized manner that is more easily understood. For example, a hospital organizational chart is a model that attempts to demonstrate the interrelationships of the various levels of the hospital's administration.

What Do You Think?

Do you consider yourself to be healthy? What factors make you healthy? What factors are indicators of illness?

What Do Nurses Do?

Although a model tends to be more concrete than a theory, they both help explain and direct nursing actions. This use of a systematic and structured approach is one of the key elements that raises nursing from a task-oriented job to the level of a profession that requires judgment and knowledge to make informed decisions about patient care. With the use of a **conceptual model**, nurses can provide intelligent and thoughtful answers to the question, "What do nurses do?" Consider the scenario involving Mr. X, summarized in the corresponding quote.

Without an understanding of the underlying dynamics involved, the nurses might themselves become sarcastic and scold the patient about his behavior or simply minimize their contact with him. This type of response will not improve Mr. X's health status. If, however, the nurses knew about and understood the dynamics of grief theory, they would realize that Mr. X is probably in the anger stage of the grief process. This understanding would direct the nurses to allow, or even to encourage, Mr. X to express his anger and **aggressiveness** without condemnation and to help him deal with his feelings in a constructive manner. Once Mr. X gets past the anger stage, he can move on to taking a more active part in his care and thus improve his health status. The **patient goals** would then be achieved.

If a researcher were to stop 10 people at random on the street and ask the question, "What do nurses do?" the researcher would likely get 10 different answers, but the confusion about nurses' activities extends far beyond the public at large. What if the researcher asked 10 hospital administrators, 10 physicians, or even 10 nurses the same question? The answers would probably vary almost as much as the answers from laypersons.

Professional Practice Model

With the development of the Magnet Recognition Program whereby health-care organizations can earn Magnet status by meeting requisite criteria, the American Nurses Credentialing Center reinforced the need for professional practice models (PPMs). For an institution seeking Magnet status, the PPM needs to provide an "overarching conceptual framework for nurses, nursing care and interprofessional patient care." The PPM is a way to describe in a pictorial way all the iterations, values, beliefs, and activities that go into producing high-quality patient outcomes. It must be evaluated annually to ensure that it is current with the institution's practices.[2]

The Iowa Project (Nursing Interventions Classification)

In an attempt to identify exactly what it is that nurses do, J. C. McCloskey and G. M. Bulechek, two nurse researchers at the University of Iowa, have been conducting an ongoing research project since 1990 to develop a **taxonomy** of the **interventions** that nurses use in their practice (Box 3.1). This project began as the Iowa Project but is now called the Nursing Interventions Classification (NIC).[3–4] The NIC is maintained by the University of Iowa College of Nursing. The classification system is published in book and eBook form and is also accessible

---

Box 3.1 **What Constitutes Care?**

At first glance, it would seem that everybody knows that nurses take care of patients. But what constitutes care? A study conducted by the faculty of the University of Iowa, called the Nursing Interventions Classification (NIC), has identified 565 tasks or interventions for which nurses are responsible in their care of patients. Not all nurses carry out all 565 of these tasks all the time, but during an average career, a nurse would likely be involved in the majority of these tasks. Although this project was undertaken in 1990, it remains the benchmark study. Since the original study, several additional studies have reaffirmed the findings of the initial Iowa Project, and researchers have undertaken projects to use the data generated by the NIC in actual patient-care situations. It now forms the basis for the classification of patients in health-care institutions.

This project is an excellent example of how a nursing theory led to a research project that developed information that nurses can use in their daily practice. On the principle that nursing interventions are specific actions that a nurse can perform to bring about the resolution of a potential or actual health problem, the NIC identifies and classifies nursing interventions. It also ranks those interventions according to the number of times a nurse is likely to perform one during a working day. The goal was to develop a nursing information system that could be incorporated into the current information systems of all clinical facilities. By using the NIC system, hospital administrators, physicians, nurses, and even the public should be better able to recognize and evaluate the multiple interventions that nurses are responsible for in their daily work.

It is generally acknowledged that nurses, as the largest single group of health-care providers, are essential to the welfare and care of most patients. Yet, in an age of health-care reform, nurses are finding it increasingly difficult to delineate the specific contributions they make to health care. If nurses are unable to define the care they provide, how can the reformers, politicians, and public identify the unique contribution made by nursing?

Unfortunately, many of the contributions that nurses make to health care are currently invisible because there is no method of classification for them in the computerized database systems now in use. Commonly used nursing interventions such as active listening, emotional support, touch, skin surveillance, and even family support cannot be measured and quantified by most current information systems.

The large number of interventions used daily by nurses demonstrates the complex and demanding nature of the profession. The breadth and depth of knowledge and skills demanded of nurses on a daily basis are much greater than are found in many other health-care professions. One study found that nurses working in general medical-surgical units during a 6-month period were likely to care for 500 patients with more than 600 individual diagnoses (many patients have multiple diagnoses). These researchers also found that the physical demands of the work were actually less difficult and tiring than dealing with the emotional and technical demands of handling the huge amounts of information generated by the care given.

Sources: G. Bulechek, J. McCloskey, Nursing interventions classification (NIC), *Medinfo*, 8 Pt 2: 1368, 1995, https://pubmed.ncbi.nlm.nih.gov/8591448; M. Vera, Nursing diagnosis guide and list: All you need to know to master diagnosing, Nurseslabs, 2022. https://nurseslabs.com/nursing-diagnosis.

from a nurse's phone on a number of apps. NIC's focus has shifted from identifying what nurses do to a system of communication, or standardized language, among nurses and between nurses and other health-care team members. It has become an important element in health-care informatics.

A Classification System

The NIC addresses an ongoing need for nurses to be able to identify and quantify what they do. In the current era of concern for high-quality health care, this need has become even more acute. The first results, published in 1992, categorized and ranked 336 interventions that nurses use when they provide care to patients. By 1996, nearly 100 additional interventions (433) had been categorized and ranked. Researchers also investigated which nursing interventions are commonly used by nurses in specialty settings. Forty specialty areas responded, and the researchers were able to develop a table that lists what core skills are used by each specialization.

The NIC is currently in its seventh edition (2018), and the College of Nursing anticipates publishing updated editions approximately every 5 years. It now contains 565 interventions within a taxonomy of seven domains (physiological: basic; physiological: complex; behavioral; safety; family; health system; and community) and 30 classes of interventions.

Research into nursing intervention classification systems is ongoing and, in addition to providing a system of communication, has served as the foundation of several methods to define nursing practice and measure the outcomes of patient care. The need to increase patient satisfaction and achieve successful outcomes of nursing care is a key element in the Affordable Care Act (ACA), which was passed in 2010. Although Congress attempted to do away with the ACA completely, the act survived the effort. Congress did manage to chip away at some of the provisions, but they were almost totally restored when a new administration was elected in 2020. Even more than in the past, these elements will be the basis of reimbursement for health-care providers.

Using the NIC as a starting point, the Work Complexity Assessment (WCA) was developed so that nurses could identify specific interventions they routinely perform for various patient populations. Taking the process one step further, the Nursing Outcomes Classification system closes the loop by providing a means for nurses to evaluate whether the outcomes were achieved.[6]

Although initially used to help nurses with the delegation of duties to unlicensed personnel by linking skills with performance requirements, WCA is now an important tool in the improvement of the quality of nursing care. When nurses analyze the care they provide and actually look at the various interventions they use, they increase their understanding of both the methods and rationales for care. WCA also fits nicely into the use of evidence-based practice when nurses share with other nurses what they have learned about improving care.

> **The need to increase patient satisfaction and achieve successful outcomes of nursing care is a key element in the Affordable Care Act (ACA), which was passed in 2010. . . . Even more than in the past, these elements will be a basis of reimbursement for health-care providers.**

This type of research helps identify the important contributions made by nursing to the health and well-being of patients. It also demonstrates the complex and demanding nature of the nursing profession. Much of the public, and even many physicians and nurses, do not really understand what nurses do for patients on a daily basis. Using classification systems aids in clarifying what nurses bring to patient care, makes what they do measurable, and validates the importance of the nursing profession.

Nursing Competencies

One way in which the nursing profession identifies what nurses do is by looking at **competencies**. In nursing, *competence* is often defined as the combination of skills, knowledge, attitudes, values, and abilities that support the safe and effective practice of the nurse. Nurses practice competently when they have mastered a range of skills and decision-making processes demonstrated in the care of patients. All the major nursing organizations have developed lists of competencies for nurses. These are usually general, broad statements rather than catalogs of specific skills. (See "Issues Now: The Pew Commission Final Report" in this chapter.)

Nursing competencies first came under close scrutiny because of the large number of medication and other types of errors in the health-care setting that have led to numerous patients being injured or killed. The Institute of Medicine's (IOM, now the Health and Medicine Division of the National Academies of Sciences, Engineering, and Medicine) document on the future of nursing contains recommendations and lists of competencies for nursing school graduates to help improve the quality of care. The **Quality and Safe Education for Nurses (QSEN)** project, built on the IOM recommendations, has developed a framework for nursing schools' curricula (see more about IOM competencies and QSEN in Chapter 4).

Nursing researchers have attempted to develop specific lists of skills based on the general competency statements from the various nursing organizations. These skills lists help differentiate the various levels of nursing practice.

KEY CONCEPTS COMMON TO NURSING MODELS

Although nursing models vary in terminology and approach to health care, four concepts are common to almost all of them: patient or client (individual or collective), **health**, environment, and nursing. Each nursing model has its own specific definition of these terms, but the underlying definitions of the concepts are similar.

Patient

The concept of patient (or client) is central to all nursing models because it is the patient who is the primary recipient of nursing care. Although *patient* usually refers to a single individual, it can also refer to small groups or to a large collective of individuals (e.g., for community health nurses, the community is the patient). The use of *patient* became unpopular for a number of years because of its origin from the Latin word *pati*, which means to "suffer." However, it seems to be making a return to usage in professional publications.

A Complex Relationship

The concept of patient has changed over the years as knowledge and understanding of human nature have developed and increased. A patient constitutes more than a person who simply needs **restorative care** and comes to a health-care facility with a **disease** to be cured. Patients are now seen as complex entities affected by various interrelating factors, such as the mind and body, the individual and the **environment**, and the person and the person's family. When nurses talk about patients, the term *biopsychosocial* is often used to express the complex relationship between the body, mind, and environment. These elements are at the heart of preventive care that has been an emphasis of professional nursing since the time of Florence Nightingale. The prevention of disease and promotion of health are key provisions in the health-care reform bill passed in 2010 that opened the door for nurses to practice to the full extent of their licenses.

> " *Although nursing models vary in terminology and approach to health care, there are four concepts that are common to almost all of them: patient or client (individual or collective), health, environment, and nursing.* "

Modeling a Healthy Patient

A patient, in many of the nursing models, is not required to have an **illness** to be the central element of the model. This is also one of the clearest distinctions between medical models and nursing models. Medical models tend to be restrictive and reactive, focusing almost exclusively on curing diseases and restoring health after the patient becomes ill. Nursing models tend to be proactive and **holistic**. Like medical models, they are certainly concerned with curing disease and restoring a patient's health, but they also focus on preventing disease and maintaining health. A healthy person is just as important to many nursing models as the person with a disease.

Health

Like the concept of patient, the concept of health has undergone much development and change over the years as knowledge has increased. Traditionally, health was thought of as an absence of disease. A more current, realistic view is that of health as a continuum, ranging from a completely healthy state in which there is no disease to a completely unhealthy state, which results in death. At any given time in our lives, we are located somewhere along the health continuum and may move closer to one side or the other, depending on circumstances and health status.[7]

Health is difficult to define because it varies so much from one individual to another. For example, a 22-year-old bodybuilder who has no chronic diseases perceives health differently than does an 85-year-old who has diabetes, congestive heart failure, and vision problems. The perception of health also varies from among cultures and at different historical periods within the same culture. In some past cultures, a sign of health was pale white skin, whereas in recent American culture, a dark bronze tan was considered a sign of health—although research has shown how harmful ultraviolet light is to the skin.

Environment

Environment is another element in most current nursing models. Nursing models often broaden the concept of environment from the simple physical environment to elements such as living conditions, public sanitation, and air and water quality. Factors such as interpersonal relationships and social interactions are also included.

Some internal environmental factors that affect health include personal psychological processes, religious beliefs, sexual orientation, personality, and emotional responses. It has long been known that individuals who are highly self-motivated and internally goal directed (i.e., type A personality) tend to develop ulcers and have myocardial infarctions at a higher rate than the general population. Medical models, which are primarily illness oriented, may not consider personality types treatable. Nursing models that consider personality as one of the environmental factors affecting health are more likely to attempt to modify the individual's behavior (internal environment) to decrease the risk for disease.

Like the other key concepts found in nursing models, the concept of environment is consistent within a particular model's overall structure. Nursing models try to show how various aspects of environment interrelate and how they affect the patient's health status. In addition, nursing models treat environment as an active element in the overall health-care system and assert that positive alterations in the environment will improve the patient's health status.

Nursing

The culminating **concept** in all the various nursing models is nursing itself. After consideration of what it means to be a patient, what it means to be healthy, and how the environment influences the patient's health status (either positively or negatively), the concept of nursing delineates the function and role of nurses in their relationships with patients that affect the patient's health.

Historically, the profession of nursing has been interested in providing basic physical care (i.e., hygiene, activity, and nourishment), psychological support, and relief of discomfort. Modern nursing, although still including these basic elements of patient care, has expanded into areas of health care that were only imagined a generation ago.

Patient as Partner

In the modern nurse–patient relationship, the patient is no longer the passive recipient of nursing care. The relationship has been expanded to include patients as key partners in curing and in the health-maintenance process. In conjunction with the nurse, patients set goals for care and recovery, take an active part in achieving those goals, and help in evaluating whether those actions have achieved the goals.[8]

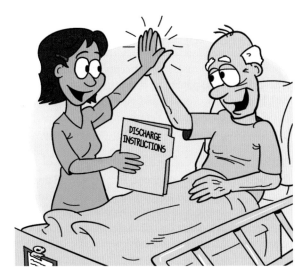

Partnerships with patients equal successful recoveries.

What Do You Think?

How do you define nursing? What competencies are important for you to practice safely when you graduate?

Because of the broadened understanding of environment, several nursing models include manipulation of environmental elements that affect health as an important part of the nurse's role. The environment may be directly altered by the nurse with little or no input from the patient, or the patient may be taught by the nurse to alter the environment in ways that will contribute to curing disease, increasing comfort, or improving the patient's health status.[9]

Four Key Concepts

To analyze and understand any nursing model, it is important to look for these four key concepts: patient, health, environment, and nursing. These concepts should be clearly defined, closely interrelated, and mutually supportive. Depending on the particular nursing model, one element may be emphasized more than the others. The resultant role and function of the nurse depend on which element is given greatest emphasis.

GENERAL SYSTEMS THEORY

A widely accepted method for conceptualizing and understanding the world and what is in it derives from a systems viewpoint. Generally understood as an organized unit with a set of components that interact and affect each other, a system acts as a whole because of the interdependence of its parts.[10] As a result, when part of the system malfunctions or fails, it interrupts the function of the whole system rather than affecting merely one part. The terminology and principles of systems theory pervade U.S. society. Humans, plants, cars, governments, the health-care system, the nursing profession, and almost anything that exists can be viewed as a system.

> *The culminating concept in all the various nursing models is nursing itself. After consideration of what it means to be a patient, what it means to be healthy, and how the environment influences the patient's health status (either positively or negatively), the concept of nursing delineates the function and role of nurses in their relationships with patients that affect the patient's health.*

A Basis in Thought

Although **general systems theory** in its pure form is rarely, if ever, used as a nursing model, its process and much of its terminology underlie many nursing models. Elements of general systems theory in one form or another have found their way into many textbooks and much of the professional literature. General systems theory often acts as the unacknowledged **conceptual framework** for many educational programs. An understanding of the mechanisms and terminology of general systems theory is helpful in providing an orientation to understanding nursing models.

Manageable Fragments

General systems theory, sometimes referred to simply as **systems theory**, is an outgrowth of an innate intellectual process. The human mind has difficulty comprehending a large, complex entity as a single unit, so it automatically divides that entity into smaller, more manageable fragments and then examines each fragment separately. This is similar to the process of deductive reasoning in which a single complex thought or theory is broken down into smaller, interrelated pieces. All scientific disciplines, from physics to biology and the social sciences (e.g., sociology and psychology), use this method of analysis.

Reassembling the Fragments

Systems theory takes the process a step further. After analyzing or breaking down the entity, systems theory attempts to put it back together by showing how the parts work individually and together within the system. This interrelationship of the parts makes the system function as a unit. Often, particularly when the system involves biological or sociological entities, the system that results is greater than the sum of its parts.

For example, a human can be considered to be a complex biosocial system. Humans are made up of many smaller systems, such as the endocrine system, neurological system, gastrointestinal system, urinary system, and so forth. Although each of these systems is important, in and of themselves they do not make a human. Many animals have the same systems, yet the human is more than the animal and more than the sum of the systems.

A Set of Interacting Parts

Although the early roots of general systems theory can be traced as far back as the 1930s, Ludwig von Bertalanffy is usually credited with the formal development and publication of general systems theory around 1950.[11] His major achievement was to standardize the definitions of the terms used in systems theory and make the concept useful to a wide range of disciplines. Systems theory is so widely applicable because it reflects the reality that underlies basic human thought processes.

Very simply, a system is defined as a set of interacting parts. The parts that compose a system may be similar or may vary a great deal from each other, but they all have the common function of making the system work well to achieve its overall purpose.

> *Systems theory is so widely applicable because it reflects the reality that underlies basic human thought processes.*

A school is a good example of how the dynamics and connections of a system work. A school as a system consists of several units, including buildings, administrators, teachers, students, and various other individuals (e.g., counselors, financial aid personnel, bookkeepers, and maintenance persons). Each of these individuals has a unique job but also contributes to the overall goal of the school, which is to provide an education for the students and to further the development of knowledge through research.

All systems consist of four key parts: the system itself (whether it is open or closed), input and output, throughput, and a feedback loop.

Open and Closed Systems

A system is categorized as being either open or closed. Very few systems are completely open or completely closed. Rather, they are usually a combination of both.

Open Systems

Open systems are those in which relatively free movement of information, matter, and **energy** into and out of the system exists. In a completely open system, there would be no restrictions on what moves in and out of the system, thus making its boundaries difficult to identify. Most systems have some control over the movement of information, energy, and matter around them. This control is maintained through the semipermeable nature of their boundaries, which allows some things in and keeps some things out, as well as allowing some out while keeping others in. This control of input and output leads to the dynamic equilibrium found in most well-functioning systems.

Closed Systems

Theoretically, a **closed system** prevents any movement into and out of the system. In this case, the system would be totally static and unchanging. Probably no absolutely closed systems exist in the real world, although some systems may tend to be closed to outside elements. A stone, for example, considered as a system, seems to be almost perfectly closed. It does not take anything in or put anything out. It does not change very much over long periods. In reality, though, it is affected by several elements in nature. It absorbs moisture when it is damp, freezes when cold, and becomes hot in the summer. Over long periods, these factors may cause the stone to crack, break down, and eventually become topsoil.

Systems with which nurses deal frequently are relatively open. Primarily, the patient can be categorized as a highly open system that requires certain input elements and has output elements too. Other systems that nurses commonly work with (e.g., hospital administrators and physicians) are generally considered to be open, although their degree of openness may vary widely.

Input and Output

The processes by which a system interacts with elements in its environment are called **input** and **output**. *Input* is defined as any type of information, energy, or material that enters the system from the environment through its boundaries. Conversely, *output* is defined as any information, energy, or material that leaves the system and enters the environment through the system's boundaries. The end product of a system is a type of output that is not reusable as input. Open systems require relatively large amounts of input and output.

Throughput

A third term sometimes used in relationship to the system's dynamic exchange with the environment is **throughput**. Throughput is a process that allows the input to be changed so that it is useful to the system.

For example, most automobiles operate on some form of liquid fossil fuel (input) such as gasoline or diesel fuel. However, going to the gas station and pouring liquid fuel on the roof of the car will not produce the desired effects. If the fuel is put into the gas tank, it can be transformed by the carburetor or fuel-injection system into a fine mist, which when mixed with air and ignited by a spark plug burns rapidly to produce the force necessary to propel the car. Without this internal process (throughput), liquid fuel is not a useful form of energy.

Feedback Loop

The fourth key element of a system is the **feedback loop**. The feedback loop allows the system to monitor its internal functioning so that it can either restrict or increase its input and its output and maintain the highest level of functioning.

Positive Feedback

Two basic types of feedback exist. Positive feedback leads to change within the system, with the goal of improving the system. For example, students in the classroom receive feedback from the teacher in several ways; it may be through direct verbal statements such as "Good work on this assignment" or through examination and homework grades. Feedback is considered positive if it produces a change in a student's behavior, such as motivating him or her to study more, spend more time on assignments, or prepare more thoroughly for class.

Negative Feedback

Negative feedback maintains stability—that is, it does not produce change. Negative feedback is not necessarily bad for a system. Rather, when a system

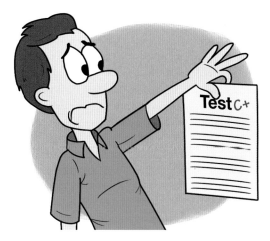

Improve test scores by learning the test-taking tips.

has reached its peak level of functioning, negative feedback helps it maintain that level. For example, if a person on a weight-loss regimen has reached the target weight, he or she knows what type of diet and exercise is needed to stay at the ideal weight. Negative feedback—in the form of numbers on the bathroom scale—indicates that no changes in diet or exercise patterns are required.

The feedback loop is an important element in systems theory. It makes the process circular and links the various elements of the system together. Without a feedback loop, it is virtually impossible for the system to have any meaningful control over its input and output.

Feedback loops are used at all levels in a hospital. Nurses get feedback about the care they provide from both patients and supervisors. The hospital administration gets feedback from patients and accrediting agencies. Physicians get feedback from patients, nurses, and the hospital administration. Since the passage of the ACA with its emphasis on quality of care, feedback from patients about the care they received while in health-care facilities is an important part of the facilities' economic survival. Systems theory is present, if sometimes unseen, in almost all health-care settings. Professional nurses need to be able to understand and identify the components of systems theory when they are encountered to improve their nursing practice and quality of care.

NURSING THEORIES AND MODELS

A Hierarchy

Nursing theories and models are arranged into a hierarchical system. At the top are the *grand theories and models*, which are highly theoretical and contain broad general concepts and suppositions that demonstrate and mirror what the author has observed in their own experience of nursing care. These provide a broad way of conceptualizing nursing care and practice in almost all setting and situations. The abstract nature of these theories or models makes them difficult to test through empirical nursing research, so they are difficult to translate into daily nursing care without significant modification.

The second level of nursing theories or models are referred to as *middle-range nursing theories or models*. They differ from the grand models in that their scope is much narrower and they are much more concrete. Consequently, they are easier to translate into a theory-based daily nursing practice. Because they are less complex, they usually deal with a limited number of variables, and more to the point, they are more amenable to scientific research testing. They serve as a way to connect some of the high-level abstract thinking found in grand models with the nurse's everyday practice.

Third are the *nursing practice theories or models*. These have an even narrower scope and less abstraction than the middle-range theories and are generally limited to a particular situation or set of circumstances. They provide the rationales for specific nursing interventions and help guide the nurse in developing goals and outcomes for a specific patient or community. Nursing students almost always use practice theories when they are developing care plans for their assigned patients.

Borrowed or shared nursing theories or models use knowledge from other sciences and disciplines and incorporate it into a theory or model that focuses primarily on nursing. The borrowed knowledge may come from psychology, medicine, systems analysis, and so forth. These borrowed or shared theories can be found at all three levels of nursing theories or models. Some borrowed theories include Nightingale,

Roy, and Orem. Some nursing theories that do not borrow from others include Neuman, Watson, Parse, and Peplau.

Nursing is always striving to develop a unique body of knowledge. Does that fact make borrowed or shared theories less valuable than original theories? Not necessarily. The key factors to look for are as follows: (1) Is the knowledge being used harmonious with nursing knowledge? (2) Can the knowledge be placed in a nursing context where it becomes a part of a nursing framework? (3) Has the knowledge been modified or used in a way that can guide nursing practice? and (4) Does the knowledge advance nursing knowledge? If the answer is yes to all four elements, then the theory or model is usually deemed a valuable contribution to nursing.[12]

GRAND THEORIES OR MODELS

At least 15 published nursing models (or theories) are considered grand and are used to direct nursing education and nursing care (Box 3.2). These models are called *grand* or sometimes *broad-range theories* because they have a broad or comprehensive scope and are at a high level of abstraction. They are difficult to test or retest in practice, but they form the underpinnings of many of the middle-range theories. Grand theories usually have three general areas of focus: human needs, process of interaction, and the process of unity of care.[13]

> *The feedback loop is an important element in systems theory. It makes the process circular and links the various elements of the system together.*

The nursing models discussed here were selected because they are the most widely accepted and are good examples of how the concepts of patient, health, environment, and nursing are used to explain and guide nursing actions. Discussion of these theories is not intended to be comprehensive but rather to provide an overview of the main concepts of the nurse theorist. It is important to understand the terms used in the theories as defined by their authors and to see the interrelationship between the elements in each theory as well as the similarities and differences among the various models.

The Roy Adaptation Model

As developed by Sister Callista Roy, the Roy adaptation model of nursing is very closely related to

Box 3.2 **Partial List of Grand Theories in Nursing**

Behavioral system model—Dorothy E. Johnson

Conservation model—Myra Estrine Levine

Emancipated decision making in health care—Ruth A. Wittman-Price

Goal attainment model—Emogine M. King

Health as expanding consciousness—Margaret Newman

Humanistic nursing—Josephine Paterson and Loretta Zderad

Interpersonal relations model—Hildegard E. Peplau

Modeling and role modeling theory—Helen C. Erickson, Evelyn M. Tomlin, and Mary Ann P. Swain

Nursing process theory—Ida Jean Orlando

Philosophy and theory of transpersonal caring—Jean Watson

Roy adaptation model—Sister Callista Roy

Science of unitary human beings—Martha E. Rogers

Self-care theory—Dorothea Orem

Theory of human becoming—Rosemarie Rizzo Parse

Transcultural nursing (formerly culture-care)—Madeleine Leininger

---

systems theory.[14] The main goal of this model is to allow the patients to reach their highest level of functioning through the process of adaptation.

Patient

The central element in the Roy adaptation model is man (a generic term referring to humans in general, or the patient in particular, collectively or individually). Man is viewed as a dynamic entity with both input and output. As derived from the context of the four modes in the Roy adaptation model, the patient is defined as a biopsychosocial being who is affected by various stimuli and displays behaviors to help adapt to the stimuli. Because the patient is constantly being affected by stimuli, adaptation is a continual process.[14]

Inputs are called *stimuli* and include internal stimuli that arise from within the patient and stimuli coming from external environmental factors such as physical surroundings, family, and society. The output in the Roy adaptation model is the behavior that the patient demonstrates as a result of stimuli that are affecting him or her.

Output, or behavior, is a very important element in the Roy adaptation model because it provides the **baseline data** about the patient that the nurse obtains through assessment techniques. In this model, the output (behavior) is always modified by the patient's internal attempts to adapt to the input, or stimuli. Roy identifies four internal adaptational activities that patients use, called the *four adaptation modes*:

1. The physiological mode (using internal physiological process)
2. The self-concept mode (developed throughout life by experience)
3. The role function mode (dependent on the patient's relative place in society)
4. The interdependence mode (indicating how the patient relates to others)

Health

In the Roy adaptation model, the concept of health is defined as the location of the patient along a continuum between perfect health and complete illness. In this model, health is rarely an absolute. Rather, "a person's ability to adapt to stimuli, such as injury, disease, or even psychological stress, determines the level of that person's health status."[14] For example, a patient who broke her neck in an automobile accident and was paralyzed but who eventually went back to college, obtained a law degree, and became a practicing lawyer would, in the Roy adaptation model, be considered to have a high degree of health because of the ability to adapt to the stimuli imposed.

Environment

The Roy adaptation model's definition of environment is synonymous with the concept of stimuli. The environment consists of all those factors that influence the patient's behavior, both internally and externally. This model categorizes these environmental elements, or stimuli, into three groups: (1) focal, (2) contextual, and (3) residual.

Focal stimuli are environmental factors that most directly affect the patient's behavior and require most of their attention. Contextual stimuli form the general physical, social, and psychological environment from which the patient emerges. Residual stimuli are factors in the patient's past, such as personality characteristics, past experiences, religious beliefs, and social norms, that have an indirect effect on the patient's health status. Residual stimuli are often very difficult to identify because they may remain hidden in the person's memory or may be an integral part of the patient's personality.

Nursing

In the Roy adaptation model, nursing becomes a multistep process, similar to the **nursing process**, to aid and support the patient's attempt to adapt to stimuli in one or more of the four adaptive modes. To determine what type of help is required to promote **adaptation**, the nurse must first assess the patient.

Assessment

The primary **nursing assessments** are of the patient's behavior (output). Basically, the nurse should try to determine whether the patient's behavior is adaptive or maladaptive in each of the four adaptational modes previously defined. Some first-level assessments of the patient with pneumonia might include a temperature of 104°F, a cough productive of thick green sputum, chest pain on inspiration, and signs of weakness or physical debility, such as the inability to bring in wood for the fireplace or to visit friends.

> *In the Roy adaptation model, nursing becomes a multistep process, similar to the nursing process, to aid and support the patient's attempt to adapt to stimuli in one or more of the four adaptive modes.*

A second-level **assessment** should also be made to determine what type of stimuli (input) is affecting the patient's health status. In the case of the pneumonia patient, this might include a culture and sensitivity test of the sputum to identify the invasive bacteria, assessment of the patient's clothes to determine whether they were adequate for the weather outside, and an investigation to find out whether any neighbors could help the patient upon discharge from the hospital.

Analysis

After performing the assessment, the nurse analyzes the data and arranges them in such a way as to be able to make a statement about the patient's adaptive or maladaptive behaviors—that is, the nurse identifies the problem. In current terminology, this identification of the problem is called a **nursing diagnosis**. The problem statement is the first part of the three-part PES (problem–etiology–signs and symptoms) formulation that completes the nursing diagnosis (Fig. 3.1).

Setting Goals

After the problem is identified, goals for optimal adaptation are established. Ideally, these goals should be a collaborative effort between the nurse and the patient. A determination of the actions needed to achieve the goals is the next step in the process. The focus should be on manipulation of the stimuli to promote optimal adaptation. Finally, an evaluation is made of the whole process to determine whether the goals have been met. If the goals have not been met, the nurse must determine why, not how, the activities should be modified to achieve the goals.[11]

The Orem Self-Care Model

Dorothea E. Orem's model of nursing is based on the belief that health care is each individual's own responsibility. The aim of this model is to help patients direct and carry out activities that maintain or improve their health. Orem's model is also referred to as the *self-care deficit* model or theory because it focuses on identifying and remediating where the patient falls short in their self-care.[15]

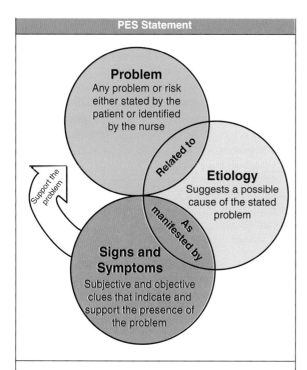

PES Statement

Problem
Any problem or risk either stated by the patient or identified by the nurse

Related to

Etiology
Suggests a possible cause of the stated problem

Support the problem

As manifested by

Signs and Symptoms
Subjective and objective clues that indicate and support the presence of the problem

Together, these components make up the *PES* (**P**roblem, **E**tiology, **S**igns/symptoms) statement, which is demonstrated below.

***Pain**, acute, may be **related to surgical wound**, as manifested by **facial grimacing**, **increased heart rate**, and **verbal complaints** of pain at the incision site.*

Figure 3.1 Together, these components make up the **PES** (**p**roblem–**e**tiology–**s**igns and symptoms) statement: Pain, acute, may be related to *surgical wound*, as manifested by *facial grimacing, increased heart rate*, and *verbal complaints* of pain at the incision site.

Patient

As with most other nursing models, the central element of the Orem model is the patient, who is a biological, psychological, and social being with the capacity for self-care. *Self-care* is defined as the practice of activities that individuals initiate and perform on their own behalf to maintain life, health, and well-being. Self-care is a requirement for maintenance of life and for optimal functioning.

Health

In the Orem self-care model, health is defined as the person's ability to live fully within a particular physical, biological, and social environment, achieving a higher level of functioning that distinguishes the person from lower life forms.

Quality of life is an extremely important element in this model of nursing. A person who is healthy is living life to the fullest and has the capacity to continue that life through self-care. According to Orem, an unhealthy person is an individual who has a self-care deficit. Based on this definition, not only adults with diseases and injuries but also children, elderly persons, and people with disabilities could be considered unhealthy if they are not able to carry out one or more of the key health-care activities. These activities have been categorized into six groups:

1. Air, water, and food
2. Excretion of waste
3. Activity and rest
4. Solitude and social interactions
5. Avoiding hazards to life and well-being
6. Maintaining healthy mental status while practicing universal self-care

Self-care

In the Orem model, self-care is a two-part concept. The first type of self-care is called *universal self-care* and includes those elements commonly found in everyday life that support and encourage normal human growth, development, and functioning. Individuals who are healthy, according to the Orem model, carry out the activities listed in order to maintain a state of health. To some degree, all of these elements are necessary activities in maintaining health through self-care.[16]

The second type of self-care, called *health deviation self-care*, comes into play when the individual is unable to conduct one or more of the six self-care activities. Health deviation self-care includes those activities carried out by individuals who have diseases, injuries, physiological or psychological stress, or other health-care concerns. Activities such as seeking health care at an emergency department or clinic, entering a drug **rehabilitation** unit, joining a health club or weight-control program, or going to a physician's office fall into this category.

Environment

Environment, in the self-care model, is the medium through which patients move as they conduct their daily activities. Although less emphasized in this model, the environment is generally viewed as a negative factor in a person's health status because many environmental factors detract from the ability to provide self-care. Environment includes social interactions with others, situations that must be resolved, and physical elements that affect health.

Nursing

The primary goal of nursing in the Orem model is to help the patient conduct self-care activities in such a way as to reach the highest level of human functioning. Because there is a range of levels of self-care ability, three distinct levels, or systems, of nursing care are delineated and are based on the individual's ability to undertake self-care activities. As patients become less able to care for themselves, their nursing care needs increase.

Wholly Compensated Care

A person who is able to carry out few or no self-care activities falls into the wholly compensated nursing care category in which the nurse must provide for most or all of the patient's self-care needs. Examples of patients who require this level of care include comatose and ventilator-dependent patients in an intensive care unit, patients in surgery and the immediate recovery period, women in the labor and delivery phases of childbirth, and patients with emotional and psychological problems so severe as to render them unable to conduct normal activities of daily living (ADLs).

Partially Compensated Care

Patients in the partially compensated category of nursing care can meet some to most of their self-care needs but still have certain self-care deficits that require nursing intervention. The nurse's role becomes one of identifying these needs and carrying out activities to meet them until the patient reaches a state of health and is able to meet the needs personally. Examples of patients who need this level of nursing care include postoperative patients who can feed themselves and do basic ADLs but are unable to care for a catheter and dressing and patients with newly diagnosed diabetes who have not yet learned the technique of self-administered insulin injections.

Supportive Developmental Care

Patients who are able to meet all of their basic self-care needs require very few or no nursing interventions. These patients fall in the supportive developmental category of nursing care in which the nurse's main functions are to teach the patient how to maintain or improve health and to offer guidance in self-care activities and provide emotional support and encouragement.

What Do You Think?

Based on your experiences with the health-care system, write your own definition of a patient (patient). What factors led you to this definition?

Also, the nurse may adjust the environment to support the patient's growth and development toward self-care or may identify community resources to help in the self-care process.[16] Conducting prenatal classes, arranging for discharge planning, providing child screening programs through a community health agency, and organizing aerobic exercise classes for postcoronary patients all are nursing actions that belong in the supportive developmental category of care.

> *The primary goal of nursing in the Orem model is to help the patient conduct self-care activities in such a way as to reach the highest level of human functioning.*

A Three-Step Process

In the Orem model, nursing care is carried out through a three-step process. Step 1 determines whether nursing care is necessary. This step includes a basic assessment of the patient and identification of self-care problems and needs. Step 2 determines the appropriate nursing care system category and plans nursing care according to that category. Step 3 provides the indicated nursing care or actions to meet the patient's self-care needs.

Step 3—the provision of nursing care (**implementation** phase)—is carried out by helping the patient through one or a combination of five nursing methods:[12]

1. Acting for or doing for another person
2. Guiding another person
3. Supporting another person (physically or psychologically)

4. Providing an environment that promotes personal development
5. Teaching another person

Orem, by focusing on the individual's ability to perform self-care, was many years ahead of her time. Current trends in health care reinforce her belief that individuals can take responsibility for care of themselves and others. The capacity for self-care is a key premise of the ACA and the more than 8,000 apps that are available that deal with self-care. It might even be referred to as "Digital Orem."

The King Model of Goal Attainment

The current widely accepted practice of establishing health-care goals for patients and directing patient care to meet these goals has its origins in the King model of goal attainment developed by Imogene M. King. It is also called the King intervention model.[16]

The King model also notes that nursing must function in all three systems levels found in the environment: personal, interactional, and social. The primary function of nursing is at the personal systems level, where care of the individual is the main focus. However, nurses can effectively provide care at the interactional systems level, where they deal with small to moderate-sized groups in activities such as group therapy and health-promotion classes. Finally, nurses can provide care at the social systems level through such activities as community health programs. In addition, the role of nursing at the social systems level can be expanded to include involvement in policy decisions that have an effect on the health-care system as a whole.

Patient

As in other nursing models, the focal point of care in the King model is the person or patient. The patient is viewed as an open system that exchanges energy and information with the environment—a personal system with physical, emotional, and intellectual needs that change and grow during the course of life. Because these needs cannot be met completely by the patient alone, interpersonal systems are developed through interactions with others, depending on the patient's perceptions of reality, communications with others, and transactions to reduce stress and tension in the environment.

Environment

Environment is an important concept in the King model and encompasses a number of interrelated elements. The personal and interpersonal systems or groups are central to King's conception of environment. They are formed at various levels according to internal goals established by the patient.

Personal Systems

At the most basic level are the personal systems, where an interchange takes place between two individuals who share similar goals. An example of such a personal system is a patient–nurse relationship.

Interpersonal Systems

At the intermediate level are the interpersonal systems that involve relatively small groups of individuals who share like goals, such as a formal weight-loss program in which the members have the common goal of losing weight. Human interactions, communications, role delineation, and stress reduction are essential factors at this level.

Social Systems

At the highest level are social systems, which include the large, relatively homogeneous elements of society. The health-care system, government, and society in general are some important social systems. Common goals of these social systems are organization, authority, power, status, and decision. Although the patient may not be in direct interaction with the social systems, these systems are important because the personal and interpersonal systems necessarily function within larger social systems.

Invoking the principle of **nonsummativity**, whenever one part of an open system is changed, all the other parts of the system feel the effect. For example, a decision made at the governmental level to reduce **Medicare** or **Medicaid** payments may affect when and how often a patient can use health-care services such as doctor's office visits, group therapy, or emergency department care. The King model also includes the external physical environment that affects a person's health and well-being. As the person moves through the world, the physical setting interacts with the personal systems to either improve or degrade the patient's health status.

Health

Viewed as a dynamic process that involves a range of human life experiences, health exists in people when they can achieve their highest level of functioning. Health is the primary goal of the patient in the King model. It is achieved by continually adjusting to environmental stressors, maximizing the use of available resources, and setting and achieving goals for one's role in life. Anything that disrupts or interferes with people's ability to function normally in their chosen roles is considered to be a state of illness.

Nursing

The King model considers nursing to be a dynamic process and a type of personal system based on interactions between the nurse and the patient. During these interactions, the nurse and the patient jointly evaluate and identify the health-care needs, set goals for fulfillment of the needs, and consider actions to take in achieving those goals. Nursing is a multifaceted process that includes a range of activities such as the promotion and maintenance of health through education, the restoration of health through care of the sick and injured, and preparation for death through care of the dying.[16]

The process of nursing in the King model includes five key elements considered central to all human interactions:

1. Action: A sequence of behaviors involving mental and physical activities
2. Reaction: The resulting behaviors produced by the process of action
3. Interaction: The patient and nurse communicating together to establish goals
4. Transaction: A life situation in which perceivers and things perceived are encountered and entered into as active participants
5. Feedback: Change that occurs as a result of the interaction and transaction process

With some modifications, the King model has been successfully implemented in a variety of health-care settings ranging from rural clinics to acute urban care centers. Its focus on the one-on-one interaction between the nurse and the patient is at the heart of all nursing practice. Establishing goals *with* the patient rather than *for* the patient raises the success level of the interventions and promotes better outcomes.

> ❝ *For King . . . nursing is a multifaceted process that includes a range of activities such as the promotion and maintenance of health through education, the restoration of health through care of the sick and injured, and preparation for death through care of the dying.* ❞

The Watson Philosophy and Theory of Transpersonal Caring or Model of Human Caring

Although the concept of caring has always been an important, if somewhat obscure, element in the practice of nursing, the Watson model of human caring defines caring in a detailed and systematic manner. In the development of her model, Jean Watson used a philosophical approach rather than the systems theory approach seen in many other nursing models. Her main concern in the development of this model was to balance the impersonal aspects of nursing care that are found in the technological and scientific aspects of practice with the personal and interpersonal elements of care that grow from a humanistic belief in life. Watson is also one of the very few theorists who openly recognizes the patient's and family's spiritual beliefs as an essential element of health.[17]

Patient

The concept of patient or patient in the Watson model is developed closely with the concept of nursing. The individuality of the patient is a key concern. "The Watson model views the patient as someone who has needs, who grows and develops throughout life, and who eventually reaches a state of internal harmony."[17]

The patient is also seen as a gestalt, or a whole entity, who has value because of inherent goodness and capacity to develop. This gestalt, or holistic, view of the human being is a recurring theme in the Watson model; it emphasizes that the total person is more important to nursing care than the individual injury or disease process that produced the need for care.

Environment

Environment in the Watson model is a concept that is also closely intertwined with the concept of nursing. Viewed primarily as a negative element in the health-care process, the environment consists of those factors that the patient must overcome to achieve a state of health. The environment can be both external (physical and social elements) and internal (psychological reactions that affect health).

Health

Health, for Watson, is a high level of overall physical, mental, and social functioning; a general adaptive-maintenance level of daily functioning; and the absence of illness, or the presence of efforts leading to the absence of illness. To be healthy, according to the Watson model, the individual must be in a dynamic state of growth and development that leads to reaching full potential as a human. As with other nursing models, health is viewed as a continuum along which a person at any point may tend more toward health or more toward illness.[17]

Illness, in the Watson model, is the patient's inability to integrate life experiences and the failure to achieve full potential or inner harmony. In this model, the state of illness is not necessarily synonymous with the disease process. If the person reacts to the disease process in such a way as to find meaning, that response is considered to be healthy. A failure to find meaning in the disease experience leads to a state of illness.

Issues Now

The Pew Commission Final Report

Projected estimates of the nursing shortage based on data collected by the U.S. Bureau of the Census Current Population Survey, Division of Nursing, the Pew Commission, and the Buerhaus and Staiger data collection agency in 1998 are now considered woefully inadequate. According to the Bureau of Labor Statistics (2017), by 2022 the nursing shortage could be much worse, with as many as 1 million nursing positions unfilled. Some say the worst shortage may be regional in nature. The Pew Commission's final report addresses the competencies that nurses in the future will need.

Twenty-One Competencies for the 21st Century

1. Embrace a personal ethic of social responsibility and service.
2. Exhibit ethical behavior in all professional activities.
3. Provide evidence-based, clinically competent care.
4. Incorporate the multiple determinants of health in clinical care.
5. Apply knowledge of the new sciences.
6. Demonstrate critical thinking, reflection, and problem-solving skills.
7. Understand the role of primary care.
8. Rigorously practice preventive health care.
9. Integrate population-based care and services into practice.
10. Improve access to health care for those with unmet health needs.
11. Practice relationship-centered care with individuals and families.
12. Provide culturally sensitive care to a diverse society.
13. Partner with communities in health-care decisions.
14. Use communication and information technology effectively and appropriately.
15. Work in interdisciplinary teams.
16. Ensure care that balances individual, professional, system, and social needs.
17. Practice leadership.
18. Take responsibility for quality of care and health outcomes at all levels.
19. Contribute to continuous improvement of the health-care system.
20. Advocate for public policy that promotes and protects the health of the public.
21. Continue to learn and help others to learn.

(continued)

Issues Now (continued)

The Pew Commission also identified five key areas for professional education:

1. Change professional training to meet the demands of the new health-care system.
2. Ensure that the health profession workforce reflects the diversity of the nation's population.
3. Require interdisciplinary competence in all health professionals.
4. Continue to move education into ambulatory practice.
5. Encourage public service of all health-professional students and graduates.

   The changes that will occur over the next decade may take some health-care professionals out of their comfort zone, but they will also open a vista of opportunities for those willing to look creatively into the future. Nursing has to recognize that it will grow only to the extent that it is able to contribute to the needs of an evolving health-care system. These needs will change with time. The Pew Report, although broad in scope, provides the nursing profession with a blueprint for dealing with these changes as they occur. It is a call to action that nurses and the nursing profession need to hear.

Sources: *Gaines K. What's really behind the nursing shortage. Nurse.org, 2022. https:/nurse.org/articles/nursing-shortage-study; J. P. Bellack and E. H. O'Neil, Recreating nursing practice for a new century: Recommendations of the Pew Health Professions Commission's Final Report,* Nursing and Health Care Perspectives, *21(1):14–21, 2000; U.S. Department of Health and Human Services, Health Resources and Services Administration, National Center for Health Workforce Analysis,* National and regional supply and demand projections of the nursing workforce: 2014–2030, *2017; B. Donaho, The Pew Commission Report: Nursing's challenge to address it,* ANNA Journal, *24(5):507–512, 1997.*

Nursing

Watson makes a clear distinction between the science of nursing and the practice of curing (medicine).[12] She defines nursing as the science of caring in which the primary goal is to assist the patient to reach the greatest level of personal potential. Watson believes that holistic health care is central to the practice of caring in nursing. She defines nursing as a human science of persons and human health–illness experiences that are mediated by professional, personal, scientific, esthetic, and ethical human transactions. The practice of curing involves the conduct of activities that have the goal of treatment and elimination of disease.[17]

   The process of nursing in the Watson model is based on the systematic use of the scientific problem-solving method for decision making. To best understand nursing as a science of caring, the nurse should hold certain beliefs and be able to initiate certain caring activities.

Values

Basic to the beliefs necessary for the successful practice of nursing in the Watson model is the formation of a humanistic, altruistic system of values based on the tenet that all people are inherently valuable because they are human. In addition, the nurse should have a strong sense of faith and hope in people and their condition because of the human potential for development.

Caring

According to Watson's caring model, several activities are important in the practice of nursing. These include establishing a relationship of help and trust between the nurse and the patient; encouraging the patient to express both positive and negative feelings with acceptance; manipulating the environment to make it more supportive, protective, or corrective for the patient with any type of disease process; and assisting in whatever way is deemed appropriate to meet the basic human needs of the patient.[17]

The Johnson Behavioral System Model

By integrating systems theory with behavioral theory, Dorothy E. Johnson developed a model of nursing that considers patient behavior to be the key to preventing illness and to restoring health when illness occurs. Johnson holds that human behavior is a type of system in itself that is influenced by input factors from the environment and has output that in turn affects the environment. The more nurses understand about human behavior, the better they can position themselves to grasp how others see, interpret, and adapt to their various environments.[18]

Patient

Drawing directly on the terminology of systems theory, the Johnson model describes the person, or patient, as a behavioral system that is an organized and integrated whole. The whole is greater than the sum of its parts because of the integration and functioning of its **subsystems**. In the Johnson model, the patient as a behavioral system is composed of seven distinct behavioral subsystems. In turn, each of these seven behavioral subsystems contains four structural elements that guide and shape the subsystem.

Security

The first behavioral subsystem is the attachment, or affiliate, subsystem. Its driving force is security. For the most part, the type of activity that this subsystem undertakes is inclusion in social functions, and the behavior that is observed from this subsystem is social interaction.

Dependency

The second behavioral subsystem is dependency; its main goal is to help others. The primary type of activity involved is nurturing and promoting self-image. The observable behaviors that are a result of this activity include approval, attention, and physical assistance of the person.

Taking In

The third behavioral subsystem is the ingestive subsystem. Its motive is to meet the body's basic physiological needs of food and nutrient intake. Correspondingly, its primary activity is seeking and eating food.

Eliminative Behavior

The fourth behavioral subsystem is the eliminative; its goal is removing waste products from the system. Its primary activity is means of elimination, which is observed as the behavior of expelling waste products.

Sexual Behavior

The fifth behavioral subsystem is sexual behavior, which is found in the Johnson model's description of the person. The sexual subsystem has gratification and procreation of the species as its goals. It involves the complex activities of identifying gender roles, undergoing sexual development, and participating in sexual activity. It manifests itself in courting and mating behaviors.

Self-Protection

The sixth behavioral subsystem is the aggressive subsystem; its main goal is self-preservation. All of the actions that individuals undertake to protect themselves from harm, either internal or external, derive from this subsystem and are shown in actions toward others and the environment in general.

Achievement

The seventh, and final, behavioral subsystem is achievement. Exploration and manipulation of the environment are the objectives of this subsystem. Gaining mastery and control over the environment is the primary activity; it can be demonstrated externally when the individual shows that learning has occurred and higher-level accomplishments are being produced.[18]

As with all open systems, the behavioral system that makes up the person seeks to maintain a dynamic balance by regulating input and output. This regulation process takes the form of adapting to the environment and responding to others. However, the Johnson model sees human behavior as being goal oriented, which leads the person to constant growth and development beyond the maintenance of a mere steady state.

> *The Johnson model sees human behavior as being goal directed, which leads the person to constant growth and development beyond the maintenance of a mere steady state.*

Health

According to the Johnson model, a state of health is achieved when balance and a steady state exist within the behavioral systems of the patient. Under normal circumstances, the human system has enough inherent flexibility to maintain this balance without external intervention. At times, however, the system's balance may be disturbed to such a degree by physical disease, injury, or emotional crisis as to require external assistance. This out-of-balance state is the state of illness.

Environment

In the Johnson model, the environment is defined as all those internal and external elements that have an effect on the behavioral system. These environmental elements include obvious external factors, such as air temperature and relative humidity; sociological factors, such as family, neighborhood, and society in general; and the internal environment, such as bodily processes, psychological states, religious beliefs, and political orientation.

All seven behavioral subsystems are involved with the patient's relationship to the environment through the regulation of input and output. The patient is continually interacting with the environment in an attempt to remain healthy by maintaining an internal dynamic balance.

Nursing

In the Johnson model, nursing is an activity that helps the individual achieve and maintain an optimal level of behavior (state of health) through the manipulation and regulation of the environment.[18] Nursing has functions in both health and illness. Nursing interventions to either maintain or restore health involve four activities in the regulation of the environment:

1. Restricting harmful environmental factors
2. Defending the patient from negative environmental influences
3. Inhibiting adverse elements from occurring
4. Facilitating positive internal environmental factors in the recovery process

As a professional, the nurse in the Johnson model provides direct services to the patient. By interacting with, and sometimes intervening in, the multiple subsystems that are found in the patient's environment, the nurse acts as an external regulatory force. The goal of nursing is to promote the highest level of functioning and development in the patient at all times.

Nursing actions include helping the patient act in a socially acceptable manner, monitoring and aiding biological processes that are necessary for maintaining a dynamic balance, demonstrating support for medical care and treatment during illness, and taking actions to prevent illness from recurring. In this model, nursing makes its own unique contribution to the health and well-being of individuals and provides a service that is complementary to those provided by other health-care professionals.

The Neuman Systems Model, or Health as an Expanding Consciousness

As envisioned by Betty Neuman, the health-care systems model focuses on the individual and their environment and is applicable to a variety of health-care disciplines apart from nursing. Drawing from systems theory, the Neuman model also includes elements from stress theory with an overall holistic view of humanity and health care.[19]

> *In the Johnson model, nursing is an activity that helps the individual achieve and maintain an optimal level of behavior (state of health) through the manipulation and regulation of the environment.*

Patient

In this model, the patient is viewed as an open system that interacts constantly with internal and external environments through the system's boundaries. The patient-system's boundaries are called *lines of defense* and *resistance* in the Neuman model and may be represented graphically as a series of concentric circles that surround the basic core of the individual. The goal of these boundaries is to keep the basic core system stable by controlling system input, the penetration of the defense boundaries by elements of the environment that are negative to the system.[19]

Neuman classifies these defensive boundaries according to their various functions. The internal lines of resistance are the boundaries that are closest to the basic core and thus protect the basic internal structure of the system. The normal lines of defense are outside the internal lines of resistance; they protect the system from common, everyday environmental stressors. The flexible line of defense surrounds the normal line of defense and protects it from extreme environmental stressors. The general goal of all these protective boundaries is to maintain the internal stability of the individual.

Health

Health, then, in the Neuman model is defined as the relatively stable internal functioning of the patient. Optimal health exists when the patient is maintained in a high state of wellness or stability.

As in other nursing models, health is not considered an absolute state but rather a continuum that reflects the patient's internal stability while moving from wellness to illness and back. It takes a considerable amount of physical and psychological energy to maintain the stability of the person who is in good health.

The opposite of a healthy state, illness, exists when the patient's core structure becomes unstable through the effects of environmental factors that overwhelm and defeat the lines of defense and resistance. These environmental factors, whether internal or external, are called **stressors** in this model.

Environment

The environment is composed of internal and external forces, or stressors, that produce change or response in the patient. Stressors may be helpful or harmful, strong or weak. Understanding the connection between the patient and the environment allows nurses to make better clinical decisions, to offer support that is unique to the patient and their family, and to increase the chance of success in aiding the patient to return to a state of wellness.[19]

Stressors are also classified according to their relationship to the basic core of the patient-system. Stressors that are completely outside the basic core are termed *extrapersonal* and are either physical, such as atmospheric temperature, or sociological, such as living in either a rural or an urban setting. *Interpersonal* stressors arise from interactions with other human beings. Marital relationships, career expectations, and friendships are included in this group of interpersonal stressors. Those stressors that occur within the patient are called *intrapersonal* and include involuntary physiological responses, psychological reactions, and internal thought processes.

Nursing

The nurse's role in the Neuman model is to identify at what level or in which boundary a disruption in the patient's internal stability has taken place and then to aid the patient in activities that strengthen or restore the integrity of that particular boundary.[19] The Neuman model expands the concept of patient from the individual to include families, small groups, the community, or even society in general.

Identifying Stressors

Nursing's main concern in this model is either to identify stressors that will disrupt a defensive boundary in the future (prevention) or to identify a stressor that has already disrupted a defensive boundary, thereby producing instability (illness).[19] The Neuman model is based on the nursing process and identifies three levels of intervention: primary, secondary, and tertiary.

Types of Intervention

The main goal of a **primary intervention** is to prevent possible symptoms that could be caused by environmental stressors. Teaching patients about stress management, giving immunizations, and encouraging aerobic exercise to prevent heart disease are examples of primary interventions.

A **secondary intervention** is aimed at treating symptoms that have already been produced by stressors. Many of the actions that nurses perform in the hospital or clinic (e.g., giving pain medications or teaching a patient with cardiac disease about the benefits of a low-sodium diet) fall into this secondary intervention category.

A **tertiary intervention** seeks to restore the patient's system to an optimal state of balance by adapting to negative environmental stressors. Teaching a patient how to care for a colostomy bag at home after discharge from the hospital is an example of a nursing activity at the tertiary level. It occurs after the patient has received a secondary intervention and offers support to the patient so that they can continue to recover or prevent further deterioration in health.

What Do You Think?

Which of these grand theories appeals to you most? Why? How would you apply it to an actual patient you have seen in the clinical setting or to a sick family member?

TRENDS FOR THE FUTURE IN NURSING THEORY

Although the search for the perfect nursing model continues, the emphasis in recent years has shifted from developing new theories to applying existing theories to nursing practice. Also, modern theorists seem to be more interested in expanding existing nursing theories by including such concepts as cultural diversity, spirituality, family, and social change rather than starting over from the beginning. A good example of this trend is the cultural meaning–centered theory that was published by Mendyka and Bloom. This theory expands the King model by adding a cultural perspective and a learner-centered component.[20]

A More Recent Theory

One of the more recent of the established grand nursing theories is the human becoming theory proposed by Rosemary Rizzo Parse. Although her original work started in 1981, a more developed form of her theory was published in 1987.[21–22] Parse's theory stresses the elements of experience, personal **values**, and lifestyle choices in the maintenance of health.

A Matter of Choice

In this theory, the practice of nurses focuses on quality of life as it is described and lived by the patient. Offering an alternative to both the conventional biomedical approach found in medical-oriented models and the biopsychosocial-spiritual approach of many nursing theories and models, Parse's human becoming theory of nursing rates the quality of life from each patient's own viewpoint as the goal of the practice of nursing. The name of this theory was changed from "man-living-health" theory to the "human becoming theory" in 1992.[21]

In Parse's theory, the patient can be any person or family who is concerned with the quality of their life situation. The patient is viewed as an open, whole being who is influenced by past and present life experiences. The ability to make free choices is essential in this theory. The patient, through choices they make, interacts with the environment to influence health either positively or negatively.[22]

For example, during the COVID-19 pandemic, a large number of persons refused to receive the COVID vaccination for reasons ranging from the fear of receiving injected nanobots that would allow them to be tracked by the National Intelligence Agency (NIA) to doubts that the vaccine had been adequately tested. These choices influenced many patients' health in that after vaccinations became widely available, the vast majority of patients hospitalized and on ventilators or who died were the unvaccinated.[23] Their choices also were believed to affect the health of those they came in contact with and spread the virus to.

This scenario reinforces Parse's contention that health is an ongoing process. Because patients make free choices, their health status is continually unfolding. In addition, health is determined by lived experiences, synthesis of values, and the way the patient lives.[24]

Finding Meaning

The main role of nursing in the Parse model is to guide patients in finding and understanding the meaning of their lives. Once the patient chooses a healthy life situation, the nurse can further increase the quality of the patient's life and improve their health status. The ability to change the patient's health-related values is an important skill for nurses to master in this model.[24]

Parse does not specifically define the concept of environment in relationship to her theory. It seems to be any health-related setting, but it can also be expanded to include past and present experiences.

MIDDLE-RANGE THEORIES AND MODELS

Middle-range theories and models (Box 3.3) have been present in nursing research for many years. More than 50 are identified as middle range, although many more fit into the category.[25] A **middle-range theory** is a set of relatively concrete concepts or propositions that lie between a minor working hypothesis found in everyday nursing practice theories and a well-developed grand nursing theory, like those previously discussed.[25] Middle-range models develop from middle-range theories, although not all middle-range theories have a model.

Middle-range theories can be classified into three major categories. **Middle-range descriptive theories** are created and tested using descriptive research method, and they can be either qualitative or quantitative in design. An example of a middle-range descriptive theory is Peplau's theory of interpersonal relations. (For more information on nursing research, see Chapter 24.)

Middle-range explanatory theories postulate the relationships between or among two or more concepts. Explanatory theories describe why the relationship exists and the degree to which one concept is related to another concept or affects the other concept. These theories are produced and tested using correlational research that is usually quantitative in design. An example of a middle-range explanatory theory is Pender's health promotion model.[22]

Box 3.3 Partial List of Middle-Range Theories

Acute pain management theory—Myra Huth and Shirley Moore

Advancing technology, caring, and nursing—Rozzano C. Locsin

Cultural brokering theory—Mary Anne Jezewski

Framework of systemic organization—Marie-Louise Friedemann

Health belief model—Blanche Mikhail

Health promotion model—Nola Pender

Nurse as wounded healer—Marion Conti O'hare

Quality of nursing care theory—June H. Larrabee

Synergy model—American Association of Critical-Care Nurses

Theory of caring—Kristen M. Swanson

Theory of comfort—Katharine Kolcaba

Theory of the deliberative nursing process—Ida Orlando

Theory of group power within organizations—Christina Sieloff

Theory of maternal role attainment—Ramona Thieme Mercer

Theory of self-transcendence—Pamela Reed

Theory of uncertainty in illness—Merle Mishel

Theory of unpleasant symptoms—Elizabeth R. Lenz and Linda C. Pugh

Uncertainty in illness—Merle Mishel

Woman's anger theory—Sandra Thomas

Middle-range predictive theories actually attempt to predict the relations between concepts rather than just explaining them. These theories attempt to identify how changes in one element affect other elements. Testing of this type of theory uses experimental research models and quantitative designs. Orlando's theory of the deliberative nursing process is an example of a middle-range predictive theory.[25]

Middle-range theories generally contain only a few basic ideas or concepts that researchers are attempting to prove or illustrate. They do not have a large number of **variables** and tend to focus on one or two

problems that are linked, like the grand theories, to human beings, environment, health care, or nursing. They are less abstract than the grand theories and are much more easily applied to practice hypotheses. However, when several middle-range theories are used to investigate the same or similar concepts over a period of time, they can be woven together to reinforce or even form the fabric of a new grand nursing theory.[25]

Middle-range theories should be socially significant, meaning that they deal with people or populations with health-care conditions. They should also have theoretical significance, meaning that they develop a new set of facts or data that adds to the theoretical knowledge base of nursing. The whole movement toward **evidence-based practice (EBP)** depends on this type of research. Middle-range theories often form the **theoretical framework** for a research project. The results of these research projects act to provide firsthand information that informs the theory, which can then expand its concepts and range. These expanded middle-range theories, then, suggest new questions and provide ideas for more research. The relationship among the three elements—theory, research, practice—becomes reciprocal, expanding knowledge in all three.[25]

Two Middle-Range Nursing Theories

Formulated in 1987, Nola Pender's **health promotion** model is widely used as the theoretical framework for research on prenatal care and pregnancy. The model is based on her conceptualizations of Orem's self-care model. Pender proposes that several key factors provide the primary motivation for individuals to adopt behaviors that maintain and improve their health.[26] These factors include the person's perception of

- How important it is to be healthy.
- How much control they have over their health.
- How much control they have over the health-care system.
- What it means to them to be healthy.
- What their current health status is.
- What the benefits and barriers are to health improvement.

The goal of the individual is to move toward a balanced state of positive health and well-being.[27] Health is up to the individual, not the health-care system; although the health-care system can be an important part, it will always be secondary to the individual.

Kristen M. Swanson's theory of caring, first published in 1991, was inspired by the writings of Watson and by Swanson's own experiences as a nurse providing care for patients and families. As she observed how patients used their internal strengths to overcome their illnesses and transition to a state of health, Swanson began to see a pattern of how patients who successfully made the transition to wellness related to other individuals and how those individuals affected the final health status of the patient.[28]

As the elements of the theory became more defined, Swanson conducted three studies that reinforced the underlying assumptions of her theory. The data from these three studies were used to better clarify the key concepts of her theory: person, environment, health/well-being, and caring actions. Based on additional research, Swanson was able to develop instruments to measure key concepts and identify concrete interventions to use in implementing her theory of caring.[29] She identified five "caring processes" that are essential to the successful transition to health experienced by patients: knowing, being with, doing for, enabling, and maintaining belief.[29]

The role of the nurse in the theory of caring is to guide the patient through discussions of their experiences so that they believe their problems are understood by the nurse. Through these discussions, patients are kept informed with key information, their needs are met, their lives are validated, and the nurse's belief in the patient's ability to move toward wellness is expressed. The anticipated outcome is that the patients are better able to integrate their sufferings and losses into their lives.[28] Although originally studied in the perinatal setting, the theory of caring has been adapted to many other health-care settings, including critical care, mental health, public health, hospice, gerontology, and oncology.

Some other middle-range theories that are commonly used in nursing research include Mishel's uncertainty in illness theory, Reed's self-transcendence theory, Thomas's women's anger theory, Jezewski's cultural brokering theory, and Huth and Moore's acute pain management theory.[22]

Practice-Level Nursing Theories (Nursing Practice Theories) (Micro-Range Theory)

Theories categorized in this level are the most focused. They deal with situation-specific concepts that are very narrow in scope and home in on a specific patient population. They have a low level of abstraction, if any. They provide the frameworks for nursing interventions and predict outcomes of specific nursing actions. The size of these theories is small, and they analyze only a narrow part of an action. Examples of nursing practice theories are the theory of barriers and facilitators, and targeting patients with heart failure.[22]

> *When several middle-range theories are used to investigate the same or similar concepts over a period of time, they can be woven together to reinforce or even form the fabric of a new grand nursing theory.*

New Challenges to Nursing Theory

As with any developing science, nursing will continue to change and respond to the dynamic trends of society. Older nursing models will be either replaced by new ones or modified to include developing concepts. One of the hallmarks of a sound nursing theory or model is its flexibility and ability to adapt to new discoveries.

An increasing number of **independent nurse practitioners** and other advanced practice nurses are testing nursing theories as they have never been tested before. The theories that are flexible, realistic, and usable in practice will survive and remain as the pillars of professional nursing.[24] Those that are too theoretical or rigid will fall by the wayside and become mere footnotes in nursing texts.

Conclusion

As nursing takes its rightful place among the other helping professions, nursing theory takes on additional importance. Nursing theories and models are the systematic conceptualizations of nursing practice and how they fit into the health-care system. Nursing theories help describe, explain, predict, and control nursing activities to achieve the goals of patient care. By understanding and using nursing theory, nurses can better incorporate theoretical information into their practice to provide new ways of approaching nursing care and improving nursing practice.

The development of nursing theory and models indicates a maturing of the profession. As the knowledge associated with the profession increases and becomes unique, more complex, and better organized, the general body of nursing science knowledge also increases and EBP becomes a reality. When nursing becomes a well-developed body of specialized knowledge, it will be fully recognized as a separate scientific discipline and take its rightful place as a true profession.

CRITICAL-THINKING EXERCISES

Mrs. M is an 88-year-old woman who has been a resident of St. Martin's Village, a lifetime care community, since her husband died 8 years ago. Her health status is fair. She has adult-onset diabetes controlled by oral medication and a scar from a tumor behind her left ear that was removed surgically. The wound from this tumor removal has never healed completely, and it has continuously oozed a serous fluid, requiring a dressing.

At St. Martin's Village, Mrs. M has her own apartment, which she maintains with minimal assistance. She receives one hot meal each day in a common dining room and has access to a full range of services such as a beauty shop, recreational facilities, and a chapel. She is generally happy in this setting. She has no immediate family nearby, and the cost of the facility was covered by a large, one-time gift from her now-deceased husband. Recently, she is becoming increasingly weak and has difficulty walking; attending activities, including meals; and changing the dressing on her ear. The nurse at St. Martin's Village is sent to evaluate this patient.

• Select two nursing models and apply their principles to this case study. Make sure you include the concepts of patient, health, environment, and nursing.

NCLEX-STYLE QUESTIONS

1. Why are theories and models important to the profession of nursing?
   1. They describe the interventions nurses use to care for patients.
   2. They provide a conceptual structure for understanding nursing care and practice.
   3. They help nonmedical people understand what nurses do.
   4. They distinguish between the competencies required of ADNs and BSNs.

2. What key concepts are commonly found in nursing theories and models? **Select all that apply**.
   1. Patient
   2. Environment
   3. Health
   4. Nursing
   5. Feedback

3. _____ theories or models have a narrow scope, are concrete rather than abstract, and provide rationales for specific nursing interventions.

4. General systems theory is the theoretical basis for many nursing theories and models. What aspect of general systems theory is most comparable to the key concept of nursing in nursing theory?
   1. Input
   2. Output
   3. Throughput
   4. Feedback loop

5. According to Sister Callista Roy's model, what is the best measure of a person's health status?
   1. The person's ability to perform self-care
   2. The person's ability to adapt to the stimuli imposed on them
   3. The person's ability to engage in the dynamic process of the nurse–patient relationship
   4. The person's ability to integrate life experiences and achieve their full potential

6. What distinguishes a middle-range theory from a grand theory of nursing?
   1. Middle-range theories have a large number of variables, while grand theories have only a few.
   2. Grand theories should be socially significant, while middle-range theories have theoretical significance.
   3. Middle-range theories, not grand theories, form the theoretical framework for EBP research projects.
   4. There are fewer middle-range theories than there are grand theories.

7. What is the goal of Orem's self-care model of nursing?
   1. To return the patient to a disease- or illness-free state
   2. To allow the patient to reach their full potential as a human

3. To return the patient to a state of balance that does not require external intervention
4. To help the patient direct and carry out activities that maintain or improve their health

8. One key concept of nursing theories is that of environment. What theme related to environment is present across several grand nursing theories?
   1. Environment, both internal and external, can negatively affect a person's health.
   2. Environment cannot be changed and must be adapted to.
   3. Changing one's environment is an act of self-care.
   4. Nursing interventions include helping the patient change their environment.

9. In what way is the human body a system, according general systems theory?
   1. The human body takes in food (input) and excretes waste (output).
   2. The human body is an open system, which is why pathogens can make us ill.
   3. The human body has a feedback loop that signals when we have had enough to eat.
   4. The human body functions as a set of interacting parts that work together to achieve an overall purpose.

10. Which factor has had the greatest effect on the rise of middle-range nursing theories?
    1. The increasing numbers of research-focused PhD-level nurses
    2. The rise of EBP as the gold standard for care
    3. The rejection of the grand theories for being out of touch with bedside care
    4. The changing requirements of graduate schools of nursing

References

1. Melnyk B, Fineout-Overholt E. *Evidence-Based Practice in Nursing & Healthcare: A Guide to Best Practice* (4th ed.). Philadelphia: Wolters Kluwer, 2019.
2. Fawcett J, Gigliotti E. Using conceptual models of nursing to guide nursing research: the case of the Neuman systems model. *Nursing Science Quarterly*, 14(4):339–345, 2021. https://doi.org/10.1177/089431840101400411
3. Butcher H, Bulechek G, McCloskey Dochterman J, Wagner M. *Nursing Interventions Classification (NIC)* (7th ed.). St. Louis, MO: Elsevier, 2018.
4. Bulechek G, Butcher H, McCloskey Dochterman J. *Nursing Intervention and Classification (NIC)* (5th ed.). St. Louis, MO: Mosby/Elsevier, 2008.
5. Vera M. Nursing diagnosis guide and list: All you need to know to master diagnosing. Nurseslabs, 2022. https://nurseslabs.com/nursing-diagnosis/
6. Johnson M, Maas M. The Nursing Outcomes Classification. *Nursing Care Quality*, 12(5):9–20, 1998. https://doi.org/10.1097/00001786-199806000-00005
7. Seven dimensions of health. MD-Health.com, 2022. https://www.md-health.com/Dimensions-Of-Health.html
8. Molina-Mula J, Gallo-Estrada J. Impact of nurse-patient relationship on quality of care and patient autonomy in decision-making. *International Journal of Environmental Research in Public Health*, 17(3):835, 2020. https://doi.org/10.3390/ijerph17030835
9. Nursing theorist analysis: The environment theory. NursingAnswers.net, June 22, 2020. https://nursinganswers.net/essays/nursing-theorist-analysis-the-environment-theory.php
10. General systems theory and historical influences on nursing essay. Ivy Panda, April 11, 2022. https://ivypanda.com/essays/general-systems-theory-and-historical-influences-on-nursing/
11. Rodgers B. The evolution of nursing science. In JB Butts & KL Rich (Eds.), *Philosophies and Theories for Advanced Nursing Practice* (3rd ed., pp. 19–54). Burlington, MA: Jones & Bartlett Learning, 2018.
12. Nelson D. What is the relationship between nursing theory and nursing practice? The Health Board, 2022. https://www.thehealthboard.com/what-is-the-relationship-between-nursing-theory-and-nursing-practice.htm
13. Grand nursing theories. Daeman Library, n.d. https://libguides.daemen.edu/NurTheory/grand-theories
14. The nursing process and the Roy adaptation model [slide deck]. 2015. https://www.yumpu.com/en/document/read/38034189/the-nursing-process-and-the-roy-adaptation-model
15. Hartweg D. Metcalfe S. Orem's self-care deficit nursing theory: Relevance and need for refinement. *Nursing Science Quarterly*, 35(1):70–76, 2022. https://doi.org/10.1177/08943184211051369
16. Gonzalo A, King, I. Theory of goal attainment. Nurselabs, 2023. https://nurseslabs.com/imogene-m-kings-theory-goal-attainment/
17. Petiprin A. Watson's philosophy and science of caring. Nursing-Theory.org, n.d. https://nursing-theory.org/theories-and-models/watson-philosophy-and-science-of-caring.php
18. BetterHelp Editorial Team. What is human behavior? Theories, definition, and types. BetterHelp.com, October 4, 2022. https://www.betterhelp.com/advice/behavior/what-is-human-behavior-theories-definition-and-types/
19. Hannoodee S, Dhamoon A. Nursing Neuman Systems Model. *StatPearls* [Internet], 2021. https://www.ncbi.nlm.nih.gov/books/NBK560658/
20. The importance of a learner-centered approach. HARAPPA, June 18, 2021. https://harappa.education/harappa-diaries/learner-centered-approach/
21. Petiprin A. Parse's human becoming theory. Nursing-Theory.org, n.d. https://nursing-theory.org/theories-and-models/parse-human-becoming-theory.php
22. Alligood M. *Nursing Theorists and Their Work*. St. Louis, MO: Elsevier, 2022.
23. Gore D. Latest CDC data: Unvaccinated adults 97 times more likely to die for COVID-19 than boosted adults. https://www.factcheck.org/2022/scicheck-latest-cdc-data-unvaccinated-adults-97-times-more-likely-to-die-from-covid-19-than-boosted-adults/
24. Harris J. The healthspan revolution: How to live a long, strong and happy life. Theguardian.com, 2023. https://www.theguardian.com/lifeandstyle/2023/mar/28/healthspan-revolution-how-to-live-long-strong-happy-life
25. Peterson S, Bredrow T. *Middle Range Theories: Application to Nursing Research and Practice* (5th ed.). Philadelphia, PA: Wolters Kluwer, 2020.
26. Petiprin A. Pender's health promotion model. Nursing-Theory.org, n.d. https://nursing-theory.org/theories-and-models/pender-health-promotion-model.php
27. Wayne G. Nursing theories and theorists: The definitive guide for nurses. Nurselabs, 2023. https://nurseslabs.com/nursing-theories/
28. McKelvey M. Finding meaning through Kristen Swanson's caring behaviours: A cornerstone of healing for nursing education. Pubmed, 2018. https://pubmed.ncbi.nlm.nih.gov/29490829
29. Hagedom S, Quinn A. Theory-based nurse practitioner practice: Caring in action. *Topics in Advanced Practice Nursing eJournal*, 4(4), 2004. https://www.medscape.com/viewarticle/496718_3

The Process of Educating Nurses

4

Joseph T. Catalano

Learning Objectives

After completing this chapter, the reader will be able to:

- Explain why the Institute of Medicine (IOM) competencies are important to nursing education and how they improve quality of care
- List the six Quality and Safety Education for Nurses (QSEN) competencies and their relationship to nursing education
- Compare the major differences among the diploma, associate degree nursing, and bachelor of science in nursing educational programs
- Discuss at least three types of advanced nursing degrees
- Distinguish between the different types of doctoral degrees available to nurses
- Explain the concept of advanced practice for nurses
- Discuss the significance of the doctorate in nursing practice for advanced practice nurses
- Identify and explain the importance of interprofessional education for nurses and future nursing practice

EDUCATIONAL PATHWAYS

Unlike many other professions, nursing has several related but unique educational pathways that lead to licensure and professional status. The current system of nursing education creates confusion about nursing not only among the public but also among nurses. Perhaps the belief that "a nurse is a nurse is a nurse" developed because, even though registered nurses (RNs) may be trained in educational programs that vary in length, orientation, and content, the graduates all take the same licensing examination and, superficially, all seem able to provide the same level of care.

PARADIGM SHIFTING

The current profession of nursing faces many difficult challenges and extraordinary opportunities. Future trends in health care are being driven by several powerful government and societal forces that are producing an inevitable reshaping of health-care delivery. For many years, nurses were an invisible element in the health-care system; however, the COVID-19 pandemic brought nurses out of the dark and into the light. Pictures and stories on nightly news programs showed nurses providing the lion's share of patient care and placing themselves at the highest risk of contracting the virus when emersed daily in the health crisis. The pandemic reshuffled most elements of the health-care system, with nurses being affected the most because they compose up to 80 percent of health-care workers. The demand for the skills nurses had learned in their education programs were at their highest in history.[1]

Traditionally, nursing education was somewhat insulated from the forces of change; however, because of the COVID-19 pandemic, nursing educators have been made to recognize that graduates need to be prepared with high levels of flexibility, critical thinking, knowledge, and skills that are in tune with a health-care system that can change overnight. The most powerful of these forces of change are

- A health-care system that is unprepared for major health crises.
- Health-care reform that will increase the availability of health care to more diverse patients who previously were shut out of the health-care market.
- The wider use of capitated **managed care** for financing coverage and a market-driven system.
- The increasing age and diversity of the U.S. population.
- The shortage of nurses.
- The shortage of qualified nursing faculty.
- The rapid leaps forward in health care and information technology.
- The government's attempts to increase health-care coverage for uninsured citizens.

In the 2020 report of the Bureau of Labor Statics (the most recent at time of print), 61 percent of the 3,080,00 employed RNs worked in acute care hospitals, and that trend appears likely to continue well into the future.[2] Hospitals have attempted to slow the drain of nurses to other employment settings by seeking Magnet status certification, which identifies the facility as being "nurse friendly" and a place where the nurse turnover rate is low.[3] The other 40 percent of nurses are employed in a wide variety of settings, including private practice, public health agencies, **home health-care**, primary nursing, school-operated nursing centers, **ambulatory care centers**, insurance and managed-care companies, education, and health-care research. There is also an ever-growing group of **emerging health occupations** that have not yet been officially recognized by professional organizations.[2]

What Do You Think?

Is there a Magnet hospital in your area? If you have clinical rotations there, is there any difference between the care at the Magnet and a non-Magnet facility? How about the attitudes of the nurses and the overall facility atmosphere?

What Nursing School Graduates Must Know and Be Able to Do

It has always been a challenge for nursing educators to decide how much and what nursing students need to learn before they graduate. Some of the curricular content is dictated by the **licensure examination**, but high-quality nursing programs recognize that this test knowledge is the minimum required for safe practice at an entry level. The health-care marketplace demands more than the minimum. In this regard, the consumers of the products of nursing education—that is, the health-care entities that hire nursing school graduates—have had an important if somewhat unstructured role in determining curricular content.

The Pew Study

The Pew Health Professions Commission Study, or Pew Report, was published in the late 1990s. It was the first comprehensive study to systematically address which competencies nursing students should possess upon graduation.[4] A few of the 21 recommendations for all schools preparing health-care professionals are

> *Nursing educators are continually challenged to evaluate whether the graduates of their programs are adequately prepared to meet the demands of all areas of care.*

- Expanding the scientific basis of the programs.
- Promoting interdisciplinary education.
- Developing cultural sensitivity.
- Establishing new alliances with managed-care companies and government.
- Increasing the use of **computer technology** and interactive software.

The Pew Report also recommends a **differentiated practice** structure to simplify and consolidate the titles that are used for the different practitioner levels so that there is just one title for each level. While the Pew study was in its final stages, the Institute of Medicine (IOM) became interested in the data it was producing and began its own parallel study, which is one of today's driving forces for quality health care.

Nursing educators are continually challenged to evaluate whether the graduates of their programs are adequately prepared to meet the demands of all areas of care. Nursing educators also need to evaluate whether their own educational and skills preparation is sufficient to meet the needs of diverse health-care settings.

Required Skills and Knowledge

In an attempt to structure the input from the hospitals and other facilities who hire new graduate nurses, a study was conducted to survey administrators who worked at hospitals, home health-care agencies, and nursing homes. They were asked to rank 45 skills or knowledge-based competencies they expected to see in the baccalaureate-level graduate nurses they hired. The results showed a mix of skills and knowledge competencies that were most sought after. Those that ranked the highest included

- Teaching patients **health promotion** and prevention.
- Teaching patients about how lifestyle affects health.
- Effectively supervising less-educated staff.
- Effectively delegating and monitoring staff.
- Efficiently organizing routine daily tasks.
- Safely administering medications.
- Having competency using computer databases and charting.
- Having the ability to organize nursing care for 6 to 10 patients at the same time.

" Health-care technology has advanced so rapidly in recent years that it has put a strain on both the faculty teaching nursing students and the students attempting to master it. "

Overall, the expectations for new graduates cluster around the ability to initiate and adapt to change, use **critical thinking** in problem-solving, attain a basic level of skills, and be able to communicate with patients and staff. It is interesting to note that the basic competencies have not changed much since Florence Nightingale organized her first nursing school. Like her students, current students still need to master basic skills, communicate effectively, and solve patient care issues.

The Institute of Medicine Competencies and the Future of Nursing

In 2010, a report by the American Nurses Association (ANA) and the Constituent Member Associations (CMA) moved the discussion to a new level by outlining the key messages from the IOM's report on the future of nursing.[5] This report is part of an ongoing project aimed at using evidence-based practice (EBP) to advance the nursing profession so that nursing can keep pace with health-care reform activities. Although not entirely new, the four key messages from the report are the following:

- *Nurses should practice to the full extent of their education and training.* A fundamental element of this goal is to revise states' nurse practice acts by removing unnecessary scope-of-practice restrictions. The 111th Congress promoted this issue in various health-care settings, but it fell by the wayside after the Trump administration took over in 2017. The issue again received attention with a new administration in 2020.
- *Nurses should achieve higher levels of education and training through an improved education system that promotes seamless academic progression.* The goals for this competency included increasing the number of RNs with baccalaureate degrees to at least 80 percent by 2020, up from 50 percent in 2010. Unfortunately, baccalaureate-degree nurses in 2020 accounted for only 64.2 percent of nurses.[6] The second goal was to double the number of nurses with doctorates by 2020. With the advent of the doctor of nursing practice (DNP) degree, this goal has been achieved. In 2010, there were 532 nurses with a PhD and 1,282 nurses with a DNP (total 1,814). By 2020, these numbers had risen to 759 doctor of philosophy (PhD) nurses and 9,158 DNP recipients (total 9,917).[7] The remaining goals are difficult to measure and include increasing the number of nurses committed to lifelong learning, increasing the diversity of nurses to better meet the needs of an increasingly diverse U.S. population, expanding residency programs, and focusing on easing the transition into practice. All of these are fundamental to the progression of newly licensed nurses into successful professionals.
- *Nurses should be full partners with physicians and other health professionals in redesigning health care*

in the United States. For a long time, nurses have needed expanded opportunities to demonstrate their leadership and management skills as key members of the health-care team. In collaboration with physicians and other team members, nurses need to be involved in redesigning the health-care system through such activities as conducting research, improving practice environments, developing care systems, and improving quality of care.

- *Effective workforce planning and policy-making require better data collection and an improved information infrastructure.* Collaboration between national, state, and local initiatives in collecting and analyzing data can make the data more useful to all health-care providers.
- *Nursing education has long strived to be relevant and vibrant in a rapidly changing health-care system.* The shift in recent years to a consumer-driven health-care system is shaping what nurses need to be able to accomplish in their practice.

Out of these guiding principles, the IOM developed five key competencies that nursing students must be able to achieve upon graduation:

1. Patient-centered care
2. Interdisciplinary teamwork
3. EBP
4. Quality improvement (QI)
5. Informatics

Because of society's demands for an increased level of safety and high-quality nursing care, nursing education institutions began using the IOM competencies to develop the **Quality and Safety Education for Nurses (QSEN)** competency model for nursing curricula.[8]

Quality and Safety Education for Nurses Competencies Guide for Nursing Curriculum
Current leaders in nursing education have built on the Nightingale, Pew, and IOM principles and developed the QSEN competencies to help guide what is being taught in nursing programs. However, health-care technology has advanced so rapidly in recent years that it has put a strain on both the faculty teaching nursing students and the students attempting to master it.

The push for an improved nursing curriculum began with recognition of the large numbers of medication and medical errors that occur in today's health-care system. These errors lead to the injury and death of as many as 90,000 patients per year. Driven by community and professional concerns, the Robert Wood Johnson Foundation undertook a three-phase project to improve the quality and safety of patient care by focusing nursing education on student competency. The project, QSEN, is built on the five competencies developed initially by the IOM.[8]

Phase I began in 2005 with a $590,000 grant to the University of North Carolina at Chapel Hill School of Nursing. The goal of Phase I was to develop the theoretical foundations for QSEN, including student competencies; the knowledge, skills, and abilities (KSAs) necessary to maintain a safe health-care system; and measurable outcomes for graduates of nursing programs.

> **" *Nurses of the future will need to practice with self-reliance, independence, and flexibility. They will be required to have well-developed decision-making skills on the basis of critical-thinking ability, a working knowledge of community resources, and computer and technical competencies.* "**

A thorough and extensive set of KSAs was developed for each competency for undergraduate students. In addition, Phase I established an electronic resources center, supported by the grant, which contains materials on patient safety and quality initiatives.

With Phase I still ongoing, Phase II kicked off in 2007 with the goals of developing KSAs for graduate students and developing QSEN-based curricula in 15 selected schools. The 15 pilot schools explored the difficulties in implementing QSEN in their programs.

Phase III began in 2009 and is ongoing. The goals of Phase III are:

- Developing nursing faculty knowledge and skills in teaching QSEN competencies.
- Writing textbooks that include the six competencies.

- Working with licensing, accreditation, and certification agencies to develop standards that reflect QSEN competencies.
- Developing ongoing innovative methods to implement QSEN.

The overarching goal of Phase III is to develop a culture of safety in the health-care system that is so ingrained in health-care providers that they will practice safety without even thinking about it. It will be in development for many years to come. Many of the pilot schools have published information about their experiences implementing QSEN as their curricular model. Overall, the conversion seems to be going smoothly and successfully.[6]

One issue troubling some nursing leaders is that the QSEN competencies are based on a model developed by the IOM (i.e., a medical model). All agree on the need for quality and safety measures to reduce harm to patients, and QSEN certainly meets that need. However, for many years, the American Association of Colleges of Nursing (AACN)'s *Essentials of Baccalaureate Education for Professional Nursing Practice* has been the gold **standard** for nursing program outcomes. Is there a clearcut advantage in using the QSEN competencies over the *Essentials* as a curricular model?[9]

Some nursing leaders believe that by conforming to QSEN-based curricula, they will transform the professional identity of nursing into something other than nursing. What about the competencies of caring, integrity, and patient advocacy? What about research and scholarship? Where does prevention—a key nursing role since the time of Florence Nightingale—fit in? Those who support QSEN believe that if a nurse is providing safe, high-quality care, then caring and integrity are already included. Others believe that a seventh competency, "professional person," should be added to include those aspects of nursing that make it unique and separate from the medical profession[8] (see Table 4.1).

It has always been a challenge to measure competency in the health-care professions. The current interest in positive patient outcomes as a measure of performance reinforces the need to better measure competency. It is by no means a new issue. The **Competency Outcomes Performance Assessment (COPA)** model, developed in the early 1990s, has been used by medical schools and some schools of nursing to validate the skills and knowledge of their graduates. It is designed to promote competency for clinical practice at all levels. With a few modifications, the COPA

Table 4.1   Competency/Outcome Comparison: IOM, QSEN, AACN Essentials

IOM Competencies	QSEN Competencies	AACN Essentials
Patient-centered care	Patient-centered care	Liberal education for baccalaureate generalist nursing practice
Interdisciplinary teamwork	Teamwork and collaboration	Basic organizational and systems leadership for high-quality care and patient safety
EBP	EBP	Scholarship for EBP
QI	QI	Information management and application of patient-care technology
Informatics	Safety informatics	Health-care policy, finance, and regulatory environments
		Interprofessional communication and collaboration for improving health outcomes
		Clinical prevention and population health
		Professionalism and professional values
		Baccalaureate generalist nursing practice

AACN = American Association of Colleges of Nursing; EBP = evidence-based practice; IOM = Institute of Medicine; QI = quality improvement; QSEN = Quality and Safety Education for Nurses.

Sources: *Update on the AACN Essentials. AACN, 2023.* https://www.aacnnursing.org/essentials/latest-updates; *Nursing education competencies. NLN, 2022.* https://www.nln.org/education/nursing-education-competencies.

model fits well with QSEN and can be used as the evaluation tool for graduates of these schools. It can be used in both schools of nursing that have competency-based curricula and schools that have more traditional curricula to enhance student learning and make curricular revisions appropriate for the demands of the health-care system of today and of the future.

NURSES OF THE FUTURE

Nurses of the future will need to practice with self-reliance, independence, and flexibility. They will be required to have well-developed decision-making skills on the basis of critical-thinking ability, a working knowledge of community resources, and computer and technical competencies. Just as important, they will need to deliver high-quality care and patient education while working within the constraints of a managed-care system with tight cost-control measures.

Will nursing education ever be able to prepare a graduate who fulfills all the qualities required of nurses of the future? Nursing education responds with a yes, but only with curricular revisions that provide graduates with the tools to continue to learn as they advance in their careers.

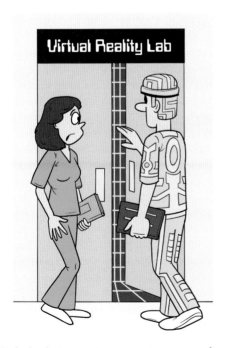

A holodeck is coming soon to your school.

Hospital Skills and More

Hospital-based acute care nursing practice will always have an important place in any health-care system. Highly skilled acute care nurses will always find a place to practice. It is generally accepted that the older population requires more health care of all types—acute, chronic, and community based. Although the current system experienced a decrease in the use of acute care beds, a gradual reverse in this trend is beginning as the baby boomers become the senior citizens who require more care for acute problems.

Paradigm shifting in nursing education does not need to be an either/or proposition. It is sometimes felt that nursing education is either acute care focused or community focused. Nursing education needs to combine the two so that the graduate can practice with competence in either or both settings. The skills are similar, but the emphasis may be different. Although some hospital skills are being done by non-nurses at a cheaper cost, nursing education must still teach such important skills as critical thinking, therapeutic relationship, **primary care**, and **case management**, as well as how to be comfortable with a consumer-driven health-care system.

Critical Thinking

Critical thinking has been an important element in nursing practice for many years. It is generally recognized as the ability to use basic core knowledge and decision-making skills in resolving situations with a relatively small amount of data and a high degree of risk and ambiguity. Critical thinking is the basis for clinical judgment used by nurses in making decisions about patient care and is a key part of the nursing licensure examination. Nursing has long been concerned with the ability to make good judgments and decisions about patient care.

At a fundamental level, the nursing process is a type of critical thinking. Unfortunately, in the health-care system of the future, a nurse's critical-thinking skills will have to go far beyond those of the basic nursing process. Nursing education will need to prepare students for more advanced critical thinking by exposing them to real-life situations that require the use of creativity, intuition, analysis, and deductive and inductive reasoning. These situations are introduced in the classroom as case studies and are reinforced in the clinical setting through guided experiences and mentoring.

Issues Now

e-Nursing Education

The nursing shortage is expected to get worse. Projected shortages for nurses range from 200,000 to 800,000 over a 10-year period from 2022 to 2032. Compounding the nursing shortage is a lack of nursing faculty qualified to educate new nurses. Many faculty are past retirement age, and it is difficult to attract new staff due to the relative low wages in education as compared to hospitals and the private sector for nurses with similar degrees. However, e-nursing education, which is now being used by most nursing programs, is seen as the solution to the shortage of nursing faculty.

Most nursing schools have steadily increased their online learning opportunities to the point where many programs are now totally online. Full immersion into e-nursing education requires not only a total acceptance of technology but also a shift in fundamental thought processes and teaching methodologies. Both nursing students and nursing instructors are already experiencing several key technologies.

"Intelligent" assistive health-care devices have spurred the growth of new industries that did not exist even 5 years ago. Artificial limbs that respond to computer-mediated signals from the brain are being used by those with amputations. Smart 3D printers are making body parts such as blood vessels that can be used to repair arteries and veins. Older adults and those with mobility problems are being helped by intelligent walkers to ambulate and to change position from sitting to standing and vice versa. Nursing education needs to keep pace with these developments by teaching students how to use these devices and how to educate patients in their use.

All nursing faculty are aware that current and future nursing students are not like students of the past, even the recent past. They are referred to as "Generation Z" (age 9 to 24) and the upcoming "Generation Alpha," or "Gen A" (age 0 to 9), who will be in nursing programs within 10 years. The average Gen Z student spent their early childhood playing with their parents' mobile phones or tablets and received their first mobile phone around age 10. All they have known is a world that is hyperconnected with smartphones as the primary method of communication. They spend, on average, 3 hours a day on some form of mobile device, although for some students that number is much higher.

Using computers is second nature to these students, so they do not respond well to sitting in lecture classes. They like to be more interactive, and they adapt readily to new technologies. They are masters at electronic multitasking and are nonlinear in their thought processes. The challenge for nursing educators is to develop and use technologies that keep these students engaged while ensuring that they master the vast amount of material required to practice nursing safely in today's complex health-care environment.

Several educational software companies have developed simulators and electronic learning games that address this need. One example is the Interactive Community Simulation Environment for Community Health Nursing, otherwise known as the Community Health Nursing Serious Game, which is based on the **modular Synthetic Training Research Evaluation and Extrapolation Tool (mSTREET)** platform to deliver computerized virtual training. In the game, students can investigate and respond to a variety of settings as they walk through the streets of a virtual city. The same mSTREET platform can be used for other health-care settings. Students will be able to walk into the room of an intensive care patient and observe and manipulate the machines connected to the patient, such as a ventilator, cardiac monitor, cooling blanket, and other commonly used devices.

Serious games technology (SGT) uses virtual reality to take learning one step beyond simulation. A number of serious games (SG) have been developed in recent years that teach clinical reasoning and improve students' knowledge of the care involved in treating patients with COVID-19 and the administration of medications. Students using SGT have the advantage of total participation in health-care scenarios, ranging from counseling sessions for patients with psychiatric disorders to advanced life support resuscitation of a patient in cardiac arrest. Combined with simulation technology, virtual reality allows students to use the equipment they will see in the work setting.

Issues Now (continued)

Wireless technology provides new learning opportunities and techniques. Access to the Internet through cellular networks allows anyone to access a whole world of information, from e-mail to video streaming. Students enrolled in online programs can now access them from almost any place where they can make a cell phone call. Publishing companies offer textbooks in electronic form (e-texts). Incorporated into these books are interactive exercises, videos, and simulation activities. Students can now read their textbooks on one of the many tablets available on the market today.

What will the nursing classroom of the future look like? It is a sure bet that the whole experience will be different. In reality, there may be no centrally located classrooms at all. Classroom lectures and interactive discussions will be conducted electronically over wireless devices from nursing educators. The way students learn will not be as important as what they learn, and learning will be measured through outcome testing. Nursing education will be asynchronous and available to anyone anywhere. It has been proposed that sometime in the future there may be only one nursing program for the whole country that is located in the cloud and totally online. That possibility certainly requires major paradigm shifting!

Sources: *O. Petit dit Dariel, T. Raby, F. Ravaut, M. Rothan-Tondeur, Developing the Serious Games potential in nursing education,* Nursing Education Today, *33(12):1569–1575, 2020, https://doi.org/10.1016/j.nedt.2012.12.014; J. Arellano, Three challenges to 3D printers in health care, Cybernet, April 5, 2022, https://www.cybernetman.com/blog/3-challenges-to-3d-printing-in-healthcare; Kasasa, Boomers, Gen X, Gen Y, Gen Z, and Gen A explained. Kasasa Exchange, July 6, 2021, https://www.kasasa.com/exchange/articles/generations/gen-x-gen-y-gen-z.*

The Therapeutic Relationship

Therapeutic relationship skills have long been stressed by mental health nursing faculty as a key element in the treatment of psychiatric problems. In reality, therapeutic relationship skills are essential for all nurses to fulfill their roles as health-care providers and healers. Although these skills are currently being taught in a limited and focused way in most nursing schools, they need to be expanded to involve **directed services** and relationship-centered nursing care.

Trust Is Essential

Relationship-centered nursing care is patient focused and revolves around the patient's trust in, value of, and understanding of the nurse's skills and role in the healing process. The patient must be able to feel comfortable with the nurse and share their own understanding of both illness and health.

Follow-up Care

Currently, in some **licensed practical nurse (LPN)** and **licensed vocational nurse (LVN)** programs offering the associate degree in nursing, clinical experiences consist of one-time, 8-hour provision of care for an acutely or chronically ill patient. Little time is spent in follow-up care. However, many bachelor of science in nursing (BSN) programs and some associate degree nursing (ADN) programs have expanded clinical experiences to include **discharge planning** and follow-up home health-care experiences.

To meet the demands of the future health-care system, all nursing education programs must be able to develop learning experiences for students that involve care for selected individuals or families over extended periods of time, perhaps ranging from several weeks to several semesters.

Case Management

Care management is a general term that refers to a method of coordinating care either with an individual patient or on a systemwide basis. Case management in a health-care system driven by the demand for better-quality, cost-effective care usually is associated with coordinating care for individual patients as they move from one level to another through the health-care system. Case management is now a certified specialty; however, there is a lack of qualified nurses trained in case management. Almost all the proposals for revisions in the health-care system include the **case manager** as an important element in the overall management of care (see Chapter 27).

(text continues on page 73)

Issues in Practice

No-Loan Nursing School

Unless you are independently wealthy or come from a wealthy family, when you thought about going to college for your nursing degree, you probably worried about how you were going to pay for it. The first thought many students have is, "I guess I'll have to take out a big loan." Not so fast! I attended a hospital diploma program, a diploma to bachelor of science in nursing (BSN) program, a master of science in nursing (MSN) program, and a PhD program and never took out 1 cent in loans. You can do it too. Here's how:

Outline a Basic Budget

There's an old saying that goes, "How can you get there if you don't know where you are going?" We all know that the first step in the nursing process is assessment. Figuring out how much money you are going to need is the assessment phase of the money-for-college process. Make a list or flow sheet of all the expenses you can think of, or ask someone who has gone to this college about what it costs (parents can be a good resource). A visual representation is an excellent way to watch what you are spending. A quick search of the Internet will yield several useful budget sheets.

As a new student, you will have to estimate several unknowns. Track all your expenses by writing them down or recording them in your phone—every penny you spend. This takes a little effort, but you will be surprised by the results. After the first semester of the first year is completed, you will have a more solid idea of what your actual expenses are. Update your original budget.

Some expenses you can be pretty sure about because they are listed on the college's Web page, such as tuition, laboratory fees, supplies, dormitory costs, and meal costs if you are staying in a dorm. (Many larger colleges require all freshmen to live in a dorm.) Unknown expenses are things like books (figure $700 to $1,000 per semester), travel expenses, laboratory coats and uniforms, and entertainment. If you are renting a house or an apartment off campus, you need to calculate rent, groceries, utilities, and transportation to and from campus. Some expenses remain the same each month, while others can vary quite a bit, such as your heating costs during the winter. Try to calculate every expense at its highest. The most important thing about budgeting is actually following it religiously. Spending hours working on a detailed budget is a waste of time if you end up blowing half of it on a new digital sound system.

Scholarships and Grants

Now that you know how much money you will need, it is time to figure out where to get it. There is a lot of money out there in the form of scholarships and grants, and much of it goes unclaimed every year. One of my strategies was to apply for every scholarship I could find. Back when I was going to nursing school, there weren't nearly as many scholarships as there are now, and they were a lot harder to find without the Internet. I managed to get three pretty good scholarships out of about eight I applied for, and they paid for most of my education.

You may think that all scholarships are based on grade point average (GPA), but that is nowhere near the truth. Many are based on public service that you may have performed during high school. Were you a member of your church's youth group performing projects that helped the needy? Did your high school have a public service requirement? Other scholarships are based on your ethnic heritage, where your parents work, and especially your major. Many large corporations and hospital systems know about the nursing shortage and are willing to help fund students in nursing schools. There are scholarships based on gender, age, second career, and no particular criteria at all. Once you go online, you're going to be surprised at the money floating around just waiting to be applied for!

Issues in Practice (continued)

Remember to look close to home. Many church organizations have money available through grants. Grants are like scholarships; but because some institutions, like churches, are listed as **not-for-profit**, the law does not allow them to give out scholarships. They are usually smaller sums, say $1,000, but that covers your books for a semester. Some grants, as well as scholarships, are ongoing and can be renewed year after year—if you keep your GPA up! Many state nurses associations offer—and advertise—several grants available for nursing students, but typically, few students apply for them. Those who do, of course, get the grants. Be creative in your search.

Most scholarships or grants require you to fill out an application. Make sure your application looks neat and professional and that you fill in all the blanks. If it is a paper application, you might want to make a copy and fill that out as a practice application. You can print an online application and fill it in as a template for typing in the online form later. If a question does not apply to you, write "Nonapplicable" in the blank. Watch the deadlines. Some of the bigger scholarships have early deadlines so that decision-makers have time to evaluate all the applicants. Make several copies of the documents that scholarships usually ask for, including transcripts from every high school and college you have attended, test scores (SAT, ACT, etc.), financial aid forms, financial information (tax returns, etc.), proof of eligibility (birth certificate, passport, etc.), and so forth. Prepare a **résumé** that you can print or attach electronically to the application.

Some scholarship applications require you to write an essay. Do not panic, and do not automatically eliminate the scholarship. Just follow a few simple pointers:

1. *Stick to the topic you are asked to write about.* Common topics include the following: Why do you want to be a nurse? Who was the person who most influenced you? What event in your life most affected your decision to be a nurse? What is your favorite book, and why? and What do you think is the number one issue in health care today?
2. *Follow the rules or guidelines meticulously.* If the guidelines specify 750 words, do not write a 753-word essay. Otherwise, the reviewers will likely just discard it. If the guidelines call for double-spaced, 12-point, Times New Roman font, make sure you follow the instruction exactly. Never use a script font to write any kind of document. It is hard to read!
3. *Try to be original.* Telling stories is a good technique to make an essay interesting. Never use trite or worn-out statements, such as "I'm a people person" or "I was as hot as a pistol!"
4. *Keep the essay personal.* Write it in the first person *(I, me, my)* unless instructed not to. Whoever reviews the essay really wants to know how you think and feel about issues. Quoting famous authors or dropping names of famous people you know is never appropriate.
5. *Avoid vague statements by using concrete details.* For example, "I helped an old man in the grocery store" is vague, whereas the following is clear: "Mr. Byrd, an elderly neighbor of mine, knocked over a can display in the grocery store. Together, we restacked the cans into a near-perfect pyramid."
6. *Have a person who writes and speaks English well review your essay.* Ask him or her *not* to go easy on it! Misspellings, poor sentence structure, and grammatical errors make a poor impression. Have this person read your application as well, looking closely for such mistakes. You may have to rewrite your essay several times before you feel confident the review committee will find it acceptable.
7. *Can you use the same essay for more than one application if the applications ask for the same information?* This point is a little tricky. You cannot plagiarize yourself unless the material has been published, so strictly speaking, it would not be illegal to use the same essay more than once. The likelihood of the same people reviewing essays for two different scholarships is very small; however, if that should happen, you would likely lose both scholarships.

(continued)

Issues in Practice (continued)

Letters of recommendation are usually required, and if not, scholarship committees usually will ask for the names, addresses, phone numbers, and e-mail addresses of three people who know you. Make sure you ask the people before you list them as references. Also, they should be people who know you well and have a little status (teacher, pastor, employer, principal). Letters of recommendation should focus on characteristics such as how quickly you learn, your grades (if they are good), your work ethic, how you interact with others, and maybe a major achievement during high school.

Make a copy of all the paperwork you are going to submit, and put it in a separate manila envelope in a safe place for later reference. Date and keep track of all the applications you send. Submitting duplicate applications is not effective!

When should you send your application in? There is some disagreement on this point. Some say as early as possible, others say just before the deadline. The one thing everyone agrees on is that it must be in before the deadline.

Pay Out of Pocket During the Semester

If you work full time or even part time during the summer before you start college, you can save up a considerable amount of money. It is unlikely that it will be enough to pay for a full year of college, but along with other money from scholarships or grants, it could be enough to get you through. You can also work part time during the semester. Many colleges have work-study positions, and health-care facilities like to hire nursing majors on a part-time basis as secretaries and aides. I had a variety of part-time jobs during the school year and summers. I worked with my brother, who is an electrician; I mopped floors and cleaned toilets at the apartment building I lived in; and during the summers, I worked as an orderly at my training hospital. The jobs did not pay a lot, but along with my scholarship money, I earned enough to get me through without starving!

Employer Tuition Reimbursement

When you are looking for a job, look for employers who might help you pay for college. There are two ways they do this: first, they may give you the money before you start classes; second, and more commonly, after you finish the semester and bring them your grade sheet showing you passed, they will reimburse you for your expenses. Some facilities require you to work for them for 2 to 4 years after you graduate. Of course, if the employer is a health-care facility, you are guaranteed a job when you graduate! Also, the experience will make you more marketable, and you can add it to your résumé.

Take Classes Part Time

This tactic does not really lower the cost of your education, but it allows you to work more and earn more money to avoid loans. Taking classes part time works best for advanced degrees where many of the programs are either online or tailored for the part-time student. It does mean that completing the program will take longer. Taking classes during the summer helps you complete a part-time program faster. This is how I got through graduate school.

Take More Hours

You may or may not be able to take more hours depending on the rules of the college you are attending. At the college I attended for my diploma to bachelor of science degree, tuition was the same for 16 hours as for 21 hours of classes. It was pretty brutal taking 21 hours a semester and working full time, but I completed a 2-year program in 18 months. It saved the cost of a whole semester. Even increasing your number of hours each semester by two or three can shorten your program significantly over eight semesters.

The Military Option

All branches of the U.S. military are always looking for nurses. Once you sign up, they pay for nearly all expenses, and you have a guaranteed job as a commissioned officer when you graduate. Not only do they pay for tuition, books, and fees, they also give you a stipend (money) for living expenses. After you graduate

Issues in Practice (continued)

and work for them for a few years, they will pay for your graduate education too. It is a really good deal for anyone thinking about the nursing profession.

I Think I Still Need a Loan

So, you have added up all the numbers, and it looks like you are going to be several thousand dollars short. Guess you will need a loan. What is the next step?

You already have the basic information figured. You know how much college is going to cost, and you know how much money you have on hand or can obtain from scholarships and work. If you subtract how much money you can get your hands on from what it costs for college, you will have a good idea of how much you need to borrow.

Where should you borrow from, and what is the process? The first thing to keep in mind is to never borrow any more than you need. Every penny you borrow has interest attached to it. Never use a private loan. Private loans have much higher interest rates than federal loans; and when it comes time to repay them, they are very inflexible.

There are many online resources with information about student loans and loan repayment programs. In 2022, President Joe Biden signed into law a student loan/debt forgiveness program of up to $10,000 for each student who met the repayment criteria and up to $20,000 for students who went to college under Pell Grants. In addition, because of the grave nursing shortage, nurses are also eligible for student loan forgiveness under the Expanded Public Loan Forgiveness program.

A Growing Need

With the changes introduced into the health-care system by the Affordable Care Act (ACA), the need for case managers increased. However, like the ACA's future, the role of case managers is in question. Currently, case managers do not have to be RNs; however, with the increased complexity of health-care technologies and the demands for improved outcomes, RNs have the knowledge and skills to fulfill the role. Perhaps the ideal situation for case management would be to have a **health-care team**, with both an RN and a social worker coordinating all aspects of the patient's care.

> *With the changes introduced into the health-care system by the Affordable Care Act (ACA), the need for case managers increased. However, like the ACA's future, the role of case managers is in question.*

follow-up, health-care practices, and developmental stages.

The knowledge and thinking required by an effective case manager go far beyond what is currently required of new graduates. Nurses must be able to understand the immediate disease process and the long-term outcomes and factors that influence the disease. Case managers must also practice health-focused nursing and primary levels of intervention. Decisions must be made about care from a broad **database** as well as from an understanding of the patient's abilities, knowledge level, and even financial status.

Nursing education will be severely challenged to provide experiences to prepare students for this role. Students must be allowed to experience the authority, accountability, and responsibility of guiding a patient's health care over an extended period. It might be beneficial to combine the learning experiences mentioned earlier

A Wide Range of Skills

As case managers, nurses are responsible for developing clinical pathways and for directing and guiding the overall health care of a specific group of patients. Case management includes overseeing the patients' care while they are in the hospital and following them through their rehabilitation at home, long-term in establishing the therapeutic relationship with the managed-care experience.

The Consumer in Authority

A consumer-driven health-care system is the nurse's dream—and nightmare. Many widely used nursing models or theories claim to be patient centered, which translates into being consumer driven. Yet, when these models are put into practice, the care given is more provider driven than anything else.

Care as Requested

A patient/consumer-driven health-care system means that the care given and the outcomes are both determined by the consumer. The nurse must be able to accept the authority of the group or community as a determinant of health care. The nurse's role becomes one of a partner in guiding, implementing, and overseeing ways to deliver requested health care for a given community.

Many nursing programs, particularly baccalaureate programs, include a course in community health and home health-care nursing. Often, a requirement of this course is to have the students perform a community survey in which they determine the needs of the community as they perceive them. Many of these courses have been modified so that the students learn the community members' perceptions of their own needs.

Paradigm shifting is never easy. Major paradigm shifts in thinking and acting are even more difficult. Nursing education is currently dealing with a huge paradigm shift. How educators are meeting these challenges will, to a large extent, shape the future of professional nursing.

AMERICAN NURSES ASSOCIATION POSITION PAPER ON EDUCATION FOR NURSES

After evaluating the changes that occurred in the health-care system during the 1950s and studying the projected educational needs for nurses, the ANA published a paper in 1965 that took a stand on an issue that was, and still is, highly controversial. Although written almost 60 years ago, this document is still relevant to many of the issues in nursing education today.

After World War II, there was an explosion of scientific and technological knowledge used in health care. The educational level of the population was also increasing, resulting in greater public demand for higher-quality health care. In reevaluating the nature and scope of nursing practice and the type and quality of education needed to meet these new demands, the ANA reached the conclusions that are presented in its position paper.

A Changing Role for Hospitals

Hospitals recognized that they would no longer retain their traditional role of preparing nurses for practice. Even though pressure to move nursing education from hospital-based diploma schools to institutions of higher education had been building for some time, in the mid-1960s, 75 percent of the graduating nurses were from hospital-based diploma programs.[10]

Colleges Under Pressure

Colleges and universities were pushed to quickly develop undergraduate and graduate curricula for increasing numbers of nursing majors. The relatively few baccalaureate programs in existence at the time were generally small, and institutions found it difficult to expand the programs rapidly. It also became evident that a clear distinction between technical and professional programs needed to be made.

The Debate Continues

To this day, the ANA remains firmly committed to its stand that all nursing education should be housed in institutions of higher learning. Almost 60 years have elapsed since this statement was made, and the profession of nursing is still trying to reach a consensus on the issue of basic educational preparation for entry into practice.

The Future of Nursing (FON) set an ambitious goal of increasing the number of graduates from BSN programs to 80 percent by 2020. Although the interim report of the FON in 2016 showed an increase of only 3 percent between 2010 and 2014 (49 to 51 percent), the absolute numbers were more impressive. Approximately 150,000 nurses graduated from BSN programs in 2010, and the number for 2014 was approximately

> *" A consumer-driven health-care system is the nurse's dream—and nightmare. "*

173,000, an increase of 23,000. As of 2020, the goal still remains unmet with only 62.4 percent of nurses holding baccalaureate degrees.[6]

Over the past few years, several states have been looking at the BSN-in-10 proposal for legislation that would require graduates from ADN programs to obtain their BSN degrees within 10 years after graduating from the ADN program. Because of the strong lobbying efforts against this proposal on the part of the ADN programs, there has been almost no movement on its implementation. In addition, the current nursing shortage due to the COVID-19 pandemic has put any attempt to push this plan forward on an indefinite hold.[9]

Defining a Profession

A similar resolution defining **entry into practice** was proposed by the ANA in 1985, but it also met strong opposition and was never enacted. In 1996, the AACN presented its own position paper emphasizing the belief that the baccalaureate degree should be the minimal requirement for entry into the nursing profession. The discussion remains ongoing with seemingly little hope for resolution. The most influential reasons these proposals have not been adopted are economic, not conceptual. Although some experts believe it is time to leave the old debate behind and work toward developing a better-educated profession in general, many others see the issue as important to the definition of nursing as a profession.

DIPLOMA SCHOOLS

The Nightingale School of Nursing was a diploma school in the strict use of the term. When nurses graduated from this school, they were given a certificate or diploma noting their graduation, but no academic degree. They were also listed in a "register" in case someone might wish to check on their qualification, hence the name registered nurse. The first graduates from the Nightingale School soon began to establish their own schools of nursing based on the Nightingale model and adhered to her philosophy of nursing education. These were also diploma schools.[10]

An Improvement in Care

After an initial period of uncertainty and trepidation, both physicians and hospital administrators began to recognize that when the education of nurses improved, so, too, did the overall quality of the care provided by their hospitals. They also understood that these types of schools that were closely associated with hospitals could provide a source of free or inexpensive labor in the form of nursing students.

Diploma schools sprang up throughout Europe; and in time, each hospital had its own school of nursing. Many of Nightingale's principles and concerns about nursing education were abandoned during this period of growth.

Catching Up to Europe

In the United States, developments in nursing education, as with health care in general, lagged behind those in Europe. It was not until the mid-1870s that the first school of nursing was established in the United States. This was a diploma school attached to the New England Hospital for Women.[10]

As in Europe, the idea of diploma schools quickly caught on. Within 10 years, almost every large hospital in the United States had its own diploma school of nursing. These schools had very little in common with the Nightingale School of Nursing. There was no uniformity in curriculum, length of program, or requirements. To guarantee adequate enrollment, uneducated and impoverished candidates were again being recruited.

> *In early hospital-based diploma schools of nursing, hospitals used the student nurses as a major source of free labor for their facilities. There was little or no classroom or theoretical study.*

A Source of Cheap Labor

In early hospital-based diploma schools of nursing, hospitals used the student nurses as a major source of free labor for their facilities. There was little or no classroom or theoretical study. The students learned exclusively by hands-on experience during their 12- to 14-hour, 7-day-a-week work shifts.

Most of the students were young, single women recruited just after they graduated from high school. They were confined to dormitories on the hospital property. The dormitories were monitored closely by a housemother who enforced the rigorous rules of behavior covering all aspects of the students' lives and dismissed students for even minor infractions of the rules. The early diploma schools of nursing were organized and administered on a model that was similar to the strictest of the religious orders.

Submission to Authority

The nurses who graduated from these schools were proficient in basic nursing skills and could assume positions in the hospital where they were trained or in-home nursing, where they worked on a case-by-case basis without any additional orientation or education. Because of the 24-hour-a-day, 7-day-a-week socialization process administered by these schools, diploma graduate nurses tended to be very submissive to authority and willing to carry out any duty to please the physician, administrator, or head nurse. Before the advent of licensure examinations and standardization of practice, nurses from diploma schools were often limited to employment in their own training institutions or in-home health-care settings.

A Move Toward Accreditation

Diploma schools of nursing remained relatively unchanged in the United States until 1949, when the National Nursing Accrediting Service, working under the guidance of the National League for Nursing (NLN), became the licensing body for all schools of nursing that voluntarily sought accreditation. The first formal accreditation of nursing schools occurred in the early 1950s. In 1952, the NLN assumed accrediting responsibilities for all schools of nursing. In 2013, the name of the Commission was changed to the Accreditation Commission for Education in Nursing (ACEN); and in 2015, the ACEN endorsed academic progression programs in nursing in cooperation with the Robert Wood Johnson Foundation Academic Progression in Nursing (APIN) program and the Future of Nursing: Campaign for Action. It is important to note that the ACEN is the only nationally recognized accrediting agency for nursing education programs and schools, both postsecondary and higher degree, which offer a certificate, diploma, or a recognized professional

> **The early diploma schools of nursing were organized and administered on a model that was similar to the strictest of the religious orders.**

degree including clinical doctorate, master's, baccalaureate, associate, diploma, and practical nursing programs in the United States and its territories, including those offered via distance education.[11] Accreditation by a nationally recognized accrediting agency has always been and remains a voluntary undertaking.

Outcome Criteria

To be accredited by the ACEN, schools of nursing had to meet specific **outcome criteria** and teach specific content in their curricula. Many of the diploma schools of nursing could not or would not submit to these criteria and eventually closed. Some of the requirements for the schools that did choose to comply with the ACEN included the following:

- Implementing a 3-year course of study meeting the criteria established by the state board of nursing using only faculty with baccalaureate or higher degrees in nursing
- Developing a philosophy and demonstrating how that philosophy was implemented through learning objectives, course objectives, and outcome criteria
- Showing an adequate pass rate on the state board examination or National Council Licensure Examination (NCLEX)[11]

A Jump in Expense

One of the key factors that all state boards of nursing were concerned about was that the school should be able to demonstrate that students were not being used as unpaid hospital personnel while they were in their education and training programs. When students could no longer be used as free labor, diploma nursing schools became very expensive to the hospitals, whereas previously they were virtually free.

Not only did the hospitals still have to pay for the room and board of the students, but they also now had to hire and pay additional staff because the students could no longer be included in the overall staff numbers. Due to the overwhelming financial burden to the hospitals, even more diploma schools closed. The schools that stayed open were forced to increase their tuition rates, which made nursing schools just as expensive as programs granting academic degrees.

CONVERTING THE CURRICULUM

During the 1960s and 1970s, many diploma schools became associated with universities and converted their curricula into degree-granting programs. According to recent data published by the National Academy of Medicine, approximately 95 accredited diploma programs remain open in the United States. They are of universally high quality and meet all the standards necessary for ACEN accreditation. The main emphasis remains on preparing nurses who are highly competent in technical nursing skills through extensive hands-on practice in the clinical setting, but elements of leadership, humanities, and general sciences are also included in the classroom setting.[12]

PRACTICAL/VOCATIONAL NURSING

The practical/vocational nurse has been a part of the health-care system in the United States for more than 100 years. Although the earliest formal schools of practical/vocational nursing were started around 1890, informal training programs for this level of nursing probably existed well before that time—for example, in the Young Women's Christian Association (YWCA), particularly in New York City. What is the difference between an LVN and an LPN? They are almost identical because they are both entry-level into nursing. LVNs and LPNs both provide basic-level nursing care to patients and work under the supervision of nurses with more advanced titles, such as RNs, and physicians. The main difference between the two is where they work. An LVN works in the state of California or Texas. Every other state uses the title of LPN.[13]

A Useful Trade

These programs accepted uneducated girls who had migrated from rural areas and farms to the cities in search of employment and taught them a useful trade with which they could support themselves. With no regulation or accreditation for the early practical/vocational nurse programs, there were wide variations

in the quality, length, and focus of what was being taught. Generally, the students were taught to provide home care, similar to that given by **private duty nurses**, for patients ranging from newborns to elderly and invalid individuals.

The number of **practical nursing programs** gradually increased during the next 50 years. Graduates of these 3-month programs were beginning to find employment in hospitals and nursing homes as well as in areas of private duty. During the nurse shortage after World War I, many hospitals found that these relatively undereducated nurses, after receiving on-the-job training in the hospital, could function at a fairly high level of skill and at a much-reduced cost. Soon, the number of these unlicensed nurses increased.

Compulsory Licensure

By the late 1930s, the ANA saw the need to regulate the quality of the practical/**vocational nursing programs** to protect public safety. It was not until 1938 that the state of New York took seriously the ANA's recommendation for compulsory licensure for practical/vocational nurses and enacted the first law requiring such licensure. In 1960, all practical/vocational nurses were required to pass a licensure examination before they could practice.

> *Continuing the discussion and efforts to bring about collaborative agreement on nursing education is a goal that the profession must work toward.*

The Importance of Technique

Although education for LPNs/LVNs varies slightly from one state to another, there are some common characteristics. Most of the programs are from 9 to 12 months and are measured in clock hours rather than academic hours. They are often offered in hospitals, high schools, vocational schools, and trade schools, although some forward-looking programs are conducted in community colleges and even in universities.

Orientation of the curricula in these programs is highly technical and emphasizes the learning of skills in the hospital or nursing home setting, with less emphasis on theoretical knowledge. Because they are **technicians**, it is much more important for practical/vocational nurses to learn *how* to do something rather than *why* they are doing it.

Filling a Shortage

The stated scope of practice for the practical/vocational nurse involves providing care for patients in hospitals, nursing homes, or the home setting for those who have stable conditions. LPNs/LVNs are to be under the supervision of an RN or another licensed **provider**.

However, in the real world, LPNs/LVNs are often required to provide care well outside their scope of practice, leaving them in legal limbo and vulnerable to lawsuits. They often function in leadership roles or provide care in acute settings with highly unstable patients. LPNs/LVNs are often hired when there are shortages of RNs to fill the gaps in patient care.[13]

Many associate degree RN programs have developed a ladder curriculum whereby an LPN/LVN can go back to school for a shorter period, often receiving credit for years of experience, complete the program in 1 year, and then take the RN licensure examination.

ASSOCIATE DEGREE NURSING

The **associate degree nursing program** was developed by Mildred Montag as a temporary solution to the nursing shortage experienced after World War II.[10] Originally designed to prepare students for technical nursing practice, the 2-year ADN programs were offered through community colleges with an emphasis on developing the skills necessary to provide high-quality bedside care in less time than BSN programs required.

Technical Orientation

In 1952 at Teachers College, Columbia University, Montag conducted a successful pilot program for ADNs to prepare technical nurses who could assist professional nurses. It demonstrated that community college–based programs could attract large numbers of students, prove cost effective, and produce skillful technical nurses in half the time required for BSN programs.[10]

Which Exam to Take?

Early on, there was some heated debate concerning licensure and titling for this group of nurses. The technical orientation of the curriculum was very similar to that found in programs that prepare LPNs, but the location of the programs in the community college setting and the increased theoretical orientation seemed to elevate these programs to a higher educational plane. It was finally decided that the ADN graduates should take the RN licensure examination rather than the LPN/LVN examination.[13]

A Proven Track Record

The emphasis on technical skills of the ADN programs met a need in the health-care system of the 1960s and 1970s. By the early 1980s, there were more than 800 ADN programs across the United States; as of 2016, the number was more than 1,000, with more than 66,000 students; and in 2021, there were some 1,275 ADN programs, although not all of them are accredited by a national agency.[14] Graduates from these programs exceeded the number of graduates from all the diploma, BSN, and LPN/LVN programs combined.

Although it is possible to complete the requirements for an ADN in 2 academic years, most programs take at least 3 years to complete for a new student who has no prior college credit.[13] ADN graduates have a proven track record for providing safe bedside care for patients from the first day they are hired. They function well as team members and, after a period of orientation, can assume responsibility for the care of patients who are more acutely ill.

> *ADN graduates have a proven track record for providing safe bedside care for patients from the first day they are hired.*

BACCALAUREATE EDUCATION

Early attempts at college-level nursing programs sometimes took the form of "prenursing" courses over a 1- or 2-year period that prepared students to enter upper-division schools of nursing. Generally acclaimed as the first university program to be completely conducted in the higher education setting, the University of Minnesota School of Nursing was opened in 1909. In 1923, the Yale School of Nursing began accepting students; it is considered the first autonomous college of nursing in the United States.[10]

A Slow Increase

The development of schools of nursing in the university and college setting was a gradual process that extended over several decades. Only a few collegiate nursing programs were established during the years when the diploma programs were expanding. Some of these early collegiate programs were a hybrid of college-level classes and diploma-school clinical experiences that still granted only a diploma rather than an academic degree.

The number of university-based nursing programs gradually increased over the years, and by the beginning of World War II, there were 76 programs granting baccalaureate degrees in nursing. These programs tended to specialize in preparing nurses for public health nursing, teaching, administration, and supervisory positions in hospitals. Although all of these programs included a **clinical component**, the emphasis was more on theoretical knowledge, development of critical thinking, decision-making skills, and leadership.

Universities in general enjoyed rapid growth immediately after World War II, and higher education nursing programs expanded along with the universities. Many military nurses, prepared by the Cadet Nurse Corps during World War II, went back to school under the GI Bill to complete their baccalaureate degrees, thus providing the framework for current ADN to BSN programs.

Education for a Profession

During this rapid growth period, these **baccalaureate degree nursing programs** were plagued with problems similar to those found in the diploma programs during their own rapid expansion period. Primarily, the lack of uniformity in content, curriculum, and even the length of programs was problematic. It was difficult to find qualified faculty because most of the nurses at this time had received their education in diploma programs. No doctorate degrees existed in nursing, few nurses had master's degrees, and only a smattering of nurses had baccalaureate degrees.

During the late 1940s and early 1950s, it was clearly necessary to start stratifying nursing education programs into technical levels and professional levels.

> *During the late 1940s and early 1950s, it was clearly necessary to start stratifying nursing education programs into technical levels and professional levels. It became apparent that all health-care professionals should have, at minimum, a baccalaureate degree.*

It became apparent to most nursing leaders that all health-care professionals should have, at minimum, a baccalaureate degree.[15]

The NLN and other accrediting agencies began to develop strict criteria for the accreditation of baccalaureate nursing programs. These criteria included courses in general education, general sciences, humanities, and language as well as specific nursing courses. They required a certain number of hours to be spent in the clinical setting practicing nursing skills, a faculty prepared at the master's degree level, and the availability of laboratory and library facilities for the students. Faculty-to-student ratios were limited, particularly in the clinical setting, and outcome criteria were required for the students.[15]

Different Approaches

Although all university-level baccalaureate degrees in nursing have the same number of required credit hours and educational requirements, there are three avenues for attaining this degree: professional and full academic degrees, discussed here, and ladder programs, discussed in the next section.

The Professional Degree

The BSN degree fulfills the criteria of a professional degree. It meets the overall requirements for a college baccalaureate degree (120 to 124 credit hours, 65 hours of nursing major, and most of the general education requirements) but does not meet all the general education requirements for an academic bachelor of science (BS) degree. Although a professional degree is usually obtained in a traditional college setting, it can also be obtained through an **external degree** program in which the student has to meet the criteria for the BSN.

The Full Academic Degree

The second approach is found in programs that offer a BS degree with a major in nursing (also mistakenly called a BSN degree). This degree is a full academic college degree and guarantees that the person holding it has met all of the general education, science, and major subject requirements. In 2021, there were 990 baccalaureate nursing programs in the United States, although not all of them are accredited by a nursing accrediting agency. A third avenue that may be pursued is sometimes called the career ladder, or RN to BSN program.[15]

LADDER PROGRAMS

Career ladder, educational ladder, **articulation**, or educational mobility programs have become increasingly popular as a result of an interest in **upward mobility**, educational articulation, and **career mobility**.

Upward Mobility

A ladder program allows nurses to upgrade their education and move from one educational level to another with relative ease by granting credit for previous coursework and experience and without loss of credits from previous education.

Each ladder program is developed according to the philosophy of the particular nursing school, may use any one of a number of curricular patterns, uses one of several means of **advanced placement** or credit granted for previous education, and must meet ACEN accreditation standards.

Ladder programs take several different forms. Some provide a **competency-based education** that allows the students to proceed at their own pace as long as they fulfill required educational outcomes. Ladder programs have become increasingly popular as colleges move toward Web-based courses and programs.

> *Should the BSN-in-10 proposal ever gain a toehold, there will be more than enough spaces for students coming from ADN programs.*

The Associate Ladder

The LPN/LVN to ADN ladder allows individuals who have been licensed as LPNs/LVNs to take a minimal number of courses in an associate degree program to obtain their ADN and then take the NCLEX-RN to become licensed as RNs. Programs vary widely as to how many credits they will accept from the LPN/LVN programs and how many courses the students take to complete the degree. Some of the requirements for number of hours are out of the control of the nursing programs because they have been established as general education requirements of the college or are state regent's requirements. LPN/LVN and ADN programs are highly compatible because of the similarity of curricula and the technical orientation of both types of programs.

The Baccalaureate Ladder

Some LPN/LVN to BSN ladder programs either allow LPNs/LVNs to challenge a number of courses, particularly when the LPN/LVN program is located in an associate degree–granting facility, or to grant students credit for nursing courses on the basis of previous experience and demonstrated competency. Students who enter these types of ladder programs usually spend more time in school than those in the LPN/LVN to ADN programs. In addition to meeting the requirements of the BSN, they also have to meet the general education requirements for a baccalaureate degree and complete 120 to 124 hours of college-level courses. One problem in developing these types of ladder programs is that many states' boards of regents do not recognize courses taken at the vocational-technical level as higher education courses and therefore will not transfer them into the college setting. One way around this requirement is for students to take challenge examinations in both general education courses and nursing courses. Once the students pass the test, they are granted college-level credit for the course. These examinations tend to be difficult and are really a type of outcome-based learning. However, they do not require the student to attend classes and are much cheaper than a regular college course.

Two Plus Two: RN to BSN

Nursing education has seen a marked increase in the number of ADN to BSN, associate to baccalaureate (ATB), and diploma to BSN ladder programs, sometimes called **two plus two (2 + 2) programs**, although this terminology has mostly fallen out of use in current educational jargon, and these programs are generally called RN to BSN programs. These programs admit individuals who are already licensed as RNs but who have either a diploma or an associate degree.[15]

RN to BSN programs may take several different forms. Upper-division baccalaureate programs have no unlicensed students and are designed exclusively to meet the educational needs of students who are already RNs. Most of these programs have adopted a totally online format: students take all of the classes on their home computers, with only minimal requirements for class attendance on campus. These types of classes work particularly well for students who work full time and may have family responsibilities.

Other programs accept ADN or diploma graduates in addition to unlicensed students as students. These schools often have separate programs for ADNs or diploma RNs that allow them to take examinations to prove educational knowledge and nursing proficiency (**challenge examinations**) in specific classes, thus granting credit for their nursing experience. The RNs then take advanced-level nursing courses, such as community health/home health care, leadership, and critical care, which are not commonly found in diploma or ADN programs. Many of these programs are also online.

The ATB program is similar to the RN to BSN discussed previously. However, in the ATB program, the ADN program partners with several universities. The student chooses the university partner where they want to complete the BSN and then applies to both the BSN and the ADN programs. The student is then enrolled in both programs at the same time and takes a few courses at the university partner throughout the 2-year associate degree program. Once the student completes the ADN and passes the NCLEX-RN, they go right into the university and complete courses for the BSN. With this partnership approach, the ATB program takes approximately 3 years.

On completion of the degree requirements, these nurses are granted a baccalaureate degree. Some of these programs have an **open curriculum** that allows students to enter and leave the program freely. There are more than 762 of these programs according to the AACN's 2021 Annual Survey, and the number continues to grow.[16] The capacity to accept ADN graduates into these completion programs is almost unlimited. Should the BSN-in-10 proposal ever gain a toehold, there will be more than enough spaces for students coming from ADN programs.

Fast-Track Options

Some nursing programs have gotten creative in their attempt to educate nurses at the baccalaureate level. One approach is to place students who have a BS or BA degree in another major, such as biology or English, in fast-track programs that allow them to obtain their nursing degree in 1 or 2 years. In many ways, these programs are similar to the RN to BSN programs, but they also teach the basic nursing skills that ADN graduates already have.

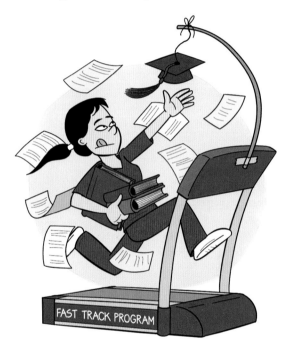

Fast Track Programs are challenging!

The Master's Ladder or Bridge Program

A growing trend in educational ladder programs is the ADN to MSN programs, now commonly called *bridge programs*. These programs are a way to accelerate the process for associate nurses to attain a post-graduate MSN degree in a reduced amount of time. This type of program allows students to transfer the credits earned by completing their ADN program directly to the MSN program. However, the path from an ADN to an MSN degree requires the completion of a BSN degree before a student can actually be enrolled in a conventional MSN degree program. The length of these programs varies from school to school, and most are completely online, often allowing students to work at their own pace.[17]

MASTER'S AND DOCTORAL-LEVEL EDUCATION

The baccalaureate degree is considered a generalist degree that exposes students to a wide range of subjects during the 4 years spent in college. The master's degree, on the other hand, is a specialist's degree.[17] Students who pursue a master's degree concentrate their study in one particular subject area and become expert in that given area.

Master's Degree Programs

Master's degree in nursing programs have been in existence almost from the time baccalaureate-level nursing programs were started. Some early and current nursing leaders have stated that the master's degree in nursing should be the entry-level degree for the profession.[19] The early master's degree in nursing programs were designed for students who had baccalaureate degrees in other majors, such as biology, and wanted to become nurses. After completion of an additional 36 to 42 credit hours in nursing courses only, these students were awarded the MSN and could then take the licensure examination for RNs.

Experience Required

Today, most master's degree in nursing programs prefer RNs who have a baccalaureate degree, although the ADN to MSN program is gaining popularity. In the past, many of these programs required at least 1 year of clinical practice after the BSN and an additional 36 to 46 college credit hours. Most students who enter master's degree programs attend classes on a part-time basis while they work and may take up to 5 years to complete the requirements. Many universities have recognized this trend and have tailored their programs to meet the needs of these part-time students. Universities now offer master of science (MS) degrees almost completely online as well as distance education in the evening and on weekends or 1-day-a-week programs. There are more than 631 accredited

master's degree programs in nursing in the United States.[16]

There are several available areas of study for those pursuing master's degrees in nursing. Some of the more popular areas include nursing administration; community health; psychiatric mental health; adult health; maternal–child health; **gerontology; rehabilitation** care; nursing education; and some more advanced areas of practice, such as certified registered nurse anesthetist (CRNA), pediatric nurse practitioner (PNP), **family** nurse practitioner (FNP), geriatric nurse practitioner (GNP), women's health nurse practitioner (WHNP), and certified nurse midwife (CNM).[16]

Many of these programs require the student to pass a comprehensive written or oral examination. Some courses require the student to write an extensive research thesis before graduation, although some programs are now requiring a published journal manuscript in lieu of the thesis.

> *Some early and current nurse leaders have stated that the master's degree in nursing should be the entry-level degree for the profession.*

Professional and Academic Degrees

There are two basic types of the master's degree in nursing. The MSN is the professional degree, and the MS with a major in nursing degree (MS nursing) is the formal academic degree.[17] In practice, however, little differentiation is made between the two. Almost all master's programs are accredited and require the applicant to have at least a 3.0 grade point average and to demonstrate academic proficiency by achieving a satisfactory score on the Graduate Record Examination (GRE) or the Miller Analogies Test before admission, although some programs are opting out of this requirement. The GRE is also used to recommend remedial coursework needed to correct deficiencies before the master's program is undertaken.[18]

What Do You Think?

Have you ever been to an advanced practice nurse for health care? How would you rate the quality of that care? If you have not been to an advanced practice nurse, would you consider going to one for care? Why or why not?

Doctoral Programs

In the evolution of the various levels of education, the baccalaureate degree is a generalist's degree, the master's degree is a specialist's degree, and the academic doctoral degree is a generalist's degree, although at a much higher academic level than the baccalaureate degree. The major purpose of early doctoral degrees was to prepare the individual to conduct advanced research in a particular area of interest. Nurses holding these degrees conduct much of the research used in EBP. To apply for a doctoral program, the applicant must be an RN with some experience and generally hold a master's degree in nursing.

The future for doctoral degrees in nursing looks bright, and these degrees are increasingly being required in employment settings. Currently, there are 149 research-focused doctoral programs and 407 doctor of nursing programs in the United States. Often, these two programs are offered in the same university.[16]

A Wide Range of Choices

There is a wide range of available doctoral degrees for nurses. The PhD is the most accepted academic degree and is designed to prepare individuals to conduct research. The doctor of education (EdD) degree is considered a professional degree, although in many programs there is little difference between the courses of study taken by EdD and PhD candidates. The PhD focuses primarily on research, whereas the EdD focuses more on administration in the educational setting. The classes and research credits differ somewhat between the two degrees.[19]

Academic Doctorates

Almost all PhD in nursing programs have an additional focus on education because most PhD graduates will be teaching nursing in institutions of higher education. Nurses with PhDs learn about administration in higher education, classroom teaching, curriculum development, and the evaluation process. Some programs require "nursing student teaching" for their candidates during their capstone courses to evaluate their teaching methodologies and techniques.[19]

Professional Practice Doctorates

Since the 1970s, doctoral programs for nurses have been developed to stress the clinical rather than the academic nature of nursing. These programs include the doctor of nursing science (DNSc, DNS) and the doctor of science in nursing (DSN), whose graduates are educated to be nurse scientists and who are substantially influencing the health-care system. These nurse scientists function as leaders in the clinical setting, perform research, act as analysts in both the private sector and health-care setting, and work in health-care informatics.

The doctor of nursing in education (DN or ND) degree is for the person with a BS or an MS in a field other than nursing who wants to pursue nursing as a career. It is a generalist's degree at a basic level of education. Its graduates focus on advanced practice specialties as well as evidence-based research, and the degree usually requires 3 to 5 years of full-time classes either online or in person.

The DNP degree was first granted almost 40 years ago at Case Western University. However, at that time, very few schools of nursing granted it, and there was a great deal of confusion about what the degree was and what nurses holding it could do. A small number of nurses opted for the degree. Graduates of a DNP program are prepared for a range of clinical activities including leadership in clinical care delivery, research, and organization supervision. Although DNP graduates are not, strictly speaking, academic doctorates, they often end up teaching and even directing schools of nursing. The DNP is now considered as the terminal degree for advanced practice nurses, and the number of graduates has greatly increased.[19] Many universities now offer the DNP in conjunction with the curriculum for becoming a nurse practitioner. In recent years, there has been some discussion of making the

> *In the evolution of the various levels of education, the baccalaureate degree is a generalist's degree, the master's degree is a specialist's degree, and the doctoral degree is a generalist's degree, although at a much higher academic level than the baccalaureate degree.*

DNP degree the basic entry-level degree required for the profession of nursing.

An additional degree for nurses who wish to pursue a career in higher education is the doctor of nursing education (DNEd) degree; however, it is considered a professional, not an academic, degree. Few nursing schools still offer this degree since the advent of the DNP. The corresponding academic degree is the EdD, which is available at many universities.

More Programs, Tough Requirements

There has been rapid growth in the number of programs across the United States offering doctorate level programs to accommodate the wide range of doctoral degrees in nursing. Despite the increase in these programs, only 11.2 percent offer a research-focused doctorate and 14.1 percent the DNP.[19]

The requirements for all doctoral education degrees are similar, even though the specific degrees being sought may be different. The student must have attained a master's degree and must have achieved a satisfactory score on the GRE. Often, candidates must go through an admission interview and preprogram examination before they can be formally admitted to the program. Research doctoral programs are at least 60 college credit hours in length, require many statistics and research courses, and often have a residency requirement. Before the doctoral degree can be granted, the student must successfully complete both oral and written comprehensive examinations and must write a doctoral dissertation that explains how to conduct a major research project.

Almost all students in these programs now pursue their degrees on a part-time basis while they are working full time, whereas few others opt to attend classes full time, often completing the program in 3 to 4 years. Many programs have gone to a totally online format. Some programs require that the individual complete all the requirements within 10 years. Although this may seem like a long time, it is not unusual for the dissertation process itself to take 2 to 3 years.[19]

Leaders in the Profession

Nurses with master's or doctoral degrees are regarded as leaders in the nursing profession. Many of the larger hospitals in the United States require their unit managers and supervisors to have master's degrees and their directors of nursing or vice presidents of nursing to have doctorates. Of course, in baccalaureate programs, the minimal requirement for teaching is the master's

degree, and the doctorate is preferred. Nurses with these advanced degrees provide direction and leadership for the profession through their publications, research, and theory development. As health-care delivery becomes more complicated, facilities will require larger numbers of nurses with advanced degrees.

EDUCATION FOR ADVANCED PRACTICE

Advanced practice is one of those often-misused terms in nursing that add to the public's confusion about educational levels of those in the profession. The advanced practice registered nurse (APRN) certification has become the recognized credential for nurses receiving a master's degree in a specialized expanded practice role. It is also sometimes referred to as **expanded role** or *expanded practice*. Nurses who obtain certification are allowed to practice at a higher and more independent level, depending on the nurse practice act of their individual state. Advanced practitioners diagnose illnesses, prescribe medications, conduct physical examinations, and refer patients to specialists for more intensive follow-up care. These nurses practice under their own licenses as **independent practitioners** but often work closely with a physician so that they can quickly refer patients who have medical problems that lie outside their scope of practice.[20]

Historically, an amendment to the New York Nurse Practice Act in 1988 was the first legislative act legally establishing a separate scope of practice and title protection for nurse practitioners (NPs). Ever since New York's NP amendment, there has been confusion regarding which of the advanced nursing practice categories are included within the scope of practice, particularly CNSs, CNLs, CNMs, and CRNAs. This confusion, especially in psychiatric mental health nursing and nurse anesthesia, is related to the legal interpretations of the NP amendment. The resultant debate about this issue has led to a clearer definition and understanding of the term *advanced practice registered nurse*, which was finally defined by the APRN Consensus Model and is now accepted by 39 state boards of nursing.[10]

The Nurse Practitioner

The NP levels of nursing are most widely accepted as advanced practice areas for nursing. These include the PNP (acute or primary care), the FNP, the neonatal nurse practitioner (NNP), the GNP (acute or primary care), WHNP, and the psychiatric mental health nurse practitioner (PMHNP).

Although CRNAs and CNMs do not carry the nurse practitioner title, they are the oldest of the advanced practice specialties for nurses and have been well accepted in the medical community for many years. The other advanced practice nurses experience varying levels of acceptance from physicians. However, the COVID-19 pandemic highlighted the glaring need for nurses with higher education and advanced practice skills in providing the care that saved lives. Many physicians who were working side by side in intensive care units (ICUs) and emergency departments (EDs) across the country with APRNs saw firsthand their high levels of skills, knowledge, and caring.[1] Moreover, the public in general likes the care they receive from advanced practice nurses. All states now have granted some type of **prescriptive authority** to NPs. Currently, most NP programs are offered in major universities, requiring students to complete the master's degree before allowing them to take the certification examination.[20]

The Clinical Nurse Specialist

Another level of nursing that falls under the umbrella of advanced practice is the **nurse specialist**, or **clinical nurse specialist** (CNS). The CNS provides care in a specialty area that is identified by the type of patient population requiring care, the level of care the patient needs, the clinical setting, and the type of disease process. These specialists focus on one primary discipline, which includes but is not limited to teaching, mentoring, and advising less prepared nurses; diagnosing patient health problems; developing facility or departmental policies and procedures; ordering and analyzing tests for patients; and assessing patient outcomes for quality levels.[21]

Education for the CNS student includes attaining graduate-level nursing education (MSN or DPN) and completing additional general training to prepare them to practice independently. This includes finishing an additional 500 hours of supervised clinical with the population with which they want to work. After completion of the educational requirement, the student can apply for various CNS certifications, such as adult health, pediatric health, and others, through organizations such as the American Nurse Credentialing Center (ANCC) and the AACN.[21]

The Clinical Nurse Leader

Although the clinical nurse leader (CNL) role has been around since 2015, it is still in a state of development as a role that APRNs can assume. The clinical nurse leader gathers data, assesses treatment actions, and uses the information to improve care outcomes. In conjunction with multidisciplinary teams composed of physicians, pharmacists, social workers, CNSs, case managers, and NPs, the CNL's mission is to identify ways to improve the quality of patient care. Rather than focusing on management or administrative responsibilities, they focus totally on patient care. Goals of the CNL include shortening the length of patient stays, lowering admission and readmission rates, reducing health-care-related errors such as falls and medication errors, and introducing cost-saving measures that do not decrease the quality of care.

Education for the CNL is similar to that for the CNS. A nurse wishing to become a CNL must initially earn an MSN degree from an accredited program. This level of education is required for the CNLs because they must be able use their high levels of clinical skills at the point of care and use their knowledge base to serve as a resource for the rest of the patient-care team. Few programs offer a master of science CNL program, and those that do require advanced courses in pathophysiology, clinical assessment, and pharmacology. After completion of the program, the nurse may obtain the CNL certification from the Commission on Nurse Certification.[22]

> *This level of education is required for CNLs because they must be able use their high levels of clinical skills at the point of care and use their knowledge base to serve as a resource for the rest of the patient-care team.*

The Scope of Advanced Practice

Although all three roles—the NP, the CNS, and the CNL—are advanced practice nurses, CNSs differ from NPs and CNLs in their respective scopes of practice. Nurse specialists usually focus their efforts on research, patient and nurse education, and consulting with management. NPs generally provide primary patient care, and CNLs more often work in conjunction with a multidisciplinary team to improve care outcomes by encouraging the use of evidence-based changes.

The future career opportunities for APRNs are numerous and bright, according to the major nursing organizations and the government's Bureau of Health Care Occupations.[20,12] Many NPs work for county health departments, for rural clinics, and on Native American reservations; others work in hospitals, with physicians in private practice, and in rehabilitation centers. Some have even established their own independent clinics. APRNs often provide primary health-care services in areas where there is a lack of primary care physicians. Although many of these areas are traditionally rural, inner-city areas also often need this type of health care. With the passage of the ACA in 2010, the opportunity for APRNs grew and is likely to grow again now that the Biden administration is reinvesting in primary health care. Health-care reform often requires that a patient seeking entry into the health-care system be evaluated by a primary health-care practitioner before referral to a specialized practitioner. Although the family practice physician, or general practitioner, is the still the most common primary health-care provider to evaluate the patient, NPs also function in this role, sometimes at a higher level of skill.[12]

DNP for the APRN?

As the number of nursing schools granting the APRN increased and the number of APRNs grew, nursing leaders began to question whether all these NPs were prepared to meet the complexities of today's health-care system. Nursing leaders noticed that, unlike dentists, physical therapists, or pharmacists, APRNs had no terminal degree. A *terminal degree* is a degree for which no higher level of education is available. It is important to remember that the DNP is a *degree*, and not a practice role, like the NP title. Generally, a particular degree is needed to fulfill requirements of a particular role; for example, the BSN is needed to fulfill the role of the RN, or an MSN is needed to fulfill the role of educator in a nursing program. Because of the high level of skills and

knowledge required for APRNs, many of whom can practice independently, it would seem logical that a terminal degree focusing on practice expertise should be required for entry into the APRN level.[20]

Is the Master's Enough?

Out of the doctoral degrees discussed in this chapter, the DNP seems best suited to meet the requirements of a terminal practice doctoral degree. As a result, the AACN decided in 2004 that all advanced practice nursing master's degrees should transition to the DNP by the year 2015.[223] Although this goal has not yet been reached, there has been an explosion of DNP programs across the country, and the number of nurses with DPN degrees has increased tremendously. Currently, practicing APRNs would not be affected, except to be exempted into the new status. More than 50 other nursing organizations and societies have endorsed the proposal. However, questions linger.[23]

> ❝ *Most college and university administrators do not understand the difference between a PhD and a DNP. To them, a doctoral degree is a doctoral degree is a doctoral degree.* ❞

Does It Make Sense?

Those who favor the transition to the DNP point out that practitioners need the highest levels of education to care for patients in today's complex and demanding health-care system. Requiring the DNP is the only way to guarantee safe, high-quality care. Granting accreditation to all APRNs at the DNP level would provide better consistency in both the educational requirements and the titling of what is now a confusing array of programs and certifications. Those in favor also argue that current master's APRN programs have added so much practice and theoretical content in an attempt to keep current with the practice setting that they are almost at the doctoral level anyway.[22] Almost all professional practice specialty areas, except for nursing, now require a terminal degree. The DNP would seem the logical degree to demonstrate the high skill levels, knowledge, and expertise for nurses.

Those who do not support the DNP degree ask, How does the degree improve the practice of the APRN? and Doesn't adding another degree only make it more confusing for the public? Although no research has been conducted so far, it would be interesting to ask currently practicing APRNs if they believe they are practicing at the top levels of skills and knowledge and if an additional degree will make them "better." An additional degree does not necessarily make a higher-quality APRN. Many nurses now have a DNP but are not practicing APRNs.[23]

Then there is the question of cost. It is obvious that adding additional courses to an APRN program so that the nurse can attain the DNP would also increase the cost; however, when the two programs are folded in together, the added cost is not really apparent. Also, if a program converts an MSN to a DNP and offers only the DNP, the additional cost may again be hidden.[23]

The Long-Term Effect

The bigger objection to the DNP degree is its long-term effect on nursing education. The PhD has been the gold standard for nursing education since the beginning of college-level nursing baccalaureate degrees. Deans and chairpersons of nursing programs had to hold a PhD to earn accreditation from a national organization. Currently, at many schools, nurses holding the DNP degree are being appointed to dean and chairperson positions. Also, nurses with the DNP are now being considered as faculty with a terminal educational degree. The intent is not to imply that any particular individual is unqualified for their job. However, because the DNP is advertised as a "practice" degree and not an educational degree, the DNP programs are not providing the content required for teaching or administering nursing programs. Most non-nursing college and university administrators do not understand the difference between a PhD and a DNP. To them, a doctoral degree is a doctoral degree is a doctoral degree. They do recognize how difficult it is to find nurses with any type of post-master's degree, so finding a nurse with any kind of doctorate is like finding hidden treasure.[23]

Some feel that the long-term impact on nursing education could be disastrous. In the short term, the negative effects are muted because all programs still have a mix of PhD and master's in nursing education faculty along with DNP faculty. However, as time goes on and the current aging PhD population is replaced by DNP deans and faculty, the expertise and knowledge in areas such as curriculum development, evaluation, and teaching methodologies will be lost. Also, because much of the research currently used as the basis for EBP is conducted by PhD-prepared nurses, over time the profession will lose the ability to

maintain its body of knowledge at a rate and quality that matches the growth in technology and in medical and nursing knowledge.[23]

There is also the question of titling in the clinical setting. In a physician-centric health-care system such as exists in the United States, physicians in general, particularly those with MD after their names, would prefer that they be the only ones addressed as "doctor" when in clinical areas. However, the word *doctor* is a title that comes from a Latin word that means "teacher" and refers to someone who has earned a doctorate degree from a university, including but not limited to the MD degree. Professors with a PhD have been called doctor since the 13th century in England, long before those in the medical community began using the title.[24] There have been many attempts over the years by the various medical associations around the country to limit the use of the title doctor to MDs, DOs, medical students, residents, dentists, optometrists, and veterinarians. As recently as April 2022, a bill was sponsored by the Oklahoma Medical Association to strictly limit the use of the title of doctor to MDs only. Through the efforts of the Oklahoma Nurses Association and others, the bill was defeated. A similar bill was also put before the Florida legislature that would prohibit the use of the title doctor by advanced practice nurses with DNPs or PhDs. This bill was also defeated.[25] However, when nurses with advanced degrees are addressed as "doctor" in the clinical setting by nursing students or other nurses, it does cause some confusion among patients. The confusion is usually quickly remedied with a brief explanation; however, the discussion will continue.[24]

The changeover to the DNP seems to be a certainty. It is extremely important for students who are thinking about obtaining advanced nursing degrees to consider the direction of their professional future. If they are truly interested in clinical practice as a lifelong career of primarily patient care, the DNP is the degree to obtain. However, if they are even considering a career in education at some point in the future, the MSN in nursing education and the PhD are the way to go.[23]

INTERPROFESSIONAL EDUCATION

Interprofessional education is defined as "two or more students from different professions learning about, from and with each other to enable effective collaboration and improve health outcomes."[26] It also goes by other names, such as *transprofessional* and *interdisciplinary education*. Although interprofessional education has been an incidental part of nursing education for many years, it was first formally recognized as an element in health-care education in 1972 at the first IOM conference. There, more than 120 leaders in many areas of health care—such as nursing, nutrition, physical therapy, pharmacy, dentistry, and medicine—recognized the necessity of learning centers to conduct interdisciplinary learning to improve the real-world outcomes for the well-being of patients.

More recently, along with the recognition that medication errors were a leading cause of injury and death for hospitalized patients, The Joint Commission (TJC or JC) also noted that the poor communication and lack of teamwork among health-care professionals were major contributors to the increased number of medication and other errors in the hospital setting. They surmised that increasing the communication skills between health-care professionals and promoting a spirit of teamwork would decrease errors and improve the quality of care.[27]

In 2011, in response to JC findings, the AACN assembled a blue-ribbon panel (Interprofessional Education Collaborative Expert Panel [IECEP]) to study how nursing, in conjunction with other health-care disciplines, could integrate teaching and learning to improve health-care outcomes. Their findings noted four key competencies related to interprofessional education efforts:

1. Values and ethics for interprofessional practice
2. Roles and responsibilities
3. Interprofessional communication
4. Teams and teamwork

They recommended that these competencies be emphasized throughout nursing and other professional health-care curriculums.[28]

The Medical Home

Passage of the ACA in 2010 further stimulated interest in interprofessional education. One of the new concepts to approach health care from this perspective is the patient-centered medical home (PCMH) approach. The PCMH focuses its interdisciplinary efforts on producing better outcomes for chronically ill and high-risk patients in the primary care arena. It takes the emphasis placed on primary care in the ACA and expands it to all areas of health care. The key components of the PCMH model include

- Expanded accountability for the management of chronic disease.
- Joint efforts by acute and public health-care professionals to address prevention issues.
- Making the maintenance of healthy environments the responsibility of health-care professionals in all settings.

Although part of the emphasis in nursing care since the time of Nightingale, the PCMH includes a community component along with the individual patient. In the PCMH, nurses coordinate care for patients and their families with cooperation from other health-care professionals in both urban and rural settings.[29] The future of the PCMH model of care looks bright now that ACA is back on track for additional funding under the Biden administration.

New Models of Interprofessional Nursing Education

Over the past several years, new models for nursing education have been developed that are built around interdisciplinary education. Three models in particular use a framework in which interprofessional interaction is a key component.

The D'Amour and Oandasan model combines four key components: (1) health professional education, (2) interprofessional collaborative practice, (3) patient needs, and (4) community-oriented care.[30] This model is linear in design and links the four concepts in much the same way as the systems model.

The World Health Organization (WHO) developed a *Framework for Action on Interprofessional Education and Collaborative Practice* that focuses on curriculum and the education process but also includes institutional support, the culture of the workplace, and the many environmental elements that affect collaborative practice.[34] Some of the key factors in this model that drive interprofessional practice include

- Meeting local health needs.
- Consolidating fragmented health-care practices.
- Addressing present and future health-care needs.
- Eliminating shortages in the health-care workforce.

- Encouraging collaborative practice.
- Working toward an improved health-care system.

The model's goal is to produce a well-integrated health-care workforce that will improve the overall quality of health care.[31] The WHO model is not designed as a framework for a nursing curriculum but rather can be included as one element in a more detailed design.

Again, in response to the push from the ACA for a more comprehensive view of health-care needs, the Commission on Education of Health Care Professionals in the 21st Century developed a model that focuses on social accountability and social equality. They noted that current health-care education is fragmented and does not really respond to the needs of all populations. Similar to the other two models, this model sees the need for integration of public health into the overall picture of health care. The model satisfies many needs in both the education and the health-care systems. These include patient and population needs, patient and population demands, the actual provision of health care, labor market pressure for health-care workers, and the actual supply of health-care workers. This model considers the current education system for health professionals a "silo," where the members interact only with themselves. Interprofessional or transprofessional education will teach professionals to be collaborative and effective members of teams that are nonhierarchical, thus promoting better patient care.[32]

> *In response to the push from the ACA for a more comprehensive view of health-care needs, the Commission on Education of Health Care Professionals in the 21st Century developed a model that focuses on social accountability and social equality.*

Research Shortage

Only a few studies have been conducted that demonstrate the positive effects of interprofessional education for nurses and provide a limited EBP base. These studies are often hard to conduct, demonstrating the difficulty in implementing interprofessional education as a standard feature of health-care curricula.

Many of the studies focus on only one or two IECEP competencies at a time, which leads to an incomplete picture of interprofessional education's effectiveness. However, the results have been encouraging, particularly in the areas of teamwork and communication. Students involved in interprofessional research projects showed an increased awareness of patient safety, particularly when they were caring for several patients with complex problems. In working with medical students, nursing students gained knowledge about when the physician should be notified, and conversely, medical students gained a clearer understanding of the need for more precise communication. Overall, communication became more effective with the members of the interdisciplinary team.[33]

More studies are needed to develop a solid foundation of real-world evidence-based knowledge that supports the extensive changes required to fully integrate interprofessional learning into the nursing curriculum. The benefits include decreasing errors in care, improving the quality of care, and increasing the satisfaction of **health-care practitioners**.

Conclusion

In today's rapidly changing health-care environment, there is an ever-increasing need for health-care professionals who are educated to practice at the highest levels.[1] It is imperative that the schools educating future nurses be responsive to the changes, challenges, and demands of an increasingly sophisticated and technologically advanced health-care system. Nursing education is an important part of a much larger network of health-care systems, including the service and practice sector, government and regulatory agencies, and licensing and credentialing institutions. All of these interact with each other and together form the health-care system.

The nursing profession has, over the years, developed many different types of education programs in an attempt to meet the demands of a growing health-care system. Some of the programs developed for

Issues Now

BS Degree = Lower Death Rates

Nurse educators have been insisting for many years that patient outcomes will be better when more nurses have baccalaureate degrees. However, health-care policymakers and hospital administrators have not fully bought into the concept, as evidenced by their hiring practices. Part of the problem lies in the lack of empirical evidence that supports the supposition.

Over the past decade, only a few studies were conducted that demonstrated improved patient outcomes when the nurses caring for patients were educated at the baccalaureate level. Some studies even showed no significant improvements. However, a study conducted between 1999 and 2006 in 134 hospitals across Pennsylvania examined discharge data from postoperative patients and demonstrated that the BS degree does make a difference.

Conducted under the auspices of the Pennsylvania School of Nursing's Center for Health Outcomes and Policy Research, the researchers found that hospitals that increased the number of nurses with baccalaureate degrees by 10 percent or more had reductions in the death rates of postoperative patients by 2.12 for every 1,000 undergoing surgery. In addition, there was a reduction of 7.47 deaths for every 1,000 patients who experienced either operative or postoperative complications. Although the study demonstrated a strong correlation between the increased number of baccalaureate RNs and the reduced death rates, it did not claim causality. A national study in 2010 reached the same conclusion that when more BS-prepared RNs were present to provide care, better outcomes were achieved and fewer medical errors occurred.

The research design eliminated the effect of other variables such as staffing levels, nurses' years of experience, and variations in staff skill levels in affecting the outcome data. The research findings indicate that the reductions in death rates may be due to better assessment and monitoring of postoperative patients by BS-prepared nurses. They were able to detect subtle changes in patients' conditions that were the first indicators of a deteriorating condition and then quickly initiate actions to reverse the decline.

This type of research is in line with the IOM's call for higher education levels for RNs. The research project was funded by grants from the Agency for Healthcare Research and Quality, the National Institutes of Health's National Institute of Nursing Research, and the Robert Wood Johnson Foundation.

Sources: *BSN by 2020: Where are we now?* University of New Mexico, 2020, https://hsc.unm.edu/nursing/programs/bsn/rn-bsn/; A. Androus, *Do BSN-educated nurses provide better patient care?* Registered Nursing.org, 2022. https://www.registerednursing.org/articles/do-bsn-educated-nurses-provide-better-patient-care/

specific needs that no longer exist should be examined for their usefulness and viability in today's advanced health-care atmosphere. Perhaps their resources could be rechanneled to programs that are more in tune with current needs. Students should carefully evaluate programs they might enter and decide which one best meets their career goals.

Meanwhile, nursing education continues to develop innovative approaches to help nurses meet the demands for more education, more technical skills, and more leadership ability. The ladder programs are a good example. By recognizing the dynamic state of nursing education and implementing changes that respond to or even anticipate changes in the health-care system, the nursing profession will continue as one of the pillars of the health-care system.

Educators in nursing have begun to recognize that it is impossible to teach nursing students everything they need to know in the short time allowed for formal education. The demands of the changing health-care system will make that goal even more difficult. However, it may not be necessary to teach nursing students everything. It is more important to teach these students the thinking, decision-making, and management skills that will allow them to adjust to an ever-changing and developing health-care system.

CRITICAL-THINKING EXERCISES

• Discuss why the current educational system for nurses leads to confusion over the role and scope of practice for nurses.
• The literature reports that there will be a nursing shortage well into the 21st century. What aspects of health-care reform are likely to produce changes in nursing education? Identify possible changes that may occur in nursing education because of the projected nursing shortage. Will these changes be beneficial or harmful to the profession of nursing?
• Are nurses holding the DNP degree better practitioners than those with an MSN? Defend your position.

NCLEX-STYLE QUESTIONS

1. Which Institute of Medicine (IOM) competency is demonstrated by the nurse and the respiratory therapist coordinating care of a patient hospitalized with an exacerbation of COPD?
   1. Patient-centered care
   2. Interdisciplinary teamwork
   3. Evidence-based practice
   4. Quality improvement
2. Which statement BEST describes the relationship between the IOM competencies and the QSEN competencies?
   1. The IOM competencies are based on a medical model; the QSEN competencies are based on a nursing model.
   2. Only the IOM competencies address safety; the QSEN competencies do not.
   3. Only the IOM competencies are included in up-to-date nursing textbooks.
   4. The IOM competencies were used to create the QSEN competencies to guide the development of nursing curricula.
3. Alonzo wants to become an RN and is trying to decide between an ADN program and a BSN program. Which of the following is an advantage of the ADN? **Select all that apply**.
   1. Lower schooling costs
   2. Earlier entry into the workforce
   3. An easier form of the NCLEX-RN
   4. Just as much prestige as a BSN
   5. An emphasis on skills training
4. Ashley, an ADN, wants to pursue a degree that will allow her to provide advanced nursing care to the patients in the nursing home where she works. Given Ashley's interest and training, which of the following is her BEST option?
   1. MSN nurse practitioner
   2. PhD
   3. EdD
   4. DNP
5. The _____ program prepares doctoral students to conduct the research that supports evidence-based nursing practice.
6. What are the effects of having multiple paths to entering the nursing profession? **Select all that apply**.
   1. More options are available to students.
   2. More respect exists between nursing colleagues.
   3. Multiple paths cause confusion among the public.
   4. The NCLEX-RN becomes an equalizer.
   5. Multiple paths cause confusion among nurses.
7. Carla tells her supervisor that she wants to become an advanced practice nurse. Which statement of Carla's indicates a need for more information?
   1. "When I am certified, I will be able to write some prescriptions."
   2. "When I finish my MSN, I will be an advanced practice nurse."
   3. "When I am advanced practice nurse, I will continue to care for patients."
   4. "Training as an advanced practice nurse is specialized."

8. What main concern do nursing educators have about the DNP degree?
   1. The DNP program is not as rigorous as the PhD program.
   2. The DNP program will divert students from MSN programs.
   3. The DNP program is a practice degree, not a teaching or administration degree.
   4. The DNP program will cost significantly more than a PhD program.
9. Which factor was primarily responsible for the shift away from diploma schools of nursing?
   1. The cost to hospitals of running diploma schools became too high.
   2. Nurses trained in diploma schools were not as proficient as others.
   3. Women were no longer limited in the types of professions they could choose.
   4. Accreditation standards were developed that diploma schools could not or would not meet.
10. What factor motivated the inclusion of interdisciplinary teamwork as an IOM competency?
    1. Poor communication and lack of teamwork led to burnout and high staff turnover.
    2. Poor communication and lack of teamwork among health-care workers contributed to errors.
    3. Good communication and teamwork improve job satisfaction among health-care workers.
    4. Good communication and teamwork improve patient-satisfaction scores.

References

1. Pearce K. COVID-19 ushers in decades of change for nursing profession. Johns Hopkins University, 2020. https://hub.jhu.edu/2020/10/19/nursing-changes-covid-19
2. U.S. Bureau of Labor Statistics. s.v. Registered nurses. *Occupational Outlook Handbook*, September 8, 2022. https://www.bls.gov/ooh/healthcare/registered-nurses.htm
3. Rodriguez-Garcia, Carmels M, et al. Original research: How magnet hosptial status affects nurses, patients, administration and organizations: A systematic review. *AJN* 120(7): 28–38, July 2020. https://journals.lww.com/ajnonline/fulltext/2020/07000/original_research__how_magnet_hospital_status.31.aspx
4. Cunningham R. New PEW report stirs dialogue on future nursing workforce needs. *Medical Health*, 52(17):1–4, 1998.
5. Stringer H. IOM Future of Nursing report card: Progress after 10 years. Nurse.com, July 1, 2019. https://www.nurse.com/blog/2019/07/01/iom-future-of-nursing-report-card-progress-after-10-years
6. The American Association of Colleges of Nursing (AACN). Fact sheet: Nursing shortage. American Association of Colleges of Nursing, October 2022. https://www.aacnnursing.org/News-Information/Fact-Sheets/Nursing-Shortage
7. Campaign for Action. Number of people receiving nursing doctoral degrees annually. *The Future of Nursing 2030 Draft Action Plan Campaign for Action*, September 15, 2021. https://campaignforaction.org/resource/number-people-receiving-nursing-doctoral-degrees-annually/
8. Kelly Vana P, Vottero B, Altmiller G. *Quality and Safety Education for Nurses: Core Competencies for Nursing Leadership and Care Management* (3rd ed.). New York, NY: Springer, 2023
9. The essentials: Core competencies for professional nursing education. AACN, 2021. https://www.aacnnursing.org/Portals/42/AcademicNursing/pdf/Essentials-2021.pdf
10. Wyatt L. *A History of Nursing*. Glouestershire UK: Amberly Publishing, 2019.
11. History of nursing accreditation. Accreditation Commission for Nursing Education, 2021. https://www.acenursing.org/about/acen-history-of-accreditation/
12. Flaubert J, Menestrel S, Williams D, Wakefield M (Eds.). *The Future of Nursing 2020–2030, Charting a Path to Achieve Health Equity*. Washington, DC: National Academies Press, 2021.
13. The future of the associate degree in nursing program. NursingLicensure.org, 2022. https://www.nursinglicensure.org/articles/adn-program-future/
14. Associate degree in nursing (ADN). Nursing Explorer, 2021. https://www.nursingexplorer.com/adn
15. BSN programs. Nursing Explorer, 2021. https://www.nursingexplorer.com/bsn
16. Highlights from AACN's 2021 annual survey. American Association of Colleges of Nursing, 2021. https://www.aacnnursing.org/Portals/42/Data/Survey-Data-Highlights-2021.pdf
17. ADN to MSN bridge programs. MSN Degree, 2022. https://www.msndegree.org/msn-degree-programs/adn-to-msn-degree-programs/
18. Abalihi O. Effect of multiple entry levels into nursing practice and professionalism. [Doctoral dissertation, Walden University], 2019. https://scholarworks.waldenu.edu/cgi/viewcontent.cgi?article=9053&context=dissertations
19. DNP and PhD programs. Nursing Explorer, 2021. https://www.nursingexplorer.com/doctoral
20. Advanced practice registered nurse (APRN). American Nurses Association, 2022. https://www.nursingworld.org/practice-policy/workforce/what-is-nursing/aprn/
21. Clinical nurse specialist. Top Nursing, 2022. https://www.topnursing.org/career/clinical-nurse-specialist/
22. Clinical nurse leader. Top Nursing, 2022. https://www.topnursing.org/career/clinical-nurse-specialist/

23. What is a DPN and is it worth it? Nursing.org, 2022. https://nurse.org/articles/how-to-get-a-dnp-is-it-worth-it/

24. The use of the title "dr." Texas Nurse Practitioner, July 20, 2020. https://www.texasnp.org/news/517996/The-Use-of-the-Title-Dr-.htm

25. Briggs E. Legislative update: "The Doctor Title bill" by any other name. . . . Florida Coalition of Advanced Practice Nurses, November 22, 2019. https://aprnadvocacy.com/legislative-update-the-doctor-title-bill-by-any-other-name/

26. What is interprofessional collaboration in health care? CliniConx, March 31, 2022. https://cliniconex.com/blog/interprofessional-collaboration-in-healthcare/

27. Young G. Implementing competency-based interprofessional education in historically black colleges and universities. *Journal for Nurse Practitioners*, 18(8):886–888, 2022. https://doi.org/10.1016/j.nurpra.2022.03.001

28. National patient safety goals. The Joint Commission, n.d. https://www.jointcommission.org/standards_information/npsgs.aspx

29. Lyon M, Ches A, Rossier M, Rosenbaum S. *The Affordable Care Act, Medical Homes, and Childhood Asthma: A Key Opportunity for Progress*. George Washington University School of Public and Health Services, 2022. https://publichealth.gwu.edu/departments/healthpolicy/DHP_Publications/pub_uploads/dhpPublication_67550887-5056-9D20-3DD02730276FFC88.pdf

30. Metersky K, Schwidn J. Interprofessional care: Patient experience stories. *International Journal of Person Centered Medicine*, 5(2), 2015. https://doi.org/10.5750/ijpcm.v5i2.528

31. De Marchis E, Doekhie K, Willard-Grace R, Olayiwola J. The impact of the patient-centered medical home on health care disparities: Exploring stakeholder perspectives on current standards and future directions. Pubmed, 2019. https://pubmed.ncbi.nlm.nih.gov/29920148/

32. Home care regulatory resources. National Association for Home Care and Hospice, 2022. https://www.nahc.org/resources-services/regulatory-operational-resources/home-care-regulatory-issues/

33. Provine A, Davidson H, Waynick-Rogers P, Cole S, Rosentiel D, Lofton R, Hilmes MA. Quality improvement projects conducted by interprofessional teams of learners: Implementation and impact. *Journal of Interprofessional Care*, 2022. https://doi.org/10.1080/13561820.2022.2060195

The Evolution of Licensure, Certification, and Nursing Organizations

5

Joseph T. Catalano

Learning Objectives

After completing this chapter, the reader will be able to:

- Identify the purposes and needs for nurse licensure
- Distinguish between permissive and mandatory licensure
- Explain why institutional licensure is unacceptable in today's health-care system
- Evaluate the importance of nurse practice acts
- Analyze the significance of professional certification
- Identify the key elements of the licensure, accreditation, certification, and education (LACE) model
- Discuss the long-term effects of the consensus model for APRN regulation

MEETING EXPECTATIONS

Almost from the inception of nursing, societal needs and expectations have been the driving forces behind the establishment of the standards that guide the profession. In the early days of nursing, when health care was relatively primitive and society's expectations of nurses were low, there was little demand for regulations or controls over and within the profession. However, as technology and health care have advanced and become more complex, there has been a corresponding increase in societal expectations for nurses. All nurses now accept **licensure** and **certification** examinations as a given in today's health-care system. Where did these examinations come from, and what do they mean to the profession? This chapter explores the answers to these questions.

Rather than looking on the evolving health-care system, growing information technologies, redesigned health-care organizations, and increasing **health-care consumer** demands with fear and trepidation, nurses should consider this an exciting time of growth and opportunity. In today's health-care system, nurses have an almost unlimited number of ways to provide new and creative nursing care for clients in all settings. For example, the COVID-19 pandemic brought a number of regulatory restrictions to the forefront, particularly scope-of-practice rules for advanced practice nurses and the way they perform their roles. The pandemic became a transformational time for the profession of nursing, rearranging many aspects of the health-care system. Because nurses comprise some 80 percent of all health-care professionals, their skills and knowledge were recognized as never before.[1]

The pandemic caused society's needs and expectations to change, and as a result, regulations and **standards** of nursing practice also changed, redefining how nurses practice. Through their professional nursing organizations, nurses can help shape health-care regulations that establish the most freedom to provide effective care while maintaining the goal of protecting the public. It is likely that, in the future, state boards of nursing will look very different, just as the profession of nursing will differ from that of its past.

THE DEVELOPMENT OF NURSE PRACTICE ACTS

A nurse practice **act** is state legislation regulating the practice of nurses that protects the public, defines the scope of practice, and makes nurses accountable for their actions. **Nurse practice acts** establish state boards of nursing (SBNs) and define specific SBN powers regarding the practice of nursing within the state. Rules and regulations written by the SBN become **statutory laws** under the powers delegated by the state **legislature**.

Regulatory Powers

Although nurse practice acts differ from one state to another, the SBNs have many powers in common. These are considered regulatory powers because they provide the SBN with control over nurses according to rule, principle, or law. By legislative act, all SBNs have the power to grant licenses, approve nursing programs, establish standards for nursing schools, and write specific regulations for nurses and nursing practice in general in that state.

Of particular importance is the SBNs' power to take disciplinary actions such as to deny or revoke nurse licenses (Box 5.1).[2]

Additional functions of SBNs include

- Defining nursing and the scope of practice.
- Ruling on who can use the titles of registered nurse (RN) and licensed practical nurse/licensed vocational nurse (LPN/LVN).
- Setting up an application procedure for licensure in the state.
- Determining fees for licensure.
- Establishing requirements for renewal of licensure.
- Determining responsibility for any regulations governing expanded practice for nurses in that particular state.

The Need for Licensure

Imagine what the quality of health care would be if anyone could walk into a hospital, claim to know how to care for clients, and be given a job as a nurse. This situation might sound impossible in today's health-care system, but in the past, it was the norm rather than the exception.

Throughout the last half of the 19th century and the first half of the 20th century, rapid growth in

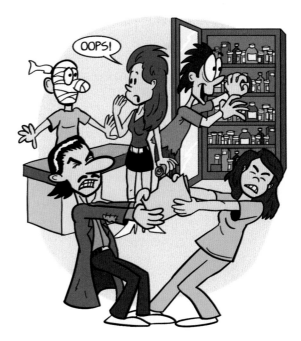

Without licensure, health care would be chaos!

health-care technology moved the primary source of health care out of the home and into hospitals. However, individuals who were qualified to provide hospital-level care were in short supply. There were wide variations both in the abilities of those who claimed to be nurses and in the quality of the care they provided. Paradoxically, nursing leaders who had always advocated some type of **credentialing** for nurses to ensure competency found that their attempts to initiate registration or licensure met with strong opposition from physician groups, hospital administrators, and practicing nurses themselves.

Early Attempts at Licensure

The idea of registering nurses had been in existence for a long time, starting with Florence Nightingale, who was the first to establish a formal list, or register, for graduates of her nursing school. In the United States and Canada, there was widespread recognition of the need for some type of credentialing of nurses as far back as the mid-1800s. The first organized attempt to establish a credentialing system was initiated in 1896 by the Nurses Associated Alumnae of the United States and Canada (later to become the American Nurses

Box 5.1 **Reasons the State Boards of Nursing May Revoke a Nursing License**
• Conviction for a serious crime • Demonstration of gross negligence or unethical conduct in the practice of nursing • Failure to renew a nursing license while continuing to practice nursing • Use of illegal drugs or alcohol during the provision of care for clients or use that carries over and affects clients' care • Willful violation of the state's nurse practice act

Box 5.2 **Key Points in the New York State Licensure Bill (1904)**
• Established minimum educational standards • Established the minimum length of basic nursing programs at 2 years • Required all nursing schools to be registered with the state board of regents (who oversee all higher education) • Established a state board of nursing (SBN) with five nurses as members • Formulated rules for the examination of nurses • Formulated regulations for nurses that, if violated, could lead to the revocation of licensure

Source: L.D. Dietz, *History and Modern Nursing*, Philadelphia, PA: FA Davis, 1963.

Association [ANA]). As with other early attempts at licensure, it was met with resistance and eventually failed.[3]

Several early American nursing leaders, including Lillian Wald and Annie Goodrich, recognized the inconsistent quality of nursing care and the need for licensure to protect the public. In 1901, after an extensive and lengthy campaign to educate the public, physicians, hospital administrators, and nurses themselves about the need for licensure, the International Council of Nurses passed a resolution that required each state to establish a licensure and examination procedure for nurses. It took 3 more years before the state of New York, through the New York Nurses Association, developed a licensure bill that passed the legislature (Box 5.2). Other states that followed New York's lead were North Carolina, New Jersey, and Virginia. Although these states had bills that were weaker than New York's nurse practice act, passage of such legislation was considered a major accomplishment for several reasons[3] Women did not even have the right to vote in general elections at the time these bills were passed. In addition, few licensure requirements and regulations of any type existed during this period in the United States, even for the medical profession.

The Importance of Licensure Examinations

The thought of having to take an examination that determines whether or not one can practice nursing can make even the best student anxious. Adding to the tension is that the examination is given outside of the academic setting, by computer, and is created by individuals other than the students' teachers. (See Chapter 28 for a detailed discussion of NCLEX-RN, CAT, now called the Next Generation NCLEX-RN [NGN-RN].)

A Measure of Competency

However, some type of objective method is necessary to prove that the individual is qualified to practice nursing safely; otherwise, the public is not protected from unqualified practitioners. Early attempts at creating **licensure examinations** for nurses were met with strong resistance. Although all states had some form of licensure examination by 1923, the format and length of the examinations varied widely. Some states required both written and practical examinations to demonstrate safety of practice; others added an oral examination.

Although licensure was and is a state-controlled activity, the major nursing organizations in the United States eventually realized that, to achieve consistency of quality across the country, all nurses needed to pass a uniform examination. The ANA Council of State Boards of Nursing was organized in 1945 to oversee development of a uniform examination for nurses that could be used by all SBNs.

The NGN-RN

The National League for Nursing Testing Division developed a test that was implemented in 1950. Originally, the test was simply called the State Board

Examination, but it was renamed the National Council Licensure Examination (NCLEX) in 1987. In 1994, the computerized version of the examination was implemented—the National Council Licensure Examination Computerized Adaptive Testing for Registered Nurses (NCLEX-RN, CAT). In 2023, the format of the questions and type of knowledge assessed was changed, and the name of the examination became the Next Generation NCLEX-RN or NextGen NCLEX-RN or NGN-RN. Currently, because everyone knows the examination is computerized, *CAT* is no longer used in reference to the test.[4]

The Enhanced Nurse Licensure Compact

Licensure for nurses has undergone a recent major change. The mutual recognition model for nursing licensure was a regional agreement among some states, which allowed RNs licensed in one state to practice nursing in other states that belonged to the agreement. These local agreements have been replaced by the Enhanced Nurse Licensure Compact (eNLC). On July 20, 2017, the 26th state joined, meeting the requirement for the eNLC enactment to be signed into law. The Interstate Commission of Nurse Licensure Compact Administrators (ICNLCA), the governing body of the eNLC, implemented the eNLC on January 19, 2018. The eNLC compact has been enacted or has pending legislation in 24 of the original NLC states. Eight more states have legislation waiting for approval prior to becoming members of the eNLC. Two more states and the Virgin Islands have ratified the eNLC and are awaiting enactment. As of January 11, 2023, 39 states and territories fully ratified the eNLC. Guam allowed nurses to apply for multistate license in 2022. Ohio implemented eNLC starting January 1, 2023.[5] The COVID-19 pandemic not only pushed the eNLC movement forward by allowing nurses to practice in states where there was a greater shortage; it also proved the value of nurses who could travel unimpeded by SBN rules to other states.[1]

> ❝ *Through their professional nursing organizations, nurses can help shape health-care regulations that establish the most freedom to provide effective care while maintaining the goal of protecting the public.* ❞

What the eNLC Means for Nurses

Nurses who obtain an eNLC license are allowed to practice nursing in person or via telehealth in both their home state and other eNLC states. All applicants for a multistate license must meet the same licensing requirements, which include federal and state criminal background checks, which may be biometric. At the time of publication of this book, the member states of the eNLC include Alabama, Arizona, Arkansas, Colorado, Delaware, Florida, Georgia, Guam, Idaho, Indiana, Iowa, Kansas, Kentucky, Louisiana, Maine, Maryland, Mississippi, Missouri, Montana, Nebraska, New Hampshire, New Jersey, New Mexico, North Carolina, North Dakota, Ohio, Oklahoma, Pennsylvania, South Carolina, South Dakota, Tennessee, Texas, Virgin Islands, Utah, Vermont, Virginia, Wisconsin, West Virginia, and Wyoming. The eNLC applies only to RNs for almost all states, except Pennsylvania, which allows both RNs and LPNs to practice in that state from other eNLC states. Several more states have legislation pending that would make them members, and the ICNLCA will continue to work until all 50 states belong to the compact.[5]

REGISTRATION VERSUS LICENSURE

The terms *registration* and *licensure* are often used interchangeably, although they are not synonymous. They serve a similar purpose, but some technical differences exist.

Registration

Registration is the listing, or registering, of names on an official roster after certain preestablished criteria have been met. Before mandatory licensure by the states became the norm, the only way a health-care institution could find out whether an applicant had met the standards for the position was by calling the applicant's school to see if the person had graduated or passed an examination. The school would tell the institution whether the applicant's name appeared on the official roster or register—hence the origin of the term *registered nurse*. With the advent of state board examinations, an institution merely has to contact the SBN to find out whether the individual is registered or licensed. In many states, this process can be conducted online.

Licensure

Licensure is a legal action conducted by the state through the enforcement powers of its regulatory boards to protect the public's health, safety, and welfare by establishing professional standards. Licensure for nurses, as for other professionals who deal with the public, is necessary to ensure that everyone who claims to be a nurse can function at a minimal level of competency and safety. There are several different types of licensure.

Permissive Licensure

Permissive licensure allowed individuals to practice nursing as long as they did not use the letters *RN* after their names. Basically, permissive licensure protected only the "registered nurse" title but not the practice of nursing itself. Although most early licensure laws were permissive, all states now have mandatory licensure. Under a permissive licensure law, anyone could carry out the functions of an RN, regardless of educational level, without having to pass an examination that indicates competency.

Health-care administrators supported the concept of permissive licensure because it allowed them to employ less-educated and lower-paid employees rather than the more highly educated and better-paid RNs. However, they also recognized that the quality of care decreases when the education level of health-care providers is lower.

What Do You Think?

Should permissive licensure be reestablished because it will help reduce the cost of health care? Why? Why not?

Mandatory Licensure

Mandatory licensure requires anyone who wishes to practice nursing to pass a licensure examination and become registered by the SBN. Because different levels of nursing practice exist, different levels of licensure are necessary. At the technical level, the individual must pass the LPN/LVN examination; at the professional level, the individual must pass the RN examination.

Mandatory licensure forced SBNs to distinguish between the activities that nurses at different levels could legally perform. The scope of practice defines the boundaries for each of the levels: advanced practice registered nurse (APRN), RN, and LPN/LVN. As more levels of nursing education (e.g., the associate degree in nursing [ADN]) have been added, however, lines dividing the different scopes of practice have become blurred. In the current health-care system, it is not unusual to find LPNs/LVNs performing activities that are generally considered professional.

A particularly confusing element in today's health-care system is the use of unlicensed individuals to provide health care. The advent of certified nursing assistants (CNAs) and unlicensed assistive personnel (UAP) has led to widespread use of such individuals in all health-care settings. Although they must be supervised by an RN or LPN/LVN, these individuals are sometimes illegally assigned nursing tasks much more advanced than their levels of training. Even though permissive licensure is no longer legal, CNAs and UAP appear to fall under an unofficial type of permissive licensure.

Institutional Licensure

Although universally rejected by every major nursing organization, **institutional licensure** has become a reality for many other types of health-care workers, such as respiratory therapists and physical therapists.

Cut Corners, Cut Costs, Cut Quality of Care

Institutional licensure allows individual health-care institutions to determine which individuals are qualified to practice nursing within general guidelines established by an outside board. A back-door approach to allowing institutional licensure has been to allow **foreign graduate nurses** and nurses who are licensed in foreign countries to work in specific institutions without taking the U.S. licensure examination. They are sometimes categorized as nursing assistants or nursing technicians; however, within the clinical setting, they often perform RN-level skills. Hospital administrators realize that the quality of care is unlikely to be the same as with nurses licensed in the United States, but they believe the savings in lower wages to foreign nurses offset any decreases in quality care. Up to this point, bills that support this action have been stopped by the state nursing organizations before they could become law. Institutional licensure has been proposed periodically over the years as an alternative to governmental licensure.

During the peak years of the COVID-19 pandemic, the demand for foreign-born RNs was so extreme that it created a backlog in excess of 5,000 of qualified nurses awaiting clearance to work in the United States.[6] Before these nurses could seek a nursing work visa to enter the country, they were required to meet all the health, educational, examination, and licensure requirements of the states where they were seeking employment. A number of international nurse-recruiting agencies vetted foreign-born nurses to make sure they were properly documented. The primary impediment to getting these nurses into this country was in obtaining final visa approval. Even before the pandemic, the Trump administration had put strict limits on visa applications.[6] After international nurses were offered and then accepted jobs, they were required to attend a final interview to obtain a visa from the State Department. Many of the embassies where interviews were conducted were closed at the peak of the pandemic or had only very limited interview staff available. Although the backlog ebbed as the pandemic eased in the United States, in many of the countries from which the nurses were trying to leave, hospitalization and infection levels still remained high.

Up to 77 percent of international nurses working in the United States come primarily from three countries: the Philippines, Jamaica, and India, although substantial numbers also come from Thailand, Kenya, Ghana, and Nigeria. It is interesting to note that up to 90 percent of the international nurses employed in the United States hold a bachelor of science in nursing or similar degree while only 56 percent of the American nurses they work with have the same education level. International nurses also enter high-stress health-care settings such as intensive care units or emergency departments with more practical experience than American nurses. While many American nurses are leaving the profession because of high stress levels and long hours, international nurses are satisfied with their jobs. Rather than being employed by the hospitals they are working in, most international nurses remain in the employment of the recruiting agency that brought them to the United States. The hospitals pay the employment agency, which in turn pays the nurses. Wages of up to $200 an hour are not uncommon. After a period of time, the hospital may seek to hire the international nurse as part of their regular staff, and the nurse may seek permanent resident status.[7]

A Lack of External Control

Probably the most critical problem with institutional licensure is the lack of any external control to determine a minimal level of competency. The designations of RN and LPN/LVN would be virtually meaningless under institutional licensure. These nurses would not be under the control of a state **licensing board** and thus would not be held to the same standards of practice as nurses who were licensed by the states.

A second problem is that nurses who wished to move to a new place of employment would have to undergo whatever licensure procedure the new institution had established before being allowed to work there. Currently, nurses who move from one state to another can obtain **licensure by endorsement** by having the state recognize their nursing license from the original state of licensure. This process is generally referred to as **reciprocity**.

CERTIFICATION

At first glance, it may appear that there is not much difference between certification and licensure. Strictly defined, licensure can be considered a type of legal certification. However, in the more widely accepted use of the term, certification is a granting of credentials to indicate that an individual has achieved a level of ability higher than the minimal level of competency indicated by licensure.[3] As technology increases and the health-care environment becomes more complex and demanding, nurses are finding a need to increase their knowledge and skill levels beyond the essentials taught in their basic nursing courses.

Certification acknowledges the attainment of increased knowledge and skills and provides nurses with a means to validate their own self-worth and competence. All certification attaches an increased level of legal liability. Individuals who are certified in any area are held to a higher standard of ability congruent with their increased level of knowledge. Even CNAs have an increased level of potential liability. Some certification also carries with it a legal status, similar to licensure, but in many cases, certification merely indicates a specific professional status. The public, employers, and even nurses have difficulty understanding what certification means.

Another element that adds confusion to the understanding of the process of certification is that many groups can offer certification. These are usually professional specialty groups like the National Association of Pediatric Nurse Associates and Practitioners (NAPNAP) and the American Association of Critical-Care Nurses (AACN), but they can also be national organizations like the National League for Nursing (NLN) or the ANA.

Individual Certification

The most common type of certification is called *individual certification*. When a nurse has demonstrated attainment a certain level of ability above and beyond the basic level required for licensure in a defined area of practice, that nurse can become certified. Usually, some type of written and practical examination is required to demonstrate this advanced level of skill.

The ANA has its own certifying organization, the American Nurses Credentialing Center (ANCC), that offers widely recognized certifications in more than 40 areas. Almost all nurses with individual certification are required to maintain their skills and competencies through **continuing education** and a specified number of **continuing education units** (CEUs). Recertification may be achieved by completing CEUs or retaking the certification examination.

Organizational Certification

Organizational certification is the certification of a group or health-care institution by some external agency. It is usually referred to as **accreditation** and indicates that the institution has met standards established either by the government or by a nongovernmental agency. Often, the ability of the institution to collect money from insurance companies or the federal government depends on whether the institution is certified by a recognized agency. Most hospitals are accredited by **The Joint Commission** (formerly the Joint Commission on Accreditation of Healthcare Organizations, or JCAHO) as a minimum level of accreditation. Almost all baccalaureate and master's degree programs are accredited by one of the two national nursing accrediting organizations, and many of the associate's degree programs are also accredited. To work for any health-care facility run by the federal government (military, Indian Health Service, Veterans Administration), nurses must be graduates of accredited programs.

Advanced Practice

Some state governments may either award or recognize certification granted to nurses in areas of advanced practice. In these cases, the certification becomes a legal requirement for practice at the APRN level. Depending on the individual state's nurse practice act, nurses thus certified fall under regulations in the state's practice act that control the type of activities nurses may legally carry out when they perform advanced roles.[4]

For example, many states recognize the position of nurse **midwife** as an advanced practice role for nurses. In these states, a nurse midwife may practice those skills allowed under the nurse practice act of that state after obtaining certification. Generally, nurse midwives are allowed to conduct prenatal examinations, do prenatal teaching, and deliver babies vaginally in uncomplicated pregnancies. They usually are not allowed to perform cesarean deliveries or other procedures that are surgical in nature. If they do perform procedures outside their scope of practice, they leave themselves open to lawsuits and loss of licensure.

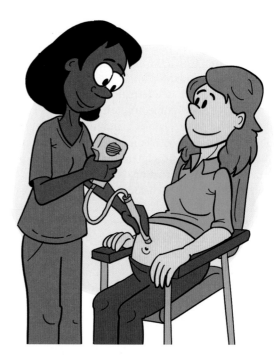

"It looks like you are having twins."

Varying Standards

In 1978, an independent certification center was proposed to establish uniform criteria and standards and to oversee all certification activities. This proposal received strong opposition from physicians and health-care administration groups for many years.

Some states recognize almost all certifications and have provisions in their nurse practice acts to help guide these practices. Other states have very little legal recognition of certification levels and thus few guidelines for practice. This confusion results from so many organizations offering certification in different areas. In some advanced practice specialties, such as nurse practitioner, two or more organizations may offer certification for the same title. The standards for qualifying for certification vary among organizations, and the method of determining certification may also be different.

A More Significant Role

The passage of the Affordable Care Act (ACA) of 2010 identified APRNs as extremely valuable assets in the health-care system of the future. APRNs are in the perfect position to successfully move the country's health-care system into the 21st century. The ACA recognizes APRNs as equal partners in providing health care at multiple levels, but particularly in the area of primary care. In 2013, the ANA recommended that the Centers for Medicare and Medicaid Services (CMS), which is the organization that pays for health-care services, must offer plans on state health insurance exchanges that include a minimum number of APRNs in each plan's network of health-care providers. That minimum number would be set in each state and should be equal to 10 percent of the number of APRNs recorded in the state as independently billing Medicare Part B. Of the approximately 355,000 APRNs in 2022, almost 291,000 are billing Medicare Part B independently.[5]

Unless the ACA is repealed, APRNs will play an ever-larger role in the rapidly evolving health-care system of the future. What that role will be depends on how well governmental organizations and the public understand the contributions of nurse practitioners and how hard APRNs work to meet the Institute of Medicine's report recommendations that nurses must practice to the fullest extent of their education and at the top of their licenses.

APRN CONSENSUS MODEL: LACE

As discussed previously, the legal regulation and licensure of America's 355,000 APRNs (2022 data) is inconsistent and lacks standard definitions. Some states certify them as advanced practice nurses but do not have a separate license; other states recognize

a licensing level for them but use different titles. If an APRN living in one state moves to another state, their scope of practice may be different, and the licensing process and title may also be different.

A Blueprint for the Future?

To address these and related APRN issues, in 2008 the APRN Consensus Work Group and the National Council of State Boards of Nursing (NCSBN) APRN Advisory Committee issued a report on the **licensure, accreditation, certification, and education (LACE)** of APRNs. This statement addresses the lack of common definitions regarding APRN practice, the ever-increasing numbers of specializations, the inconsistency in credentials and scope of practice, and the wide variations in education for APRNs.[6] The goal was to implement the consensus model for APRN regulation in all states by 2015. In 2013, all national regulatory, educational, credentialing, and professional associations agreed to promote the application of the model. In addition, 16 states completed implementation of the model, and several other states were in various stages of making the model part of their nurse practice act. As of 2018, only 41 states had fully implemented the APRN consensus model, with several other states strongly considering it. Work will continue until all states have adopted it.

Definition and Roles

The APRN Consensus Work Group and the NCSBN Advisory Committee developed a uniform definition of the APRN role. According to their final report, an APRN is a nurse

1. who has completed an accredited graduate-level education program preparing him/her for one of the four recognized APRN roles;
2. who has passed a national certification examination that measures APRN role and population-focused competencies and who maintains continued competence as evidenced by **recertification** in the role and population through the national certification program;
3. who has acquired advanced clinical knowledge and skills preparing him/her to provide direct care to patients, as well as a component of indirect care; however, the defining factor for **all** APRNs is that a significant component of the education and practice focuses on direct care of individuals;

Issues Now

Health-Care Reform and Advanced Practice Nurses–Who's Driving the Bus?

Those who favor health-care reform see it as a giant step toward increasing health-care coverage for some 56 million Americans who either have no coverage or have only limited coverage. Those who oppose it see it as a giant step toward socialization and an era of big government control. Either way, it is here now, and one of the many issues that need to be worked out is the role of APRNs and how they will be regulated in the future. If the ACA is revoked, the role of the APRN in the health-care system will become even less clear.

Although nursing as a profession has consistently been ranked number one among the most trusted professions, the public still seems to have a very narrow view of what nurses can really do and the contributions they can make to health care. The role of APRN is even more obscure to the public, except for people who receive their care. For many years, APRNs have been quietly asserting their role as autonomous practitioners amid confusing state regulations, multiple certifications, licensure issues, and political squabbling.

The American Medical Association (AMA) has always viewed APRNs as a threat to their scope of practice and even their livelihood, although study after study has shown this to be untrue. Their main concern on paper is the educational preparation of APRNs, and they have devoted significant research funds to comparing the education of APRNs to the education of medical doctors. Of course, it is the obligation of all professions to examine their preparation techniques and reflect on their growth and scope of practice.

The AMA has long held the belief that diagnosing, prescribing, and performing high-level clinical skills is the exclusive domain of physicians. APRNs, who graduate from accredited institutions of higher education and are certified by national organizations and licensed by their states, have shown that they, too, can successfully and safely carry out formerly exclusive physician practice areas, and usually more economically.

Professional nursing groups need to establish their own regulations to promote and achieve the outcomes of their profession. It is essential that all nurses, not just APRNs, control their own scope of practice and make their own decisions on how best to provide care for their clients. As health-care reform is fully implemented over the next several years, increasing numbers of clients will be seeing health-care providers for the first time. This situation is particularly suited for the skill set that APRNs bring to the table.

So, is there a rivalry between physicians and nurses? The answer is no. They each have their own practice acts and scopes of practice. Both nurses and physicians will need the educational and skills preparation to work together to deal with the large influx of new clients in the near future. Will there be tensions between the two groups at the legislative and professional levels? As the situation exists today, it is hard to imagine otherwise. However, the nursing profession must stand its ground and vigorously guard against allowing other groups to regulate and define APRN practice. The ANA and most of the state nursing organizations closely monitor legislation that deals with nursing practice. When a different health-care group tries to change the scope of practice for nurses, they send out a warning so that members can respond by contacting the appropriate legislators.

Sources: *AMA successfully fights scope of practice expansions that threaten patient safety. AMA, 2023. Retrieved from: ama-assn.org/practice-management/ scope of practice/ama-successfuly-fights-scope-of-practice-expantions-threaten; Nurse practitioner career overview. Nurses Journal, 2023. https://nursejournal .org/nurse-practitioner/.*

4. whose practice builds on the competencies of registered nurses (RNs) by demonstrating a greater depth and breadth of knowledge, a greater synthesis of data, increased complexity of skills and interventions, and greater role autonomy;

5. who is educationally prepared to assume responsibility and accountability for health promotion and/or maintenance as well as the assessment, diagnosis, and management of patient problems, which includes the use and prescription of pharmacologic and non-pharmacologic interventions;

6. who has clinical experience of sufficient depth and breadth to reflect the intended license; **and**

7. who has obtained a license to practice as an APRN in one of the four APRN roles: certified registered nurse anesthetist (CRNA), certified nurse-midwife (CNM), clinical nurse specialist (CNS), or certified nurse practitioner (CNP). [emphases in original][5]

Some APRNs who have been in practice for many years are concerned that they will no longer be able to practice when the new requirements are implemented. The language of the consensus model includes a process called *grandfathering*, which allows nurses to continue the same level of practice as long as they maintain an active license. The benefit of the model is that it would permit nurses to move to another state and still practice at the same level. However, it is up to each individual APRN to be knowledgeable about legislative issues that may affect their practice, monitor any additional requirements a state may add, and work to have the grandfathering language included in their state's practice act update.[7]

Titles for APRNs

The APRN consensus model requires that advanced practice nurses use the designation *APRN* after their name and follow it with a specified role. For example, an advanced practice nurse who is also a certified nurse practitioner would sign their name and then write *APRN, CNP* after it. The particular group of clients or specialty may also be included; for example, *APRN, CNP, pediatrics*, or just a capital *P*. Nurses who are prepared and licensed in more than one role would include all the relevant roles. Employers of APRNs retain the responsibility for verifying the nurse's education and license.

Education for APRNs

Although there has been some movement by higher education for consistency in APRN programs, there remains a wide variation in length and requirements for the programs. The APRN consensus model expects that any educational program for advanced practice be preapproved by accrediting entities *before* the students enter the program. This will guarantee that the students will have met the prerequisites for licensure and certification upon graduation. The programs will have to meet established educational standards so that students can sit for national certification examinations when they graduate. Actually, these standards already exist, although not all programs currently meet them.[8]

Nurses currently in APRN educational programs need to keep up with proposed changes as they are applied to these programs. This begins with being aware of proposed legislation because the changes will first take place at the SBN and legislative levels. Generally, SBNs allow nursing programs 2 years to implement required changes after they become part of the practice act. It is imperative that students talk with the professors and the deans of their programs about how modifications will affect them. Again, the purpose of preapproval is to make sure the graduates meet the eligibility requirements for certification and licensure.

Even though specialization in areas such as **oncology**, nephrology, or **palliative** care do not fall into one of the four population focus areas of the APRN consensus model, nurses can still specialize in these areas. There are several ways to achieve this specialized education. Nurses can finish a preapproved APRN population-focused program, become certified and licensed, and then pursue additional education in the specialty of choice. Another option is to attend a program that prepares nurses for the population-focused APRN and the specialty they wish to pursue at the same time. When the nurses graduate, they can take the certification/licensure examination for the APRN and then the certification examination for their specialty of choice. It is important to remember that specialty areas of practice are identified by professional organizations and are not specifically regulated by SBNs. The professional organizations establish the competencies for the specialization and usually have a separate certification examination and other requirements.[9]

The APRN consensus model does not require a program to offer a doctor of nursing practice (DNP) degree; however, the AACN has recommended that entry-level training for an APRN be moved to the DNP. A master's degree still is the basic requirement. Programs that have the option to offer the DNP must meet the requirements for the APRN as outlined in the model. Although nursing education has fallen short of the 2015 goal for the DNP as the terminal degree for advanced practice, the AACN will continue to pursue this goal.[9]

LACE

LACE is not the same as the APRN consensus model but rather an outgrowth of the process to put the model into practice. LACE serves as a means for those who are seeking to adopt the APRN consensus model to debate the concepts, requirements, and methods of execution. It is more inclusive and asks for input from parties who may be affected by changes in the legal status of APRNs or the scope of their practice, such as community groups, medical associations, and hospitals. The ultimate goal of LACE is to provide a general consensus for the implementation of the APRN consensus model.[10]

While states move forward on legislation to implement the APRN consensus model, it is important for nurses to watch for other proposed legislation and practices that politicians, medical associations, and health-care institutions are initiating.

NURSING ORGANIZATIONS AND THEIR IMPORTANCE

The establishment of a professional organization is one of the most important defining characteristics of a profession. An association is a group of people banding together to achieve a specific purpose. By working together for a specific purpose, an association or organization amplifies its impact; and by developing a strategic plan, it focuses that impact to achieve certain results. Many professions have a single major professional organization to which most of its members belong and several specialized suborganizations that members may also join. Professions with just one major organization to which most of their members belong generally have a great deal of political power.

Strength in Numbers

Nurses need and use power in every aspect of their professional lives, ranging from supervising unlicensed personnel to negotiating with the administration for increased independence of practice. An individual nurse has relatively little influence over nursing standards and practices, but as a group, nurses' power to influence their profession increases exponentially. The dedication to high-quality **nursing standards** and improved methods of practice by the major nursing organizations has led to improved care and increased benefits to the public as a whole.[11]

> *An individual nurse has relatively little influence over nursing standards and practices, but as a group, nurses' power to influence their profession increases exponentially.*

Speaking With One Voice

National nursing organizations need the participation and membership of all nurses in order to claim that they are truly representative of the profession. A large membership allows the organization to speak with one voice when making its values about health-care issues known to politicians, physicians' groups, and the public in general.

The National League for Nursing

The NLN is also a strong force in community health nursing, occupational health nursing, and nursing services activities. It was the first national nursing organization to provide accreditation for nursing programs at all levels.

Purposes

The primary purpose of the NLN is to maintain and improve the standards of nursing education. Its bylaws state that its purpose is to foster the development and improvement of hospital, industrial, and public health; other organized nursing services; and nursing education through the coordinated action of nurses, allied professional groups, citizens, agencies, and schools so that the nursing needs of the people will be met.

Membership

Although membership is open to individual nurses, the primary membership of the NLN comes in the form of agency membership, usually through schools of nursing. One of the major functions of the NLN, through the organization formerly known as the National League for Nursing Accrediting Commission (NLNAC) but renamed the Accreditation Commission for Education in Nursing (ACEN), is to accredit schools of nursing through a self-study process. The schools are given a set of criteria, or **essentials for accreditation**, and are then required to evaluate their programs against these criteria. After the evaluation report is written and sent to the ACEN, site representatives visit the school to verify the information in the report and see whether the school has met the criteria. If the school meets the evaluation criteria, it is accredited for up to 8 years.

Accreditation of a nursing school by the ACEN indicates that the school meets national standards. In some work settings, a nurse must be a graduate of an ACEN-accredited school of nursing before they can be hired or accepted into many master-level nursing programs.

Other services and activities that the NLN carries out include testing; evaluating new graduate nurses; supplying career information, continuing education workshops, and conferences for all levels of nursing; publishing a wide range of literature and DVDs covering current issues in health care; and compiling statistics about nursing, nurses, and nursing education.

The American Association of Colleges of Nursing

The AACN was established to help colleges with schools of nursing work together to improve the standards for higher education for professional nursing. It serves the public interest by assessing and identifying nursing programs that engage in effective educational practices.

Purposes

The AACN, through the Commission on Collegiate Nursing Education (CCNE), has developed standards for the accreditation of baccalaureate schools of nursing and is poised to become a major accreditation agency, competing with the NLNAC. The AACN has developed and published a set of guidelines for the education of professional nursing students that is widely used as the theoretical basis for baccalaureate curricula.

Membership

Only deans and directors of programs that offer baccalaureate or higher degrees in nursing with an upper-division nursing major are permitted membership in the AACN.

The American Nurses Association

The ANA grew out of a concern for the quality of nursing practice and the care that nurses were providing. In the early part of the 20th century, when the ANA was organized, there was little or no regulation for the requirements to practice as a nurse. ANA took some of the first steps in developing standards for the profession.

Purposes

The major purposes for the existence of the ANA, as stated in its bylaws, include improving the standards of health and access to health-care services for everyone; improving and maintaining high standards for nursing practice; and promoting the professional growth and development of all nurses, addressing concerns such as economic issues, working conditions, and independence of practice.[7]

In 2012 and 2013, the ANA underwent a major structural reorganization. The ANA board of directors was reduced from 16 to 10, and all of the standing committees were disbanded. The traditional house of delegates that convened every other year was restructured into a membership assembly model that reduced the representation at the convention to two elected members and one appointed member from each state. Voting in the ANA Membership Assembly is by weighted vote, and the members meet once a year.[12] The goal of the restructuring was to streamline the organization and make it more responsive to a rapidly changing health-care system and society. Committees are now formed when needed to address a particular issue and then disbanded after the issue is resolved. For example, the Code of Ethics for Nurses was updated, so a committee was formed to deal with the changes that need to be made.

Membership

Membership in the ANA also changed with the restructuring. Currently, it is limited to 52 constituents:

50 state organizations; Washington, DC; and Puerto Rico. An individual joins a state organization and through the state organization indirectly is a member of the ANA. Certain discounts in membership are offered for new members and new graduate nurses. Various levels of membership are available for nurses who work part time or who are retired. The ANA makes every effort to encourage individual nurses to join the organization. The proposed changes to the governance and membership structure would not require nurses to join their states first. Rather, they would become direct members of the ANA. Unfortunately, most nurses do not belong to this potentially powerful, politically active, and very influential organization.

Each state has the opportunity to determine what is needed from each member to run the state association; the amount of the dues that is sent to ANA is predetermined. Although dues are relatively expensive (they change a little from year to year but are about $200 per year), the ANA offers various plans for payment, such as three equal payments over the course of a year or monthly payroll deductions, which make membership affordable for most nurses.

Other Services

When nurses pursue advanced education and levels of practice, as many are doing today, the ANA ANCC is essential for testing and certification of many of these practice levels. Although other organizations offer advanced practice certification, without the ANCC, there would be even less standardization for and less recognition of these practitioners by the public, physicians, and lawmakers.

Entry Into Practice

Another important issue that the ANA has been involved in is the entry-level education requirement for professional nurses. The ANA has supported the baccalaureate degree as the minimum educational requirement for nurses since 1958. The ANA is always in the forefront of the debate over **entry into practice**, which has continued into the 21st century.[13]

Standards of Practice

Additional functions carried out by the ANA include the establishment and continual updating of standards of nursing practice. These standards are the yardstick against which nurses are measured and held accountable by courts of law. The ANA also established the official code of ethics that guides professional practice.

Legislation

Many of the political and economic activities of the ANA are carried out in the halls of legislatures and offices of legislators. The ANA Political Action Committee (ANA-PAC) is one of the most powerful in Washington, DC. (See Chapter 18 for a more detailed discussion.) Such activities have a profound effect on the role that nurses play and will continue to play in health care well into the 21st century.

Successful PAC activities require money and the power of a large, unified membership. The ANA-PAC seeks to influence legislation about nurses, nursing, and health care in general. It has been and will be a strong voice in the formulation of current national health-care reform.

The National Student Nurses' Association

The National Student Nurses' Association (NSNA) is an independent legal corporation established in 1953 to represent the needs of nursing students. Working closely with the ANA, which offers services, an official publication, and close communication, the NSNA consists of state chapters that represent student nurses in those particular states.

Purposes

The main purpose of the NSNA is to help maintain high standards of education in schools of nursing, with the ultimate goal of educating high-quality nurses who will provide excellent health care.[11] The ideas, concerns, and needs of students are extremely important to nursing educators. Most nursing programs have committees in which students are asked to participate, including **curriculum** development and evaluation techniques. It is important that students belong to these committees and actively participate in the committees' activities.

Membership

Membership consists of all nursing students in registered nurse programs. Students can join at the local, state, or national level or at all levels if desired. Dues are low, with a discount for the first year's membership.

Other Services

In addition, the NSNA is concerned with developing and providing workshops, seminars, and conferences that deal with current issues in nursing and health care, with a wide range of subjects, from ethical and legal concerns to recent developments in pharmacology, test-taking skills, and professional growth. Student nurses who belong to the NSNA and who take an active part in its functions are much more likely to join the ANA after they graduate. Professional identity and professional behavior are learned. By beginning the process during the formal school years, student nurses develop professional attitudes and behaviors that they will likely maintain for the rest of their careers.

Benefits for Students

Many benefits exist for student nurses who belong to the NSNA. Several scholarships are available to members of organization. Members receive the official publication of the organization, *Imprint*, and the *NSNA News*, which keep student nurses current on recent developments in health care and nursing.

Student members also have political representation on issues that may affect them now or in the future. Some of these issues include educational standards for practice, standards of professional practice, and health insurance. The NSNA is also concerned with the difficulty that many nursing students from minority groups experience in the educational process. The Breakthrough Project is an attempt by the NSNA to help such students enter the nursing profession.

Practicing Professionalism

Student nurses who join the NSNA experience firsthand the operation, activities, and benefits of a professional organization. In schools with active memberships, the NSNA can be a very exciting and useful organization for students.

Many NSNA chapters are involved in community activities that provide services at a local level and allow the student to practice "real" nursing. These services include providing community health screening programs for hypertension, lead poisoning, vision, hearing, and birth defects; setting up information and education programs; giving immunizations; and working with groups concerned with drug abuse, child abuse, drunken driving, and teen pregnancy. All nursing students should be encouraged to belong to this organization.

The International Council of Nurses

Membership in the International Council of Nurses (ICN) consists of national nursing organizations, and the ICN serves as the international organization for professional nursing. The ANA is one member among 104 nursing associations around the world. Each member nation sends delegates and participates in the international convention held every 4 years. The quadrennial conventions, or congresses, are open to all nurses and delegates from all nations.

The goal of the ICN is to improve health and nursing care throughout the world. The ICN coordinates its efforts with the United Nations and other international organizations when appropriate in the pursuit of its goals.

Some issues that have been the focus of concern of the ICN are the social and economic welfare of nurses, the changing role of nurses in the present health-care environment, the challenges being faced by the various national nursing organizations, and how government and politics affect the nursing profession and health care. Overseeing the ICN is the Council of National Representatives. This body meets every 2 years and serves as the governing organization. ICN headquarters is located in Geneva, Switzerland.

Sigma Theta Tau

Sigma Theta Tau is an honors organization that was established in colleges and universities to recognize individuals who have demonstrated leadership or made important contributions to professional nursing. It is international, and candidates are selected from among senior nursing students or graduate or practicing nurses.

The organization has its headquarters in Indianapolis, where it has a large library open to members to use for scholarly activities and research. It also boasts the first online nursing journal, which can be accessed by any nurse with a computer anywhere in the world. Local chapters of Sigma Theta Tau collect and distribute funds to nurses who are conducting nursing research. The organization also holds educational conferences and recognizes those who have made contributions to nursing.

Grassroots Organizations

A growing trend in contemporary nursing has been the formation of grassroots nursing organizations. In reality, all nursing organizations start as the grassroots efforts of local nursing groups that are trying to solve a particular problem. Over time, these small grassroots organizations become more structured, larger, and eventually national or international when they spread to other areas across the country or around the world. Unfortunately, the large organizations tend to lose sight of the fundamental issues they were originally formed to solve, or they are unable to deal effectively with local problems.

Working to Bring About Change

Grassroots organizations usually have relatively small memberships; are localized to a town, city, or sometimes a state; and attempt to solve a problem or deal with an issue that the members feel is not being adequately handled by a large national organization. They may be created as a completely new and separate organization, or they may break away from a larger, established group. Because all the members of grassroots organizations are passionately concerned about only one or two issues at a time that affect them directly, they tend to work hard to effect change and can bring a great deal of concentrated power to bear on people, such as legislators, who make the decisions about the issues.

Grassroots groups use a number of techniques that are often frowned upon by the more established organizations to attain their goals. In addition to the traditional techniques of writing letters, sending e-mails, and calling legislators, members of grassroots groups actively seek media attention, march on capitol buildings and state houses, introduce resolutions, and testify before committee hearings. Their success varies from issue to issue and location to location.

Successful Grassroots Efforts

Two examples of successful grassroots efforts are found in California and Pennsylvania. The California Nurses Association decided to break away from the ANA because it was not addressing some key state issues such as length of hospital stays, reduction in professional nursing staffs, and preoccupation with profit. The grassroots group in Pennsylvania formed a completely new organization, the Nurses of Pennsylvania (NPA), and focused their energies on the trend to replace licensed RNs with unlicensed technicians, sometimes called *downskilling*.

> *In reality, all nursing organizations start as the grassroots efforts of local nursing groups that are trying to solve a particular problem.*

Special-Interest Organizations

The historical origins of special-interest organizations in nursing are even older than those of the main national organizations. For example, the Red Cross, established in 1864, is one of the oldest special-interest organizations that nurses have been involved with.

Why Do They Exist?

Most specialty organizations in nursing were founded when a group of nurses with similar concerns sought professional and individual support. These organizations usually start out small and informal, then increase in size, structure, and membership over several years. There were relatively few of these organizations until 1965, when an explosion in specialty organizations in nursing took place. During the next 20 years, almost 100 new organizations were formed, with the associated effect of diminishing membership levels in the ANA.

Clinical Practice

Specialty organizations are usually organized according to clinical practice area. Organizations exist for almost every clinical specialty and subspecialty known in nursing, such as obstetrics/gynecology, critical care, operating room, emergency department, and occupational health, as well as less known areas such as flight nursing, urology, and cosmetic surgery.

Education and Culture

Another focal area for these organizations is education and ethics. Organizations such as the AACN and the Western Interstate Commission for Higher Education fall into this category. Often, organizations focus on the common **ethnic group** or cultural or religious backgrounds of nurses. The National Association of Hispanic Nurses and the National Black Nurses Association represent this type of specialty organization.

Education and Standards

Although many of these organizations promote the personal and professional growth of their membership, they also carry out many other activities. Particularly important among these activities is establishing the **standards of practice** for the particular specialty area. As much as the ANA establishes overall standards of practice for nursing in general, the specialty organizations establish standards for their particular clinical areas. Providing educational services for their members is another important activity of specialty organizations. Conferences, workshops, and seminars in the clinical area represented are important venues for nurses to keep current on new developments and to maintain high standards of practice.[7]

Should They Matter to You?

How many of these specialty nursing organizations are there? No one really knows. Many such organizations are informal and run by volunteers. Organizations are continually being formed, and others are being disbanded.

Should nurses belong to these organizations? Of course they should. But to maximize nursing's political clout, nurses should also belong to the ANA. Many of the larger specialty organizations have recognized this fact and have established close ties with the ANA. The ANA is well aware of the membership bleed-off from the specialty organizations and has initiated efforts to become more involved in the specialty nursing areas.

Before nurses join a specialty organization, they should determine whether its purposes are at odds with those of the ANA. Many of the large specialty organizations have their own lobbyists in both state and national legislatures. Because the legislators really do not know the differences between the various nursing organizations, they can easily become confused over health-care issues if they are receiving pressure from two nursing groups representing opposing sides of the same issue. Consequently, legislators may simply surmise that the professional opinions of those in the industry are too contradictory to consider and vote on an important issue without regard to nurses and nursing.

The tendency toward specialization has led to an ever-increasing number of nursing organizations, each focusing on a particular practice field within the profession. This trend has diluted the unity and ultimately lessened the power that nursing as a profession can exert in health-care issues. Although it is important to recognize the complexity of today's health-care system and the pluralism inherent in nursing, consensus of opinion on major issues is essential if nursing is to have any influence on the future of the profession.

The challenge for nurses in the future is to use the diversity in the profession as a positive force and to unite as a group on important issues. Awareness of earlier development of nursing organizations provides a perspective for the current situation and can act as a framework for planning the future.

What Do You Think?

What type of power does the individual nurse have? Cite examples of individual nurses who have used their power to effect changes in health care and nursing.

Issues in Practice

Juanita, an RN at a large inner-city hospital, has been working on her off hours as a volunteer in a storefront clinic to treat the indigent and underserved population of that part of the city. The clinic clientele is primarily Mexican American, as are the majority of the 20 nurses working at the clinic. Because all the nurses, including a family nurse practitioner, volunteer their time and receive no pay, the small private grant that Juanita had managed to secure was adequate to cover the cost for rental of the building, basic supplies for the clinic, and a few medications. However, the grant is about to run out and is nonrenewable.

Juanita first tried to obtain money from the hospital to keep the clinic going, but she was told that the hospital was having its own financial problems because of managed care demands and could not spare any money. At a staff meeting of the nurses from the clinic, the nurses decided to band together and form a grassroots organization called the Storefront Clinic Nurses to focus their efforts on obtaining funds to keep the clinic open. They printed and passed out flyers, called local and city politicians, encouraged the patrons of the clinic to talk to people they knew, and even called the local television station for an interview about their plight.

(continued)

Issues in Practice (continued)

Although most of the nurses' efforts went unrewarded, a large pharmaceutical company became aware of their plight and wanted to provide the clinic a sizable financial stipend as well as free medications for a period of at least 5 years. In addition to its philanthropic interests, the pharmaceutical company wanted to gather long-term data about a newly developed antihypertensive medication. The company would provide the medication free to the clients at the clinic, the majority of whom had some degree of hypertension; all the nurses had to do was take and record the clients' blood pressure readings and complete "reported side effects" forms on each client. Client identifier codes, rather than names, would be used to maintain confidentiality. Juanita, as the group's coordinator, would be responsible for coordinating and preserving the data.

Although Juanita saw it as an answer to her prayers, she was concerned about the medication project. The pharmaceutical company said that no research consent forms were needed because the medication had already been through clinical trials and had received approval by the Food and Drug Administration. Juanita called another meeting of her nurses to discuss the issue. Without the grant, the clinic would close; but if they accepted the grant, they would have to participate in a medication research project that made Juanita feel uncomfortable.

Questions for Thought
1. What are the main issues in this case study?
2. What ethical principles are being violated? What is the ethical dilemma that Juanita is facing?
3. Are there any other solutions to this problem?

Conclusion

Nursing, in its journey toward professionalism, has been propelled and shaped by its nursing organizations, which were the main vehicles for the development of educational and practice standards, initiation of licensure, promotion of advanced practice, and general improvement in the level of care nurses provide. From their beginnings, nursing organizations have served as channels of communication among nurses, consumers of health care, and other health-care professionals. In many cases, the nursing organizations have focused the power of the profession to influence important health policies that affect the whole nation.

Licensure and certification are both methods of granting credentials to demonstrate that an individual is qualified to provide safe care to the public. Without proof of competency, the profession of nursing would become chaotic, disorganized, and even dangerous.

CRITICAL-THINKING EXERCISES

- Develop a strategy for increasing the membership of the ANA.
- A labor union is attempting to organize the nurses at your hospital. Is it better for the professional nursing organization to represent the nurses? Why or why not?
- A new graduate nurse is working in the intensive care unit (ICU) of a large hospital. She wants to join a nursing organization but has a limited amount of money to spend. Her coworkers in the ICU want her to join the AACN, but she would also like to join the ANA. Basing her decision on economic and professional issues, which organization should she join?
- Compare and contrast certification and licensure. Should certification be legally recognized? Justify your answer.

NCLEX-STYLE QUESTIONS

1. What is the purpose of nurse licensure?
   1. To justify higher nursing salaries
   2. To protect the public from unqualified nurses
   3. To increase enrollment at accredited nursing schools
   4. To allow nurses with a single license to practice in multiple states
2. Why is a mandatory license preferable to a permissive license?
   1. A mandatory license indicates that the nurse has received advanced nursing training.
   2. Mandatory licensure signifies that the nurse is an RN, not an LPN/LVN.
   3. A mandatory license blurs the scope of practice between the different levels of nursing.
   4. Mandatory licensure requires the nurse to pass a licensure examination and be registered by the state board of nursing.
3. What are the negative aspects of institutional licensure in today's health-care system? **Select all that apply**.
   1. The quality of the nursing care delivered is not as good.
   2. There is no agreed-upon measure of minimal level of competency.
   3. It keeps staffing costs down by using less qualified nurses.
   4. It is not transferable to another facility or state.
   5. It allows nurses licensed in foreign countries to avoid taking the U.S. licensure examination.
4. A _____ is state legislation regulating the practice of nurses that protects the public, defines the scope of practice, and makes nurses accountable for their actions.
5. What is a downside of professional certification in nursing?
   1. Certification acknowledges the attainment of increased knowledge and skills.
   2. All certification attaches an increased level of legal liability.
   3. The public, employers, and even nurses have difficulty understanding what certification means.
   4. Many different professional groups can offer certification.

6. What issues related to APRNs does the LACE statement address? **Select all that apply**.
   1. The lack of common definitions regarding APRN practice
   2. The inconsistency from state to state in credentials and scope of practice
   3. The increasing number of APRN specialization
   4. The wide variations in education for ARNPs
   5. The overlapping scope of practice between physicians and APRNs
7. Which of the following was accomplished with the consensus model?
   1. A uniform definition of the APRN role
   2. A requirement that APRN programs offer a DNP degree
   3. Requiring the use of "APRN" after a practitioner's name
   4. Establishing 10 APRN roles or areas of practice
8. Why was a national nursing licensure examination developed despite that licensure is controlled by state boards of nursing?
   1. Some states refused to implement licensure examinations for nurses.
   2. Individual state examinations varied widely, and consistent quality could not be ensured.
   3. Nurses pushed for a national examination so that they could practice in different states.
   4. The ANA demanded a national examination to exert more control over state boards of nursing.
9. What is the primary concern the AMA has with the growing role of nurse practitioners?
   1. Infringement on physicians' scope of practice and livelihood
   2. Endangering patient safety
   3. Lack of evidence-based practice
   4. Confusion about professional roles
10. If the Affordable Care Act is repealed, what will be the most likely effect on APRNs?
    1. The number of APRNs will increase significantly.
    2. The educational requirements for APRNs will become stricter.
    3. The scope of practice for APRNs will expand greatly.
    4. The role of APRNs in primary care will be reduced.

References

1. Pearce K. COVID-19 ushers in decades of change for nursing profession. Johns Hopkins University, October 19, 2020. https://hub.jhu.edu/2020/10/19/nursing-changes-covid-19

2. What is the role of the state board of nursing? *NurseJournal*, 2021. https://nursejournal.org/resources/what-is-the-role-of-the-state-board-of-nursing/

3. Wyatt L. *A History of Nursing*. Pittsburgh, Amberley Publishing, 2019.

4. 2023 NCLEX-RN Test plan. NCSBN, 2023. ncsbn.org/publication/2023-nclex-rn-test-plan

5. NP Fact Sheet. AANP, 2022. Retrieved from: aanp.org/all-about-nps/np-fact-sheet

6. Gaines K. Compact nursing state list 2023. Nurse.org, 2023. https://nurse.org/articles/enhanced-compact-multi-state-license-enlc/

7. Elhi N. Short-staffed and COVID-battered, U.S. hospitals are hiring more foreign nurses. Health News from NPR, January 6, 2022. https://www.npr.org/sections/health-shots/2022/01/06/1069369625/short-staffed-and-covid-battered-u-s-hospitals-are-hiring-more-foreign-nurses

8. Merelli A. There's one group of nurses in America who don't hate their job. Quartz, December 5, 2021. https://qz.com/2097686/foreign-nurses-working-in-the-us-are-happier-than-american-nurses/

9. Deering M. Nurse practitioner career overview. NurseJournal, November 4, 2023. https://nursejournal.org/nurse-practitioner

10. Legal differences between certification and licensure. National Registry of EMTs, 2022. nremt.org/Document/certification_licensure

11. Greggs-McQuilkin D. Why join a professional nursing organization? *Nursing*, 35(suppl 19):19, 2005. https://doi.org/10.1097/00152193-200509001-00006

12. Membership assembly. American Nurses Association, n.d. http://www.nursingworld.org/FunctionalMenuCategories/AboutANA/Leadership-Governance/Membership-Assembly

13. Clarke S. The BSN entry into practice debate. *Nursing Management*, 47(11):17–19, 2016. https://doi.org/10.1097/01.NUMA.0000502806.22177.c4

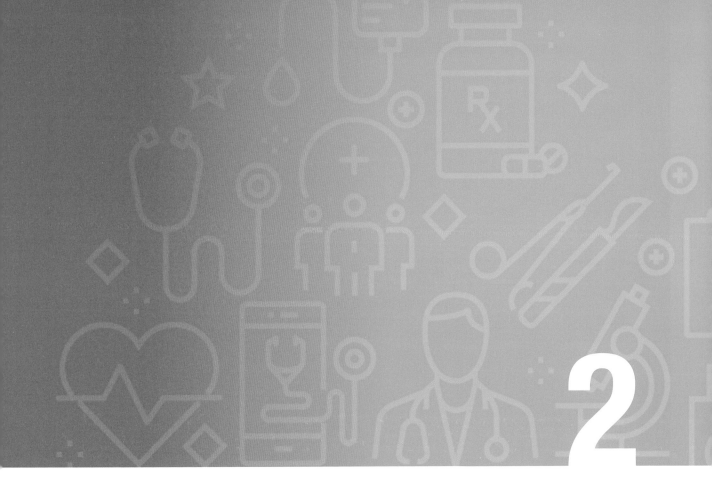

2

Making the Transition to Professional

6

Ethics in Nursing

Joseph T. Catalano

Learning Objectives

After completing this chapter, the reader will be able to:

- Discuss and analyze the difference between law and ethics
- Define the key terms used in ethics
- Discuss the important ethical concepts
- Distinguish between the two most commonly used systems of ethical decision making
- Apply the steps in the ethical decision-making process

A LEARNED SKILL

Nurses who practice in today's health-care system soon realize that making ethical decisions is a common part of daily nursing care. However, experience shows that in the full curricula of many schools of nursing, the teaching of ethical principles and ethical decision making gets less attention than the topics of nursing skills, core competencies, and electronic charting. As health-care technology continues to advance at a rapid pace, nurses will likely find it increasingly difficult to make sound ethical decisions. Many nurses feel the need to be better prepared to understand and deal with the complex ethical problems that keep evolving as they attempt to provide care for their patients.[1]

Many individuals confuse ethics with social norms, religious beliefs, or the legal system. Some simply believe ethics are the same as morals. Although elements of ethics may be found in all of these places, ethics itself is a standalone set of concepts and principles that guide humans in general, and professionals in particular, in making decisions about what types of behaviors will help or harm other members of society. Ethics generally presents broad concepts to guide decision making and does not have specific rules such as are found in moral systems.

Ethical decision making is a skill that can be learned. The ability to make sensible ethical decisions is based on an understanding of underlying ethical principles, ethical theories or systems, a decision-making model, and the profession's code of ethics. This skill, like others, involves mastery of the theoretical material and practice of the skill itself. This chapter presents the basic information required to understand ethics, the code of ethics for nurses, and ethical decision making. It also highlights some of the important **bioethical issues** that challenge nurses in the current health-care system.

FOUR CATEGORIES

As a part of a philosophical system, ethics is generally divided into levels or categories:

Metaethics: The abstract, overarching philosophical way of understanding ethics. One of the most important questions that philosophy in general addresses is that of epistemology, or how we know that we know. In ethics, this question is refined to, *How* do we know what is right and wrong? It also seeks to answer the question, What is truth? It is concerned with the meaning of ethical language and explaining the fundamental meaning of the words. The discussion of the ethical terms that follows is actually a metaethics approach to understanding ethics. Without metaethics, it is almost impossible to take the next step to normative ethics.

Normative Ethics: The use of the concepts and principles discovered by metaethics to guide decision making about specific actions in determining what is right or wrong when interacting with other people. Normative ethics tends to be more prescriptive than metaethics and forms the basis for theories and systems of ethics. Both the codes of ethics and the deontological **ethical system** find their underpinnings in metaethics and normative ethics.

Applied Ethics: The application of the theories and systems of ethics developed by normative ethics to real-world situations. Applied ethics is broken into specialized fields such as health-care ethics, legal ethics, bioethics, and business ethics. This is the category of ethics that is used most by nurses and other health-care providers. It is used in resolving ethical dilemmas.

Descriptive Ethics: A bottom-up approach to ethics that starts with what society is already doing ethically and develops ethical principles based on the observed actions of people rather than starting with ethical principles and applying them to society such as normative ethics does. There are no preset values in descriptive ethics except for the consistent ethical decisions that are already being made by the majority of members of society. It is also sometimes called *comparative ethics* and forms the basis for situational ethics and the utilitarian system of ethics. Although widely used in politics, economics, and business, it creates additional issues for health-care providers when applied to difficult health-care decisions.[2]

IMPORTANT DEFINITIONS

In Western cultures, the study of ethics is a specialized area of philosophy, the origins of which can be traced to ancient Greece. In fact, certain ethical principles articulated by Hippocrates still serve as the basis for many of the current debates. Like most specialized areas of study, ethics has its own language and uses terminology in precise ways. The following are some key terms that are encountered in studies of health-care ethics.

> *" Values are usually not written down; however, at some time in their professional careers, it may be important for nurses to make lists of their values. "*

Values

Values are ideals or concepts that give meaning to an individual's life. Values are derived most commonly from societal norms, religion, and family orientation and serve as the framework for making decisions and taking action in daily life. People's values tend to change as their life situations change, as they grow older, and as they encounter situations that cause value conflicts. For example, before the 1950s, pregnancy outside of marriage was unacceptable; unmarried women who were pregnant were shunned and generally separated from society. Today this situation is more widely accepted, and it is not uncommon to see pregnant high school students attending classes.

Values are usually not written down; however, at some time in their professional careers, it may be important for nurses to make lists of their values. This **value clarification** process requires that nurses assess, evaluate, and then determine a set of personal values and prioritize them. This will help them make decisions when confronted with situations in which the patient's values differ from the nurse's values.

Value conflicts that often occur in daily life can force an individual to select a higher-priority value over a lower-priority one. For example, a nurse who values both career and family may be forced to decide between going to work and staying home with a sick child.[2]

Morals

Morals are the fundamental standards of right and wrong that an individual learns and internalizes, usually in the early stages of childhood development. An individual's moral orientation is often based on religious beliefs, although societal influence plays an important part in this development. The word *moral* comes from the Latin word **mores**, which means "customs" or "values."

Moral behavior is often manifested as behavior in accordance with a group's norms, customs, or traditions. A moral person is generally someone who responds to another person in need by providing care and who maintains a level of responsibility in all relationships.[3] In many situations in which moral convictions differ, it is difficult to find a rational basis for proving one side right over the other. For example, animal rights activists believe that killing animals for sport, their fur, or even food is morally wrong. Most hunters do not even think of the killing of animals as a moral issue at all.

What Do You Think?

What type of value conflicts have you experienced in the past week? How did you resolve them? Were you satisfied with the resolution, or did it make you feel uncomfortable?

Laws

Laws can generally be defined as rules of social conduct made by humans to protect society, and these laws are based on concerns about fairness and justice. The goals of laws are to preserve the species and promote peaceful and productive interactions between individuals and groups of individuals by preventing the actions of one citizen from infringing on the rights of another. Two important aspects of laws are that they are enforceable through some type of police force and that they should be applied equally to all persons.

Ethics

The term *ethics* has its origins in the Greek word *ethos*, which is generally translated as "quality" or "character." It is a branch of traditional Western philosophy known as *moral philosophy* that studies moral behavior in humans and how humans should act toward each other individually and in groups.

Ethics, as a system of beliefs and behaviors, goes beyond the law, which has as its primary underlying principle the preservation of society.[3] Ethics is more focused on the quality of the society and its long-term survival. Similar to the legal system, ethical systems are only needed when there is a group of people living together. A hermit living alone in a cave on a mountain does not need laws or ethical systems. Primitive societies that were composed of a small number of individuals had to have some basic laws for survival, such as not killing each other, and some basic ethical principles, such as **distributive justice**—for example, all members of the tribe get the same amount of food. As a society increases in size and becomes more complex, a need for more laws and a stronger ethical system ensues.

A System of Morals

Ethics are declarations of what is right or wrong and of what ought to be. Ethics are usually presented as systems of value behaviors and beliefs; they serve the purpose of governing conduct to ensure the protection of an individual's rights. Ethics exist on several levels, ranging from the individual or small group to the society as a whole. The concept of ethics is closely associated with the concept of morals in the development and purposes of both. In one sense, ethics can be considered a system of morals for a particular group. There are usually no systems of enforcement for those who violate ethical principles;[3] however, repeated and obvious violation of ethical precepts of a code of ethics by professionals can result in disciplinary action by the profession's licensing board.

A code of ethics is a written list of a profession's values and standards of conduct. The code of ethics provides a framework for decision making for the profession and should be oriented toward the daily decisions made by members of the profession.

A Dilemma

An **ethical dilemma** is a situation that requires an individual to make a choice between two equally unfavorable alternatives. The basic, elemental aspects of an ethical dilemma usually involve conflict of one individual's rights with those of another, conflict of one individual's obligations with the rights of another, or combined conflict of one group's obligations and rights with those of another group.[4]

Principles in Conflict

By the very nature of an ethical dilemma, there can be no simple correct solution, and the final decision must often be defended against those who disagree with it. For example:

A patient went to surgery for a laparoscopic biopsy of an abdominal mass. After the laparoscope was inserted, the physician noted that the mass had metastasized to the liver, pancreas, and colon, and even before the results of the tissue biopsy returned from the laboratory, the physician diagnosed metastatic cancer with a poor prognosis. When the patient was returned to his room, the physician told the nurses about the diagnosis but warned them that under no circumstances were they to tell the patient about the cancer.

When the patient awoke, the first question he asked the nurses was, "Do I have cancer?" This posed an ethical dilemma for the nurses. If they were to tell the patient the truth, they would violate the principle of fidelity to the physician. If they lie to the patient, they would violate the principle of veracity or telling the patient the truth.

> *By the very nature of an ethical dilemma, there can be no simple correct solution, and the final decision must often be defended against those who disagree with it.*

KEY CONCEPTS IN ETHICS

In addition to the terminology used in the study and practice of ethics, several important principles often underlie ethical dilemmas. These principles include autonomy, justice, fidelity, beneficence, nonmaleficence, veracity, standard of best interest, and obligations.

Autonomy

Autonomy is the right of self-determination, independence, and freedom. It refers to patients' rights to make health-care decisions for themselves even if the health-care provider does not agree with those decisions.

As with most rights, autonomy is not absolute; and under certain conditions, limitations can be imposed on it. Generally, these limitations occur when one individual's autonomy interferes with another individual's rights, health, or well-being. For example, patients generally can use their right to autonomy by refusing any or all treatments. However, in the case of contagious diseases (e.g., tuberculosis) that affect society, the individual can be forced by the health-care and legal systems to take medications to cure the disease. The individual can also be forced into isolation to prevent the disease from spreading. Consider the following situation:

June, who is the 28-year-old mother of two children, is brought into the emergency department (ED) after a tonic-clonic–type seizure at a shopping mall. June is known to the ED nurses because she has been treated several times for seizures after she did not take her antiseizure medications. She states that the medications make her feel "dopey" and tired all the time and that she hates the way they make her feel.

Recently, June has started to drive one of her children and four other children to school in the neighborhood carpool once a week. She also drives 62 miles each way on the interstate twice a week to visit her aging mother in a nursing home. The nurse who takes care of June this day in the ED knows that the state licensing laws require that an individual with uncontrolled seizures must report the fact to the department of motor vehicles (DMV) and is usually ineligible for a driver's license. When the nurse mentions that she has to report the seizure, June begs her not to report it. She would have no means of taking her children to school or visiting her mother. She assures the nurse that she will take her medication no matter how it makes her feel.

The ethical issue in this case study is a conflict of rights and obligations. June has a right to autonomy to determine whether she will take her medication and whether she will self-report having seizures to the DMV. The nurse has an obligation to recognize and honor June's autonomy, but she also has an obligation to maintain public safety, including reporting June's seizures. This is a classic case of an ethical dilemma. Does June's right to autonomy supersede the nurse's obligation to public safety? Do the legal issues involved in the situation affect the ethical decision the nurse makes? How would you decide?

Justice

Justice is the obligation to be fair to all people. The concept is often expanded to what is called *distributive justice*, which states that individuals have the right to be treated equally regardless of race, gender, sexual orientation, marital status, medical diagnosis, social standing, economic level, or religious belief. The principle of justice underlies the first statement in the American Nurses Association (ANA) Code of Ethics for Nurses (2015): "The nurse in all professional relationships practices with compassion and respect for the inherent dignity, worth, and uniqueness of each individual, unrestricted by considerations of social or economic status, personal attributes, or the nature of health problems."[5]

What Do You Think?

All laws are ethical. Do you agree or disagree with that statement? Discuss the relationship between laws and ethics and give reasons why you agree or disagree.

Distributive justice sometimes includes ideas such as equal access to health care for all. As with other rights, limits can be placed on justice when it interferes with the rights of others.[2] For example:

A middle-aged homeless man who was diagnosed with type 1, insulin-dependent diabetes mellitus demanded that Medicaid pay for a pancreas transplant. His health record showed that he refused to follow the prescribed diabetic regimen, drank large quantities of wine, and rarely took his insulin. The transplantation would cost $108,000, which is the total cost of immunizing all the children in a state for 1 year. Should he receive the transplant?

Fidelity

Fidelity is the obligation of individuals to be faithful to commitments made to themselves and to others. In health care, fidelity includes the professional's faithfulness or loyalty to agreements and responsibilities accepted as part of the practice of the profession. Fidelity is the main support for the concept of accountability, although conflicts in fidelity might arise from obligations owed to different individuals or groups. For example:

A nurse who is just finishing a very busy and tiring 12-hour shift may experience a conflict of fidelity when he is asked by a supervisor to work an additional shift because the hospital is short-staffed. The nurse has to weigh his fidelity to himself against fidelity to the employing institution and against fidelity to the profession and patients to do the best job possible, particularly if he feels that his fatigue would interfere with the performance of those obligations.

> *Fidelity is the main support for the concept of accountability, although conflicts in fidelity might arise from obligations owed to different individuals or groups.*

Beneficence

Beneficence, one of the oldest requirements for health-care providers, views the primary goal of health care as doing good for patients under their care. In general, the term *good* includes more than providing technically competent care for patients. Good care requires that the health-care provider take a holistic approach to the patient, including the patient's beliefs, feelings, and wishes, as well as those of the patient's family and significant others. The difficulty in implementing the principle of beneficence is in determining what exactly is good for another and who can best make the decision about this good.[3]

Consider the case of the man involved in an automobile accident who ran into a metal fence pole. The pole passed through his abdomen. Even after 6 hours of surgery, the surgeon was unable to repair all the damage. The man was not expected to live for more than 12 hours. When the man came back from surgery, he had a nasogastric tube inserted, so the physician ordered that the patient should have nothing by mouth (NPO) to prevent depletion of electrolytes.

Although the man was somewhat confused when he awoke postoperatively, he begged the nurse for a drink of water. He had a fever of 105.7°F. The nurse believed the physician's orders to be absolute and thus repeatedly refused the patient water. He began to yell loudly that he needed a drink of water, but the nurse still refused his requests. At one point, the nurse caught the man attempting to drink water from the ice packs that were being used to lower his fever. This continued for the full 8-hour shift until the man died. Should the nurse have given the dying man a drink of water? Why or why not? Or is it not that simple?

Again, the ethical dilemma in this situation is a conflict of rights and obligations. The patient has a right to self-determination (autonomy) that would certainly include the right to have a drink of water. The nurse has an obligation of beneficence to do good for the patient. The nurse also has an obligation to carry out the physician's orders. However, is withholding water, which is an essential nutrient for life, really doing good for the patient? On the other hand, the nurse is fulfilling the obligation to follow the physician's order, which may be based on the physician's belief that withholding water is good for the patient because giving it will harm the patient in some way or quicken his death. If the nurse believes that the physician is wrong, does the nurse's judgment supersede the physician's?

What would you do? Is there something else the nurse could have done, such as calling to ask the physician to change the order? Are physician's orders always absolute, even when they seem to be causing harm to the patient?

Nonmaleficence

Nonmaleficence is the requirement that health-care providers do no harm to their patients, either intentionally or unintentionally. In a sense, it is the opposite side of the concept of beneficence, and it is difficult to speak of one term without referring to the other. In current health-care practice, the principle of nonmaleficence is often violated in the short term to produce a greater good in the long-term treatment of the patient. For example, a patient may undergo painful and debilitating surgery to remove a cancerous growth to prolong their life.[4]

By extension, the principle of nonmaleficence also requires that health-care providers protect from harm those who cannot protect themselves. This protection from harm is particularly evident in groups such as children, the mentally incompetent, the unconscious, and those who are too weak or debilitated to protect themselves. In fact, very strict regulations have developed around situations involving child abuse and the health-care provider's obligation to report suspected child abuse. (This issue is discussed in more detail in Chapter 7.)

Veracity

Veracity is the principle of truthfulness. It requires the health-care provider to tell the truth and not to intentionally deceive or mislead patients. As with other rights and obligations, limitations to this principle exist. The primary limitation occurs when telling the patient the truth would seriously harm (principle of nonmaleficence) the patient's ability to recover or would produce greater illness. Although the principle of veracity is not a law, it is one of the basic foundations for the trusting relationship between nurse and patient that underlies any successful therapeutic relationship.

A Right to Know

Health-care providers often feel uncomfortable giving a patient bad news, and they hesitate to give patients difficult information regarding their condition. But feeling uncomfortable is not a sufficient reason to avoid telling patients the truth about their diagnosis, treatments, or prognosis. Although veracity is an obligation for nurses, it is a right of patients to know the information about their conditions.

One common situation in which veracity is violated is in the use of placebo medications. At some point during their careers, most health-care providers will observe the placebo effect among some patients. Sometimes, when a patient is given a gel capsule filled with sugar powder and it seems to relieve the pain, the placebo has the same effect as a narcotic but without the side effects or potential for addiction. Of course, if the patient is told that it was just a sugar pill (veracity), it would not have the same effect. How should nurses feel about this practice?[6]

Costly Errors

Another issue that has come into the public eye is the number of deaths caused by medical errors.

Issues in Practice

Ethical Issues During a Pandemic

Regina had wanted to be a nurse since she was a little girl. She had been a volunteer at the local hospital during her high school years and worked as a nursing assistant while getting her BS degree in nursing at the University Hospital School of Nursing. The nurses working in the critical care areas had always fascinated her. She was impressed at their knowledge and skill levels and seeming ability to solve all types of difficult patient care problems.

After finishing nursing school, Regina was hired for the intensive care unit (ICU) at the University Hospital. It was a four-pod ICU with 12 beds in each pod. She learned quickly and obtained all the certifications she could get in the critical areas. By her sixth year working in the ICU, she had become one of the most skilled and knowledgeable nurses on the pod, often being sought for her knowledge by other nurses.

An otherwise healthy 46-year-old man was admitted to the ICU with atypical respiratory symptoms— high fever, cough, loss of sense of smell and taste, and difficulty breathing. His oxygen saturation (PO_2) was low: 85 percent on room air (normal = 90 to 100). After some basic tests, he was diagnosed with pneumonia. Because the physicians were not sure what the causative organism was, the patient was placed on basic respiratory isolation, which required everyone to wear a mask and wash hands when entering his room.

Even on high concentrations of O_2 by mask, the patient's PO_2 kept dropping. His attending physician decided he needed to be intubated with an endotracheal tube and connected to a ventilator. About the time they connected him to the ventilator, two more patients came in with almost identical symptoms. Then several more arrived with the same symptoms. The nurses had not received much information from management about what was going on; however, the news media were beginning to talk about a new type of coronavirus that was highly lethal with an almost 90 percent death rate. One whole pod (12 beds) was now filled with patients with these symptoms. Almost all of these patients were connected to ventilators, which were starting to be in short supply.

Finally, based on information from the Centers for Disease Control and Prevention (CDC), the World Health Organization (WHO), and additional test results, the patients were diagnosed with COVID-19. There was little information about treatment, but the disease was classified as a highly contagious one that required the highest levels of personal protective equipment (PPE) and isolation measures. These measures included shoe covers, liquid-proof gowns, hair covers, and N-95 masks for anyone entering the patient's room. The items were to be discarded immediately after leaving the room, followed by good hand washing. The hospital was quickly running short of PPE as well as ventilators.

Regina knew the reasoning behind these precaution measures and accepted their use, helping other nurses with the physical and psychological limitations imposed by them. When all the ICU pods became full of COVID-19 patients and they began to spill over on to other units, the hospital went to a one-nurse-one-room policy to save on dwindling supplies of PPE. This policy required that just one nurse, called the inside-nurse, enter a patient's room wearing all the required PPE and stay there, except for one break, for the whole shift. That nurse would provide all patient care, including respiratory, phlebotomy, and any other care usually provided by others on the team.

Communication became a major problem, so instead of trying to yell back and forth through closed glass doors while wearing masks, the nurses came up with a plan to use "door-notes." Using erasable markers, they would write to each other on the glass doors. Although writing backwards was tricky, the notes could be erased using paper towels.

(continued)

Issues in Practice (continued)

One shift, Regina was working as the inside-nurse caring for a 72-year-old man who had become unresponsive and had been connected to a ventilator for 2 weeks. She noted that his urine output had dropped to almost zero, indicating kidney failure, and that his skin had become a yellowish-orange color, indicating liver failure. From experience with previous patients, Regina knew this one was going into organ shutdown, and she was pretty certain he would die within a week, even with all the extraordinary treatments he was receiving.

The patient's attending physician tapped on the door and wrote: "How is he doing?" Regina held up the vital sign sheet so that he could see. He shook his head. Then the physician wrote "Take him off the ventilator and connect him to a T-tube at 100% O_2." Regina was confused. She had switched many patients over from ventilators to T-tubes to wean them from ventilators when their conditions were improving. But T-tubes provide no respiratory assistance to the patient. This patient was not improving, and he needed all the respiratory assistance he could get. She wrote back on the window "Why? He will die if I do that!"

Regina knew that the patient would likely be dead within a week anyway, but with only the T-tube, he probably wouldn't last the night. The physician wrote back, "I know, but we need the ventilator for a 29-year-old mother of three who has a good chance for survival."

Regina slowly turned around and looked at the patient she had been caring for on and off for 3 weeks. Like many patients with COVID-19, he didn't have an advance directive. He wasn't married, and as far as could be determined, he had no living relatives. What should she do? Having been brought up in a religious home, Regina felt that following the physician's order would seem like killing this man. Her nursing education had taught her the difference between active and passive euthanasia, and this seemed a lot like active euthanasia, which legally could be equated to homicide. On the other hand, keeping the ventilator from the young woman who had a good chance of living might kill her.

Questions for Thought

• Using the ethical decision-making model (Figure 6.1), work though the steps of the process and make a decision about what Regina should do.
• What are the key ethical principles involved in this situation?
• Are there any statements in the ANA Code of Ethics that may help resolve this dilemma?
• What would be the consequences of refusing the physician's request?

According to 2020 data, the last year available at the time of publication, medical errors caused approximately 120,000 deaths per year and were the third leading cause of death in the United States. Of this number, 4,000 to 7,000 deaths were due to medication errors. Nurses are often involved in these incidents.[7] If a nurse knows that another nurse or physician has made a medical error, what is the nurse's ethical obligation to reveal this information? Some believe that if there is no injury to patients, the error need not be revealed; however, the reporting of errors or near errors has become a quality-control issue in the prevention of medical mistakes. (See Chapter 14 for more details.)

Consider the following case study from the viewpoint of the principle of veracity:

Tisha S, a senior nursing student, was acting as the team leader during her final clinical experience. Jamie D, a close friend of Tisha's, was one of three junior nursing students on Tisha's team that day. Because of some personal problems, Jamie had been late and unprepared for several clinical experiences. She was informed by her instructor that she might fail unless she showed marked improvement during clinical training.

Claire B, a 64-year-old woman with diabetes and possible renal failure, was one of Jamie's

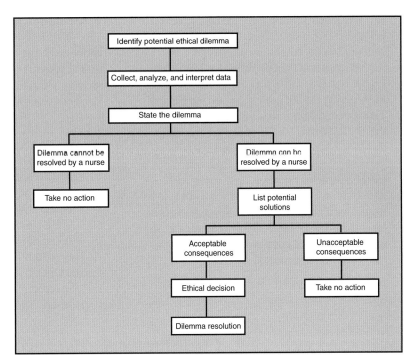

Figure 6.1 Ethical decision-making algorithm. (Adapted with permission from Catalano JT. Ethical decision making in the critical care patient. *Critical Care Nursing Clinics of North America.* 1997;9(1):45–52.)

Issues in Practice

A Question of Distributive Justice

Jessica B was diagnosed with acute lymphocytic leukemia at age 4. She is now 7 years old and has been treated with chemotherapy for the past 3 years with varying degrees of success. She is currently in a state of relapse, and a bone marrow transplant seems to be the only treatment that might improve her condition and save her life. Her father is a day laborer who has no health insurance, so Jessica's health care is being paid for mainly by the Medicaid system of her small state in the Southwest.

The current cost of a bone marrow transplant at the state's central teaching hospital is $1.5 million, representing about half of the state's entire annual Medicaid budget. Although bone marrow transplants are an accepted treatment for leukemia, this therapy offers only a slim chance for a total cure of the disease. The procedure is risky, and there is a chance that it may cause death. The procedure will involve several months of post-transplant treatment and recovery in an intensive care unit far away from the family's home and will require the child to take costly antirejection medications for many years.

The family understands the risks and benefits. They ask the nurse caring for Jessica what they should do.

Questions for Thought

1. How should the nurse respond?
2. Does the nurse have any obligations to the Medicaid system as a whole?

---

patients. Mrs. B was having a 24-hour urine test to help determine her renal function. After the test was completed later that afternoon, she was to be discharged and treated through the renal clinic. Jamie understood the principles of the 24-hour urine test and realized that all the urine for the full 24 hours needed to be saved, but she became busy caring for another patient and accidentally threw away the last specimen before the test ended. She took the specimen container to the laboratory anyway.

At the end of the shift, when Jamie was giving her report to Tisha, she confided that she had thrown away the last urine specimen but begged Tisha not to tell the instructor. This mistake meant that the test would have to be started over again, and Mrs. B would have to spend an extra day in the hospital. Out of friendship, Tisha agreed not to tell the instructor, rationalizing that they had collected almost all the urine and she was going to be treated for renal failure anyway. When the instructor asked Tisha for her final report for the day, she specifically asked if there had been any problems with the 24-hour urine test.

In this case, it is pretty clear that Jamie's and Tisha's obligation to veracity significantly outweighs Tisha's obligation of friendship to Jamie. The reporting of medical errors is important in identifying areas in the system that need to be corrected. In this case, the instructor should have supervised the student more closely.

Standard of Best Interest

Originally designed as a standard of surrogate decision making, the standard of best interest was first used by courts for making end-of-life decisions regarding incompetent patients. Using the standard of best interest requires that a good faith decision is made about what treatments or actions would lead to the best results for the patient after considering all the relevant information. The decision must be made in accordance with ethical and medical standards. This is generally considered a quality-of-life issue and is strongly opposed by groups who advocate for right to life at any cost.

The Patient's Wishes

Standard of best interest describes a type of decision made about a patient's health care when the patient is unable to make the informed decision. The standard of best interest is used on the basis of what health-care providers and the family decide is best for that individual. It is very important to consider the individual patient's expressed wishes, either formally in a written declaration (e.g., a living will) or informally in conversation with family members.

A Designated Person

Individuals can also legally designate a specific person to make health-care decisions for them in case they become unable to make decisions for themselves. The designated person then has what is called durable power of attorney for health care (DPOAHC), or the attorney-in-fact (AIF), which gives the designated person even broader powers in decision making.[8] The person signing the affidavit for the DPOAHC must be mentally competent, and the person acting as the attorney must be over 18 years of age. The Omnibus Budget Reconciliation Act (OBRA) of 1990 made it mandatory for all health-care facilities, such as hospitals, nursing homes, and home health-care agencies, to provide information to patients about the living will and DPOAHC (see Box 6.1 for a DPOAHC affidavit).

In determining what is in the patient's best interest, the DPOAHC, in consultation with medical professionals, should consider:

- the patient's current level of physical, sensory, emotional, and cognitive abilities.
- the level of pain resulting from the patient's disease process, treatments, or termination of the treatment.
- how much loss of dignity and humiliation the patient will experience as a result of the illness and/or treatments.
- the patient's life expectancy and chance for recovery both with and without the treatment.
- all the treatment options available to the patient.
- the risks, side effects, and benefits of each of the treatment options.

The standard of best interest should be based on the principles of beneficence and nonmaleficence.

> *Using the standard of best interest requires that a good faith decision is made about what treatments or actions would lead to the best results for the patient after considering all the relevant information.*

Box 6.1 Sample Affidavit for Durable Power of Attorney for Health Care

State of _____

County of _____

Before me, the undersigned authority, personally appeared (Durable Power of Attorney for Health Care) ("Affiant") who swore or affirmed:

Affiant is the Attorney named in the Durable Power of Attorney executed by _____ ("Principal") on _____, 20__.

   To the best of Affiant's knowledge after diligent search and inquiry:

The Principal is not deceased, has not been adjudicated incapacitated or disabled; and has not revoked, partially or completely terminated, or suspended the Durable Power of Attorney; and

A petition to determine the incapacity of or to appoint a conservator for the Principal is not pending.

   Affiant agrees not to exercise any powers granted by the Durable Power of Attorney if Affiant attains knowledge that it has been revoked, partially or completely terminated, suspended, or is no longer valid because of the death or the adjudication of incapacity of the Principal.

   Pursuant to the provisions of *[state of residence]* CODE ANN. *[insert appropriate legal code number]*, an affidavit executed by the Durable Power of Attorney stating the above is conclusive proof of the nonrevocation or nontermination of the power of attorney.

_____
Affiant

Sworn to and subscribed before me on _____, 20__.

_____
Notary Public

My Commission Expires: _____

Source: T. Takacs, Understanding and using powers of attorney, Takacs McGinnis Elder Care Law, 2017.

Unfortunately, when patients are unable to make decisions for themselves and no DPOAHC has been designated, the resolution of the dilemma can be a unilateral decision made by health-care providers.[8] Health-care providers making a unilateral decision that disregards the patient's wishes implies that the providers alone know what is best for the patient; this is called *paternalism*.

Obligations

Obligations are demands made on an individual, a profession, a society, or a government to fulfill and honor the rights of others. Obligations are often divided into two categories: legal and moral.

Legal Obligations

Legal obligations are those that have become formal statements of law and are enforceable under the law. For

instance, nurses have a legal obligation to provide safe and adequate care for patients assigned to them.

Moral Obligations

Moral obligations are those based on moral or ethical principles that are not enforceable under the law. In most states, for example, no legal obligation exists for a nurse on a vacation trip to stop and help an automobile accident victim.

Rights

Rights are generally defined as something owed to an individual according to just claims, legal guarantees, or moral and ethical principles. Although the term *right* is frequently used in both the legal and ethical systems, its meaning is often blurred in daily use. Individuals sometimes mistakenly claim things as rights that are really privileges, concessions, or

Issues in Practice

The nurse, Karen, is caring for a critically ill patient in the surgical intensive care unit (ICU) after radical neck surgery. The patient is connected to a ventilator and is on a sedation protocol with continuous IV infusion of midazolam (Versed), a powerful sedative that requires constant monitoring and titration to maintain the required level of sedation. During the night shift, the nurse discovers that the medication bag is almost empty, and the pharmacy, which is closed, did not send up another bag. Karen looks the medication up in a drug guide and proceeds to mix the drip herself. The night charge nurse is busy supervising a cardiac arrest situation out of the ICU and is unavailable to double-check how the medication was mixed.

Inadvertently, the nurse mixes a double-strength dose of the medication. Thirty minutes after she hangs the new drip, the patient's blood pressure is 44/20 mm Hg. The patient requires a saline bolus and a dopamine drip to stabilize the blood pressure. The family is notified that the patient has "taken a turn for the worse" and that they should come to the hospital immediately. In backtracking for the cause of the hypotension, the nurse realizes that she has mixed the sedative double strength and reduces the rate by half.

When the family arrives, the patient's blood pressure has started to return to normal. They ask the nurse what happened and why their mother was on the new IV medication.

Questions for Thought
1. Should the family be told about the error?
2. Who should tell them? The nurse? The physician?
3. What approach should be used?
4. What ethical principles are involved in resolving this dilemma?

Source: *T.H. Gallagher, D. Studdert, W. Levinson. (2007). Disclosing harmful medical errors to patients.* New England Journal of Medicine, 356*(26), 2713–2719,* *https://doi.org/10.1056/NEJMra070568*

freedoms. Several classification systems exist in which different types of rights are delineated. Three types of rights—welfare, ethical, and option—include the range of definitions.

Welfare Rights

Welfare rights (also called **legal rights**) are based on a legal entitlement to some good or benefit. These rights are guaranteed by laws (e.g., the **Bill of Rights** of the U.S. Constitution, Amendments to the Constitution), and violation of such rights can be punished under the legal system. For example, citizens of the United States have a right to equal access to housing regardless of race, gender, sexual orientation, or religion. After the *Roe v. Wade* decision in 1973, the right to have an abortion became legally protected under the legal system. Anyone attempting to prevent a woman from having an abortion could be arrested and punished under the law for a human rights violation. In 2022, the U.S. Supreme Court, through its approval of a state law of Florida, effectively reversed *Roe*.[9]

Ethical Rights

Ethical rights (also called **moral rights**) are based on a moral or ethical principle. Ethical rights usually do not need to have the power of law to be enforced. In reality, ethical rights are often privileges allotted to certain individuals or groups of individuals. Over time, popular acceptance of ethical rights can give them the force of a legal right.

An example of an ethical right in the United States is the belief in universal access to health care. In the United States, it is really a long-standing privilege with many citizens left without health care, whereas in many other industrialized countries, such as Canada, Germany, Japan, and England, universal health care is a legal right.

Option Rights

Option rights are rights that are based on a fundamental belief in the dignity and freedom of humans. These are **basic human rights** that are particularly evident in free and democratic countries, such as the

United States, and much less evident in totalitarian and restrictive societies, such as Iran. Option rights give individuals freedom of choice and the right to live their lives as they choose, but within a given set of prescribed boundaries. For example, people may wear whatever clothes they choose, as long as they wear some type of clothing in public.

ETHICS COMMITTEES

Physicians, nurses, and other staff members often encounter ethical conflicts they are unable to resolve on their own. In these cases, the interdisciplinary ethics committee can help the health-care provider resolve the dilemma. An increasing number of health-care facilities, particularly hospitals, have instituted ethics committees that make their consultation services available to health-care providers.

The people who belong to ethics committees vary somewhat from one institution to another, but almost all include a physician, a member of administration, a registered nurse (RN), a clergy person, a philosopher with a background in ethics, a lawyer, and a person from the community. Members of ethics committees should not have any personal agenda they are promoting and should be able to make decisions without prejudice on the basis of the situation and ethical principles.[3]

Depending on the institution, the scope of the ethics committee's duties can range widely, from very limited activity with infrequent meetings on an ad hoc basis to active promotion of ethical thinking and decision making through educational programs. Other common functions of ethics committees include evaluating institutional policies in light of ethical considerations, making recommendations about complex ethical issues, and providing education programs for medical and nursing schools as well as the community. It is extremely important that nurses participate in these committees and that the ethical concerns of the nurses are recognized and addressed.

Although ethics committees usually work in the background, during the peak of the COVID-19 pandemic, they were thrust into the spotlight. Because of a shortage of life-saving equipment, particularly the ventilators that kept critically ill patients breathing, ethics committees sometimes had to make decisions about who would be connected to a ventilator and live and who would not receive one and likely die.[10]

ETHICAL SYSTEMS

An ethical situation exists every time a nurse interacts with a patient in a health-care setting. A system of ethics is a formal method for making decisions about difficult ethical situations. Ethical systems provide the nurse a way to make decisions in resolving questions of how humans interact with each other by defining concepts such as good and evil, right and wrong, and how the nurse should act in certain situations. Nurses continually make ethical decisions in their daily practice, whether or not they recognize it.

> *Over time, popular acceptance of ethical rights can give them the force of a legal right. An example of an ethical right in the United States is the belief in universal access to health care. In the United States, it is really a long-standing privilege. . . .*

Although there are several different areas of ethics, nurses are most likely to encounter normative ethics and applied ethics, particularly where they intersect with bioethical issues. **Normative ethics** deals with practical questions that require a choice between actions. **Applied ethics** helps nurses determine what is permitted or obligated by their legal status as a nurse. These two become **bioethics** when nurses attempt to make decisions concerning a patient's life and death, quality of life, life-sustaining and life-altering technologies, and biological science in general. The two systems that are most directly concerned with ethical decision making in the health-care professions are utilitarianism and deontology. In resolving ethical questions, nurses often use just one of these two systems, or they may use a combination of several ethical systems.[3]

Utilitarianism

Utilitarianism (also called **teleology**, *consequentialism*, or *situation ethics*) is the ethical system of doing what is considered most useful. As a type of normative ethics, utilitarianism defines *good* as happiness or pleasure. This system is associated with two underlying principles: the greatest good for the greatest number and the end justifies the means. Because of these two principles, utilitarianism is sometimes subdivided into rule utilitarianism and act utilitarianism.

Rule Utilitarianism

According to rule utilitarianism, the individual draws on past experiences to formulate internal guidelines that are useful in determining the greatest good. In practice, true followers of utilitarianism do not believe in the validity of any system of rules or guidelines because they believe that the rules can change depending on the circumstances or situations surrounding whatever decision needs to be made.

Act Utilitarianism

With **act utilitarianism**, the particular situation in which a nurse is placed determines the rightness or wrongness of a particular act. Situation ethics is probably the most publicized form of act utilitarianism. Joseph Fletcher, one of the best-known proponents of act utilitarianism, outlines a method of ethical thinking in which the situation itself determines whether the act is morally right or wrong. Fletcher views acts as good to the extent that they promote happiness and bad to the degree that they promote unhappiness.

Abortion, for example, is considered ethical in this system in a situation in which a single mother on welfare with four children unintentionally becomes pregnant a fifth time. The argument can be made that the greatest good and the greatest amount of happiness would be produced by aborting this unwanted pregnancy. An

---

Issues in Practice

When to Tell

A 48-year-old woman was scheduled for a below-the-knee amputation due to complications from diabetes. She was admitted to the preoperative area, signed a number of surgical permits, and was given her preoperative sedative medication. Because patients undergoing this type of surgery usually lose a significant amount of blood, several units of blood had been typed and cross-matched and placed on standby for her. After she was moved to the operating room and anesthetized, the nurse anesthetist rapidly administered the first unit of blood in preparation for the anticipated blood loss during surgery.

The circulating nurse was checking the paperwork before the beginning of the operation and noticed that there was no consent signed for the administration of blood products. In examining the chart further, she noted that "Jehovah's Witness" was written under the Religion section. The Jehovah's Witness religion does not allow blood transfusions or transplantation of any tissue or organs. The circulating nurse told the nurse anesthetist about the patient's religion, and his response was, "Holy cow—I can't believe this is happening!"

The family did not know about the blood transfusion, and obviously the patient, who was under anesthesia, did not know she had received a unit of blood. The nurse anesthetist announced that it was not his fault because he was never told about the patient's religion and was not going to tell the family or patient about the mistake. The circulating nurse felt that because she did not administer the blood, she should not be the one to inform the family. The unit manager was called in, and the consensus was that she should be the one to reveal the information because she was ultimately responsible for what occurred in the surgical unit. Her feeling was that because no physical harm was done to the patient, the whole incident should just be kept quiet.

Questions for Thought

1. Using the ethical decision-making model, work through the decision-making process for this ethical dilemma.
2. What are the key ethical principles involved in this dilemma?
3. What are the possible solutions to the dilemma and their consequences?
4. How would you resolve the dilemma? How would you defend your decision?

abortion would serve the dual purposes of reducing the financial drain on society and possibly allowing the other four children to grow up with more opportunities.

In the system of utilitarianism, the concepts of good, greatest good, and happiness have somewhat fuzzy definitions. Many equate *good* with happiness, but then that brings up the question of how one should define *happiness* (see "What Is Happiness?" for more discussion).

Because utilitarianism is based on the concept that moral rules should not be arbitrary but rather should serve a purpose, ethical decisions derived from a utilitarian framework weigh the effect of alternative actions that influence the overall welfare of present and future populations. As such, this system is oriented toward the good of the population in general and toward the individual in the sense that the individual participates in that population.

Advantages

The major advantage of the utilitarian system of ethical decision making is that many individuals find it easy to use in most situations. Utilitarianism is built around an individual's need for happiness in which the individual has an immediate and vested interest. Another advantage is that utilitarianism fits well into a society that otherwise shuns rules and regulations.

A follower of utilitarianism can justify many decisions on the basis of the happiness principle. Also, its utility orientation fits well into Western society's belief in the work ethic and a behavioristic approach to education, philosophy, and life.

Most recently, examples of the widespread use of utilitarianism in health care came about during the peak of the COVID-19 pandemic. When health care is practiced in a non-pandemic environment, the general philosophy is to try to save everyone. But the COVID-19 pandemic created situations similar to what are found in mass-casualty events, where a triage system is used to make decisions about patients' care and survival. Using emergency triage, decisions are made in the field or emergency department about

who will and who will not receive treatment; the decisions are based on the assessment of who is likely to survive and who is likely to die and the amount of life-saving equipment available. Emergency triage is the ultimate example of utilitarianism in the health-care setting. So many people became critically ill during the pandemic that the business-as-usual model of health care became overwhelmed and normal systems began to break down. In such an out-of-control scenario, the usual ethical assumptions about who should get treated collapsed in the face of scarce medical resources, both equipment and personnel, and the real threat of public disorder. The usual guiding ethical principle that the first to arrive should be the first to receive care gave way to the triage-like principle to save those who are most likely to recover and to save those who are most important to society (the greatest number for the greatest good). Not all health-care providers working the front lines of the pandemic agreed.

However, even during a pandemic, the indispensable duties to respect and care for others and for self does not change. One negative element noted in using the triage method of treatment during the pandemic was that the obligation for justice for minority groups, the poor, and the disadvantaged was violated more often than for everyone else.[10]

> *"Health-care providers making a unilateral decision that disregards the patient's wishes implies that the providers alone know what is best for the patient; this is called paternalism."*

Telling a Sad Truth?

The follower of utilitarianism will support a general prohibition against lying and deceiving because ultimately the results of telling the truth will lead to greater happiness than the results of lying. Yet truth-telling is not an absolute requirement to the follower of utilitarianism. If telling the truth will produce widespread unhappiness for a great number of people and future generations, it would be ethically better to tell a lie that will yield more happiness than to tell a truth that will lead to greater unhappiness.

Although such behavior might appear to be unethical at first glance, the strict follower of act utilitarianism would have little difficulty in arriving at this decision as a logical conclusion of utilitarian ethical thinking.

Disadvantages

Who Decides?

Some serious limitations exist in using utilitarianism as a system of health-care ethics or bioethics. An immediate question is whether *good* and *happiness* refer to the average good and happiness of all or the total good and happiness of a few. Because individual good and happiness are also important, one must consider how to make decisions when the individual's good and happiness conflict with those of the larger group.

More fundamental is the question of what constitutes happiness. Similarly, what constitutes the greatest good for the greatest number? Who determines what is good in the first place? Is it society in general, the government, governmental policy, or the individual? In health-care delivery and the formulation of health-care policy, the general guiding principle often seems to be the greatest good for the greatest number. Yet where do minority groups fit into this system?

Also, the tenet that the ends justify the means has been consistently rejected as a rationale for objectionable actions. It is generally unacceptable to allow any type of action as long as the final goal or purpose is good. For example, the Nazis in the 1930s and 1940s used this aphorism to justify killing 11 million Jews and other minorities in gas chambers and concentration camps. They also justified brutal human experimentations and many other actions that would be viewed by others to be considerably less than good. Minorities rarely fare well under a utilitarian system.

What Is *Good*?

What is good can take different forms. There are things that would seem to be absolutely good, such as life, honesty, health, and justice. People would seek to have as much of these good things as possible. However, the majority of good things—money, pleasure, comfort, relaxation, freedom from fear or pain, and just freedom in general—are more provisional. Doing everything possible to maximize the good of a majority of a society likely compromises the good of some of its members.

As discussed earlier, a classic example of the greatest good for the greatest numbers can be found in emergency situations where there are a large number of victims. The triage system is used to literally choose who receives vital health care and who is merely made comfortable until they die. All nurses are educated in how to use this system during their basic education and quite often are placed in this decision-making role. They are supposed to make decisions on the basis of medical criteria of high-priority victims, who are most likely to survive if given care, and low-priority victims, who will not benefit from care but instead only deplete limited resources needed by others and die anyway. But what decision should the nurse make if the president of the United States is one of the victims who clearly fits the low-priority classification? Or maybe one of the low-priority victims is the nurse's mother or son? Similarly, imagine a nurse comes home from work and finds his house on fire with both his child and grandmother inside. There is time to get only one person out. Which one does he choose?

The other difficulty in determining what is good lies in the attempt to quantify such concepts as *good, harm, benefits*, and *greatest*. This problem becomes especially acute in regard to health-care issues that involve individuals' lives. For example, an elderly family member has been sick for a long time, and that course of illness has placed great financial hardship on the family. It would be ethical under utilitarianism to allow this patient to die or even to euthanize the patient to relieve the financial stress created by the illness.

If the principle is the greatest good for the greatest number, who decides what the greatest good is? Does

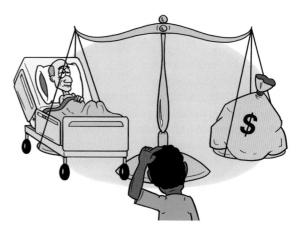

Today's health care attempts to balance costs with patient outcomes.

the greatest number determine it? Or does each individual need to decide?

What Is Happiness?

Some who use the utilitarian ethical system equate good with happiness. But what do they mean by happiness? Fletcher defined *happiness* as the happiness of the greatest number of people, yet the happiness of each person also is to be considered. Other philosophers equate happiness with "subjective well-being" (i.e., how people feel about themselves). The only way to measure it is by asking people to report how satisfied they feel with their own lives and how much positive and negative emotion they are experiencing. The more positive emotions a person is experiencing, the happier the person is. Others define happiness as a virtue, good fortune, pleasure, contentment, joy, pride, or gratitude.

Maslow saw happiness as extraordinary moments, known as peak experiences, profound episodes of love, understanding, or rapture, during which a person feels more whole, alive, self-sufficient, and yet a part of the world. The highest level of self-actualization or what produces real happiness, in Maslow's hierarchy of human needs, is self-centered.[3] Maslow's concept of happiness does not include service to others or the common good unless it somehow enriches the individual.

Utilitarianism as an ethical system is highly self-centered in its focus. As a health-care decision-making process, the greatest good element requires use of an additional principle of distributive justice as an ultimate guiding point. Unfortunately, whenever an unchanging principle is combined with this system, it negates the basic concept of pure utilitarianism.

Pure utilitarianism, although easy to use, does not work well as an ethical system for decision making in health care because of its arbitrary, self-centered nature. In the everyday delivery of health care, utilitarianism is often combined with other types of ethical decision making in the resolution of ethical dilemmas.[10]

> *" Another advantage is that utilitarianism fits well into a society that otherwise shuns rules and regulations. A follower of utilitarianism can justify many decisions on the basis of the happiness principle. "*

Deontology

Deontology is a system of ethical decision making based on moral rules and unchanging principles. It focuses on the relationship between **duty** and the **morality** of human actions. This system is also termed the *formalistic system*, the *principle system of ethics*, or *duty-based ethics*. A follower of a pure form of the deontological system of ethical decision making believes in the ethical absoluteness of principles *regardless of the consequences of the decision*. For example, an active shooter enters a church and starts shooting the church members. The church is named the Right to Life of All God's Creatures, and all the members literally and fundamentally believe in the Seventh Commandment: Thou shalt not kill. They interpret it to mean that they must never kill any living creature, ranging from an ant to a human. One of the members who is standing behind the shooter has access to a heavy candlestick with which he could hit the shooter on the head. For fear that he might kill the shooter, the church member decides not to pick up the candlestick and allows the shooter to kill the entire congregation.

The Categorical Imperative

Strict adherence to an ethical theory in which the moral rightness or wrongness of human actions is considered separately from the consequences is based on a fundamental principle called the *categorical imperative*. It is not the results of the act that make it right or wrong but the principles by reason of which the act is carried out. These fundamental principles are ultimately unchanging and absolute and are derived from the universal values that underlie all major religions. Focusing on a concern for right and wrong in the moral sense is the basic premise of the system. Its goal is the survival of the species and social cooperation.

Unchanging Standards

Deontology is based on the belief that **standards** exist for the ethical choices and judgments made by individuals. These standards are fixed and do not change when the situation changes. Although the number of standards or rules is potentially unlimited, in reality—and particularly in dealing with bioethical issues—many of these principles can be grouped together into a few general principles.

These principles can also be arranged into a type of hierarchy of rules and include such maxims as the following: People should always be treated as ends and never as means; human life has the highest value; one is always to tell the truth; above all in health care, do no harm; humans have a right to self-determination; and all people are of equal value. These principles echo such fundamental documents as the Bill of Rights and the American Hospital Association's Patient's Bill of Rights.

Advantages

The deontological system is useful in making ethical decisions in health care because it holds that an ethical judgment based on principles will be the same in a variety of given similar situations regardless of the time, location, or particular individuals involved. In addition, deontological terminology and concepts are similar to the terms and concepts used by the legal system.

The legal system emphasizes rights, duties, principles, and rules. Significant differences, however, exist between the two. Legal rights and duties are enforceable under the law, whereas ethical rights and duties usually are not. In general, ethical systems are much wider and more inclusive than the system of laws that they underlie. It is difficult to have an ethical perspective on law without having it lead to an interest in making laws that govern health care and nursing practice.

Disadvantages

The deontological system of ethical decision making is not perfect. Some of the more troubling questions include the following: What do you do when the basic guiding principles conflict with each other? What is the source of the principles? Is there ever a situation in which an exception to the rule will apply?

Although various approaches have been proposed to circumvent these limitations, it may be difficult for nurses to resolve situations in which duties and obligations conflict, particularly when the consequences of following a rule end in harm or hurt being done to a patient. In reality, there are probably few pure followers of deontology, because most people will consider the consequences of their actions in the decision-making process.

APPLICATION OF ETHICAL THEORIES

Ethical theories do not provide recipes for resolution of ethical dilemmas. Instead, they provide a framework for decision making that the nurse can apply to a particular ethical situation.

A Framework for Decisions

At times, ethical theories may seem too abstract or general to be of much use to specific ethical situations. Without them, however, ethical decisions may be made without reasoning or forethought and may be based on emotions. Most nurses, in attempting to make ethical decisions, combine the two theories presented here.

> *Ethical theories do not provide recipes for resolution of ethical dilemmas. Instead, they provide a framework for decision making that the nurse can apply to a particular ethical situation.*

What Do You Think?

Identify a situation in which you were faced with an ethical dilemma. Which system of ethical decision making did you use? Why did you select that system?

Nursing Code of Ethics

A code of ethics is generally a written statement or list of the ethical principles that govern a particular profession. Codes of ethics are presented as general statements and thus do not give specific answers to every possible ethical dilemma that might arise. However, these codes do offer guidance to the individual practitioner in making decisions.

A Lengthy Development Process

Although the term *code of ethics* is relatively new to health care, nurses have a long tradition of using ethical principles and basic values to guide the practice of the profession, starting with the writings of Florence Nightingale. Nightingale reflected the values of the society of her time and the place of women in that society. Her writings emphasize the need to follow the physician's orders and the desire that nurses remain pure and inviolate as they carry out their duties in tending for the sick.

The history of the development of the current code of ethics is as follows:

- 1893—Nightingale Pledge: Although the Nightingale Pledge was written by Lystra E. Gretter and a committee at the Farrand Training School for Nurses in Detroit, Michigan, it was still called the Nightingale Pledge in recognition of the founder of modern nursing. The pledge is a statement of the ethics and principles that the nursing profession at that time held as important. It emphasizes keeping the nurse away from immoral and harmful situations and the need to seek out and treat the ill in any setting without regard for their social status (distributive justice). It also included the need to maintain confidentiality.
- 1926—The *American Journal of Nursing* (AJN), the official publication of the ANA, published a document that looked very much like a code of ethics but was not given that name. It was *not* accepted by the ANA as an official document or statement of ethics for nurses.
- 1935—The Nightingale Pledge was revised by adding a statement about nurses needing to help physicians and dedicating their lives "in service of human welfare."
- 1940—The AJN again published a list of statements that could be used to guide the ethical practice of nurses. Still not called a code of ethics, it was adopted by the National League for Nursing as a "statement of ethical principles."
- 1950—The ANA's statement of ethical principles began to look even more like a code of ethics, but it still was not being called a code of ethics. Several revisions were made to include some of the rapid technological development of the postwar period.
- 1960—The statement of ethical principles was revised with an emphasis on the independence of practice for nurses. It still was not being called a code of ethics.

- 1968—The statement of ethical principles was again revised, making a distinction between public and private nursing. It still was not being called a code of ethics.
- 1985—A major revision of the statement of ethical principles was conducted to more accurately reflect the rapid growth in technology and society and to demonstrate that the profession of nursing was also growing to keep pace with the changes. It included statements about the need for all nurses to follow ethical principles, to be aware of bioethical issues, and to acknowledge their social and international responsibilities. Although officially not called a code of ethics, many in the profession began referring to it as such; and after a short time, it was generally accepted as a code of ethics.
- 2001—The ANA Code of Ethics for Nurses was developed from the previous statements of ethical principles. The ANA identified it as a framework for ethical decision making, and it included new statements on patients' rights, focusing on patients' right to self-determination.
- 2011—The ANA approved the need for a new revision to be more reflective of society's changing values. A call was put out for a revision panel.
- 2015—Revisions of the 2011 code were accepted, and it became the current code of ethics (see the current code of ethics at https://www.nursingworld .org/practice-policy/nursing-excellence/ethics/ code-of-ethics-for-nurses/).

A Periodic Review

Ideally, codes of ethics should be reviewed periodically to address changes in values and technological advances in the profession and society as a whole. Although codes of ethics are not judicially enforceable as laws, consistent violations of the code of ethics by a professional in any field may indicate an unwillingness to act in a professional manner and will often result in disciplinary actions that range from reprimands and fines to suspension of licensure.

Clearly Stated Principles

The ANA Code of Ethics has been acknowledged by other health-care professions as one of the most complete. It is sometimes used as the benchmark against which other codes of ethics are measured. Yet a careful reading of this code of ethics reveals only a set of clearly stated principles that the nurse must apply to actual clinical situations. The ANA Code of Ethics is highly deontological in its construction and wording. It provides overarching principles that are almost universally accepted.

For example, the nurse involved in resuscitation will find no specific mention of **no-code orders** (also called *do not resuscitate [DNR]* orders) in the ANA Code of Ethics. Rather, the nurse must be able to apply general statements to the particular situation. For example:

> The nurse . . . practices with compassion and respect for the inherent dignity, worth, and uniqueness of every individual, unrestricted by considerations of social or economic status, personal attributes, or the nature of health-care problems.[5]

> The nurse is responsible and accountable for individual nursing practice and determines the appropriate delegation of tasks consistent with the nurse's obligation to provide optimum patient care.

The ANA Code, 2015

The 2015 Code of Ethics restates and reinforces the basic values and commitments that have been and remain essential to the profession of nursing. Traditional ethical principles such as confidentiality, veracity, justice, beneficence, and autonomy are reemphasized. The nurse is still expected to practice with cooperation, wisdom, compassion, honesty, courage, and respect for the patient's privacy. However, the 2015 code, in response to changing health-care practices, defined the boundaries of duty and loyalty. Ethical challenges, such as cost containment, delegation, and information technology, require nurses to look at health care from new perspectives.

The 2015 code supports nurses in their attempts to upgrade their employment conditions and work environment through measures such as collective bargaining. The 2015 code addresses and supports

nurses who are involved in whistle-blowing when dealing with health-care team members who may be chemically impaired or otherwise incompetent in practice. It also supports nurses in their right to refuse to practice in treatments that violate their beliefs.[10]

The 2015 code also expands nursing duties beyond individual nurse–patient interactions. It recognizes that professional nurses now work in multiple practice areas; therefore, they are responsible for developing and using their knowledge in these expanded areas through research and collaborative practice.

The 2015 code includes elements of the sweeping changes in health care such as the Affordable Care Act and the APRN Consensus Model. The 2015 code is a different type of code from those of the past. It is in electronic form and contains links embedded in the text to references, ethical situations, and other places where nurses can click on hyperlinks to find additional information to help guide their ethical decision making. Visit the ANA's Web site to see the revised code with interpretive statements.

> " *In the fast-paced world of social media, people often "tweet" before they think, which can lead to violations of professional standards and nursing ethics.* "

A GROWING ETHICAL QUANDARY

In the fast-paced world of social media, people often "tweet" before they think, which can lead to violations of professional standards and nursing ethics. Platforms such as Twitter, Instagram, LinkedIn, Facebook, and YouTube can be valuable to nurses in their personal lives. In their professional careers, these tools can improve and speed up communications with the health-care team, relay changes in patients' conditions, and generally improve the quality of health care. However, it is very easy to accidently post inappropriate content.

The ANA Code of Ethics and other standards of practice apply to nurses when they are on social media as well as when they are working in the clinical setting. Because social media is primarily a means of communication, the standard of care that is most applicable is the Health Insurance Portability and

Accountability Act (HIPAA) that deals with breaches of patient privacy and confidentiality. All the HIPAA rules that apply to charting and verbally revealing information to other members of the health-care team or to private individuals also apply to social media.

Violations of HIPAA regulations include, but are not limited to, posting pictures of patients without their permission, sending messages about patients to people not authorized to have the information, making fun of patients or their families, contacting patients or former patients by social media, posting pictures of other employees, posting negative information about the facility or coworkers, accessing personal social media while on duty, advertising through social media, and posting anything offensive. Even attempting to obtain professional advice from a provider about the patient's care or condition without the patient's permission can trigger a HIPAA violation.

Although, strictly speaking, they may not be HIPAA violations, activities such as posting complaints about coworkers, administrators, or facility policies can be considered ethical violations and unprofessional behaviors. Personal posts, depending on content, can be considered unprofessional, particularly **bullying**, unprofessional photos, comments about being at a party where illegal drugs or alcohol are being used, or any type of violence. Once these are posted, they are very difficult or even impossible to remove from the Internet. Anyone can report a nurse for a HIPAA violation or unprofessional behavior, even years after the action took place.

For violations of HIPAA regulations, nurses can be terminated, lose their licenses, receive significant fines, and even be jailed. For both HIPAA violations and unprofessional behavior, nurses will be reported to the board of nursing in their state of practice. Even if the behavior is not a HIPAA violation, unprofessional conduct almost always results in a hearing at the board of nursing, some action on the nurse's license, and termination of employment.

Nurses can help protect themselves by using extreme caution before posting anything on social media. If there is any concern at all that what is going to be posted might violate HIPAA regulations, do not do it! Nurses who are angry should wait at least 24 hours before posting. And always THINK, THINK, and THINK again before posting anything on social media.[11]

THE DECISION-MAKING PROCESS

Nurses, by definition, are problem solvers, and one of the important tools that nurses use is the nursing process. The nursing process is a systematic step-by-step approach to resolving problems that deal with a patient's health and well-being.

Although nurses deal with problems related to the physical or psychological needs of patients, many feel inadequate when dealing with ethical problems associated with patient care. Nurses in any health-care setting can, however, develop the decision-making skills necessary to make sound ethical decisions if they learn and practice using an ethical decision-making process.

Modeling the Nursing Process

An ethical decision-making process provides a method for nurses to answer key questions about ethical dilemmas and to organize their thinking in a more logical and sequential manner. Although there are several ethical decision-making models, the problem-solving method presented here is based on the nursing process. It should be a relatively easy transition from the nursing process used in resolving a patient's physical problems to the ethical decision-making process for the resolution of problems with ethical ramifications.

The chief goal of the ethical decision-making process is to determine right and wrong in situations in which clear demarcations are not readily apparent. This process presupposes that the nurse making the decision knows that a system of ethics exists, knows the content of that ethical system, and knows that the system applies to similar ethical decision-making problems despite multiple variables. In addition to identifying their own values, nurses need an understanding of the possible ethical systems that may be used in making decisions about ethical dilemmas.

The following ethical decision-making process is presented as a tool for resolving ethical dilemmas (Fig. 6.1).

Step 1: Collect, Analyze, and Interpret the Data

Obtain as much information as possible concerning the particular ethical dilemma. Unfortunately, such information is sometimes very limited. Among the important issues are the patient's wishes, the patient's family's wishes, the extent of the physical or emotional problems causing the dilemma, the health-care provider's beliefs about health care, and the nurse's own orientation to issues concerning life and death.

What Do You Think?

Identify a health-care-related ethical situation that is currently in the news. What are the key elements of the dilemma? Discuss how to resolve it with your classmates.

Many nurses, for example, face the question of whether to initiate resuscitation efforts when a terminally ill patient is admitted to the hospital. Health-care providers often leave instructions for the nursing staff indicating that the nurses should not resuscitate the patient but should instead merely go through the motions to make the family feel better, which is sometimes referred to as a **slow-code order**.[12] The nurse's dilemma is whether to make a serious attempt to revive the patient or to let the patient die quietly. Important information that will help the nurse make the decision might include the following:

- The mental competency of the patient to make a no-resuscitation decision
- The patient's desires
- The family's feelings
- Whether the health-care provider previously sought input from the patient and the family
- Whether there is a living will or DPOAHC

Many institutions have policies concerning no-resuscitation orders, and it is wise to consider these during data collection. After collecting information, the nurse needs to bring the pieces of information together in a manner that will give the clearest and sharpest focus to the dilemma. In practice today, written slow-code orders are considered illegal; health-care providers do not write them but may suggest them to the nurse.

Step 2: State the Dilemma

After collecting and analyzing as much information as is available, the nurse needs to state the dilemma as clearly as possible. In this step, it is important to identify whether the problem is one that directly involves the nurse or is one that can be resolved only by the patient, the patient's family, the health-care provider, or the DPOAHC.

Recognizing the key aspects of the dilemma helps focus attention on the important ethical principles. Most of the time, the dilemma can be reduced to a few statements that encompass the key ethical issues. Such ethical issues often involve a question of conflicting rights, obligations, or basic ethical principles.

In the case of a no-resuscitation order, the statement of the dilemma might be "the patient's right to death with dignity versus the nurse's obligation to preserve life and do no harm." In general, the principle that the competent patient's wishes must be followed is unequivocal. If the patient has become unresponsive before expressing his or her wishes, the family members' input must be given serious consideration. Additional questions can arise if the family's wishes conflict with those of the patient.

> *Recognizing the key aspects of the dilemma helps focus attention on the important ethical principles. Most of the time, the dilemma can be reduced to a few statements that encompass the key ethical issues.*

Step 3: Consider the Choices of Action

After stating the dilemma as clearly as possible, the next step is to attempt to list, without consideration of their consequences, all possible courses of action that can be taken to resolve the dilemma. This brainstorming activity may require input from outside sources such as colleagues, supervisors, or even experts in the ethics field. The consequences of the different actions are considered later in this chapter.

Some possible courses of action for the nurse in the resuscitation scenario might include the following:

- Resuscitating the patient to the nurse's fullest capabilities despite what the health-care provider has requested
- Not resuscitating the patient at all
- Only going through the motions without any real attempt to revive the patient
- Seeking another assignment to avoid dealing with the situation
- Reporting the problem to a supervisor
- Attempting to clarify the question with the patient
- Attempting to clarify the question with the family
- Confronting the health-care provider about the question
- Consulting the institution's ethics committee

For nurses who are unsure about which issues can be referred to the ethics committee, the facility's policy and procedure manual can give direction.

Step 4: Analyze the Advantages and Disadvantages of Each Course of Action

Some of the courses of action developed during the previous step are more realistic than others. The identification of these actions becomes readily evident during this step in the decision-making process, when

---

Issues Now

On July 26, 2017, a horrific motor vehicle crash in Utah left William Gray with burns over 50 percent of his body. Gray was hauling a load of sand in northern Utah when a pickup truck speeding away from police crossed the center line and hit his truck head-on, causing an explosion. State police had been trying to pull over the pickup driver after several people called 911 to report he was driving recklessly. Gray was not suspected of wrongdoing.

Gray was brought to the University of Utah Health Center accompanied by police detective Jeff Payne. Gray was unconscious at the Salt Lake City hospital when Nurse Alex Wubbels was asked to draw his blood by Payne several hours after the crash. The pickup driver, Marcos Torres, 26, had died at the scene of the crash, and Utah police routinely collect blood evidence from everyone involved in fatal crashes, particularly looking for any alcohol or drugs in the driver's system.

Nurse Wubbles was now faced with an ethical dilemma. She understood that all patients have the right to self-determination and that it is impossible for an unconscious patient to grant permission. In addition, she knew that the hospital policy required a warrant, patient consent, or consent from a designated decision-maker. On the other hand, she recognized her obligation to follow the directions of an official of the police department. Other nurses had drawn blood in similar situations. Payne said it would help protect Gray from prosecution.

Although Wubbles refused, Payne insisted that she draw the blood or she would be arrested. Wubbles argued that it was not ethical and not in line with hospital policy and quoted the policy to him. Payne became angry and frustrated and forcibly handcuffed her on charges of resisting arrest and failure to comply with the orders of a law officer. She was roughly dragged outside, placed in a police car, and held until her lawyer got her released. Later, all charges against Wubbles were dropped, and Payne was fired from the police department.

Wubbles stated: "We're supposed to be on the same team, and that is to help provide a safe and secure situation for those that can't provide it for themselves," she said. "And [police] are supposed to be a source of help, not the source that tears that down."

Sources: *D. Olsen, The ethical and legal implications of a nurse's arrest in Utah,* American Journal of Nursing, *118(3): 47–53;* Associated Press, *Cop who forcibly arrested nurse for refusing to draw blood is fired,* New York Post, *October 10, 2017, https://nypost.com/2017/10/10/cop-who-forcibly-arrested-nurse-for-refusing-to-draw-blood-is-fired.*

the advantages and the disadvantages of each action are considered in detail. Along with each option, the consequences of taking each course of action must be thoroughly evaluated.

Consider whether initiating a discussion might anger the health-care provider or cause distrust of the nurse involved. Both these responses may reinforce the attitude of the nurse's submission to the health-care provider and could create difficulty in continuing to practice nursing at that institution. The same result may occur if the nurse successfully resuscitates a patient despite orders to the contrary. Failure to resuscitate the patient has the potential to produce a lawsuit unless a clear order for no resuscitation has been given. Presenting the situation to a supervisor may, if the supervisor supports the health-care provider, cause the nurse to be considered a troublemaker and thus have a negative effect on future evaluations. The same process could be applied to the other courses of action.

When considering the advantages and disadvantages, the nurse should be able to narrow the realistic choices of action. Other relevant issues need to be examined when weighing the choices of action. A major factor would be choosing the appropriate code of ethics. The ANA Code of Ethics should be part of many patient-care decisions affected by ethical dilemmas.

Step 5: Make the Decision and Act on It

The most difficult part of the process is actually making the decision, following through with action, and then living with the consequences. Decisions are often made with no follow-through because nurses are fearful of the consequences. By their nature, ethical dilemmas produce differences of opinion, and not everyone will be pleased with the decision.

In the attempt to solve any ethical dilemma, there will always be a question of the correct course of action. The patient's wishes almost always supersede independent decisions on the part of health-care professionals. A collaborative decision made by the patient, health-care provider, nurses, and family about resuscitation is the ideal situation and tends to produce fewer complications in the long-term resolution of such questions.

Step 6: Accept the Consequences of the Decision

It is likely that there may be consequences to the decision you make. In an ethical dilemma, there are always two opposing opinions, and they are usually strongly held by both sides. A resolution that is contrary to the beliefs of a person or group that is powerful or rich will often produce threats such as "I'll have your job" or "I'm going to sue you!"

Conclusion

The nursing profession has a long history of using ethical principles to guide its practice. Although society and society's values change and evolve over time, there are a number of unchanging ethical principles that nurses have been following since the development of modern nursing. These principles include maintaining confidentiality, treating the sick and injured regardless of their state in life, preventing injury, and doing good for patients. In the current era of concern for quality of care and economic responsibility in health care, nurses need to have a clear and comprehensive understanding of ethics and ethical principles. They must also know how to apply those principles in their daily professional setting so that they can practice nursing ethically to the very best of their ability.

By definition, ethical dilemmas are difficult to resolve. Rarely will a nurse find ethical dilemmas covered in policy, procedure, and protocol manuals; but nurses can develop the skills necessary to make appropriate ethical decisions. The key to developing these skills is the recognition and frequent use of an ethical decision-making model and application of the appropriate ethical theories to the dilemma. As an orderly approach in solving the often disorderly aspects of ethical questions encountered in nursing practice, the decision-making model presented in this chapter can be applied to almost every type of ethical dilemma. Although each situation is different, ethical decision making based on ethical theory can provide a potent tool for resolving dilemmas found in patient-care situations.

CRITICAL-THINKING EXERCISES

- Ask the facility where you work or have clinical rotations what code of ethics it uses. How does it differ from the ANA Code of Ethics?
- Ask your faculty what code of ethics is used for your evaluation.
- Compare and contrast ethics with laws by delineating the purposes, scopes, and methods of enforcement of each.
- Distinguish between the two types of obligations.
- Compare the three categories of rights.
- Analyze the following ethical dilemma case study using the ethical decision-making process:
  1. What are the important data in relation to this situation?
  2. State the ethical dilemma in a clear, simple statement.
  3. What are the choices of action, and how do they relate to specific ethical principles?
  4. What are the consequences of these actions?
  5. What decision can be made?

Bill L, a veteran ED nurse, called the resident physician about a patient just admitted to the ED after a fall from a ladder. The patient, a 52-year-old man, had been fixing his roof when the accident occurred. He had suffered a minor head injury, a twisted ankle, and a badly bruised arm. He also had a long history of asthma and heavy smoking. Not long after his admission to the ED, the patient became cyanotic, dyspneic, and semiconscious. By the time the resident physician arrived, the nurse had prepared the patient for endotracheal intubation and had already notified the personnel in the medical intensive care unit (MICU) that they would be receiving this patient.

After a hasty evaluation of the patient, the resident decided to perform an emergency tracheostomy before transporting the patient to the MICU. While performing the tracheostomy, the physician severed a major blood vessel, and the patient hemorrhaged profusely. After several tense minutes, the endotracheal tube was inserted, and the patient was quickly transported to the MICU. The patient remained cyanotic and had great difficulty breathing. Shortly after the patient left the ED, the nurse realized that the oxygen tank connected to the patient was empty. The patient never regained consciousness and died 3 days after admission. His death was due to respiratory failure and not to the injuries sustained in the fall.

When the patient's wife came to the unit to collect the deceased's belongings, the nurse was torn between telling her about the mistakes that were made in the treatment of her husband and remaining silent.

- What are the key ethical principles involved in this situation?
- Are there any statements in the ANA Code of Ethics that may help resolve this dilemma?
- What would be the consequences of informing the patient's wife of the truth?
- What are the consequences of not informing her?

NCLEX-STYLE QUESTIONS

1. What is a similarity between laws and ethics?
   1. They are both enforceable by police authorities.
   2. They are both needed when a group of people live together.
   3. They are both focused on how a society should function.
   4. They are both concerned with the basic survival of a group.

2. _____ are meaningful ideals that are derived from societal norms, religion, and family orientation and serve as the framework for making decisions and taking action in daily life.

3. Gerard, an RN, is caring for Mr. Sweeney, a 75-year-old cancer patient in an infusion center. Mr. Sweeney tells Gerard that he will not continue his chemotherapy after this treatment; he wants to travel during the time that remains. Gerard tells his patient that he (Gerard) will get in trouble with his supervisor if Mr. Sweeney discontinues treatment. Which ethical principle is Gerard violating? **Select all that apply**.
   1. Autonomy
   2. Justice
   3. Fidelity
   4. Beneficence
   5. Nonmaleficence
   6. Veracity

4. Which of the following examples demonstrates the ethical principle of justice?
   1. A med-surg nurse provides an equal amount of an analgesic to each of her patients.
   2. A family practice NP spends an equal amount of time with each patient he sees.
   3. A mother-baby nurse gives all of her patients high-quality care.
   4. A pediatric nurse gives more nursing care to patients whose parents are not able to stay with them.

5. A new nurse observes that a patient's respiratory rate has increased from 16 bpm at the beginning of shift to 28 bpm near the end of shift. The nurse does not know how to interpret this finding, and instead of discussing it with a more experienced colleague, the nurse prepares to leave work. Fifteen minutes later, the patient codes. What ethical principle did the nurse violate?
   1. Justice
   2. Fidelity
   3. Veracity
   4. Nonmaleficence

6. Clinic manager Stacy explains to the providers in her organization that if they stop accepting patients with renal failure, who require complex case management, they can provide primary care services to many more patients. What ethical system underlies Stacy's recommendation?
   1. Utilitarianism
   2. Deontology
   3. Normative ethics
   4. Bioethics

7. Matthew believes absolutely that nurses must do nothing to speed a patient's death. Matthew's hospice patient Mrs. Albright is in severe pain from bone cancer, and her prescribed opioid medication is barely helping. Despite Mrs. Albright's cries for someone to bring her relief or death, Matthew, feeling heartbroken for his patient, administers only the prescribed dose of medication. What type of ethical system is Matthew using to guide his decision making?
   1. Utilitarian
   2. Deontological
   3. Normative
   4. Bioethics

8. Place the steps of the ethical decision-making process in the order they should be done.
   1. State the dilemma.
   2. Collect, analyze, and interpret the data.
   3. Analyze the advantage and disadvantages of each course of action.
   4. Consider the choices of action.
   5. Accept the consequences of the decision.
   6. Make the decision and act on it.

9. Mr. Vazquez has end-stage kidney failure. In his chart, he has a copy of his living will specifying that no heroic live-saving measure be taken and a DNR signed by his physician. Mr. Vazquez codes, and his family members demand that the health-care team begin resuscitation efforts. What is this situation an example of?
   1. Nonmaleficence
   2. Metaethics
   3. An ethical system
   4. An ethical dilemma

10. What should the designated power of attorney and medical professionals consider when determining the best interests of a patient who is unable to make autonomous health-care decisions?
   1. The cost of various treatment options
   2. The patient's life expectancy and chance for recovery with and without treatment
   3. The convenience of the patient's family and friends
   4. The patient's religious affiliation

References

1. The value of ethics in nursing. Arkansas State University, April 4, 2022. https://degree.astate.edu/articles/nursing/value-of-ethics-in-nursing.aspx

2. Carlson K. Nurses and vulnerable populations: Ethics and social justice. Nurses USA, n.d. https://nursesusa.org/article_nurses_and_vulnerable_populations.asp

3. Butts J. *Nursing Ethics: Across the Curriculum and Into Practice.* Burlington, MA: Jones & Bartlett Learning, 2022.

4. What are ethical dilemmas? DRK-Schluechtern, May 2, 2022. https://drk-schluechtern.de/en/questions/what-are-ethical-dilemmas-pdf/

5. American Nurses Association. *Code of Ethics for Nurses With Interpretive Statements.* Silver Spring, MD: American Nurses Association, 2015. https://www.nursingworld.org/practice-policy/nursing-excellence/ethics/code-of-ethics-for-nurses

6. Hanna J. How to ethically harness the power of the placebo effect. MDLinx, April 13, 2022. https://www.mdlinx.com/article/how-to-ethically-harness-the-power-of-the-placebo-effect/7hpXVDVB1jWF8Dr75yC2wC

7. Medical error statistics. My Medical Score, 2020. https://mymedicalscore.com/medical-error-statistics/

8. Durable power of attorney for healthcare. Drugs.com, 2022. https://www.drugs.com/cg/durable-power-of-attorney-for-healthcare-decisions.html

9. Megerian C. What's next for abortion rights after Supreme Court leak? PBS, May 3, 2022. https://www.pbs.org/newshour/politics/whats-next-for-abortion-rights-after-supreme-court-leak

10. Jia Y, Chen O, Xiao Z, Bian J, Jia H. Nurses' ethical challenges caring for people with COVID-19: A qualitative study. *Nursing Ethics*, 28(1):33–45, 2021. https://doi.org/10.1177/0969733020944453

11. 6 HIPAA-regulated entities report email account breaches and the exposure of PHI. *HIPAA Journal*, May 2, 2022. https://www.hipaajournal.com/6-hipaa-regulated-entities-report-email-account-breaches-and-the-exposure-of-phi/

12. Advanced directives vs do not resuscitate orders. Elder Law Care, April 29, 2022. https://www.apracticewithpurpose.com/advance-directives-vs-do-not-resuscitate-orders/

7

Bioethical Issues

Joseph T. Catalano | Sarah T. Catalano

Learning Objectives

After completing this chapter, the reader will be able to:

- Discuss the key health-care ethical principles involved in
  - Abortion
  - Genetic research
  - Fetal tissue research
  - Organ donation and transplantation
  - Use of scarce resources
  - Assisted suicide
  - COVID-19 and vaccinations
  - Children's issues
  - Elder abuse
- Discuss the nurse's role in these ethical dilemmas
- Analyze and make a thoughtful ethical decision in a complex situation

THE CLIENT'S WELL-BEING

In the recent history of nursing, numerous biomedical and ethical **dilemmas** have arisen. Historically, the nursing profession has been acutely aware of and concerned with moral responsibility and ethical decision making. This awareness and concern are reasons that nursing is consistently ranked the most ethical profession in national polls. The nursing code of ethics and its frequent revisions demonstrate the profession's concern with providing ethical health care.

The study of ethics is one of the key fields in philosophy. Ethics has evolved throughout the history of human beings and is still evolving. It directs how humans survive, live, and even thrive in a society. Humans need direction on how they ought to treat each other, how they ought to act, what they ought to do, and the reasons for actions. All humans deal with ethical issues on a daily basis. Every encounter with another person presents a potential ethical situation. Ethical rules not only protect people from harm but also help human societies grow and prosper.

The earliest nursing codes of ethics made obedience to the physician the nurse's primary responsibility. Revisions of the code throughout the years have reflected changes in the values in society and the advancement of technology in health care. The 2001 Code of Ethics for Nurses recognized that the primary responsibility of the nurse was the client's well-being. This change in emphasis reflected the profession's increased self-awareness, independence, and growing accountability for its actions. Unfortunately, this new attitude also heralded an era of increased tension, self-doubt, and ethical confusion for nurses.

The 2015 Code revisions emphasize individual responsibility, patient safety, ethical practice, and high-quality care. The revised Code addresses evolving issues, some of which were not even present in 2001, such as the use of social media, which threatens patient privacy; technologies that are right out of science fiction; emerging levels of nursing professionals and their ability to collaborate with others; social justice issues of universal health care, immigration, and poverty; and the recognition that poor health care in other countries can affect the health status of the United States. By examining the issues and identifying the key moral and ethical conflicts, nurses are able to accept their moral responsibilities and make informed ethical decisions.

In the course of their careers, nurses are likely to encounter any number of ethical dilemmas. Although a complete analysis of every issue is beyond the scope of this book, some common situations and their important ethical features are presented as examples of ways to analyze such dilemmas and to make informed decisions. The resolution of ethical dilemmas is never an easy task, and it is likely that some will disagree with whatever resolution is reached.

USE OF SCARCE RESOURCES IN PROLONGING LIFE

In these days of huge federal budget deficits and attempts to control them by shrinking the health-care budget, money for health care is becoming more difficult to obtain. It is recognized that most public money allocated for health care is spent during the last year of life for many elderly clients. Expensive procedures, therapies, technologies, and care are provided to terminally ill individuals to extend their lives by a few days or even a few hours. It is not unusual to spend as much as $5,000 to $10,000 a day on a terminally ill client receiving care in an intensive care unit (ICU).

Preserving Life at Any Cost

The traditional belief has been that life should be preserved at all costs and by any means available. In fact, many health-care providers feel uncomfortable when cost considerations are mentioned regarding treatments for terminally ill clients. Yet, in the context of current problems in society, such considerations are both economic and ethical realities. The necessity of conserving resources has forced society, through governmental action, to face this issue.

All proposed health-care plans, including the Patient Protection and Affordable Care Act and the Health Care and Education Reconciliation Act of 2010, take into consideration some type of cost-control measures related to restricting payment for client care for all patients, not just terminally ill ones. In addition, the **hospice care** movement and a growing number of physicians and other health-care professionals support **palliative** care for persons with

a terminal illness. Palliative care provides pain relief and comfort measures but does not try to prolong the person's life.

In reality, the American health-care system has been rationing care to some degree for many years. People who are not covered by health insurance often do not seek health care until they are at the point where it will do little good or will be extremely expensive. People receiving Medicaid or Medicare may shy away from seeking health care because of restrictions placed on it. Individuals who are covered by insurance often have limits on how much care their insurance company is willing to pay for.

The Ethics of Tube Feeding

The long-standing controversy over tube feedings periodically comes to public attention when the media become involved in cases such as those of Terri Schiavo, Karen Quinlan, and Nancy Cruzan. Tube feeding is a relatively simple procedure used in all areas of health care, from feeding premature infants in the neonatal intensive care unit to maintaining elderly postoperative clients under the supervision of home health-care staff. In addition, it is a way of maintaining nutrition and hydration, two of the most basic needs of life. Some nurses who work with terminally ill clients may believe that once a feeding tube has been inserted, it cannot be removed for any reason because that would constitute active euthanasia, or mercy killing.[1] But is that belief justified in all circumstances?

Should Care Be Restricted?

The use of public funds for health care is an ethical issue that revolves around the principle of distributive justice. In this context, distributive justice requires that all citizens have equal access to all types of health care, regardless of their income levels, race, gender, religious beliefs, or diagnosis. Many complex issues are involved in this dilemma.[2]

Following are examples of how the United States is already rationing health care:

Preauthorization requirements
Requiring a referral from the patient's primary care
    physician before seeing a specialist
Medication formularies
Step therapy for prescription medications
Restrictive provider networks in HMOs and EPOs

Issues in Practice

Mrs. Ada Floral, who is 82 years old, had just suffered a massive stroke that rendered her unresponsive. Her large family—consisting of her husband of many years, three sons, and two daughters—was very upset. Although she was breathing on her own, she had no voluntary movements and seemed to be completely paralyzed. Magnetic resonance imaging (MRI) showed a large area of bleeding around the midbrain and brain stem. Her pupils were constricted and unresponsive. The physician explained that the prognosis was extremely grave and that the likelihood of Mrs. Floral's survival was minimal.

However, the family members all agreed that "everything" should be done, so the physician reluctantly initiated aggressive medical therapy with IV glucocorticoids, osmotic diuretics, antihypertensives, and physical therapy. After a week, there was no change. The family wondered whether Mrs. Floral might be "starving to death" and asked the physician to have a feeding tube inserted and feedings started.

One month later, the still-unresponsive Mrs. Floral is being cared for at home by her family with the supervision of the local hospice and home health-care program. She is off all IV medications; however, she is receiving some medications, a commercially prepared feeding, and water through the feeding tube. Some of the family members are beginning to question whether they did the right thing by insisting that everything be done, and they wish to remove the feeding tube so that Mrs. Floral can die a peaceful and dignified death. Other family members feel that if they give permission for the tube's removal, they would be killing their mother and could not live with the guilt.

The hospice nurse in charge of the case has discussed the issue with the family. She, too, believes that once a feeding tube has been placed, it should not be removed, even if all the family agrees on its removal. She feels that it is not an issue a family can simply change their minds about. Although she is in frequent contact with Mrs. Floral's health-care provider, she has not mentioned that the family is thinking about removing the feeding tube in fear that the provider might agree.

Questions for Thought
1. Is the hospice nurse correct in her belief about the removal of the feeding tube?
2. When do tube feedings stop being beneficial to clients?
3. What ethical principles could be used for removing the feeding tube in this case?
4. What constitutes a death with dignity?

Waiting lists for organ transplant
Cost sharing
Increasing deductibles
Copayments
Health insurance premiums[2]

These issues go far beyond the questions of who gets what type of care and where and how the care takes place. Although **universal health-care coverage** was not mandated for all Americans by the passage of the Health Care Reform Act, coverage was expanded significantly. By expanding Medicaid health-care coverage to millions of low-income citizens, the Affordable Care Act would allow them to have health coverage with no monthly premium and very low out-of-pocket costs. But some states have refused to expand their Medicaid programs, creating a coverage gap for their poorest residents.[2]

The question remains: Is it fair that some individuals (taxpayers) pay for the health care of others? Should individuals who contribute to their own poor state of health by driving without seatbelts or refusing to exercise be provided with the same type of care as those who do not put themselves at risk? Who is going to make the decisions about who gets expensive treatment such as organ transplantations, experimental medications, placement in ICUs, or life-extending technologies?

The use of criteria such as age, potential for a high-quality life, and availability of resources for determining who receives life-extending technologies is gaining wider acceptance, but is this a valid ethical position? Because nurses are often involved in situations in which terminally ill clients are brought to the hospital for their final hours or days, nurses need to serve an active role in helping formulate policies concerning end-of-life care.

What Do You Think?

Do all U.S. citizens have a right to health care? How can that be achieved? On what ethical principle(s) do you base your position?

GENETICS AND GENETIC RESEARCH

Genetics is the branch of science that studies genes, heredity, and variation in living organisms. Although genetics originally focused on understanding the process of trait inheritance from parents to offspring, the science of genetics is now being used to alter and grow genetic material. Humans have been altering the genetics of plants and animals since the dawn of agriculture. These early gene-altering practices were "natural" in that they required selective breeding of one animal with another or crosspollination of one plant with another. After 1900, the ability to alter genetic material in the laboratory to produce organisms that differ greatly from their original form became more widespread. Scientific and popular literature is filled with reports of new ways to identify and change the genetic material of all types of living creatures. Recently, there has been a surge in interest in using DNA analysis to trace a person's ancestral origins through direct-to-consumer genetic testing. There are also tests by which biogenetic companies can analyze DNA for the presence of 121 potential genetic disorders.

The Future Is Now

Currently, genetically altered bacteria (e.g., *Escherichia coli*) are used to produce various medications, including a purer form of insulin. Genetically altered corn now grows in very hot, dry places and is resistant to most insects. Abnormal genes that indicate individuals who are at risk for various types of cancer, Alzheimer's disease, Parkinson's disease, celiac

disease, bipolar disorder, and others have been identified. Artificial bacteria are produced in the laboratory by chemically generating DNA segments and then assembling them into larger structures. The process is called *homologous recombination* and has been used experimentally for several years to repair damaged chromosomes in yeast. Animal trials are being conducted wherein damaged genes that produce disease are removed and replaced with healthy genes.

Homologous recombination is viewed by scientists as the first step to understanding how life developed on earth and eventually as a way to create designer bacteria that can produce everything from medicines to biofuels. Detractors fear the development of bioweapons that will not have any antidotes and may spread worldwide, devastating the entire population of Earth.

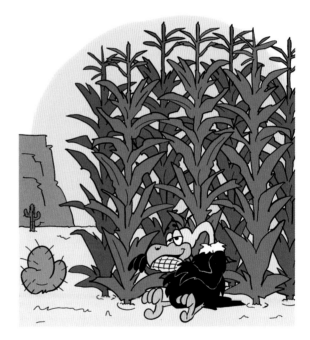

Genetic engineering produces insect and heat-resistant crops.

Gene Replacement (Augmentation) Therapy

Gene replacement therapy in humans has been studied by scientists since 1990. Approved for the first time in the United States in 2017, gene replacement therapy was used to treat a rare, inherited form of vision loss. Genetic diseases are often caused when a gene is altered or missing and the source of an important protein is diminished or absent. Using a new, working gene to replace the function of a non-working or missing gene, gene replacement therapy provides the blueprint for the body to construct the missing or deficient protein that the body needs.

Formed in a laboratory and then packed in a delivery vehicle called a vector, which can be some type of non-infectious virus, the replacement gene is carried by the vector into the nucleus of specific cells. Depending on the vector used, the gene may become part of the cell's RNA or DNA, or it may stay separate. Either way, it starts to make the protein that is missing or in short supply. This type of gene therapy has been used to treat cystic fibrosis and similar disorders. Many experimental gene replacement therapies are currently being investigated in clinical trials.

Gene Addition Therapy

Gene addition therapy, unlike gene replacement therapy, involves adding a brand-new gene to the genetic sequence rather than just replacing a gene that is already there. The therapy begins outside the patient's body, using the patient's own cells, and is given as a one-time treatment. The risk of complications such as rejection and allergic reactions is greatly reduced. The patient's stem cells are harvested in a hospital and then have new genetic information introduced into them using a modified virus. At this point, the modified cells carry functional copies of the appropriate gene. After several doses of high-potency chemotherapy that create space in the bone marrow for the modified cells, the new cells are given to the patient by way of transfusion. Because of severe suppression of the immune system, the patient remains in reverse-isolation in the hospital while transfused cells multiply in the patient's body and produce new cells with the functional gene.[2]

Gene addition therapy is used for more serious diseases such as cancer or heart failure where there are multiple causes for the disease and a single treatment

> " *The use of criteria such as age, potential for a high-quality life, and availability of resources for determining who receives life-extending technologies is gaining wider acceptance, but is this a valid ethical position?* "

modality or correcting one specific mutation is not sufficient to cure the disease. The treatment has also been used when the usual treatment for serious infectious diseases has not been successful. Gene addition therapy adds a new gene into the body that takes aim at the specific underlying causes of the disease.[3]

Gene Inhibition Therapy

Gene inhibition therapy involves the introduction of a gene "stopper" into the body, which halts the production of the disease-causing protein. It corrects the protein's poisonous effect by turning off, or "quieting," a mutated or damaged gene that produces a toxic protein or too much of a protein. It targets mutant messenger RNA (mRNA), similar to the natural process used by the body's immune system to target damaged genetic material and eliminate it. Using gene inhibition requires the delivery of specific genetic material that will prevent the reading of the instructions for the production of the toxic protein and stop its manufacture. When the toxic protein production is reduced or stopped, the disease should end. One of the strategies is the use of clustered regularly inter-spaced short palindromic repeat (CRISPER) genome editing. By using a guide RNA that can precisely identify the DNA or RNA sequence that is producing the toxic protein, the process can be adapted to halt the toxin production.[4]

Suicide (Suicidal) Gene Therapy

Suicide gene therapy is specially designed to treat and, hopefully, cure cancer. This therapy works by allowing the immune system to begin to identify the cancer cells as an invasive foreign protein and forcing cancer cells to self-destruct after being attacked by the patient's own immune cells. Patients are given, by injection or transfusion, a modified genetic material that produces a toxic product or protein that induces a strong immune response against that cell that leads to cell death. In cancer, it is necessary to kill the invasive cell; however, standard chemotherapy drugs damage both healthy and cancerous cells. Suicide gene therapy attacks only the cancer cells, leading to fewer side effects. This therapy delivers genes that convert initially harmless drugs into highly toxic ones, but only within tumor cells. Initially used for treatment of pleural mesothelioma, it has also been shown to be effective with other cancers such as glioma, prostate cancer, and ovarian cancer. In theory, suicide gene therapy could be used for most types of cancer, and research to increase its effectiveness is ongoing.[5]

There is not enough room in this text, nor is it within its scope, to go into greater detail about the rapidly expanding world of genetic therapies. In recent years, volumes have been written on the variations in gene therapy and its uses. Although nurses are not likely to become directly involved in gene therapy research, it is possible that they will be providing care for these patients and even administering genetic medications. Knowledge of basic terminology is a must.

In 21st century society, the belief that scientists should be allowed to do whatever they are capable of doing is so commonly accepted that few questions are asked about the ethics of genetic engineering and research. As with most scientific research and techniques, the techniques of genetic engineering are ethically neutral. Procedures such as refining recombinant DNA, gene therapy, altering germ cells, and cloning other cells are neither good nor bad in themselves. However, the potential for misuse of these procedures is so great that it may permanently alter or even destroy the human species.

Ethics of Genetic Research

Several ethical issues need to be considered when genetic engineering and research are being conducted, including the safety of genetic research, the legality and morality of genetic screening, and the proper use of genetic information. In 2008, the Genetic Information Nondiscrimination Act (GINA) was passed to help guide health-care workers in the use of genetic information and the protections for clients under the law. However, the law has several major limitations and does not protect all clients in all situations. A final rule was issued in 2016 that deals with the amount and type of genetic information that an employer can release to an employee's spouse. Other laws regulating genetic research have been proposed to prevent the production of a supervirus or superbacterium that could exterminate the entire human population.[6]

In 1996, the cloning of Dolly the sheep sent shockwaves through the scientific world. Most ethicists agreed, after considerable discussion, that the act of cloning an animal was probably ethical but had great potential for abuse, especially when used with humans. Jump forward to 2018, and the world was shocked again to find out that a scientist in China had use the CRISPR gene-editing method to alter the DNA of two babies while they were still embryos. Nonidentical twin girls were born from the process, violating many ethical rules established years before limiting or preventing this kind of human DNA editing. Also known as *germline editing*, the altered genetic characteristics implanted into these children can be passed on to their offspring. Almost all ethicists agree that China's experiment was grossly thoughtless, irresponsible, immoral, and illegal. This type of germline editing of genes can potentially be used to create "super soldiers" of the future who are bigger, stronger, and more resistant to injury. As occurs in many fields, experimentation in genetics is turning science fiction into scientific fact.[8]

Mandatory Screening

With current technology, it is possible to detect genetic patterns in newborn infants that are linked to breast and colon cancer, heart disease, Huntington's disease, and Parkinson's disease. Recently, home genetic testing kits that cost as little as $100 have become available. The consumer swabs their mouth and sends the sample to the laboratory specified in the kit. The results are returned in about 3 weeks, and all results are supposed to be confidential; however, in the age of electronic information, *confidentiality* is a nebulous term. The advantage to insurance companies, which may obtain these results or screen individuals as early as infancy for costly and potentially lethal diseases later in life, is obvious: these individuals could be excluded from health and life insurance coverage, thus saving the insurance companies a great deal of money. This practice was made illegal under the Affordable Care Act (ACA), but it is unclear if this restriction will remain if the ACA is repealed.

What Do You Think?

What are your views about genetic research? What restrictions, if any, would you place on this type of research? Are these restrictions plausible or enforceable?

Although this practice is unethical, the concept of mandatory genetic screening is not unrealistic. Because it requires just one blood sample from a person at some point during that person's life, it is possible that this type of screening could be done even without the individual's knowledge or consent with a sample of cord blood at birth.

Informed Consent

Informed consent is permission granted by a person with full knowledge of the risks and benefits of what is being done. The basic questions are these: Do parents violate the right of informed consent if they give permission to have genetic testing performed on their newborn and have the results released to an insurance company? Do insurance companies violate informed consent if they somehow obtain the information without the knowledge of the client? (Informed consent is discussed in detail in Chapter 8.)

Confidentiality

Confidentiality is at great risk of being violated by genetic screening. The confidentiality, trust, and fidelity that exist between the health-care provider and the client have been the basis of the therapeutic relationship since nursing began.

It is possible that individuals may be denied employment because of the results of genetic testing. In this time of the information superhighway and vast computerized databases, very little of a client's health history remains confidential.[8] Do people really know what happens to their DNA samples after they are sent in to trace their ancestors? It is a fairly common practice for companies to sell lists of their customers' names to other companies. Recently, various state and federal law enforcement agencies have compiled DNA databases for identifying criminals.

What is the problem with doing that? Many citizens view using DNA samples to identify criminals as a good thing, regardless of how the samples are obtained. Also, the armed services use DNA to identify fallen service members when there is no other way to identify them. However, the ethical dilemma is this: Is it worth violating many citizens' right to privacy in order to identify a small subset of people who are criminals? What if the government decided to take DNA samples from all newborns and keep them on file just in case that child becomes a criminal or a service member later in life? Is it more ethical to forego a means of positive identification in order to preserve the right to privacy?

Emotional Impact

An important ethical implication for nurses is the emotional impact that genetic information may have on the client. Knowledge of the possible long-term outcome of one's health, particularly if that knowledge is negative, may cause a client **anxiety**, or the person may become depressed or suicidal. Nurses must further hone their teaching and counseling skills to assist clients in dealing with the implications of this type of information. For example, a woman requests genetic testing from her primary care physician to assess her risk for breast cancer. Before ordering laboratory work, the physician discusses the possible results of the test and listens to the woman's concerns. When she learns that she carries the breast-cancer gene, the woman is understandably upset; however, she is also ready to explore options for lowering her risk of actually developing breast cancer.

Obstetric and pediatric nurses have been involved with genetic screening procedures for years. Some of the most important information obtained from prenatal testing deals with the genetic composition of the fetus. Typically, genetic testing of a fetus is not conducted unless one of the routine prenatal screening tests suggests an anomaly. It is important that the mother understand how the test will be conducted, the type of information it may yield, and any risks involved to herself or the fetus. Only then can she give informed consent for this procedure. Sometimes genetic abnormalities are not revealed until after a baby is born. Pediatric nurse practitioners may observe abnormalities in the infant during follow-up well-child examinations that indicate a genetic defect. These children are then referred to a genetic clinic for testing.

> *" The confidentiality, trust, and fidelity that exist between the health-care provider and the client have been the basis of the therapeutic relationship since nursing began. "*

Self-Determination

Nurses have a strict ethical obligation to refuse to participate in mandatory, involuntary screening programs and are strictly prohibited from revealing genetic test results to unauthorized individuals. Forcing testing on clients who are strongly opposed to finding out information about their genetic status is clearly a breach of those clients' right to self-determination. However, as much as the current practice of routine screening for tuberculosis, hepatitis, and blood lead levels promotes the general health of the population, so does screening for genetic diseases. Clients can and should be educated about the benefits of genetic testing, but those who are strongly opposed to such genetic screening must be allowed the option to refuse it to maintain their right to self-determination.

Promise or Threat?

Now that the human genome has been decoded, a whole new world of possibilities—both positive and negative—has been opened for health-care providers. The impact of the Human Genome Project, cloning research, and related genetic procedures is on par with the discovery of bacteria and antibiotics. The potential now exists for the cure of almost all known diseases, ranging from viral infections to cancer to the regeneration of spinal cord nerves.

On the other side of the issue, there is the potential for the development of superviruses that could wipe out our entire population. Even without human intervention in its genetics, the COVID-19 virus killed more than 1 million people in the United States, despite the development of effective vaccines. Nurses need to inform themselves about developments in genetic research and call their governmental representatives when they believe science is moving into dangerous areas.[9]

The Human Genome Project was expanded in 2013 to include decoding the genetic sequence of a great ape. The purpose is to examine the genetic structure of these animals, which are about 98 percent identical genetically to humans, to see if there is a possibility of using animal DNA to repair or replace human DNA. There have also been attempts to alter animal DNA by inserting human DNA fragments into it so that the animal organs would not be rejected if transplanted into a human. This research is ongoing at a rapid pace, and many believe it may hold the cure for cancer and many other diseases that currently stump scientists and health-care providers.

Abortion

Abortion is the termination of pregnancy before the fetus becomes viable. With the advances in neonatal care and technology, some babies born as early as 24 weeks can survive and eventually leave the hospital. Abortions that occur spontaneously—that is, without any outside intervention—are called *miscarriages* before 20 weeks and *stillbirths* after 20 weeks. When the termination of the pregnancy occurs due to outside intervention, it is called an *induced abortion*. An elective abortion is an induced abortion that is performed when the woman elects not to continue the pregnancy.

> *" The potential now exists for the cure of almost all known diseases, ranging from viral infections to cancer to the regeneration of spinal cord nerves. "*

A Polarizing Issue

Few issues evoke as strong an emotional reaction as abortion. Because of abortion's religious, ethical, social, and legal implications, nearly everyone has an opinion about it, and there seems to be little middle ground. Many people either support a woman's right to choose or oppose abortion completely. Others would allow abortion in limited cases, such as when a pregnancy results from rape or incest, when the fetus has a defect incompatible with life outside the womb, or when continuing the pregnancy would endanger the life of the mother. In politics, abortion has become a central issue, and the outcomes of some elections may well be decided by the candidates' positions on the law that supports the practice.

What Do You Think?

Do you support or reject the practice of elective abortion? Or do you favor some middle ground? On what ethical principles do you base your belief?

A Woman's Right to Choose

Elective abortion is the voluntary termination of a pregnancy before 24 weeks of gestation. An elective abortion may be either therapeutic or self-selected. A therapeutic abortion is one performed in consultation with and on the recommendation of a psychiatrist or other physician, based on the conclusion that the woman's health or psychological state would be damaged otherwise.

Self-selected abortions are those performed solely at the request of the woman. In the case of *Roe v. Wade* in 1973, the Supreme Court made elective abortion legal in the United States, but the ethical basis and moral status of this decision remain controversial. A careful reading of the court's decision in *Roe v. Wade* reveals that the justices made no decision about the ethics or morality of elective abortion. Rather, the court said that, according to the U.S. Constitution, all people have a right to determine what they can do with their bodies (i.e., the right to self-determination) and that such a right includes termination of a pregnancy.

Over the past several years, a number of states enacted laws that, while not outlawing abortion, created so many obstacles to obtaining one that the effect is virtually the same. Women from these states who want to have an abortion must travel to other states where the laws are less restrictive.

The constitutionality of stricter state abortion laws was further tested when in 2022 the U.S. Supreme Court upheld Mississippi's ban on abortion after 15 weeks of gestation in the case of *Dobbs v. Jackson Women's Health Organization*. The arguments discussed neither the morality or ethics involved nor the central premise of *Roe v. Wade* that a woman has a right to determine what she can do with her own body. Rather, the decision merely upheld the principle that states have a right to make their own laws. However, there was a broader ripple effect across the nation that allowed other states to immediately enact their own restrictions on abortion. The Supreme Court's draft decision to overturn *Roe v. Wade* was leaked several weeks before the Court announced its decision. At that time, up to 27 states had already passed "trigger laws" that would automatically ban or severely limit abortion in the event that *Roe* was overturned. The end result of this decision is a patchwork of abortion-restricting laws that vary among states.

Women's organizations throughout the country protested the decision with little effect.[10]

Only a minority of Americans wanted *Roe* overturned. In 2022, a poll conducted by the Associated Press-NORC Center for Public Affairs Research showed that 57 percent of Americans believed abortion should be legal in all or most cases.[10]

A Conflict of Rights?

The fundamental issues at the heart of the abortion debate center on the question of when life begins and the right of freedom of choice. Those who argue against abortion believe that life begins at the moment of conception and therefore hold that abortion is an act of killing. Proponents of women's right to choose argue that the fetus is not fully human until it reaches the point of development when it can live outside the mother's body (i.e., the age of viability, about 24 weeks). From a deontological standpoint, abortion represents a basic conflict of rights. On one hand, a woman's rights to privacy, self-determination, and freedom of choice are at issue. In the United States, these rights are fiercely held and are considered to be issues of **public policy** and **constitutional law**. These rights form the basis of the *Roe v. Wade* decision.

The other side of the abortion dilemma is the fetus's right to life. In most Western civilizations, particularly those that are based on Judeo-Christian beliefs, the casual and intentional taking of a human life is strongly prohibited. Life is the most basic good because without it there can be no other rights. In general, the right to life is considered to be the most profound of the rights and is absolute in most situations.

When attempting to resolve the ethics and morality of abortion, these two conflicting rights need to be weighed against each other. Nurses may care for clients who are making decisions about having an abortion. They may sometimes be asked to participate in the procedure itself. What is the nurse to do?

Where Your Values Fit In

In practice, ethical issues are always affected by the health-care provider's moral values. In the dilemma over abortion, nurses must analyze their own values and perceptions of their roles to make the best decisions. As human beings, nurses are entitled to their personal opinions about a woman's right to choose and are free to believe whatever they wish. However, professional nursing ethics requires nurses to be care-givers and advocates for their clients. What impact do nurses' personal beliefs have on their ability to care and advocate for clients? How can a nurse avoid influencing a woman's decision about abortion? Can a nurse ethically and legally refuse to assist with abortions? Should the client's reason for wanting an abortion, how she became pregnant (e.g., birth-control failure, rape, incest), or her stage of pregnancy (i.e., first or second trimester or later) have any influence on the nurse's decision?

The 2022 Supreme Court decision to override the 1973 constitutional decision of *Roe v. Wade* by appealing to the states' rights doctrine added another layer to the decision-making process. In the states with strict antichoice laws, the act of having an abortion or participating in the procedure is now illegal. Nurses who aid in the abortion procedure can be fined or even imprisoned if caught, even if their ethical decision supports a woman's self-determination.[10]

These questions are not easily answered, but examining the underlying ethical principles—autonomy, beneficence, nonmaleficence—involved in the issue may help defuse some of the emotional impact that often surrounds this topic. As in all complicated ethical dilemmas, the nurse needs to remember that the client must receive competent, high-quality care regardless of the nurse's personal values or moral **beliefs**.

> *In practice, ethical issues are always affected by the health-care provider's moral values. In the dilemma over abortion, nurses must analyze their own values and perceptions of their roles to make the best decisions.*

USE OF FETAL TISSUE

Fetal tissue is markedly different from mature tissue in that it is in an early formative period of development. Fetal cells have unique properties that cannot be replaced by mature cell types. Advantages of these cells include little or no specialization, quicker reproduction, and less resistance to new environments, which reduces rejection issues.

Fetal tissue research first started in the 1930s and has been conducted ever since. Traditional fetal tissue research was generally limited to taking living cells from aborted fetuses and transplanting them into people who have chronic or severe diseases. The development of vaccines, including the vaccines for polio, rubella, measles, chickenpox, adenovirus, and rabies, has been a result of fetal tissue research. More recently, this research has shown that the Zika virus can cross the mother-placenta barrier, and it has been used to develop and test vaccines for treating diseases such as influenza, dengue fever, HIV/AIDS, and hepatitis B and C. Ongoing research using cells derived from fetal tissue includes work on neurodegenerative diseases such as Parkinson's, Alzheimer's, and amyotrophic lateral sclerosis (ALS), as well as spinal cord injury, stroke, retinal disease, rheumatoid arthritis, cystic fibrosis, hemophilia, and age-related macular degeneration. The fetal or stem cells that are currently being used in some vaccination production are replicated from cells that are many generations in the past. Although some people objected to the COVID-19 vaccination because it contained material from aborted fetal cells, none of the current vaccines use that process in their production.[11]

Growing Tissue on Demand

In the late 1990s, fetal tissue research was another hot-button issue with right-to-life proponents. Laws have been passed and revised many times, almost since the research began, that alternately restrict and broaden research. The fact is that fetal tissue research has always been an ethically controversial issue, which makes for passionate arguments on both sides. Many states have current laws restricting the use of fetal tissue, although they vary from highly restrictive to moderately permissive.[11]

Artificial Conception

From 1997 to 2000, the Human Genome Project added a new twist to this research. Rather than using tissue from aborted fetuses, scientists are now growing their own fetal tissue in the laboratory through **artificial insemination** and in vitro fertilization procedures. These test-tube fetuses are then dissected. Various fetal tissues are used for genetic and other types of research. The legal system became aware of the potential abuses of these procedures and has passed legislation to control their use, including limiting the age of in vitro fetuses to 6 weeks. After 6 weeks, such fetuses have to be destroyed.

Stem Cell Research

Stem cell research is a closely related issue. Stem cells are the very early cells present in the developing fetus that have not yet begun to differentiate—that is, all the cells are identical and contain all the genetic material needed to reproduce an individual identical to the fetus. Stem cells can be stored for up to 23 years. When used, they are separated and then placed in an environment where they will form more stem cells; the genetic material from the stem cell can be removed and replaced, or the genetic material can be removed, manipulated, and then replaced. Recent federal administrative acts have lifted many of the restrictions put in place by the George W. Bush administration. However, the types of government-funded research that can be conducted are still tightly restricted. There are no restrictions on privately funded stem cell research.[12]

For a number of years, research in stem cell technology has demonstrated that umbilical cord blood contains significant levels of stem cells. Because the placenta and umbilical cord are discarded after a baby is born, this source of stem cells would seem to lack the ethical implications of in vitro fertilization and embryonic research, which require the destruction of embryos. However, several ethical questions to consider are the following: Who owns the placenta and umbilical cord after the baby is born? Does the mother own it? Should she receive payment for it? Is it the baby's? Or is it just considered medical waste, like a tumor that has been removed?

> *Some diseases currently being treated with adult stem cell therapy include osteoarthritis, rheumatoid arthritis, multiple sclerosis, other autoimmune diseases, leukemias and hematopoietic diseases, peripheral vascular disease, diabetes, heart failure, and other degenerative disorders.*

Adult stem cell research has yielded a new source of stem cells without the ethical issues that swirl around fetal stem cells. Bone marrow, fat, and peripheral blood can provide a source of stem cells in adults; however, unlike fetal stem cells that can produce a whole new person, adult stem cells can produce only certain tissues. After the stem cells have been extracted, they are sent to the laboratory where they are examined for quality and then processed before being returned to the patient. Adult stem cells found in bone marrow or fat lack differentiation and have the ability to grow into different types of cells, including nerve cells, liver cells, heart cells, and cartilage cells. They also have the characteristic of "homing," which allows them to move to areas of damaged tissues by themselves and repair the damage. Some diseases currently being treated with adult stem cell therapy include osteoarthritis, rheumatoid arthritis, multiple sclerosis, other autoimmune diseases, leukemias and hematopoietic diseases, peripheral vascular disease, diabetes, heart failure, and other degenerative disorders. All stem cell therapies currently are considered experimental.[12]

The Source of the Material

Even a superficial consideration of these procedures necessarily raises many important ethical issues. The source of the genetic research material is basic to the ethics of this type of research. In the past, much of the material came from elective abortions.

Potential for Abuse

Because of the immaturity and lack of differentiation of cells during the first trimester of pregnancy, the best fetal tissue comes from fetuses aborted during the second trimester. Most scientists agree that second-trimester fetuses have well-developed nervous, cardiovascular, gastrointestinal, and renal systems and are capable of feeling pain. Even though fetal tissue research has not led to an increase in abortions, the potential for abuse exists.

Paying for Fetuses?

Another consideration is whether fetal tissue research scientists are behaving ethically if they pay others to collect and send them aborted fetuses. If payment is being made for aborted fetuses, it would seem to violate both the laws that prevent payment for organs used in transplantation and the moral respect for humanity. Questions also arise concerning who is giving permission for the use of these aborted fetuses. Does anyone really "own" them?[11]

In Vitro Fertilization

Another important ethical issue concerns the use of in vitro fertilization (IVF) as a source for fetal tissue. Many religious groups question the morality of IVF itself. Even if IVF is considered ethical for procedures such as surrogate motherhood, is it ethical to create fetuses that are going to be used only for research and transplantation? From whom are the ova and sperm coming? Have these donors given permission for such use of their tissues? What, if any, rights belong to a fetus that is created in a test tube and will never be viable?

The Nurse's Role

The 1988 directive, which was extended indefinitely in 1990 to prevent the Department of Health and Human Services from using federal money for fetal tissue research, was amended in 2001 to allow this type of research on a very limited basis with federal funding. This regulation was reinforced by the Obama administration in 2009. Local biomedical ethical panels can make decisions about this type of research. Many of these panels, which consist mainly of research scientists, have ruled in favor of continuing research.

Nurses have an important role in issues involving fetal tissue research. Nurses who are employed in facilities where elective abortions are performed must become aware of the issues involved in fetal tissue research. They also should know where the aborted fetuses are taken and how they are disposed of.

Nurses should remain informed about developing procedures and techniques regarding fetal tissue research; they should support legal and ethical efforts to control its abuses.

CORD-BLOOD BANKING

The potential use of the stem cells present in umbilical cord blood to treat disease has been steadily gaining public awareness and acceptance since the late 1990s. It is worth noting that embryonic (pluripotent) stem cells come from fetal tissue, whereas cord blood supplies hematopoietic stem cells. Umbilical cord stem cells reside in the umbilical cords of newborn babies. Human umbilical cord tissue (HUCT) stem cells, like all postnatal cells, are considered to be "adult" stem cells. These stem cells are responsible for the development of red blood cells, white blood cells, and platelets, thereby making cord blood a viable treatment option for blood and immune system diseases, cancers, and congenital defects.[13]

> *The American Academy of Pediatrics advises against private cord-blood storage unless there is a family history of specific genetic diseases.*

Nurses caring for clients who are soon-to-be parents may encounter questions regarding cord-blood banking, and it is important to remember there are two options to present to parents. Public cord-blood banks accept donations that can be used for anyone in need. For the most part, public cord-blood banking is accepted by the general medical community, provided the entities involved follow the stringent guidelines set in place to allow the donated cord blood to be added to a public **registry**. The National Marrow Donor Program maintains a list of public regional cord-blood banks on its website.[13] It is important to note that most public cord-blood banks do not charge processing or storage fees, and once cord blood is donated to a public bank, the family has no way to access the unit should it be needed again in the future.

Another option families have is a private cord-blood bank, which can store the donated blood with a link to the donor so that the unit can be accessed again if it is needed. Private banks charge processing and storage fees as well as "biological insurance" premiums, so it is important to note that choosing to store cord blood in a private bank is a personal decision best made by both parents.[5] In addition, many private cord-blood banks use coercive marketing campaigns designed to play on the fears of expectant parents.

Like transplantable human tissues, corneas, and bone, cord blood and cord-blood banks are regulated by the Food and Drug Administration (FDA)'s Code of Federal Regulations under Title 21, Section 1271. All cord-blood banks, both public and private, must comply with strict testing, storage, processing, and preservation guidelines.

Ethics in Cord-Blood Banking

The medical community has varying opinions regarding cord-blood banking; however, the general consensus is that public cord-blood banking, because of its altruistic nature and low cost to the donors, is more widely accepted than private cord-blood banking.[13] In fact, the American Academy of Pediatrics advises against private cord-blood storage unless there is a family history of specific genetic diseases.[6] Generally, autologous (self-to-self) transplants are discouraged because autologous cord-blood samples may not be able to effectively treat some diseases. For example, if a child develops leukemia, it is possible cells containing the same defect also would be present in the autologous transplant. In cases where a disease develops, the donated sample may not be enough to treat the disease. Private banks will store samples, but it is estimated that up to 75 percent of all cord-blood samples do not contain enough stem cells to treat a small child.[13]

Nurses should encourage parents interested in cord-blood banking to read the fine print before signing any contracts regarding processing and storage of their infant's cord blood. The contracts of many of the largest cord-blood banks contain ambiguities that allow future uses of the cord blood that are not explicitly approved by the donor and the parents and do not provide the donors with reasonable ownership privileges.[13]

ORGAN TRANSPLANTATION

Despite widespread public and medical acceptance of organ transplantation as a highly beneficial procedure, ethical questions still remain. Whenever a human organ is transplanted, many people are involved, including the donor, the donor's family, medical and nursing personnel, and the recipient and recipient's family. Transplantation is one of the few health-care fields in which actions taken by a group of medical professionals in one part of the country affect their counterparts in another part of the country.

Society as a whole is affected by organ transplantation, mainly because of the high cost of the procedures, which usually are covered by federal funding from taxes or reimbursement from private insurance, which in turn increases insurance premiums. Whether it is presented in a national news program, a popular medically oriented television series, or a movie where organ donation is the primary focus, organ donation has more exposure now than in decades past. Also on the increase is the illegal purchase of organs on the black market.[14] This popular exposure increases awareness of the need for organ donation and calls attention to people or groups of people who are affected by every aspect of donation and transplantation. Each one of these persons or groups has rights that may directly conflict with the rights of others.

> *Whenever a human organ is transplanted, many people are involved, including the donor, the donor's family, the medical and nursing personnel, and the recipient and recipient's family.*

The Good of the Donor

Currently, the three primary sources for organ and tissue donations are living related donors; living unrelated donors; and deceased donors, formerly called **cadaver donors**. Transplantation centers and organizations involved in obtaining organs and tissues have developed complex procedures to cope with the ethical and legal issues involved in transplantation. Despite these efforts, some ethical uncertainties still surround the issue of organ transplantation.

When the Donor Is a Child

Living pediatric organ donors exemplify a particularly sensitive issue. For example, when one sibling donates a kidney to another sibling, the procedure poses some serious risk for both donor and recipient. Parents are required to give consent for medical procedures for their children. By legal definition, a child younger than 18 years of age cannot give informed consent to such a procedure. However, it can be argued that ethically the donor child, as a participant, should have input in making such a decision. At what age should a child have a say in the decision? Can a child be forced, for example, to donate a kidney even if they refuse? (See the discussion of children's ethics later in this chapter.)

One situation that illustrates this dilemma is that of a teenage girl who developed leukemia. The only way to save her life was to find a bone marrow donor who matched her genetic type. When no donor could be found, the parents decided to have another baby in the hope that the bone marrow of the second child would match that of the first child. After the baby was born, it was found that the bone marrow did indeed match, and when the child was old enough to donate safely, the bone marrow was taken from the younger child and transplanted into the older child. In Pennsylvania, a 10-year-old girl with pulmonary hypertension needed a bilateral lung transplant and was being kept off the adult transplant list due to the Under 12 Rule. This rule states that children under 12 years of age cannot be placed on the adult transplant list. The case was referred to a judge to decide whether the rule should be waived in this particular situation.

> *" Transplantation centers and organizations involved in obtaining organs and tissues have developed complex procedures to cope with the ethical and legal issues involved in transplantation. "*

The judge placed an **injunction** against the Under 12 Rule and allowed the child to be placed on the adult transplant list in addition to the child list. This ruling allowed for the exception to be immediately applied to 12 other children. Ultimately, the Under 12 Rule was lifted by organ procurement and transplant networks. Hospital transplant teams can now seek permission from these networks to list a patient age 11 years or younger, who meets certain criteria, on the child and adult waiting lists for donor lungs.

What Do You Think?

How would you have decided this case if you were the judge? If you decided in favor of the children, where does distributive justice fit in? Should adults be allowed to be on the child lung transplant list also? Give a rationale for your decision.

When Does Death Occur?

Despite the best efforts of the medical and legal communities to establish criteria for death, some ethical questions still linger about what constitutes death. Because organs for transplantation such as the heart, lungs, and liver should ideally come from a donor whose heart is still beating, some clinicians fear that there will be a tendency for physicians to declare a person dead before death actually occurs. Many people also mistakenly believe that if they indicate they would like to be organ donors and become sick or injured and admitted to the hospital, physicians will not work as hard to save their lives.

The most commonly used criterion for determining death in deceased donors is death by neurological criteria, formerly called **brain death**.[15] The definition of death by neurological criteria in conjunction with organ donation is very clear, and health-care professionals use proven procedures to test for and determine death by neurological criteria. Because death by neurological criteria is defined by the complete cessation of function of the brain stem, brain death can be declared even when an electroencephalogram (EEG) shows continued cortical brain activity.

Brain death is not a coma or persistent vegetative state because both of these still have brain stem activity. Brain death must be determined by one or more physicians who are *not* associated with the transplant team or a potential organ recipient. Some causes of brain death include but are not limited to severe head trauma such as a gunshot wound, automobile accident injury, or severe blow to the head; a cerebrovascular incident such as a ruptured aneurism or arteriovenous malformation; long-term anoxia of the brain from drowning, choking, or cardiac arrest; blood clots in the vascular system of the brain or tumors that cut off the blood supply to the brain. Some researchers and health-care professionals struggle with the perceived ramifications of this determination of death. Should some other criteria be examined in conjunction with the neurological criteria for death?[15]

Since 2006, the use of organs from non-heart-beating donors who have suffered a cardiac arrest, also known as donation after cardiac death (DCD), has become more readily accepted by the transplantation community as a viable alternative to narrowing the donation gap. It is interesting to note that after the heart has stopped beating, the brain continues to function for 4 to 6 minutes, so strictly speaking, these patients are not brain dead. DCD organ donation has its own set of ethical and legal considerations. Typically, only kidneys are recovered and transplanted from a DCD donor. However, with the advent of new technologies and procedures, progressive transplantation programs have been successfully transplanting DCD livers and lungs.[15]

Selecting the Recipient

One of the most difficult ethical issues involved in organ transplantation is the selection of recipients. Because far fewer organs are available than the numerous people who need them, the potential ethical dilemmas are great. To give some perspective of the disparity of need versus availability, as of May 2022, 106,043 people were listed on the transplant waiting list, whereas only 40,000 organ transplants were performed in the previous 12 months. On average, 17 people die each day in the United States waiting for an organ transplant, and one donor can save eight lives.[16]

Legislating Donation

The **Uniform Anatomical Gift Act**, passed in 1968, made the donation of organs, eyes, and tissue for transplantation a legal transaction involving a pre-specified recipient. Later legislation prohibited pre-specification of recipients by creating a federal entity to regulate the transplantation industry and made the sale of human organs illegal. This legislation, the National Organ Transplant Act, created the United Network for Organ Sharing (UNOS) to regulate organ allocation and maintain the national organ transplant waiting list. UNOS created a database of all people wait-listed for an organ and listed potential recipients using a prioritized computerized algorithm designed to ensure each recipient will benefit the most from a transplant. Transplant professionals create match-run lists for organ allocation based on the database and algorithm when a donor organ becomes available.[16]

In addition, each organ has its own requirements for allocation, and a match-run list for transplantation is generated according to the individual allocation policies for each organ. Important criteria for ranking potential recipients include stage of disease process, length of time spent waiting, tissue and blood type compatibility, size matching, and geographic proximity to the donor. The UNOS allocation policy is designed to provide organs for clients who have the greatest need as well as the best projected outcome for a successful transplantation. Despite widespread public beliefs, the amount of money a potential recipient has or the amount of publicity generated by a recipient and their family does not have any bearing on the way organs are allocated.

> *Important criteria for ranking potential recipients include stage of disease process, length of time spent waiting, tissue and blood type compatibility, size matching, and geographic proximity to the donor.*

Forty-eight states have passed first-person consent (or donor designation) laws, with the remaining states in the development stage. These laws are strictly upheld by local organ recovery agencies.[16] However, not all states have identical laws, and obtaining a donation from a person who is not in the state where they died can be difficult. Federal legislation known as the revised Uniform Anatomical Gift Act (UAGA) was designed to ensure the donor's wishes are honored at the time of death. This piece of legislation has created a myriad of ethical and legal issues, but all transplantation organizations agree that not accepting the donation from a medically suitable donor is a violation of this law. In addition, failure to honor client wishes, in this case the donor's, may result in a risk management issue for the hospital in question. Recent revisions of the UAGA have strengthened the law to make the donor's wishes override all opposition and have given permission for organ procurement professionals to proceed with donation in the face of disapproving family members, many of whom threaten litigation. A position paper from the National Organization for Transplant Professionals states, "From an ethical perspective, not accepting the donor's gift is a violation of their autonomy and a disregard for their wishes to help those in need."[17]

At least 25 countries in Europe have gone to an opt-out, or presumed consent, model for obtaining organ donations. With this system, all people, upon death, are presumed to be an organ donor unless they have indicated that they do not want to be a donor. In these countries, the organ donation rate has exceeded 90 percent, whereas in the United States, the rate struggles to reach 15 percent. Several states, such as Texas, Connecticut, and New York, have considered passing presumed-consent-for-donation laws, but the legislatures seem reluctant to move forward without federal support, which so far has not been strong.[17]

The Nurse's Responsibility

All states have passed laws requiring health-care workers to refer all potential organ donors to the local organization responsible for organ recovery. One important function of nurses in the organ donation process is to recognize and refer potential donors to the local organ procurement organization. Referral rates of potential organ donors within hospitals are tracked and reported to agencies such as The Joint Commission and the Centers for Medicare and Medicaid Services. Many nurses, particularly those who work in emergency departments and critical-care units, care for clients who are potential organ donors. Such nurses should note that the referral of a client to the organ procurement organization for evaluation should not be viewed in any way as giving up on the client.

Organ donation professionals do not become involved in care of the client until after death has been declared by a physician or other designated health-care professional. Nurses should not hesitate to make a referral for fear that it is too soon or not appropriate. A referral is simply a notification of a client who meets or may meet criteria for organ donation. It is up to organ recovery professionals to determine whether the client is medically suitable for donation and to facilitate the donation process.

When Should I Refer?

Although the exact requirements for referral vary by geographical service area, in general, clients meeting the following criteria should always be referred to the local organ procurement organization for evaluation for organ donation:

- Severe neurological insult or injury (i.e., hemorrhagic stroke, ruptured aneurism, head trauma such as from gunshot wounds or motor vehicle accidents, and anoxic brain injury resulting from significant cardiac downtime)
- Glasgow Coma Scale score of 4 or less
- Intubated (on a ventilator) with a heartbeat
- When brain death evaluation is scheduled
- Before terminal extubation of a client meeting any of the above criteria[17]

> *One important function nurses perform in the organ donation process is to recognize and refer potential donors to the local organ procurement organization.*

Nurses are involved in all stages of organ recovery and transplantation. Operating room nurses may help in surgical procedures to recover organs from a deceased donor and prepare the organs for transport and eventual transplantation into a recipient's body. Other nurses provide the postoperative care for clients who have received a transplant. Home health-care nurses give the follow-up care to such clients at home. Many organ recovery agencies also train nurses to maintain the potential for organ donation in their clients and to deal with family members of potential donors in a compassionate, professional manner.

Obtain Permission Gently

On the other side, the families of potential organ donors are usually distraught about the sudden and traumatic loss of a loved one. They are vulnerable to psychological manipulation. The emotionally fragile state of a trauma victim's family members predisposes them to feelings of guilt and grief. Health-care providers should avoid appealing to these emotions or becoming coercive when obtaining permission for organ donation. Providers are welcome, in appropriate situations, to discuss donation with a potential donor's family. However, discussing organ, tissue, and eye donation and obtaining consent for these activities is generally best left to professionals who work exclusively for organ procurement organizations and have had training in communicating with distraught patients. They are specially trained, have time to spend with the families, and can make the organ donation process a positive experience for both the donor's family and the health-care professionals involved.

Nurses should avoid making statements or giving nonverbal indications of their approval or disapproval of potential recipients. Generally, neither the donor nor the family plays any part in selecting a recipient, and the identity of the recipient is carefully guarded by organ recovery professionals.

At times, organ recovery professionals can facilitate a process called *directed donation* whereby a donor's family can indicate a particular recipient. Whether this process is successful depends on several factors, including geographical proximity, tissue and blood type compatibility, and whether the potential recipient is listed and has completed all the prerequisite tests to receive the organ. In cases in which directed donation is desired but not possible, the donated organs are allocated according to UNOS policy.[18]

> *Generally, neither the donor nor the family plays any part in selecting a recipient, and the identity of the recipient is carefully guarded by organ recovery professionals.*

Vascular Composite Allographs

Vascular composite allograph (VCA), also called composite tissue allotransplantation (CTA), is a category of transplantable tissues such as skin, blood vessels, muscles, nerves, bone, and connective tissue. Although organ donation is done within a clinical setting, tissue and eye retrieval can take place in such venues as hospital morgues, funeral homes, and specialized recovery suites anywhere from 12 to 24 hours after cardiac death has occurred. Many families are approached regarding tissue and eye donation after they have left the hospital, if a death has occurred in a hospital, or on the arrival of the decedent's body at the funeral home. Recovery of donated tissue and corneas takes place in a sterile setting, and recovered tissues are often shipped to processors for storage and later dispersal.

Tissue and eye donation differs from organ donation in several respects. First, donated human tissue is regulated by the FDA as a medical implant or device and is subject to stringent quality-control guidelines. Donated tissue undergoes rigorous testing before implantation to ensure the safety of the recipients. Tissue recovered from one cadaver can potentially be implanted in up to 2,500 recipients, so testing for biohazards and infectious disease is of the utmost priority in tissue recovery and dispersal.

Second, recovered tissue typically does not have a predetermined recipient waiting on the other end for a transplant. Donated tissue, particularly bone, can be processed and stored for up to 10 years after recovery. Two exceptions to this rule are donated corneas, which can be transplanted up to 12 hours after recovery, and heart valves, particularly those recovered from children. Heart valves from pediatric donors go to pediatric recipients because heart valves must be implanted in a recipient heart of similar size.

Vascular Composite Allographs Expanded

Bohdan Pomahač, a Czech plastic surgeon who has performed four face transplants at Boston's Brigham and Women's Hospital, has said, "There's [almost] nothing [about the human body] that could not be replaced by transplantation."[19] As of 2022, more than 40 face transplants had been performed, 86 percent of which were successful.[20] As of 2022, more than 120 successful hand and 100 uterine transplants had been conducted worldwide.[21] There would likely have been more, but the COVID-19 pandemic severely restricted elective surgeries in 2020 and 2021. For many years, there was little or no regulation of these types of transplants. However, in 2014, the U.S. government announced that VCAs—which include penises, uteruses, hands, faces, and limbs—would be categorized and treated just like the transplantation of any other tissue and regulated by the FDA.

There are a number of ethical issues involved with VCAs. Signing a general consent to donate or indicating it on a driver's license does not give blanket permission to obtain any and all body parts. Generally, special permission is required of the donor or the donor's designated spokesperson. A bigger question is how to maintain allocation procedures and waiting lists for these less-commonly transplanted body parts. Currently, waiting lists for faces, hands, feet, and other body parts tend to be localized and a direct donation from one person to another. But it is not too much of a stretch to believe that these types of procedures can go nationwide in the near future.

A third ethical factor is the cost because none of these body-part transplants are covered by insurance. A hand, foot, or penis transplant costs $500,000 to $600,000 plus a lifetime follow-up cost of antirejection medications of another $500,000. A face transplant runs more than a million dollars. These costs are currently being absorbed by the large hospitals where the surgeries are performed under the heading of research and publicity. Facilities may try to recoup these costs in the form of higher room fees and other hospital-associated costs. The early follow-up research on VCA patients has shown that their life expectancy may be shortened by as much as 25 years due to the high doses of antirejection medication they must take.[20]

Discussions between UNOS and multiple federal agencies started in 2020 but failed to develop any new regulations for transplantable tissues. However, in 2023, the Biden administration presented a plan to break up UNOS and modernize the system to shorten patient waiting times, address racial inequities, and reduce the number of usable organs wasted because of slow processes. The plan also seeks funding to develop genetically altered animals to develop organs and tissues that are human compatible. This plan would provide more competition, increase transparency of the process, and reduce the death rate of patients waiting for organs. Tissue and limb transplants are also addressed in the new plan.[21]

The government regulates kidney, heart, and other organ transplants with waiting lists. What's next? Face and hand transplant waiting lists? The nationwide system is intended to match and distribute body parts and ensure donor testing to prevent deadly infections. It is a big step toward expanding access to these radical operations—especially for wounded troops returning home. More than 1,500 troops have lost an arm or leg in Afghanistan and other wars.[22] Transplantation of body parts may be one solution to these types of injuries.

"These body parts are starting to become more mainstream, if you will, than they were 5 or 10 years ago when they were first pioneered in this country," said Dr. James Bowman, medical director of the Health Resources and Services Administration, the government agency that regulates organ transplants.[22]

New Body Parts From a Test Tube?

New experimental technologies are aimed at replacing humans as a source of organs for transplantation. In most cases, use of animal tissues and organs is not currently a viable option. The protein structures of animal organs are so different from that of humans that the human immune system identifies them as a foreign substance and tries to destroy (reject) them as it would a bacterium or virus. Advances in decoding and understanding the animal genome have the potential to alter animal DNA so that it much more closely matches human DNA and therefore would not be rejected.

Scientists have grown a range of body structures that have been successfully tested in animals. For a number of years, researchers have been "growing" human tissues and organs in the laboratory. Skin cells harvested from a person are placed in a special growth medium in a dish and will, within a few days or weeks, grow a new layer of skin. This process is currently being used for burn victims to grow new skin that is grafted onto third-degree burn areas of their bodies. Because the source of the skin is from the victims themselves, the DNA is a perfect match with no chance of rejection.

The porcine, or pig, genome is very similar to the human genome, and in January 2022, a pig heart was transplanted into a 57-year-old man who could not receive a human heart due to his poor physical condition. He survived for only 2 months because the pig heart contained the porcine cytomegalovirus, which was undetected before the procedure. Due to the high doses of immunosuppressive medications the man was on, the virus could not be repressed.[23]

Research continues on the use of pig tissues for human transplantation through alteration of the genetic structure of the tissues to render them even more similar to human tissue. Pigs are being used to grow human organs in a two-stage process. CRISPR gene editing is used in the first stage to identify and remove a gene from a human organ. The second stage involves combining human stem cells that can develop into any organ with the CRISPR gene and then injecting the genetic combination into the pig embryo. The embryo is then implanted into a sow (female pig). The theory is that a human organ would grow inside the pig embryo and later be removed and implanted in a human who needs it. However, animal-rights groups as well as a few religious groups have ethical objections to this process for using human stem cells in this way and for using pigs as biological incubators for human organs.[23]

Scientists have been able to grow human ears on the backs of mice that were implanted with cells from a human donor ear. Researchers have also recently been able to grow miniature human organs, known as *organoids*, that are being used to study human organ function and structure at its earliest stages of development. Some of the tissues that have been cultivated include fallopian tube, brain, cardiac, nephron, alveolus, and hepatic cells. This research uses both stem cells and cells from developed human organs. Scientists have not yet been able to grow full-sized organs that could be used for transplant, but can that development be far off?[23] Again, animal-rights groups as well as a few religious groups object on the ethical grounds of using human stem cells in this way and of using mice to incubate human organs because the process usually kills the mice.

Bioprinting

The newest health-care technology comes from the world of electronics. Available on the market today are 3D printers. Also known as *additive manufacturing*, **3D printing** is a process of making a copy of a three-dimensional solid object of almost any shape or form from a digital model on a computer. In normal printing, a layer of ink is deposited on paper. In the 3D printing process, layers of material are laid on top of each other until a replica of the computerized shape is "printed." To print a shape, the 3D printer reads the design from the computer and then lays down successive layers of liquid, powder, paper, or sheet material to build the form in a series of cross-sectional layers. The process is currently being used in architecture, construction, and industrial design and in the automotive, aerospace, military, and engineering industries. It has also been used to fashion jewelry, eyewear, educational material, and geographic information systems. The most common material used in the printing process is a form of plastic polymer, although other materials can be used if in the right form for the printer.

In the health-care industry, some items already being used in surgical procedures and dentistry are being manufactured by the 3D printing process. However, the race to "print" human tissues and organs has already left the starting line. The major problem of how to print acceptable human tissue using the 3D printer's layering process (**bioprinting**) is the "ink." Dumping a glob of cells into a printer cartridge and squirting them through tiny nozzles onto a page is highly impractical. Two Swedish scientists took on this challenge and, in 2016, developed a substance called *Cellink*, which is also the name of the company that manufactures it. It is the first standardized bioink, and it is manufactured primarily from a material called *nanocellulose alginate*, which is extracted in part from seaweed.[24]

The bioprinting process starts by using a computer program to make a virtual representation of the organ or tissue to be reproduced, and then a printer builds it layer by layer. In some organs, a pre-prepared scaffold or skeleton may be required to maintain the organ's structure until it is finished, when it may or may not be removed. However, one major problem researchers encountered after developing a usable ink was the printer itself. Injection of the ink through tiny nozzles damaged cells and did not work. An American company developed a laser that deposits cells one by one, at a rate of 10,000 cells per second, without any damage to the cells. This machine is similar to an inkjet printer and works by successively layering microdrops of cells on a surface. It has been given the name *4D bioprinting*, with the fourth dimension being time. The laser-assisted bioprinting technology can print an organ one cell at a time. This process allows scientists to control the interaction between the cells and their environment to print tissues with the biological properties they want.

A new technology called *bioprinting-on-chip* is a method for constructing scaffolds, or frameworks, on which new tissues can grow. Organ-on-a-chip models that duplicate the structural, microenvironmental, and physiological activities of human organs are input into a computer that controls the bioprinter. Bioprinting has been able to create organ-on-a-chip models that allow for the building of a microenvironment with any number of 3D forms ranging from soft tissues like skin to hard organs like kidneys. However, there are limitations in the bioprinter's ability to replicate human tissue and organs. The soft scaffolds produced by 3D printing are problematic in growth and manipulation when implanted into animals.[24]

Until now, only small patches of tissue and parts of lung, liver, and heart tissue have been printed, at great cost. The pioneers in this field believe that whole organs that are suitable for transplant will be available in 10 years. One wonders if someday scientists will attempt to print an entire human being. However, once this problem is solved, there will be no more ethical or legal issues involved in obtaining organs for transplant.[24] Or would there?

THE RIGHT TO DIE

The right-to-die issue is an extension of the right to self-determination issue discussed in Chapter 8. It also overlaps with the issues of **euthanasia** and assisted suicide. Health-care providers often become involved in the end-of-life decision-making process when clients are irreversibly comatose, vegetative, or suffering from a terminal disease. The choices that the families of such clients face are either death or the extension of life using painful and expensive treatments.[25]

What Is Extraordinary?

One of the difficulties in resolving right-to-die issues is understanding the terminology used. Often, clients who have living wills state that they want no extraordinary treatments if they should become comatose or unable to make decisions involving health care. But what constitutes extraordinary treatments? A general definition of ordinary treatments includes any medications, procedures, surgeries, or technologies that offer the client some hope of benefit without causing excessive pain or suffering.

By this definition, extraordinary treatments (sometimes called *heroic measures*) are those treatments, medications, surgeries, and technologies that offer little hope for curing or improving the client's condition. Although these general definitions provide some guidelines for making decisions about ordinary and extraordinary treatments, discerning the nature of the specific modalities remains difficult.

Ventilation

For example, a ventilator is a machine that assists a client's breathing. In ICUs, it is a common mode of treatment for many types of clients, including postoperative clients, clients with cardiac and respiratory diseases, and victims of trauma. During the peak of the COVID-19 pandemic, ventilators became one of the single-most effective modes of treatment to keep the most severely ill patients alive. Prior to the pandemic, ventilators were almost always restricted to ICUs where highly trained nurses cared for the patients connected to them. However, during the pandemic, patients who were infected with COVID-19 and were on ventilators were moved to other areas of the hospital and cared for by non-ICU nurses.[26] Does the ventilator's widespread and frequent use make it an ordinary mode of treatment? Many would say yes, whereas others would say it is still extraordinary because of its invasive nature and complicated technology.

> *In reality, the American health-care system has been rationing care to some degree for many years.*

Cardiopulmonary Resuscitation

Another issue often included in the right-to-die debate is that of codes and do not resuscitate (DNR) or allow natural death (AND) orders, depending on the part of the country or the physician's preference. Cardiopulmonary resuscitation (CPR) is widely taught to both health-care providers and the general public. It is often used to treat clients who have suffered heart attacks and gone into cardiac arrest as well as clients suffering from electrical shock, drowning, and traumatic injuries.

With the widespread dissemination of **automated external defibrillators (AEDs)**, high-level hospital care has been brought to the street. An AED is a portable, easy-to-use medical device that sends an electric shock through the chest wall to the heart of a victim who has no pulse. It is used primarily to stop an irregular heart rhythm (dysrhythmia), which may facilitate the restoration of a normal cardiac rhythm. It can also restart a heart that has stopped from a condition called sudden cardiac arrest (SCA). The AED literally "talks" the user through the steps so that just about anyone can use it. Its use, however, presumes that the victim does not have a DNR in place and does wish to be resuscitated. Little has been said about the ethics involved in AED use.[27]

In the hospital setting, the nursing staff is obligated to perform CPR on all clients who do not have a specific DNR order. This obligation can lead to situations in which terminally ill clients may be subjected to CPR efforts on several different occasions before it no longer is effective and they die.

Advance Directives

As an issue of self-determination, it is essential that the client's wishes about health care be followed. All client communication to the nurse about desires for future care should be documented. If possible, the client should be encouraged to designate an individual to act as a moral surrogate—a designated decision-maker—should the client become unable to make their own decisions. The expressed desires about future medical care are known as *advance directives*. They are the best means to guarantee that a client's wishes will be honored.

A Formal Document

Advance directives, in the form of a living will or durable power of attorney for health care (DPOAHC), can and should specify which extraordinary procedures, surgeries, medications, or treatments can or cannot be used. These directives are often formal documents that need to be witnessed by two individuals who are not related to the client (Box 7.1). Living wills are also known as *personal directives* or *advance decisions*. A number of websites have been developed that allow the person who wants an advance directive to merely fill in the blanks on the computer and print it in a few minutes.[27]

As useful as advance directives are in helping clients decide on future care, clients often are unable to anticipate all the possible types of treatments that are available and could become necessary. For example, an elderly client with a long history of cardiovascular disease specified in his living will that he did not want CPR performed and did not want a ventilator. When his heart developed a potentially lethal dysrhythmia that rendered him unresponsive, his physician decided to use electrical cardioversion because this mode of treatment was not specifically forbidden by the client's living will. Strictly speaking, the physician did not violate the letter of the living will, but did he violate its spirit? Similarly, would the administration of a potent and potentially dangerous IV antidysrhythmic medication be in violation of the client's living will?

Box 7.1 Checklist for Evaluating a Client's Living Will Document

1. Statement of intention: The document was written freely when the client was competent.
2. Statement of when the document goes into effect: Usually when the client is no longer able to make own decisions.
3. Section specifying general health-care measures to be excluded from care.
4. Open section for specific measures (ventilators, pacemakers, etc.) and any other specific instructions concerning care.
5. Proxy statement (sometimes called *durable power of attorney*): Optional, but a strong addition. Allows another person to make decisions in situations not anticipated in the living will. (Check your state law concerning details of proxy selection.)
6. Substitute proxy: Optional. Specifies who can make decisions if first-choice proxy is not available.
7. Legal statement that the proxy or proxies may make decisions.
8. Witness selection statement: Many states require that witnesses not be related to or members of the health-care team.
9. Signature and date: Document must be signed and dated by the client. Some states have very specific regulations concerning how long the will is valid. It may range from a few months to 5 years.
10. Legal signatures of witnesses (required).
11. Notary seal, if required by state law. State laws differ on notary seal requirement. It is usually required if a proxy is selected.

A Legal Requirement

Advance directives, which include living wills, are now a required part of the health care of all clients. The Omnibus Budget Reconciliation Act of 1990 requires that all hospitals, nursing-care facilities, home health-care agencies, and caregivers ask clients about advance directives and provide information concerning living wills and DPOAHC to help clients make informed health-care decisions.[28] However, the federal law mandates only the requirements and not the directives to implement the law. The actual implementation of the law is left to the individual states. Because of the law's vagueness, a great deal of confusion exists, particularly with regard to living wills.

In 2017, House Bill 410 (Protecting Life Until Natural Death) was passed by the U.S. Congress. This bill amends the Omnibus Budget Reconciliation Act of 1990 (title XVIII [Medicare] of the Social Security Act) to exclude from Medicare coverage advanced-planning services, with the exception of certain hospice-related services that may include advising on end-of-life or advance care planning. Under this bill, hospitals that receive federal funds (almost all of them) no longer have to talk to patients about advance directives.[29]

Nurses serve an important role in ensuring that clients understand the implications of their choices pertaining to decisions that may prolong their lives during medical emergencies. Because of their front-line position as caregivers within the health-care system, nurses must understand this role, specifically as it pertains to living wills.

Ethical Difficulties of Living Wills

In 2009, Barack Obama became the first U.S. president to announce publicly that he had a living will, and he encouraged others to obtain their own living wills. His announcement followed widespread misunderstanding of a provision in the ACA that proposed reimbursement for health-care-provider time spent in talking to clients about advance directives. (See Chapter 19 for more detail about the ACA.)

> ❝ *The expressed desires about future medical care are known as advance directives. They are the best means to guarantee that a client's wishes will be honored.* ❞

What Did the Client Know?

Although a living will seems to be a simple solution to a complex care situation, nurses need to understand some ethical difficulties are inherent in its use. Primary among these ethical difficulties is the question of the client's level of knowledge of potential and future health-care problems at the time the will was formulated. Because living wills are often formulated long before they are used, there may later be serious questions about how informed the person was about the disease states and treatment modalities that might later affect care. If there is any indication that the person did not understand the full implications of future therapies or potential medical problems, the validity of the living will is in question.

In addition, living wills reflect a client's condition at a particular time during their life. Almost everyone knows or has heard about a person who was very near death and yet survived and went on to live a normal life. As life situations change, living wills need to be updated to ensure that the actions taken by health-care providers are the actions the client really wishes.

A Moral Conflict

A second ethical difficulty for nurses encompasses the principles of beneficence and nonmaleficence. The principle of beneficence states that a health-care professional's primary duty is to benefit or do good for the client. The principle of nonmaleficence states that health-care providers should protect the client from harm. It is sometimes difficult to determine whether the primary duty is to produce benefit or prevent harm.

When evaluated from the beneficence and nonmaleficence viewpoints, living wills seem to violate the principle of providing benefit to the client. This perception makes many health-care providers ethically uncomfortable. In some situations, the implementation of a living will might actually involve the termination of some modes of treatments already in use. Termination of treatments would seem to constitute harm to the client.

Issues in Practice

In their practice, nurses may encounter elderly clients who function independently at home and have not officially or legally been declared incompetent but whose behavior might indicate that they are unable to make rational decisions about their care. Consider the following situation:

A 74-year-old client, Buster Mack, had been a long-haul truck driver for most of his life and was still driving his big rig into his 60s. He had been in relatively good health until 5 years earlier, when he was diagnosed with lung cancer. A lobectomy was performed at that time, and he was treated with follow-up radiation and chemotherapy, but the cancer had slowly metastasized to the bone. His current hospitalization was because of a syncopal episode witnessed by a neighbor in the front yard of Mr. Mack's home, where he lives by himself.

During the admission assessment, the nurse observed that Mr. Mack had trouble focusing on the questions, and often the answer was unrelated to the question or in the form of a long rambling account of something that happened many years ago. Although he knew he was in a hospital (he could not remember the name), he had no idea where it was or what the date was. His demeanor was cooperative and pleasant, and he laughed easily when the nurse joked with him. He could not remember whether he had any family left living, although the name and address of a son in a distant city were listed on the old records.

Mr. Mack signed all the admission papers and consent forms placed in front of him for a number of neurological tests. His health-care provider was fearful that the cancer might have spread to his brain and wanted to do an MRI, spinal tap, and brain scan. The MRI and brain scan showed a small tumor in an area of the brain where it could be removed rather easily. Mr. Mack's provider, in consultation with a neurosurgeon, felt that an immediate craniotomy with removal of the tumor was required. After explaining the procedure to Mr. Mack, the surgeon placed the consent-to-operate form on his over-the-bed table and gave him a pen. He promptly signed and gave it back.

Later that day, during her shift assessment, the nurse checked on Mr. Mack. The neighbor who had found him unconscious was visiting at the time. When the nurse asked Mr. Mack whether he was ready for the surgery scheduled for the next morning, he had a blank look on his face. On further questioning, the nurse concluded that Mr. Mack had no idea what was going to happen to him the next day. The neighbor, who helped Mr. Mack with his bills and other paperwork at home, stated, "He'll pretty much sign anything that you put in front of him." At this point the nurse felt that Mr. Mack was incapable of making an informed decision about the craniotomy.

The nurse called both the primary health-care provider and the neurosurgeon about her observations. She was told bluntly that the consent had been signed and that they were going to operate on Mr. Mack the next day for his own good. If she wanted what was best for the client, she would just drop the issue.

Questions for Thought
1. Should the nurse just drop the issue?
2. Is there anything she could do to resolve the problem?
3. What ethical principles are involved with this situation?

In either case, respecting a living will might appear to health-care providers to be a violation of their duty to help clients and preserve life. Nurses, as well as other health-care providers, often experience a sense of frustration when they are not allowed to use all the skills they have learned to preserve life.

Lack of Clarity

A third difficulty nurses and other health-care workers may have with living wills is their formulation and legal enforcement. In general, the language used in the standard living will document is broad and vague. Living wills are often not specific enough to include all the forms of treatments that are possible for the many types of illnesses that might render a person incompetent to make decisions. Health-care providers may have little direction as to the care they are to give if the circumstances at the time the living will was formulated are significantly different from the declared wishes of the client.

Furthermore, unless the particular state has enacted into law a special type of living will called a *natural death act*, the living will has no mechanism of legal enforcement. Also, when a client travels from one state to another, the legal effect of the living will may be in question. Does the nonresident state have an obligation to honor it?

In two states, a living will is considered only advisory, and the health-care provider has the right to comply with it or treat the client as the provider deems most appropriate. In Massachusetts, the living will is not officially recognized as a legal document; however, Massachusetts does recognize health-care proxies. Michigan actually has no state law at all for living wills but accepts the decision of a designated patient advocate for health care.[25]

There is no legal protection for nurses or other health-care practitioners against criminal or civil liability in the execution of living wills in states without a natural death act. Once a valid living will exists, it becomes effective only when the person who formulated it meets the qualifications for the natural death act. In most states, the individual must be diagnosed as having a terminal condition in which the continuation of treatment and life support would only prolong the client's dying process, but there is no clear consensus on the definition of *terminal condition*.

A Guide for the Care Provider

Despite all these difficulties, living wills are still a good way for a client to make health-care wishes known to providers. Documents that are specific about treatment modalities, written in a legal format, and signed by two or more witnesses tend to be treated with respect. Because the laws on advance directives vary widely among states, there is no standard advance directive whose language conforms

exactly with all states' laws. It is easy to download any particular state's form by going to the National Hospice and Palliative Care Organization's website.

Nurses can help clients plan ahead for their care should they become unable to make decisions for themselves. Although the nurse should not make decisions for the client, the nurse can provide important information about the various treatment modalities that the client is considering. The nurse also can help clients clarify their wishes and guide them through the process of formulating an advance directive (Fig. 7.1).

Ethics of Vaccinations

Although disagreement over vaccinations has existed for many years, the COVID-19 pandemic brought it to the forefront due to the lethal nature of the virus. Simply stated, the question became, Is there an ethical obligation to receive a COVID-19 vaccination? At the time of this writing, the U.S. death toll from COVID-19 infections had just crossed the one million mark. Until the recent pandemic, the Spanish flu epidemic of 1918 was the deadliest pandemic in U.S. history, killing more than one-fourth of the country's population. In the early 20th century, there was little understanding of the public health measures needed to control a severe viral outbreak. The use of measures such as wearing masks, isolation, public distancing, quarantine, hand washing, and good personal hygiene prevented the COVID-19 death rate from getting any higher than it was. In fact, it is projected that without these measures, the death rate for the COVID-19 pandemic might have been as high as 81 million in the United States.[29] And of course, there was no vaccine for the Spanish flu.

There are two basic ways a person achieves a relatively high degree of protection from a highly contagious disease such as COVID-19: one is by being vaccinated, and the other is by catching and experiencing the disease. Both confer what is called *active immunity*.[30]

Herd Immunity

A person may avoid catching an infectious disease because of something called *herd immunity*. Herd

> " *Although the term euthanasia simply means a "good" or peaceful death, it has taken on the connotation of some type of action that produces death.* "

INSTRUCTIONS	**PENNSYLVANIA DECLARATION**
PRINT YOUR NAME	I, _____, being of sound mind, willfully and voluntarily make this declaration to be followed if I become incompetent. This declaration reflects my firm and settled commitment to refuse life-sustaining treatment under the circumstances indicated below. I direct my attending physician to withhold or withdraw life-sustaining treatment that serves only to prolong the process of my dying, if I should be in a terminal condition or in a state of permanent unconsciousness. I direct that treatment be limited to measures to keep me comfortable and to relieve pain, including any pain that might occur by withholding or withdrawing life-sustaining treatment.

CHECK THE OPTIONS WHICH REFLECT YOUR WISHES	In addition, if I am in the condition described above, I feel especially strongly about the following forms of treatment:
	    I ( ) do ( ) do not want cardiac resuscitation.
	    I ( ) do ( ) do not want mechanical respiration.
	    I ( ) do ( ) do not want tube feeding or any other artificial or invasive form of nutrition (food) or hydration (water).
	    I ( ) do ( ) do not want blood or blood products.
	    I ( ) do ( ) do not want any form of surgery or invasive diagnostic tests.
	    I ( ) do ( ) do not want kidney dialysis.
	    I ( ) do ( ) do not want antibiotics.
	
	I realize that if I do not specifically indicate my preference regarding any of the forms of treatment listed above, I may receive that form of treatment.

ADD PERSONAL INSTRUCTIONS (IF ANY)	Other instructions:
© 2000 **PARTNERSHIP FOR CARING, INC.**	

Figure 7.1 Sample advance directive. Because the laws on advance directives vary widely among states, there is no standard advance directive whose language conforms exactly with all states' laws. (Reprinted with permission of Partnership for Caring, formerly Choice in Dying, 200 Varick Street, New York. For more information, visit http://www.caringinfo.org.)

immunity exists when a high enough percentage of the population has developed antibodies to the infective source so that the disease is no longer widespread in the population. Scientists disagree somewhat on what the exact percentage should be. For the flu, most agree that around 90 percent of the population having antibodies will convey herd immunity, while with the COVID-19 virus and its variants, that number may range between 75 percent to 95 percent. Obviously, the higher the percentage, the greater the herd immunity.

The ethics of vaccinations includes concepts of herd immunity, public good, and vaccination refusal.

An ethical situation exists whenever a person chooses to vaccinate or not to vaccinate themselves or to have their children vaccinated or not.[30] Moral values involved in vaccination are related to very basic ethical principles. However, there are complex reasons and explanations why people choose not to vaccinate themselves or their children.[31]

Anti-vaxxers; Vaccine Denialist; Vaccine Hesitators

You may hear people refer to all those who refuse vaccinations as anti-vaxxers, but that label is often used in error. Only individuals who refuse all vaccinations for any and all possible reasons can be said to be anti-vaccination. Another group, vaccine denialists, deny the effectiveness or safety of some or all vaccines. They may also have moral or religious views that are incompatible with the use of vaccines. Another group are the vaccine hesitators, who do not refuse vaccination in principle but are ultra-cautious about particular vaccinations. They question whether some vaccines are really safe and/or effective.[31] A large percentage of people who refused the COVID-19 vaccine probably fall into this last group.

Recent psychological research into the phenomenon of why people refuse lifesaving vaccinations supports the idea that many individuals who make the decision to refuse or postpone these vaccinations use a type of illogical reasoning or predisposed choice rather than a perceptive decision-making process.[32] A predisposed choice can be defined as an internalized prejudice or bias that leads a person to make unsubstantiated decisions or choices. This same psychological research has revealed two internalized thought processes that lead to faulty reasoning about vaccines. One, omission bias, views the outcome of not receiving the vaccine (either getting the disease or being lucky and missing it) as a better outcome than getting the vaccine and perhaps having side effects. The second one, naturalness bias, exists when the individual has an extreme belief that only natural products or substances should enter their bodies. They consider vaccines to be synthetic substances because they are manufactured in a laboratory.[33] In truth, most vaccines, including the COVID-19 vaccines, contain the same natural viruses that cause the disease, only these viruses have been killed. Killed viruses produce the same antigens as live viruses but are unable to produce the disease.

Ethical Dilemmas

As with almost all the ethical issues found in health-care decisions, the ethical dilemma that exists with vaccinations is a conflict between autonomy (self-determination; the right of the individual to make decisions about their own care) and best interest (the obligation to make a decision for someone who is unable to make the decision for themselves) or distributive justice (the obligation to make a decision that is best for the general population). Adults can refuse a vaccination because they can make decisions for themselves under the principle of self-determination. Even if the vaccination is in the adult's own best interest, they cannot be forced to be vaccinated. However, self-determination is not an absolute right; for example, all efforts are taken to prevent a person from committing suicide. It can be argued that a child's best interest is to be protected against any type of harm, including infectious diseases, particularly ones that can produce death.[32] Therefore, it would appear a parent has an ethical obligation, based on the child's best interest, to have the child vaccinated, thereby protecting the child's health. But what about the parents who argue that it is *not* in the best interest of their child to have them vaccinated? Other parents may argue that even if the vaccination is in a child's best interest, as the child's decision-maker, the parent still has the right to make independent choices about what is given to their children. The ethical issue here is a conflict between a child's best interest and the parents' right to make autonomous choices about their child's health.[30]

Distributive Justice

Another ethical dilemma exists when there is a conflict between the individual's autonomy and distributive justice (the health of the public at large). There is an old saying about rights: "Your right to swing your fist ends where my nose begins." Ethically, exercise of autonomous decisions, even about a person's body, can be constrained when they cause harm to other individuals or groups. For example, I own an automatic firearm and have a right to shoot it in my state; however, that right ends when I'm at a grade school. Therefore, the question becomes, Does a person have a right to refuse vaccination for themselves or their children even when this choice would expose other people to preventable, potentially life-threatening infectious diseases?

The concept of distributive justice is also ethically relevant because protection of the community from infectious diseases is a matter of both communal and individual responsibility. Fulfillment of a collective obligation such as herd immunity can be achieved only when each individual accepts their share of the process. Therefore, there is an individual obligation to support the communal well-being. It can be argued that this shared or group obligation produces an individual obligation that applies to every individual member of the community. In other words, the communal requirement of herd immunity obligates the individual to participate in the vaccination process.[33]

Another factor involved in distributive justice is the cost, both monetary and societal, of a person contracting COVID-19 because they are unvaccinated. In 2022, the cost for long-term care in the ICU of a patient with COVID-19 could run to well over $100,000.[29] Up until 2022, the majority of this cost was being paid by insurance companies and several government-assistance programs, with little out-of-pocket expense on the part of the patient. However, in 2022, these programs were being phased out, and insurance companies were no longer waiving copays of virus-related hospitalizations. The high cost of treating COVID-19 meant that the government could not spend money on other health-care-related problems in the general population. In addition, patients who contracted the disease either died or could not work for a long period of time, thus removing them from society. Both elements violate the principle of distributive justice.

So Why Do People Get Vaccinated?

Reasons people give for receiving the COVID-19 vaccination include the following:

- They believe that they and their children need to be protected from a potentially lethal virus through vaccination.
- They believe that there is a duty to protect other members of the community against diseases.
- They believe that there is a moral obligation to get a vaccination.
- They believe that one more person vaccinated (themselves) really does contribute to herd immunity.
- From a utilitarian standpoint, they believe that it is the greatest good for the greatest number.[30]

Responsibility for Harm

Ethicists would argue that an unvaccinated individual is both causally and morally responsible for the harm caused to another person if that person should receive the infectious disease from the unvaccinated person.[30] However, in the early stages of a pandemic when relatively few individuals are vaccinated, it may be hard to establish direct causality of illness unless the unvaccinated individual was in close proximity to the group, such as a family member or coworkers in an office. Over the two peak years of the COVID-19 pandemic, many individuals who were interviewed on TV news programs apologized for not getting a vaccination; they believed that their COVID-19 infection caused a severe illness or even death to a family member.[33]

Is It Fair?

Another ethical value involved in the vaccination argument is the principle of fairness. Everybody likes to be treated fairly. But what is fairness? Fairness can be understood from a deontological viewpoint as objective and realistic behavior in harmony with accepted rules or principles. The key identifiers of the ethical principle of fairness include impartiality, respect, and stewardship among individuals or the community and how they relate to others in the community.[34] Justice and fairness are closely intertwined, and, in some respects, fairness forms the basis for justice. This justice-fairness link is often seen in the legal system, where all people are supposed to be treated equally under the law and similar punishments are to be applied for similar crimes.

From a teleological point of view, fairness supports the belief that an ethical choice concerning vaccinations is one that benefits as many members of the community as possible. It reinforces the concept of the greatest good for the greatest number. It matters little whether or not the actual result of the individual choice has much of an effect on the attainment of the communal goal, such as herd immunity. The principle of fairness connects group and individual responsibilities because fairness is not primarily about the impact of an individual's behavior but about spreading both the benefits and costs across the whole community.[35] Therefore, the principle of fairness asks that individuals contribute whatever activities they are reasonably able to do in order to accomplish the group responsibilities and goals. Both fairness and justice create an ethical obligation for every individual member of a community to be vaccinated unless there are medical reasons that would make vaccination dangerous, such as being immunosuppressed or having other contraindications.[35]

Still Low Vaccination Numbers

Despite the ethical arguments that all individuals should be vaccinated except for those who have health restrictions precluding vaccinations, vaccination rates in several states remain as low as 51 percent, with a national fully vaccinated rate of only 68 percent.[32] The minimal threshold to achieve herd immunity for the COVID-19 virus hovers around 75 percent, including individuals who have been infected with the virus and recovered. However, research has shown that the immunity of the infected-recovered group is relatively short-term (several months) and that as a group they are more than twice as likely to get reinfected with a variant strain.[33] Because of ongoing public resistance to receiving the COVID-19 vaccination and inability to achieve herd immunity, it is projected that the pandemic will continue episodically for years to come, particularly in states with low vaccination rates.

EUTHANASIA AND ASSISTED SUICIDE

After 2022, when the U.S. Supreme Court upheld states' rights to ban abortions, effectively overturning *Roe v. Wade*, some groups turned their attention to other ethical issues, particularly, eliminating transgender rights (see Chapter 21), euthanasia, and prisoner executions. These groups have for many years resisted any attempts to legalize euthanasia or assisted suicide in any form. They find it hypocritical that individuals who oppose abortion would support euthanasia and execution. Their argument is that the right to life includes all human life. These advocates believe that the acceptance of abortion indicates a devaluation of the respect for life at its beginning, which inevitably leads to a devaluing of life at its end. When fetuses became disposable, they argue, it is a simple jump to the elderly and infirm becoming disposable.[36] Although the term *euthanasia* simply means a "good"

or peaceful death, it has taken on the connotation of some type of action that produces death. A distinction needs to be made between passive and active euthanasia. Passive euthanasia usually refers to the practice of allowing an individual to die without any extraordinary intervention. This umbrella definition includes practices such as DNR orders, living wills, and withdrawal of ventilators or other life support.

Active Euthanasia

Active euthanasia usually describes the practice of hastening an individual's death through some act or procedure. This practice is also sometimes called *mercy killing* and takes many forms, ranging from use of large amounts of pain medication for terminal cancer clients to use of poison, a gun, or a knife to end a person's life.

> *The central issue that Kevorkian raised was whether it is ever ethically and legally permissible for health-care personnel to assist in taking a life.*

The Case of Dr. Kevorkian

Assisted suicide—brought to public attention by Dr. Jack Kevorkian, a Michigan physician who publicly practiced it for many years—can be considered a type of active euthanasia or mercy killing. The central issue that Kevorkian raised was whether it is ever ethically and legally permissible for health-care personnel to assist in taking a life. In most states, the practice is illegal. The legal definition of homicide—bringing about a person's death or assisting in doing so—seems to fit the act of assisted suicide. In the past, there has been a great deal of hesitation on the part of the legal system to prosecute persons who are involved in assisted suicide and on the part of juries to convict physicians who participate in the activity.

A Killing on TV

In the fall of 1998, Kevorkian raised the legal and ethical stakes. On a nationally broadcast network news show, *60 Minutes*, he not only admitted to administering a lethal medication to a client without the client's assistance but also played a videotape that showed the whole episode.

The client, who had Lou Gehrig's disease (amyotrophic lateral sclerosis), had requested that

Kevorkian help him end his life. The client had signed a **consent** form and release and was even given an extra 2 weeks to "think about it." The client waited for only 3 days before making his final request for the lethal medication.

Under Michigan law, Kevorkian could have been charged with **manslaughter** or even first-degree murder. Kevorkian admitted that his **motivation** for the act was to be tried under these laws as a test case for active euthanasia. Two weeks after the tape was broadcast, he was arrested on a charge of first-degree murder. However, he believed that a jury would never convict him. The jury found him guilty of second-degree murder, and he served 10 years of a 25-years-to-life prison term. He was released on probation in 2007 and died on June 3, 2011. This verdict reinforced the belief that mercy killing or assisted suicide is always ethically wrong.

The unfortunate fallout from Kevorkian's conviction is that many health-care providers have become even more reluctant to write DNR orders or comply with clients' or families' wishes to allow clients to be removed from life support.[36]

An Issue of Self-Determination

The fundamental ethical issue in these situations is the right to self-determination. In almost every other health-care situation, a client who is mentally competent can make decisions about what care to accept and what care to refuse. Yet, when it comes to the termination of life, this right becomes controversial.

A Last Act of Control?

Supporters of the practice of assisted suicide believe that the right to self-determination remains intact, even with regard to the decision to end one's life. Suicide may be the last act an individual has to control their own fate. Supporters of assisted suicide believe that medical personnel should be allowed to assist clients in this procedure, just as they are allowed to assist clients in other medical and nursing procedures. They also believe that it is up to the individual to decide their death, not the government or religious institutions and their ideologies.[37]

Death With Dignity Laws

Several states have passed laws permitting assisted suicide, but these states have very strict guidelines. Assisted suicide, also called physician-assisted suicide or medical aid in dying, allows someone to take their own life with someone else's assistance, usually a doctor. Assisted suicide occurs when someone helps a person with a terminal illness, such as cancer, take their own life to avoid suffering.[25]

Nine states with death with dignity laws, also called "right to die" states, allow assisted suicide for adults with terminal illnesses. After they meet certain criteria, they can receive a prescription medication to assist in their death.

The conditions include the following:

• Patient must be an adult who is mentally competent.
• Because of the patient's illness, they must have fewer than 6 months to live.
• They must have resident status in the state where they will receive the medication.
• The terminal diagnosis, prognosis, mental competence, and voluntariness of the patient's request must be confirmed by two physicians.
• Although the time span varies somewhat from state to state, the patient must wait for two periods of time: one between the oral request for the medication and another between the time when they receive the prescription and the time when it is filled to allow them time to change their minds.
• In all right to die states, it is illegal for the physician to give the medication directly to the terminally ill patient.[25]

Federal law allows states to make their own laws regarding assisted suicide. However, assisted suicide is legal in nine states:

• California
• Colorado
• District of Columbia
• Hawaii
• Maine
• New Jersey
• Oregon
• Vermont
• Washington

In Montana and New Mexico, although their legislatures have not passed right to die laws, their states' supreme courts made it legal through court rulings.

An Unacceptable Practice?

Those who oppose assisted suicide find these arguments unconvincing. Legally, ethically, and morally, suicide in U.S. society has never been an accepted practice. Health-care staff goes to great lengths to prevent suicidal clients from injuring themselves. In addition, individuals in the terminal stages of a disease, who are overwhelmed by pain and depressed by the thought of prolonged suffering, might not be able to think clearly enough to give informed consent for assisted suicide. Also, because the termination of life is final, it does not allow for spontaneous cures or for the development of new treatments or medications.

Nonmaleficence is the obligation to do no harm to clients. Whether assisting in or causing the death of a client violates this principle is most likely to be an issue that will continue to be debated for some time. The American Nurses Association (ANA) and other nurses' organizations oppose assisted suicide as a policy and believe that nurses who participate in it are violating the code of ethics. For similar reasons, the ANA opposes nurses participating in executions of convicted criminals.

ETHICS INVOLVING CHILDREN

Although children are universally acknowledged as the hope of the future, many children remain poorly fed, inadequately clothed, in substandard housing, and educated below a minimal standard. They are in dire need of all types of health care. Even in affluent countries such as the United States, children are held in cages on the southern border. In countries undergoing invasions and the devastation of war, such as Ukraine, children are experiencing homelessness, violence, and starvation. Conditions such as these increase the incidence of child neglect and child abuse.[41]

The Power of Parents

Our society generally acknowledges the tremendous decision-making power that parents have on behalf of their children; however, there are limits to how parents may decide to act. These limits are sometimes obvious, as in cases of physical abuse and cruelty to children; however, they may also be less conspicuous, such as in cases of neglect or decisions about withholding medical care for religious reasons. Health-care professionals often find themselves trying to make decisions about the appropriateness of a parent's actions toward a child.

The legal and ethical factors surrounding the decisions that health-care providers must make about child health issues are complicated and sometimes contradictory, ranging from laws about reporting suspected abuse to obtaining permission for treatment. This section focuses on child abuse and the ethical issues that it creates for nurses and on the issues of informed consent as it pertains to children.

Issues involving children have always been an important consideration in our society. Whereas the political attention seems to focus on education, drug and alcohol abuse, and child health-care issues, ethical concerns in **pediatrics** are never forgotten and often serve as the unspoken basis for the more visible issues.

Child health ethical issues are numerous and diverse, ranging from mass screening for diseases to withholding permission for treatment.

Child Abuse Case Study

Emily, who is 8 months old, was brought to the hospital by her 17-year-old unemployed mother, who stated that the baby refused to eat at home and vomited a lot. Emily was very small for her age and was below the growth curve for weight. She was also neurologically introverted and showed little interest in her surroundings. She slept a great deal of the time. She was admitted to the hospital with a diagnosis of nonorganic failure to thrive.

During her stay in the hospital, Emily ate well and gained a significant amount of weight. Her neurological status also improved.

One nurse suspected that this was a case of neglect (a form of child abuse) and suggested to the physician that CPS be notified to evaluate the case. The physician resisted because there was not enough evidence to make a definitive case, and he thought that it was unfair to the parents to make such a claim. The other nurses felt that by reporting the case they would lose the trust of the mother and cause her to avoid health care for Emily in the future. They also cited a case in which nurses and the hospital were sued when they reported a teenage mother for neglect; the accusation later proved to be false.

Emily was sent home after 3 weeks but was readmitted 1 month later with the same complaints of poor feeding. She had lost weight since her discharge from the hospital, and she was again neurologically

Issues in Practice

Nurses Legally Protected for Reporting Child Abuse

A newborn was admitted to the nursery with signs of drug withdrawal and tested positive for cocaine, although the mother denied using the drug before delivery. Hospital personnel are required by law to report suspected child abuse, and illegal drugs in the circulatory system of a newborn is one of the indicators for mandatory reporting. On the basis of this finding, the nurses in the newborn nursery filed a report with the local child protective services (CPS), which investigated the case.

CPS removed the child from the home shortly after discharge from the hospital. The mother went to court a few days after the child was removed to plead her case before a family court judge. The judge upheld the decision to remove the child. The mother then became even more irate, still insisting she had not used cocaine, and filed a lawsuit against the hospital, the physicians, the nurses, and CPS. She cited that these entities were conspiring to keep her from exercising her constitutional rights.

Over the past decade, courts have been recognizing the integrity of the family and are beginning to make rulings that support it as a constitutional right. Because of this trend, the mother's lawyer felt that the case had merit and might result in a ruling in her favor with a large punitive settlement.

Looking at all the evidence, the higher court decided that there had been no attempt on the part of the hospital and staff to deprive the mother of her constitutional rights: the mother had been given the opportunity to plead in a lower court shortly after the child's removal from the home. The court upheld the nurses' requirement to report suspected child abuse and their immunity from civil lawsuits for carrying out their obligations in good faith.

Questions for Thought

1. Did the court violate the mother's rights? What makes you think so?
2. Current laws require the mandatory removal of an infant from its mother when the infant tests positive for an illegal drug. Is there any alternative way to address this situation? What suggestions do you have?
3. Common law seems to be moving in the direction of "giving the child back." Do you think this trend is moving in the right direction? Why or why not?

Source: Stewart v. Jackson County, *2009 WL 2922940 S.D. Miss., September 8, 2009.*

---

withdrawn. The physician still refused to notify CPS because of the lack of hard evidence. He thought that the available data did not warrant an investigation and possible removal of the child from the home. The nurse still believed that the mother should be reported on the basis of suspicions that could be substantiated legally.

Ethics Regarding Child Abuse

There is a general legal requirement in all states that suspected child abuse must be reported by health-care providers and by anyone who suspects that child abuse has occurred.[38] Abuse is more obvious when the child has physical injuries that do not fit the medical history or are atypical for the age group. However, in cases of neglect, the evidence may be very minimal or even nonexistent. Often, nurses and health-care providers who specialize in the care of children rely on their experience in making decisions to report or not report suspected abuse.

A conflicting ethical principle sometimes forgotten in the reporting of suspected child abuse is the family's right to privacy and self-determination. It is an equally fundamental right that Emily's parents be allowed to live their lives according to their own values, free from intrusions.

Decisions about reporting suspected child abuse or neglect rest on the underlying ethical principles of beneficence and protection of the best interests of the child. It is always difficult to decide how far ranging these concerns for "best interest" should be. However, when the child is a client in the hospital, beneficence usually outweighs fidelity and veracity.

Physicians tend to focus on solving the immediate problem. Nurses have a more holistic viewpoint and tend to see children in relationship to their environments and to the environments of the parents.

Resolving the Dilemma

How is the nurse going to resolve this dilemma? Should the nurse report the case and go against the physician's decision? Should the nurse just defer to the physician's greater medical knowledge? Should the nurse submit the problem to the hospital ethics committee? Are there any other possible options for action in this case?

It is likely that the physician's decision about this case was correct. Rather than remove the baby from the mother, CPS would likely institute home monitoring to ensure that the baby is cared for properly. Therefore, how can the ethical obligations for the best interest of the child be met?

One very plausible solution is to monitor the child closely through frequent follow-ups, either at the provider's office or at the local health department.[39] In addition, a follow-up and home evaluation could be arranged through a home health-care agency, which could also make available other community resources to help in Emily's care. If the infant continued to fail to gain weight, or if it was later determined that Emily's mother was indeed unable to care adequately for her, the case could then be referred to CPS.

The role of the nurse who cares for the very young or abused child is one of client advocate. These children need help and protection, and at times, for their very survival, must be taken out of an abusive or neglectful home setting. Nurses need to be aware of and use all the resources available in these situations, including the police, CPS, welfare, and home health-care agencies.

Informed Consent and Children Case Study

Peter, one of a pair of 7-year-old identical twins, developed severe bilateral glomerulonephritis after a streptococcal (strep) throat infection. The renal involvement was so severe that it did not respond to any medical treatment, and both of his kidneys had to be removed. Paul, Peter's identical twin, was evaluated for kidney donation and, as expected, matched on all six antigens as well as blood type and size. Paul seemed to understand what had happened to his brother and agreed to donate one of his kidneys to keep his brother alive.

However, the children's parents were having some trouble agreeing on whether Paul should donate a kidney to Peter. The twins' mother felt that the donation and transplantation should be permitted because it would indeed help keep Peter alive and would also make Paul feel that he was an important part of the process. She argued that if Peter ever did die, Paul would be overcome with guilt knowing that he could have saved his brother but did not.

The twins' father was not as certain about the transplantation procedure. He thought that Paul was too young to make a truly free decision of that type and that he did not really understand the serious nature of a kidney removal operation. He thought that Paul, because he was so young, might have been unduly influenced by subtle yet powerful pressures from his family. No one had directly told Paul that he *must* donate one of his kidneys, yet the fact that his brother's survival might well depend on his decision could have had a major effect on his willingness to donate. Because Peter was being maintained on dialysis and seemed to be doing fairly well, the twins' father thought that he should be put on the transplant list to see whether a suitable nonrelated donor could be found.

The nurses on the unit where Peter was being cared for were equally divided about whether the transplantation should be performed. At various times during Peter's lengthy stay in the hospital, they had all been asked by the parents, usually one parent at a time, whether or not they should go ahead with the transplantation.

Case Study Analysis

Does a 7-year-old child have sufficient rational decision-making ability to decide to donate a kidney to his brother? If, after careful assessment of the child, the answer is yes, then under the rights-in-trust doctrine, the right to self-determination can be turned over to the child, and he can make his own decision.

If the answer is no, the child should not be permitted to donate the kidney.

Other ethical theories can be brought to bear on this decision. From a utilitarian viewpoint, the child should be allowed to donate the kidney because it would provide the greatest good or happiness for the greatest number of people. Similarly, love-based ethics, or the Golden Rule system of ethical decision making, would also support the donation on the grounds that Paul identifies closely with his brother and appears to understand the issues involved in donation. However, from an egoistic or beneficent viewpoint, because the transplantation has little benefit for the donor and will surely cause pain and place him at risk for postoperative complications, the operation should not be permitted.

As with many ethical dilemmas, there is no perfect answer to this situation. The best that can be done is to ensure that the parents and children have as much necessary information as possible and to support their decisions (Box 7.2).

By recognizing the rights of children as individuals, we also recognize their importance to society. However, parents and health-care professionals also have the duty to nurture, support, and guide children as they grow into adolescence and adulthood.

Nurses who work with children are challenged to support their independence by encouraging them to be responsible for and participate in their own health care.

Ethical Principles Regarding Child Health Care

One important difference between adults and children that always needs to be considered in ethical decisions about child health care is that children are dependents. As dependents, they generally are not attributed the right to self-determination that is fundamental to adult decision making.

A Three-Way Relationship

Whenever an ethical dilemma involves child health-care issues, a three-way relationship develops involving the child, the health-care professional, and the parents. Generally, the parents have the primary role in deciding health-care issues for their underage, dependent children on the basis of what they consider to be in the child's best interests.

Current routine child health practices reinforce this principle. Young children are given immunizations and medications, have blood drawn for tests, and even

---

Box 7.2 Determining the Greatest Good

Sherry is an RN who works for a rehabilitation center that deals mainly with developmentally delayed children. For several years, Sherry has been following the case of Margie N, who is now 8 years old and has Down syndrome. Margie has made slow but steady progress in achieving basic motor and cognitive skills but still requires close supervision of all activities and care for all basic hygiene needs. Margie is still not advanced enough to participate in group activities at the center's day clinic.

Mrs. N, Margie's mother, a 42-year-old widow, has been providing a high level of care for Margie at home as well as meeting the child's demands for love and attention. Recently, Mrs. N was diagnosed with systemic lupus erythematosus (SLE), which has displayed as its primary symptoms severe joint pain and stiffness. During the past several months, Mrs. N has been finding it increasingly difficult to care for Margie because of the progressive nature of the SLE.

Mrs. N is trying to make a decision about long-term care for Margie. She trusts Sherry's judgment completely and often relies on the information and teaching given by the nurse to make changes in Margie's care. Sherry is uncertain about what advice she should give. She recognizes that the high level of care and comfort provided by Mrs. N has been an essential part in the advances Margie has made up to this point, but she also recognizes that Mrs. N may soon reach a point where she can no longer provide care. It seems that to do what is good for Mrs. N (i.e., place Margie in an institution) would be harmful to Margie, whereas to do what is good for Margie (i.e., leave her at home) would be harmful to Mrs. N. What is the best course of action in this situation? Are there any alternative solutions to this dilemma?

have operations such as tonsillectomies or myringotomies, all without anyone asking for their permission. This exemption to the principle of self-determination in children is based on the belief that young children do not yet have the capacity to make fully rational decisions. Yet the final expectation for children is that at some point in their lives they develop the capacity to make informed, correct decisions. The primary questions then become, When do they develop this capacity for rational decision making? and How should they be treated until they develop this capacity?

Safeguarding the Child's Rights

The legal system has fixed the age for rational decision making at age 18 years. Children who are younger than 18 years of age, with a few exceptions, require the permission of the parent for any and all medical procedures. Children older than 18 years of age can make their own decisions about health care.

The difficulty with fixing an age is that it is arbitrary and does not reflect the reality of the individual child's development. From experience, it can be observed that many children who are 9 or 10 years old exhibit rather advanced and adultlike decision-making skills, whereas other "children" who may be 18 or 19 years of age display a marked lack of this ability.

> *Whenever there is an ethical dilemma involving child health-care issues, a three-way relationship develops involving the child, the health-care professional, and the parents.*

However, the more serious question is, How should underage children be treated? One solution is to deny, because of their age, that they have rights and then treat them as being incompetent by bringing to bear paternalistic, best-interest interventions. Another approach is to say that children do have the same rights as adults except that these rights are temporarily suspended until the child is sufficiently mature to exercise them. This is called *rights-in-trust*, and the rights are turned over to the child at the appropriate time. So, when is the appropriate time?

One way to proceed is to turn over all the rights to the child at the same time—for example, when the child reaches 18 years of age. A more vigilant manner is to gradually release individual rights as the child grows older and is prepared to exercise them. In either case, appropriate adults, including nurses, have the role of safeguarding the child's rights and acting as guardians, protectors, and advocates of the children under their care.

ETHICAL ISSUES IN ELDER ABUSE

Almost all the ethical principles involved in cases of child abuse also apply to cases of elder abuse. Because of the rapidly increasing numbers of elderly persons who require additional physical care and monitoring due to altered levels of cognition brought on by various types of dementia, elder abuse is on the rise. Consider the following case study.

Case Study

Bruce, a 72-year-old man in the early stages of Parkinson's disease, lives at home with his wife, who cares for him, cooking, washing clothes, helping him with his medication, and doing other household chores. Bruce is mobile, alert, and oriented most of the time. His wife dies suddenly of a heart attack, leaving him alone to care for himself in his rather large house. The nearest family members are several states away, and Bruce refuses to move closer to them.

Because he usually burns the food he attempts to cook for himself, Bruce begins eating in a small family restaurant down the street from his home. He enjoys his daily chats with Misty, a waitress in her early 30s. After several weeks, Bruce considers Misty a friend and asks her to move in with him. She agrees.

The arrangement seems to be going well for the first few weeks until Misty is caught trying to sell some watches from Bruce's expensive pocket-watch collection. Bruce is shocked and angry when the police show up at his door to report the theft. Misty pleads for forgiveness, telling Bruce she really needs the money to pay off some loans that have come due. Despite learning that Misty has a criminal record for petty theft and writing bad checks and is out on bail,

Bruce forgives her and bails her out for this latest offense.

Misty's parole officer is suspicious of the living arrangement and requests that Bruce have a cognitive evaluation before Misty can return to the home. Bruce is found to be mildly demented but capable of understanding the implications of his decisions. Bruce marries Misty a few weeks later, and they resume the living arrangement they previously had.

Bruce has not been seen outside the house for approximately a month, when suddenly Misty physically kicks him out. He stumbles down the street to the restaurant, where the staff find him shaking, severely disoriented, and with bruises on his face and over his upper body. Adult protective services (APS) are called, and Bruce is taken temporarily to an assisted living facility for his own protection, where it is found that he has not taken his anti-Parkinson's medications for several weeks.

Bruce's daughter is called and travels to his hometown from another state. She has the situation investigated by APS, who find the house in shambles, many of the furnishings sold, and evidence that Bruce had been tied down in bed. Misty's bail is revoked from the previous charges, and she is returned to jail. New charges of assault and battery are filed against Misty, and the marriage is annulled.

The ethics of elder care focus on preventing unnecessary suffering and maintaining the highest quality of life possible for the longest time. Conflicts of values between individuals and between individuals and institutions lead to ethical dilemmas. The challenge for nurses is to identify and explore the underlying issues and value conflicts that produce these dilemmas.

For elderly persons, retaining their autonomy and self-determination is likely on the top of their list of important ethical issues. These principles are based on the ability of a person to make a free and informed decision without pressure or coercion.

Only the individual can delegate their own autonomy to another person, although it can be taken away by force or coercion. However, assessing autonomy and self-determination in elderly clients can be challenging. Basically, it requires determining a person's decision-making capacity, including the capacity to understand what is being decided and, more important, to appreciate the consequences of the decision. Assessing autonomy is particularly difficult when a person seems fully oriented one day and completely disoriented the next. The modern health-care system is set up to err on the side of safety rather than independence, so a person with varying levels of orientation may be placed in a facility where they can be monitored and cared for appropriately.[40]

In order for a decision to be truly autonomous, there must not be any duress (pressure, coercion, threat, persuasion) to make the decision in one direction or the other, and the person must be able to express the consequences of the decision clearly. Internal factors, such as pain, depression, psychiatric illness, or medication effects and side effects, can decrease the person's decision-making capability. It is important to remember that physical weakness does not necessarily imply the lack of mental ability. The ability to make decisions cannot be judged only on the basis of physical decline and disability.

Nurses working with elderly clients need to be especially mindful of the ethical principles of beneficence and nonmaleficence. The ethical principle of beneficence rests on the belief that what is being done for an elderly person is in the person's best interest. The promotion of a patient's well-being and stability should direct clinical decisions. The principle of doing no harm is the basis for nonmaleficence. Its negative, malfeasance, produces negligence, or failure to act in the patient's best interests. Unfortunately, intrusive beneficence or nonmaleficence can, even with the best intentions, turn into paternalism. Paternalism is the belief that the health-care provider's decisions are better than the patient's, thereby limiting the freedom of another person (usually against their will) with the justification that it will prevent harm and improve

> *For elderly persons, retaining their autonomy and self-determination is likely on the top of their list of important ethical issues.*

the person's condition. There is a fine line between beneficence and paternalism, which again rests on the person's decision-making ability.[40] For example, is convincing a reluctant elderly client to take a medication because "it will improve how you feel" a form of coercion and paternalism? Some believe that paternalism can be either weak or strong and that weak paternalism, such as convincing a patient to take a pill, is probably not an ethical violation.

Abuse experienced by older adults is often complicated when it occurs within the family or with an intimate partner. Older adults sometimes struggle with social, cultural, financial, religious, or relationship pressures that force them to continue to live with their abusers.[40] All health-care providers have a duty to protect vulnerable populations, including older adults, and to report suspected abuse. However, it can be difficult to intervene successfully in all abusive situations. Nurses must carefully assess the ethical implications of intervention from the perspective of the older adult, being particularly sensitive to the older adult's decision-making ability and need for independence.

Conclusion

Ethical issues are a factor in the daily practice of all nurses. Any time a nurse comes in contact with a client, a potential ethical situation exists. In today's world, with rapidly advancing technology and unusual health-care situations, ethical dilemmas are proliferating. Nurses can be prepared to deal with most of these dilemmas if they keep current with the issues and are able to follow a systematic process for making ethical decisions. At some point, difficult decisions must be made, and we should not avoid making them. Ethical decision-making does not ensure that everyone involved in a dilemma will be happy with the decision. However, if the decision is made after thoughtful analysis and on the basis of sound ethical principles, it can usually be defended.

CRITICAL-THINKING EXERCISES

CASE STUDY IN ETHICS

Analyze the following case study using the ethical decision-making process given in Chapter 6, Figure 6.1.

Sally Jones, RN, a public health nurse for a rural health department, was preparing to visit Mr. Weems, a 58-year-old client who was recently diagnosed with chronic bronchitis and emphysema. Mr. Weems was unemployed as a result of a farming accident and had been previously diagnosed with hypertension and extreme obesity. Ms. Jones was making this visit to see why Mr. Weems had missed his last appointment at the clinic and whether he was taking his prescribed antibiotics and antihypertensive medications.

As Ms. Jones pulled into the driveway of Mr. Weems's house, she noticed him sitting on the front porch smoking a cigarette. She felt a surge of anger, which she quickly suppressed, as she wondered why she spent so much of her limited time teaching him about the health consequences of smoking.

During the visit, Ms. Jones determined that Mr. Weems had stopped taking both his antihypertensive and antibiotic medications and rarely took his expectorants and bronchodilators. He coughed continuously, had a blood pressure of 196/122 mm Hg, and had severely congested lung sounds. Mr. Weems listened politely as Ms. Jones explained again about the need to stop smoking and the importance of taking his medications as prescribed. She also scheduled another appointment at the clinic in 1 week for a follow-up.

As she drove away to her next visit, Ms. Jones wondered about the ethical responsibilities of nurses who provide care for clients who do not seem to care about their own health. Mr. Weems took little responsibility for his health, refused to even try to stop smoking or lose weight, and did not take his medications. She wondered whether there was a limit to the amount of nursing care a noncompliant client should expect from a community health agency. She reflected that the time spent with Mr. Weems would have been spent much more productively screening children at a local grade school or working with mothers of newborn infants.

- What data are important in relation to this situation?
- State the ethical dilemma in a clear, simple statement.
- What are the nurse's choices of action, and how do they relate to specific ethical principles?
- What are the consequences of these actions?
- What decisions can the nurse make?

NCLEX-STYLE QUESTIONS

1. Briana is thinking about purchasing a home genetic-testing kit. What reasonable concerns might she have about using such a kit? **Select all that apply**.
   1. Who will have access to her genetic information?
   2. How will the information be used?
   3. Is she prepared for the emotional impact of negative genetic information?
   4. Will the test hurt?
   5. Can her genetic information be used to clone her without her consent?

2. Umbilical cord blood is a rich source of stem cells. Which of the following is an ethical issue associated with the use of cord blood for medical research?
   1. It requires embryos to be created in vitro.
   2. Embryos must be destroyed to harvest the stem cells.
   3. The ownership of the placenta and umbilical cord is in question.
   4. Hospitals can collect cord blood without obtaining consent.

3. Raquel, an RN, has strong ethical beliefs against abortion. Her client Marisol, whose pregnancy test just came back positive, has asked Raquel to tell her what a medical abortion is. Which of the following is the most ethical response for Raquel to give?
   1. "I can't discuss that with you. You will need to ask the doctor."
   2. "Any kind of abortion is wrong. Here is some information about adoption."
   3. "A medical abortion uses two different medications to terminate a pregnancy. The first medication causes the lining of the uterus to break down; the second causes contractions to expel the tissue."

   4. "Think about all the couples who are struggling to conceive!"

4. _____ are transplantable tissues such as skin, blood vessels, muscles, corneas, nerves, bone, and connective tissues that can be retrieved from 12 to 24 hours after cardiac death has occurred.

5. Which principle of nursing ethics would support a terminally ill patient's right to die on his or her own terms?
   1. Provision 1.1, Respect for Human Dignity
   2. Provision 1.4, The Right to Self-Determination
   3. Provision 2.1, Primacy of the Patient's Interests
   4. Provision 5.1, Duties to Self and Others

6. In the period between 2019 and 2021, some nurses refused to care for patients diagnosed with severe COVID-19. What ethical principle of nursing did these nurses breach?
   1. Provision 1.2, Relationships with Patients
   2. Provision 2.4, Professional Boundaries
   3. Provision 3.1, Protection of the Rights of Privacy and Confidentiality
   4. Provision 3.4, Professional Responsibility in Promoting a Culture of Safety

7. Which statement about health-care rationing is true?
   1. Under the ACA, rationing of health care is conducted by "death panels."
   2. Palliative care is a way to limit the health-care options of a terminally ill person.
   3. Health care is already rationed for individuals who contribute to their own poor health by smoking, drinking, overeating, or taking illicit drugs.
   4. Triage at a disaster scene is an example of health-care rationing; limited resources are allocated to those most likely to survive.

8. Mr. Jefferson is a 66-year-old male whose adult daughter has encouraged him to make an advance directive. At his next doctor's appointment, Mr. Jefferson asks the nurse to explain what an advance directive is. Which statement by Mr. Jefferson indicates the need for additional teaching?
   1. "So an advance directive made in one state may not be fully enforceable in another state."
   2. "Once I sign my advance directive, I can't change my mind about the heroic measures I will allow."
   3. "The advance directive lists which heroic measures I do and do not agree to allow medical personnel to perform."
   4. "I don't need to hire an attorney in order to create a legal advance directive."

9. Aaron, an RN in the emergency department, is caring for a 7 year old who has been injured in a motor vehicle accident. The ED physician has ordered a unit of packed red blood cells (PRBCs) for the child. However, the family are Jehovah's Witnesses, and the parents refuse to let their child receive blood products. What is Aaron's ethical responsibility in this situation?
   1. Aaron must alert the physician to the parents' refusal so that alternative interventions can be ordered to stabilize the child.
   2. Aaron must call security to restrain the parents while he administers the blood transfusion.
   3. Aaron must attempt to persuade the parents that the blood transfusion is necessary.
   4. Aaron must tell the parents that he is giving their child an artificial blood expander, not a unit of PRBCs.

10. Nurses regularly face ethical dilemmas on the job. What steps should nurses take to ensure that they are acting as ethically as possible? **Select all that apply**.
    1. Know the Code of Ethics for Nurses.
    2. Strictly follow the facility's policy and procedures manual.
    3. Identify and articulate their own personal ethics and their source.
    4. Make the best interests of the client the priority.
    5. Defer to a more experienced colleague.

References

1. Ramirez C, Dahlin C. Discontinuing medically administered nutrition. *American Nurse*, April 29, 2022. https://www.myamericannurse.com/discontinuing-medically-administered-nutrition-manh/

2. Davis E. How healthcare rationing in the United States affects even you. Verywell Health, April 24, 2022. https://www.verywellhealth.com/how-health-care-rationing-in-the-us-affects-even-you-1738482

3. How does gene addition work? GTnetwork, n.d. https://genetherapynetwork.com/gene-replacement/how-does-gene-addition-work/

4. Overview of gene inhibition therapy. GTnetwork, n.d. https://genetherapynetwork.com/gene-replacement/gene-inhibition-therapy/overview-of-gene-inhibition-therapy/

5. Marchese S. Mesothelioma clinical trial matches treatment to genetic profiles. Asbestos.com, February 28, 2022. https://www.asbestos.com/news/2022/02/28/mesothelioma-trial-genetic-profiles/

6. Berkman B. Genetic Information Nondiscrimination Act (GINA). National Institute of Health, 2022. https://www.genome.gov/genetics-glossary/Genetic-Information-Nondiscrimination-Act

7. Greely H. *CRISPR People: The Science and Ethics of Editing Humans*. Cambridge, MA: MIT Press, 2021

8. Lea D, Williams J, Donahue P. Ethical issues in genetic testing. *Journal of Midwifery Womens Health*, 50(3):234–240. https://doi.org/10.1016/j.jmwh.2004.12.016

9. Li M, Wang H, Tian L, Pang Z, et al. COVID-19 vaccine development: Milestones, lessons and prospects. *Signal Transduction & Targeted Therapy*, 7, 2022. https://doi.org/10.1038/s41392-022-00996-y

10. Megerian C. What's next for abortion rights after Supreme Court leak? PBS News, May 3, 2022. https://www.pbs.org/newshour/politics/whats-next-for-abortion-rights-after-supreme-court-leak

11. Hengstschlager M, Rosner M. Embryoid research calls for reassessment of legal regulations. Stem Cell Research and Therapy, 2021. https://stemcellres.biomedcentral.com/articles/10.1186/s13287-021-02442-2

12. Stem cell. National Human Genome Research Institute, 2022, https://www.genome.gov/genetics-glossary/Stem-Cell

13. The complete guide to cord blood banking: Pros, cons, costs and basics. Health Prep, n.d. https://healthprep.com/technology-health/the-complete-guide-to-cord-blood-banking-pros-cons-costs-and-basics

14. Buying and selling organs for transplantation in the United States: Are body parts considered property? *MedScape Education*, 2003. https://www.medscape.org/viewarticle/465200_3

15. What is brain death? Yes, Therapy Helps, 2022. https://en.yestherapyhelps.com/what-is-brain-death-is-it-irreversible-12462

16. Organ Procurement and Transplant Network. Home page, 2022. https://optn.transplant.hrsa.gov

17. Symons X, Poulden B. An ethical defense of a mandated choice consent procedure for deceased organ donation. *Asian Bioethics Review*, 14(3):259–270. https://doi.org/10.1007/s41649-022-00206-5

18. Gracon A. What are organ donation requirements? Ochsner Health, April 27, 2022. https://blog.ochsner.org/articles/what-are-organ-donation-requirements

19. Plastic surgeon Bohdan Pomahač visited the faculty of medicine MU. Masaryk University Faculty of Medicine, September 22, 2021. https://www.med.muni.cz/en/news/plastic-surgeon-bohdan-pomahac-visited-the-faculty-of-medicine-mu

20. Peters B. What to expect from a face transplant. Verywell Health, June 8, 2022. https://www.verywellhealth.com/face-transplant-4843553

21. Stolberg, S. G. U.S. Organ Transplant System, Troubled by Long Wait Times, Faces an Overhaul. *The New York Times*, March 22, 2023. https://www.nytimes.com/2023/03/22/us/politics/organ-transplants-biden.html

22. Fitzpatrick S, Brogan D, Grover P. Hand transplants, daily functioning, and the human capacity for limb regeneration. *Frontiers in Cell Development Biology*, 10:812124, 2020. https://doi.org/10.3389/fcell.2022.812124

23. Paleia A. The pig heart that was transplanted to a human was infected with a pig virus. Interesting Engineering, May 6, 2022. https://interestingengineering.com/pig-heart-transplanted-human-virus

24. How 3D bioprinting technology is revolutionizing the healthcare industry. Delveinsight, May 4, 2022. https://www.delveinsight.com/blog/3d-bioprinting-in-the-healthcare-industry

25. Voluntary assisted dying. End of Life Law in Australia, 2022. https://end-of-life.qut.edu.au/assisteddying

26. Treston C. COVID-19 in the Year of the Nurse. *Journal of the Association of Nurses AIDS Care*, 2020. https://doi.org/10.1097/JNC.0000000000000173

27. Behring S. What is an advance directive? Health Line, April 28, 2022. https://www.healthline.com/health/what-is-an-advance-directive

28. H.R.410 - 115th Congress (2017-2018). Protecting Life Until Natural Death Act (2017, January 25). https://www.congress.gov/bill/115th-congress/house-bill/410

29. Hacket M. Average cost of hospital care for COVID-19 ranges from $51,000 to $78,000, based on age, November 5, 2020. https://www.healthcarefinancenews.com/news/average-cost-hospital-care-covid-19-ranges-51000-78000-based-age

30. Giubilini A. Vaccination ethics. *British Medical Bulletin*, 137(1):4–12. https://doi.org/10.1093/bmb/ldaa036

31. Yan H. COVID-19 vaccine myths. CNN News, 2021. https://www.cnn.com/2021/07/19/health/covid-vaccine-myths-debunked/index.html

32. US Coronavirus vaccine tracker. USA Facts, n.d. https://usafacts.org/visualizations/covid-vaccine-tracker-states/

33. Bort R, Take it from them: Americans hospitalized with COVID regret not getting the vaccine. Rolling Stone, 2021. https://www.rollingstone.com/politics/politics-features/covid-hospitalizations-unvaccinated-regret-1206032/

34. Fairness and philosophy. The Fairness Institute. https://fairnessfoundation.com/fairnecessities/full/fairness-and-philosophy

35. Blake D. What are the most important ethical issues? LanguageHumanities.org, 2022 https://www.languagehumanities.org/what-are-the-most-common-ethics-issues.htm

36. Assisted suicide states 2023. World Population Review, n.d. https://worldpopulationreview.com/state-rankings/assisted-suicide-states

37. Sleeper effect. Psychology, n.d. https://psychology.iresearchnet.com/social-psychology/social-influence/sleeper-effect/

38. Children's rights. Government Officials of Sweden, June 2, 2022. https://www.government.se/government-policy/childrens-rights/

39. Gluck S. Mandatory reporting of child physical abuse. Healthy Pace, November 19, 2008. https://www.healthyplace.com/abuse/child-physical-abuse/mandatory-reporting-of-child-abuse

40. What are the ethical issues in elder health care? MDhealth.com, n.d. https://www.md-health.com/Ethical-Issues-In-Healthcare.html

41. Christensen T. What are Good Samaritan Laws? My Law Questions, 2022. https://www.mylawquestions.com/what-are-good-samaritan-laws.htm

Nursing Law and Liability

8

Mary Evans | Tonia Aiken

Learning Objectives

After completing this chapter, the reader will be able to:

- Distinguish between statutory law and common law
- Differentiate civil law from criminal law
- Explain the legal principles involved in
  - Unintentional torts
  - Intentional torts
  - Quasi-intentional torts
  - Informed consent
  - Do-not-resuscitate (DNR) and allow-natural-death (AND) orders
- Describe the trial process
- List methods to prevent litigation
- Identify legal considerations in delegation

THE LEGAL SYSTEM

For many nurses, the mere mention of the word *lawsuit* provokes a high level of anxiety. At first glance, the legal system often seems to be a large and confusing entity whose intricacies are designed to entrap the uninitiated. Many nurses feel that even a minor error in client care will lead to huge settlements against them and loss of their nursing license. In reality, even though the number of lawsuits against nurses has been increasing since the early 1990s, the number of nurses who are actually sued in court remains relatively small. However, many cases are settled out of court, often before any official legal action has been taken.

It is important to remember that the legal system is just one element of the health-care system. Laws are rules to help protect people and to keep society functioning. The ultimate goal of all laws is to promote peaceful and productive interactions among the people of that society.

An understanding of basic legal principles will augment the quality of care that the nurse delivers. In our litigious society, it is important to comprehend how the law affects the profession of nursing and the individual nurse's daily practice.

SOURCES OF LAW

There are two major sources of laws in the United States: statutory law and common law (Box 8.1). Most laws that govern nursing are state-level statutory laws because licensure is a function of the state's authority.

Statutory Law

Statutory (legislated) law consists of laws written and enacted by the U.S. Congress; the state legislatures; and other governmental entities such as cities, counties, and townships. Legislated laws enacted by the U.S. Congress are called federal **statutes**. State-drafted laws are called *state statutes*. Individual cities and municipalities have legislative

Box 8.1 Division and Types of Law

Statutory Law and Common Law
I. Criminal law
  A. Misdemeanor
  B. Felony
II. Civil Law
  A. Tort law
    1. Unintentional tort
    2. Intentional tort
    3. Quasi-intentional tort
  B. Contract law
  C. Treaty law
  D. Tax law
  E. Other

bodies that draft **ordinances**, codes, and regulations at their respective levels.

The laws that govern the profession of nursing are statutory laws. Most of these laws are written at the state level because licensure is a responsibility of the individual states. These laws include the nurse practice act, which establishes the state board of nursing, the scope of practice for nurses, individual licensure procedures, punitive actions for violation of the practice act, and the schedule of fees for nurse licensure in the state.

Common Law

Common law is different from statutory law in that it has evolved from the decisions of previous legal cases that form a **precedent**. These laws represent the accumulated results of the **judgments** and decrees that have been handed down by courts of the United States and Great Britain through the years.

Common law often extends beyond the scope of statutory law. For example, no statutes require a person who is negligent and causes injury to another to compensate that person for the injury. However, court decisions that have addressed the same legal issues, such as negligence, over and over have repeatedly ruled that the injured person should receive compensation. The way in which each case is resolved creates a precedent, or pattern, for dealing with the same legal issue in the future. The common laws involving negligence or malpractice are the laws most frequently encountered by nurses.

Common law, or case law, is law that has developed over a long period. The principle of *stare decisis* requires a judge to make decisions similar to those that have been handed down in previous cases if the facts of the cases are identical. Common-law decisions are published in bound legal reports. Generally speaking, common law deals with matters outside the scope of laws enacted by the legislature.

DIVISIONS OF LAW

In the U.S. legal system, there are many divisions in the law. One example is the difference between criminal law and civil law, either of which may be statutory or common in origin.

Criminal Law

Criminal laws are concerned with providing protection for all members of society. When someone is accused of violating a criminal law, the government at the county, city, state, or federal level imposes a punishment that is appropriate to the type of **crime**. Criminal law involves a wide range of **malfeasance**, from minor traffic violations to murder.

Although most criminal law is created and regulated by the government through the enactment of statutes, a small portion falls under the common law. Statutes are developed and enacted by the legislature (state or federal) and approved by the executive branch, such as a governor or the president. Criminal law is further classified into two types of offenses: (1) **misdemeanors**, which are less serious criminal offenses, and (2) **felonies**, which are serious criminal offenses.

In the criminal law system, an individual accused of a crime is called the *defendant*. The case is brought by the "State" (also called "the people"), wherein the prosecuting attorney represents the people of the city, county, state, or federal jurisdiction who are accusing the individual of a crime. The burden of proof of a crime rests with the state. A **criminal action** is rendered when the person charged with the crime is brought to trial and convicted. Penalties or sanctions are imposed on the violators of criminal law and are based on the scope of the crime. They can involve a range of punishments, from community service work and fines to imprisonment and death.

Criminal cases can be tried before a judge or jury. In a jury trial, there must be unanimous agreement among the jurors before a guilty or not guilty decision is rendered. The jury may consist of 6 or 12 people. A mistrial occurs when the jury cannot agree on a decision (a "hung jury"), and the defendant may or may not be tried again depending on the judge's decision to dismiss the case with or without prejudice. If it is dismissed with prejudice, the defendant cannot be tried again for the same crime. A decision of not guilty does not necessarily mean that the defendant is innocent but that the prosecution did not have enough evidence to convince the jury of the defendant's guilt beyond a reasonable doubt.

Jury nullification occurs when the jury ignores the law and the facts presented and issues a verdict of not guilty. Judges and prosecutors do not like jury nullification, but it is one of the powers granted to juries by the Ninth Amendment of the Constitution. Jury nullification is the people's most important veto power under our constitutional system and represents real decentralization of political power. When the jury vetoes in the judicial system, it is the only time citizens ever vote on the application of a real law in real life.

Although the right to a trial by jury is guaranteed by the Constitution, a defendant may opt to have a trial by judge, or bench trial. In cases that are highly charged emotionally, such as the trial of police officers for shooting an unarmed man, the jury may have strong feelings attached to their verdict, even if they swear under oath during *voir dire* (jury selection process) that they are neutral in their feelings about the defendant. With a trial by judge, the facts of the case can be presented, and emotions are less likely to enter into the final verdict. A judge may also nullify a verdict if they believe that the jury's application of the law was inappropriate, too punitive, or too strict.

> *The most common violation by nurses of the criminal law is failure to renew nursing licenses. In this situation, the nurse is practicing nursing without a license, which is a crime in all states.*

What Do You Think?

Do you know anyone who has filed a malpractice suit or a health-care provider who was the defendant in a malpractice suit? What was the situation that caused the case? How was it resolved? If you have never been involved with a malpractice suit or do not know anyone who has, how would you feel if a lawsuit were to be brought against you?

The Nurse's Involvement

Nurses can become involved with the criminal system in their nursing practice in several ways. The most common violation by nurses of the criminal law is failure to renew nursing licenses. In this situation, the nurse is practicing without a license, which is a crime in all states.

Nurses also become involved with the illegal diversion of drugs, particularly narcotics, from the hospital. This is a more serious crime, which may lead to imprisonment.

On December 26, 2017, former registered nurse (RN) Ronda Vaught, 38, injected the paralyzing drug vecuronium instead of the sedative midazolam (Versed) into 75-year-old Charlene Murphey after Murphey was admitted to the intensive care unit (ICU) with a brain bleed. At a jury trial in 2022, Vaught was found guilty of criminally negligent homicide, a lesser offense than the original charge of reckless homicide. The state judge sentenced her to 3 years' probation, and she lost her license to practice nursing. This case was somewhat unusual in that medication errors are usually settled in a tort proceeding, and nurses are usually not charged or punished for crimes associated with the error. However, because the expert witness testified that Vaught's error was an egregious violation of the standard of care, the prosecution believed that a criminal trial was appropriate.[1] Other recent cases involving intentional or unintentional deaths of clients and assisted suicide cases have also led to criminal action against nurses.

Civil Law

Nurses are much more likely to become involved in civil lawsuits than in criminal violations. **Civil laws** generally deal with the violation of one individual's rights by another individual. The court provides the forum that enables these individuals to have their disputes resolved by an independent third party, such as a judge or a jury of the defendant's peers. A decision made by a jury in a civil case does not have to be unanimous but requires only three-fourths agreement (8 out of a 12-member jury). In civil cases, the **burden of proof** rests with the plaintiff. The court finds either for the plaintiff or for the defendant rather than guilty or not guilty. If it finds for the plaintiff, the punishment is always a monetary award rather than jail or prison.

The individual who brings the dispute to the court is called the **plaintiff.** The formal written document that describes the dispute and the resolution sought is called the **complaint.** The individual against whom the complaint is filed is the defendant, who, in conjunction with his or her attorney, prepares the **answer** to the complaint. Civil law has many branches, including contract law, treaty law, tax law, and tort law. It is under tort law that most nurses become involved with the legal system.

Tort Law

A **tort** is generally defined as a wrongful act committed against a person or the person's property independently of a **contract.** A person who commits a tort is called the **tortfeasor** and is **liable** for **damages** to those who are affected by the person's actions. Derived from the Latin *tortus* (twisted), *tort* is a French word for "injury" or "wrong." Torts in the health-care setting can involve several different types of actions, including a direct violation of a person's legal rights or a violation of a standard of care that causes injury to a person. Torts are classified as unintentional, intentional, or quasi-intentional.

Unintentional Torts

Unintentional tort is an umbrella term that includes any type of unplanned event or mistake that leads to injury, property damage, or financial loss by a person. The person who caused the incident did so by mistake and typically because they were not being alert or careful. For example, Stella orders a salad for lunch at a local restaurant. During the early morning process of grating a large block of cheese to be used on top of the salads during the day, Chuck, the sleepy kitchen worker, had accidentally dropped a clear plastic container into the grating machine without noticing. After eating lunch, Stella becomes violent ill and has

> *Because of their professional status, nurses are held to a higher standard of conduct than the ordinary layperson.*

to go to the hospital, where shreds of plastic are found in her gastrointestinal system. Chuck has committed an unintentional tort because of his inattention to the grating of the cheese. Chuck did not *intend* to make anyone sick, but injury still occurred.

Negligence

Negligence is the primary form of unintentional tort. It is generally defined as the **omission** of an act that a reasonable and prudent person would perform in a similar situation or the commission of something a reasonable person would not do in that situation.[2] For example, Don has been invited to Paul's house on Sunday to watch the big football game. On his way up the front steps of Paul's house, Don trips on a toy left there by one of Paul's children, falls down the steps, and hits his head on the concrete sidewalk, suffering a fractured skull and memory loss. Paul is liable for negligence because a reasonable and prudent person in the same situation would have removed the toy from the step.

Nonfeasance is a type of negligence that occurs when a person fails to perform a legally required duty.[2] For example, Kelly Anne is a flag person on a road construction site. Her job is to direct vehicles around a large, deep hole in the road that the road crew is going to fill. A cold wind begins to blow, and Kelly Anne feels chilled. Because the road looks empty as far as she can see, she runs to her nearby car to get her jacket. In the meantime, a car speeds around the corner and drives headfirst into the hole that the driver did not see. The driver is injured, and his car is totaled. Kelly Anne has committed an act of nonfeasance both because she failed to direct the driver around the hole in the road (negligence) and because she had a *legally required duty* to stay at her post because of her agreement with the paving company to act as a flag person.

Malpractice

Malpractice is a type of negligence for which professionals can be sued (professional negligence). Because of their professional status, nurses are held to a higher standard of conduct than the ordinary layperson. The standard for nurses is what a reasonable and prudent *nurse* would do in the same situation. RNs nurses must use the skill, knowledge, and judgment they have learned through their education and experience.[3]

For instance, it is reasonable and prudent that the nurse would put a pair of nonslip shoes or nonskid slippers on a client's feet before taking the client for a required walk, to prevent slipping and falling on the hard hospital floors. One day, the nurse is in a hurry and forgets to put nonskid footwear on a client. A spot on the floor is wet, which causes the client to slip and fall, fracturing a hip. Can the nurse be sued for professional negligence (malpractice) for forgetting to have the client put on nonslip footwear before going for the walk? See if this example fits the four elements that are required for a person to make a claim of malpractice:

1. A **duty** was owed to the client (professional relationship).
2. The professional violated the duty and failed to conform to the standard of care (breach of duty).
3. The professional's failure to act was the **proximate cause** of the resulting injuries (causality).
4. Actual injuries resulted from the breach of duty (damages).[2]

If any of these elements is missing from the case, the client will probably not be able to win the lawsuit (Box 8.2).

Professional Misconduct

Malpractice is more serious than mere negligence because it indicates professional misconduct or unreasonable lack of skill in performing professional duties. Malpractice requires the existence of a professional standard of care and proof that the nurse clearly deviated from that standard of care. A professional **expert witness** is often asked to testify in a malpractice case to help establish the standard of care to which the professional should be held accountable.

A case from South Dakota presents an example of nursing malpractice. The nurse failed to question the physician's order to discharge a client when she discovered the client had a fever. In this case, a supervisory nurse provided expert testimony and reported to the judge that the general standard of care for nurses is to report a significant change in a client's condition, such as an elevated temperature. It is the nurse's responsibility to question the health-care provider's order as to appropriateness of discharge.

Box 8.2 Malpractice Considerations

Nursing malpractice is based on the legal premise that a nurse can be held legally responsible for the personal injury of another individual if it can be proved that the injury was the result of negligence. Nursing malpractice is based on four elements: (1) duty, (2) breach of duty, (3) causation (the "but for" test), and (4) damage or injury.

Inappropriate work assignment and inadequate supervision are a breach of duty and could be the basis for finding a nurse's actions to be negligent. Failure or breach of duty to delegate is established by proving that a reasonably prudent nurse would not have made a particular assignment or delegated a certain responsibility or that supervision was inadequate under the circumstances.

The act of improper delegation of tasks or inadequate supervision must be evaluated in light of the "but for" test related to the injury. If the person who performed the injurious act had not been assigned or delegated to perform the task or had been adequately supervised, the injury could have been avoided. Consequently, the nurse is not being held liable for the negligent act of [the nurse's] subordinate *but for the lack of competence in performing the independent duties of delegation and supervision*.

Off-Site Consideration

Registered nurses who practice in public health, community, or home-care settings must rely frequently on written or telephone communication when delegating patient care duties to assistive personnel. The nurse who must supervise from off-site has a particular duty to assess the knowledge, skills, and judgment of the assistive personnel before making assignments. Regular supervisory visits and impeccable documentation will help the registered nurse ensure that care provided by assistive personnel is adequate.

Source: G. Guido, *Legal and Ethical Issues in Nursing* (7th ed.), Upper Saddle River, NJ: Pearson Prentice Hall, 2020, 66–69.

The records on this case indicated that the client's elevated temperature was charted after the physician had completed his rounds. The nurse did not notify the physician of the client's fever, and the client was subsequently discharged. The client was readmitted a short time after discharge and died in the hospital. The nurse was found negligent. The court held that negligence can be determined by failure to act as well as by the commission of an act.

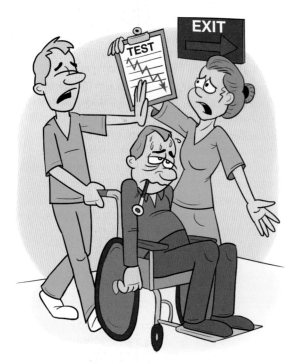

Does this patient look ready to be discharged?

Many other types of actions by nurses can produce malpractice lawsuits. Following are some of the more common actions:

- Leaving foreign objects inside a client during surgery
- Failing to follow a hospital standard or protocol
- Not using equipment in accordance with the manufacturer's recommendations
- Failing to listen to and respond to a client's complaints
- Not properly documenting phone conversations and orders from health-care providers

- Failing to question health-care provider orders when indicated (e.g., too large medication dosages, inappropriate diets)
- Failing to clarify poorly written or illegible health-care provider orders
- Failing to assess and observe a client as directed
- Failing to obtain a proper informed consent
- Failing to report a change in a client's condition, such as vital signs, circulatory status, and level of consciousness
- Failing to report another health-care provider's **incompetency** or negligence
- Failing to take actions to provide for a client's safety, such as not cleaning up a liquid spill on the floor that causes a client to fall
- Failing to provide a client with sufficient and appropriate education before discharge[3]

If the Nurse Is Liable
If a nurse is found guilty of malpractice, several types of action may be taken. The nurse may be required to provide monetary compensation to the client for general damages that were a direct result of the injury, including pain, suffering, disability, and disfigurement. In addition, the nurse is often required to pay for special damages that resulted from the injury, such as all involved medical expenses, **out-of-pocket expenses**, and wages lost by the client while the client was in the hospital.

Optional damages, including those for emotional distress, mental suffering, and counseling expenses that were an outgrowth of the initial injury, may be added to the total settlement. If the client is able to prove that the nurse acted with conscious disregard for the client's safety or acted in a malicious, willful, or wanton manner that produced injury, an additional assessment of punitive or exemplary damages may be added to the award. These fines are added as a warning to other nurses not to repeat the behavior that led to the injury. Because malpractice is a tort action and not a crime, no probation or jail time can be adjudicated.

Intentional Torts

An **intentional tort** is generally defined as a willful act that violates another person's rights or property. Intentional torts can be distinguished from malpractice and acts of negligence by the following three

Issues in Practice

Case Study

Consider the following situation:

Mr. Fagin, a 78-year-old client, was admitted from a nursing home for the treatment of a fractured tibia after he fell out of bed. After the fracture was reduced, a fiberglass cast was applied, and Mr. Fagin was sent to the orthopedic unit for follow-up care. While making her 0400 rounds, the night charge nurse, an RN, discovered that Mr. Fagin's foot on the casted leg was cold to the touch, looked bluish purple, and was swollen approximately one and a half times its normal size. The nurse noted these findings in the client's chart and relayed the information to the day-shift nurses during the 0630 shift report.

The charge nurse on the day shift promptly called and relayed the findings to Mr. Fagin's physician. The physician, however, did not seem to be concerned and only told the nurse to "keep a close eye on him, and don't bother me again unless it is an absolute emergency." A short time later, Mr. Fagin became agitated, complained of severe pain in the affected foot, and eventually began yelling uncontrollably. The charge nurse called the emergency department (ED) physician to come check on the client. The ED physician immediately removed the cast and noted an extensive circulatory impairment that would not respond to treatment. A few days later, Mr. Fagin's leg was amputated. His family filed a malpractice lawsuit against the hospital, the physician, and both the night and day charge nurses.

Questions for Thought

1. Are all the elements present in this case for a bona fide malpractice lawsuit?
2. What could have been done to prevent this situation from happening?
3. How should nurses deal with reluctant or hostile health-care providers?

requirements: (1) the nurse must intend to bring about the consequences of the act, (2) the nurse's act must be intended to interfere with the client or the client's property, and (3) the act must be a substantial factor in bringing about the injury or consequences.

The most frequently encountered intentional torts are assault, battery, false imprisonment, abandonment, and intentional infliction of emotional distress. With intentional torts, the injured person does not have to prove that an injury has occurred, nor is the opinion of an expert witness required for adjudication. Punitive damages are more likely to be assessed against the nurse in intentional tort cases, and some intentional torts may fall under the criminal law if there is gross violation of the standards of care.

Gross negligence, also called willful misconduct, is a wanton and reckless violation of one or more standards of care. Gross negligence is somewhat hard to define but is one of those things, as in the Vought

case, that people know when they see it. Ordinary negligence and gross negligence differ in degree of inattention, while both differ from willful and wanton conduct, which is conduct that is reasonably considered to cause injury.[4] Gross negligence is carelessness that displays complete and reckless disregard for the safety or lives of others. It is so great that it almost appears to be a conscious violation of other people's rights to safety.[5] For example, Vince Johnson has severe right lower abdominal pain and is taken to the hospital where he is diagnosed with appendicitis. He goes for emergency surgery for removal of his appendix. Because of a crowded surgery schedule, he is worked in between already scheduled clients. In the recovery room, he discovers the surgeon has confused him with the next scheduled client and has amputated his left foot instead of removing his appendix. The surgeon and hospital staff in this case have committed gross negligence, as any reasonable person would see that the first step of the surgical team should be to

Issues in Practice

Nurse Malpractice in Client Fall

At a hospital in Washington State, a client with a recent leg amputation was still partially sedated after surgery. The nurse assigned to his care was called away from the room and failed to raise the bed rails. The client attempted to get out of bed, fell, and was injured.

The client sued the hospital for negligence. Using the hospital's own policies and procedures manual, the client's lawyer pointed out the requirement that satisfactory precautions be taken to restrain disabled or sedated clients.

The nurse's lawyer based the defense on the argument that the nurse was following the physician's **standing orders** to allow the client to ambulate postoperatively to hasten recovery and prevent complications.

The court agreed with the client and concluded that the nurse had an obligation, based on the hospital's policy and procedures, to assess the client's physical and mental condition. Nurses have an obligation not to leave clients unattended in an unsafe bed configuration.

All lawsuits alleging health-care provider negligence require expert witness testimony. Without this, courts will almost always dismiss a negligence case decided by a lay jury, even when it is as obvious as a fall from bed. In this case, the expert testimony not only supported the lawyer's contention that the hospital's policy and procedures upheld the suit but also emphasized the point that clients recently returned from surgery are disoriented from anesthesia and should never be left alone unless the bed rails are raised to their full upright position.

When the case was appealed, the court of appeals wrote the following ruling:

A lawsuit against a hospital for negligence does not necessarily have to involve medical malpractice committed by a physician. A hospital's nurses have their own independent legal duties in assessing and caring for their patients.

A hospital is not relieved of its own legal liability for negligence just because the hospital's staff nurses followed the health-care provider's orders. That is, a hospital's nursing staff cannot necessarily rely on standing orders for a patient to be up and out of bed and leave the bed rails down.

A patient freshly out of surgery who is taking pain and sedative medications must be evaluated continually by the staff. The patient's present physical and mental state is all that matters. The nurses may have to disregard standing orders and instead follow the hospital's policies and procedures for a restraint in the form of raised bed rails when necessary to ensure the patient's safety.

Questions for Thought

1. Do you agree with the jury's decision against the nurse? Why?
2. The nurse has a legal and ethical obligation (fidelity) to follow the health-care provider's order. Is there ever a situation when the nurse can ignore an order?
3. Under what legal principle was the hospital held liable for the nurse's actions?
4. What other actions might the nurse have taken, besides putting up the bed rails, to prevent the patient from falling?

Source: Greenberg v. Empire Health Services Inc., *2006 WL 1075574 Wash. App., April 25, 2006.*

identify the client who is about to be operated on. The second step should be to confirm the type of surgery the client needs or at least realize they were amputating a healthy limb.

Assault and Battery

Assault is the unjustifiable attempt to touch another person or the threat of doing so. **Battery** is actual harmful or unwarranted contact with another person without their consent. Battery is the most common intentional tort seen in the practice of nursing.[3]

For a nurse to commit assault and battery, there must be an absence of client consent. Before any procedure can be performed on a competent, alert, and normally oriented client, the client must agree or consent to the procedure being done. Negligence does not have to be proved for a person to be successful in a claim for assault and battery.

A common example of an assault and battery occurs when a nurse physically restrains a client against the client's will and administers an injection against the client's wishes.

False Imprisonment

False imprisonment occurs when a competent client is confined or restrained with intent to prevent them from leaving the hospital. The use of restraints alone does not constitute false imprisonment when they are used to maintain the safety of a confused, disoriented, heavily medicated, or otherwise incompetent client. In general, mentally impaired clients can be detained against their will only if they are at risk for injuring themselves or others. The use of threats or medications that interfere with the client's ability to leave the facility can also be considered false imprisonment.

Intentional Infliction of Emotional Distress

Intentional infliction of emotional distress is another common intentional tort encountered by the nurse. To prove this intentional tort, the following three elements are necessary: (1) the conduct exceeds what is usually accepted by society, (2) the health-care provider's conduct is intended to cause mental distress, and (3) the conduct actually does produce mental distress (causation). Any nurse who is charged with assault, battery, or false imprisonment is also at risk for being charged with infliction of emotional distress.

A 1975 case, *Johnson v. Women's Hospital*, is an example of infliction of emotional distress. A mother wished to view the body of her baby, who had died during birth. After she made the request, she was handed the baby's body, which was floating in a gallon jar of formaldehyde.[3] The *Johnson* case demonstrates a clear lack of respect shown to the mother. If the mother in this delicate situation had been treated with dignity and respect, the lawsuit would have been avoided.

Client Abandonment

Because of the ongoing nursing shortage, **abandonment** of clients has become an important legal and ethical issue for health-care providers. Abandonment occurs when there is a unilateral severance of the professional relationship with the client without adequate notice and while the requirement for care still exists. The nurse–client relationship continues until it is terminated by mutual consent of both parties.[3]

From an ethical standpoint, the issue of abandonment falls under the umbrella of the ethical principle of beneficence. From the legal view, client abandonment can be considered an intentional tort, **breach of contract**, or in some cases in which injury occurs, malpractice. The key phrase to keep in mind when discussing client abandonment is *without adequate notice*. If the client knows that the nurse's shift is scheduled to end at 7 p.m., the client and the hospital both have adequate notice.

During the peak years of the COVID-19 pandemic, the nursing shortage was so extreme that it was difficult for nurses to provide even minimally adequate care for the many critically ill patients on their units. Many patients who survived the ordeal of having the virus complained that they felt abandoned and, in fact, were often left alone for long periods of time.[5] Although many patients may have felt that they were abandoned when left alone in isolation rooms for extended periods of time, it is highly unlikely their situations would fit the definition of abandonment. The nurse assigned to their care may have left them to care for other patients but did not leave them without adequate notice. Also, these patients were likely connected to monitors that were being watched outside their rooms to detect changes in their conditions. It would seem that rather than experiencing abandonment, these patients were experiencing lone-liness and social isolation because they could not have visitors.

It is not uncommon for nurses in today's health-care system to be approached by nursing supervisors telling them, "Everyone else called out, so you will have to work a double shift or you could be charged with client abandonment." In this case, the abandon-ment becomes the hospital's responsibility, not the nurse's. Nurses sometimes feel uncomfortable about going on strike because it seems to imply client aban-donment; however, if there is adequate notice about the strike and if the facility has had time to make arrangements for care or discharge of clients, there is no client abandonment. The growing practice of emergency client diversion, occurring when facili-ties can no longer safely care for emergency clients because of lack of space or staffing, can potentially fall under the legal definitions of abandonment.

Quasi-Intentional Torts

A **quasi-intentional tort** is a mixture of unintentional and intentional torts. It is defined as a voluntary act that directly causes injury or distress without intent to injure or to cause distress.[3] A quasi-intentional tort does have the elements of volition and causation without the element of intent. Quasi-intentional torts usually involve situations of communication and often violate a person's reputation, personal privacy, or civil rights (Box 8.3).

Defamation of Character

Defamation of character, which is the most common of the quasi-intentional torts, is harmful to a person's reputation. Defamation injures a person's reputation by diminishing the esteem, respect, good will, or con-fidence that others have for the person. It can be espe-cially damaging when false statements are made about a criminal act or an immoral act or when there are false allegations about a client's having a contagious disease. When a statement about a person is obviously not true, it is called defamation per se.[6] Examples include the two situations that follow.

In *Schessler v. Keck* (1954), a nurse was found liable for defamation of character when she told a friend that a client for whom she was caring was a caterer and was being treated for syphilis. Even though the statement was false, when the information became public, it destroyed his catering business.

Box 8.3　**Registered Nurse Licensure**

The legislature of each state enacts laws that govern the practice of nursing. The purpose of licensing law is to ensure that the public is pro-tected from unqualified practitioners by developing and enforcing regulations that define who may practice in the profession, the scope of that prac-tice, and the level of education for the profession.

A fundamental premise of nursing practice is that a professional nurse is personally respon-sible for all acts or omissions undertaken within the scope of practice. The American Nurses Association defines delegation as "the transfer of responsibility for the performance of an activ-ity from one person to another while retaining accountability for the outcome."[4] In addition, the nurse is responsible for the adequate supervision of a task delegated to a subordinate. If the nurse fails to delegate appropriately or supervise adequately, any injuries resulting from the acts of the subordi-nate may result in licensure ramifications. The state licensing board may take disciplinary actions.

In another case, the father of a 6-year-old child was questioned by a nurse about suspected sexual abuse when the child was treated for the third time for a urinary tract infection. Another nurse at the nurses' station, believing that the father was out of earshot, com-mented that the father looked like a pervert and child abuser. The father became upset by the comment and went to a lawyer who filed a defamation suit and viola-tion of the HIPAA law against the nurse who made the unsubstantiated comment. No other evidence existed that the child had been sexually abused. Opinions should always be backed up by clinical proofs and substantiated data. It is obvious that in this case, the nurse had no hard evidence for her supposition about the father.[6]

Defamation includes **slander**, which is spoken communication in which one person discusses another in terms that harm that person's reputation. **Libel** is a written communication in which a per-son makes statements or uses language that harms another person's reputation. To win a defamation lawsuit against the nurse, the client must prove that the nurse acted maliciously, abused the principle of **privileged communication**, and wrote or spoke a lie.[6]

Medical record documentation is a primary source of defamation of character. Through the years, the client's chart has been the basis of many defamation lawsuits. Discussion about a client in the elevators, cafeteria, and other public areas can also lead to lawsuits for defamation if negative comments are overheard.

In today's information overloaded society, anyone can write or say pretty much anything they want on the Internet and social media. People write what they think and feel online where nothing is private, and it is common for former patients, disgruntled or unhappy patients, former employees, or others with a grudge to spout untruths about individuals or institutions. It is often called *cyber defamation* when the information that people are writing or saying on mobile devices rises to the level of defamation. Lawyers and potential plaintiffs are well aware of the amount of money awarded by juries in defamation cases. It is not unusual for plaintiffs to receive awards in the millions of dollars because of defamation. Unlike most health-care tort cases, which may drag on for years, defamation cases are expedited and heard much sooner because defamation immediately downgrades the individual's reputation and often results in loss of income.[6]

Invasion of Privacy

Invasion of privacy is a violation of a person's right to protection against unreasonable and unwarranted interference with one's personal life. To prove that a nurse has committed the tort of invasion of privacy, the client must show that (1) the nurse intruded on the client's seclusion and privacy, (2) the intrusion is objectionable to a reasonable and prudent person, (3) the act committed intrudes on private or published facts or pictures of a private nature, and (4) public disclosure of private information was made.[3] Examples of invasion of privacy include using the client's name or picture for the sole advantage of the health-care provider, intruding into the client's private affairs without permission, giving out private client information over the telephone, and publishing information that misrepresents the client's condition. Because of the Health Insurance Portability and Accountability Act (HIPAA) of 1996, health-care providers have become more aware than ever of the issue of confidentiality in the health-care setting.[7]

Breach of Confidentiality

Confidentiality of information concerning the client must be honored. A breach of confidentiality results when a client's trust and confidence are violated by public revelation of confidential or privileged communications without the client's consent.[7]

> *Examples of invasion of privacy include using the client's name or picture for the sole advantage of the health-care provider, intruding into the client's private affairs without permission, giving out private client information over the telephone, and publishing information that misrepresents the client's condition.*

Privileged Communication
Privileged communication is protected by law and exists in certain well-defined professional relationships—for example, physician–client, psychiatrist–client, priest–penitent, and lawyer–client. Privileged communication ensures that the professional who obtains any information from the client cannot be forced to reveal that information, even in a court of law under oath. Nurses do not have privileged communication with clients. However, they can be bound, by extension, under the seal of privileged communication if they are in a room with a physician when the client reveals personal information.

Most breach of confidentiality cases involve a physician's revelation of privileged communications shared by a client. Nurses who overhear privileged communication or information, however, are held to the same standards as a physician with regard to that information.

Privileged client information can be disclosed only if it is authorized by the client. In accord with the HIPAA regulations, all health-care facilities must have specific guidelines dealing with client information disclosure. Disclosure of information to family members violates HIPAA regulations unless the client is under 18 years of age or gives permission for the disclosure. For instance, a client may not wish to disclose to a family member a specific diagnosis, such as cancer. If this is the case, the nurse should honor this request; otherwise, it is considered a violation of HIPAA regulations.[8]

Electronic Pitfalls

Use of computerized documentation and **telemedicine** has led to several lawsuits based on breach of confidentiality and malpractice. (See Chapter 17 for examples.) The current widespread practice of texting on portable wireless electronic devices has also opened up a new world of possible confidentiality violations.[8] The HIPAA regulations on communication are the government's attempts to force the legal system to keep pace with the use of computers and electronic record-keeping. Cases exist in which medical records have been lost because of computer failure; however, there have been an increasing number of cases where institutions that provide health care or collect and store data from health-care entities have been hacked, producing massive loss or release of personal patient information.

In 2022, the U.S. District Court for the Central District of California filed a class-action lawsuit against SuperCare Health, Inc., which is a respiratory-care provider. Allegedly, the company was hacked for the personal and health information of its patients. Lead plaintiff, Hamid Shalviri, alleges that SuperCare committed negligence and breach of implied contract. Because of SuperCare's negligence, the suit alleges that the company allowed the invasion of privacy of more than 300,000 current and former patients' personal and health information, leading to the compromise of patient names, addresses, dates of birth, health insurance, and medical records. The suit also alleges violations of the California Confidentiality of Medical Information Act.[7]

> *Because of the rapid proliferation of lawsuits since the 1990s, there is now a higher probability that a nurse, at some time in their career, will be involved either as a witness or as a party to a nursing malpractice action.*

FACING A LAWSUIT

Because of the rapid proliferation of lawsuits since the 1990s, there is now a higher probability that a nurse, at some time in their career, will be involved either as a witness or as a party to a nursing malpractice action. Knowledge of the litigation process increases nurses' understanding of the way in which their conduct is evaluated before the courts.

The Statute of Limitations

A malpractice suit against a nurse for negligence must be filed within a specified time. This period, called the **statute of limitations**, generally begins at the time of the injury or when the injury is discovered and lasts until some specified future time. In most states, the limitation period lasts from 1 to 6 years, with the most common duration being 2 years. However, in cases involving children, the statute of limitations extends until the person reaches 21 years of age. If the client fails to file the suit within the prescribed time, the lawsuit will be barred.[3]

The Complaint

Filing the suit (also called the *complaint*) with the court begins the litigation process. The written complaint describes the incident that initiated the claim of negligence against the nurse. Specific allegations, including the amount of money sought for damages, are also stated in the **legal complaint**. The plaintiff, who is usually a client or a family member of a client, is the alleged injured party, and the defendant is the person or entity being sued (i.e., the nurse, health-care provider, or hospital). The first notice of a lawsuit occurs when the defendant (nurse) is officially notified or served with the complaint. All defendants are accorded the right of **due process** under constitutional law.

The Answer

The defendant must respond to the allegations stated in the complaint within a specific time frame. This written response by the defendant is called the *answer*. If the nurse had liability insurance at the time of the negligent act, the insurer will assign a lawyer to represent the defendant nurse. In the answer, the nurse can outline specific defenses to the claims against them.

The Discovery

After the complaint and answer are filed with the court, the discovery phase of the litigation begins. The purpose of discovery is to uncover all information relevant to the malpractice suit and the incident in question. The nurse may be required to answer a series of questions that relate to the nurse's educational background and emotional state, the incident that led to the lawsuit, and any other pertinent information. These written questions are called **interrogatories**.

In addition, the plaintiff's lawyer may request documents related to the lawsuit, including the plaintiff's medical records, **incident reports**, electronic communications, address books or lists of contacts, the institution's policy and procedure manual concerning the specific situation, and the nurse's job description. The plaintiff is also required to disclose information as part of the discovery process, including the plaintiff's past medical history.

The Deposition

The next step in the process is the taking of a deposition from each party in the lawsuit, as well as any potential witnesses, to assist the lawyers in the trial preparation. A **deposition** is a formal legal process that is recorded by a court reporter. A deposition is the taking of an oral statement of a witness under oath before trial. It has two purposes: to find out what the witness knows and to preserve that witness's testimony. The intent is to allow both parties to learn all the facts before the trial so that no one is surprised at trial. Depositions are usually wide ranging in scope and often include information not allowed in a trial, such as **hearsay** testimony. In some cases, videotaped depositions may be used. Nurses can prepare for a deposition by keeping some key points in mind (Box 8.4).

The deposition **testimony** is reduced to a written document called an **affidavit** for use at trial. If a witness during the trial changes testimony from that given at the deposition, the deposition can be used to contradict the testimony. This process is called *impeaching the witness*. Impeaching a witness on a

specific issue can create doubt about that witness's credibility and can thus weaken other areas in the witness's testimony. In some situations, witnesses can later be charged with **perjury** if it is proved that they gave false testimony under oath.

The Trial

The **trial** often takes place years after the complaint was filed. Once **jurisdiction** is determined, the *voir dire* process, more commonly called *jury selection*, begins. After jury selection, each attorney presents opening statements. The plaintiff's side is presented first. Witnesses may be served with **subpoenas** that require them to appear and provide testimony.

Each witness or party is subject to direct examination, cross-examination, and redirect examination. Direct examination involves open-ended questions by the attorney. Cross-examination is performed by the opposing lawyer, and questions are asked in such a way as to elicit short, specific responses. The redirect examination consists of follow-up questions to address issues that were raised during the cross-examination.

After both parties have presented their case, the lawyers deliver their closing arguments. The case then goes to a jury or a judge for deliberation. If the facts are not in dispute, the judge may render a **summary judgment**. If either party is not satisfied, the decision or ruling made about the case can be appealed. The party appealing the decision is called the **appellant**. There is almost always an appeal if a large sum of money is awarded to the plaintiff.

Monetary Awards

The primary reason clients sue health-care providers, nurses, and hospitals is to recover monetary compensation and other associated costs against the person or institution that harmed the client; the secondary reason is to prevent additional malpractice by the defendant. Generally, when lawyers are evaluating a case as a potential malpractice suit, they look for the person or institution that has "deep pockets" (i.e., the one that is backed by a large source of income or that maintains a high-payout insurance policy). Lawyers will generally refuse a case if there is not a good probability of substantial monetary rewards. There are several types of awards that a plaintiff may seek when a favorable decision is rendered by the jury:

Box 8.4　Giving a Deposition

1. Do not volunteer information. Give only enough information to answer the question.
2. Be familiar with the client's medical record and nurse's notes.
3. Remain calm throughout the process, and do not be intimidated by the lawyers.
4. Clarify all questions before answering; ask the lawyer to explain the question if you do not understand. (You can do this with every question a hostile lawyer is asking.)
5. Do not make assumptions about the questions.
6. Do not exaggerate answers.
7. Wait at least 5 seconds after a question is asked before answering it to allow objections from other lawyers.
8. Tell the truth—you are under oath, and lying is the crime of perjury.
9. Do not speculate about answers.
10. Speak slowly and clearly, using professional language as much as possible.
11. Look the questioning lawyer in the eye as much as possible.
12. If unable to remember an answer, simply state, "I don't remember" or "I don't know." You cannot just refuse to answer unless it reveals confidential information.
13. Think before answering any question (also a reason to wait 5 seconds before answering).
14. Bring a résumé or curriculum vitae (CV) to the deposition in case it is requested.
15. Request a break if you are tired or confused.
16. Avoid becoming angry with the lawyers or using sarcastic language with them.
17. Avoid using absolutes (e.g., *always, never, no one, everybody, none*) in your answers.
18. If a question is asked more than once, ask the court recorder to read the previous answer.
19. Answer questions verbally instead of using body language such as nodding the head, using facial expressions, or changing position.
20. Avoid starting answers with "Well, to be honest with you. . . ."
21. Pleading your right against self-incrimination under the Fifth Amendment is allowed in a civil lawsuit if you somehow become a co-defendant. But use this carefully and only with advice of your lawyer.
22. Watch out for compound and trick questions that may set you up for answers you did not intend to provide. For example, "When did you stop abusing your patients?"
23. Do not let the lawyer put words in your mouth. For example, "So you would say Dr. Cutter was overly eager to operate on patients that really didn't need surgery?"
24. Do not bring notes, diaries, or any other documents unless thoroughly reviewed by the defendant's lawyer. They can be used as additional evidence against the defendant, if harmful.
25. Dress professionally (no scrubs unless the deposition is in the hospital during your shift), speak professionally, and act professionally at all times. (No smoking.)
26. Be sure to read over the deposition just before the trial.
27. Avoid starting answers with "I think that . . ." statements. Better to say, "The evidence shows. . . ."

Sources: K.C. Wagner, D. Hunter-Adkins, R. Clifford, Questions & answers. Effective preparation of the expert witness for deposition, *Journal of Legal Nurse Consulting*, 19(4):26–29, 34, 2009; Indest G. Preparing for a deposition for nurses. The Health Law Blog, 2018. https://www.thehealth lawfirmblogs.com/preparing-for-a-deposition-for-nurses/#:~:text=Preparing%20for%20a%20Deposition%20for%20Nurses%201.%20Dress,a%20 deponent%20during%20a...%203.%20Tell%20the%20.

Compensatory damages, also called *actual damages,* are awards that cover the actual cost of injuries and economic losses caused by the injury. These include all medical expenses related to the injury and any lost wages or income that resulted from extended hospitalization or recovery period.

General damages are monetary awards for injuries for which an exact dollar amount cannot be calculated. These awards include pain and suffering, loss of companionship, shortened life span, loss of reputation, and wrongful death. Some state legislatures have recently passed new tort reform laws that severely limit or completely eliminate general damage awards.

Punitive damages, also called *exemplary damages,* are awarded in addition to compensatory and general damages when the actions that caused the injury to the client were judged to be willful or malicious or demonstrated an extreme measure of incompetence and gross negligence. The primary purpose of punitive damages is to "punish" the plaintiff and deter them from ever acting in the same way again. These awards are almost always extremely large, usually in the millions of dollars, and quickly gain the attention of other health-care providers to avoid the same types of actions. Some states have recently passed tort reform laws to limit punitive awards to much smaller amounts (less than 10 percent of a usual award) in the belief that it will bring down the cost of malpractice insurance and, hopefully, the overall cost of health care.

Treble damages allow the judge, in certain instances, to triple the actual damage award amount as an additional form of punitive damages. Not all states allow judges this decision-making power; and it, too, has been opposed by legislatures advocating tort reform.

Normal damages can be awarded when the law requires a judge and jury to find a defendant guilty but no real harm happened to the plaintiff. The award is usually very small, generally in the sum of $1,000.

Special damages are awarded to the plaintiff for out-of-pocket expenses related to the trial. It would cover the expenses of taking a taxi back and forth to the courthouse, use of special assistive equipment, and special home health-care providers not covered under actual damages.

It is easy to understand why most malpractice suits are settled out of court by insurance companies. The expenses for lawyers and lengthy trials quickly become astronomical, and there is never any certainty about the way a jury will decide. On the plaintiffs' side, although the money they receive from the insurance company may be significantly smaller than the award they might get from a jury, they get the money immediately rather than having to wait through a long appeals process that could take years.

POSSIBLE DEFENSES TO A MALPRACTICE SUIT

Laws dealing with the awarding of damages vary from one state to another. The amount awarded also depends on the types of injuries sustained. Generally, the more severe the injuries, the greater the award because of the higher cost of treatment.

Contributory Negligence

In a state with contributory negligence laws, plaintiffs are not allowed to receive money for injuries if they contributed to those injuries in any manner. For example, a nurse forgot to raise the bed rail after administering an injection of a narcotic pain medication to a postoperative client but instructed the client to turn on the call light if he wanted to get out of bed. The client fell while attempting to go to the bathroom; because he did not use the call light, he contributed to his own injuries and thus could not receive compensation.

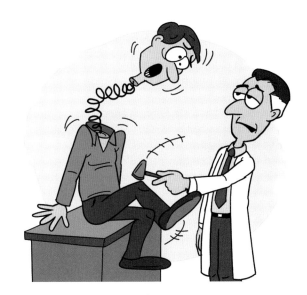

"I suppose this means another malpractice suit."

Comparative Negligence

In a state with comparative negligence laws, the awards are based on the determination of the percentage of fault by both parties. For example, in the aforementioned case, if $100,000 was awarded by the jury, it may be determined that the nurse was 75 percent at fault and the client was 25 percent at fault. In that case, the client would receive $75,000. In general, if the client is 50 percent or more at fault, no award will be made. Evidently, determination of these types of awards is highly subjective, and an **appeal** about the decision is almost always made to a higher court.

Case Study

Ms. Gouge, a 44-year-old client who weighed 307 pounds, was admitted to a large university medical center ED with complaints of chest pain and disorientation and a blood pressure of 208/154 mm Hg. She also displayed aphasia, hemiplegia, and loss of sensation and movement on her right side.

After an MRI scan of the head, it was discovered that she had an inoperable cerebral aneurysm. In addition to appropriate medical treatment for blood pressure and circulation, her family physician told her that she had to lose a significant amount of weight. The nurse in the physician's office instituted a weight loss teaching plan for Ms. Gouge, planned out a calorie-restricted low-fat diet, and gave her a large amount of information about a healthy diet and a DVD of low-impact aerobic exercises. At a follow-up visit 1 month later, Ms. Gouge weighed 315 pounds.

Six months later, Ms. Gouge's aneurysm ruptured, leaving her in a vegetative state. Ms. Gouge's family filed a lawsuit against the physician and his office nurse, claiming that they had failed to institute proper and appropriate preventive measures and that they had failed to inform the client of the seriousness of her condition.

Did the nurse's decisions or actions contribute to the filing of this suit? Is there any contributory negligence? What is the nurse's role in defending against this suit? What might the nurse have done to prevent the suit in the first place?

Assumption of Risk

When the client signs the informed consent form for a particular treatment, procedure, or surgery, it is implied that the client is aware of the possible complications of that treatment, procedure, or surgery. Under the assumption-of-risk defense, if one of those listed or named complications occurs, the client has no grounds to sue the health-care provider. For example, a common complication from hip replacement surgery is some loss of mobility and range of motion of the affected leg. Even if a client, after having a hip replaced, is able to walk only using a walker, they still do not have any grounds for a lawsuit.

Good Samaritan Act

All 50 states and the District of Columbia now have Good Samaritan laws, although the laws vary among states. Written initially to protect physicians only, most laws now include other health-care providers such as nurses, emergency medical technicians, and paramedics. The laws usually do not protect health-care providers who are on duty in a health-care facility or ambulance. The Good Samaritan laws were written because health-care providers were sometimes hesitant to provide care at the scene of accidents, in emergency situations, or during disasters because they feared lawsuits. The **Good Samaritan Act** is designed specifically to protect health-care providers in these situations. A health-care professional who provides care in an emergency situation cannot be sued for injuries that may be sustained by the client if that care was given according to established guidelines and was within the scope of the professional's education. Legally, Good Samaritan laws do not require a health-care provider to render aid; however, there may be an ethical obligation.[9]

For example, a nurse finds a person in cardiac arrest on the sidewalk and administers CPR to revive the person. In the process, she fractures several of the client's ribs. The client would not be able to sue the nurse for the fractured ribs if the CPR was administered according to established standards.

However, Good Samaritan laws do have some limitations. While they cover nurses from liability for ordinary negligence, they do not cover nurses for grossly negligent acts in the provision of care or for acts outside the nurse's level of education. For example, in the case of a person choking on a piece of meat, the nurse initially attempts the Heimlich maneuver but without success. As the person loses consciousness, the nurse decides to perform a tracheostomy. The client survives but can sue the nurse for injuries from the tracheostomy because this is not a normal part of a nurse's education.

Although there has been some impetus for Obligation to Treat, or Bad Samaritan, laws, only three states, Minnesota, Rhode Island, and Vermont, have enacted these laws. These laws essentially establish a duty to help those in need and apply to everyone, not just health-care providers. These laws are very difficult to enforce and generally apply only if the person rendering aid to a victim can do so without placing themselves in harm's way.[9]

Unavoidable Accident

Sometimes accidents happen without any contributing causes from the nurse, hospital, or health-care provider. For example, a client is walking in the hall and trips over her own bathrobe. She breaks an ankle. There were no puddles on the floor or obstacles in the hall, and the client was alert and oriented. Because no one is at fault, there are no grounds for a lawsuit.

Defense of the Fact

Defense of the fact is based on the claim that the actions of the nurse followed the standards of care or that even if the actions were in violation of the standard of care, the actions themselves were not the direct cause of the injury.[3] For example, a nurse wraps a dressing too tightly on a client's foot after surgery. Later, the client loses his eyesight and blames the loss of vision on the nurse's improper dressing of his foot. The two events had nothing to do with each other.

Going through the litigation process can produce high levels of anxiety. Placing every aspect of the nurse's conduct under scrutiny in a trial is very stressful. All aspects of the alleged negligent act will be examined and re-examined. Often, events that happened years before can be brought in to establish a "pattern of behavior." Every word of the nurse's notes and the medical record will be closely analyzed and questioned. Nurses can survive the litigation process with the help of good attorneys and by being honest and demonstrating that they were acting in the best interests of the client. From this viewpoint, it is easy to see the importance of carrying nursing liability insurance.

ALTERNATIVE DISPUTE FORUMS

Although most lawsuits against nurses are settled through the court system, there are other methods of settling them. Because of the large number of cases and the resultant overload of the judicial system, different ways of resolving disputes have become increasingly more common. These alternative forums are being used for many types of conflict and are seen more frequently in the areas of torts, contracts, employment, and family law. Mediation and arbitration are the most commonly used alternatives to trial.

Mediation

Mediation is a process that allows each party to present their case before a mediator, who is an independent third party trained in dispute resolution. The mediator listens to each side individually. This one-sided session is called a *caucus*. The mediator's role is to find common ground between the parties and encourage resolution of the challenged matters by compromise and negotiation. The mediator aids the parties in arriving at a mutually acceptable outcome. The mediator does not act as a decision-maker but rather encourages the parties to come to a "meeting of the minds."

> " *Health-care providers are sometimes hesitant to provide care at the scene of accidents, in emergency situations, or during disasters because they fear lawsuits. The Good Samaritan Act is designed specifically to protect health-care providers in these situations.* "

Arbitration

Arbitration, in contrast, allows a neutral third party to hear both parties' positions and then make a decision or ruling on the basis of the facts and evidence presented. Arbitration, by agreement or by statutory definition, can be binding or nonbinding. **Arbitrators** or mediators are often retired judges who work on an hourly fee basis or are practicing attorneys. In the family law area, they are frequently social workers or specially trained mediators. Negligence and malpractice issues are frequently resolved through arbitration and mediation.

COMMON ISSUES IN HEALTH-CARE LITIGATION

Nurses need to be aware of certain situations in the routine provision of care that constitute legal minefields. If the nurses are aware of these sensitive situations, they can exercise an extra degree of caution to make sure they are meeting standards of care and not violating a client's rights.

Informed Consent

Informed consent is both a legal and an ethical issue. Informed consent is the voluntary permission by a client or by the client's designated proxy to carry out a procedure on the client. Clients' claims that they did not grant informed consent before a surgery or invasive procedure can and do form the basis of a significant percentage of lawsuits.[10]

Although these lawsuits are most often directed against health-care providers and hospitals, nurses can become involved when they provide the information but are not performing the procedure. The person who is performing the procedure has the responsibility to obtain the informed consent. However, some health-care providers habitually give the nurse the consent form and ask the nurse to "get the client to sign this." Informed consent can be given by a client only after the client receives sufficient information on:

- Treatment proposed.
- Material risk involved (potential complications).
- Acceptable alternative treatments.
- Outcome hoped for.
- Consequences of not having treatment.

The health-care provider should provide most of this information. Nurses can reinforce the information given by the health-care provider and even supplement the material but should not be the primary or only source of information for the informed consent.[10] It is often difficult to draw a clear distinction between where the health-care provider's responsibility ends and that of the nurse begins.

What Do You Think?

Have you ever had a surgical procedure for which you signed an informed consent form? Did it meet all five criteria listed? Which ones were missing?

Exceptions to Informed Consent

There are two exceptions to informed consent:

1. Emergency situations in which the client is unconscious, incompetent, or otherwise unable to give consent.

2. Situations in which the health-care provider feels that it may be medically contraindicated to disclose the risks and hazards because it may result in illness, severe emotional distress, serious psychological damage, or failure on the part of the client to receive lifesaving treatment.

Patient Self-Determination Act

The Patient Self-Determination Act of 1990, sponsored by Senator John Danforth, is a federal law that requires all federally funded institutions to inform clients of their right to prepare advance directives. Advance directives are meant to encourage people to discuss and document their wishes concerning the type of treatment and care that they want (i.e., life-sustaining treatment) in advance so that it will ease the burden on their families and providers when it comes time to make such a decision.

There are two types of advance directives: the living will and the medical durable power of attorney (Box 8.5). The **living will** is a document stating what health care a client will accept or refuse after the client is no longer competent or able to make that decision. The medical durable power of attorney, or health-care proxy, designates another person to make health-care decisions for a person if the client becomes incompetent or unable to make such decisions.

Each state outlines its own requirements for executing and revoking the medical durable power of attorney and living wills. These documents and rules can be accessed on the state's website, generally under the "Department of Health and Human Services" or a similar designation. Any particular state's living will form can be downloaded by going to the National Hospice and Palliative Care Organization's website.

Incompetent Client's Right to Self-Determination

The courts are protective of incompetent clients and require high standards of proof before allowing a health-care provider to terminate any life-sustaining

> *Nurses can reinforce the information given by the health-care provider and even supplement the material but should not be the primary or only source of information for the informed consent.*

Box 8.5 **Common Questions About Advance Directives**

Q. Which is better—a living will or a medical durable power of attorney for health care (i.e., health-care proxy)?

A. These documents are different and allow you to do two different things. The living will states what health-care procedures you will accept or refuse after you are no longer competent or able to make that decision. The medical durable power of attorney, or health-care proxy, allows you to designate another person to make health-care choices for you.

Q. If I have a living will and change my mind, can I cancel the living will or durable medical power of attorney?

A. Yes. Each state has ways that your advance directives can be canceled or negated. Most states require an oral or written statement, destruction of the document, or notification to certain individuals, such as the physician. Again, each state's statute should be checked for the specific details required.

Q. If I have a living will in one state, is it good in all states?

A. It may or may not be, depending on that state's requirements for the living will. It is important that you have your living will checked by an attorney to determine whether it may be effective in the states in which you are traveling or working.

Q. If I have a living will and have a medical durable power of attorney, who should get copies?

A. Copies should be given to your next of kin, your primary health-care provider, and your attorney so that more than one person has a copy and knows what your intentions are. Some states allow you to register your living will with certain state agencies such as the Secretary of State. There are also national groups that allow you to register your living will with them so that there is access to it.

---

treatment for that client. Consider the following examples:

On January 11, 1983, 25-year-old Nancy Cruzan lost control of her car while driving at night. When paramedics arrived and assessed her, she had no respirations and no pulse, but after lengthy resuscitation efforts, she eventually regained a weak pulse and shallow respirations. She was admitted to the intensive care unit, and after 3 weeks of unresponsiveness, she was diagnosed as being in a persistent vegetative state (PVS). A gastrostomy feeding and hydration tube was inserted at this time to assist with nutrition and electrolyte balance. Cruzan's husband, her primary guardian and decision-maker, consented to the feeding tube.

A PVS occurs when, after a prolonged period of unresponsiveness, a client can perform a few select, involuntary peripheral nerve reflex actions on their own, such as breathing, blinking, smiling, opening their eyes, and tracking movements with the eyes. Unlike "brain death," in PVS the lower brain stem is still healthy and fully functioning, which is why clients in PVS can breathe on their own.

Clients who are brain dead have no brain function at all, of which the inability to breath is an indicator.

Five years later, Cruzan's parents asked her providers to remove the feeding tube. The hospital refused to do so without a court order, because they believed that removal of the tube would be the proximate, or nearest, cause of Cruzan's death as opposed to the remote, or most distant, cause of death, which was the car accident.

Cruzan's family filed for and received a court order for the feeding tube to be removed. The local trial court ruled that constitutionally, there is a "fundamental natural right . . . to refuse or direct the withholding or withdrawal of artificial death prolonging procedures when the person has no more cognitive brain function . . . and there is no hope of further recovery."[9] The court ruled that Nancy had effectively "directed" the withdrawal of life support by telling a friend earlier in the year of the accident that if she were sick or injured, "she would not wish to continue her life unless she could live at least halfway normally."

The state of Missouri and Cruzan's guardian ad litem both appealed this decision to the Missouri Supreme Court. A *guardian ad litem* is a court-appointed official whose sole interest is the safety and concerns of the ward of the court, in this case Cruzan.

In a 4–3 decision, the Missouri Supreme Court reversed the lower trial court's decision. It ruled that "no one may refuse treatment for another person, absent an adequate living will or the clear and convincing, inherently reliable evidence absent here."[9] Cruzan's parents then appealed again to a higher court, and in 1989, the U.S. Supreme Court agreed to hear the case.

The issue before the Supreme Court was whether the state of Missouri could use its own standard of clear and convincing proof for removal of the tube or whether a 14th Amendment due-process guarantee of a "right to die" would override the state statute. It was decided that the constitutional right would not be extended and the state procedural requirement would be allowed, at which time the burden of proof was put on Cruzan's family to show that she would not have wanted to continue living in this manner. The court held that the state had the right to err on the side of life, and the tube was left in. The Supreme Court recognized that a living will would have been sufficient evidence of Cruzan's wishes to sustain or to remove her feeding tube.

After the Supreme Court's decision, the family collected more evidence that Cruzan would have wanted her life support terminated. The State of Missouri withdrew from the case because its law had been upheld and it had won the Supreme Court decision. Without opposition from the State of Missouri, Cruzan's family went to the local Jasper County probate judge, who ruled that, based on the additional information they had collected, there was sufficient evidence that Cruzan would not have wished to live on life support. The judge issued a court order to remove the feeding tube. Eight years after she had entered a PVS, Nancy Cruzan died quietly in a bed surrounded by her family.

A few years later, another landmark case began. In 1990, a 26-year-old woman, Terri Schiavo, passed out at home due to cardiac arrest and was successfully resuscitated by emergency medical service (EMS). This case paralleled the Cruzan case in several ways. Like Cruzan, Schiavo suffered massive brain injury because of a lack of oxygen to her brain. A feeding tube was inserted for nutrition and hydration shortly after her admission to the hospital. She was diagnosed, after two and a half months without improvement, as being in a PVS. For the next 2 years, providers attempted speech and physical therapy and other experimental therapy, hoping to return her to a state of awareness, without success. At that time, Terri's husband, Michael, petitioned the Sixth Circuit Court of Florida to remove her feeding tube based on Florida law. He was opposed by Terri's parents, Robert and Mary Schindler. The court determined that Terri would not have wished to continue life-prolonging measures; and after the court ruling, her feeding tube was removed for the first time, only to be reinserted several days later.

The Schiavo case went through 14 appeals and numerous motions, hearings, and petitions from both sides in the Florida courts and five suits in federal district court. There was extensive political intervention by the Florida state legislature, Florida Governor Jeb Bush, the U.S. Congress, and President George W. Bush himself. After four denials of lower court reviews from the U.S. Supreme Court, the initial decision to remove the tube was upheld. The tube was finally removed 3 weeks after the original court ruling to have it removed. Schiavo died about 2 weeks later. Upon autopsy, her brain, just like Cruzan's, showed areas of massive degeneration due to the lack of oxygen, indicating that there had been no chance of recovery.

Several lessons can be learned from these cases. First, not much progress has been made in developing legal solutions for this type of case during the decades since the Cruzan and Schiavo cases began. Second, the legal system is poorly equipped and not the place to decide life and death ethical dilemmas. The purpose of a legal system is to provide a systematic, orderly, and predictable mechanism for resolving disagreements. The judicial function is the center of any legal system and rests upon the judgments made in deciding disputes and issuing a decision as to how the disagreement should be settled. The goal of the legal system is to ensure that laws are being followed and enforced. However, when there are no clearcut laws for certain situations, the courts are left rudderless and must attempt to decide the issues from parallel laws from other cases. Most of the time, it does not work very well. In the end, it often comes down to one judge's beliefs and attitudes about the case.

The reality is that across the United States, many times every day, life support is removed from patients who have no chance of living any kind of "normal" life. Some of these patients are brain dead and have donated their organs for transplant. Many others are like Cruzan and Schiavo in PVSs. These difficult decisions are made by family members, the health-care team, and often a pastor or priest who knows the family. The decision to remove life support is never easy; however, these decisions are made using ethical principles of which the family may not even be aware.

The Nurse's Role in Advance Directives

Because laws vary among states, it is important that nurses know the laws of the state in which they practice that pertain to advance directives, clients' rights, and the policies and procedures of the institution in which they work. With the passage of the Nurse Compact Law and the participation by a number of states so that nurses licensed in one state can work in another without obtaining that state's license, the knowledge of state laws becomes even more important. Nurses must inform clients of their right to formulate advance directives and must realize that not all clients can make such decisions.

It is important for the nurse to establish trust and rapport with a client and the client's family so that the nurse can assist them in making decisions that are in the client's best interests.[11] Nurses must also teach about advance directives and document all critical decisions, discussions with the client and client's

> *Because laws vary among states, it is important that nurses know the laws of the state in which they practice that pertain to advance directives, clients' rights, and the policies and procedures of the institution in which they work.*

family about such decisions, and the basis for the evaluation process. Also, it is essential to prevent discrimination against clients and their families based on their choices regarding their advance directives.

Nurses must determine whether clients have been coerced into making advance directive decisions against their will. Nurses need to become involved in ethics committees at hospitals or nursing specialty groups at local, state, or national levels to help clients come to a comfortable resolution about advance directives.

Do-Not-Resuscitate and Allow-Natural-Death Orders

Although instructions against resuscitation may be included in a person's advance directive, do-not-resuscitate (DNR) or allow-natural-death (AND) orders are legally separate from advance directives. For the health-care professional to be legally protected, there should be a written order indicating no code, AND, or DNR in the client's chart.

Protection for the Nurse

Each hospital should have a policy and procedure that outlines what is required with regard to a client's condition for a DNR order. The DNR order should be reviewed, evaluated, and reordered. Different facilities have established different time periods for these reviews. Nurses must also know whether there is any law that regulates who should authorize a DNR order for an incompetent client who is no longer able to make this decision. Hospitals often have policies and procedures describing what must be done and which clients fit the requirements for a DNR order. The American Nurses Association (ANA) published a position statement on nursing care and DNR decisions.[11] Although the primary responsibility for explaining a DNR order to the patient or family rests with the physician, the nurse plays a key role in clarifying and reinforcing the teaching. The position statement stresses the need for nurses to talk with clients and their families about the DNR decision so that they are fully informed when they make the decision. It includes discussing the benefits and burdens of prolonged treatments, what comfort measures are possible, the effects of symptom palliation, and the understanding that aggressive life-sustaining technology will be withdrawn if it does not meet the goals and wishes of the client and their family. Any decision about a DNR needs to be based on the client's right to self-determination in order for it to be ethical.

Nurses face many legal dilemmas when dealing with confusing or conflicting DNR orders. For example, it may be difficult to interpret a DNR order when it has been restricted—for instance, "do not resuscitate except for medications and defibrillation" or "no CPR or intubation." Often, a lack of proper documentation in the medical records indicating how the DNR decision was reached can be a critical issue if a medical malpractice case is involved and it is disputed whether the client or family actually gave consent for the order.

Many facilities have developed DNR decision sheets. A DNR sheet may record information about DNR discussions or be dated and signed by the client and those family members who took part in the discussion. It then becomes a permanent part of the medical record.

Protection for the Client

It is very important that nurses not stigmatize clients by the use of indicators for DNR orders, such as dots on the wristband or over the bed. Health-care providers' attitudes often change because they feel that the client is "going to die anyway." This abandonment can jeopardize the care of a client designated with a DNR order. However, it is also important for the nurses and staff to know whether an order is to be honored and what the policies and procedures are with regard to transfer clients and DNR orders that accompany the incoming client.[11]

Information about the DNR status of a client should be obtained during shift reports. If there has not been a periodic review, is the order still in effect? If a client is transferred from one facility to another and has a DNR order that is time limited and has not been reordered, what should a nurse do?

Professional Standards for Nursing

Professional nursing, as defined by the ANA, is made up of three components: (1) professional standards of care, (2) professional performance standards, and (3) standards of nursing practice.

Professional standards of care are the yardsticks that the legal system uses to measure the actions of a nurse involved in a malpractice suit. The underlying principle used to establish standards of care is based on the actions that would probably be taken by a reasonable and competent nurse in the same or similar circumstances. Standards of care stipulate what is appropriate treatment that is based on scientific evidence. They define diagnostic, intervention, and evaluation competencies.[12]

The standard usually includes both objective factors (e.g., the actions to be performed) and subjective factors (e.g., the nurse's emotional and mental state). Specifically, a nurse is judged against the standards that are established within the profession and specialty area of practice. The ANA and specialty groups within the nursing profession, such as the American Association of Critical-Care Nurses (AACN), publish standards of care that are updated continually as health-care technology and practices change. Recently, standards of care have become the concern of the U.S. government. The Affordable Care Act of 2010 addresses standards of care both directly and indirectly. Particular areas addressed are limiting readmissions, formation of accountable care organizations (ACOs), and the review of the quality of care provided by health-care providers and hospitals.[12]

Professional performance standards categorize the roles nurses perform in providing patients with direct care, consultation, education, and quality assurance. They establish the professional practices, ethics, and activities that members of a profession must follow. Violation of professional standards can also lead to a lawsuit but are more likely to elicit actions from the state board of nursing on the nurse's license and practice.[12] For example, a nurse at the end of a busy 12-hour shift accidently connects a feeding tube to the port of a critically ill patient's IV. The mistake is not caught for several hours, and the patient dies. The family declines to file a lawsuit because the patient was terminal anyway. The incident is reported to the board of nursing, a hearing is held, and it is determined that the nurse committed an act of gross negligence. The board's action includes revoking the nurse's license permanently and placing a report of the incident in the nurse's permanent record.

Standards of nursing practice include clinical policy statements, standard operating procedures, clinical practice protocols, and clinical procedures. They are the standards that promote and guide the professional nurse in how to practice nursing by describing the skilled level of care in each stage of the nursing process. They define assessment, diagnostic, intervention, and evaluation competencies. The main purpose of professional standards is to direct and maintain safe and clinically competent nursing practice. These standards can also become important in a lawsuit against a nurse when the nurse does not follow one of the standards and it leads to injury to the patient. Standards of practice are not absolute and can be ignored in certain situation; however, the nurse must have a very strong reason for violating the standard and must be willing to accept the consequences if something should go wrong.[12]

External Standards

The ANA has developed six standards of nursing upon which all the other standards are built:

- Thinks critically and analyzes nursing practice.
- Engages in therapeutic and professional relationships.
- Maintains the capability for practice.
- Comprehensively conducts assessments.
- Develops a plan for nursing practice.
- Provides safe, appropriate, and responsive quality nursing practice.[13]

Both external and internal standards govern the conduct of nurses. External standards include the ANA's nursing standards, the state nurse practice act of each jurisdiction, criteria from accrediting agencies such as The Joint Commission (TJC), guidelines developed by various nursing specialty practice groups, and federal agency regulations. Nurses are encountering an increasing number of incidents in which conflicts occur between institutional and professional standards—for example, in staffing ratios. These disputes are difficult to resolve and may require deliberation and decisions from

> *Nurses are encountering an increasing number of incidents in which conflicts occur between institutional and professional standards—for example, in staffing ratios.*

institutional committees. As a general rule, when a conflict exists, it is safer legally to follow professional standards.

Internal Standards

Internal standards include nursing standards defined in specific hospital policy and procedure manuals that relate to the nurse in the particular institution. The nurse's job description and employment contract are examples of internal nursing standards that define the duty of the nurse.

Criteria for Good Care

The rationale for advancing standards of care for the nurse is to ensure proper, consistent, and high-quality nursing care to all members of society. When nurses violate their duty of care to the client as established by the profession's standards of care, they leave themselves open to charges of negligence and malpractice. Until recently, nurses were held to the standards of the local community. National criteria have now replaced most **locality rule standards of care**. Individual nurses are held accountable not only to acceptable standards within the local community but also to national standards.

Although standards of care may seem to be specific, they are merely guidelines for nursing practice. Because every client's situation is different, the appropriate standard of care may be difficult to identify in a certain case. More than one course of nursing action may be considered appropriate under a proper standard of care. The final decision must be guided by the nurse's judgment and understanding of the client's needs.

The Nurse Practice Act

The nurse practice act defines nursing practice and establishes standards for nurses in each state. It is the most definitive legal statute or legislative act regulating nursing practice. Although nurse practice acts vary in scope from one state to another, they tend to have similar wording based loosely on the ANA model published in 1988. The nurse practice act provides a framework for the court on which to base decisions when determining whether a nurse has breached a standard of care.

Most state nurse practice acts define scope of practice, establish requirements for licensure and entry into practice, and create and empower a board of nursing to oversee the practice of nurses. In addition, nurse practice acts identify grounds for disciplinary actions such as suspension and revocation of a nursing license.[12]

The judicial interpretation of the nurse practice act and its relationship to a specific case provide guidance for decisions about future cases. Many state legislatures have responded to the expanded role of the nurse by broadening the scope of their nurse practice acts. For example, the addition of the term *nursing diagnosis* to many states' nurse practice acts reflects the legislature's recognition of the expansion of the nurse's role.

Although some states were beginning to include occupational roles such as nurse practitioner, **nurse clinician**, and clinical nurse specialist in their nurse practice acts, the process was inconsistent and confusing. To address this confusion, in 2008 the APRN Consensus Work Group and the National Council of State Boards of Nursing (NCSBN) APRN Advisory Committee issued a report on the licensure, accreditation, certification, and education (LACE) of APRNs. This statement addresses the lack of common definitions regarding APRN practice, the ever-increasing numbers of specializations, the inconsistency in credentials and scope of practice, and the wide variations in education for APRNs. The goal was to implement the APRN model of regulation in all states by 2015. However, by 2018, only 20 states had fully implemented this model. (For a more detailed discussion of the model, see Chapter 5.) It is important to remember that as the nurse's role expands, so does the legal accountability of the role.[15]

PREVENTING LAWSUITS

What can the nurse do to avoid having to go through the always stressful and sometimes financially and professionally devastating process of litigation? The following guidelines provide some ways to avoid a lawsuit.

Effective Communication

After many years of collecting data and analyzing sentinel and critical events, TJC concluded that miscommunication among health-care workers is the leading cause of health-care-related errors leading to injury, death, and lawsuits. TJC called for a concrete communication strategy that would provide a framework for communication between caregivers and would be easy for all health-care workers to remember. It would need to work in all situations, from end-of-shift reports to exchanges in high-pressure critical-care areas, when a nurse's immediate responses and actions could make the difference between life and death. Care expectations could be communicated in a focused, simple way that allowed all team members to understand and respond quickly. The overall goal is to develop a "culture of client safety" that would permeate any organization.[14]

Situation, Background, Assessment, Recommendation

The **Situation, Background, Assessment, Recommendation (SBAR)** system (pronounced *s-bar*) was initially developed by the U.S. Navy to improve communications on the nuclear submarine fleet. Refined and adopted by Kaiser Permanente of Colorado in the late 1990s, SBAR has been incorporated into health-care facilities and has worked its way into the nursing education system. SBAR has proven useful when a client's status changes unexpectedly. A review of client charts in these emergency situations shows how confused the communication between the health-care provider and the nurse can be. Fatigue, lack of experience, or insufficient level of nursing education often leads to the omission of key information. In this type of situation, SBAR forms an outline for the communication of critical information.[17]

Each letter in *SBAR* stands for a step in the process:

Situation: Asks the question, "What is going on?" For this step, provide the following information:
- Identify yourself, the hospital unit or health-care location, and the room number.
- Identify the client by name, age, gender, and date of birth.
- Describe the problem the client has that triggered the SBAR communication.

Background: Provides key information that will help determine what actions to take:
- Give a short summary of the client's relevant past medical history.
- Provide the client's diagnosis.

• Describe the client's current mental status, current vital signs, complaints, pain level, oxygen saturation, and physical assessment findings.

Assessment: Allows the nurse to analyze the situation and isolate the specific problem:
• Note what vital signs are outside of parameters.
• Give the nurse's clinical impressions of the client and additional concerns.
• Rank the severity of the client's condition.
• Identify specific client needs to resolve the situation.

Recommendation: Identifies what actions will resolve the situation:
• Identify what needs to be done to resolve the client's problem.
• Note how urgent the problem is and when action needs to be taken.
• Suggest what action should be taken.
• State the desired client response.[16]

Here is an example of how an SBAR communication could be used:

Situation: Hello, Dr. Nife, this is Alexis Zanetti, RN, in the step-down unit, calling about Mr. Jenkins. He is a 68-year-old male who had a femoral bypass graft done yesterday. He was undergoing cardiac monitoring according to protocol and within the last 15 minutes went from a sinus rhythm to an atrial fibrillation of 165 beats per minute.

Background: As you know, Mr. Jenkins has a history of cardiac disease, including a myocardial infarction in 2005. He has type 1 diabetes and has had several deep vein thromboses over the past 3 years. He has an IV infusion of D5 half-normal saline running at 125 mL per hour. He is complaining of some slight chest pressure. His incision site is clean and dry, and he has +2 pedal pulses in both feet.

Assessment: His blood pressure normally runs 136/76, pulse 90, respiration 18, and O_2 saturation 96 percent. His current vital signs are: blood pressure, 98/54; pulse, 165; respirations, 26; O_2 saturation, 89 percent; and urine output, 82 mL per hour. This is the first time he has complained of chest pressure, but he ranks it as only a 2 on a 1-to-10 scale. The vital sign changes all occurred shortly after the change in his cardiac rhythm. His neurological status is unchanged, and the femoral graft has not been affected by the cardiovascular changes. He has been taking sips of water by mouth and tolerating it well.

Recommendations: It appears that restoring Mr. Jenkins to normal sinus rhythm is the highest priority. What would you think about restarting him on Lanoxin, 0.25 mg, which was discontinued preoperatively? We could give it either by IV or by mouth because he is tolerating water.

In general, nurses feel uncomfortable making medical recommendations to health-care providers. Also, some providers do not handle recommendations from nurses very well. However, recommendations are part of the SBAR process, and the health-care provider can always just say no. Disguising the recommendations in the form of a question softens the impact and meets with more success.[16]

Medical Record

Charting in the medical record is the best way to display the care provided and the communication between health-care workers. It is the single-most frequently used piece of objective evidence in a malpractice suit. In preparation for the trial, the lawyers attempt to reconstruct the events surrounding the incident in a minute-by-minute timeline. The client's **chart** is the most important source for this timeline. Maintaining an accurate and complete medical record is an absolute requirement (Box 8.6).

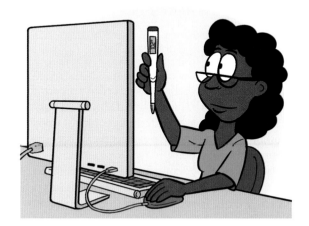

Charting vital signs ASAP is important.

In nursing and medical negligence claims, lawyers are beginning to ask whether the hospital has adopted the use of SBAR. They examine the materials used to educate the staff and any policies or procedures concerning the use of SBAR. They note

---

Box 8.6 **Some Documentation Guidelines**

Medications
- Always chart the time, route, dose, and response.
- Always chart why prn medications were given and the client response.
- Always chart when a medication was not given, the reason (client in radiology, physical therapy, etc.; do not chart that the medication was not on the floor), and the nursing intervention that followed ("Medication given when patient returned").
- Chart all medication refusals and report them to the appropriate source.
- Do not use unapproved abbreviations.

Communication With Health-Care Providers
- Document each time a call is made to a health-care provider, even if the provider is not reached. Include the exact time of the call. If the provider is reached, document the details of the message and the response.
- Read verbal orders back to the health-care provider and confirm the client's identity as written on the chart. Chart only verbal orders that you have heard directly from the source, not those told to you by another nurse or other unit personnel.

Formal Issues in Charting
- Before charting, check to be sure you have the correct client record.
- Correct any charting mistakes according to the policy and procedures of your institution.
- Chart in an organized fashion, following the nursing process.
- Document concisely and avoid subjective statements.
- Record specific and accurate descriptions.
- When charting a symptom or situation, chart the interventions taken and the client response.
- Document your own observations, not those that were told to you by another party.
- Chart frequently to demonstrate ongoing care and chart routine activities.
- Chart client and family teaching and the response.

Source: C. Cross, Importance of documentation and charting in nursing care, *Small Business Chronical*, n.d. https://smallbusiness.chron.com/importance-documentation-charting-nursing-care-80092.html

---

any mention of SBAR communication in the medical record and see whether it is recorded properly.[15] Even if the facility has not adopted SBAR as a hospital-wide communication technique, nurses who know how can use it to help protect themselves in subsequent legal actions.

Patients' charts are considered legal documents and can be used in court. The old adage "If it isn't written, it didn't happen" remains true in most situations; however, recent court trials have recognized some exclusions, such as charting by exception. Charting is a method of keeping a clinical record of the important facts about a client and how the client is progressing with regard to treatments and therapies. The client's chart generally includes information such as laboratory test results, lists of medications, radiology reports, consultation notes from other

providers, and notations from nurses and other providers documenting professional observations and nursing judgments.[16]

Charting by exception is a method of charting designed to reduce the time nurses spend carrying out clerical activities. In charting by exception, a notation is made in the chart only when there is a change in the client's condition different from the baseline or expected outcome, for example, when the client's blood pressure is above or below the normal range. Charting by exception can be compared to selecting the correct choice from a list of options. Lawyers dislike charting by exception because it allows nurses who are on trial or giving a deposition to say, "There must have been no change in the patient's condition because if there had been, I would have charted it." If the client is stable and recovering as expected, there may be very little written in the chart about their physical or mental assessments. However, some judges and juries have begun to recognize that charting by exception is a valid form of health-care record-keeping.

Trying to recall specific events from 2 to 6 years ago without the benefit of written notes is almost impossible. In general, the client record should *not* contain personal opinion, should be legible, should be in chronological order, and should be written and signed by the nurse. Although opinions have a relatively low value in legal proceedings, the documentation should indicate the nursing judgments made. An entry should never be obliterated or destroyed. If a nurse questions an order, a record must be made that the health-care provider was contacted and the order clarified.

Patient charts have other uses such as for research in developing best practices. They are reviewed by medical coders in the medical records department who look for documentation of procedures, physician visits, medication administration, nursing interventions, surgeries, and treatments. These elements are given an appropriate code so that the hospital can receive the highest payments from insurance companies and Medicare. Patient charts are also used for accreditation purposes. All health-care facilities want to be accredited by their appropriate accreditation organization. In addition to actually visiting the facility, accreditors closely review patients' charts to assess if the quality of care being provided meets the standards of the accrediting agency.[16]

Rapport With Clients

Establishing a rapport with the client through honest, open communication goes a long way in avoiding lawsuits. Treating clients and their families with respect and letting them know that the nurse really cares about them may well prevent a lawsuit. Many people are willing to forgive a nurse's error if they have good rapport and a trusting relationship with a nurse whom they believe is interested in their well-being.[14]

Current Nursing Skills

Keeping one's nursing knowledge and skills current is vital to preventing errors that may lead to lawsuits. It is better to refuse to perform an unfamiliar procedure than to attempt it without the necessary knowledge and skills. Taking advantage of in-service training, workshops, and continuing nursing education classes is an important part of maintaining the nurse's skill level.[14] Nurses must practice within their level of competence and scope of practice.

Knowledge of the Client

Recognizing the client who is lawsuit prone can help reduce the risk for litigation. Some common characteristics of this type of client include constant dissatisfaction with the care given, constant complaints about all aspects of care, and negative comments about other nurses. This client often complains about the poor care given by nurses on the previous shift and may also have a history of lawsuits against nurses.

> *Being direct, solving problems with the client, and helping the client become involved in their care are helpful in defusing this negative behavior.*

Being direct, solving problems with the client, and helping the client become involved in their care are helpful in defusing this negative behavior. Also, even more careful documentation of the care provided and the client's responses to the care can be helpful if a lawsuit is filed later.

Families can also be an important factor in lawsuits. Establishing a good relationship with family members when they are visiting, keeping them informed, recognizing that they are an important part of the recovery process, and providing them small comforts such as a cup of coffee or a soft drink while they are waiting goes a long way in softening the impact of bad news.

What Do You Think?

Think about being involved in a legal or courtroom activity as a defendant, complainant, witness, or juror. What would your role be in each situation?

LIABILITY INSURANCE

Maintaining proper liability insurance is a necessity. Nurses who do not carry liability insurance place themselves at high risk. The nurse's personal assets, as well as wages, may be subject to a judgment awarded in a malpractice action. Even if the client does not win at the trial, the litigation process, including hiring a lawyer and paying the costs of experts, can be financially devastating.

A professional liability insurance policy is a contract with an insurer who promises to assume the costs paid to the injured party in exchange for the professional paying a premium (Box 8.7). There are two types of malpractice policies: claims made and occurrence. **Claims-made policies** protect only against claims made during the time the policy is in effect. **Occurrence policies** protect against all claims that occur during the policy period, regardless of when the claim is made. Generally, the occurrence type of liability insurance offers more protection. Claims-made policy coverage can be broadened by purchasing a tail—a separate policy that extends the time of coverage.

Box 8.7 What to Look for in an Insurance Policy

The following factors should be reviewed to determine what is the best policy for your type of nursing practice:

1. Type of insurance policy (claims-made or occurrence basis).
2. Insuring agreement. The insurance company's promise to pay in exchange for premiums is called the *insuring agreement*. The insurance company agrees to pay a money award to a plaintiff who is injured by an act of omission or commission by a health-care provider who is insured by the company.
3. Types of injuries covered. The language must be scrutinized to determine whether it is broad or limiting. Some companies will agree to pay only if the insured nurse is sued for damages, which means the nurse must be sued for a money amount or award. If the nurse is sued for a specific performance lawsuit or an injunctive relief action, which means that the nurse will either have to perform something or discontinue doing something, that particular insurance policy may not be adequate. Also, most insurance policies do not cover the nurse for disciplinary actions.
4. Exclusions. Items that are not covered by a policy are called *exclusions*. It is important to review the exclusions. Some of the more common exclusions include sexual abuse of a client, injury caused while under the influence of drugs or alcohol, criminal activity, and punitive damages. Punitive damages are used to punish the defendant for egregious acts or omissions.

Who Is Covered Under the Policy

The purchaser is the named insured and can be an individual, institution, or group. Others who may be covered by the policy are nurses, employees, agents, and volunteers, among others.

Limitations and Deductions

In exchange for payment of the premium, the insurance company agrees to pay up to a certain amount on behalf of the insured. This amount is called the *limit of liability*. It is usually expressed in two ways: the amount that can be paid per incident (per occurrence) and the amount that will be paid for the entire policy year. For example, if you have a policy that states $1,000,000/$3,000,000, it means that the company will pay up to $1 million per incident and a total of $3 million per policy year. The insurance industry relies on the A.M. Best Company to evaluate both the financial size and relative strengths of insurance companies. An A.M. Best rating of A or better should be a prerequisite for purchase of any policy.

The Right to Select Counsel

Some insurance companies allow nurses to select their own attorneys to represent them in a medical negligence claim. Others retain attorneys or law firms, and the nurse does not have the opportunity to make that selection.

The Right to Consent to Settlement

Some policies allow the nurse to decide whether a case should be settled or go to trial, whereas others do not.

Some hospitals have liability insurance policies for the nurse as a part of the nurse's employment package with the institution. This hospital policy may be limited to claims arising from the nurse's employment and might not apply in a situation in which a nurse renders care outside the institution—for instance, at an automobile crash site.[17] It is preferable to have liability insurance coverage that includes all situations in which the nurse may be involved.

Some myths have grown up concerning nurse liability insurance:

MYTH 1: Nurses do not need their own insurance because their employer's policy covers them.
Most nurses believe that they are covered for malpractice by their employer's policy. But have they ever seen the policy or asked someone in human resources about what is actually covered? Most often, there are big gaps in coverage, and the policy does not cover many of the risks nurses are exposed to every day. Following are some examples of uncovered events:

- The nurse commits a mistake that is outside their scope of practice or job description.
- The mistake falls within one of the many policy exclusions (read the fine print).
- If the claim is for a large monetary settlement, the employer can (and probably will) refuse to defend the nurse.
- If the claim is filed after the nurse resigned or was terminated, the policy probably does not cover the nurse.

MYTH 2: Only physicians get sued for malpractice.
It is true that physicians face more lawsuits than do nurses; however, the trend is to also include nurses in the lawsuit or to sue nurses separately. Along with nurses being increasingly recognized as professionals comes increased individual accountability. Being accountable for their practice means nurses can and are being sued for malpractice because of their own bad acts and omissions.

MYTH 3: If a nurse has their own insurance, they are more likely to get sued.
Not true. A person's insurance status is not public information and can be discovered only *after* a lawsuit is filed. A standard practice for a plaintiff's attorney is to initially "cast a wide net" and name as many defendants as possible. Once the initial net is cast,

the attorney looks for "deep pockets" and eliminates many of those initially named. The likelihood of the plaintiff including the nurse after learning they have insurance depends on multiple factors, such as the part the nurse played in the incident or whether the nurse has large enough assets to satisfy a potential judgment (such as savings, a home, or a vacation property).

MYTH 4: A nurse can be sued only if they made an error that caused injury.
Not true. One legal truism to memorize is this: "Anyone can be sued by anybody at any time for anything." If the patient believes that the nurse is responsible for a bad outcome due to the care they provided, even if that belief is false, the nurse can be sued. Nurses can be sued by a patient who has not suffered any injury but hopes to win a settlement. This is called a frivolous lawsuit, and such suits are usually quickly dismissed by the court. Even though the lawsuit has no merit, the nurse will still have to pay the expenses of getting the suit dismissed, such as lawyer costs, court fees, and loss of time from work. An individual malpractice insurance policy will pay for these expenses and protect against the financial ruin that can result from being sued.[17]

MYTH 5: The state board of nursing (SBN) will protect the nurse from being sued.
Not true. The role of the SBN is to protect the public from unprofessional conduct of nurses (see below). The state nurses association and ANA work to keep nurses safe from a variety of actions that may be taken against the nurse's license.

Individual **indemnity insurance** coverage that is independent of the facility's policy is recommended for all nurses. With passage of the **Federal Tort Claims Act** and similar state laws, nurses who were formerly protected from lawsuits by working at federal or state health-care facilities can now be sued for malpractice just like nurses at any other facility.

REVOCATION OF LICENSE

One of the most severe punishments that a nurse can experience is revocation of the license to practice nursing. The nursing profession is responsible for monitoring and enforcing its own standards through the state licensing board. These actions may or may not be related to tort law, contract law, or criminal charges. Each state's licensing board is charged with the responsibility to oversee the professional nurse's competence.

The state's nursing board receives its authority to grant and revoke licenses from specific statutory laws. The underlying rationale for establishment of a licensing board is to protect the public from uneducated, unsafe, or unethical practitioners. If nurses fail to adhere to the standards of safe practice and exhibit unprofessional behavior, they can be disciplined by the state nursing licensing board. One of the remedies that these boards can use is suspension or revocation of a nurse's license.[18]

The Disciplinary Hearing

A disciplinary hearing is held to review the charges of the nurse's unprofessional conduct. This hearing is less formal than the trial process, and the nurse is allowed to present evidence and be represented by legal counsel at the hearing. Due process requires that the nurse be notified in advance of the specific charges being made. The question of what constitutes unprofessional conduct is an issue frequently dealt with at the disciplinary hearing. Each respective state's nurse practice act provides guidance with regard to the specifics of unprofessional conduct. The most common actions performed by a nurse that can lead to revocation of their license to practice nursing include

- Falsifying information on a nursing application or renewal application.
- Committing a felony that involves bodily harm to others.

- Working while under the influence of drugs or alcohol.
- Taking drugs from the facility for personal use.
- Pretending to be another health-care provider, such as a physician.
- Using a counterfeit nursing license.
- Forging or charting fake information in patient's charts.
- Unprofessional conduct either at work or when off duty.
- Improper use of the Internet by posting false information, information about a patient, etc.
- Violation of HIPAA standards.
- Violating standards of care by mistreating, abusing, molesting, or neglecting patients.
- Violating a pre-existing probation or suspension.
- Administering a medication without a prescription.
- Aggressing violations of the Nurses Code of Ethics.

In the case of a criminal action against a nurse, the court proceeding is allowed to be completed before the board of nursing takes action on the nurse's license.[18]

Unprofessional conduct can be reported by a nursing peer, a supervisor, a patient, or a patient's family. Many cases are dismissed before the hearing takes place if the board finds there is no support for the allegation being made against the nurse. If a hearing is necessary, it is in the best interest of the nurse not to speak to anyone about the case because those comments to a third party can be used against the nurse. As soon as the nurse becomes aware of a possible lawsuit, they should seek legal counsel as soon as possible because of the potential risk of license revocation.

Conclusion

The legal system and its effects on the practice of nursing are ever-present realities in today's health-care system. Nurses need to be aware of the implications of their actions but should not be so overwhelmed by fear that it reduces their ability to care for the client. The more advanced and specialized the nurse's practice becomes, the higher the standards to which the nurse is held. Nurses will be challenged throughout their careers to apply legal principles in the daily practice of nursing. An awareness of what constitutes malpractice and negligence will aid in the prevention of litigation.

CRITICAL-THINKING EXERCISES

Consider the following case: *Thomas v. Corso* (MD 1982). The client was brought to the hospital emergency department (ED) after being involved in an automobile accident. The ED nurse assessed and recorded the client's vital signs and a complaint of numbness in his right anterior thigh. The client was able to move the right leg, and there was no discoloration or deformity. After he was given meperidine (Demerol) for his pain, his blood pressure (BP) dropped to 90/60 mm Hg, and the nurse notified the ED physician of the change. The physician ordered the nurse to arrange for admission to the hospital, which she did.

The client was transferred to a medical-surgical unit, but he could not be placed in a room because of an influenza epidemic. He was placed in the hall next to the nurses' station for close observation. A nurse checked the client's vital signs about 20 minutes after the transfer and noted that the BP was now 70/50, respiratory rate 40, and pulse 120. His skin was cool and diaphoretic, his breathing was deep and rapid, and he was asking for a drink of water. The client also complained of pain in his leg, but the nurse did not give him more pain medication because of his blood pressure.

The nurse assessed him about 30 minutes later and found his skin warmer, although he still complained of pain and thirst. The nurse also noted a strong odor of alcohol on the client's breath. An assistant supervisor also assessed the client's condition but refused to give him any water because he had obviously been drinking alcohol. She had been told about the low blood pressure by the client's nurse but attributed it to the alcohol and pain medication combination. The nurse checked his vital signs again and found a BP of 100/89. Thirty minutes later, it was 94/70, pulse 100, and respirations 28. When the nurse next assessed the client an hour later, he had a Cheyne-Stokes respiratory pattern, no pulse, and no blood pressure. She started CPR and called a code blue, but after a lengthy attempt at resuscitation, the client died.

An autopsy was performed and showed that the client had a lacerated liver and a severe fracture of the femur with bleeding into the tissues. The coroner determined that traumatic shock, secondary to the fractured femur and lacerated liver, was the cause of death. His family sued the nurses for poor judgment and the hospital for malpractice and won.

1. What mistakes were made by the nurses in this case?
2. What legal liability did the nurses incur by their actions?
3. How can the nurses best prepare for trial in this case?
4. What actions could the nurses have taken with this client to prevent a lawsuit?
5. What are your feelings toward inebriated clients? Did the nurses' attitudes about inebriation affect their judgment?
6. Why are clients who are drunk at higher risk for injury and poor medical outcomes than other clients?

NCLEX-STYLE QUESTIONS

1. Which of the following are associated with statutory law? **Select all that apply**.
    1. Evolves from decisions of previous legal cases
    2. Develops over a long period of time
    3. Written and enacted by government bodies
    4. Includes the nurse practice act
    5. Uses precedents to inform decisions
    6. Defines criminal laws
    7. Classifies offenses as misdemeanors or felonies

2. Rochelle, an LVN in an assisted-living facility, is caring for Mrs. Whelan, a very wealthy and very difficult client. Nothing Rochelle can do is good enough or prompt enough for Mrs. Whelan, who makes one loud complaint after another. When Mrs. Whelan takes her afternoon nap, Rochelle sneaks into her room and steals her favorite gold brooch. What has Rochelle committed?
    1. A quasi-intentional tort
    2. An intentional tort
    3. An unintentional tort
    4. Malpractice

3. Jordan, an RN on a busy medical-surgical unit, just received orders to discharge Mr. Sánchez, who speaks only Spanish. The hospital's medical interpreter is busy helping another nurse with a client, so Jordan, who knows a little Spanish, decides to give the discharge instructions to the client himself. Which part of this scenario demonstrates a breach of duty?
   1. The hospital breached duty by discharging Mr. Sánchez too soon.
   2. The medical interpreter breached duty by not being available.
   3. Jordan breached duty by not waiting for the medical interpreter.
   4. Mr. Sánchez breached duty by not speaking English.

4. In order for a client to give informed consent, what information must be explained by the health-care provider? **Select all that apply.**
   1. Proposed treatment
   2. Potential complications
   3. Outcome hoped for
   4. Consequences of not having treatment
   5. Acceptable alternative treatments
   6. Estimate of the cost of the treatment

5. What is the essential difference between a living will and a do not resuscitate (DNR) order?
   1. A living will is a document stating the client's wishes for his or her end-of-life care; a DNR is an order in the client's medical record indicating the client's wishes.
   2. A living will applies only outside a hospital or other health-care facility; a DNR applies only within a hospital or other health-care facility.
   3. A living will is a legal document; a DNR is a medical document.
   4. A living will protects the client's interests; a DNR protects the interests of the health-care provider or facility.

6. In the trial process, the _____ is a formal legal process that involves the taking of testimony under oath and is recorded by a court reporter.

7. Mei-Ling, an RN, is scuba diving on vacation when another diver is badly bitten by a shark. Once they are safely in the boat, Mei-Ling notes that the bite has severed the diver's femoral artery. She quickly applies a tourniquet proximal to the bite. The diver survives, after undergoing an above-the-knee amputation. He sues Mei-Ling for malpractice. What is Mei-Ling's BEST defense?
   1. Contributory negligence
   2. Assumption of risk
   3. Unavoidable accident
   4. Good Samaritan Act

8. What is the FIRST step in a malpractice suit?
   1. The discovery
   2. The deposition
   3. The complaint
   4. The answer

9. To prevent litigation, which of the following may be employed? **Select all that apply.**
   1. Discovery
   2. Mediation
   3. Deposition
   4. Arbitration
   5. Summary judgment

10. Which of the following applies to criminal law? **Select all that apply.**
    1. A jury decision requires three-fourths (8 out of 12) agreement.
    2. Punishment can range from community service to imprisonment or even death.
    3. Contract law, tax law, and treaty law are branches of criminal law.
    4. It deals with the violation of one individual's rights by another individual.
    5. The case is brought by a prosecuting attorney.

References

1. Lamb J. Nurses travel to Nashville for Vaught sentencing. News Channel 5, May 13, 2022. https://www.newschannel5.com/news/nurses-travel-to-nashville-for-vaught-sentencing
2. McDuffey T. What is medical negligence? LegalMatch, November 7, 2022. https://www.legalmatch.com/law-library/article/what-is-medical-negligence.html
3. Guido G. *Legal and Ethical Issues in Nursing* (7th ed.). Upper Saddle River, NJ: Pearson Prentice Hall, 2020.
4. How can you prove that willful misconduct is serious? Legal Knowledge Base, n.d. https://legalknowledgebase.com/how-can-you-prove-that-a-willful-misconduct-is-serious
5. Alberty E. Patient with COVID-19 describes betrayal and abandonment. *Salt Lake Tribune*, February 4, 2022. https://www.sltrib.com/news/2022/02/04/patients-with-covid-risks/

6. Ronquillo Y, Varacallo M. Defamation. In *StatPearls* [Internet], 2021. https://www.ncbi.nlm.nih.gov/books/NBK531472/

7. Rattigan K. SuperCare Health hit with another data breach class action. Data Breach, Enforcement + Litigation, April 28, 2022. https://www.dataprivacyandsecurityinsider.com/2022/04/supercare-health-hit-with-another-data-breach-class-action/

8. Health Insurance Portability and Accountability Act (HIPAA) & Health Information Technology for Economic and Clinical Health (HITECH) Act. Microsoft Compliance, 2022. https://docs.microsoft.com/en-us/compliance/regulatory/offering-hipaa-hitech

9. West B, Varacallo M. Good Samaritan laws. In *StatPearls* [Internet], 2021. https://www.ncbi.nlm.nih.gov/books/NBK542176/

10. Henry T. Washington's high court considers new meaning for informed consent. American Medical Association, April 20, 2022. https://www.ama-assn.org/practice-management/sustainability/washington-s-high-court-considers-new-meaning-informed-consent

11. Advanced directives. Drugs.com, 2022. https://www.drugs.com/cg/advance-directives.html

12. What are the ANA standards of practice for Registered Nurses? Godwin University, 2022. https://www.goodwin.edu/enews/ana-standards-of-practice-for-nurses/

13. ANA Standards of Practice. American Nurses Association, 2022. https://www.nursingworld.org/ana/about-ana/standards/

14. Bailey T. How you can avoid getting sued. Bailey Law Firm, 2021. https://baileylawfirmsc.com/2021/06/14/how-you-can-avoid-getting-sued/

15. SBAR in nursing: How to use the SBAR method (with examples). Indeed.com, July 19, 2022. https://www.indeed.com/career-advice/career-development/sbar-nursing

16. Cross C. Importance of documentation and charting in nursing care. Small Business Chronical, n.d. https://smallbusiness.chron.com/importance-documentation-charting-nursing-care-80092.html

17. Buppert C. Questions and answers on malpractice insurance for nurse practitioners. *Topics in Advanced Practice Nursing eJournal*, 6(1), 2006. https://www.medscape.com/viewarticle/520660

18. Mitchell J. Nursing licensure: Legal requirements, revocation, suspension, and credentialing. May 16, 2016. https://study.com/academy/lesson/nursing-licensure-legal-requirements-revocation-suspension-and-credentialing.html

Reality Shock in the Workplace

Joseph T. Catalano | Leah Cullins

9

Learning Objectives

After completing this chapter, the reader will be able to:

- Describe the concept of reality shock
- Describe appropriate documents and procedures for job interviews
- List evidential artifacts used to develop professional nursing portfolios
- Define burnout and list its major symptoms
- Discuss the key factors that produce burnout
- List important elements in personal time management
- List at least four health-care practices nurses can use to prevent burnout and to improve their professional performance

WHAT IS REALITY SHOCK?

"That is not how we do it in the real world." How many times do students and new graduate nurses hear that sentence? In many ways, that sentence is correct: in nursing school, students are instructed in the ideal theoretical, research-based, and instructor-supervised practice. Although demanding physically, mentally, and emotionally, nursing school shelters students from the realities of the everyday work world where nursing practice consists of not only theory and research but also heuristic practice, human emotion and response, policies, regulations, and the push and pull of life responsibilities. Things are different in the real world. The transition from nursing student to registered nurse (RN) is often referred to as **reality shock (transition shock)**.[1]

MAKING THE TRANSITION FROM STUDENT TO NURSE

At any point in their lives, most people fulfill several different roles simultaneously. Sometimes, role conflict occurs.[2] Role conflict, sometimes called *role ambiguity*, exists when a person is unable to integrate the three distinct aspects of a given role: **ideal, perceived**, and **performed role images**. For nursing students, a significant role conflict may occur when they transition from the role of student to that of RN. In addition to reality shock, other factors can contribute to role conflict. For example, during the peak of the COVID-19 pandemic, hospitals were at full patient capacity. The nurses working at this time experienced severe stress and fatigue resulting in many leaving the profession. As more nurses left, the nursing shortage became even greater and new graduate nurses were pressed into positions of care and leadership for which they were ill prepared.[3]

Ideal Role

In the academic setting, the student is generally presented with the ideal of what a nurse should be. The ideal role projects society's expectations of a nurse. It clearly delineates obligations and responsibilities as well as the rights and privileges that those in the role can claim. Although the ideal role presents a clear image of what is expected, it is often somewhat unrealistic to believe that everyone in this role will follow this pattern of behaviors.

An Angel of Mercy

The ideal role of the nurse might require someone with superhuman physical strength and ability and unlimited stamina who possesses superior intelligence and decision-making ability, yet remains kind, gentle, caring, and altruistic, and not concerned about money. This perfect nurse can communicate with any client at any time and can function independently and know more than even the health-care provider. This angel of mercy is able to prevent egregious errors in client care while continuing to always be responsive to clients' needs and requests and carry out the provider's orders with accuracy and absolute obedience. Perceptive students soon begin to suspect that this ideal role of nurse does not exist anywhere in the real world.

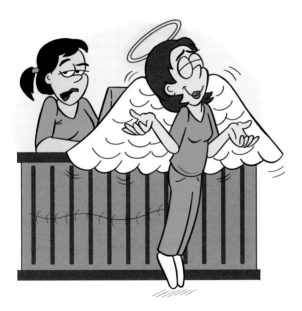

"The new nurse certainly has taken on an ideal role."

Perceived Role

The perceived role is an individual's own definition of the role, often more realistic than the ideal role. When individuals define their own roles, they may reject or modify some of the norms and expectations of society that were used to establish the ideal role. Intentionally or unintentionally, though, the ideal role is often used as the intellectual yardstick against which the perceived role is measured.

After a minimal amount of clinical experience, nursing students may realize that nurses do not possess extraordinary physical strength or intellectual ability but may continue to accept unconditionally, as part of their perceived role, that nurses must be kind, gentle, and understanding at all times with all clients and other health-care staff. The perceived role is the role with which the nursing student often graduates.

Performed Role

The performed role is defined as what the practitioner of the role actually does. Reality shock occurs when the ideal or perceived role comes into conflict with the performed role. Many new graduate nurses soon realize that the accomplishment of role expectations depends on many factors other than their perception and beliefs about how nursing should be performed. The work environment has a great deal to do with how the obligations of the role are met.

In nursing school, where students are assigned to care for one or two clients at a time, there is plenty of time to practice therapeutic communication techniques; to provide completely for the physical, mental, educational, emotional, and spiritual needs of the client; and to develop an insightful care plan. However, the realities of the workplace may dictate that a nurse be assigned to care for six to eight clients at a time. In this situation, the perceived role of the nurse may have to be set aside for the more realistic performed role, from communicator to task organizer. Meeting all of the client's physical, psychological, social, and spiritual needs becomes less possible, and the care plan becomes briefer and to the point.

Heart, Hands, and Ears
I lost a baby I wanted more than anything
   He was stillborn at 35 weeks
      You sat on the edge of my bed and listened to
      me sob when no one else would

I am only 8 and have leukemia
   The chemo shots hurt really really bad
      You sang a silly song with me while you gave
      the shot and made me laugh

I crashed my motorcycle and ripped open my leg
  It got a raging infection that required constant
  treatment
    You changed the dressing with skill and com-
    passion

I had a stroke long before I should have
  My hands no longer work the way they used to
    You taught me how to use the fork with the big
    handle and now I can feed myself

I stood by my father's bedside while the machines he
was connected to went straight line
  He was sick for a long time but I loved him with
  every fiber of my being
    You stood quietly beside me and your strength
    gave me the courage to go on

I asked you one day, "What does a nurse do?"
  I was wondering if it was something I could do too
    You answered:
    Nurses use their ears and compassion to listen
    Nurses use their hands and skills to heal
    Nurses use their hearts and souls to care
    Nurses take those who are at the crossroads of
    their lives,
    Who are battered and scarred with disease, and
    change their souls forever more with their
    hearts and their hands and their ears.

Joseph T. Catalano

Cognitive Dissonance

The difference between expectation and reality can produce what is called *cognitive dissonance* in many new graduate nurses. They know what they should do and how they should do it, yet the circumstances do not allow them to carry it out. The end result is increased apprehension. High levels of anxiety, left unrecognized or unresolved, can lead to various physical and emotional symptoms. When these symptoms become severe enough, a condition called **burnout syndrome** may result. In today's health-care climate and with the current nursing shortage, it is important that health-care agencies retain high-quality nurses and that nursing schools prepare graduates for their transition from student to nurse.

NURSING SHORTAGE CONTRIBUTES TO STRESS

A lack of qualified nurses has been present in the health-care system for so long that the term *nursing shortage* has become a truism. A 2022 survey of some 400,000 nurses showed that over a third of them plan to quit their current positions, although many intend to pursue a nursing role in a different location. During the COVID-19 pandemic, health-care facilities have been hiring traveling and per-diem nurses in much larger numbers than usual to fill nursing shortage gaps. The permanent nurses, although appreciating the additional help, by and large were not excited with this tactic. Traveling nurses, who work for the staffing agency, not the hospital, generally receive much higher wages and better benefits than the regular staff nurses. Some staff nurses believed that the quality of patient care and the morale on their units were decreased because of the lack of skills and knowledge of the traveling nurses. However, multiple recent studies about employment opportunities project that there will be a shortage of up to 1.2 million nurses by 2030.[4]

What Do You Think?

Does the nursing shortage in your region affect the health care that you can obtain at your local hospital? How can the nursing shortage be fixed?

Nurses in Demand

The demand for RNs is recognized by high school counselors and employment agencies who are seeing it as a viable career opportunity for both women and men. Enrollments in nursing schools are up; however, they are not maintaining a level sufficient to replace the nurses who are leaving the profession. In 2021, there were 278,815 first-time NCLEX-RN takers, up from 177,407 in 2020. Despite the disruption in nursing education due to the COVID-19 pandemic and the lack of qualified educators overall, the graduates maintained an 85 percent pass rate on the examination.[4]

Drops in nursing program enrollments tend to occur when the economy is strong; however, this does not seem to be the case with the current economic recovery. Enrollment in higher education in general tends to decrease during periods of strong economic growth and increase when the economy takes a downturn. In short, when the economy is strong, there are more employment opportunities, which give graduating high school students a broader spectrum of both professional and nonprofessional fields to choose from.

There are several reasons for the increased demand for RNs.

COVID-19

The COVID-19 pandemic created an upsurge in early nurse retirements that would not otherwise have occurred. The pandemic increased the stress levels of nurses due to increased numbers of critically ill patients who required the highest levels of around-the-clock care and the need to make urgent life-altering decisions. Early on in the pandemic, nurses faced a lack of personal protective equipment (PPE) to keep themselves from contracting the virus. Nurses were often called upon to participate in making life-or-death decisions for COVID-19 patients who required nonexistent ventilators.[3] Often, a nurse was the only one at the bedside of patients as they took their last breaths. Many nurses were moved from their usual departments and roles to assist with the intensive care of COVID-19 patients in totally unfamiliar units. Nurses are devoted to providing the highest levels of care for all patients; however, nurses' stress levels hit their peak when nurses were thrown into a new area of nursing they were totally unfamiliar with, especially in an area as difficult as critical care.[4] After life-saving vaccines became available, some nurses felt irritation and annoyance at taking care of critically ill patients who probably would not have been hospitalized if they had received the COVID-19 vaccine.

Aging Patient Population

On top of the COVID-19 pandemic, the population of older adults in the United States has increased and has brought an increase in age-related health-care needs. These include more chronic diseases and longer life spans that increase the demand for well-educated, highly skilled nurses (Chapter 22). The country has a larger population over the age of 65 than ever before in its history, composed primarily of baby boomers (those born between 1946 and 1964). This 65+ demographic has grown rapidly, jumping from 41 million people in 2011 to 71 million in 2019—a whopping 73 percent increase.[4] And the U.S. Census Bureau projects that number will continue to rise, reaching 73 million by 2030.[5]

Aging RN Population

It is also important to note that a high percentage of RNs who are currently working will retire within the next 10 years and therefore will not be an active part of the workforce. Baby boomers include not just patients but also nurses. Nearly half (47.5 percent) of all RNs are now over the age of 50.[4] A 2015 study predicted that more than 1 million RNs will retire from the workforce between now and 2030, taking with them their valuable accumulated knowledge and nursing experience.

Contributing Factors

A number of factors have consistently contributed to the ongoing nursing shortage, including the lack of equitable pay for equitable work; failure to recognize nurses as professionals and their contribution to the health care of patients; substandard working conditions such as short staffing, long hours, and multiple shifts; and the inability of nursing programs to accept all the qualified applicants due to an extreme shortage of qualified nursing faculties.[4]

One factor that has been mitigated to some degree is the unprofessional image of nurses portrayed in the entertainment media and believed by the public. Although the news media reports have been sympathetic to nurses on the front lines of the pandemic, their analyses have remained largely superficial. Similar to how the entertainment media presents nurses, the news media often portrays nurses as a homogenous, altruistic, and obedient group willing to put their lives on the line in the care of patients. However, there is very little real analysis about what nurses do and who they are.

The entertainment media is still falling short in portraying nurses as professional and equal partners with physicians. However, if one positive factor has come out of the COVID-19 pandemic, it is the recognition of the important role nurses play in caring for critically ill patients.

Public appreciation of the courageous members of the nursing profession was high during the pandemic.

However, the nursing profession must be able to transform recent feelings of gratitude and the current discussion about how important nurses are to the health care of the public into long-term positive actions that will distinguish nurses as highly educated, skilled, and autonomous professionals who function independently and as part of a highly skilled team. This challenge for a new recognition of the potential of nursing has never been so important given the projected shortage of nurses.[6]

COVID-19 has provided nurses the opportunity to challenge the media and public understanding of nursing and to present a realistic version of the profession that underscores all that nurses have accomplished in their clinical, educational, and leadership roles during the COVID-19 crisis.

Although the numbers vary, the Department of Health and Human Services currently anticipates a shortfall of up to 808,000 RNs by 2025. Other research and health-care groups project a nursing shortage ranging from 200,000 to 1 million nurses.[6] In 2022, the Biden administration began a massive grant program for issues related to the COVID-19 pandemic. In recognition of the important role nurses have in the health-care system and the impending shortage, many grants were made available for student loan payback, increases in nursing faculty, and improvement in nursing education in general.[7]

Periodically, some facilities try to cut costs by reducing the number of their most expensive personnel, the RNs. Most of these facilities eventually recognize that, although a reduction in RN positions may reduce costs in the short term, the long-term effects on the quality of health care are devastating. It is obvious that exchanging qualified nurses for lower-paid unlicensed technicians will eventually affect the quality of client care. With the current emphasis by The Joint Commission (TJC), the Institute of Medicine (IOM), the American Nurses Association (ANA), and the Affordable Care Act of 2010 (ACA) being placed on the delivery of quality client care, hospitals and other health-care facilities are recognizing that increasing the number of RNs they employ is the only way to increase the quality of care they provide. Unfortunately, in many areas of the country, facilities have been unable to fill their vacant RN positions.

Decentralized Care

Certain groups of nurses are in higher demand than ever; these include nurses who can practice independently in several different settings, **multiskilled practitioners**, home-care nurses, community nurses, and hospice nurses.[4] A major trend in health care that started a decade ago is to move the care out of the hospital and into the community and home settings. Provision of nursing services in these settings often requires that a nurse have at least a bachelor's degree or an even higher education. In 2021, fewer than 50 percent of all new graduate nurses graduated from bachelor's degree programs.[8]

The IOM report "The Future of Nursing: Leading Change, Advancing Health" established a goal of 80 percent baccalaureate-prepared nurses by 2020 to meet the needs of a health-care system that is constantly increasing in complexity. It is obvious that this goal was not met: the rate still hovers around 50 percent, basically unchanged since 2010.[8] The *Future of Nursing 2020–2030: Charting a Path to Achieve Health Equity* vision report does not posit any particular number for future baccalaureate-degree nurses but rather discusses "the key areas for strengthening the nursing profession to meet the challenges of the decade ahead." These key areas include nursing workforce, leadership, nursing education, nurse well-being, emergency preparedness and response, and the responsibilities of nursing with respect to structural and individual determinants of health.[9]

It is self-evident that modern-day professional nursing is becoming increasingly complex every day. However, no nurse who joined the profession in 2020 did so with the expectation that they could die while providing care to patients. Many lessons can and should be learned from the COVID-19 pandemic. The profession may never be quite the same again. It is important to remember that nursing has been advancing since Nightingale's push to move nursing education out of the grasp of physicians. Nurses must

> ❝ *The Department of Health and Human Services currently projects a shortfall of up to 808,000 RNs by 2025.* ❞

now move toward a sweeping new reality of modern nursing that has found its own voice.[8]

In the past, skill-based competencies were adequate to meet the needs of patients both in the hospital and in community settings; however, those competencies, while still important, fall short of meeting today's complex patient requirements. A graduate from a nursing program today needs to have the ability to access information, be competent in **health policy** at multiple levels, develop system improvements, use research and evidenced-based practice, build teamwork and collaboration, make complex decisions, and demonstrate leadership. The IOM report adds that baccalaureate-prepared nurses are better equipped than nurses with any other level of entry education to manage this increasing complexity in nursing care.[8]

Although most nurse practitioners are currently based in community clinics, the ACA is providing them with new opportunities to become involved in primary care and even the care of hospitalized clients. A key element in the ACA is that clients must be evaluated by a primary health-care provider before they can be referred to secondary health-care providers or specialists. During the COVID-19 pandemic, advanced practice nurses proved invaluable at the bedside, helping guide the care of staff RNs and making decisions about patient care as primary providers.[10] The advanced-practice education of nurse practitioners makes them eminently qualified to fill this role of primary health-care provider.

Certain specialty areas with a high burnout rate, such as transplant, intensive care, neonatal, oncology, and burn units, are always seeking nurses. The nursing shortage has lowered levels of work satisfaction, increased stress levels, and increased turnover rates of these nurses with highly specialized skills. Research has shown that as the perception of staffing shortages increases, so too does the number of nurses leaving these types of specialty units.[11] As with community nurses, nurses who provide care in specialty units must be able to work independently and use evidence-based practice by drawing from the large base of theoretical knowledge now available on the Internet.

Stress for nurses produces or contributes to burnout and can come from many sources. In recent years, cyberbullying has become a widespread issue. Because of the wide use of wireless technology, bullying behaviors can now occur in digital form via any number of sources such as instant messaging, e-mail, text messaging, social networking sites, and blogs. Cyberbullying has been identified by the National Council for the State Board of Nursing as a form of lateral, or nurse-on-nurse, violence. It can occur even if the post is from outside the hospital during non-work hours.

Nurses can take steps to fight cyberbullying in their workspace:

• Save evidence of bullying comments either electronically or printed.
• Present, during a private conversation, the accumulated evidence to the person who made the comments.
• Document the conversation and its outcome.
• If the cyberbullying continues, report it to the nurse manager along with copies of the evidence.
• If the behavior still continues, alert the chief nursing officer.

> *" . . . there is zero tolerance for bullying of any kind, including comments made online. "*

All nursing units should have a policy on cyberbullying, and the nurse manager needs to reinforce that there is zero tolerance for bullying of any kind, including comments made online. In its extreme form, cyberbullying can be considered the crime of harassment and involve legal authorities.[12]

The nursing profession and nursing educators need to increase their vigilance during nursing shortages to maintain the high standards of the profession and not fall into the "any warm body will do" trap. They must continue to recruit high-quality graduates and improve working conditions and salaries to keep the high-quality professional nurses they already have.

A POSITIVE TRANSITION TO PROFESSIONAL NURSING

The reality shock that new graduates often experience can be reduced to some extent. Some schools of nursing have instituted **preceptor** clinical experiences and other types of experiences during the last semester of the senior year. The main goal of preceptor clinical experience is to help the student feel more comfortable in the role of RN.

Nurse Residency Programs

The IOM has recommended that nurse residency (NR) programs be established to help new nurses make the transition from the sheltered environment of nursing school to the practice setting. NR programs concentrate on establishing solid decision-making skills in difficult patient situations, refining clinical leadership skills, and integrating the nurse's basic education and knowledge into realistic practice. Because 25 percent of new nurse graduates (prior to COVID-19) leave the profession during the first year, the NR program's goal is to be a support system to help them through that demanding time. Effective NR programs do this by reducing the new nurse's clinical workload, integrating classroom content along with clinical learning, and concentrating on critical-thinking skills in regard to patient outcomes and professional roles. NR programs help develop new nurses' skills, increase their knowledge, and aid them in providing safer client care.[13]

Researchers have calculated that it takes one or more years for new graduates to master the skills necessary to be successful in their position. Specialty units generally take longer. In the past, many hospitals used a sink-or-swim approach in which the new graduate was placed on a unit soon after graduation and expected to perform at the same level as an experienced nurse. This practice is no longer acceptable. New graduate nurses often do not possess the knowledge or skills to make a quick transition to providing competent and safe bedside care.

Without residency programs, some hospitals experience a resignation rate of new nurses ranging from 25 percent to a whopping 75 percent during their first year. A high turnover rate of nurses is equated with a high financial cost in recruiting and training more new nurses. A new graduate nurse who leaves their job within the first year will cost the institution between $27,500 and $40,000. That cost is then added to the expense of recruiting and orienting a new nurse, which has been estimated to range from a low of $8,000 to as much as $60,000 for nurses in specialty units. Some studies estimate the cost for losing and replacing a new RN to be as high as $80,000.[14]

> *In the past, many hospitals used a sink-or-swim approach in which the new graduate was placed on a unit soon after graduation and expected to perform at the same level as an experienced nurse. This practice is no longer acceptable.*

COVID-19's Effect on NR Programs

Prior to the COVID-19 pandemic, many nursing schools were already struggling to find direct-care clinical experiences for their students, and health-care facilities were having difficulties finding experienced staff nurses to supervise the new graduates in residency programs. With the onset of the pandemic, many health-care facilities closed their doors to nursing students, citing fear of liability should the students become sick, lack of PPE, and the lack of time for working with unproven learners. Similarly, NR programs all but dissolved as a transitioning and learning environment for new graduate nurses. In a very short span of time, new graduate nurse residents became full-fledged staff nurses, working 12-hour shifts and as much overtime as they could physically and emotionally handle.[15]

In the face of an ongoing nursing shortage and the unlikely prospect of hiring new nurses to meet the exploding demand for care of the new COVID-19 patients, many facilities looked inward to see if their current staff could be brought into areas where the greatest demand was predicted, such as acute care and critical care. When health-care facilities stopped performing elective procedures and reduced many other types of noncritical services, nurses employed in these areas became available to support other nurses who were caring for COVID-19 patients. Some facilities modified their staffing models to have noncritical care nurses work in public health, contact tracing infected individuals or administering vaccinations when these became available. In a process sometimes called *upskilling*, nurses from surgical units and nonacute clinics were cross-trained in the skills necessary to respond to the expected surge in intensive care units. During the peak of the pandemic, many areas of the hospital became critical care units, including medical-surgical units, oncology units, and even hallways.[16]

Suddenly, nurses who never thought they would get near a critical care unit became critical care nurses caring for patients connected to ventilators who were in strict isolation. Some facilities used their existing residency training programs to transition staff into their new roles. There are little data at the time of publication on the exit rate of nurses in NR programs. It can be anticipated that it was probably similar to that of experienced RNs who left because of the stress brought on by providing nursing care during the pandemic.[16]

Based on research done and data gathered at the peak of the pandemic, the U.S. Bureau of Labor Statistics (USBLS) estimated that approximately 500,000 experienced nurses were expected to leave the profession between 2020 and the end of 2022. In addition to the already existing nursing shortage plus the number of nurses leaving because of the pandemic, the USBLS estimated that there would be a shortage of 1.1 million nurses.[17] However, as the pandemic has begun to gradually slow and working conditions have become more tolerable, that prediction may be higher than the actual number. Some nurses are already coming back because they see what they do as a calling, not just a job. They like taking care of patients, but not in the pressure-cooker environment found during the peak of the pandemic.

Guidelines for NR Programs

The IOM has established some guidelines for NR programs. It believes it is important for state boards of nursing and state nurses associations to actively support and encourage facilities to develop programs that will ease the transition to safe clinical practice. The IOM encourages external funding for NR programs, which can be very expensive. This funding should be sought from major health-care organizations or groups that have a vested interest in improving health-care quality. Once the programs are established, they must be overseen and evaluated for effectiveness. Three key **evaluation criteria** include increased nurse retention, increased knowledge and competency of the nurses in the program, and an overall improvement in client satisfaction and outcomes.[13] The number of NR programs in the United States continues to grow despite the COVID-19 pandemic, and the results have been extremely positive. The retention rate for new nurses completing 1-year NR programs was 85.6 percent in 2021, which far exceeds the 25 percent rate for non-NR facilities. The rate was even higher for NR programs when coupled with tuition payback and sign-on bonuses. Evaluation data also showed that nurses felt a marked increase in their ability to provide safe, high-quality nursing care.[18]

Preceptorships

Students experience the role of the RN by working the same hours and on the same unit as the nurse to whom they are assigned. As students absorb the role expectations of the workplace during the preceptor experience, their perceived role expectations also change, allowing movement from the student role to that of practicing professional with less anxiety and stress.[19]

Another experience that lessens role transition shock may be an internship (sometimes called an *externship*, depending on the hospital). Internships or externships are available to students between the junior and senior years at some hospitals. These experiences allow students to work in a hospital setting as nurses' aides while permitting them to practice, with a few restrictions, at their level of nursing education. These experiences are valuable for gaining practice in skills and for becoming socialized into the professional role.

Employment in Today's Job Market

Although the health-care industry is in dire need of RNs, employers are still looking for the best of the best for the positions they have available.

What Do You Think?

Have you ever had a job interview? What did you do well during the interview? What mistakes did you make? How can you correct those mistakes in the future?

Initial Strategies

Employers are looking for graduates who can function independently, require little retraining or orientation, and can supervise a variety of less-educated and unlicensed employees. The ability to use critical-thinking skills in making sound clinical judgments is a necessity in today's fast-paced, complicated, and highly technical health-care systems.

Although these requirements may seem daunting, some strategies can be used to increase the chance of being hired. Students should take advantage of preceptor and intern or extern experiences in their junior and senior years and should attempt to meet their clinical obligations in the institution where they want to be employed. In this way, the student can evaluate the hospital closely and observe its working conditions and the type of care provided to clients.

For its part, the hospital has the opportunity to examine closely the student's knowledge, skills, personality, and ability to relate to clients and staff. The hospital benefits by getting employees who are familiar with the hospital before employment starts, thus decreasing the overall time of paid adjustment (referred to as *orientation*).

The Résumé

When nursing students think about finding a job in nursing, they may falsely assume that getting a nursing job should be easy, especially with all the talk of the current and future nursing shortage. As mentioned previously, both the USBLS and the IOM have projected a large scarcity of nurses in the next few years. However, calling this a nursing shortage is not entirely accurate. The Nursing Executive Council Advisory Board has redefined the nursing shortage as an *experience-complexity gap*, which is the mismatch between patients who are older and have more severe illnesses and recently graduated inexperienced nurses who are entering the workforce with only basic knowledge and skills. In reality, health-care facilities are seeking nurses with more experience to take the place of those nurses who are retiring or leaving the profession and taking their years of experience with them. Because of the experience gap, nurses who are just beginning their careers may find it challenging to land that first job.[20]

Today's nursing graduates who are attempting to enter the workforce are comfortable with the technology they grew up with and used during nursing school. Because they feel comfortable with online technology, many who are applying for nursing positions are using a passive approach to their job searches. They are sitting at their computers and surfing career boards, hoping that their ideal position will

> *First impressions are important. Preparing a neat, thorough, and professional-looking résumé is worth the time and effort.*

pop up and then clicking on the site to apply. Applying for a job online is fairly simple and sometimes does not even require a résumé. However, applying online increases the number of competitors for the positions and limits the applicant's opportunities.

The hidden job market should also be considered when seeking employment for the first time. The *hidden job market* consists of job positions that have never been posted formally on a website or in a nursing journal. Most commonly, these are job positions that employers attempt to fill by word-of-mouth or are open positions that employers do not want to spend money on advertising.

How does the new graduate find out about these positions? A number of strategies can be used:

- Investigate health-care facilities in the local community. Read their brochures.
- Find individuals, such as preceptors, faculty, family members, and health-care providers, who have connections with or intimate knowledge of the community facilities.
- Meet in person or via virtual meeting or phone call with the individuals and pick their brains. What methods did they use to get their job? Why do they like working there? What perks does their facility offer new graduates, such a mentorship, student-loan payback, and so on?
- Now begin to examine the facility's website for job openings that match the graduate's interests and experience. Contact the nursing recruitment department of the facility.
- Fill out an application, submit a résumé, and collect other documents the facility may require.[20]

No matter how you apply for a job, in today's job market, the **résumé** is often the institution's first contact with the nurse seeking employment, and it has a substantial effect on the whole hiring process (Box 9.1). First impressions are important. Preparing a neat, thorough, and professional-looking résumé is worth the time and effort. With a computer, such a résumé can be prepared and printed at almost no cost.

Box 9.1 Sample Résumé

Mary P. Oak
100 Wood Lane, Nicetown, PA 22222   Telephone (333) 555-1234 (H)   e-mail: moak@aol.com

Objectives
Obtain an entry-level position as a registered nurse; deliver high-quality nursing care; continue my professional development.

Skills
- Good organizational and time-management skills
- Communication and supervisory ability
- Sensitivity to cultural diversity

Education
Mountain University, Nicetown, PA
Bachelor of Science in Nursing, May 2022

Experience
Supercare Hospital, Hilltown, PA
Nursing Assistant, 2022 to present
Responsibilities: Direct client care, including bathing, ambulation, daily activities, feeding paralyzed clients, assisting nurses with procedures, charting vital signs, and entering orders on the computer.

Big Bob's Burgers, Hilltown, PA
Assistant Manager, 2015-2017
Responsibilities: Supervised work of six employees; counted cash-register receipts at end of shift; inventoried and ordered supplies.

Awards
Nursing Student of the Year, 2022
Mountain University, Nicetown, PA
Pine Tree Festival Queen, 2017
Hilltown High School, Hilltown, PA

Professional Membership
National Student Nurses Association, 2020 to present
Mountain University, Nicetown, PA

A Complete Picture

The goal of a résumé is to provide the hospital with a complete picture of the prospective **employee** in as little space as possible. It should be easy to read and visually appealing and have flawless grammar and spelling.[20] Although various formats may be used, all résumés should contain the same information. Each area of information should have a separate heading (see Box 9.1).

Many print and online guides exist for organizing the information in a résumé. Moreover, most new computers come from the factory loaded with software that can prepare résumés in different formats. Keep an electronic copy of your résumé for future use or reference. The required information includes the following:

- Full name, current address (or address where you can always be reached), telephone number (including area code), and e-mail address.
- Educational background (all degrees), starting with the most recent, naming the institution, location, dates of attendance, and degrees awarded. Usually, high school graduation information is not necessary.

- Former employers, again starting with the most recent. Give dates of employment, position title, name of immediate supervisor, supervisor's telephone number, and a short description of the job responsibilities. *Should non-health-care-related work be included in your résumé?* Very basic jobs—for example, cooking hamburgers at Big Bob's Burgers—could probably be omitted unless they fill in a large gap in your employment history. However, if the job required supervision of other employees or demonstrated some higher degree of responsibility such as developing budgets, handling money, or preparing work schedules, it should be included and described.
- Any scholarships, achievements, awards, honors, or certifications (e.g., BLS, ACLS) that you have received, along with any professional development activities in which you participated, starting with the most recent. Also note volunteer activities, especially those related to health care or community service (e.g., Red Cross).
- Professional memberships, offices held, and dates of memberships.
- Any works you have published. If both books and journal articles were published, list the books separately, starting with the most recent.

- Any military service, including branch, location, and years.
- An "Other" category, if applicable, to describe any unpublished materials produced (e.g., an internal hospital booklet for use by clients), research projects, **fellowships**, grants, and so forth.
- Professional license number and annual number for all states where you are licensed, along with the date of license and expiration date.

References

References should be included on a separate sheet of paper. Most institutions require three references. After obtaining permission from the individuals listed as references, you should make sure to have their current and accurate titles, addresses, e-mail addresses, and telephone numbers.

An individual selected as a reference must know you well in either a professional or a personal capacity, have something positive to say about you, and be in some position of authority. Nursing program directors, esteemed nursing faculty, supervisory-level personnel at a health-care facility, and health-care providers make good references. It is best not to list relatives unless the hospital is asking specifically for a personal reference.

Issues in Practice

Compassion Fatigue Among Nurses

If you no longer really care about the clients to whom you are assigned, you may be suffering from compassion fatigue. Much like burnout, compassion fatigue results from long-term stress caused by caring for those with chronic diseases or those with terminal illnesses. Nurses with compassion fatigue also experience chronic physical fatigue, emotional distress, and feelings of apathy. Nurses can recognize the condition when they become calloused, withdraw from the delivery of health care, and merely go through the motions. Unfortunately, compassion fatigue can spread to other staff and ultimately produce negative client outcomes.

The first step in preventing compassion fatigue is to take care of yourself. You need to eat right, exercise, and get plenty of rest. There is no shame in reaching out to a professional counselor for advice and help. Staying in close contact with family and friends, looking after your own spiritual needs, developing fulfilling and fun hobbies, and participating in activities that are fun and that renew your spirit are all important in dissipating the stress that leads to compassion fatigue. Also, rely on your coworkers. Working with a team you enjoy will help you stay connected with the reasons you entered the profession in the first place.

There are also courses and seminars available that can teach you ways to lower stress and deal with difficult situations. They will help you build up positive emotions to improve your attitude and enthusiasm levels.

Source: A. Redmann, Decreasing compassion fatigue and burnout in nursing through mindfulness: A quality improvement project, Sigma Repository, *May 2, 2022*, https://sigma.nursingrepository.org/handle/10755/22595.

Do not obtain letters of reference until the facility asks for them. Many facilities now use e-mail or phone references in place of letters as a time-saving method.

Résumés via Institutional Website

Many health-care facilities want prospective employees to apply for positions and submit their résumés through the institution's website rather than in person or on paper. The first step is to find the link on the institution's website that will take you to the employment application; the link will read something similar to "Prospective Employees" or "Job Opportunities" and should present an option such as "Apply for a Job." It is important that the job seeker read the instructions carefully and follow them to the letter. Comparable with the paper résumé, first impressions are important. If the person applying for a job cannot even follow the directions for applying, what kind of impression is that going to make on the human resources director? Each institution has its own format for applying. Some have boxes where a résumé can be pasted, some have a place to attach a résumé electronically, and some have a combination of the two. Others merely want the résumé attached to an e-mail and sent to a specific e-mail address.

A well-written paper résumé is a suitable place to start in creating an electronic résumé. However, the transition from a paper résumé created in a common word-processing program such as Microsoft Word is anything but smooth and seamless. Many e-mail systems, scanners, and Web browsers change how a document looks when it is opened in another system. These systems change fonts for headings, delete punctuation, and even move text around. To have the best-looking electronic résumé, it is important to use the least amount of formatting possible and a letter font that is nonproportional. Generally, such features as tables, page borders, and multiple fonts should not be used. Keeping two versions of a résumé is a good idea—a "fancier" one for submitting by mail or taking to an interview and a simpler electronic version that can be e-mailed or attached to an institute's website with minimal alterations.

The following steps for formatting an electronic résumé work with most word-processing programs and avoid giving applicant tracking systems (ATS; discussed shortly) unclear information:

1. Open the résumé in the word-processing program normally used.
2. Click FILE, then click SAVE AS, and select TEXT ONLY (which eliminates all nontext formatting).
3. Close and then reopen the résumé using the new text-only version in Notepad or a similar plain-text editor.
4. Format the text-only résumé:
   - Change to a nonproportional font (i.e., use a font where all the letters take up the same amount of line space, such as Courier Brougham, Letter Gothic, Orator, Lucida Sans Typewriter, MonoTxt, Isocteur, Lucida Console, Courier, and Monospace 821). These fonts prevent the lines of text from varying in width across the page.
   - Do not indent by using tabs. Some Web browsers don't recognize them and might move the text around on the page.
   - Keep all lines justified to the left side of the page, and use line breaks (Enter key) to separate headings and sections. Using the spacebar to indent or center text has unpredictable results when read by another browser.
   - Use ALL CAPS rather than **boldface** or *italic* to emphasize a word or words or when starting a new section of the résumé.
   - Never use accent marks, quotation marks (" "), asterisks (***), or other special characters ($#). These almost never come out like they were in the original document.
   - Write the résumé in the third person. Avoid "I" statements.
   - Target your résumé to the specific position. Do this by reading job descriptions and selecting *key words* noted in the descriptions—competencies, skills set, education, and experience. Use these keywords wherever they fit logically in your résumé.
   - Match individual experiences to key words/key skills found within the job posting.
   - Research the employer and target the résumé to the facility's values and culture.
   - Include a professional summary if you are an experienced nurse.
   - Make sure your skills and knowledge are a 100 percent match for the qualifications that are required for the position. For example, if a job listing says "BSN required" and you have an ADN, do not apply for the position—you do not meet the required qualifications for the position.

- Use standard, simple section headers such as "Work History" and "Education." Avoid section headings such as "Where I Went to School." The ATS does not understand it.
- List specific skills clearly.
- If you use acronyms and abbreviations, make sure to spell out the entire name or phrase followed by the shortened version the first time the term is used.
- Do not put information in the document header or footer. ATS will not "see" it there.
- Never use tables, graphs, diagrams, clip art, graphics, special fonts, photos, colored fonts, PDFs, or bullets. ATS are not programmed to read them.

5. Save the edited résumé as a separate document from the original.
6. Send the electronic résumé by attaching it to an e-mail, posting it on the Internet, or copying and pasting it into an institution's Web page.[21]
7. These steps should also be followed when creating a personal website or electronic portfolio.

Fighting Robots

Employers like electronic résumés because they can screen them with a résumé-reading robot (RRR). If you are on a facility's website and you click an "Apply Now" button, you can be pretty sure you are going to find a robot on the other end. The RRR is an essential part of ATS that scans the electronic résumé for key words and phrases. The employer can set up the program to find positive phrases, "knockout" phrases or words, and even disqualifying statements. Positive phrases might include "supervision of 3 aides." A knockout word might be *no* in answer to a question such as "Are you licensed in in the state of XYZ?" A disqualifying statement might be, "I have 4 DUIs on my record." The latest data indicate that up to 75 percent of employers use some form of RRR. Some are better than others at filtering data, so make sure to follow all of the tips regarding an electronic résumé.[21]

As with the paper résumé, electronic résumés should be accompanied by a separate cover document specifying what job you are applying for and why you feel qualified for the position (see "The Cover Letter"). Some sites have a "Check which job you want" box that may eliminate the need for a cover letter; however, it is a good idea to prepare a letter using the

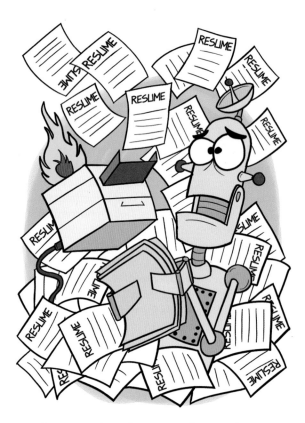

Automated applicant tracking software pre-screens electronic resumes.

preceding guidelines and make it the first page of the résumé. Doing so will cover all possibilities.

Creating a Professional Website Summary

By the time you have completed your nursing education, you probably have looked at enough websites to know which ones grab your attention and which ones you quickly skip over. Professional websites should follow some general principles, although creativity has a place as long as it is not too far out there! Then, when you e-mail a prospective employer, you can attach a link to the site. Remember that first impressions count. What should your professional Web page contain?

1. A professional posed photo of you should appear on the first page. Selfies do not make a good initial impression. Each page should have a different, related photo. A résumé page should have a candid photo of you in a work setting.

2. On the first page, use creative graphics or background photos that say something positive about you. A picture of a field of wildflowers behind the individual indicates a calm, attractive personality. A picture of a waterfall projects an image of power and direction. Be careful that the background is not so dark as to make the text hard to read.

3. Give a short summary of your personality and strengths on the home page. Use third-person descriptions. For example: "Julie's passion is to provide high-quality care to the most vulnerable of the population—premature infants and abused children." This page should also summarize your background. How did you become interested in nursing—through a specific event (e.g., a parent having cancer) or a person who inspired you? Did you have to overcome any difficult circumstances in nursing school? This page can also demonstrate your writing skills. Make sure an experienced writer or editor reviews it before you post it.

4. Write a career objectives page. This page is like a résumé, but it can be longer and is in paragraph form. You can include portfolio images of your work to demonstrate your accomplishments visually—show pictures from that in-service presentation you gave as part of the leadership class assignment. Make sure you include information about your education and employment history and a description of what you would consider the "perfect career." Describe in a few sentences what your dream job would be and why. Describe your professional objectives and why they are important to you. Do you want to go back to school to become a nurse practitioner at some point in the future? Why?

5. Include a résumé page. This page should use the standard résumé format for professional résumés. It should be no longer than one page. Make sure you update the information on this page as it changes. You will be sending an electronic copy to the employer's Web page and using the hard copy when going for an interview.

6. Include a contact page with all your contact information: address, phone numbers, and e-mail addresses. Make sure these are kept current. Include a link on the contact page to the site you created, just in case the prospective employer is not adept at previewing job candidates electronically. Also include a link back to the home page of your website.[15]

Where to Post Your Résumé

Several websites are generally recognized as locations for professional networking and job hunting. Web-savvy employers often search these sites first. Examples include the following:

1. https://www.linkedin.com. This site contains more than 5 million professional résumés and is often used by professionals to track each other. Employers can use it for finding potential employees in specific fields of expertise.

2. https://www.blogger.com. Probably the easiest of the sites to use, this site takes the user through the step-by-step process of setting up a blog in less than 30 minutes.

3. https://www.livecareer.com/resume-templates. Here you can post your résumé on up to 90 top résumé sites with just one click to get it in front of a large number of recruiters and employers all at one time. This site also offers live help by phone or chat along with résumé-building and job-searching tips.

4. https://www.wordpress.com. This site is generally used by top-level professionals, although anyone can post on it. It has some advanced features in design and content generation.[5]

The Cover Letter

A cover letter should be sent with every mailed résumé (Box 9.2). Like the résumé, it should be neatly typed without errors and should be short and to the point. Although a friendly, rambling letter might provide insight into a prospective employee's underlying personality, most personnel directors, human resource managers, and nursing directors are too busy to read through a lengthy document. The letter should be written in a business letter format, left justified, with 1-inch margins on the top, bottom, and sides. If at all possible, the letter should be addressed to a specific person. Letters beginning with "To Whom It May Concern" or "Dear Sir or Madam" do not make as favorable an impression.[20]

Organizing the Letter

The statement of interest and name of the position should constitute the opening paragraph of the letter.

Box 9.2 Sample Cover Letter

Mary P. Oak
100 Wood Lane
Nicetown, PA 22222

May 25, 2022

Mr. Robert L. Pine
Director of Personnel
Doctors Hospital
Gully City, PA 44444

Dear Mr. Pine:

I am interested in applying for the registered nurse position in the General Medical-Surgical Unit. I have 5 years of experience in providing care for a variety of clients with medical-surgical health-care problems as a nursing assistant. I completed my baccalaureate degree in nursing on May 9 and am scheduled to take the NCLEX examination on June 3. Enclosed find my résumé.

I believe that my organizational and time-management skills will be a great asset to your fine health-care facility. I work well with all types of staff personnel, and having been a nursing assistant for the past 5 years, I can appreciate the problems involved in their supervision.

Thank you very much for consideration of my résumé and application. I will call you within the next few days to arrange a date and time for an interview. Feel free to call me at home anytime, (333) 555-1234, or contact me by e-mail: moak@aol.com.

Sincerely,

Mary P. Oak
Encl.

Mention where you heard about the position as well as a date when you would be able to begin working.

The second paragraph should give a brief summary of any work experience or education that qualifies you for this position. Newly graduated nurses will have some difficulty with this part, but they should include their graduation date, the name of the school they graduated from and the director of the school's nursing program, and the prospective date for taking the NCLEX. This paragraph should also state which shifts the applicant is willing to work.

The third paragraph should be very short. It should express thanks for consideration of the nurse's résumé, a telephone number, and an e-mail address. Both the letter and résumé should be sent by first-class mail in a 9 × 12 envelope so that the résumé will remain unfolded, making it easier to handle and read.[20]

Will They Ever Answer?

Waiting for a reply can be the most difficult part of the process. Resist the urge to call the hospital too soon. Because most health-care institutions recognize the high anxiety levels of new graduates, they attempt to return calls within 1 to 2 weeks after receipt of the application. If no response is given after 3 weeks, the nurse should call the hospital to see whether the application was received. Mail does get lost. If the application has been received, the applicant should make no further telephone calls. Harassing the personnel director or nursing director about a job is not usually an effective employment strategy.

The Portfolio

Today's current work climate requires recruiters to interview, screen, and hire the most qualified person for the job in a short amount of time. The nursing shortage and a workforce that embraces career portability have created the need to often recruit and hire nurses on a moment's notice. Taking a portfolio that is articulate and polished to an interview can impress the human resources officer who is interviewing the new graduate. A portfolio provides the employer with a more detailed look at nurse's capabilities, personality, and qualifications.

Evidence of Positive Outcomes

Professional portfolios are being looked at closely by many non-artist professions to document skill qualifications, continued competency, accountability for professional development, and credible evidence to support employment claims during an interview. Nursing is one of the professions embracing this concept. If the trend continues, student nurses of today will become the next generation of the 4 million RNs in the United States who use portfolios instead of résumés to interview for jobs, become certified, maintain certifications, and demonstrate competency.[22]

Health-care employers today are looking for nurses who believe that high-quality performance on the job is more important than just having a job. Professional nurses can apply the nursing process to their own personal development and place evidence of positive outcomes in their portfolio.

Constructing a portfolio requires looking at a career as a collection of experiences, which can be grouped and reordered to match the changing direction of one's career journey. Many nursing programs are in the process of transitioning to an electronic format for producing student portfolios. A portfolio also offers an opportunity for nurses to reflect on their experiences, create new goals, design/develop and implement a plan, and then evaluate it. The portfolio supports the lifelong process of self- and career development. Although the construction of a portfolio may look like a daunting and time-consuming task, many websites exist that can take much of the confusion and leg work out of the task.[22]

Assembling a Portfolio

Once a student has decided to initiate a portfolio as a professional vehicle for showcasing their experiences, education, skill sets, accomplishments, and potential for achievement, time and effort are required to create it. However, the effort is well worth it in the long run.

Although the task might seem quite overwhelming, there are many online programs to help develop a professional-looking portfolio. The initial development of a portfolio may be somewhat time consuming, but once it is developed, keeping it current should become part of a professional's routine activities. Converting it to an electronic format is a must in today's high-tech health-care system.[22] Whether the portfolio is paper or electronic, the content and purpose are the same. Many books and online resources are available that describe the format and organization of a portfolio; an example is discussed here.

Use a Binder. One format that many experts agree on is a three-ring binder. It should include a table of contents, and the various sections should be separated by dividers.

Ask Yourself Questions. Questions to ask while you prepare to gather materials for your portfolio include: What do I want to do next in my career? Why do I think I am qualified for this job? What do I want to tell the employer about myself? Why should my employer promote me?

Interview a Professional. Once you make a decision on an employment area of interest, it is helpful to discuss the needed skills and education with someone who is currently employed in that work setting. Personal interviews can provide information about required skills or education. It is a good idea to show a draft of the portfolio to the nurse being interviewed to see if it reflects the required knowledge or if there is a need to pursue further education or skill development.

Showcase Your Education. Box 9.3 lists work samples that can be included in the portfolio. Box 9.4 lists basic categories for organizing the portfolio. Remember, these are just examples, and each nurse needs to use a format that will best showcase their education, work experience, skill sets, and accomplishments.

Use the Internet. Creating a Web version of the portfolio can enhance the application process (see earlier). Links can be created to digitize versions of portfolio information, examples of presentations, or photos of accomplishments or events. Portfolios are limited only by the nurse's imagination and access to space on the Web. Portfolios are an excellent way to impress

> *" Harassing the personnel director or nursing director about a job is not usually an effective employment strategy. "*

Box 9.3 Examples to Collect for a Professional Portfolio

1. Education and training examples
2. General work performance examples
3. Examples regarding using data or nursing informatics
4. Examples pertaining to people skills
5. Examples demonstrating skills with equipment

Items that may be collected to support these areas include, but are not limited to, the following:

Articles	Awards
Brochures	College transcripts and degrees
Drawings and designs	Forms
Flyers	Grants
Letters of commendation	Letters of reference
Manuals and handbooks	Merit reviews
Photographs	Military service and awards
Presentations	PowerPoint presentations
Proposals	Professional memberships
Résumés	Research
Technical bulletins	Scholarships
Videos	Training certificates

Box 9.4 Categories to Organize Your Professional Portfolio

1. **Career Goals:** Where do you see yourself in 2 to 5 years?
2. **Professional Philosophy/Mission Statement:** What are your guiding principles?
3. **Traditional Résumé:** Concise summary of education, work experience, achievements.
4. **Skills, Abilities, and Marketable Qualities:** Examples that support skill area, performance, knowledge, or personal traits that contribute to your success and ability to apply that skill.
5. **List of Accomplishments:** Examples that highlight the major accomplishments in your career to date.
6. **Samples of Your Work:** See Box 9.3.
7. **Research, Publications, Reports:** Include examples of your written communication abilities.
8. **Letters of Recommendation:** A collection of any kudos you have received, including from clients, past employers, professors, and so on.
9. **Awards and Honors:** Certificates of award, honor, or scholarship.
10. **Continuing Education:** Certificates from conferences, seminars, workshops, and so on.
11. **Formal Education:** Transcripts, degrees, licenses, and certifications.
12. **Professional Development Activities:** Professional associations, professional conferences, offices held.
13. **Military Records, Awards, and Badges:** Evidence of military service, if applicable.
14. **Community/Volunteer Service:** Examples of volunteer work, especially as it may relate to your career.
15. **References:** A list of three to five people who are willing to speak about your strengths, abilities, and experience; prepared letters from same.

potential employers, reach a larger employment pool, and put the Internet to work for a prospective employee.[22] Even if you have a Web portfolio, it is a good idea to bring a paper portfolio to an interview.

As discussed in the previous section, a résumé is an excellent tool for allowing the prospective health-care recruiter or employer to receive a concise overview of a potential employee in as little space as possible, and it serves as a frame of reference once the interview process is complete. A nurse who offers to share a portfolio during the interview process provides tangible evidence of skills, accomplishments, and future potential. Showing a well-prepared portfolio leaves a positive lasting impression with the interviewer and provides a foundation to build on as the nurse's career develops.

Interviews

The next important step in the hiring process is the interview. The interview allows the institution to obtain a firsthand look at the applicant and provides an opportunity for the applicant to obtain important information about the institution and position requirements. The interview often produces high levels of anxiety in new graduates who are interviewing for what might be their first real job.

Make a Good Impression

Again, first impressions are important (Box 9.5). The interview starts the moment the new graduate enters the office waiting room. Conservative business clothes that are clean, neat, and well pressed are an absolute necessity. If you are still dressing in the waiting room, it is likely to have a negative impression on the employer. A conservative hairstyle and limited accessories, jewelry, and makeup produce the best impression. Depending on the facility's policies and the part of the country in which you are planning to

work, visible body piercings, particularly in the nose septum, eyebrows, and lips, could be an issue. The same goes for visible tattoos and ear gauges. Smoking, chewing gum or tobacco, biting fingernails, or pacing nervously does not make a good first impression. *Turn off your phone and put it away!* Texting, surfing the Web, or answering e-mails during an interview is not "multitasking"; it is leaving the interviewer with a bad impression of you. The interviewer recognizes that interviews are stressful and will make allowances for certain stress-related behaviors, but do try to avoid the mistakes listed in Box 9.6.

Arriving a few minutes early allows time for last-minute touch-ups of hair and clothes and gives the applicant a chance to calm down. Carrying a small briefcase with a copy of the résumé, cover letter, references, and information about the hospital also makes a favorable impression.[23]

> *Health-care employers today are looking for nurses who believe that high-quality performance on the job is more important than just having a job. Professional nurses can apply the nursing process to their own personal development, and the evidence of positive outcomes is placed in the portfolio.*

Come Prepared

Mental preparation is as important to a successful interview as physical preparation. Most interviewers start with some small talk to put the interviewee at ease. Resist the temptation to launch into a long and rambling account of personal experiences or your life history. Next, the interviewer usually asks about the résumé or portfolio, if one is used. A quick review just before the interview is helpful so that you are familiar with the information contained in the résumé or portfolio.

Expect questions about positions held for only a short time (less than 1 year), gaps in the employment record (longer than 6 months), employment outside the field of nursing (e.g., food server, clerk), educational experiences outside the nursing program, or unusual activities outside the employment setting. Answer the questions honestly but briefly. Most personnel directors and nursing directors are

Box 9.5 **Fashion Dos and Don'ts of Interviews**

The Do List
Men
1. Do invest in a good haircut and shave or trim facial hair neatly.
2. If you use aftershave or cologne, do so sparingly (a little goes a long way).
3. Do carry a money clip or wallet and a small, plain, functional briefcase.
4. Do wear shoes that are polished and in good repair.
5. Do wear calf-length dark socks.
6. Do wear a tailored suit (blue, gray, or beige is best) with a dress shirt (lighter in color than the suit). Do wear a conservative tie.
7. Do wear minimal conservative jewelry such as a wedding ring, class ring, or cufflinks.
8. Do search the facility's Web page for its policies on visible tattoos and body piercings before the interview and attempt to comply with them.

Women
1. Do invest in a good haircut. Clean, neat, and conservative is best.
2. If you use perfume or cologne, do so sparingly (a little goes a long way).
3. Do carry a briefcase or simple (small) handbag.
4. Do wear shoes that are polished and in good repair.
5. Do wear hosiery—socks, stockings, or tights—that coordinates in color, style, and texture with your shoes and outfit.
6. Do dress conservatively in a blue, gray, or beige suit or other work-appropriate outfit.
7. Do wear minimal conservative jewelry, such as small earrings, a simple necklace, a wedding or engagement ring.
8. If you wear makeup, apply it lightly and carefully.
9. If you wear nail polish, use a conservative color and apply it carefully.
10. Do search the facility's Web page for its policies on visible tattoos and body piercings before the interview and attempt to comply with them.

The Don't List
Men
1. Don't overstuff your wallet, money clip, or briefcase.
2. Don't carry a can of smokeless tobacco in your back pocket or a pack of cigarettes in a shirt pocket.
3. Don't wear sandals, running shoes, or cowboy boots.
4. Don't wear socks that are a lighter color than your trousers.
5. Don't wear flashy colors.
6. Don't wear large earrings or display other facial piercings. Don't wear necklaces outside your shirt or rings on multiple fingers (other than a wedding ring or class ring).

Women
1. Don't wear sneakers, sandals, cowboy boots, or heels more than 1½ inches high.
2. Don't overstuff your handbag or briefcase.
3. Don't apply makeup so that it looks artificial and heavy.
4. Don't use black or dramatically colored nail polish.
5. Don't wear skimpy or low-cut outfits or fringed apparel.
6. Don't wear large, dangling earrings or display other facial piercings.

Source: Kleber R, What to wear to a nursing interview. FreshRN, 2023. https://www.freshrn.com/what-to-wear-to-a-nursing-interview-2022-guide

Box 9.6 Twenty Worst Job Interview Mistakes

1. Arriving late
2. Arriving too early (10–15 minutes is okay)
3. Dressing incorrectly (see Box 9.5)
4. Having your cell phone go off during the interview (and answering it); using your phone to text, tweet, or answer e-mails during the interview
5. Drinking alcohol or smoking before the interview
6. Chewing gum and/or blowing bubbles
7. Bringing along a friend, relative, or child
8. Not being prepared—not having an interview "dress rehearsal"
9. Calling the interviewer by his or her first name
10. Not knowing your strengths and weaknesses
11. Asking too many questions of the interviewer (a few are okay)
12. Not asking any questions at all
13. Asking about pay and vacation as the first questions
14. Accusing the interviewer of discrimination
15. Bad-mouthing your present or former boss or employer
16. Name-dropping to impress the interviewer
17. Appearing lethargic and unenthusiastic
18. Having a weak ("dead fish") or excessively firm ("bone-crusher") handshake—a medium-firm handshake is best
19. Looking at your watch during the interview
20. Losing your cool or arguing with the interviewer

busy and do not appreciate long, detailed, chatty answers. Applicants can anticipate being asked these questions:

- Why do you want this position?
- Tell me about yourself.
- Why have you selected this particular facility?
- Tell me about the time you had to handle a difficult patient during a clinical rotation.
- Why do you think you are qualified for the position?
- How did you handle the stress of nursing school? Will you use the same techniques in handling working on the units?
- What unique qualifications do you bring to the job to make you more desirable than other applicants?
- Where do you see yourself 5 years from now? Ten years from now?[23]

Practice answering these questions with another graduate. If you are not sure how to answer them or what would be the best answers, go online and find a site that lists interview questions and answers.[23] Using the portfolio will help answer some of these questions.

By showing tangible examples of qualifications and accomplishments, the interviewee can help the busy interviewer discern between actual performance and mere rehearsed answers.

> *Portfolios are an excellent way to impress potential employers, reach a larger employment pool, and put the Internet to work for a prospective employee.*

Forbidden Topics

There are a number of personal topics that prospective employers are not legally supposed to discuss, but they sometimes do anyway. These include questions about sexual orientation or habits, age, race, pregnancy status or plans for a family, marital status, personal living arrangements, **significant others**, and religious or political beliefs.

If these questions are asked, the applicant needs to consider the implications of not answering them. Although there is no legal obligation for the applicant to answer, refusal to do so or pointing out that the question should not have been asked in the first place may give the interviewer a negative impression. If the applicant answers these personal questions, which violate their right to privacy and may be discriminatory, and then is not hired for the position, there may be grounds for some type of legal action based on discrimination.

Ask Your Own Questions

At some point in the interview, usually toward the end, applicants are asked whether they have any questions. Although most do have questions, many applicants are afraid to ask. In fact, asking questions can be seen as a demonstration of independence, initiative, and intellectual curiosity—all traits that are highly valued by health-care providers. It is important that the first questions are not about salary, vacations, and other benefits. Questions that indicate interest in the institution are included in Box 9.7.

After these questions have been answered, the applicant may want to ask about salary, raises, vacations, and other benefits. Some questions that the applicant should never ask include: When will I get a promotion? When do I get my first raise? What sort of flex-time options do you have? or any question that indicates the applicant was not paying attention during the interview. It would also be wise to inform the interviewer of the dates scheduled for the NCLEX so that arrangements can be made for time off. The applicant should also ask for written material on the nurse's contract with the institution, including benefits and job descriptions. Often, the interviewer provides this information without being asked in the course of answering some of the other questions.

Take this scenario as an example: The job applicant had successfully fielded all the usual interview questions: Why do you want this job? What are your qualifications? Why should I select you over other candidates? Then the interviewer asked the question that all job applicants hate: What do you consider to be your major weakness? A good way to answer that question is to find a weakness that can be turned into a strength. The applicant might answer, "I tend to be a perfectionist and spend too much time trying to get things just right."

It is appropriate to close the interview by asking for a tour of the facility. A tour allows firsthand evaluation of the workplace and a chance to observe the staff and clients in a real work setting. The interviewer may

---

Box 9.7 Questions Interviewees Should Ask

- What is the culture of your hospital?
- What are the responsibilities involved in the position?
- What personal characteristics are you looking for in a job candidate?
- How do you measure nursing success?
- What do the nurses like best about working here?
- What skill set would best match the position for which I'm applying?
- What type of orientation and training do you have for new employees?
- How long is the probation period for new employees?
  - Who are the other staff or personnel working on this unit?
  - What is the typical client-to-staff ratio for the unit?
- How long are your shifts?
  - Are there any mandatory rotating shifts, weekend obligations, overtime, or floating?
  - Does the hospital offer opportunities for continuing education, clinical ladder, advancement, or movement to other departments?
- Please describe the facility's policies for employee health and safety.

Source: Gerencer T, Top 25 nursing interview questions and answer examples, Zety, 2022. https://zety.com/blog/nursing-interview-questions.

not be able to provide a tour at that time and may ask another individual (e.g., an administrative assistant) to take the applicant on the tour.

Beware of the Internet

Nothing Is Private

Savvy employers almost always enter the name of a prospective employee in a search engine and search for them on one or more social media platforms before an interview. Research has shown that up to 77 percent of employers look up candidates before the interview and up to 70 percent have rejected potential employees because of information found online. Some employers go even further to find out about the candidate; often they can electronically locate unflattering pictures or video sequences, ill-advised comments or tirades, and even financial information.[19]

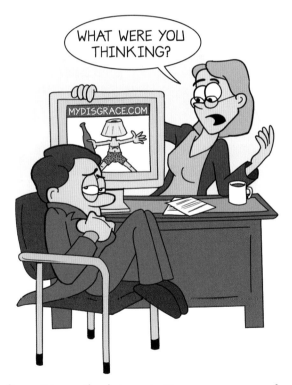

Once it's on the Internet, it never goes away!

It Never Goes Away

As a candidate for a job, especially as a new graduate, you need to be aware that the person sitting across from you at the interview desk may well have run your name through an electronic search engine and

found you through a people-finder website or on social media. New graduates should visit data-broker or people-finder websites such as Spokeo, Intellius, MyLife, or BeenVerified to see all the information listed about themselves that is available for anyone, including a human relations manager, to see. These sites get their information from a variety of sources, such as public records like real estate transactions and legal and court proceedings, and so on. They can also retrieve personal information from social media sites, warranty cards submitted for purchased products, sweepstakes entries, and pretty much any other places a person may submit their personal information.[25]

The following situation is an example of what could happen during a candidate's interview for a job. During an interview, after the candidate answered all the questions, the interviewer remarked, "I found a video segment of you on Instagram that was shot about two years ago showing you at a party appearing inebriated with very few clothes on. Would you mind commenting on that?"

Personal blogs can be deleted and eventually will become harder to access. However, the truth is that once words or images go electronic, they never completely go away. Search engines have improved to such a point that they can find information that is 5 or more years old.

Although you can use the Internet to your advantage, your presence on it can also be a disadvantage in the job market. You may feel secure and private in a chat room with your "friends," but in reality, anything you post on the Internet can end up on any number of social media platforms, video-sharing sites, or blogs. You may feel safe using a pseudonym or password protection, but these are only as trustworthy as the people who have access to your information. A jilted boyfriend or girlfriend, a friend who thinks what you said was funny, or someone with a large circle of electronic friends all have the power to reveal your most private information.[25]

You can offset negative information about yourself by generating as much positive information as possible. Eventually, the positive information will get more hits, and the negative information will be pushed to the end of the site, where people are less likely to see it. However, digital archives such as Wayback Machine can retrieve information that has been sanitized and removed from a website even years before. Remember, nobody is perfect, and all people have information they would prefer to keep secret. If negative information about you does exist online, you can try to control it by spinning it in the best way possible. If there is a large amount of negative information and pictures, you might want to spend some money and have it professionally removed by a reputation management agency such as DeleteMe, Iron Reputation, Net Reputations, or Elixir Interactive, which can scrub and wipe clean even the most incriminating and damaging materials. These sites can be expensive. DeleteMe charges $129.00 per year.[25] These companies guarantee removal of *all* unwanted content and will also monitor your website for new postings of untoward pictures or information and automatically remove it.

Business Cards—Old School?

In some circles, business cards are considered old school. Electronic business cards are now taking the place of piles of paper business cards. A popular electronic business card is vCard (https://vcardmaker.com), which can be read by many devices (e.g., iPhone) and in various formats (e.g., e-mail). The site helps you develop and make the most of the vCard.

Another site that provides paperless business cards is Smilebox (www.smilebox.com/Electronic-Card/Free). This site can create as many non-paper business cards as you want, and the cards will never run out. They can also be sent to anyone who has a computer or a mobile phone.[26]

Follow-Up

As is the case after sending a résumé, making frequent calls about the results of the interview is unwise. However, it is appropriate for the applicant to send a letter or email within 1 week after the interview to thank the interviewer for their time and express appreciation for being considered for the position (Box 9.8). The applicant should also acknowledge how much it would mean to them to become a member of the staff at such a high-quality agency or hospital but should avoid overdoing the compliments.

If the position is offered, a formal letter of acceptance or refusal should be sent to the institution. Health-care facilities will not hold positions indefinitely, and failure to accept the position formally in a timely manner may result in their offering the position to someone else.

Box 9.8 Sample Follow-Up Letter

Mary P. Oak
100 Wood Lane
Nicetown, PA 22222

June 20, 2022

Mr. Robert L. Pine
Director of Personnel
Doctors Hospital
Gully City, PA 44444

Dear Mr. Pine:
Thank you very much for considering my résumé and for the interview on June 3, 2022. I learned a great deal from the interview and from my tour of the hospital afterwards.

I am writing to let you know that I am still interested in the position and am wondering about the status of my application. If at all possible, I would appreciate it if you could either call me or write a note relating to my potential employment at your facility.

Feel free to call me at home any time, (333) 555-1234, or contact me by e-mail: moak@aol.com.

Sincerely,

Mary P. Oak

WHEN NURSES BURN OUT

Burnout syndrome has existed for many years and has been recognized as a problem that can be reduced or even prevented. A widely accepted definition of burnout is a state of emotional exhaustion that results from the accumulated **stress** of an individual's life, including work, personal, and family responsibilities. The term *burnout* is used to describe a slow, continuous depletion of energy and strength combined with a loss of motivation and commitment after prolonged exposure to high occupational stress. Examples of occupational stress include heavy workload, lack of participation or social support, injustice, uncertainty, lack of incentive, role conflicts, job insecurity, job complexity, and structural constraints.

Although the term is not often applied to students, many of the symptoms of burnout can be observed in aspiring nurses.[1]

Who Burns Out?

The people who are most likely to experience burnout tend to be hardworking, idealistic, perfectionistic, and more intelligent than average. Certain categories of jobs and careers tend to produce a higher incidence of burnout: situations and positions in which there is a demand for consistent high-quality performance, unclear or unrealistic expectations, little control over the work situation, and inadequate financial rewards. These jobs or careers tend to be very demanding and stressful with little recognition or appreciation for the work performed. Also, jobs in which there is constant contact with people (i.e., customers, clients, students, or criminals) rank high on the burnout list.

Nurses who have been working through the COVID-19 pandemic are experiencing increased symptoms of burnout. The burnout rate for nurses during the peak of the pandemic was 50 percent.[1] This all-time high burnout rate was due to a number of factors, including working longer hours, working more shifts, being continually exposed to contagious patients, being at risk of contracting the disease themselves, and watching patients die alone and being able to do little to help them.[27]

Even with the most superficial knowledge of nursing, it is easy to see that many of these elements are present in the nurse's work situation. It is possible to recognize nurses who are in the early stages of burnout by identifying some classic behaviors (Box 9.9).

Box 9.9 Symptoms of Burnout

- Extreme fatigue
- Exhaustion
- Frequent illness
- Overeating
- Headaches
- Sleeping problems
- Physical complaints
- Alcohol and/or drug abuse
- Mood swings
- Emotional displays
- Anxiety
- Poor-quality work
- Anger
- Guilt
- Depression

How It Starts

One of the earliest indications of burnout is the attitude that work is something to be tolerated rather than eagerly anticipated. Nurses in the early stages of burnout often are irritable, impatient, cynical, pessimistic, whiny, or callous toward coworkers and clients. These nurses take frequent sick days, are chronically late for their shifts, drink too much, eat too much, and often are not able to sleep.

Eventually, as their idealism erodes, their work suffers. They become careless in the performance of their duties, uncooperative with their colleagues, and unable to concentrate on what they are doing, and they display a general attitude of boredom and **apathy**. If allowed to continue, burnout may lead to feelings of helplessness, powerlessness, purposelessness, and guilt.[27]

Complications of Burnout

Nurse burnout and nursing shortages are given as the biggest single threats to patient safety in the United States. In a study in 2021, staffing shortages resulting from nurses leaving the profession led to patients having to wait longer for health care or even being turned away, despite having life-threatening emergencies. Critically ill patients had long wait times just to be triaged in emergency departments.[27] This study also found that decreases in patient safety due to increases in nurse errors were the number one result of nurse burnout. The study backed up previous studies that had found a strong correlation between nurses experiencing burnout and higher rates and spread of hospital-acquired infections, especially when nurses were working long hours and caring for too many clients at a time.

When client-to-nurse ratios are increased, there is a corresponding increase in rates of infection in hospitals. Increased client loads lead to external mental demands, such as interruptions, divided attention, and feeling rushed. The addition of just one extra client per shift per nurse was related to a 10 percent increase in rates of urinary catheter and postoperative infections. The studies demonstrated that the extra time out of the nurse's day to monitor, administer medication to, and provide care for an additional client is sufficient to reduce infection control measures such as hand washing. The researchers noted that reducing burnout by 10 percent could prevent thousands of hospital-acquired infections per year and save $41 million per hospital. By decreasing nurses' workloads, there is an increased likelihood of nurses following through on infection-control procedures, creating a better atmosphere for nurse and client safety.[28]

Nurses suffering from burnout have also been linked to increases in clinical errors, such as medication mistakes, missing treatments, and missing signs and symptoms of serious changes in condition. Burnout has also been linked to failure to complete documentation and errors in documentation.[28]

The Trauma That Keeps on Giving

Unlike a single traumatic event, no matter how horrific, COVID-19 has presented nurses with even greater workplace challenges and stress. COVID-19 might even be thought of as the trauma that keeps on giving. Even before the pandemic, nurses in many places were already experiencing the early phases of burnout. Generally, when situations on the unit causes stress to one nurse, other nurses will find ways to relieve that stress and support their colleague. However, during the pandemic, with its overwhelming workload and constant changes, nurses found it impossible to be supportive to coworkers.

Some measures used during the pandemic have seen success in at least staving off the worst of the burnout effect. "Safe-spaces" on units, where nurses can take breaks in a quiet, nonstressful environment, are one measure. The best of these spaces have comfortable massage chairs and quiet, restful music. Another strategy that met with success is the availability of mental health professionals to consult with nurses in high-stress situations both in person and via phone. Other strategies include town hall–type meetings where nurses and other health-care providers meet and discuss their problems and possible solutions to them.

Positive results of these types of actions are demonstrated through better nurse–patient relationships, fewer nurses leaving, a care team working at its peak performance, improved outcomes, and overall upgraded quality of care. Generally, improved nurse well-being is a reversal of the symptoms of burnout.[30]

Recognizing Burnout

The first step in dealing with burnout is recognizing its signs. Here are some of the key signs that a nurse may be experiencing burnout:

- Continuous physical exhaustion and excessive illnesses
- Strong feelings of being taken advantage of and unappreciated
- A feeling of impending doom when preparing to go to work
- Pulling back at work—spending as little time as possible doing tasks and communicating
- Lack of empathy for clients[11]

Despite this bleak picture, nurses do not have to fall victim to burnout syndrome. Many nurses have practiced their profession for many years, even during the peak of the COVID-19 pandemic, managed to deal with the stress, and found great personal satisfaction in what they do. These satisfied and motivated nurses have developed ways to deal with the stress of their careers while maintaining their goals and purpose as nurses.

Nurses experiencing burnout usually go through four progressive stages with some overlap between them: physical and mental exhaustion; self-shame and doubt; cynicism about work and lack of empathy for clients; and a sense of personal failure, feelings of helplessness, and an overwhelming sense of crisis.[11] Many nurses who are burning out use denial and rationalization to block recognition of burnout because it is just too painful for them to think they put so much time, money, and effort into preparing for a career they no longer want or enjoy.

It is important to realize that burnout can be halted in any one of the four phases. It does not have to progress to a crisis state. Also keep in mind that it is not the career that is producing the burnout but rather the difficulty in coping with the stresses the career is producing. Although it may not be possible to change the requirements of the profession significantly, it is possible to learn how to cope more effectively with stress.[16]

Manage Stress and Time

Although there are many schools of thought about stress- and time-management techniques, several common threads run through many of these theories. These views include setting personal goals, identifying problems, and using strategies for problem-solving.

Set Personal Goals

Goals and goal setting are an important part of client care. Nursing students—and, by extension, practicing nurses—are highly proficient in the planning stage of the nursing process, in which goal setting is the primary task. Nurses know that a good set of goals should be client centered, time oriented, and measurable and that they should write these goals with every care plan they prepare.

In their personal lives, however, these nurses may rush full tilt into one erratic day after another, subordinating their own needs to the needs of others and working long, hard hours but without accomplishing very much and feeling frustrated about it. What is the problem here? Very simply, these nurses can prepare realistic, beneficial goals for their clients, but they seem to be unable to do the same for themselves.

Long-Term Goals

Personal goals should include both long-term and short-term goals. Typically, personal long-term goals look into the future at least 10 years and include a statement about what the nurse wants to achieve during their lifetime. Some examples are going back to school to obtain an advanced degree, becoming a director of nursing, or even writing a book.

Practicing nurses who are caught up in the whirlwind of everyday life find it difficult to formulate statements about the future. One other important characteristic of long-term goals is that they need to be flexible. As life circumstances change, modifications are required.

Short-Term Goals

Short-term goals are those that the nurse expects to accomplish in 6 months to 2 years. These goals should be aimed primarily at making the nurse's professional or personal life more satisfying and fulfilling. Like long-term goals, they do not need to be related to work. Perhaps visiting a foreign country, going on a skiing trip in the mountains, or learning how to paint a picture or play the piano may be achievable in a relatively short time. In the professional realm, joining a professional organization, becoming a head nurse, or changing an outdated hospital policy are goals that can be achieved in a short time. The fact that everyone ages over time cannot be altered, but time can be used to achieve personal satisfaction in life and increase knowledge and accomplishments.

> *" Also keep in mind that it is not the career that is producing the burnout but rather the difficulty in coping with the stresses the career is producing. "*

An End Achieved

Although goal setting is an important first step in dealing with the stress that leads to burnout, any good nurse recognizes that a plan without implementation is useless. As difficult as personal goal setting may be for nurses, carrying it out may be even more difficult. Although goal achievement requires a degree of hard work and personal sacrifice, when people are working toward something they really want, the effort that it takes to achieve the end actually becomes enjoyable. This process takes a lot of work, but it becomes an exciting adventure in its own right.

Identify Underlying Problems

Another important step in dealing with burnout is to identify the problems that are producing the stress. Again, nurses are taught as students that they need to identify client problems so that they can work toward

Issues Now

Exercise is a great way to reduce and relieve stress and promote overall good health. But like most other popular activities, exercise is surrounded by a lot of beliefs and recommendations—some based on sound evidence, and others, not. Can you tell if each of the following beliefs is true or false?

Exercise Beliefs: True or False?

1. Exercise cannot turn fat into muscle.
   True: Muscle and fat are two completely different types of tissue. Exercise can increase the mass of muscle tissue and decrease the size of fat cells by burning fat as energy.

2. If you are gaining weight, it always means you are getting fatter.
   False: An increasing amount of fat will make the scale numbers go up, but it is not the only cause. If you are exercising, you may be building muscle, which has a much higher density than fat (i.e., a pound of muscle takes up less space than a pound of fat). It is possible to become leaner and healthier while at the same time gaining weight.

3. I am a woman, so I will bulk up if I lift weights.
   False: The bulging, bulky muscles that men get when they pyramid train (overwork muscles) is due primarily to testosterone. Also, that type of muscle development requires lifting weights for 6 to 8 hours a day every day. Weight training will increase muscle definition in women and help tone muscles, which in turn increases metabolism and reduces weight.

4. Running outside on a track and running on a treadmill at home both produce the same amount of stress on the joints.
   True: Running is running, and it stresses the joints no matter where it is done. There are some very expensive high-end treadmills that have extra shock-absorbing features, but even those do not completely eliminate the stress on the joints.

5. Any type of aerobic exercise will burn fat.
   True: However, the harder you exercise, the more fat you burn. It is important to build up a progressive exercise tolerance before attempting to reach the maximum level of an aerobic exercise.

6. I can eat anything I want as long as I exercise every day.
   False: Any exercise will burn a certain number of calories per session. For example, if you weigh 155 pounds and run 1 mile in 12 minutes, you will burn about 560 calories. If you stop and get an 1,100-calorie super-sized chocolate milkshake after your run, you will need to burn another 440 calories to maintain your weight.

7. Using free weights causes more injuries than using weight machines.
   It depends: Free weights are very adaptable to all body types and can be adjusted easily to accommodate a person's exercise progression. The danger with free weights arises when people do not know their limits and try to overdo the weights. Also, people tend to pay less attention to good body alignment and configuration when they use free weights. With weight machines, you are less likely to drop a weight on your toe. Weight machines also tend to force you into the proper body position for the particular exercise. The problem is that machines are based on an "average-sized" person, and if you are very large or very small, the machine may not be appropriate for you.

8. When you sweat a lot, it means you are achieving the maximum workout.
   False: As warm-blooded creatures, humans sweat to keep their internal body temperature in an acceptable range (homeostasis). Sweating may or may not be related to increasing the heart rate or burning fat. Some people have a higher metabolic rate and tend to sweat a lot even with minimal exertion. When exercising on a cold day, a person may sweat little or not at all.

Issues Now (continued)

9. No pain, no gain.

    False: The corollary to this myth is "A lot of pain, a lot of gain." Although most people do experience a small amount of discomfort or pain when they exercise vigorously, it is due primarily to the toning and stretching of the muscles. If your muscles are toned, you may not experience any pain at all with regular exercise. If you are having an excessive amount of pain, it is your body's way of telling you to stop what you are doing and take a rest.

10. Stretching after you exercise may be more beneficial than stretching before exercise.

    True: After you have exercised, the muscles and connective tissues are "warmed up" and comply more readily to being flexed and lengthened. The stretches should be slow and deliberate and held for 10 to 15 seconds while breathing deeply. Cold stretching before exercise may actually cause injuries because the connective tissues are stiff and less elastic. Many people, especially women, are hyperflexible and do not need to stretch.

Sources: *Center for Spine and Orthopedics, The science of post-workout recovery: Busting myths and spilling facts, May 24, 2022, https://centerforspineandortho.com/health-wellness/the-science-of-post-workout-recovery-busting-myths-and-spilling-facts.*

solving them. The same applies to nurses resolving their own setbacks. These issues cannot be addressed if they are ignored or unknown.

Self-Diagnosis

Formulation of a nursing diagnosis is nothing more than precisely stating a client's problem. One thing nurses realize early in the learning process is that what may appear to be an obvious problem may in reality not be a problem at all. Conversely, something that a client mentions only in passing may turn out to be the real source of the client's nursing needs. Perhaps nurses should look at their own lives and attempt to formulate nursing diagnoses that deal with their stress-related problems (setting the North American Nursing Diagnosis Association list aside).

What Do You Think?

List three tasks that you have put off today. Why did you avoid doing them? How can you get them done sooner?

For example, a new graduate nurse has just completed a shift during which they were assigned to eight complete-care clients. The new nurse had to supervise two poorly prepared nurse's aides and put in 55 minutes of unpaid overtime to complete the charting. This nurse is feeling tired, frustrated, and even a little bit guilty because of an inability to provide the type of care that they were taught in nursing school.

What is the problem? A possible nursing diagnosis might be "alterations in personal satisfaction related to excessive workload, evidenced by sore feet, headache, shaky hands, feelings of guilt, frustration, and a small paycheck."

Goals and Interventions

Now that the problem has been identified, goals and interventions can be introduced to solve the problem. The goals may range from organizing time better to refusing to take care of so many complete-care clients. Interventions, depending on the goals, can include activities such as attending a time-management seminar, talking to the head nurse, or changing a policy in the policy and procedure book.

RESPONDING TO MAJOR STRESSFUL EVENTS

Although nurses often learn how to deal with the stresses routinely found in their daily work, major traumatic events that produce overwhelming stress, such as the devastation of terrorist attacks, mass shootings, or major hurricanes and tornadoes, may leave nurses with a sense of horror, helplessness, and powerlessness in addition to the normal stress responses of shock, disbelief, anger, and grief. Nurses have several skills that help them deal with traumatic events in their workplace; however, nurses are not super-people and should not expect that they can handle all stressful events without help. The end result may well be a complex of symptoms similar to burnout syndrome, including physical symptoms, depression, and chronic anxiety.

Crisis Intervention

In response to major tragedies in recent years, the **critical incident stress debriefing** (CISD) process was developed to help health-care providers deal with major acts of violence and traumatic disasters. A *critical incident* is generally defined as a sudden and unexpected event that has a significant impact on an individual's mind, body, or emotions. Although often short term, a critical incident has the potential to cause long-term effects on the person's mental health and behavior. The American Red Cross has been instrumental in training and providing resources for local CISD teams. These teams are made up of mental health professionals specially trained in crisis intervention, stress management, and treating posttraumatic stress disorder (PTSD).[29]

To be most effective, the CISD teams need to be on site within 2 to 3 days after serious events, ranging from the death of coworkers to acts of terrorism and natural disasters. The goal of the team is to encourage the participants to verbalize their feelings and thoughts, identify and develop their coping skills, and generally lower overall grief and anxiety levels. These teams provide an intensive stress-management course compressed into a few hours or few days. Unlike a single traumatic incident, a pandemic is a prolonged event that lasts for years. Although CISD techniques may be effective, they do not work well for long-term, unrelenting stress.[29]

Posttraumatic Stress Disorder

One of the keys to working with nurses is to help them recognize that they are not expected to be able to handle all situations and that they can appropriately ask for help. Although nurses study the stress response and grieving process in school, it is sometimes hard for them to apply information about normal stress reactions to themselves. When nurses do not recognize their own problems in responding to traumatic stress, they increase their risk for developing long-term stress reactions. When they do not seek help, they can develop the symptoms of PTSD anywhere from a few days to as long as 6 months after the event.

Warning signs of PTSD include the following:

- Recurring nightmares and inability to sleep
- Intrusive and vivid flashbacks
- Prolonged depression

- High levels of anxiety
- Maladaptive coping behaviors, such as drug and alcohol abuse

The CISD session generally requires up to 3 hours. Sessions can be longer or shorter, depending on the nature of the event and number of people affected. Besides having an opportunity to express emotions, the participants are educated in some ways to reduce anxiety and promote mental and physical health. This advice includes the follow:

- Not watching televised replays of the event over and over
- Staying with friends and family as much as possible
- Avoiding unhealthy, high-fat diets
- Engaging in regular aerobic exercise as much as possible
- Avoiding excessive dependence on alcohol and drugs for sleep
- Getting back to a comfortable routine as soon as possible
- Feeling comfortable seeking professional help when it is needed

During the CISD sessions, nurses are asked for their input about the process. If the team feels it is necessary, additional referrals for long-term treatment may be recommended.

STRATEGIES FOR PROBLEM-SOLVING

Nurses already know the nursing process as a client problem-solving technique. Why not apply the same knowledge and skills to personal problems? The stress level only increases if problems are left unsolved.

Although specific problems may require specific solutions, several widely accepted methods exist to deal with the general stresses produced by everyday work and personal life. Included in these methods are activities such as recognizing that nurses are only human, improving time-management skills, practicing what is preached, and decompressing.

Time-Management Skills

In modern life, there is often not enough time to do everything that needs to be done. The key to time management is setting priorities. In the world of nursing and client care, nurses are often required to do many tasks. Multitasking, the process of doing several tasks at the same time, tends to fragment the nurse's attention and concentration.

Nurses need to recognize that only some nursing activities are essential to the safety and well-being of clients. These include performing thorough assessments and ensuring that the clients get their medications on time, that their comfort needs are met, and that accidental injuries are prevented. Beyond these actions, nurses really have a great deal of discretion in what they can do when providing care to clients.

Make Room for Fulfillment

Burnout results mainly from personal and professional dissatisfaction. If nurses feel fulfilled in what they are doing, burnout is much less likely to occur. Activities that may increase nurses' satisfaction include spending time talking with clients, learning new skills, and decreasing the anxiety of families through teaching and listening. After such activities have been identified, time should be set aside for them during the shift. The real secret in using time management to prevent burnout is for the nurse to use the time left for those nursing activities that bring the most professional and personal satisfaction.

Basic skills need to be developed to allow time during a shift for these preferred activities. The nurse must learn to delegate by letting the licensed practical nurses (LPNs) or aides do those tasks they are able to do. Many nurses graduate from nursing school with the attitude that if you want it done right, you need to do it yourself. After becoming familiar with the LPN and nurse's aide job descriptions, nurses need to give others a chance to prove themselves.[11]

Overcome Procrastination

Another necessary skill is overcoming procrastination. Most people have a natural tendency toward procrastination, particularly when unpleasant or difficult tasks are involved. The primary reasons people postpone or delay doing something are that they either do not want to begin or do not know where to begin the task. More time and energy are expended in inventing excuses for putting off tasks than would be taken in doing the tasks.

The Most Distasteful Task

The best way to overcome procrastination is to start the task, even if it is only a small step. An effective method is to select the most difficult or distasteful task to be done that day and to commit just 5 minutes to it. After 5 minutes, you can either set the task aside or continue it. Once you start the task and momentum builds, you will likely carry out the task to completion. If you do nothing else that day, at least you have completed the most difficult task.

Tasks can be prioritized by listing them in three categories. Category A tasks (e.g., assessments, passing out medications, treatments, and dressing changes) are important and need to be completed on time. Category B tasks (e.g., baths, linen changes, lunch breaks, charting) are important but can be postponed until later in the shift. Category C tasks (e.g., cleaning up, organizing the supply room) are tasks that either can be delegated or can wait until the next day.

Problems Don't Solve Themselves

For daily tasks, both pleasant and unpleasant, the best time to do them is immediately. If achievement of the plan requires delegation, it needs to be done at the beginning of the shift, not at the middle or end. Some nurses have a built-in fear of taking chances. As a result, they avoid doing things if there is a chance of failure in the hope that somehow the problem will resolve itself.

Any time an important decision is made, there is a chance that someone will disagree or that the decision will be incorrect. These types of situations need to be viewed as a challenge or an opportunity rather than a life-altering risk to be avoided. Although mistakes in health care do have the potential to be fatal, learning from mistakes is one of the most fundamental ways of increasing knowledge.

Time management, like other skills, requires some practice. Once a nurse masters this skill, their life becomes more satisfying.

Practicing What You Preach

Because nursing is oriented toward keeping people healthy as well as curing illness, nurses spend a large amount of their time teaching clients about exercising regularly; eating well; getting enough sleep; going for regular dental, eye, and physical examinations; and avoiding drinking excessive amounts of alcohol and smoking. It might make an interesting student research project to have nurses rank themselves on how well they have incorporated these health-maintenance activities in their own lives. The results would probably indicate a low overall score on the "practice what you preach" scale.

Nurses know all about healthy eating habits, but they do not translate that knowledge into feeding themselves properly. In reality, there are going to be some busy days when it is impossible to eat right; but it should be possible, on a regular basis, to follow a diet that promotes health and reduces the build-up of fat plaques in the arteries.

It is important to get enough sleep to avoid chronic fatigue. People can adjust to a state of fatigue, but it tends to decrease the enjoyment that they find in life and makes them irritable, careless, and inefficient. Most people need between 5 and 8 hours of good sleep each night. It also probably would not hurt for nurses to take a short nap during the afternoon on their days off.

The Right Kind of Exercise

Many nurses feel they get enough exercise during their busy shifts, and, in truth, the average staff nurse walks between 2 and 5 miles during each 8-hour shift. Unfortunately, this type of walking does not qualify as the type of aerobic exercise recommended for improved cardiovascular conditioning and stress relief. Exercise, in order to be beneficial, must be done consistently and must raise the heart rate above the normal range for an extended period. The short sprint-type walking involved in client care does not accomplish this goal.

Research studies compared workers' exercise habits with their psychological well-being. The results indicated that the more workers exercised, the less likely they were to experience increases in depression or burnout. Those employees who exercised at least 1.5 hours per week reduced their depression and job burnout tendency by 50 percent more than those who never worked out. The group who exercised more than 4 hours per week had the same results as those who exercised 1.5 hours per week.[13]

Further research has shown that exercise actually decreases the production of stress hormones such as cortisol and epinephrine while increasing the production of endorphins, the body's natural pain- and anxiety-relief chemicals. Physical activity acts as a strong distraction from problems. Anxiety, anger, and stress can be redirected to physical exercise and may allow a person to achieve a Zenlike state in certain cases. Going to a gym, boxing ring, running trail, biking trail, or sidewalk in the neighborhood provides a pleasant change of scenery and helps lower stress.[27]

Exercise also helps a person build up an immunity to the stress of the workplace. Studies have shown that people who exercise more tend to be less affected by the daily stress they face. Reasonable exercise also builds up the immune system, making the person less susceptible to common infections; however, excessive exercise may actually deplete the immune system.[30] Exercising with others has the additional benefit of social support. When exercise and physical activity also involve others, the positive effects are doubled by combining stress-relief activity with the enjoyment of friends. Working out with a friend improves motivation, increases happiness, and makes the workout go faster and seem less like work.

> *Tension must be released, or it will eventually cause a major explosion or (if turned inward) produce anxiety.*

Walking 1 to 2 miles a day outside of work is a beneficial, simple exercise that will improve health. Nurses can also use a wide variety of exercise equipment for those days when walking outside is undesirable. The important requirement is that the exercise be done consistently and frequently. Regular exercise not only improves the cardiovascular system but also helps improve stamina, raise self-image, and promote a general sense of well-being.

Decompression Time

The profession of nursing is stressful, even under ideal circumstances. Nurses are required to deal with other people constantly and to carry out numerous tasks that are potentially dangerous. At the end of any shift, even the most skilled and best-organized nurse has a sense of internal tension. This tension must be released, or it will eventually cause a major explosion or (if turned inward) produce anxiety.

Establish a Daily Decompression Routine

It may take a little time to discover, through trial and error, what works to reduce the tension built up during the shift. Some effective techniques include setting aside approximately 30 minutes of private, quiet time to reflect on the day's activities. Perhaps relaxing in a hot bath or sitting in a favorite recliner might meet the need for decompression. Relaxation activities, such as swimming, shopping, or even going for a drive, can help reduce tension and act as a time for decompression. Of course, stress-management techniques learned at seminars (e.g., self-hypnosis or meditation) can also be used. Finally, meeting with a nurse support group can help the nurse vent feelings and make constructive plans for solving problems.

Conclusion

Although transition shock and burnout are realities of the nursing profession, they can be reduced or even avoided altogether. Nurses should be able to recognize the causes and early symptoms of transition shock and burnout to prevent them from developing into a problem. Therefore, nurses should use techniques to prevent these disorders from becoming insurmountable obstacles. In doing so, nurses will be able to practice their profession proficiently and gain the satisfaction that only nursing can provide.

CRITICAL-THINKING EXERCISES

- Make a list of the characteristics of the "perfect nurse." Make a second list of characteristics found in nurses observed in actual practice. Discuss how and why these lists differ.
- Outline a plan for implementing a preceptor clinical experience for the senior class of a nursing program. Make sure to include how many hours of practice are required, criteria for the selection of preceptors, student objectives from the experience, and methods of evaluation.
- Write at least three long-term and five short-term personal or professional goals. Develop a realistic plan and timeframe for achieving these goals. Make sure to include what is required to achieve these goals.
- Complete this statement, using as many examples as possible: "I feel most satisfied when I am done with my shift in knowing that _____." Analyze these answers and discuss how they can be implemented in everyday practice.
- Think of at least three situations in which you were asked to do something that you really did not want to do. How did you handle these situations? How could they be handled in a more assertive manner?

NCLEX-STYLE QUESTIONS

1. Marla, a medical-surgical nurse for 10 years, is giving Jerome, a new graduate RN, advice on self-care behaviors he can use to prevent burnout. Which statement by Jerome indicates that he has understood Marla's teaching?
   1. I will decompress after a difficult shift by having a few beers with friends.
   2. I get all the exercise I need during a busy shift.
   3. I will make sure to get 8 hours of sleep each night.
   4. I can postpone my annual wellness examination because I'm a health professional.

2. Khadija, a nursing student, wants to improve her time-management skills. Which is the FIRST step she must take to better manage her time?
   1. Learn how to multitask.
   2. Set priorities.
   3. Delegate household duties to her roommates.
   4. Overcome her tendency to procrastinate.

3. Brian's unit manager suspects that Brian may be starting to experience burnout. What factors would lead the manager to this conclusion? **Select all that apply**.
   1. They work in a neonatal intensive care unit.
   2. Brian has always been a hard worker and a perfectionist.

3. Brian is a team player and assists other staff when he is able to.
4. The manager overhears Brian asking for another nurse's advice about a client.
5. The hospital has had to freeze staff salaries and cancel bonuses due to financial problems.
6. Brian requests additional training to improve his skills.

4. _____ is the transition from nursing student to registered nurse.

5. Which elements of a job search can you work on while you are in nursing school? **Select all that apply**.
   1. Creating a résumé
   2. Building a portfolio
   3. Writing a cover letter
   4. Arranging an interview
   5. Following up

6. Carli wants to include evidence of her people skills in her nursing portfolio. Which of the following is the BEST evidence for her to include?
   1. A PowerPoint presentation she gave on the importance of people skills
   2. A certificate showing completion of continuing education credits in psychology
   3. Positive performance reviews from past supervisors
   4. Thank-you letters from former clients or their family members praising Carli's ability to care for and communicate with them

7. Sue, a charge nurse on a mother–baby unit, goes to see her primary-care physician. Sue reports that she feels exhausted all the time, has difficulty sleeping, experiences frequent headaches, and feels anxious and overly emotional. Her health-care provider orders laboratory tests to rule out physical ailments. Which of the following questions would BEST help the provider assess whether Sue is feeling burned out?
   1. How are things going at work? At home?
   2. What have you tried doing to feeling better?
   3. What do you think is going on?
   4. Are you feeling burned out at work?

8. The chief nursing officer (CNO) at a large hospital is concerned about nurse burnout. The CNO announces that a new hospital-wide initiative, the Stamp Out Burnout Campaign, will be developed by a committee of hospital employees. Which of the following would help this campaign be effective? **Select all that apply**.
   1. Include nurses in the campaign committee.
   2. Make safe, adequate staffing levels a priority.
   3. Update the hospital policy and procedures documents to clarify roles and responsibilities of nursing and other personnel.
   4. Extend the preceptorship program for new graduate nurses from 3 months to 6 months.
   5. Ensure that communication from management is clear and timely.
   6. Make sure that staff nurses know they can share concerns and ideas with management, including the CNO.

9. A nursing instructor has just finished lecturing on the topic of the job-search process and is taking questions from the class. Which comment by a student indicates the need for clarification?
   1. Employers can't see what I post on social media as long I use appropriate privacy settings.
   2. I like the idea of a website portfolio rather than a heavy physical one you have to carry around.
   3. Even though I'll wear scrubs at work, it's important to dress up for the job interview.
   4. After an interview, it's a good idea to send a letter or e-mail thanking the interviewer.

10. In what way does improving one's time management help to prevent nursing burnout?
    1. Effective time management allows the nurse to complete all the necessary activities of patient care and have time to relax a little, too.
    2. Effective time management allows the nurse to do less work by delegating to an LVN/LPN or to unlicensed assistive personnel.
    3. Effective time management allows nurses to do what must be done and use the remaining time to do the nursing activities that bring them the most professional and personal satisfaction.
    4. Effective time management allows the nurse to complete client care early in the shift and then focus on professional-development activities, such as pursuing an advanced degree.

References

1. Stolzman T. New nurse reality shock and early burnout. *UNLV Theses, Dissertations, Professional Papers, and Capstones. 4268.* August 1, 2021. http://dx.doi.org/10.34917/26341205

2. Hallaran A, Edge D, Almost J, Tregunno D. New nurses' perceptions on transition to practice: A thematic analysis. *Canadian Journal of Nursing Research*, 55(1), 2022. https://doi.org/10.1177/08445621221074872

3. Mitchell G. How to make a professional transition during the COVID-19 pandemic. *American Business Association Journal*, 2021. https://www.abajournal.com/columns/article/transitioning-during-covid

4. The 2021 American nursing shortage: A data study. University of St. Augustine Health Sciences Center, May 25, 2021. https://www.usa.edu/blog/nursing-shortage/

5. U.S. Census Bureau, Population Division. Projected age groups and sex composition of the population: Projections for the United States, 2017–2060 [Excel spreadsheet].2022. https://www2.census.gov/programs-surveys/popproj/tables/2017/2017-summary-tables/np2017-t2.xlsx

6. Bennett C, James A, Kelly D. Beyond tropes: Towards a new image of nursing in the wake of COVID-19. *Journal of Clinical Nursing*, 29(15-16): 2753–2755, 2020. https://doi.org/10.1111/jocn

7. Funding opportunities specific to COVID-19. National Institute of Health Grants and Funding, 2022. https://grants.nih.gov/grants/guide/COVID-Related.cfm

8. What is the national average pass rate for the NCLEX-RN? Medical Hero, 2023. https://medicalhero.com/national-average-pass-rate-nclex-rn-exam/#:~:text=If%20you%20want%20to%20consider%20all%20the%20attendees,will%20have%20to%20reappear%20again%20for%20the%20exam

9. The Next Generation NCLEX. NCSBN.org, 2022. https://www.ncsbn.org/public-files/NCLEX_Stats_2022-Q4-PassRates.pdf

10. National Academies of Sciences, Engineering, and Medicine; National Academy of Medicine; Committee on the Future of Nursing 2020–2030; Flaubert JL, Le Menestrel S, Williams DR, et al. (Eds.). *The Future of Nursing 2020–2030: Charting a Path to Achieve Health Equity.* Washington, DC: National Academies Press, 2021. https://www.ncbi.nlm.nih.gov/books/NBK573919/

11. Kleinpell R, Myers C, Schorn M, Likes W. Impact of COVID-19 pandemic on APRN practice: Results from a national survey. *Nursing Outlook*, 69(5):783–792, 2021. https://doi.org/10.1016/j.outlook.2021.05.002

12. Nurse burnout: Risks, causes, and precautions for nurses. University of St. Augustine for Health Care, July 30, 2021. https://www.usa.edu/blog/nurse-burnout/

13. Batool I. How to identify and protect against cyber bulling. Privacy Pub, 2022. https://www.cyberghostvpn.com/privacyhub/how-to-prevent-cyberbullying/

14. Weberg D. How to find new grad nurse residency programs. Trusted Health, 2022. https://www.trustedhealth.com/new-grad/how-to-find-new-grad-nurse-residency-programs

15. Abdi N. A step-by-step guide to calculating the exact cost of turnover. *Sparkbay*, 2022. https://sparkbay.com/en/culture-blog/calculate-cost-turnover-3

16. Smith-Kimble C. How will COVID-19 affect nursing students returning to school? NurseJournal, August 29, 2022. https://nursejournal.org/articles/how-will-covid-19-affect-nursing-students-returning-to-school/

17. Chan G, Bitton J, Allgever R, Elliott D, Hudson L, Burwell P. The impact of COVID-19 on the nursing workforce: A national overview. *Online Journal of Issues in Nursing*, May 31, 2021. https://doi.org/10.3912/OJIN.Vol26No02Man02

18. Peralta P. Too little, too late: 500K nurses are leaving the bedside by the end of 2022. *Benefit News*, November 18, 2021. https://www.benefitnews.com/news/nurses-are-planning-to-quit-their-jobs-if-their-needs-arent-met-post-pandemic

19. Collins S. What is a nurse residency program? Benefits, drawbacks and qualifications. AcademiaLabs, 2022. https://academialabs.com/nurse-residency-program

20. Eley S. The power of preceptorship. *RN Journal*, 2022. https://rn-journal.com/journal-of-nursing/the-power-of-preceptorship

21. Guarniere A. How to find a nursing job. The Resume Rx, 2022. https://www.theresumerx.com/how-to-find-a-nursing-job/

22. Strazzulla P. The top 13 best applicant tracking systems (ATS)—2022. Software Reviews, 2022. https://www.selectsoftwarereviews.com/buyer-guide/applicant-tracking-systems

23. Indeed Editorial Team. How to create a job-winning portfolio for your next interview. Indeed, updated December 12, 2022. https://www.indeed.com/career-advice/interviewing/portfolio-interview

24. Rubin N. How to ace a job interview. Talk District, March 5, 2020. https://www.talkdistrict.com/how-to-ace-a-job-interview

25. Gerencer T. Top 25 nursing interview questions and answer examples. Zety, 2022. https://zety.com/blog/nursing-interview-questions

26. Gordon S. How to remove your data from people-finder sites. *Popular Science*, April 30, 2022. https://www.popsci.com/remove-data-people-finder/

27. The best business card companies. Top Consumer Reviews, 2022. https://www.topconsumerreviews.com/best-business-card-companies/detailed-reviews.php

28. Kuntapay G, Justice A, Jones A, Zhang C, Santos Jr H, Hall L. The prevalence of nurse burnout and its association with telomere length pre and during the COVID-19 pandemic. PubMed, 2022. https://pubmed.ncbi.nlm.nih.gov/35294438/#affiliation-1

29. Ojemeni J, Kalamani R, Tong J, Crecelius M. Relationship between nurse burnout, patient and organizational outcomes: Systematic review. *International Journal of Nursing Studies*, 119, 2021. https://doi.org/10.1016/j.ijnurstu.2021.103933

30. Lebow H. Critical incident stress debriefing: Addressing early signs of trauma. PsychCentral, May 13, 2022. https://psychcentral.com/health/critical-incident-stress-debriefing

3

Leading and Managing

Leadership, Followership, and Management

10

Joseph T. Catalano

Learning Objectives

After completing this chapter, the reader will be able to:

- Identify and discuss the three major theories used to explain leadership
- Define and distinguish among the three styles of leadership
- Discuss the relationship of transformational and situational theories to leadership style
- Identify the key behaviors and qualities of effective leaders
- Identify the key characteristics of effective followers
- Distinguish the differences between management and leadership
- Identify and discuss the two major theories of management

In today's health-care system, even new graduates who have an "RN" after their name will be placed quickly in positions of leadership and management.

LEADERSHIP

The old saying that "leaders are born, not made" implies that at birth a person either is a leader or is forever relegated to the rank of follower. Not many people agree with this statement. Although some people may be born with personality characteristics that make it easier for them than for others to fill the leadership role, most experts believe that almost everyone can develop leadership skills.

Many definitions of leadership refer to the ability of an individual to influence the behavior of others. When nurses exert leadership, they inspire other health-care workers to work toward one or more of several goals that include developing a teamwork spirit, providing high-quality patient care, maintaining a safe working environment, developing new policies and procedures, and increasing the power of the profession.

Some leadership theories try to explain why some people are leaders and others are not, but as yet, none covers all the possibilities. That may be because leadership requirements differ according to the situation. In the intensive care unit (ICU), for example, where quick decisions are a matter of life or death, the leader is the nurse with highly developed critical-thinking and analytical skills and the confidence to make decisions under pressure. In quality management, where the problems are often long term and complicated, the leader tends to be well organized and can methodically sift through a mountain of information and statistics to develop a policy that covers the widest range of possibilities. Several of the better-known leadership theories are discussed here.

Trait Theory

The trait theory, first developed in 1869, identifies qualities that are common to effective leaders (Box 10.1). Based on personality

Box 10.1 **Leadership Traits**

- High level of intelligence and skill
- Self-motivation and initiative
- Ability to communicate well
- Self-confidence and assertiveness
- Creativity
- Persistence
- Stress tolerance
- Willingness to take risks
- Ability to accept criticism

characteristics of many successful and failed leaders throughout history, the trait theory of leadership is used to predict how effective a person might be in a leadership role. According to the theory, when a person is compared to the list of characteristics, it can be determined whether the potential leader is likely to succeed or fail. A number of personality tests have been developed that are supposed to indicate whether a person will make a good leader.

However, these tests concentrate on the differences between leaders and followers and assume that a person who is a leader would score higher in leadership qualities than those who are followers. A deeper analysis of these tests shows that there might be only a few characteristics that really matter in determining leadership potential. Many of the traits on the test, such as height, do not have much actual value in determining leadership ability. More determinate might be traits such as good communication ability or flexibility in dealing with changes.

Some experts believe that leadership ability develops in certain situations, where some qualities are more successful in some settings and less effective in others. The question left unanswered is why everyone who has these traits is not a leader.[1]

Leadership-Style Theory

One of the best-known theories of leadership looks at three leadership styles:

1. Laissez-faire
2. Democratic
3. Authoritarian

Although these theories are discussed separately, they are a continuum of leadership style that ranges from a mostly passive approach to a highly controlling one (Table 10.1).

The Laissez-Faire Style

The **laissez-faire** (French for "leave it alone") leadership style is also described as *permissive, nondirective,* or *passive.* The laissez-faire leader allows the group members to determine their own goals and the methods to achieve them. There is little planning, minimal decision making, and a lack of involvement by the leader. This style works well in only a few settings, for example, in a research laboratory that is staffed by self-motivated scientists who know what they want to achieve and are familiar with the means of achieving it.

The laissez-faire style works best when the members of the group have the same level of education as the leader and the leader performs the same tasks as the group members. In most situations, however, laissez-faire leadership can leave people feeling lost

Table 10.1 **Comparison of Authoritarian, Democratic, and Laissez-Faire Theories**

	Authoritarian	**Democratic**	**Laissez-Faire**
Degree of Freedom	Little freedom	Moderate freedom	Much freedom
Degree of Control	High control	Moderate control	Little control
Decision-Making	Leader only	Leader and group	Group or no one
Leader Activity Level	High	High	Minimal
Responsibility	Leader	Leader and group	Abdicated
Quality of Output	High quality	High quality/creative	Variable
Efficiency	Very efficient	Moderately efficient	Variable

Source: *Adapted from D. Stanley, Followership, in* Clinical Leadership in Nursing and Healthcare: Values Into Action *(2nd ed., pp. 47–58), Hoboken, NJ: Wiley-Blackwell, 2017.*

and frustrated because of the lack of direction by the leader. When the group tries to achieve some goal, often the only input from the leader is that the group is doing it incorrectly. When faced with a difficult decision, laissez-faire leaders usually avoid making a decision in the hopes that the problem will resolve itself.

The Democratic Style

In the **democratic** (also called *supportive, participative, transformational*) leadership style, all aspects of the process of achieving a goal, from planning and goal setting to implementing and taking credit for the success of the project, are shared by the group. The democratic leadership style is based on four beliefs:

1. Every member of the group needs to participate in all decision making.
2. Within the limits established by the group, freedom of expression is allowed in order to maximize creativity.
3. Individuals in the group accept responsibility for themselves and for the welfare of the whole group.
4. Each member must respect all the other members of the group as unique and valuable contributors.

The leader using the democratic style provides guidance to the group, and all members share control. This style works best with groups whose members have a relatively equal status and who know each other well because they have worked together for an extended period. In its purist form, democratic leadership can be time consuming and inefficient in some situations, particularly when group members disagree strongly; but in the end, when a goal is achieved or a decision made, there is a strong sense of ownership and achievement by the whole group. Hallmarks of this style are trust, **collaboration**, confidence, and autonomy. Followers of this system have a high level of commitment to the institution, resulting in a strong work ethic and innovative ideas in practice.[2]

Many leaders are uncomfortable with this style of leadership because of the minimal control they have over the group. Participative leadership allows the leader more control over the final decision. After considering all the opinions of the group members, the leader makes the final decision on the basis of what is best to achieve the goal.

The Authoritarian Style

The leader with an **authoritarian** (also called *controlling, directive, autocratic*) style maintains strong control over all aspects of the group and its activities. Authoritarian leaders provide direction by giving orders that the group is expected to carry out without question. The final decision-making authority rests with the leader alone, although input from the group may be considered. Micromanagers closely monitor everything the group members do and often make on-the-spot changes when they believe they know a better way to achieve a task or goal. People who work under this style of leadership usually harbor hostile feelings that they are fearful to express, use passive-aggressive techniques to try to even the playing field, and feel oppressed and unable to use their full potential as a worker.

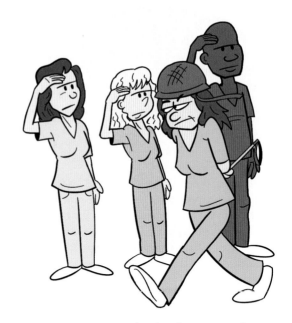

Authoritarian leadership can make staff members uneasy!

An extreme form of the authoritarian leadership style is dictatorial leadership. A leader using a dictatorial authoritarian style is called a *dictator*. This leader has no regard for the feelings and needs of the group members. Achieving the goal is the only thing that matters, and the dictator will use any means, including harsh criticism, to do so. A military mission to destroy a terrorist group by a Delta Force assault team is an example of this type of leadership.

What Do You Think?

Have you ever had to be a leader in a group? What type of leadership style did you use? How successful was the outcome of the group work?

Another type of authoritarian leadership style is the benevolent leader. The benevolent authoritarian leader uses a more paternalistic approach to achieving the goal. That leader attempts to include the group members' feelings and concerns in the final decision, but ultimately the leader makes all the decision. Some group members may feel that the benevolent leader is condescending and patronizing.

The authoritarian leadership style works best in emergency situations, when clear directions are required to save a life or prevent injury, or in situations in which it is necessary to organize a large group of individuals. Although highly efficient in achieving goals and completing tasks, authoritarian leadership suppresses the creativity of the group members and may reduce the long-term effectiveness of the group. Authoritarian leadership also reduces the motivation levels of the group and may lead to passive-aggressive behavior by the members that will further reduce the effectiveness of the group. Although some people can accept the need for the total control exerted by an authoritarian leader, most people in a long-term work relationship with this type of leader will become frustrated and even rebellious at some point. High turnover rates among the team members is almost always evident with this type of leadership.

In reality, few leaders use only one style. Most leaders use multiple leadership styles, depending on the situation. Many factors may influence what type of leadership style is used at any given time, including external regulations and requirements, the ability of the group members, the work setting, and the problem being solved. For example, a nurse manager on a hospital unit may use a highly democratic style in

most of the routine activities of the unit, but when a patient goes into cardiac arrest, she may revert to a highly authoritarian style while directing the staff through a code.

What Do You Think?

Think of the best leader you have ever worked with. What traits did that person have? Now think of the worst leader you ever worked with. What traits did that person have?

Many leadership/management theories, such as the trait theory, were developed during the Industrial Revolution to help understand how businesses worked and how leaders could make employees more productive. Most of these theories focused on ways to encourage or motivate workers who were poorly paid and often worked in substandard and dismal working conditions to be more productive. Over the years, these theories have been reworked and developed so that they are more congruent with the changes in the current work environment.

> *The old saying that "leaders are born, not made" implies that at birth a person either is a leader or is forever relegated to the rank of follower.*

Relationship–Task Orientation

One example of a more modern theory is the leadership contingency theory that was developed by Fred E. Fiedler, which posits that a leader's effectiveness is dependent on two primary elements: whether the leader is task-oriented or relationship-oriented (people-oriented).[3] Task-oriented leaders tend to focus on details, and they will not start to work on a project until they are sure they can complete it.

In contrast, relationship-oriented theories, also known as *transformational theories*, emphasize the networks formed between leaders and followers. Leaders who use this mode of leadership motivate and inspire workers by helping the group members see the importance and the positive aspects of the task. While these leaders are focused on the performance of group members, they also want each person to fulfill their potential. Leaders with this style often have high ethical and moral standards. Transformational or relationship-oriented leaders focus on creating trust and respect, and they pay attention to their employees' needs.[4] Relationship-oriented leaders will develop and work on a project as long as they have input from their workers.

The leadership-contingency theory rates leaders on whether they are oriented more toward establishing relationships or achieving assigned tasks and resolving problems, an orientation often dictated by the work setting.[3] Following are some combinations of types of leadership styles.

High Relationship–Low Task

Leaders with high relationship–low task orientations are usually well liked by their groups because of their acceptance of the group members as individuals, consideration of their feelings, encouragement, and promotion of a positive work atmosphere among all the group members. These leaders must still rely on direction, procedures, assigning responsibilities to the group, and producing high-quality work, but they pay more attention to each member's strengths, weaknesses, and professional goals, helping them achieve their full potential. They are available to staff and will counsel them when it is needed. Under a relationship-based leadership style, creativity is encouraged, good two-way communication is maintained, and teamwork is valued.[4]

The leader might also assign a specific task to one of the members who is wishing to gain more experience in a specific area of development, such as a new graduate who wants to learn how to draw arterial blood gases. A relationship-based approach fosters a more cooperative work environment where morale, efficiency, and engagement remain high. Loss of staff is not a problem because the workers enjoy greater job satisfaction.

Relationship-based leadership only becomes disadvantageous when relationship-building takes precedence over task completion. Leaders tend to become too involved with their worker's problems and issues and may sacrifice the achievement of the task when it conflicts with the feelings of the group. If the leader allows the group complete independence in decision-making with little direction as to the task at hand, the ultimate outcome will be goals that are not achieved and tasks which are not completed. Because relationship-oriented leaders place a higher value on quality of work than on volume of work, they may be inclined to procrastinate on a project rather than push

the members to complete it. The group members may view the leader as one of them rather than as a manager, and it may become difficult to correct the group members when discipline issues arise.

High Task–Low Relationship

The opposite extreme is the leader with a low relationship–high task orientation. This form of leadership is similar to the authoritarian style, where the leader does all the planning with little regard to the input or feelings of the group, gives orders, and expects them to be carried out without question.

Efficiency and job completion are the primary advantages of a task-oriented leadership approach. These leaders always hit their targets, get the job done quickly, and produce little waste of time and resources in the process. Task-oriented leaders focus almost solely on the steps they must take to achieve a particular goal. They tend to concentrate on numbers and keep tight control of all activities, allowing for little creativity. Task-oriented leaders are very hands-on in their approach to supervision, to the point of becoming micromanagers, which can be very annoying to the group members. These leaders see workers as more or less interchangeable and spend little time getting to know the strengths and weaknesses of their group members. All that is important is for the task to be done on time and for it to meet the expected standard. Once the desired procedure is developed, group members can be trained to perform that procedure, allowing leaders to delegate tasks and track progress easily. Various forms of punishment are used by task-oriented leaders, ranging from verbal put-downs to poor performance evaluations that are used to determine pay raises.

One of the primary disadvantages of task-oriented leadership is that it stifles creativity and does not allow group members to develop their skills or strengths. Instead of feeling like a valued member of a close-knit group, members often feel like a disposable cog in the machine that is chewing them up. The leader gets little or no feedback from the group, and all communication is one-way: from the top-down. This type of environment results in low morale and high turnover rates because workers find little satisfaction and lose interest in the job. If the group members become displeased with the working conditions, they may even resort to using passive-aggressive means to sabotage a project and, indirectly, sabotage the leader.

Low Relationship + Low Task Orientation = Worst Leader

The worst leader is the person with both low relationship and low task orientation. This leadership style simulates the laissez-faire style in which the leader is uninvolved, does no planning, has little concern for the group members' feelings, and accomplishes little. It tends to attract individuals who have low motivation levels and who are generally satisfied with the minimal effort they are putting out to accomplish low-quality results (i.e., lazy people). Turnover rates are usually high among team members who wish to develop their skills and increase their knowledge.

High Relationship + High Task Orientation = The Great Leader

It can be argued that perfect leaders do not exist, but great leaders certainly do. Most leaders use a combination of styles and adjust them to the circumstances. Again, think of the nurse manager who uses a high relationship–high task orientation for managing the unit in most day-to-day operations. In the cardiac arrest situation, this nurse manager may quickly change their orientation to one of low relationship–high task, guiding the team through the code until the crisis is resolved.

The best leader is the one with both high relationship and high task orientation. These leaders combine the best of both worlds: they are open to input and actively communicate with the group members, provide constructive direction, quickly resolve conflicts, and ultimately achieve creative and effective solutions to problems. In reality, a combination of both approaches is most effective, with each style being essential at varying stages of the project's development. If a leader focuses solely on tasks, the workers will likely demonstrate low morale. Conversely, focusing only on relationships can produce an atmosphere where little work is completed. The goal for an effective leader is to bring about an appropriate balance between the two leadership styles.

Because leadership usually depends on the situation in which it is used, the best leaders need to be able to apply different leadership styles as the requirements of the project develop and change.[3] For some projects, a combination of both task and relationship styles at the same time may be called for. Leaders must also be able to fine-tune their leadership styles based on the maturity, experience, knowledge, and needs of the team members and their own abilities. Task-oriented leadership can be used with success for jobs where little creativity is required, such as assembly-line or warehouse work. Relationship-oriented leadership works better in conditions where group members are highly educated and skilled and must often make their own decisions while accomplishing a task, such as patient problem-solving in health care. For example, in a psychiatric setting, relationships are key to successful treatment of the patient, and the tasks of self-realization and coping skills are achieved in the therapeutic relationship setting. On the other hand, in an immediate post-disaster environment, achieving the tasks of sorting victims into appropriate categories for treatment and keeping them alive takes precedence over strong interpersonal relationships.

The Mediocre Leader

Mediocre leaders are neither high nor low task nor high nor low relationship oriented. They attempt to walk the line between meeting the minimal tasks required to accomplish the goals of the project and minimally meeting the needs of their subordinates. Mediocre leaders attempt to maintain only enough morale to keep group members from leaving. They tend to attract mediocre group members who feel comfortable in an environment where minimal effort and just getting by are the only requirements. Neither the full requirements of the project nor the personal needs of the team are completely met. This leadership style produces average-quality work and acceptable but minimal satisfaction with workers. Unfortunately, most organizations leave leaders of this type in place because they do not rock the boat and they receive few complaints. Figure 10.1 is an adaptation of the Blake-Mouton managerial grid. It demonstrates 81 possible types of leadership style.

Although the behavior and trait theories remain popular, researchers have come to the conclusion that leadership is really a more complex process than either of those theories describe. The transformational theory, as described earlier, recognizes that multiple intangibles exist whenever people interact. Leadership characteristics such as sense of meaning, creativity, inspiration, and vision all are involved in creating a sense of mission that requires good interpersonal

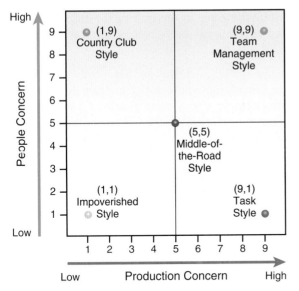

Figure 10.1 Leadership-task grid. Adapted from R. Blake, J. Mouton, *The Managerial Grid III: The Key to Leadership Excellence*, Houston, TX: Gulf Publishing Co., 1985.

relationships and rewards. Although this is true in most work settings, health care and nursing, in which care of human beings is the primary goal, require that nurses do something positive. In many health-care facilities, nursing leaders are expected to inspire excitement and commitment in nurses, who often must provide care to very ill patients in less-than-ideal circumstances.[2] This was no truer than during the COVID-19 pandemic.

More recently, the situational theory recognizes that no single approach works in all situations. Leaders need to acknowledge this and adjust their leadership style and behavior to the situation, considering the many variables that may be involved. Good leaders seem to do this instinctively, although it is a skill that can be learned. One of the key factors is the type of organization in which the group is located. The environment is always important in exercising any type of leadership. Situational leadership is a flexible leadership style designed to maximize employee potential while meeting preestablished deadlines or goals.[5]

In a situational leadership model, leadership style is matched to the group members' maturity and skill level in order to provide the most effective leadership. When matching a leadership style to a maturity or skill level, situational leaders evaluate the situation to adjust and adapt their leadership style to meet the needs of an individual or the group as a whole while keeping completion of the task in mind. This approach helps to preserve performance and produces the best results. As group members improve their knowledge and skills and gain confidence, leaders using the situational style of leadership adjust their style to thrive in the new environment.[5]

Situational leaders need to have the following leadership behaviors:

Flexibility: The linchpin of this leadership style is flexibility. Leaders must be able to consider and adjust their relationship and interactional style as the situation changes. They know there is no ideal recipe for each situation, so they monitor the environment and adjust accordingly.

Insight: Situational leaders must know the skills and knowledge levels of their group members. Insight also requires them to have a thorough understanding of the elements and complexity of the task or goals they are trying to achieve. Good assessment skills are a must for situational leaders to determine the best leadership approach that will help the group members develop and complete the task successfully.[6]

Coaching skills: When applied correctly, coaching skills help support the group members to find their own solution to a difficult problem they are confronting. It may also be an acknowledgment that the leader does not have all the answers. The situational leader as coach will monitor, support, and nurture the group as it moves through its various levels of development and maturity. The group members are motivated by the situational leader to increase their skill levels and knowledge and to succeed.[5]

Trust: See "Key Leadership Behaviors."
Problem-solving: See "Key Leadership Behaviors."

For example, if the situational leader assesses that a group member is inexperienced and has poor skills, then the leader will need to use a more directive or hands-on leadership style with that member. The group member can increase their skills through coaching from the leader and will eventually be able to take on more individual responsibilities. At some point, the team member will develop enough skills and knowledge to be able to handle some of the decision-making processes by themselves and will be delegated certain higher-level tasks. A good situational leader will adjust their leadership style according to the difficulty of the task and the skills and knowledge of the team. The ultimate goal is to build a consensus on the direction and methods the group should use to produce high-quality outcomes.[6]

KEY LEADERSHIP BEHAVIORS

Traits are characteristics that an individual possesses. Traits may or may not lead to the actions or behaviors that are required for successful leadership. It is also possible to lack leadership traits yet be able to carry out successful leadership behaviors.

Establish Trust and Cooperation Among Individuals and Groups. A trusting relationship is key to the success of a leader (or manager) on both individual and group levels. The followers must be able to trust the leader and each other.[3] Building that type of trust usually takes some time and involves individuals recognizing that the leader is honest, motivated, reliable, predictable, and consistent. Also, in the health-care setting, nurses tend to trust the individual who works hard and can perform all the required skills. Building trust and cooperation within the group can be very challenging. Effective situational leaders build relationships by compassion and support of group members. Good leaders allow the members of the group to be part of the decision-making process, which allows them to feel that the leader trusts them, thereby increasing their motivation to succeed.[6]

Personality is the sum total of a person's genetic composition and experiences. Because no two people have identical genes or experiences, each one has different needs, feelings, and orientations. Because of the many personalities and backgrounds a group brings to the work setting, they often have an inherent mistrust of those who are different from them. However, if they trust the leader, the leader can use this trust to build stable relationships within the group by recognizing the differences and directing people to their highest level of achievement.

> *The authoritarian leadership style works best in emergency situations, when clear directions are required to save a life or prevent injury, or in situations in which it is necessary to organize a large group of individuals.*

Acknowledge Good Work and Success. By providing rewards for the efforts that individuals make in achieving personal and organizational goals, the leader provides a powerful motivation for the nurse to continue working hard and being successful. These rewards do not have to be expensive or even cost anything at all. Positive verbal reinforcement is often more effective than a prize or gift. Saying, "You really did a good job taking care of that difficult patient today," or "I was impressed with how well you managed your time in taking care of those five patients," is often more of a reward than most nurses receive in a month. A birthday card or a thank-you card with a personal note is also very effective. At Christmastime, a little homemade gift and a card thanking them for all they do for the success of the unit is also very effective.

Show Respect for Individuals. Although there are some overlaps with trust and reward, showing respect for others has some key elements that are not always easy to master. Treat other people as you would want to be treated (the Golden Rule). If you want to be included in the group when they go to lunch, then include the other person. By treating others as you would want to be treated, you are acknowledging them and recognizing their needs. Be polite and courteous by saying *please*, *thank you*, and *you're welcome*. Our society seems to have adopted rudeness as its basic mode of response (see Chapter 16 for more detail). Demonstrating politeness can be contagious, and others will begin to return the courtesy. Do not make judgments about people before you really get to know them, which may take some time. People in unfamiliar situations, such as a new nurse on the unit, often respond by withdrawing from activities until they learn the routine and unwritten rules of their new surroundings. Later, they will be more open and more accepting. Show empathy and promote mutual respect. People who are respected by you will respect you in return and respect others. Never insult them or say negative things behind their backs.

Provide a Sense of Direction. Leaders need to demonstrate by their actions that they are working toward achieving goals at the personal, unit, and organizational levels. In providing a sense of direction for the group, leaders must be able to convey a vision of what can be achieved rather than how to just survive. Good communication skills are an essential element in conveying the vision to the group. Leaders must be able to show by word and deed what the vision is and why it is important for the advancement of the organization. Humans have an inborn drive to look toward the future and are attracted to individuals who have a vision of the next big thing coming down the road. Leaders who have an unwavering commitment to a greater purpose and a higher goal will attract and inspire followers to work for their goals.

Promote Higher Levels of Performance. Many factors go into promoting higher levels of performance, including rewards and motivation. One of the best ways to promote better performance is to provide individuals with more difficult challenges. Often, nurses become bored with their patient care not because it is not busy enough but because it has become routine. If leaders listen carefully to nurses, often they will discover that the nurses' desire for more challenges in a job is a fairly common concern. By providing the nurse with more challenging projects, the leader can increase that individual's performance. Also, the leader can be excited about a project and show a high level of enthusiasm in its completion. Excitement and enthusiasm are contagious and will motivate other nurses to escalate their performance.

Resolve Conflicts Successfully. The primary goal of **conflict resolution** is to facilitate a solution before matters get out of control. The main barrier to conflict resolution is that humans have a tendency to avoid overt confrontation because it makes them feel uncomfortable. The result of avoidance is that the unresolved issues continue to escalate to a point that they may no longer be resolvable. The simple solution for managing conflict between others is to encourage them to discuss the issue openly and honestly between themselves. They need to remember that everybody involved in the conflict has good intentions and truly believes they have the right answer. Leaders need to let people know up front how to go about conflict resolution. Leaders should never take sides, should never try to "solve" the conflict, and should bring the conflicting parties to the realization that it is their conflict and that they need to resolve it as professionals. (For more about conflict resolution, see Chapter 11.)

Foster Cooperation. An important goal of leadership is to foster a culture of cooperation and teamwork on the unit and in the facility. However, there is some degree of cooperation and competitiveness in every individual; few people are 100 percent cooperative or 100 percent competitive. The environment and culture of the workplace also help determine how cooperative an individual eventually becomes. If nurses who are usually cooperative find themselves in a highly competitive working environment, they are likely to become more competitive and less cooperative just to survive in the workplace. Building a culture of cooperation can be a long and difficult process, particularly when a hostile culture already exists. (See "Group Dynamics" later in the chapter.)

One key behavior that leaders can use to promote a cooperative culture is to spend more time with new employees.[2] Instead of giving the 10-minute "Hi! Nice to meet you. Here's the fifty-cent tour of the unit" introduction, leaders should sit down and talk with new employees. Ask them about their background, work habits, and competencies. Introduce them to at least six employees on the unit and have them ask their new colleagues about their backgrounds. By making this type of connection with at least six other nurses, new employees develop a sense of trust and establish essential working relationships.

> *The old question, "How do you know when you've arrived if you don't know where you are going?" is a truism that all leaders must address at some point by establishing clear goals and outcomes for the group.*

The connection also helps develop a cooperative mindset and encourages them to seek relationships beyond the initial group of six.

Reinforce Goals. The old question, "How do you know when you've arrived if you don't know where you are going?" is a truism that all leaders must address at some point by establishing clear goals and outcomes for the group. Groups who lack clear goals often feel frustrated and lost. Initially, leaders must clearly identify their goals and then continually reinforce the goals or establish new goals as the old ones are reached. Successful outcomes are a result of clear goal setting and continual reinforcement of the goals on the way to their achievement.

Develop Staff Strengths. The rapid changes and advancements in health care require nurses to continually learn and develop new skills. Through observation, a good leader can get to know what the strengths and areas for improvement are for each of the nurses on the unit. The leader can then make it known that there are learning opportunities available for those who are interested. If a nurse has a particular talent or ability or a desire to learn a new skill, the leader will support and nurture it. Another way of developing staff strengths is by cross-training a staff member with a particular strength with another staff member who may have a different strength. For example, a nurse in the ICU may be very strong in reading and interpreting electrocardiograms (ECGs) of patients but have difficulty with arterial blood gas interpretation. If paired with a nurse who can easily interpret blood gas results but is weak in ECG reading, both nurses will be able to mentor each other and improve their individual strengths. Actually, the mentoring process is very effective in developing strengths and overcoming weaknesses. The mentor can be another nurse or the nurse leader.

Lifelong learning is a goal that effective leaders seek not only for those whom they are leading but also for themselves. Leaders can function as teachers in certain settings, but a more effective means of encouraging others to continue to learn is to set a good example. It is important to recognize that learning takes place not only in a formal school-like setting but also in all those encounters and situations that affect attitudes, beliefs, and behavior.

Motivate Personnel. The ability to motivate is an essential skill for all levels of leadership. Unmotivated nurses merely go through the motions of nursing, producing low-quality care and dissatisfied patients. Motivating staff involves many of the actions discussed previously, including rewarding a job well done, showing respect, establishing reachable goals, and establishing a culture of trust and cooperation. In addition, nurse leaders can become examples of motivation by cheerfully and successfully completing their own duties and avoiding complaining and negative attitudes. Fostering pride in the achievements of the unit and the hospital as a whole can be an effective motivator. Some facilities have a "unit of the month" award system that rewards units that achieve high scores on patient satisfaction evaluations. Effective leaders also know that constantly berating or correcting other nurses for everything they do that is less than perfect quickly kills motivation and morale.[2] An overall atmosphere of encouragement and reward is a very powerful element in increased motivation.

KEY LEADERSHIP QUALITIES

No matter what style a leader favors, successful leaders have common qualities (Box 10.2):

Think Critically. The ability to think critically is a multistep process similar to the nursing process. Critical thinkers must be able to analyze data, organize and plan, and use creativity in the resolution of problems. Leaders must often make important decisions on the basis of incomplete data.

Box 10.2 Key Leadership Qualities

- Thinks critically
- Solves problems
- Has integrity
- Listens actively
- Communicates skillfully
- Is courageous
- Has ingenuity
- Demonstrates enthusiasm
- Communicates optimism
- Demonstrates perseverance
- Models well-roundedness
- Uses coping skills
- Has self-knowledge

Source: Adapted from S. Weiss, R.M. Tappen. (2019). *Essentials of Nursing Leadership and Management* (7th ed.). F.A. Davis.

Solve Problems. Being able to use the problem-solving process effectively is essential to successful leadership. Leaders in the health-care setting face problems that arise from many sources, including staffing and personnel, scheduling, and administrative, budget, and patient demands. A situational leader who supervises a group of people must be able to assess a situation or problem and quickly find a resolution. A leader with good problem-solving ability can identify when it is time to change leadership styles to complete the task.[5]

Display Integrity. For many years, nursing has been ranked as the most trusted and respected profession in the annual Gallup Poll of professions. One of the keys to this trust and respect is the integrity of the profession as it is perceived by patients and their families. The public expects nurses, as a group, to be honest, trustworthy, ethical, moral, and professional. The American Nurses Association (ANA) Code of Ethics for Nurses (see Chapter 6 for more details on the Code) is directed toward promoting and maintaining the integrity of the profession. If a group observes less than complete integrity in their leader, that person's ability to lead is markedly diminished.

Listen Actively. To be effective, leaders must be able to hear the words the person is saying, observe the body language, and interpret the underlying emotions and meaning. The experts tell us that only 7 percent of communication is verbal; 93 percent is all the other nonverbal content. Leaders often fail in their leadership roles when they do not listen to the full message of the individuals they are attempting to lead.

Communicate Skillfully. Communication is a complex process that involves an exchange of information and **feedback** (see Chapter 11 for more details on communication). Mistakes happen on both sides when the information being shared is incomplete or confusing. The best method to prevent this confusion is transparency in communication. Transparency in communication is the use of accurate, clear, and complete shared information between a sender and receiver without any filters. It requires open and honest communication that flows both ways between the leader and the followers. Transparency also mandates a level of accountability on both sides of the communication. The three key elements of transparent communication are complete disclosure of information, using clear and understandable presentation in

documents, and accurate data.[7] Transparent communication does not contain any **bias**, embellishment, or distorted facts. It limits the use of highly technical terminology, fine print, and complicated notations. The goal of transparent communication is to build a high level of trust between the leader and the team. Providing frequent and positive feedback is one of the best methods for leaders to determine how well they are communicating and how transparent the communication channels remain. It also can boost morale and improve the working environment. Effective leaders should also be able to give and use negative feedback to improve performance. If negative feedback is given in a nonthreatening and encouraging manner, those receiving it will often appreciate the chance to improve their skills.[7]

Be Courageous. Although all leaders must have the courage to maintain their convictions in the face of adversity, certain leadership positions may require a higher degree of courage. Nurses in middle management positions, such as unit managers, house supervisors, or quality control coordinators, often find themselves caught in a no-man's land between two opposing worlds. Often, staff nurses have the perception that nurse managers work for the administration.[3] For example, higher management may be attempting to implement a plan or procedure that the staff nurses strongly object to, or the staff nurses may be complaining about some issue, such as staffing, that the middle manager has little control over. The leader in this situation may need to risk offending one or the other of the groups to resolve a difficult problem.

Show Initiative. Effective leadership demands that the leader be a self-starter and have the ability to start projects without pressure from above. Often, the group relies on the leader to begin the process of completing a task or resolving a problem.

Be Energetic. *Energy* refers to the ability to do work and to display that energy in the form of enthusiasm for the work. Energy and enthusiasm are contagious. Charismatic leaders are the ones who are the most energetic and enthusiastic. The group needs to see that their leader is willing to work as hard as they are being asked to work. However, energy has to be rationed carefully to maintain the optimum levels. It is easy for a leader to burn out, particularly when the expenditure of energy seems to produce little or no tangible result.

Display Optimism. A positive attitude is also contagious. Conversely, so is a negative attitude, which often leads to discouragement and failure (Table 10.2). A leader who has an overall positive attitude and views new problems as opportunities for success will be much more successful than the leader who constantly complains about each new crisis.[8] Leaders who are optimistic give energy and attract other people who have energy. Energetic and dynamic leaders who have a positive outlook on the future will find that other people want to be around them. People are looking for leaders who radiate hope.[8]

Persevere to the End. Leaders need to be able to continue to work through difficult problems in difficult circumstances, even when others feel like quitting. Again, if the leader sets the example for the group with a "there's more than one way to skin a cat" attitude, the group will be encouraged to find new and creative solutions.

Develop Well-Roundedness. Leaders, as well as those they are leading, live multifaceted lives. It is important to develop and foster nonwork relationships with friends and family. Time at work should be balanced with recreational, spiritual, social, and cultural activities that complete the person and round out the personality. Time must also be invested in maintaining good health through proper nutrition and regular exercise, which will help prevent burnout (see Chapter 9 for more details).

Develop Coping Skills. All jobs have some degree of stress, although people in leadership positions often experience higher levels. Stress can be handled in two ways: unconsciously, through defense mechanisms, or consciously, by bringing learned coping skills into play. A more productive way to deal with stress is to use coping skills developed in dealing with past stressors to promote a positive and healthy resolution to the stress. Some people learn how to use the stress they experience to motivate them and to tap into the energy it generates to achieve a higher level of functioning.

Have Self-Knowledge. Leaders who do not know and understand themselves are less able to understand those who are working for them. Self-awareness is the beginning of self-acceptance as a thinking, feeling person who interacts with other thinking, feeling persons. Unless leaders understand and accept their motivations, biases, and perceptions, they will not be able to understand why they feel and react in certain ways to certain individuals and situations.[1]

FOLLOWERSHIP

It is obvious that leaders cannot practice leadership if they do not have any followers. Followers, much like leaders, exist in almost all social settings, both formal and informal, and not just in an organizational setting.

Followers

A follower can be viewed as a person who believes in the traditional social hierarchy of leaders and followers and then identifies as a follower in the structure. The concept of subordinate is similar except that it includes the idea of the follower having a title and a formal role in an organizational setting who reports to a supervisor or manager. Almost all leaders are also followers and subordinates at some point in their careers, often simultaneously. And many times, followers and subordinates can be leaders.

Followership can be looked at as a reciprocal, or shared, process of leadership. Followers must be willing to follow within a team and to accept their role in followership. A capable follower can help a new and inexperienced leader look good in the eyes of

Table 10.2	**Winner or Whiner—Which One Are You?**	
A Winner Says . . .	**A Whiner Says . . .**
We have a real challenge here.	This is a big problem.
I'll do my best.	Do I have to do this?
That's great!	That's nice, I guess.
We can do it.	It can't be done; it's impossible.
Yes.	Maybe, when I have some time.

Source: *Adapted from Holman, L. (1995). Eleven lessons in self-leadership: Insights for personal and professional success. Lexington, KY: Wyncom, 1995.*

higher management. As the leader learns new skills and becomes an effective leader, they can reciprocate the follower support and help them look and perform well. As the leader and followers all grow in experience and skill, the relationship grows more productive and life-affirming.[9]

Followers are not always obedient and compliant; they may also criticize and question their leader. When leaders neglect to evaluate and know who they are attempting to lead, they fail to recognize the powerful impact their followers have on their success in achieving organizational goals. Followers have a right to decide which leader they wish to follow and when they will follow. The trait approach discussed previously for leaders is also valid when considering followers (see Table 10.3).[9]

Individuals Versus Groups

Leadership viewed from the mind of the follower links the leader to the followers' perceptions of what a good leader should be and how and when to follow the directions of the leader. This perception varies from each individual and group.

When individuals look at the leader, they bring all of their experiences with past leaders into the evaluation. They base their perceptions on how well the current leader measures up to the "good leader" they experienced in the past, how the leader is managing the current situation, and what differentiates this leader from other leaders. A group brings a collection of past experiences and knowledge when considering a leader's abilities. They share their beliefs about leadership with each other and eventually negotiate a more or less unified perception of the leader's abilities.[9] If the group is cohesive in their belief that the leader is effective and has the qualities required to lead effectively, it is likely that the leader will have a high degree of success, even if one or two individuals in the group do not totally agree with the assessment. On the other hand, if the group decides the leader is not effective, the level of success will be greatly diminished.

Motivating followers is a major undertaking for any leader and is often the key to success. If followers form a positive relationship with their leader, they can potentially influence situations where they perceive the leader to be making a mistake or offer additional support if needed. They may also be able to improve circumstances for themselves and their coworkers.[9]

One method leaders can use is to understand how followers view themselves in the organizational structure. By evaluating how followers view the leader's abilities and skills and where they fit into the organization, leaders can better understand their own effectiveness. With this understanding, they can influence

Table 10.3   Types of Followers and Their Traits

Follower Type	Traits
Effective or independent	Think for themselves, are active, positive energy, independent problem-solvers, challenge the leader
Implementer	Get the job done; do not question authority
Partner or participant	Support leader but also question leader on key points
Die hard or activist	Deeply devoted to leaders or are ready to remove them from their position, willing to take risks
Survivors, pragmatics, detached, withdrawn, sheep, bystander, or passive	Wait-and-see strategy, adapt to change but do the minimum necessary to survive, do not know anything about their leaders, do not really care what the leader does, have no trust in the leader or organization, do not participate
Yes-person	Positive about leader; depends on leader for inspiration, thinking, directions, and project vision; highly supportive of leader
Individualist or alienated	Use negative energy to block leader, voice their views but do not necessarily support the leader, do not fit into the group
Impulsive	Constantly challenge authority and authority figures through rebellion, hate the status quo

Source: *D. Stanley, Followership, in* Clinical Leadership in Nursing and Healthcare: Values Into Action *(2nd ed., pp. 47–58), Hoboken, NJ: Wiley-Blackwell, 2017.*

followers to improve their self-image with the end result of increasing their motivation levels and their productivity.[9] If the followers believe they are important to the organization and their input is considered in making decisions, they will feel better about themselves and the work they are doing. As a result, they will tend to be more accepting of directions from the leader.

Although the term *follower* may have negative connotations such as inferiority, passivity, submissiveness, or laziness, in reality, followers have a great deal of power and influence over a leader's success. For followers to successfully exercise their followership role in an organization, they must avoid reinforcing the negative stereotypes associated with the term. Rather, they must take a constructive approach and view their roles as ones of co-leaders, partners, and equal participants.[9] The leader–follower relationship is an active and interpersonal process that challenges both sides to participate in better understanding their relationship to each other with an end goal of producing the best possible health-care outcomes.

MANAGEMENT

Nurses who continue employment at the same facility for any length of time will likely assume a management position at some point in their careers. These positions can range from middle management such as charge nurse or unit manager to higher-level positions such as shift supervisor or chief nursing officer. Although leadership skills are highly useful in these positions, the move to manager involves a new set of skills and behaviors that the nurse must master.[10] Sometimes the best leaders in an informal setting make terrible managers because they lack the basic management skills to fulfill the requirements of the role. Like all skills, management skills can be learned.

Unlike the study of leadership, which primarily focused on the leader, the early study of management was aimed toward influencing employees to be as productive as was humanly possible. Two schools of thought address and define management.

> " *Charismatic leaders are the ones who are the most energetic and enthusiastic. The group needs to see that the leader is willing to work as hard as they are being asked to work.* "

Time–Motion Theory

Time–motion theory developed out of the early industrial age, in which theorists concentrated on ways to complete a task most easily and efficiently. Often, their efforts resulted in increased productivity but decreased employee satisfaction. From this viewpoint, management can be defined as planning, organizing, commanding, coordinating, and controlling the work of any particular group of employees. In the time–motion approach, providing the right incentives, primarily money, is expected to increase employee productivity. Although the weaknesses of this approach make it less desirable in today's society, variations of it served as the harbingers of many of the business techniques currently in use in large organizations.

Human Interaction Theory

Early in the research into management, the limits of the time–motion approach became evident. Researchers observed that some lower-paid employee groups had higher levels of productivity than others with higher pay who were doing the same jobs. It appeared that factors such as employees' attitudes, fears, hopes, personal problems, social status in the group, and visions strongly influenced how they worked.[5] From this perspective, management can be defined as the ability to elicit from employees their commitment, loyalty, creativity, productivity, and continuous improvement.

Managers who favored the human interaction theory were required to develop a different set of management skills, including understanding human behavior, counseling effectively, boosting motivation, using efficient leadership skills, and maintaining productive communication. Just being a "nice guy" was not enough to guarantee employee cooperation and commitment. To be successful, management needed to be able to recognize and respond to employee concerns and needs, gain acceptance, and alleviate the pressures from higher administration.

It is also important to keep in mind that different management styles are necessary for different work settings. A predominantly time–motion approach may still work best in an area such as manufacturing of automobiles or washing machines. Using the same approach would be inappropriate and probably ineffective for managing a group of registered nurses (RNs) working in an ICU of a busy city hospital.

KEY BEHAVIORS OF THE NURSE MANAGER

Nurse managers often find themselves located on the organizational chart between employees and upper-level management. The functions and duties of

nurse managers depend to a great degree on how the institution defines the role. One of the first activities of a new nurse manager is to make sure they understand the job description, responsibilities, and level of authority the position has in the institution. Some of the key behaviors that have been identified as being a regular part of a nurse manager's position are listed in Figure 10.2.

In today's health-care system, nurse managers continue to move away from close supervision of the staff nurses' work to helping them complete their work safely and effectively.[10] As this role continues to

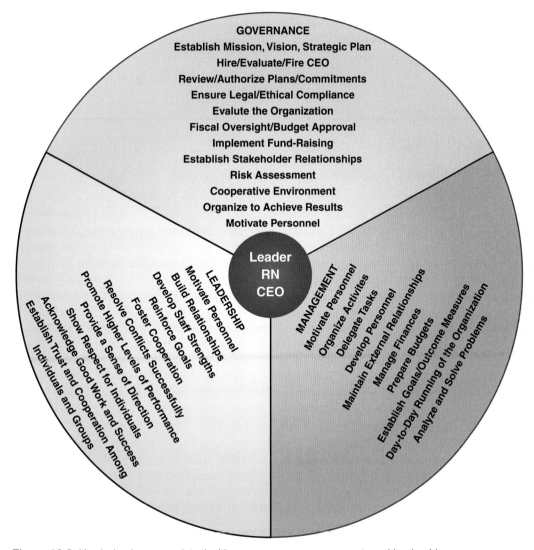

Figure 10.2 Key behaviors associated with governance, management, and leadership.

evolve, the emphasis will shift from traditional management functions to highly supportive functions, such as are seen in the leadership role.[9]

LEADERSHIP VERSUS MANAGEMENT

Several questions arise when people speak about leadership and management.

Are They the Same Thing?

Leadership can be exerted either formally or informally. Often, the most effective leaders in a group are not the ones who are officially designated as the leaders. On the other hand, managers are given the title by some higher authority and have formally designated authority to supervise a group of employees in the achievement of a task. Similarly, managers can be held formally responsible for the quality, quantity, and cost of the work that the supervised employees produce.[10]

Do Managers Need Good Leadership Skills?

The most effective managers will have highly developed leadership skills. However, by virtue of their title and position, even managers with poor leadership skills are still the official authority, although their effectiveness is reduced. Often, in groups in which the manager is not a good leader, unofficial or informal leaders emerge and exert either a strong positive or a negative influence on the group. If the informal leader is generally supportive of the manager's and administration's goals, the work group can be highly productive, and the organization's goals will be achieved. Conversely, if the informal leader's goals are opposed to those of the manager and administration, productivity may decrease to a point that higher-level management asks the manager to leave the position. Followership is as important for managers as it is for leaders.[10]

Issues in Practice

Leadership/Management Case Study

Resolving Staffing Issues

On a busy medical-surgical unit, a group of staff nurses were concerned about the process of making assignments. They believed that the usual practice of assigning nurses to a different group of patients each day eliminated any continuity of care, decreasing the quality of care and lowering morale among the staff. They agreed to meet with the nurse manager as a group to discuss ways of resolving the issues.

The meeting soon became confrontational. The staff nurses expressed a feeling of having very little autonomy in the selection of assignments. The nurse manager expressed the opinion that the nurses were being uncooperative and did not understand the problems involved in making patient assignments. She stated that her primary responsibility was to ensure provision of the best nursing care possible to all patients. The staff nurses countered that the current system was not meeting that objective as well as it might.

The staff nurses proposed a solution: after shift report, they would be allowed to select the patients they felt most qualified to care for, with the same patients reassigned to them on subsequent days until the patients were discharged. The initial response by the nurse manager was that it would be impossible to use this method in a fair and equitable manner. She also wondered what would happen if no one wanted to care for a very difficult patient and how continuity would be maintained on the nurses' days off.

Questions for Thought

1. How would nurse managers who use an authoritarian system of management resolve this issue?
2. How would nurse managers who use a laissez-faire system resolve this issue?
3. How would nurse managers who use a participative system resolve this issue?
4. What initial mistake did the nurse manager make in dealing with this problem?

(Answers are found at the end of the chapter.)

Are Good Leaders Always Good Managers?

A person who has leadership ability may not have good management skills. This phenomenon is seen in the nursing profession when a highly effective and skilled staff nurse who functions as the unofficial unit leader is taken out of that role and promoted to an official management position. Some do well; others may require additional training in management principles and skills. Some never quite master the skills needed for management.

Management and leadership skills complement each other.[10] A good manager will have mastered all the key behaviors listed above for a good leader.

Additional skills nurse managers are expected to master include staffing the unit for optimal coverage (see "Two Key Tasks of Managers"); developing a unit budget (see "Two Key Tasks of Managers"); recruitment of new staff; mentoring novice nurses; formally evaluating staff performance; developing new-nurse orientation; maintaining a safe work environment; and ensuring the facility's quality-of-care goals are met. In addition, nurse managers also serve as the representative of the staff nurses they supervise and sometimes are expected to dialog with the top management on behalf of these nurses. The day-to-day chores of a nurse manager may include maintaining an appropriate inventory of medical supplies and equipment, maintaining a positive work environment, and researching new evidence-based care practices that can be integrated into the staff's daily activities to improve the quality of patient care.[10]

As with all skills, nurse-management skills can be learned and require practice and experience to be developed fully. Even new graduate nurses can be effective leaders within their nursing roles. As they gain experience and develop new skills, their ability and opportunities to provide leadership will also increase. Learning and improving skills in one area will increase the abilities in the other.

GOVERNANCE IN THE HEALTH-CARE SETTING

Although nurses are usually not involved in high-level governance activities, there is a considerable amount of overlap among the skills involved in governance, management, and leadership. Governance is mentioned here briefly, although a more thorough discussion can be found in Bonus Chapter 30.

As with most complex concepts, there are several definitions of *governance* that often depend on the setting. Governance in the political setting has a different direction and set of expectations than governance in a nursing organization. Governance in large organizations is usually conducted by a board of directors; however, in smaller organizations, the governance role may fall to the chief executive officer (CEO) or president of the organization.[11] In the health-care delivery setting, *governance* can be defined as the process of decision making at the top levels of an organization that ensures that the organization achieves its goals and produces high-quality outcomes by defining expectations, delegating power to key personnel, and overseeing the administrative process.

The annual survey of hospital CEOs conducted in 2021 by the American College of Healthcare Executives (ACHE) to identify their three primary concerns showed that overwhelmingly the number one issue was personnel shortages. This concern was number one for the first time since 2004. Financial concerns were bumped to second place from being the number one concern for many years. Among personnel shortages, CEOs were most concerned with RNs, followed by technicians and therapists. The biggest financial concern was the increasing costs for staff, supplies, and general operation expenses. The concern that ranked third was patient safety and quality outcomes that affected reimbursement for medications and patient care costs.[11] Governance, a broader concept than management, involves making decisions at a higher level that

- Determines expectations.
- Grants power to individuals.
- Establishes performance standards.
- Maintains consistent management.
- Sets cohesive policies and processes.
- Provides organizational guidance.

Similar to leadership and management, certain key behaviors are associated with the exercise of governance. Figure 10.2 demonstrates the relationship of the key behaviors associated with governance, management, and leadership. As the behaviors move toward the middle of the wheel, they become more similar and have more overlap. A nurse who is an informal leader on a nursing unit may also engage in management and governance behaviors without knowing it. The circle of responsibility is a flexible structure, much like an elastic band, that can expand, contract, and move in any direction. For the nurse manager, the circle of responsibility completely surrounds the behaviors listed for management and many of the behaviors for leadership, but it also includes some of the governance behaviors. It is important to note that motivation is a key behavior for all three levels because if followers are not motivated, many of the other key behaviors become difficult, if not impossible, to achieve.

TWO KEY TASKS OF MANAGERS

The day-to-day running of the unit is one of the important tasks with which managers are charged. In addition to activities such as solving problems, developing personnel, and delegating tasks, managers need to master the skills of budget preparation and planning for staffing of the unit.

Budget Preparation

One of the tasks assigned to most nurse managers is creating budgets for their units, usually with a yearly budget that is then broken down into monthly budgets to better monitor the cash flow. The concept of a budget is rather simple. There are two key elements: income and expenses. The goal of creating a budget is to pay all the expenses while not exceeding the amount of income. For the nurse manager, a budget is a plan that helps control expenses and uses money in the most efficient and effective way possible.[12] Of course, this process becomes more complicated as the number of sources of income and number of expenses increase.

Although there are many different types of budgets, the one the nurse manager develops is generally referred to as an *operational* or *operating budget*. An operational budget helps the nurse manager manage the unit to produce the highest quality care in the most economical manner possible. It details the expenses for the usual maintenance and activities of the year. It is commonly a line-item budget where activities or items that require funding are listed line by line.

> *Often, in groups in which the manager is not a good leader, unofficial leaders emerge and exert either a strong positive or a negative influence on the group.*

Much like the patient care plan that all nurses are familiar with, the budget has similar elements: problem identification, use of standards, and projected outcomes. A well-developed budget keeps the individual unit—and by extension, the whole facility—out of financial jeopardy.[12]

Key Elements

In developing a successful budget, the nurse manager must keep in mind some key elements and principles. First, the budget should focus on the goals of the institution yet remain realistic. Limited resources are a reality of the current world of health care. Each item in a budget should be evaluated to see if it will achieve the objectives of the facility in the most economical manner.

Second, the nurse manager must always work within the historical context of past budgets. A budget serves as a predictor of future expenses, given that it is developed a year before it is actually implemented. By looking at past budgets, nurse managers can better identify areas where there were problems with expenditures.[14]

For example, past budgets may not have predicted the steep rise in costs for the replacement of essential equipment used by a unit when it breaks down. Future budgets must take this into consideration, or the budget will be inadequate for the expenses.

Third, all facilities use a standardized format for budgets. The nurse manager must become familiar with this format to increase the efficiency and quality of planning for the institution. Computer skills are required, as budget forms are all computerized on spreadsheets[14] and often contain charts and tables the nurse manager must learn how to manipulate.

Fourth, budgets are not static. Over the course of the time period when they are implemented, they must be evaluated and updated. Quite often, institutions have predetermined timeframes for evaluation, such as quarterly or semiannually.[13] The goal is to compare the projected budget with the actual expenditures. By doing this comparison, adjustments can be made in the budget to produce the best results.

Budget Types

Operational budgets can take several different forms. Two types of operational budgets include the fixed, or static, budget and the flexible budget. Most health-care institutions use the traditional fixed, or static, budget, which is intended to remain constant throughout the year, regardless of any changes to the organization's needs or operations. Producing a fixed budget is generally a less complicated process than creating a flexible one, and often the next year's budget is based on the past year's except for changes in the dollar amounts. However, a fixed budget has difficulty dealing with unexpected changes or unanticipated needs. Sometime managers try to build in a small "cushion" of extra money to try to compensate for probable cost increases.

On the other hand, a flexible budget is designed to change together with variables like patient volume, increases in labor costs, and unanticipated needs. The flexible budget is dynamic in nature, making it more complicated to produce than a fixed budget. However, its flexibility and adaptability are enormous advantages when considering the ever-fluctuating needs of health-care organizations.[13]

An incremental or historical budget takes the budget from the previous year and adds or deletes money from the various items listed. Also, new items may be added or old items that are no longer appropriate can be deleted. Most nurse managers work with this type of budget.

Performance-based budgeting is built on the belief that traditional methods of budgeting are too simple to account for all the variations in the budgeting process and cannot be adapted to ongoing changes. Performance-based budgets are totally outcome oriented and allocate resources to achieve certain organizational goals and objectives. For performance-based budgeting to succeed, well-defined key performance indicators must be developed prior to the process. Without the ability to measure outcomes, performance-based budgeting cannot succeed. Although the method has been tried in some health-care settings, defining performance indicators becomes very complicated, and most facilities have dropped this method of budgeting.[14]

Another type of budgeting that was popular for a time but is now rarely used is zero-based budgeting. Unlike the incremental budgets that use past experiences to predict the future, zero-based budgets require the nurse manager to start from the beginning each time a budget is created. In zero-based budgeting, there is no baseline sum that is automatically approved.[14] Rather, each expenditure item in the budget must be justified and approved each time the budget process is repeated. The nurse manager must adjust expenditures for each item either up or down according to the amount of funding available. Because the items in most unit budgets remain consistent over time, nurse managers who were required to use zero-based budgeting found that after the first year of time-consuming development of rationales for each item, they could reuse the rationales in the next year's budget, thereby turning it into an incremental budget with justifications.

It is important to note that each facility has its own particular type of budget requirements and forms. One of the steepest learning curves for nurse managers is the budgeting process.

> ❝ *One of the steepest learning curves for nurse managers is the budgeting process.* ❞

Required Skills

Although it is well beyond the scope of this text to provide a detailed presentation of the budgeting process, there are some skills that nursing students and nurses can learn to better prepare themselves for the nurse manager role as budget designer. These skills include the following:

- Learning basic budget and financial terminology
- Understanding the key elements of a budget
- Manipulating the data on the computerized budget spreadsheets
- Developing strong working relationships with the finance and billing departments
- Monitoring and analyzing the variables in the unit's budget[12]

Although nurse managers often approach the budget process with fear and dread, budget development is a skill that can be learned much like the clinical skills they already possess.

Through mastery of the budget process, nurse managers also develop the skills to be change agents for their organization and leaders to their staffs.

Planning for Staff Coverage

Another area of nursing management where there is a steep learning curve is planning for staffing of the unit. Somewhat like budgeting, the basic concepts behind staffing are deceptively simple: have enough people to meet the needs of patients and the goals and outcomes of the facility. Almost all nurses have up-close and personal experiences with staffing, usually when their units are short staffed or they are asked to work extra shifts because someone called out. New nurse managers soon learn that developing staffing plans is much more complex.

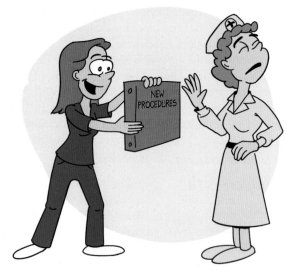

"I already know all those procedures."

Staffing is also highly dynamic and essential to the overall financial health of an organization. It affects almost every aspect of functioning in health care, including achieving institutional goals, ensuring quality of care and safety of patients, and delivering care goals.[14] The ANA recognized the importance of staffing a number of years ago. In 2005 and updated in 2012, it published the *ANA Principles of Staffing* as a guide for nurse managers in determining safe and efficient staffing levels. In 2019, it released another update to the *ANA Principles of Staffing*, but this one focuses on flexibility in staffing rather than on fixed ratios.[15] It has long been realized that nurse staffing is more than mere numbers and that other factors are relevant to staffing, such as "a nurse's level of experience, knowledge, education, and skillset, as well as patient-specific factors such as acuity and intensity."[15] The ANA's flexibility guidelines assert the position that nurse staffing must correctly match nurse qualifications and numbers to patient needs. Nurses should also have a role in staffing decisions, which would improve patient outcomes and quality of care and would increase nurse satisfaction with their work resulting in lower rates of nurse burnout, turnover, exhaustion, and mistakes.

Since the original publication of the ANA's document, there has been a tremendous increase in published literature about the effects of staffing on morbidity and **mortality**, medication and care errors, successful patient outcomes, and the effects of different types of staff on patient well-being. Although this body of literature has contributed substantially to the evidence-based practice databases, some nagging questions remain: How do you determine just the right number of staff? How can appropriate staffing be measured? How do you track staffing on a day-to-day basis?[15]

Staffing During a Pandemic

Even before the COVID-19 pandemic, health-care leaders recognized that there was a nursing shortage and that poor staffing levels would lead to poor quality of care and poor patient outcomes. The nursing shortage became particularly obvious during mass casualty events or extreme emergency situations such as tornadoes, earthquakes, bus accidents, or mass shootings. However, these events were generally short-lived, and hospital administrators could easily shuffle nursing staff around in their facilities or call in off-duty nurses for short periods of patient coverage. The nursing units with the greatest needs were identified and additional nurses supplied to them on a shift-by-shift basis.

The pandemic radically challenged health-care leaders' use of the usual methods of handling short staffing problems Not only were hospital leaders ill prepared for the pandemic and its large numbers of critically ill patients, but they also had to face new challenges that they had never seen before. More nurses than ever were calling out because of fear of contracting the virus. The pool of per-diem staff and/or traveling nurses, often used to fill in the staffing gap, dried up overnight. Training part-time staff used on less acute units was difficult to accomplish in a short period of time. Recruiting and hiring new staff came to a near standstill, and because of infection transmission rules, the only job interviews were done via remote online conferences. As ICUs became full and as critically ill patients were moved to other areas of the hospital, no department was immune from staffing shortages.

Actions Taken

One of the first actions taken to meet the nursing shortage in critical care areas was to halt all elective surgeries, thereby creating a pool of highly experienced nurses, often with critical care training, who could be moved to the critical care areas. This action also conserved precious personal protective equipment (PPE) that was in short supply at the beginning of the pandemic. Units that had patients who could be treated on an outpatient basis, such as oncology, moved patients out and moved their nurses to the critical care areas.[16] Many of these nurses were less than pleased with the relocation.

The next outreach was to retired nurses. Although many nurses hold off retiring until they are almost to the point of not being able to work, retired nurses represent a pool of nurses who have vast levels of experience. Early in the pandemic, nursing students were not allowed in acute care facilities due to fears of liability if they contracted the virus. Some hospitals recognized that senior-level students represented a group that had learned at least a minimal set of skills in their school and training programs. By working side by side with seasoned professionals, students would have a chance to hone their real-life nursing skills such as critical thinking, clinical judgment, team dynamics, and higher-level skills such as caring for patients on ventilators or cardiac monitors.[16]

> *Some hospitals recognized that senior-level students represented a group that had learned at least a minimal set of skills in their school and training programs.*

Preventing Pandemic Burnout

However, nurses who had been on the front line of the COVID-19 pandemic from its beginning, risking their own health and well-being to care for others, were starting to burn out and leave the profession at an alarming rate. A report from The Joint Commission (TJC) in 2021, based on a survey of 2,000 nurses, showed that fear of getting sick and of bringing the virus home remained the top worries for nurses. Facilities soon realized that new and creative methods were necessary if they were to maintain staffing levels during the pandemic.[16]

First, facilities needed to keep the highly skilled nurses they already had on staff. Although nurses were becoming physically exhausted, that was not the primary reason they gave for leaving the profession. Rather, as shown in TJC's report, the primary reasons were emotional and mental. Nurse leaders who were successful in keeping attrition rates lower were good at considering their team members' mental and emotional well-being. Providing occasions for staff self-care and showing appreciation for their hard and dangerous work became even more important in mitigating the constant stress of caring for critically sick patients who were likely to die anyway. One facility improved its staff's mental well-being by allowing them to use more PPE than the minimum needed, even during the PPE shortage. Staff were allowed to wear a new gown for each patient, change masks during the shift, and wear donated cloth hats from the community. These measures helped the staff feel more protected and lowered the levels of fear of contracting the virus.[16]

Another facility developed an emotional support team made up of clergy members and mental health professionals with whom staff could share their issues such as feeling anxious, overwhelmed, or depressed. Staff would be given time during their shifts to talk with the support team. Another facility set up a "respite area" in one of the waiting rooms with televisions, lounge chairs, and food. They also hired a health coach with whom the staff could schedule individual sessions. Appreciation efforts that leaders used include setting up a virtual appreciation board on the facility's computer system and hanging signs and balloons at the staff entrance to let the team know they were valued. Snacks and boxed lunches were provided by the facility's volunteer group and the community to show support for the nurses.[17]

Trust First

Other techniques that help in retaining staff include building trust between the hospital administration and the staff. This was true initially in the pandemic and remains true today. So much was initially unknown about the virus, except that it was highly contagious and killed people in large numbers. Hospitals were getting mixed messages from the Centers for Disease Control and Prevention (CDC) and the National Institutes of Health (NIH) about what measures should be taken to protect staff. That uncertainty was conveyed to the staff, resulting in the development of a high-level mistrust between staff and management. Employees need to trust that their facility is being transparent about the safety of where they are working.[16] To build trust, management needs to lead by example. Nurse managers who expect their team to come in and take care of critically ill patients had better be there too, giving advice and teaching inexperienced nurses.

Although flexibility in scheduling has always been a consideration in maintaining adequate staffing, during the pandemic it became a massive issue. With the closing of schools and day care centers, lack of childcare required flexibility in work schedules. Managers had to find a way to accommodate nurses' schedules, or the nurses would just not show up for work. Facilities with flexible scheduling kept their nurses on the floor when they were needed. Although management theory shows that money is not really a motivator (see "Motivational Theory"), some facilities offered bonus pay for staff working additional hours. For nurses who went from a two-income household to a single-income household, the option to work extra shifts was attractive. For management, these nurses closed temporary gaps in staffing shortages and were more cost effective than bringing in traveling nurses.[17]

The reality remains that things will never go back to the way they were before the pandemic. The measures leaders learned to use in managing staffing during the pandemic must become the new normal for their staffing issues in the future. Using creative strategies is the only way to retain staff and to recruit the highest-skilled nurses from nursing schools.

> *" Facilities with flexible scheduling kept their nurses on the floor when they were needed. "*

Nurses are problem solvers. Nurse managers must embrace the belief that there is a solution to every problem. Nurses showed resiliency during COVID-19 and have the ability to face any adversity in the future.[16]

The pandemic is not the only factor that is contributing to staffing shortages. There is a steep rise in the number of elderly patients seeking health care as the baby-boomer generation ages. Patients tend to be sicker yet are allowed shorter hospital stays than in the past, which decreases the time nurses have to educate their patients, which in turn leads to a higher number of readmissions. The national nursing shortage is having and will continue to have a profound effect on staffing issues—the U.S. Bureau of Labor Statistics predicts that more than 275,000 additional nurses are going to be needed from 2020 to 2030—a growth rate of approximately 9 percent. Other experts project there will be up to 800,000 vacant nursing positions by 2030.[18] With its emphasis on access to care, the Affordable Care Act (ACA) is projected to inject some 22 million newly insured patients into the health-care system between 2019 and 2024.[18] Well-educated RNs will be required to produce the high-quality outcomes required by the ACA.[17]

Is There a Perfect Staffing Ratio?

Although better patient safety, outcomes, and satisfaction have been shown when nurse-to-patient ratios have increased,[21] only California has actually passed nurse-to-patient ratio laws. Eight states—Connecticut, Illinois, Minnesota, Nevada, Ohio, Oregon, Texas, and Washington—have proposed legislation for hospitals and other agencies to enact if and when laws are passed.[19]

Research since the initiation of mandatory ratios has demonstrated mixed results in patient safety and improved care. Although there appear to be minimum ratios that increase safety and the quality of care in certain settings, the research has yet to show what the optimum ratios might be.[19] H.R. 5052 (115th): Safe Staffing for Nurse and Patient Safety Act of 2018 was introduced as a separate bill and did not receive a single vote in Congress. In 2022, nurse-to-patient ratio legislation was reintroduced by Senator Sherrod Brown (D-OH) and Representative Janice Schakowsky (D-IL) that would mandate minimum nurse-to-patient ratios at hospitals across the country. Although this legislation passed in the House of Representatives, it is currently stuck in the Senate and is unlikely to pass there. In addition, many nurse leaders do not believe that lawmakers should be mandating what health-care professionals should and should not be doing.[19] Inflexible mandated nurse-to-patient staffing ratios are an inert and an unproductive method of staffing that guarantees neither high-quality care nor nurses' satisfaction.

Nurse leaders have long realized that safe and effective staffing levels are built on a multifaceted set of factors such as unit type, patient acuity (how sick the patient is and how complicated the care), layout of the unit (how far the nurse must travel between patients), ancillary support (how many lesser trained personnel the RN has to work with), and the education and experience of the nurses. Using a one-size-fits-all approach to patient care, which is found in mandated nurse staffing ratios, takes the variables out of the equation and is generally used by higher management to set the ceiling on the number of nurses at any given time, even if more nurses are needed. Nurse managers and the nurses themselves are the best qualified to determine workable staffing levels to meet the needs of the patients on their units.[21]

The ANA asserts that a number of major problems must be solved before there can improved nurse-to-patient ratios:

- Eliminating the nursing shortage by building up a satisfactory supply of nurses and nursing students in the pipeline
- Eliminating toxic work environments through safety and empowerment
- Changing public policy to one that backs health-care outcomes and quality
- Changing state laws so that all nurses are able to practice at the top of their education and their licensure

What Is a Nurse Manager to Do?

What can new nurse managers do to better prepare themselves for the challenges they face in attempting to staff their units to deliver safe and high-quality care? Much like preparing for the budgeting process, learning the basic terminology, becoming familiar with the spreadsheets and technology, and understanding the principles of staffing will go a long way to prepare the nurse manager. The other important factor is to remember that those who are staffing the unit are real people, not just numbers to be filled in on a table. They have individual personalities, inflated or deflated egos, worries, families, personal problems, health problems, and financial needs. A considerable amount of a facility's resources is dedicated to hiring, developing, and retaining staff in such diverse areas as human resources, continuing education, legal consultants, and multiple layers of management.

> " *The other important factor is to remember that those who are staffing the unit are real people, not just numbers to be filled in on a table. They have individual personalities, inflated or deflated egos, worries, families, personal problems, health problems, and financial needs.* "

Although each facility will have variations in its staffing policies and procedures, the following basic human-relations skills will greatly aid the new nurse manager:

- Demonstrate leadership skills. Make a decision and stick with it unless it is proven to be incorrect. Then admit the mistake and make another, hopefully better, decision and stick with that one. Staff soon lose respect for a weak and indecisive leader and eventually will no longer follow.
- Interact with staff at work. Managers who are out on the floor observing and helping when an extra hand is needed are much more in tune with their staff's skills and abilities (and shortfalls). Staff tend to do a better job if they know the nurse manager is nearby.
- Do not interact with staff outside the work setting. The nurse manager is the person who makes the

hard decisions. Although everyone likes to be liked as a friend, being too friendly with staff decreases the manager's ability to lead. Staff can be very manipulative of friends who are also managers. Also, there is a tendency to develop a group of favorite nurses, which makes the ones who are not in the group feel left out.

• Secure social media privacy. Social media sites are great for sharing personal information with friends; however, if staff can access the manager's accounts, they are privy to image-altering information. Was that the nurse manager at the party dancing on the bar? The image does not engender respect.[2]

Maintaining optimal nurse-to-patient ratios is a task that nurse managers must face 24 hours a day, 7 days a week, 365 days a year. It never stops, it never gets easier, and it never goes away. Despite the challenges, nurse managers can master the skills required for safe staffing. They are not alone. The ANA and other organizations are working to develop safe staffing guidelines that nurse managers can use to meet staffing needs. It is essential that they know of these resources and can access them when dealing with facility administrators.

MOTIVATIONAL THEORY

Motivational theory can be defined as the ability to influence the choices people make among a number of possible choices open to them or to produce one behavior out of a choice of several. It encompasses the biological, emotional, social, and intellectual forces that stimulate behavior. Motivation is the *why* or driving force behind human behavior.[22]

Psychologists recognize two basic types of motivation: intrinsic and extrinsic. Intrinsic motivation drives choice due to internal rewards; that is, the motivation to make the choice comes from within the person because it produces some feeling that is naturally fulfilling to the person. Extrinsic motivation is the offering or application of some reward or punishment that the person will either choose or avoid.[22] For example, what factors would motivate a new graduate nurse to work at one hospital when there are four facilities offering them a job? External motivators might include that pay and benefits are better in one facility than another. Maybe one facility is closer to home and requires less driving. Perhaps the shifts are better, and the

facility does not require mandatory overtime. Internal motivators might include that the new graduate knows people who are already working there and would feel more comfortable working near them. Perhaps the graduate's grandmother and mother worked at the facility, and the graduate would like to continue the legacy.

Motivation can be broken down into three elements:

Initiation includes making the choice to start a behavior—for example, a new graduate beginning a new job at a hospital.

Perseverance refers to exerting the continual energy required to achieve the behavior even if there are obstacles to overcome. To continue the preceding example, the unit the graduate is assigned to is consistently short staffed, and the patient load per nurse is high.

Strength is shown in the intensity and determination that the person puts into making the behavior successful over time. Despite the work atmosphere being difficult, the new graduate remains on the unit and works toward changing the environment to one that is more satisfying.[22]

Several theorists have attempted to explain the motivational phenomenon. Probably the best known is Abraham Maslow, who developed the hierarchy of needs theory. (For more information on Maslow's theory, see Chapter 12.) Although nursing students are taught and use this theory to deal with patient needs, the theory also has applications in the realm of leadership and management. Maslow believed that human needs are arranged in a hierarchy from the most basic and essential to the more complex. Most basic are the physiological and safety needs, and until these are met in at least a satisfactory fashion, the person is less likely to deal with the higher needs such as social relationships, self-esteem, and self-actualization.[2]

For example, if a nurse is not being paid a salary that meets the needs for food, housing, and clothing, those needs, rather than delivering high-quality patient care, become the nurse's primary concern. Realistically, needs are never fully met, but they have to be accommodated to a degree to which the person feels comfortable enough to move up in the levels of the needs hierarchy.

Motivation–Hygiene Theory

Another theory that has become popular is Herzberg's motivation–hygiene theory. Although there are some similarities between Maslow's and Herzberg's theories, particularly in their applications, Herzberg believes that people have two different categories of needs that are fundamentally different from each other.[2]

Hygiene Factors

The first category is referred to as *needs dissatisfiers*, or hygiene factors. According to Herzberg, if these needs are not met, the person feels dissatisfied with their job and focuses more on the environment than the work that is supposed to be performed. Hygiene factors are related to the work environment and include, for example, salary and benefits, job security, status in the organization, work conditions, policies, and relationships with coworkers.[2]

Hygiene factors are also related to the conditions under which the work is performed and not to the work itself. They only serve as negative motivators—when they are not met, work productivity is reduced. However, if they are satisfied, there is no guarantee that increased productivity and higher-quality performance will result.

> *Hygiene factors are also related to the conditions under which the work is performed and not to the work itself. They only serve as negative motivators— when they are not met, work productivity is reduced.*

Needs Motivators

The second category of needs, according to Herzberg, is called *satisfiers*, or needs motivators. Unlike the hygiene factors, satisfiers focus primarily on the work. Some of the more important satisfiers that have been identified include elements that expand the work challenges and scope, such as career advancement, increased responsibility, recognition for achievements, and opportunities for professional growth. The satisfiers can have both a positive and a negative motivational impact. If they are satisfied, they can encourage workers to increase their productivity and deliver higher-quality work. If they are not satisfied, they often have the opposite effect.

Motivation in the Hospital Setting

Herzberg concludes that employers must satisfy the hygiene factors as a minimum requirement before there can be any increase in productivity. In reality, most of the motivators used by hospitals and other health-care entities, such as reinforcements or punishments, are extrinsic in nature. Although these types of motivators do work in most settings, the true goal of a highly competent nurse manager is to also have intrinsic motivation among workers. Behaviors that intrinsically motivate come with their own rewards, which create positive emotions within the individual. When people participate in an activity for its own sake rather than to receive external reward or avoid some external punishment, they are demonstrating intrinsic motivation.[22] These nurses will attempt to do their best in caring for patients because they are using their skills and knowledge, thereby increasing their self-actualization and fulfillment.

Nurse managers can use several methods to help increase intrinsic motivation:

Challenging workers: Achieving uncertain and sometimes difficult goals with some personal meaning increases self-esteem and provides the nurse with performance feedback.

Allowing workers control: Generally, nurses do not have much control over their working environment. When they are allowed, even to a small degree, to have some input into what they are doing, it gives them a sense that they are doing what they want to do.

Cooperating with others: A sense of satisfaction occurs when a nurse helps another nurse in performing a difficult task or accomplishing a goal. Allowing nurses to work in teams increases this intrinsic motivation.

Competition with others: Intrinsic motivation can be increased in situations where the nurse can compare their performance to that of others. The nurse manager needs to be cautious and use competition minimally because too much competition can create a toxic work environment and sabotage trust.

Activating curiosity: When something in the work environment catches the nurse's attention or when some skill makes the nurse want to learn more, internal motivation is increased. This is why programs to promote job enrichment are often effective in upgrading the achievements, roles, and satisfaction of employees.

Recognizing achievements: All people appreciate having their accomplishments recognized by others, particularly by their managers. Recognition provides them with a sense of meaning, progress, and competence when they have done something new, which is the very definition of intrinsic motivation. Reading thank-you cards from appreciative patients to the group during report can also create a team sense of intrinsic motivation.[23] The use of this type of positive reinforcement cannot be underestimated. Even small appreciative gestures go a long way in helping staff feel that the job they are doing is appreciated.

Using Both

The best managers use a combination of intrinsic and extrinsic motivation, avoiding the punishment element at all costs. A good example of this combined motivation strategy in the hospital setting is the career or **clinical ladder** program. These programs allow nurses to advance in the profession without having to move into management positions for which they are unprepared. Clinical ladder programs provide nurses with the recognition for achievement and the opportunity for advancement (intrinsic motivators), along with the chance to advance in their knowledge and skills coupled with a promotion that supplies a financial reward (extrinsic motivators). It also allows them to remain in direct patient care, which is actually a combination of both extrinsic and intrinsic motivators.

Motivation During the Pandemic

Maintaining motivation in nursing teams on any given "busy" day is a difficult task. Motivating them when every day is chaos that pushes them to their limits seems insurmountable. Facing the pandemic, nurse leaders were challenged with the reality of overcrowded units, shortages of PPE, anxious staff, and continually changing information on how to contain the disease.

Initial methods used by nurse leaders to motivate during COVID-19 included extrinsic measures such as providing meals for nurses who could not leave the floor to eat, snacks on the unit to maintain energy during long shifts, and coffee in large volumes, which is many nurses' drug of choice. Many facilities offered monetary bonuses for nurses who worked extra shifts, allowed flexibility in shift times to accommodate childcare, and set up Go Fund Me accounts for health-care workers.[23] However, as discussed earlier, extrinsic motivators only go so far and are what Herzberg refers to as hygiene factors.

During the pandemic, health-care staff were experiencing new pressures that resulted in intense emotions and anxiety. Good leaders soon recognized that extrinsic motivators were not going to stop feelings of distress, loneliness, and fear.[24] They quickly recognized that intrinsic motivators were the key to maintaining staff morale. Although risk of becoming ill when providing care was not new to any nurses, when fellow staff members became ill from the virus and were quarantined, making the staffing shortage worse, they became acutely aware of just how risky the disease could be. Nurses working in critical care areas were accustomed to having a few "wins" whenever they managed to get an acutely ill patient past their illness and keep them alive. However, no matter how much care they were given, almost all patients who were critically ill with COVID-19 virus died.

One of the first actions a nurse leader or manager can take to support motivation is to have a positive attitude themselves *at all times*.[23] A positive attitude is not something that a person can turn on for work and then turn off when at home. Rather, it is—or should be—a permanent part of the personality. The leader should expect negative comments and attitudes from the staff. They will express multiple complaints and an overwhelming sense of fear, anxiety, and other emotions.[24] Staff should be allowed the time to be honest and express whatever they are feeling. The leader's response is to politely listen. However, the leader's role is not to commiserate with staff nor to minimize their feelings, but to acknowledge the emotions the staff members are experiencing and that it is acceptable to express them (see Chapter 11). A good leader will acknowledge that they, the leader, may not have all the answers to staff member's questions but that the leader does have the ability to confidently tackle every single issue. The leader might even let staff know that they have the same feelings, too, and talk about how to handle them.

Another important intrinsic motivator is to let staff know that they are not alone in caring for these patients. The leader must show their staff that they too are ready to work by wearing their scrubs, answering call bells, helping staff move patients, and in general making themselves present to the staff at key times.[23]

Trapped

Because of the highly contagious nature of the virus, nurses who were completely covered in PPE were often literally trapped in a small ICU room with the door closed tightly, a patient on the verge of dying, and any number of monitors and machines that were constantly beeping and making other alarm noises. Many nurses experienced isolation almost to the point of sensory deprivation. Early in the pandemic, because of the shortage of PPE, these health-care providers had to spend hours at a time in that setting.[24] Good nurse leaders monitored these nurses closely, and when they showed signs of problems such as dizziness, excessive perspiration, loss of coordination, or sensitivity to light, the leaders removed them immediately from that environment. Providing a calm, dimly lit, quiet space with a relaxing chair provided a relief from their sense of isolation. As PPE became less scarce, limiting shut-in time to 1 hour became the norm. Providing radio headsets to nurses so that they could communicate with staff and managers outside the room also lessened the sense of isolation.[24]

Providing positive feedback and recognition for difficult skills that are mastered is one of the best intrinsic motivators. Positive feedback in the form celebrating accomplishments both big and small should be used as much as possible. This was demonstrated in some facilities when patients who had been on a ventilator for months survived and finally left the hospital. The nurse manager needs to let staff know

that they are doing incredible work. Recognition can be done in person, by email or messages to their phones, or through bulletin boards.[23] Whatever its form, recognition must be appropriate and sincere; otherwise, it rings hollow and sounds contrived. Including staff (see "Participation in the Change Process") in unit-based decisions is also an intrinsic motivator.

Following is a list that can be used at the end of the shift or at home to lower the tensions that have developed during the shift.

I. Before you leave the floor, check to make sure your coworkers are doing okay and that none of them needs additional help in completing their assignments.

II. When you get home:
- Review in your mind the day that you had—but don't obsess over it.
- Identify the one situation that was most troubling during the shift, and let it go.
- Think about at least three things that went well during the shift.
- Perform deep-breathing exercises for several minutes.
- Obtain your drink of choice, sit back in a cozy chair, put up your feet, and relax and revitalize.[23]

> " *Providing a calm, dimly lit, quiet space with a relaxing chair provided a relief from their sense of isolation.* "

It is important for RN leaders, even those who are not in a designated management role, to understand and be able to use motivation techniques at any time in any situation. The ability to motivate is one of the keys to success in leadership at any level, and the success of RNs is often assessed by the job performance of people on the health-care team they are supervising. Successful motivation is the door to successful leadership because the people who can motivate others are the people who can make things happen in an organization.[22]

MAKING CHANGES SUCCESSFULLY

The goal of education and growth is always to produce change in the individual. Motivating people to change is one of the most challenging and most important functions of leadership. Simply stated, *change* is the process of transforming, altering, or becoming different from what was before.[25] It is important to remember that change is an ongoing process and does not occur all at once. Although the COVID-19 pandemic may have seemed to prove this theory wrong, in general, it is impossible to produce successful major changes in one step. If the change is broken down into smaller elements and enacted over time, it has a better chance of being successful. Even changes that were required by the onslaught of critically ill patients during the pandemic took almost a full year to be successfully integrated and adopted. And challenges from the pandemic remain that will require more changes.[26]

The process of change can seem daunting, and many people find change hard to accept. Although change is a constant in health care and nursing, it is surprising how resistant nurses can be to even minor changes in their work environment. On the other hand, many nurses accept change as a positive development and become drivers of change.[27] Change can produce many emotions, ranging from excitement

and anticipation to stress, fear, and anxiety. How people deal with change can affect how they respond to the environment and communicate with others. At minimum, change makes most people feel uncomfortable. Any change can be simultaneously positive and negative. During the process of learning new skills, treatments, or techniques, most people feel a sense of accomplishment at the same time that they feel afraid of making mistakes, being judged by others, or being labeled as slow learners.

Fear of the Unknown

Imagine a new graduate nurse starting their first day at work, very excited about the new experience and the potential for career development. However, at the same time, the nurse is worried about being accepted into the group, being able to practice what was learned in nursing school, and being able to learn the new skills required by the unit. Almost everyone has a sense of dread when moving away from activities with which they are comfortable. Setting realistic personal goals and timelines for learning new information helps reduce fear and stress when making major changes.[27]

The Need to Take Risks

Change can have both positive and negative effects. Often, staff will initially resist change and fight to prevent it, but once they go through the process, they would never go back to the old way of doing things. All change involves some risk taking, and some people are better than others at risk taking.

Internal or External Forces?

Two primary forces bring about change: external forces that originate from outside the person or organization and internal forces that start from within the individual or organization. A prime example of external change is what happens when government agencies pass down new rules and regulations that affect the delivery of health care. One example is when the CDC or NIH required certain types of PPE to be worn during the COVID-19 pandemic. An example of internal change would be a hospital increasing salaries or requiring mandatory overtime from a group of nurses.[25]

Successful Change

Successful change rests on the manager's ability to include three key variabilities that have a major

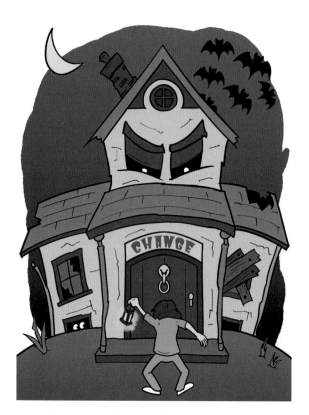

Change is always a little frightening!

Issues in Practice

Succeeding in Making Changes
Consider the following case study:

After analyzing the needs of the patients and the nursing workload of a busy medical unit, the unit manager decided to change the work shift times. In addition to the standard 7 a.m. to 3 p.m., 3 p.m. to 11 p.m., and 11 p.m. to 7 a.m. shifts, she decided to add a 5 a.m. to 1 p.m. shift to increase coverage during the busiest period of the shift. The RN assigned to the new shift recognized the benefits to the unit and to patients; thus, she accepted and supported the change with few objections. Also, the change in shift times allowed her to alter her personal schedule so that she could take extra courses toward her master's degree at a local college. For the RN, the change in shifts was a positive experience.

However, the licensed practical nurse (LPN) assigned to this new shift was upset with the change. She was a late sleeper and did not want to come in so early. She liked the shifts the way they were and did not see any advantages to changing them.

After the new shift was initiated, the LPN was usually 15 to 30 minutes late, called in sick frequently, and was grumpy and hard to talk to when she did come in to work. For this LPN, the change was negative and unacceptable.

influence the effectiveness of change: being prepared for change, participating in the change process, and recognizing the benefits of the change.[27] These three elements are interrelated and dependent on each other, much like the metaphor of the three-legged stool. Take away one of the legs, and it falls down. For example, the nurse manager may have done an excellent job planning for change and involving the team in the process, but if the change itself does not benefit the team or patients, its likelihood for success is minimal.

Being Prepared for Change
Change can be planned or unplanned. Planned change, sometimes called *anticipatory* or *developmental change*, is more productive and occurs when there is a directed and designed implementation of a particular set of predetermined steps that complete a goal.[27] Because planned change is premeditated and chosen consciously, it is not as threatening or intimidating as unplanned changed. When changes are clearly communicated before they are implemented, it allows for preparation of the team and greatly increases the success rate for changes.[28] Change can affect all

aspects of an organization, including policies, goals, organizational philosophy, work environment, and even physical structures. Planned change can be used for all sorts of projects, ranging from the minor to the most complex. Some examples include the introduction of new employee health-care benefits, changes in the incentive system, new equipment and technologies, new guidelines to improve team communication, and requirements to advance the team's technical proficiency.

When planning for change, the speed at which the intended change takes place factors into its success. In general, a relatively measured rate of change works best because it allows all members of the team to prepare for each aspect of the change and participate in it. A too-rapid rate of change can overwhelm team members so that they are unable to keep up with it, resulting in confusion and increased anxiety levels. This problem was common in the early stages of the COVID-19 pandemic when health-care personnel were required to change some aspect of their care environment each day.[25] Health-care professionals do not do well with changes that are executed suddenly and without prior communication. It makes them feel powerless and uninformed. On the other hand, change that is too slow and drags on over an extended period of time may cause the team to lose interest and even revert back to pre-change behaviors. Similarly, postponing the date for the change can drain team energy and lead to disappointment.[27]

Planned change works best when it is well organized, proceeds at a steady pace, and has a definite date for achievement. There is a level of excitement that raises energy levels when a change is near completion.

Unplanned change, sometimes called *reactive change* or *happened change*, occurs when a sudden problem or emergency forces the team or organization to respond to a situation for which they were unprepared.[28] Unplanned change is generally due to outside factors that put stress on the facility. These changes can be minor, but sometimes they can involve projects that are large in scope and highly complex. The responses by hospitals to the large numbers of COVID-19 patients is a prime example of unplanned change. Other examples include changes in staffing because of nurses who call in sick, patients who experience cardiac arrest, major disasters, or even equipment failures, such as when the electricity fails or a water main breaks.

Participation in the Change Process

Changes that originate from those who work in the health-care environment themselves have the highest rates of success and seldom meet with resistance from the health-care team. These types of changes are sometimes called *bottom-up* changes and are often the source of the most useful ideas. Health-care professionals are the most educated about what they do on a daily basis, which places them in the best position to recognize relevant difficulties and begin working toward their resolution.[27] That is why it is important that management listen and respond to the ideas presented by the team members. Open communication at all times is the key to success.

For changes that originate at the management level to succeed, the team must be involved from the start.

Being part of the change process early on and being involved throughout the process reduce the team's fear of the unknown, their anxiety, and their suspicion, thereby boosting the chance of success.[28]

Although active participation by the team throughout the process enhances success, there are some factors that can produce difficulties. One of the most common is the inability to communicate with the hierarchy of management. In large hospital systems, the top management is generally not in the facility and may even be a long distance away. Most staff-level employees do not have open channels of communication to top management levels. Generally, the unit's nurse manager or perhaps a shift supervisor are the team's only spokesperson who can go to periodic management-level meetings to express concerns.

Another element that reduces the chances of successful change is when changes are initiated by high-level administrators who are financial controllers or economists.[28] These administrators tend to evaluate the health-care system from only the financial aspect. They lack knowledge about the actual care that the floor-level staff provide. Changes initiated by the "bean counters" tend to be related to reductions in supplies or staff, which generally make staff angry. For example, requiring the reuse of PPE during the pandemic was a definite way to save on the costs of equipment, but it was seen by nurses and other health-care workers as crude and unacceptable.[25] The most successful health-care organizations have found ways to open channels of communication between staff-level employees and top management.

Recognizing the Benefits of the Change

When changes benefit neither the staff nor the patients they care for, the changes can appear meaningless and unwarranted. The team will resist changes that they do not understand, that are not coherent or based on sound causal thinking, or that seem to have no good purpose.[28] The team needs to believe that any attempted change has real value to them or

> **❝ Being part of the change process early on and being involved throughout the process reduce the team's fear of the unknown, their anxiety, and their suspicion, thereby boosting the chance of success. ❞**

their patients (or both) and that it will ultimately be beneficial for everyone. Changes should not be initiated because some top manager has decided they would like to see it made. Motivation for change is increased when health-care professionals perceive that the change focuses on and displays benefits for the patient.[27] Changes have a higher degree of completion if the team considers them to be well thought out. It is also important that managers are active participants in the change process and are respected by their employees.

A Driving Force for Change

Nurses often take on the role of the change agent—that is, the one who brings about the change (Box 10.3). All change requires the ability to overcome resistance to change (called *restraining forces*) by a driving force that pushes toward change. When the driving and restraining forces are equal, no change occurs, and the status quo is maintained.

Change can occur only when the driving force is greater than the resisting force.[9] Those who want to change have a tendency to push, but those who are being asked to change tend to push back to maintain things as they are. It is important when attempting to implement change to identify the restraining forces and ways to overcome them. Habit, comfort, chaos, and inertia are the four most common restraining forces pushing back on the forward movement of change.

As demonstrated by the COVID-19 pandemic, disorder and chaos have become permanent elements in workspace change. Nurse leaders who fear chaos and work to untangle its threads are, in reality, restraining change.[29] Good nurse leaders realize that growth and advancement are about building new care structures, and often new structures ascend from chaotic beginning. Nurse leaders in today's health-care systems are focused on excellence in care and good outcomes instead of the process of change itself and task completion. By adjusting to the chaos of change in the work setting, the nurse leader produces a framework for converting from a pre-pandemic process focus to a post-pandemic acceptance of the intricacy of change.[29]

Incrementalism is the process of making change a little at a time. It is characterized by gradualism in which there is no substantial departure from a previous policy. This process is easier to get workers to follow because it produces no substantial change.[28] The successful nurse leader needs to be able to identify when incremental types of changes are being proposed and to fight to prevent them, focusing instead on real changes that maintain quality patient care. The nurse leader as the agent of change is able to broaden their understanding to one that is interdisciplinary and more inclusive, to view the patient as a complete population, and to be focused on the full continuum of life, envisioning the increasing need for care of patients with chronic diseases.[29] Only in this way can the nurse leader foster accountability and multidisciplinary cooperation and model new behaviors in a chaotic and ever-changing work environment.

GROUP DYNAMICS

All successful leaders and managers understand and are able to use the principles of group dynamics. A group exists when three or more people interact and are held together by a common bond or interests.

The power of the group over an individual's behavior should never be underestimated. Groups establish and exert their power through a set of unique behaviors or norms that their members are expected to follow.[30] These norms may be formal or informal, written or unwritten, promulgated or merely understood. Unfortunately, in most nursing units, the norms are often not clearly expressed, yet they may be used as judgment tools or standards for evaluating work behaviors. When new nurses begin work on a particular unit, they must quickly learn the unwritten

---

Box 10.3 Characteristics of an Effective Change Agent

- Is well organized
- Identifies restraining forces
- Is able to motivate
- Demonstrates and maintains commitment to change
- Develops trusting relationships
- Responds to feedback and negotiation
- Is goal directed
- Communicates well
- Maintains optimistic attitude

unit norms and identify the informal leaders to function effectively.

A Common Goal

Groups are open systems that interact with the environment to achieve a goal. The individuals who make up the group are its subsystems and interact with each other and with the environment. Group dynamics provide the principles that underlie team building, which is essential to the success of nursing units. Establishing and sharing common goals is the starting point for successful team building.

When the common goal is to help one another, effective team building results. Members of the team respond most positively when they feel included in the decision making and when they realize that their input is valued by the other team members.[30] It is important that the leader always ask team members for their ideas about the goal that the team is working toward. A strong team spirit is crucial to the success of the team.

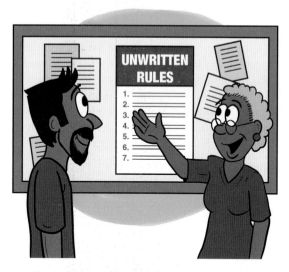

Unwritten rules can be more powerful than the policy and procedure manual.

Unwritten Rules

As with most elements in leading successfully, group dynamics may be positive or negative. Nurses who do not learn and who fail to display the expected group behaviors may be ostracized from the group, thus making the work environment psychologically uncomfortable and perhaps even physically difficult.[31] For example, nonconforming nurses may find that there is no one around when they need help ambulating an unsteady patient. A particular nursing unit staff may have a strong team approach. If a new nurse is highly independent and prefers to work alone, they may not fit in and may experience hostility or sarcasm from the other nurses on the unit.

Going Against the Group

Consider the following scenario demonstrating group dynamics:

The ICU is responsible for on-call coverage in the recovery room for unscheduled postoperative patients on the evening shifts, night shifts, and all of the weekend shifts. There is no formal written policy, but coverage has traditionally been handled on a voluntary, rotating basis.

Because coverage is voluntary, one of the ICU nurses has decided that he no longer wants to be on call. He is the only member of the ICU staff who does not take call. Soon after he announces his decision, he begins to sense anger and experience alienation from his peers. He is very knowledgeable, has highly developed nursing skills, and provides consistently high-quality care to assigned patients on his regular shifts. However, on his semiannual peer evaluation, he receives low ratings from his coworkers because of the informal call coverage standard and expectations. The unit nurses feel that he is no longer a team player.

The nurse becomes angry because he feels that the use of unclear, unwritten standards is an unfair way to evaluate his ability as a nurse. He soon finds that the other ICU nurses accidentally "forget" to invite him to group functions. He also seems to be assigned the most difficult and largest number of patients during any given shift, seemingly to compensate for not taking call.

Group dynamics involve many factors, including methods of communication, professional behaviors, professional growth, flexibility, problem-solving, participation, and competition.[31] As with all interactions between people, communication is of the utmost importance.[30] Imbedded in the communication process, but not always recognized, are patterns of interaction between the group members. Leaders need to be aware of these patterns and able to change them when necessary. Several types of common interaction patterns include the following:

- *The Maypole:* A leader-centric interactive type of communication that is primarily between the leader or central figure (the Maypole) and only one member of the group at a time.
- *The Round Robin:* Members communicate as a group with the leader by taking turns talking one at a time (leader-centric).
- *The Hot Seat:* The exchange of ideas or feelings is between the leader and one person only while the rest of the group keeps quiet (leader-centric).
- *The Free Floating:* Communication is initiated from the group, and all the members take on the obligation to communicate (group-centric).

Free-floating communication is the most effective in group work. It permits the group members to interact with each other spontaneously and willingly. However, the group leader needs to be cognizant that group-centered communication may lead to emotional bonding among the members and the development of groupthink. In addition, the group may go off on tangents that have little or nothing to do with work they are attempting to achieve.[31] In this case, the group leader may need to modify the interaction pattern to bring the group back on task.

The ability to understand and use the elements of group dynamics and group interactions has a direct relationship to the behaviors, cooperation, and effectiveness of the team. Often, when a team labels an individual member as "difficult," it most likely means that the individual is not following one or more of the informal, unwritten group norms. (For more information on difficult behavior, see Chapter 12.)

A Common Understanding

It is evident that the team will function smoothly only when the members understand their roles and the roles of the other members. A good team leader explains each member's role in accomplishing the goal and prepares them with the information and physical resources they need to succeed. When team members do not comprehend their roles and what is required of them, it is usually a sign of a poorly trained leader.[30] Team members recognize an inadequate leader quickly, leading to group dynamics that may become toxic and chaotic. Their roles identify their places on the team and establish what is expected from each member. To be successful, the leader must establish the belief that all the roles are of equal importance in achieving the goals or purposes of the group.

Mutual Support

Team members need to realize they are not merely responsible for their own roles but also must support the roles of the other members. Although the leader establishes the goals to be achieved, it is important that the team members be allowed to achieve their tasks in ways that are most appropriate for them, particularly in the case of self-motivated professionals such as nurses.[31]

> *Establishing and sharing common goals is the starting point for successful team building.*

Reward for Achievement

Ongoing or complicated projects require a long-term commitment that is sometimes difficult to maintain. Effective team leaders are good at finding milestones, accomplishments along the way, that the team can celebrate and enjoy. It allows the team members to feel good about what they have achieved to this point and motivates them to accomplish more in the future. A good leader also recognizes the accomplishments of others and rewards them appropriately. Often, even simple statements of praise can be very much appreciated.

Identity and Trust

Finally, establishing a sense of team identity and trust completes the group dynamic and team-building process. Some degree of creativity may be required for establishing team identity, ranging from similar uniforms to buttons or pins. Trust allows the team members to be more open to communications from other members and more willing to take risks. Trust empowers the members, allowing them to make independent decisions and promoting the smooth functioning of the team (Table 10.3).

COMPETITION

Competition can be a very powerful element in group dynamics. Depending on how it is channeled, expressed, and used, competition can be a positive or negative force within the group.[31] The various forms of competition can be individual, team, or unit focused.

Peer Evaluation

A common expression of competition in the group setting is peer evaluations. For peer evaluations to be a positive form of competition, the unit must decide ahead of time on the norms and expectations that they value and then design an objective measurement tool to evaluate whether the individual is meeting the norms. Each individual being evaluated must be aware of the criteria before the evaluation is conducted. The evaluation team must be educated on evaluation techniques and must be as objective and professional as possible.

In the health-care setting, it is important for all professionals, unit groups, and management to promote competition in a positive, progressive, and supportive environment. When competition is channeled positively, it leads to new and creative ideas, better programs, increased growth, more productive interactions, and higher-quality patient care (Table 10.4).[30]

When the competition is negative, it often produces failures, depression, sabotage, unit turf conflicts, decreased productivity, and lower-quality care. Consider the following case:

The competition on a nursing unit turned negative: the nurses on the 7 a.m. to 3 p.m. shift began competing with the nurses on the 3 p.m. to 11 p.m. shift in order to appear more knowledgeable about patient care to the nurse manager. To "look better," the nurses on the 7 a.m. to 3 p.m. shift intentionally withheld selected patient laboratory test results during shift report.

As a result of this action, several tests scheduled for the 3 p.m. to 11 p.m. shift were not done, angering the physicians, potentially threatening the safety of the patients, and making the nurses on the 3 p.m. to 11 p.m. shift appear incompetent. In addition, the nurses on that shift had to complete several incident reports on the errors that occurred on their shift.

One informal component the unit manager uses to evaluate the staff nurses' performance is the number of incident reports that a nurse must file. The more incident reports, the poorer will be the nurse's performance evaluation. To the unit manager, the nurses on the 7 a.m. to 3 p.m. shift seemed to be more competent because of the seemingly poor care on the

> « *Nurses who do not learn and who fail to display the expected group behaviors may be ostracized from the group, thus making the work environment psychologically uncomfortable and perhaps even physically difficult.* »

Table 10.4 Dos and Don'ts of Effective Change Agents	
Dos	**Don'ts**
Do develop a sense of trust.	Don't have a hidden agenda.
Do establish common goals.	Don't be unpredictable.
Do facilitate effective communication.	Don't miss or reschedule meetings frequently.
Do establish a strong team identity.	Don't use threats or bluffs to manipulate members.
Do contribute as much as possible.	Don't volunteer to be the recordkeeper.
Do find reasons to celebrate and recognize accomplishments.	Don't follow the rest of the crowd.

3 p.m. to 11 p.m. shift, indicated by a large number of incident reports that were being given. However, when the nurses on the 3 p.m. to 11 p.m. shift discovered what had really happened, they devised several ways to "get even" with the nurses on the 7 a.m. to 3 p.m. shift.

CARE-DELIVERY MODELS

Nowhere are the elements of group dynamics reflected better than in the nursing units of a hospital or health-care facility. The organizational structure found in the nursing units of a facility reflects how the nursing department interacts with coworkers and participates in the delivery of patient care. Various models may be used in the delivery of nursing care. Many health-care facilities have made a transition from one model to another and may even incorporate several different models at the same time.[32] The nurse must recognize which model is being used as well as its strengths and weaknesses. These models include functional nursing, team

nursing, primary care nursing, and modular nursing (Table 10.5).

Functional Nursing

Functional nursing has as its foundation a task-oriented philosophy: each person performs a specific job that is narrowly defined according to the needs of the unit. The medication nurse, for example, focuses on administering and documenting medications for the assigned group of patients.

In this organizational unit, the nurse manager is called the *charge nurse*, whose main responsibility is to oversee the various workers. Charge nurses are also appointed for each shift to manage the care during that time. This model relies on ancillary health workers, such as nurses' aides and orderlies. Some believe this model fragments care too much. Because many people have specific tasks, coordination can be difficult, and the holistic perspective may be lost.[10] Although this care-delivery style was slowly being phased out prior to the pandemic, when nurses

> *The ability to understand and use the elements of group dynamics has a direct relationship on the behaviors, cooperation, and effectiveness of the team.*

Table 10.5	**Comparison of Common Patient-Care Models**		
Model	**Nurses Are Called**	**Description**	**Where Model Is Used**
Functional	Charge nurse Medical nurse Treatment nurse	Nurses are assigned to specific tasks rather than specific patients.	Hospitals Nursing homes Nurse consultants Operating rooms
Team	Team leader Team member	Nursing staff members are divided into small groups responsible for the total care of a given number of patients.	Hospitals Nursing homes Home care Hospice
Primary care	Primary nurse Associate nurse	Nurses are designated either as the primary nurse responsible for patients' care or as the associate nurse who assists in carrying out the care.	Hospitals Specialty units Dialysis Home care
Modular	Care pair	Nurses are paired with less-trained caregivers. Generally involves cross-training of personnel.	Hospitals Home care Transport teams
PPC	Nurse leader	Nurses are distributed according to the acuity of the patients on the unit.	Hospitals

and resources were in short supply, this method was used in many facilities with great success.[16] It works well in emergency situations.

Team Nursing

Team nursing has a more unified approach to patient care, with team members functioning together to achieve patient goals. It too was used with a high degree of success during the pandemic. The team leader functions as the person ultimately responsible for the patients' well-being. More cohesiveness is present among the members of the team than is found in the functional model. Rather than having a narrow task to accomplish, team members focus on team goals under the coordination of the team leader. The team conference provides for effective communication and follow-up among team members and is the key to successful team nursing. The quality of care may suffer with team nursing if the team is not cohesive, and there may be fragmentation of care.[32]

Primary Care Nursing

The primary care nursing model gives nurses the opportunity to focus on the whole person. The **primary care nurse** provides and is responsible for all of the patient's nursing needs.

The nurse manager in this model becomes a facilitator for the primary care nurses. Primary care nurses are self-directed and concerned with consistency of care. The primary care model is similar to the case management model, which has one nurse providing total care for one or more patients. Many home health-care agencies use this method of assigning an RN to work with an individual or family for the duration of the services rendered. Although this model of care is highly effective in meeting patients' needs and produces a quality of care unmatched in the other models, many institutions reject it because it is too costly.[32]

Modular Nursing

Modular nursing, also called *patient-focused care*, is one model that was developed in response to professional nursing personnel shortages and to the downsizing of professional nursing staffs. This model is based on a decentralized organizational system that emphasizes close interdisciplinary collaboration.

Redesigning the method of nursing care delivery takes much planning and input from the various departments involved, such as nursing, respiratory therapy, physical therapy, radiology, laboratory, and dietary.

Important aspects of modular nursing include relying on unlicensed assistive personnel (UAPs), also called *unit service assistants*, for providing direct care, grouping patients with similar needs, developing **relative intensity measures**, and emphasizing team concepts in small groups that remain constant.

Strong, Explicit Leadership Required

Cross-training of personnel is another important aspect of modular nursing. For example, using this system, respiratory therapists provide respiratory treatments but also help patients to the bathroom and turn bedridden patients. Nurse managers in this system are responsible for providing explicit job descriptions, maintaining the work group's cohesiveness, carefully monitoring each staff person's abilities, delegating tasks as appropriate, and evaluating the effectiveness of care.[32]

The role of UAPs is one area of the patient-focused care model that needs more definition, particularly in relation to the RN's accountability and responsibilities in supervising these workers. State boards of nursing across the country are considering possible changes in nurse practice acts necessitated by the use of UAPs.

Benefits of the modular care delivery model include decreased staffing cost and greater autonomy of cross-trained personnel. The nurse manager must be a strong leader for this model of care delivery to succeed. Consistent collaboration between the nurse manager and physician is of utmost importance in planning patient care.

Progressive Patient Care (PPC)

The PPC model involves the organized grouping of patients according to their degree of sickness and level of reliance on nursing care instead of the way most facilities group patients now, which is based on medical specialty, disease process, injury, or gender.

In the PPC model, medical and nursing care are organized according to the degree of illness and care requirements in the hospital. PPC is a system whereby hospital facilities can use their staff and equipment

> *Leadership can be exerted either formally or informally. Often, the most effective leaders in a group are not the ones who are officially designated as the leaders.*

to better meet the individual requirements of each patient. PPC has been defined as "the right patient, in the right bed, with the right services, at the right time."[32]

With the PPC model, critically ill patients are placed in intensive care units (ICU), while the majority of patients, approximately 60 percent, are placed in intermediate care units. Patients in the recovery phase of their illness or surgery are placed in convalescent or self-care units. Under this model, the outpatient surgery and procedure unit has a few beds for patients who need to stay overnight. If the facility has the space, it could contain a long-term care unit. The highest concentration of RNs, other highly trained staff, and the most complex equipment are located in the ICU areas. Fewer RNs but perhaps more ancillary staff are employed in the intermediate care area, similar to what is currently found on most medical-surgical units. RNs supervise care, but most of the care being given by LPNs and nursing assistants.[32]

Conclusion

Over the years, there has been one constant in the changing health-care system: the RN is still expected to provide leadership and management skills to direct and ensure the highest quality of health-care given to patients. Both leadership and management require a set of skills that can be learned. Nurses who learn these skills will become successful managers and the leaders of the health-care system in the future.

Successful leaders and managers understand and often combine the best aspects of the many theories that deal with leadership and management. Knowledge of one's strengths and weaknesses provides the basis for confident and productive leadership. Developing effective leadership and management skills is a lifelong process. Learning from books and articles, as well as from other successful nurse managers, presents an opportunity for professional and personal growth.

Issues in Practice

Jill, a registered nurse, was recently appointed as the evening charge nurse on a busy postsurgical unit. She has been an active participant in the hospital's quality-assurance committee for the past 2 years since her graduation. One of the issues the committee identified as a problem was the higher-than-average surgical wound infection rate on Jill's unit. After some research, Jill determined that a major component of the high infection rate was the procedures that were used when changing postoperative dressings.

After obtaining permission from the unit manager and hospital education director, Jill developed new procedures for dressing changes, incorporating the most current research. She presented the changes in a short in-service program to the unit personnel and explained the changes several times to each of the three shifts to make sure that all the nurses and staff on the unit were familiar with the new changes. The expectation was that there would be a 25 percent reduction in wound infections after the new procedures had been used for 1 month.

At the end of the first month of using the new dressing change procedures, the postoperative wound infection rate showed no improvement over the previous month's rate. At the monthly staff meeting, Jill discovered that the LPNs on the unit were refusing to use the new procedures because they "took too much time," and they had reverted to the procedures they had always used before.

Questions for Thought
1. What was the style of leadership and management that Jill used when attempting to initiate the dressing change procedures?
2. Other than the stated reason, why do you think the LPNs did not want to use the new procedures?
3. How can Jill increase the level of compliance by the LPNs on the unit?
4. What is the role of the unit manager in initiating the new dressing change procedures?

CRITICAL-THINKING EXERCISES

- Look at the list of key qualities of a leader in Figure 10.1. Make a list of the qualities that you believe you already have and the qualities that you need to develop.
- Table 10.3 lists the types of followers and their characteristics. What type of follower are you? Can you improve your followership skills? How?
- Have you ever been in a management position? Identify some of the issues you faced. Are they similar to the issues listed in the book? How did you resolve them?
- Develop a practice budget for yourself and for your family.
- Are you a winner or a whiner? (See Table 10.2.) Be honest!

Source: D.K. Whitehead, S.A. Weiss, R.M. Tappen. (2019). *Essentials of Nursing Leadership and Management* (7th ed.). F.A. Davis.

ANSWERS TO QUESTIONS IN CHAPTER 10

ISSUES IN PRACTICE: LEADERSHIP/ MANAGEMENT CASE STUDY (PAGE 266)

1. Nurse managers who use the authoritarian system would maintain their position that the proposed plan was unworkable. Relying on their position of authority, they would insist that the nurses continue to use the established system of assignment. Any staff nurse who felt they could not work under this system could seek reassignment to another unit.
2. Nurse managers using the laissez-faire system would allow the nurses to try out the proposed system as they wanted. If any problems resulted from it, the nurses would have to figure out how to resolve the problems themselves.
3. Nurse managers using the participative system would recognize that there is always some common ground between themselves and the staff nurses. It is important to identify the common points and then work toward resolving the areas of disagreement. For example, the nurse manager could work with the staff nurses to develop a set of criteria for assignments that would be agreeable to all parties and ensure the quality of patient care. The nurse manager would then retain the ability to assign patients but would be using criteria that were developed by the staff. In the end, staff cooperation and morale would increase, as would the continuity and quality of care being provided by the unit.
4. The initial mistake the nurse manager made was meeting with the staff nurses as a group. The staff nurses would have done better to select one or two representatives to bring their issues to the nurse manager. Using this approach eliminates the "mob mentality" that sometimes develops with large groups. It also forces the staff nurses to identify the specific issues they want to resolve.

NCLEX-STYLE QUESTIONS

1. Natalie, a well-liked nurse manager, demonstrates that she values her team members and their contributions to the unit's success. Moreover, their unit consistently has lower rates of hospital-acquired infections and readmissions than any other unit in the hospital. Which major theory of leadership is this an example of?
   1. Trait theory
   2. Leadership-style theory
   3. Relationship–task orientation
   4. Benevolent leadership

2. Roger, a charge nurse, believes in giving the RNs on his unit maximum control of planning and decision making for the unit. After all, they are highly trained professionals. What is Roger's leadership style?
   1. Laissez-faire
   2. Democratic
   3. Authoritarian
   4. Benevolent

3. Tyesha is an authoritarian style of leader. Which of the following is an example of her leadership style?
   1. Tyesha insists that all nurses in her unit participate in the decision-making process to maximize buy-in of policy changes.
   2. Tyesha expects her team members to take professional responsibility and resolve their own conflicts as much as possible.
   3. Tyesha asks team members to share concerns about a new fall-reduction policy being considered. Then, she announces that their unit will implement the policy effective immediately.
   4. Tyesha encourages her team members to take responsibility for themselves and for the whole unit.

4. Bill has just been made a unit director at his facility, and he wants to be an effective leader. Which of the following behaviors and qualities should he incorporate in his professional style? **Select all that apply**.
   1. Problem-solving
   2. Acknowledging good work
   3. Fostering cooperation among team members and generally
   4. Reinforcing unit goals
   5. Focusing exclusively on his new responsibilities
   6. Having himself and promoting among the unit team a sense of optimism

5. Michelle thinks of her nurse manager, Carla, as her mentor in personal and professional life. Carla is exactly the kind of leader and person Michelle hopes to be one day, and Michelle will argue with anyone who questions Carla's authority. Which kind of follower is Michelle?
   1. Effective
   2. Partner
   3. Implementer
   4. Yes-woman

6. According to _____ theory, no single leadership approach works in every scenario or with all types of employees.

7. A nursing leadership class is discussing the differences between management and leadership. Which statement made by a student would indicate that she needs to review these concepts again?
   1. Management is a formal relationship, but leadership can be informal.
   2. Managers must have leadership skills, or else they will not be promoted.
   3. Someone who has leadership ability may not have good management skills.
   4. Managers, not leaders, are responsible for the quality, quantity, and cost of the work that their employees produce.

8. A nursing home is experiencing high turnover of its nursing staff. During exit interviews, departing nurses cite low pay and too few unlicensed assistive personnel as their main reasons for leaving. According to Herzberg's motivation–hygiene theory, what is causing the nurses' dissatisfaction?
   1. Needs motivators
   2. Physiological and safety needs
   3. Hygiene factors
   4. Lack of self-esteem

9. Miguel is a nurse manager in a cardiac ICU. Which of the following is most likely to be his primary leadership style?
   1. Democratic
   2. Laissez-faire
   3. Authoritarian
   4. Motivational

10. Allegra has always been a charismatic nursing leader in her unit, motivating her coworkers with her optimism and enthusiasm. Recently promoted to the position of nurse manager, Allegra is struggling to master budgeting and planning for staff coverage. How should Allegra handle the situation?
    1. Delegate the budgeting and staff-coverage planning to someone else on her team.
    2. Request training as soon as possible in the managerial skills she needs to develop.
    3. Join the team for drinks after work and ask them to be patient a little longer.
    4. Admit that she is a leader, not a manager, and request a demotion.

References

1. Traits of a leader and explanation behind the trait theory of leadership. Black Sheep Community, 2022. https://www.theblacksheep.community/trait-theory-of-leadership/

2. Weiss S, Tappen R, Grimley K. *Essentials of Nursing Leadership and Management* (7th ed). F.A. Davis, 2019.

3. Habas C. Task vs. relationship leadership theories. *Chron*, September 4, 2020. https://smallbusiness.chron.com/task-vs-relationship-leadership-theories-35167.html

4. Cherry K. Transformational leadership. Verywell Mind, 2022. https://www.verywellmind.com/what-is-transformational-leadership-2795313

5. Herrity J. Situational leadership theory: Definition, styles and maturity levels. Indeed, 2021. https://www.indeed.com/career-advice/career-development/situational-leadership-theory

6. Cherry K. Leadership styles and frameworks you should know. Verywell Mind., November 14, 2022. https://www.verywellmind.com/leadership-styles-2795312

7. Transparent communication. Michigan State University, 2022. https://workplace.msu.edu/transparent-communication/

8. Michael. Optimism in leadership. LeadershipGeeks.com, 2022. https://www.leadershipgeeks.com/optimism-in-leadership/

9. Rigglo R. In praise of followship. Psychology Today, 2023. https://www.psychologytoday.com/us/blog/cutting-edge-leadership/202303/in-praise-of-followership

10. Ansary AS. 55 Examples of leadership and management styles in nursing. CareerCliff, May 26, 2022. https://www.careercliff.com/leadership-and-management-styles-in-nursing/

11. Governance, boards and healthcare leadership. Consumer Health Ratings, 2022. https://consumerhealthratings.com/healthcare_category/governance-boards-and-healthcare-leadership/

12. What are the steps in preparing a budget? AccountingTools, May 15, 2022. https://www.accountingtools.com/articles/what-are-the-steps-in-preparing-a-budget.html

13. Rundio A. Budget development for nurse managers. Sigma, 2020. https://nursingcentered.sigmanursing.org/features/top-stories/budget-development-for-the-nurse-manager

14. Rundio A. *An Overview of the Nurse Manager's Guide to Budgeting and Finance* (3rd ed.). Sigma Publishers, 2021.

15. Brusie C. ANA updates nurse staffing guidelines to support flexibility. Nurse.org, December 4, 2019. https://nurse.org/articles/nurse-staffing-ana-guidelines/

16. Nuru B. Six techniques to address staffing challenges in the midst of COVID-19. RecruitingDaily, 2020. https://recruitingdaily.com/six-techniques-to-address-staffing-challenges-in-the-midst-of-covid-19/

17. The Joint Commission. Voices from the pandemic: Health care workers in the midst of crisis. *Sentinel Event Alert*, 2021. https://www.jointcommission.org/-/media/tjc/documents/resources/patient-safety-topics/sentinel-event/sea-62-hcws-and-pandemic-final-1-28-21.pdf

18. Kear T, Walz D. Solutions to shortage are complex, but require nurses lead the efforts. Healio, May 18, 2022. https://www.healio.com/news/nephrology/20220502/solutions-to-shortage-are-complex-but-nurses-first-need-respect-control-of-destiny

19. Wong M. Nurse-to-patient ratios are a patient safety issue. Physician Patient Alliance for Health Safety, 2022. https://ppahs.org/2022/05/nurse-to-patient-ratios/

20. Joyce R. H.R. 5052 (115th): Safe Staffing for Nurse and Patient Safety Act of 2018. GovTrack, 2022. https://www.govtrack.us/congress/bills/115/hr5052

21. Bailey R. High registered nurse staffing levels tied to lower mortality rates. *Practice Management News*, June 1, 2022. https://revcycleintelligence.com/news/high-registered-nurse-staffing-levels-tied-to-lower-mortality-rates

22. Cherry K. What is intrinsic motivation? Verywell Mind, September 14, 2022. https://www.verywellmind.com/what-is-intrinsic-motivation-2795385

23. Vaidya A. 5 Nurses on motivating teams during the pandemic. Becker's Hospital Review, April 15, 2020. https://www.beckershospitalreview.com/nursing/5-nurses-on-motivating-teams-during-the-pandemic.html

24. Kose S, Gezainci E, Goktas S, Mural M. The effectiveness of motivational messages to ICU nurses during the COVID-19 pandemic. *Intensive Critical Care Nursing*, 69, 2021. https://doi.org/10.1016/j.iccn.2021.103161

25. Jingxia C, Longling Z, Qiantao Z, Weixue P, Xiaolian J. The changes in the nursing practice environment brought by COVID-19 and improvement recommendations from the nurses' perspective: a cross-sectional study. *BioMedical Central Health Services*, 22: 754, 2022. https://doi.org/10.1186/s12913-022-08135-7

26. Celestine N. What is behavior change in psychology? 5 models and theories. PositivePsychology.com, August 14, 2021. https://positivepsychology.com/behavior-change/

27. Nilsen P, Seing I, Ericsson C, Birken SA, Schildmeijer K. Characteristics of successful changes in healthcare organizations: An interview study with physicians, registered nurses and assistant nurses. *BioMedical Central Services Research*, 20, 2020. https://doi.org/10.1186/s12913-020-4999-8

28. Importance of change management in helathcare: Common mistakes. Medical Advantage, 2023. https://www.medicaladvantage.com/blog/change-management-in-healthcare/

29. O'Reilly M. Change and change again—Nurse leaders in the new millennium. Medscape, 2022. https://www.medscape.org/viewarticle/568013

30. Understanding group dynamics for group work practice. Newagesocialwork, May 20,2022. https://newagesocialwork.com/understanding-group-dynamics-for-group-work-practice/

31. How to improve group dynamics for teams. Talenteria.com, October 29, 2021. https://www.talenteria.com/news/how-improve-group-dynamics-teams

32. Theory and models of nursing care delivery. Current Nursing, 2021. https://currentnursing.com/nursing_theory/models_of_nursing_care_delivery.html

Communication, Negotiation, and Conflict Resolution

11

Joseph T. Catalano

Learning Objectives

After completing this chapter, the reader will be able to:

- Explain the importance of understanding communication in the workplace
- Discuss the factors that can interfere with good communication
- Identify the important elements in assertive communication
- Discuss the impact of assertive communication
- Distinguish between aggressive and assertive communication
- Define verbal, paraverbal, and nonverbal communication and give an example of each
- List and discuss five verbal communication blockers
- Describe conflict resolution and tools used in the process
- List and explain the key elements of negotiation
- Compare and contrast arbitration and mediation

THE NURSE AS COMMUNICATOR

Communicating well is a skill that every nurse needs to master. However, much like the skills of leadership and management, not every nurse is born with a natural talent for communicating. Every day, nurses interact with numerous individuals who may come from a diverse educational and socioeconomic backgrounds and different cultures.

Good communication skills are vital to effectively address many of the problems encountered in everyday life. Television personalities, instructors, and psychologists promote improved communication skills as the answer to parental, marital, financial, and work-related problems. The nursing profession recognizes communication as one of the cornerstones of its practice. Nurses must be able to communicate with patients, family members, health-care providers, peers, and associates in an effective and constructive manner to achieve their goals of high-quality care. Good communication is also essential for good leadership and management.[1]

In today's rapidly evolving health-care system, registered nurses (RNs) are called on to supervise a growing number of unlicensed assistive personnel (UAP). One of the keys to good supervision is the ability to communicate to people what they must do to provide the required care and, often, how the care should be given. And supervision is not always easy. Many of the people whom nurses supervise have limited training and may not have the theoretical and technical knowledge base of the nurse. Nurses may also encounter resistance to delegation or direction. However, nurse supervisors can be and often are held legally responsible for the actions of those individuals who work under their direction.

UNDERSTANDING COMMUNICATION

Communication is an interactive sharing of information. It requires a sender, a message, and a receiver. **Encoding** is the process of turning thoughts into either verbal or written communication. **Decoding** is the process of turning communication into thoughts. For example, a person (the sender) may realize that they are lost and encode the following message to a nearby street vendor: "I'm looking for 410 Banks Street. Is that near here?" The street vendor (the receiver) receives the message by hearing the words that are spoken (verbal communication) and decoding them mentally back into thoughts in order to make meaning. The vendor then encodes a response: "Yes, make a right turn at the next street. A few buildings down from the corner is 410."

Several factors can interfere with the communication process. On the sender's side, these can be factors such as unclear speech, convoluted and confused message, monotone voice, poor sentence structure, inappropriate use of terminology or jargon, or lack of knowledge about the topic. On the receiver's side, factors that may interfere with communication include lack of attention, prejudice and bias, preoccupation with another problem, or even physical factors such as pain, drowsiness, or impairment of the senses.

For example, a staff nurse is in a mandatory meeting where the unit manager is discussing a new policy that will be starting the following month. However, the nurse is thinking about an important heart medication that her patient is to receive in 5 minutes. The nurse's primary concern is to get out of the meeting in time to give the medication. After the meeting, the nurse has only a minimal recollection of what was said because she did not decode the information well. The following month, when the new policy is started, the staff nurse is confused about what she should do and makes several errors in relation to the policy.

Patients who come to a health-care facility for care are physically ill and often emotionally drained. They are dealing with a variety of emotions such as anger, fear, helplessness, and hopelessness. These types of emotions are psychological defense mechanisms that aid them in controlling their new environment, adjusting to their new circumstances, and feeling safer. Effective communication requires understanding that the perceptions, emotions, and participation of both the sender and the receiver are interactive and have an effect on the transmission of the message. Nurses often encounter situations that require messages to be clarified to ensure accurate decoding.[2] The following is an example of patient teaching that requires a return demonstration:

A nurse completed a teaching session to a patient who was being sent home with a T-tube to drain off excess bile after surgical removal of gallstones from the common bile duct. After the nurse finished his instructions, he asked the patient whether he understood how to empty the drainage bottle and measure the drainage. The patient looked very confused, but mumbled, "Yes," while shaking his head. The nurse recognized that although the verbal response was positive, the nonverbal responses indicated that the patient really did not understand. The nurse surmised that further explanation or demonstration was required for this patient to decode the message properly. The nurse then asked the patient to perform each step in the process of emptying the drainage bottle as he talked the patient through the process. (For more detail on patient teaching, see Chapter 23.)

Nurses should recognize the many barriers to clear communication and the benefits of clear communication. Barriers are different from communication blockers, discussed later in the chapter. Once the barriers to communication are identified, they can be overcome, and the benefits of clear communication will follow. These barriers and the benefits that result when they are overcome are outlined in Box 11.1.

COMMUNICATION STYLES

There are five predominant styles of communication: assertive, nonassertive (passive), aggressive, passive-aggressive, and manipulative. Individuals develop their communication styles over the course of their lives in response to many personal factors. Although most people have one predominant style of communication, they can and often do switch or combine styles, depending on the situation in which they find themselves.[3] For example, a unit manager who uses an assertive communication style when supervising the staff on her unit may revert to a submissive style when called into the nursing director's office for her annual evaluation. Recognizing which communication style a person is using at any given time, as well as one's own style, is important in making communication clear and effective.

Assertive Communication

Assertive communication is the preferred style of exchanging information or ideas in most settings.

Box 11.1 Barriers to and Benefits of Clear Communication

Barriers	Benefits
• Unclear or unexpressed expectations	• Clear expectations
• Confusion	• Understanding
• Retaliation	• Forgiveness
• Desire for power	• Recognized leadership
• Control of others	• Companionship
• Negative reputation	• Respect
• Manipulation	• Independence
• Low self-esteem	• Realistic self-image
• Biased perceptions	• Acceptance
• Inattention	• Clear direction
• Mistrust	• Trusting relations
• Anger	• Self-control
• Fear or anxiety	• Comfort
• Stress	• Motivation or energy
• Insecurity	• Security
• Prejudice	• Increased tolerance
• Interruptions	• Increased knowledge
• Preoccupation	• Concentration

Box 11.2 Assess Your Assertiveness

The following questions can help you assess how assertive you are in communication. Find a quiet place and, thoughtfully and honestly, write your answer to each question. When you are finished, look back through your answers to see if you can identify any patterns. Are you already an assertive communicator? Or do fears or faulty perceptions keep you from being as assertive as you could be? What area(s) can you work on to become more assertive?

• Who am I, and what do I want?
• Do I believe I have the right to want it?
• How do I get it?
• Do I believe I can get it?
• Have I tried to be assertive with a person I am having difficulty communicating with?
• Am I letting my fears and perceptions cloud my interactions?
• What is the worst that can happen if we communicate?
• Can I live with the worst?
• Will communications have a long-term effect?
• How does it feel to fear alienation or rejection?

It involves interpersonal behaviors that permit people to defend and maintain their legitimate rights in a respectful manner that does not violate the rights of others. Assertive communication is honest and direct and accurately expresses the person's feelings, beliefs, ideas, and opinions. Respect for self and others constitutes both the basis for and the result of assertive communication. It encourages trust and teamwork by communicating to others that they have the right to and are encouraged to express their opinions in an open and respectful atmosphere. Disagreement and discussion are considered to be a healthy part of the communication process, and negotiation is the positive mechanism for problem-solving, learning, and personal growth.[3]

Assertive communication always implies that the individual has the choice to voice an opinion, sometimes forcefully, or to not say anything at all. One of the keys to assertive communication is that the individual is in control of the communication and is not merely reacting to another's emotions.[3] Use the self-assessment in Box 11.2 to evaluate your current level of assertiveness.

Rules for Assertiveness

Anyone can learn to use an assertive communication style and develop assertiveness. When first developing this skill, people often feel frightened and overwhelmed. However, once individuals become comfortable with assertiveness, it helps reinforce their self-confidence and becomes an effective tool for communication. There are a few rules to keep in mind while developing assertiveness along with an assertive communication style:

• It is a learned skill.
• It takes practice.
• It requires a desire and motivation to change.
• It requires a willingness to take risks.

- It requires a willingness to make mistakes and try again.
- It requires an understanding that not every outcome sought will be obtained.
- It requires strong self-esteem.
- Self-reward for change and a positive outcome is essential.
- Listening to self is necessary for identifying needs.
- Constant re-examination of outcomes helps assess progress.
- Role-playing with a friend before an important interaction builds skill and confidence.
- Goals for assertiveness growth need to be established beforehand.
- Assertiveness requires recognition that change is a gradual process.
- Others should be allowed to make mistakes.

Personal Risks of Assertive Communication

There are always personal risks involved in learning new skills or in attempting to change behavior. Learning assertive communication is no exception. People often fear that they may not choose the "perfect" assertive response. However, even seasoned assertive communicators may err from time to time because every encounter is unique, involving different people and situations. The person who is new to assertive communication needs to recognize that it is a skill that takes practice.

I Win, You Win

Being assertive does not mean that a person will always get their way; it is likely the individual will handle some situations better than others. Remember that the goal of assertive communication is to prevent an "I win, you lose" situation and to encourage an "I win, you win" outcome.[4] A win-win goal is achieved when both parties have the ability and willingness to negotiate even though they do not get all they want. However, there may be situations when personal goals are not achieved. Following are some questions to consider when this occurs:

- How do I feel about not getting what I wanted?
- Did I express my opinion clearly? Why not? How could I make it clearer?

- Did I do the best I could do? How could I have done better?
- Was I in control when responding to the situation? When did I lose control? What should I have done to regain control?
- Did I stay focused on the issues? What side issues distracted me? How could I have avoided distractions?
- Did I allow the situation to get personal? Did the other person initiate the personal attack? How could I have redirected it away from the personal?
- Was what I asked for under my control? If not, why did I ask for it? What would have been more realistic?

Reviewing these questions and analyzing the answers will help when you attempt to be assertive in future communications. For example, if the answer to the second-to-last question was yes, then during the next communication, you can make a special effort to avoid personal attacks during the encounter. Learning to communicate assertively is a process of continual improvement.

Impact of Assertive Communication

Another risk of changing to an assertive communication style is the impact that it can have on those who know the person best. Sometimes a person's family, friends, peers, and coworkers become barriers to change and growth. These individuals may feel uncomfortable with the person's new, assertive communication style because they are accustomed to the person's old communication style and behaviors, which developed over a long period of time. They can no longer anticipate and depend on the person's responding and reacting in the usual way.[5] In addition, they will have to develop new communication patterns of their own to match the changes caused by assertive communication.

Sometimes family, friends, peers, and coworkers become so uncomfortable that they may try to sabotage the person's attempts at assertive communication. For example, a coworker may say to the person who is attempting to be assertive, "Who died and left you in charge?" It is important to recognize why and when these sabotage efforts occur and to remember that

> **" A win-win goal is achieved when both parties have the ability and willingness to negotiate even though they do not get all they want. "**

Box 11.3 Rights and Responsibilities of Assertiveness

Rights

- To act in a way that promotes your dignity and self-respect
- To be treated with respect
- To experience and express your thoughts and feelings
- To ask for what you want
- To say no
- To change your mind
- To make mistakes
- To not be perfect
- To feel important and good about yourself
- To be treated as an individual with special values, skills, and needs
- To be unique
- To have your own feelings and opinions
- To say "I don't know"
- To feel angry, hurt, and frustrated
- To make decisions regarding your life
- To recognize that your needs are as important as others'

Responsibility

- To slow down and make conscious decisions before you act

Box 11.4 Assertive Communication Suggestions

- Maintain appropriate eye contact.
- Convey empathy; stating your feelings does not mean sympathizing or agreeing.
- Keep your body position erect, shoulders and back straight.
- Speak clearly and audibly; be direct and descriptive.
- Be comfortable with silence.
- Use gestures and facial expressions for emphasis.
- Use appropriate location.
- Use appropriate timing.
- Focus on behaviors and issues; do not attack the person.

assertiveness is an internal, personal process. Everyone has a right to change, and it must be respectfully communicated to others that their support for these changes is important.

It is also important to know and periodically review the rights and responsibilities of assertiveness to help reinforce the assertive communication process. The rights and responsibilities of assertiveness are listed in Box 11.3.

Practicing and reinforcing your assertiveness skills is especially useful when preparing for an anticipated conflict negotiation or a confrontational meeting. Although confrontation always produces some anxiety, it also has the potential to be highly productive. Box 11.4 provides suggestions for developing assertive communication.

Using appropriate methods of communication in conjunction with an assertive communication style enhances the communication and understanding by both parties. Communication builders are important in developing an assertive communication style.

Submissive Communication (Passive or Nonassertive)

When people display submissive (passive) behavior or use a submissive communication style, they allow their rights to be violated by others. Their requests and demands are surrendered to others without regard to their own feelings and needs. Many experts believe that submissive behavior and communication patterns are a protective mechanism that helps insecure people maintain their self-esteem by avoiding negative criticism and disagreement from others. In one-on-one situations, they are often considered good listeners because of their failure to speak.

Outwardly, they usually do not display their concern for their own unfulfilled needs or even their rights. Individuals with a submissive communication style internalize their responses to events that are humiliating, hostile, and upsetting to them. As a result, they become internally angry but do not channel their anger into more productive responses, and it just builds up inside them until the inner emotional tension reaches a boiling point. Once this point is reached, the person with a passive style of communication is disposed to emotional eruptions and sometimes violent negative reactions. These outbursts display a higher level of emotion and are of higher intensity than the comments or events that triggered them. The outburst in turn makes the person feel embarrassed and humiliated, thus making them even more submissive in their communication. A vicious circle develops of submissiveness, outbursts, and submissiveness.[3]

The submissive communicator, because of some event or condition during their development, is unable to use assertive communication. In addition, they may have difficulty using any type of communication, verbal or nonverbal. Much like the speech of a depressed person, when the submissive person does talk, it will be slowly, in a soft tone with a very quiet voice. The submissive person uses the soft tone/quiet voice to make the listener attend more closely and offer reinforcement.[1] The submissive communicator may also adopt other depressive indicators, such as feeling out of control, hopeless, and helpless.

When they do speak, other than in outburst mode, it is very stressful for them, and they will allow others to interrupt and speak over them. In response, rather than saying, "Please don't interrupt me" or "I'm speaking now, please wait your turn," they will stop speaking altogether. They find it difficult to maintain any type of eye contact and display a defensive body posture when in the group setting. Individuals with the submissive communication style feel nervous and troubled all the time. They strongly believe that other people think what they are saying has no value, do not like what they are saying, or will not pay attention to what they have to say. When asked by the discussion leader what they are thinking, they will often respond with "I don't know" or "Nothing worth talking about."[3]

What Do You Think?

Recall a recent exchange with someone (e.g., friend, instructor, parent, health-care provider) in which you felt you "lost" the exchange. How did you feel? How did you respond? How could using an assertive communication style have helped?

Rather than being in control of the communication or relationship, the person is trading their ability to choose what is best for the avoidance of conflict. Every communication by a submissive person becomes an "I lose; you win" situation. However, subconsciously, it is more of "You may think you win, but I really am winning because I'm avoiding conflict or rejection, which is what I really want."

Aggressive Communication

Sometimes there is a very fine line separating assertiveness from aggressive behavior and communication.[4] Whereas assertive communication permits individuals to honestly express their ideas and opinions while respecting another's rights, ideas, and opinions, aggressive communication strongly asserts the speaker's legitimate rights and opinions with little or no regard or respect for the rights and opinions of others. It easily becomes a communication blocker (see later discussion).

In aggressive communication, the exchange of information is unidirectional and directly opposes the basic goal of communication, which is an exchange of information. An aggressive communicator sends messages to the receiver without the intent of receiving any reply or informative feedback. The sender focuses only on their message, and the views, opinions, and feelings of the receiver are not considered important. The sender often sends the message with the most strength and highest intensity possible.[4]

Although the aggressive communicator may express their views by vulgar words, a loud voice, or even shouting when in an agitated state, these are not the only types of exchanges they use. In reality, the aggressive communicator often expresses themselves more coolly, but with the same type of message. They often dominate the conversation so that there is little time left for other group members to express themselves.[4] One key in recognizing an aggressive communicator is that they do not listen or pay attention when others are trying to communicate. This is not only the lack of active listening (see later) but a complete deficiency of any attention and understanding of the other speakers' dialogue. Because of the lack of listening, the aggressive communicator totally disregards the ideas of other members of the group.[3]

Unlike assertive communication, the aggressive communicator has no intention of reaching any compromises or receiving information from other group members. Their only purpose is to get their particular message across and achieve their personal goals. By humiliating the other members of the group, they take control of the conversation and manipulate others to fulfill their own fundamental needs. Aggressive communicators have a low tolerance for frustration when communicating with others. They have a tendency to interrupt others who are speaking because they believe the speakers are less intelligent than they are. When things do not go their way, they blame other members of the group, which produces an atmosphere of negativity and a toxic environment.[5]

In addition to not listening and to pushing their own personal goals, the aggressive communicator has a complete lack of empathy and does not care about the effects of their messages on the rest of the group. The group's emotions, feelings, or views take a back seat to their own personal agenda. Because of the lack of empathy, the communications within the group become stressed and tense, leaving the group feeling cold and provoked.[4] When aggressive communication is used to humiliate, dominate, control, or embarrass the other person or lower that person's self-esteem, it creates an "I win; you lose" situation. The other person may perceive aggressive behavior or communication as a personal attack. Aggressive behavior and communication are viewed by some psychologists as a protective mechanism that compensates for a person's own insecurities; other mental health professionals view it as a form of bullying. By demeaning someone else, the aggressive person feels superior and inflates their fragile self-esteem.[4]

Aggressive communication can take several forms, including screaming, sarcasm, rudeness, belittling jokes, and even direct personal insults. Aggression is an expression of the speaker's negative feelings of power, domination, and self-esteem. Although aggressive people may appear to be in control, in reality they are merely reacting to the situation to protect their self-esteem.[5]

Passive-Aggressive Communication

Passive-aggressive communication takes the worst of both aggressive communication and passive communication and combines them into an indirect, unclear, and often confusing communication style. The passive-aggressive communicator circuitously expresses feelings of resentment, bitterness, or anger all the time. Although this communication type has similarities to submissive communication, passive-aggressive communicators do not allow their rights to be directly violated by others. Also, passive-aggressive communicators do not surrender their requests and demands to others without regard to their own feelings and needs. In the submissive communication style, the person avoids expressing their opinions and emotions on any topic. Similarly, passive-aggressive communicators appear on the surface submissive and even accommodating during a group exchange; but in reality, they are talking to themselves internally and will whisper negative ideas to another member in the group while the leader is talking. For example, "They don't know what they're talking about" or "Boy, is this change going to be a bust."

Because they are trying to control and/or deflect their anger, the passive-aggressive communicator causes frustration or anger in the group, which will intensify conflict unless the leader handles it appropriately. They are also very accomplished at pushing group members' buttons, especially the leader's.

Passive-aggressive communicators will think of how to get payback and sabotage others in the group, particularly individuals they feel have slighted or insulted them, even if it was unintended. Examples of passive-aggressive communication include being obstinate by sulking during meetings, arguing minor points frequently and excessively, not completing an assignment on purpose so that the group work cannot be completed, doing the assignment incorrectly, or procrastinating.[5] On rare occasions, similar to the aggressive communicator, they will have a loud outburst that is directed toward an individual they feel has been particularly "mean" to them.

A passive-aggressive communicator may decide to remain aloof, isolated, or indifferent to others in the group because they feel alienated and estranged in the presence of others. They feel powerless and remain unfulfilled and ill-tempered throughout their lives. Because the underlying issues that produced this behavior are buried deep in their psyche, passive-aggressive communicators are unable to express their

> ❝ *The passive-aggressive communicator is circuitously expressing feelings of resentment, bitterness, or anger all the time.* ❞

primary or basic problems directly, and therefore, they cannot resolve them or develop healthy and effective coping mechanisms. Their personal relationships tend to be poor in quality, and they have difficulty maintaining long-term interpersonal relations and a usual social life.[6] Because passive-aggressive behavior is listed as a type of personality disorder, they may need professional help to overcome their issues.

Other examples of passive-aggressive communication include "You didn't tell me that assignment was due today," "That's not my problem," and "I don't want to talk about this now (or ever)."

Manipulative Communication

Manipulative communication is a method of sending a message whose intent is to control and influence others to satisfy the sender's own underlying needs. Manipulative communicators use cunning and astute messages to scheme and design situations that maximize their advantage.[3] Unlike the passive-aggressive communicator who uses their communication to indirectly express bitterness and anger, the manipulative communicator does not usually want revenge on other team members and will be more direct in their communication. One of the most common methods they use to manipulate others is to play the part of a victim so that other people will feel sorry for them and are more likely to grant their wishes. They initially hide their underlying wants and needs, attempting first to get others to feel sympathy for them. Once they have others feeling sorry for them, the manipulative communicator openly expresses what they want or need from the group.[3]

Manipulative communicators' nonverbal or body language attempts to show them as helpless and weak, thereby trying to make the group feel pity and sympathy for them. However, they actually plot out situations in advance to take control of group interactions and members of the group by using deception. They have no concept of how their behavior impacts the rest of the group, and left unchecked, they can destroy the whole group dynamic.

Other methods manipulative communicators use to control the group may include the expression of false physical appearances and emotions, such as crying, in an attempt to increase group members' sense of guilt or obligation to them.[3] Much like the passive-aggressive communicator, they have poor coping mechanisms for dealing with their daily lives as well as poor to nonexistent social lives. Upon closer examination, they are disposed to the development of personality disorders and dysfunctional interpersonal skills.[5]

Other types of manipulative communicators are commonly known as the "yes-person" or the "brown-noser." In order to get into their good graces, the yes-person agrees with everything the leader says and never contradicts or opposes them. They are not trying to control the group or the message but rather are attempting to obtain the leader's good will. They do what they are told to do without question.

The brown-noser, on the other hand, uses overt compliments, flattery, fawning, or even subservience to gain the approval and attention of others, particularly of the group leader. This person attempts to gain an elevated status or advantage that they can use later, such as an increase in pay, promotion, or acceptance by the group. Because the leader is the ultimate target of the brown-noser's aims, they will do almost anything to gain the leader's approval. In reality, they are trying to short-cut the normal process for advancement by buttering up the leader so that they can get their way.[3] Astute leaders quickly pick up on what these individuals are attempting to do and will stop their actions. However, some leaders find the yes-person's lack of opposition and the brown-noser's compliments to be flattering and will allow the behaviors to continue. Other, less flattering names for the brown-noser include ass-kisser, suck-up, toady, or the leader's pet. Others in the group often find the brown-noser's activities and praises disagreeable and may become irritated by them.[6] Ultimately, the brown-noser will be ostracized from the group.

What the Different Communication Styles Might Say

Assertive: "I believe we should make this change, which will help the whole group."

Submissive: "I don't know. You seem to be pushing change on me. It's scary!"

Aggressive: "What you said is stupid. No one wants to do that! I have a better idea."

Passive-Aggressive: "Whatever." (Whispers, "I can't wait to get out of here.")

Manipulative: "Oh, I've been feeling so depressed lately, I don't know if I can handle change now."

Unfortunate Reality

When highly educated, highly skilled, and highly motivated workers are placed in a position in which they have little power, authority, or input in their work environment and in which assertive communication is rebuffed, they may revert to some less-than-desirable types of behavior or communication in an attempt to gain acknowledgment, appreciation, and the ability to be professional. This is especially true when other figures in their work environment seem to have the ultimate power to make decisions. These workers will resort to playing the passive-aggressive game with those who are in power or management. They do not actually become a passive-aggressive personality as described earlier, but they use passive-aggressive techniques to help them complete their tasks and produce high-quality work. For example, they may have a great idea for improving a situation, but they will let the authority figure believe it is that person's idea

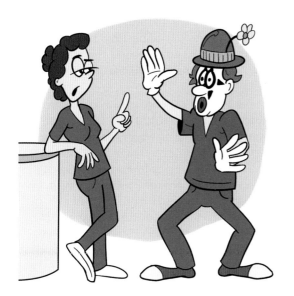

"You really need to work on your verbal skills."

Verbal, Paraverbal, and Nonverbal Communication

There are three primary methods of communication: verbal, paraverbal, and nonverbal. **Verbal** communication is either written or spoken and constitutes only about 7 percent of the communicated message.

Nonverbal communication makes up another 93 percent of communication and includes body language, facial expressions, gestures, physical appearance, touch, and spatial territory (personal space). **Paraverbal** communication is the tone, pitch, volume, and diction used when delivering a verbal message. *How* people say something is often more important than what they say.[3] A sentence can have a completely different meaning depending on the emphasis placed on different words. Paraverbal communication makes up about 38 percent of the nonverbal communication and is often considered part of nonverbal communication.[7] When a sender's verbal, paraverbal, and nonverbal messages are congruent, the message is more easily decoded and clearly understood. For example, the aggressive communicator's verbal expressions, body language, and paraverbal communications are generally highly congruent. A tense facial expression accompanied by frowning and fixed, penetrating eyes displays their challenging assertiveness and sense of superiority. Often, the intensity of the gaze forces team members to avoid eye contact and look away to avoid the discomfort it produces. The aggressive communicator uses an intimidating posture, such as leaning in toward the other person, which is accompanied by forceful and frequent arm and hand gestures to magnify feelings of intimidation.[4]

Violating the personal space (see later) of others in the group adds to the atmosphere of confrontation. All of these nonverbal elements are congruent with the paraverbal techniques of the aggressive communicator, including not pausing or allowing silences, using a forceful and raised voice, and speech that is excessively fast and does not allow for interruptions. They are often fluent verbally and accomplished speakers.[6] Verbal elements of the aggressive communicator include the use of absolutes, such as "You're always wrong," and imperatives, such as "It is absolutely necessary that we use my plan now!" They rarely begin statements with "I" but use the accusatory "You" to start. Other verbal components include criticizing the thoughts and expressions of others in the group and even using threatening expressions to prevent others from expressing themselves freely. When contradicted by another member of the group, the aggressive communicator will respond with a "machine-gun" style questioning technique in which they ask multiple questions of the questioner in rapid succession, blocking any attempt for a response.[3]

If the sender's verbal, paraverbal, and nonverbal messages are incongruent (i.e., don't match), the actual message is harder to decode. In such cases, the receiver tends to rely on the paraverbal and nonverbal messages. It is relatively easy for people to lie with words, but paraverbal and nonverbal communication tend to be unconscious and more difficult to control.

For example, the nurse suspects that the mother of a newborn infant may be experiencing postpartum depression. The nurse asks the mother how she feels about her new baby. The mother responds in a quiet, very slow monotone (paraverbal message), "I'm so happy I have this baby" (verbal message), while looking down at her feet in a slouched-over posture with her arms folded (nonverbal message). The mother's verbal, paraverbal, and nonverbal communication are incongruent. The words she uses indicate she is happy, but the paraverbal and nonverbal signs indicate that she is sad and depressed. The observant nurse concludes that more assessment for depression is required.

FACTORS THAT AFFECT COMMUNICATION

People are always communicating something, verbally, paraverbally, or through body language, and there is often a degree of overlap among the three. Some of the things people do and say help build communication, but other actions or words break communication down. Anything done or said that interferes with communication is called a *communication blocker*. Actions and speech that encourage and build communication are called *communication builders* and are often referred to as *therapeutic communication techniques*. Other factors, such as the environment the communication is taking place in, stress levels of the parties communicating, and the emotional states of the sender and receiver can also block effective communication.[7]

A simple mnemonic, or memory aid, to facilitate communication is SOLER:

- Sit **s**quarely
- Use **o**pen posture
- **L**ean in slightly toward the patient
- Maintain **e**ye contact
- **R**elax[8]

Nonverbal Communication

Nonverbal communication is the transmission of messages by body language, facial expressions, gestures, personal space, and body position. Successful decoding of nonverbal communication depends on the receiver's ability to observe and evaluate the clues that are being presented all the time whether the person is aware of it or not. Nonverbal communication provides valuable information about the person or people in the group, such as how they might be feeling that day, how the sender's message is being accepted, or what might be a better method in approaching the group. Developing the skill of being observant and interpreting nonverbal commination signs is very useful for nurses in dealing with patients, other nurses, and even physicians.[8] For example, the nurse manager is attempting to present to the staff nurses a new method for changing dressings on chest tubes. While explaining the use of the new type of packaged dressing, the manager looks up at the group and observes that most of the faces are frowning and have furrowed brows with tight lips. The manager should stop at this point because, although the group has not said anything, their nonverbal communication is that they either confused by the explanation or annoyed with the proposed change. The manager should say something like, "I can see that there may be some questions about this procedure and why we are changing it. I'd like to hear your thoughts."

Nonverbal Communication Builders

Eye contact. In general, in North American culture, using eye contact while communicating is a sign of interest in the person and what they are saying. However, there is a need to be cautious using it. Eye contact can turn into a staring contest that says, "I'm trying to dominate you." And eye contact has other meanings and uses in other cultures. Some indigenous peoples believe that direct eye contact is an attempt to take the other person's spirit. In other groups, direct eye contact may be seen as a sign of hostility and aggression or as a sexual invitation.

Stop what you're doing. Paying attention to the other person indicates that they are more important than the task you were doing and encourages better communication. Putting the smartphone down and turning it off is important for the health-care provider to build trust in communication.

Nod the head. Nodding while the other person is speaking indicates you are listening closely to what is said and that you either agree with the person or accept what they are saying. Shaking the head can also be used as a communication builder if it is used when the person is describing a difficult situation they have experienced.

Positive facial expressions. Smiling or looking surprised at appropriate times while the other person is speaking indicates that what the other person is saying is being accepted. The eyes are often the most expressive part of the face, indicating joy, approval, excitement, or sadness.

Sitting or standing in close proximity. Being relatively close to the person speaking shows that they have your full attention and actually makes speaking easier. Leaning toward the speaker also achieves this purpose. However, this technique should be used with some caution. Violating a person's **personal space** (about 18 to 24 inches in North America) may make the person feel uncomfortable. If they back away, then you are too close. Personal space also has a cultural component. People from some regions and cultures require a larger personal space than do people who experience close proximity in their everyday lives and typically require much less personal space.

Open posture, directly facing. An open posture, which means arms and legs are uncrossed and the feet are flat on the floor, while directly facing the speaker, says, "I am open to what you are saying—your thoughts are important to me."[9]

Listening empathically. Pay attention to the emotional content of the message. When the speaker attends and responds to the person's emotions, the person feels heard and understood at a deep level.

Light touch. Touching the other person's shoulder, arm, or hand, particularly if they are communicating sadness, distress, or grief, can send a message of reassurance; however, be cautious using touch as a communication technique. Touch should be used only to express support, comfort, and positive emotions.[9] Cultural taboos, power differentials between the toucher and the person being touched, as well as individual preferences, influence how a touch can be interpreted or misinterpreted. Male caregivers need to

be extremely careful using any sort of physical contact with women. Many Americans simply dislike being touched by people they do not know well.

Paraverbal Communication

Paraverbal (paralingual) communication is the transmission of a message through the nonverbal or nonlanguage elements of speech. These include the rapidity, pitch, inflection, cadence, volume, and more of speech. Similar to nonverbal messages, paraverbal communication requires the listener to pay close attention to these clues in order to understand the whole message.[9] Because it places stronger weight on the way a person sends their messages, paraverbal communication emphasizes the production rather than the content of the words or messages. Because it is formed in the subconscious part of the brain of the speaker where there is less control over its production, it tends to be more honest than the verbal communication of the same person. Paraverbal communication includes the collection of all the signs involved in a person's voice intonation such as the way a person controls or adjusts their voice that makes the sounds produced louder or softer, faster or slower, histrionic or expressive. The speaker who does not have voice intonation sends a message that sounds flat and monotonous, causing the listeners to lose attention and become tired or bored. Paraverbal communication uses tone, pitch, volume, and the speed of speech to produce an interesting and intelligible message.[9]

> *When the speaker attends and responds to the person's emotions, the person feels heard and understood at a deep level.*

Paraverbal Communication Builders

Silence. It might seem to contradict the concept of communication, but silence can be a highly effective communication builder. It is said that "nature abhors a vacuum and will try to fill it with something." Silence is a communication vacuum, and most people will not let it go on for more than a few seconds. Waiting for the other person to speak can be very uncomfortable for both parties; however, it provides the speaker with a chance to think about what they intend to say. How long is too long? There really is no "correct" answer to that question, but using a verbal prod such as "Tell me what you are thinking about" can offer the other person an opening to speak.

In addition, skilled speakers can master the use of the sudden pause in their presentations. This is particularly useful in long, technical presentations where listeners have a tendency to lose interest. The pause will cause them to look up and re-engage with the speaker.

Pitch. Pitch is the auditory quality of sound that is based on the number of sound waves that are contained in an interval of one second, called a *cycle per second*. The more waves contained in a one-second cycle, the higher the frequency or pitch. When there are few waves in a one-second cycle, there is a lower frequency or pitch to the sound. If a person is using a higher pitch, it may indicate excitement, anger, anxiety, pain, or distress. For example, when a person is scared or suddenly injured, they may produce a shrill, high-pitched sound. However, a high-pitched voice can also indicate friendliness and cheerfulness, for example, when meeting a relative or friend at the airport.

On the other hand, a lower pitched voice can convey the gravity of the message, the authority of the speaker, trust, and virility. For example, when a father tells a child in a very low-pitched voice, "Pick up your room now!" the child is likely to do as they are told. Research has shown that individuals with deeper voices have more successful careers. When a person with a deep voice speaks, they command more attention than a speaker with a high-pitched voice. The individual with a deep voice does not have to shout to get and maintain the attention of coworkers because their voice conveys that they are the leader.[11]

By relaxing the throat and vocal cords and employing the diaphragm when speaking, a person can change the pitch of their voice, using both high pitch and low pitch, which will maintain listeners' interest.[10] Pitch modulation can take some practice and possibly a voice coach.

Tone. Tone mixes a number of different pitches (inflections) to give the speaker's messages meaning. Speaking with multiple inflections in the voice prevents the message from sounding monotonous, dull, or flat. The mood of the speaker's message can also be shaped and built by the tone of their voice. A soft, gentle tone produces a mood of calmness and relaxation; whereas, when the speaker talks in a severe or harsh tone, it may produce a mood of anxiety or fear. A measured tone with multiple appropriate inflections will best engage the listener in the presentation.[3]

When communicating with agitated or hostile individuals who are speaking loudly or aggressively, a calm, soothing tone, in particular, can ease the situation. It is important not to respond to a loud or aggressive individual in kind. A calm, even tone conveys the message that the speaker is in control of the situation and that the person who is upset also needs to gain control of their emotions. An assertive tone expresses urgency and a need to respond, particularly in emergency situations. An aggressive or hostile tone usually indicates anger and frustration.[9]

Volume. Volume is the intensity of sound measured in a unit called the *decibel* (dB). The volume of the voice can affect how another person perceives the message. For example, a person who typically speaks in a loud voice (high volume) may cause listeners to become distant and alienated; this type of person is often viewed as domineering or antagonistic. However, it is not unusual for a speaker to increase their volume to stress particular words and thoughts or to convey an increase in emotional intensity. Contrast that to the soft-spoken (low volume) individual who may be interpreted as shy or timid. Listeners quickly lose interest in that person's presentation because they cannot hear the speaker. However, using a sudden decrease in speech volume is a technique speakers use to add suspense or sustain attention in the presentation.[12]

A speaker who can regulate their volume to meet the needs of the listeners will encourage meaningful communication and demonstrate that they are an effective interpersonal communicator. Also, the volume of speech should mirror the nature of the message. If the building is on fire, the speaker's message "FIRE!" would be made with a loud volume and a high-pitched tone.

One technique to use when speaking to a larger group is to outwardly project the voice rather than just raising the volume. Projection means supporting the voice with more breath, which comes from the use of the diaphragm in speaking, not from the upper airway. This method is used by trained singers. Effective speakers project to those in the back row rather than just audience members in the front row. This helps the speaker develop a strong voice that contains nuances of tone and pitch rather than just loudness.[13]

Volume, pitch, and tone are often used together to transmit a message. Using the example of the building being on fire, the person transmitting the message is probably yelling, which is a combination of loud volume, high pitch, and a severe tone. Listeners are not likely to ignore or misunderstand the message. Contrast that to the speech of a severely depressed patient, which is very low volume, almost to the point of being inaudible, and very low pitched with a quiet, cool tone. It requires well-developed listening skills to hear the message the patient is sending.

Verbal Communication

Verbal communication is the use of spoken and written language to send information to a listener or reader. Verbal communication skills include speaking and writing abilities and the delivery and reception of messages both spoken and written. Verbal communication skills are important because they enable a person to build relationships with other people through positive interactions. These skills allow a person to convey a sense of self-assurance and enable the group to better understand the information that is being relayed. When a person communicates plainly, it helps them succeed in a variety of situations, such as interacting with groups, giving instructions, relaying information, sharing project developments, negotiating, and interviewing for jobs.[13]

Verbal Communication Builders

Speaking clearly. Good articulation occurs when a speaker talks with their jaws and lips open so that each sound that is made is clear and crisp. Speakers who are in the habit of talking through clenched teeth or with little movement of their lips are difficult to understand. They may also become inaudible because the sounds they are making stay in their mouths rather than being projected to the listener. It is important to enunciate the ends of words clearly; however, in certain regions of the country, particularly the deep south, dropping the ends of words is common.[13]

Encouraging words. Short responses or interjections, such as "Okay," "Right," "Mmm-hmm," and "Tell me more," say to the speaker, "I'm paying attention," and encourage them to keep talking.

Asking open-ended questions. These are questions that cannot be answered by a simple yes or no or by one- or two-word answers. They encourage the person to continue speaking. Examples include questions such as "What is this person doing that makes you feel inferior?" and requests such as "Tell me about what made you angry" and "Describe the situation in which you felt anxious."

Use "I" rather than "You" messages. People are less likely to perceive a communication as a personal attack when the conversation begins with an explanation of a personal view of the situation or even how feelings were affected. An example of an "I" message is, "I had a hard time hearing the ED nurse's report because you were humming so loudly." The same meaning conveyed as a "you" message might look like this: "You made it hard for me to hear the report with your loud humming!"

Asking clarification questions. This type of question seeks more information and helps the speaker elaborate upon what they have already said. Questions such as "Could you explain that a little more? I didn't quite get what you were saying" and "I'm a little confused about your last statement. Can you give me an example?" are nonconfrontational and make the person feel that you really desire to understand.

Reflecting feelings and emotions. This response should be used when there is a mismatch between what the person is saying and what their body language is saying. Always believe the body language; it cannot lie. Reflection often combines observations and questions such as "You say you feel fine, but there are tears in your eyes, and your voice is shaking. Are you feeling sad?" and "Does talking about that make you angry? I notice that your jaws and hands are clenched."

Verbal modeling. This is a method of communication in which the listener duplicates the tone, pitch, and volume of the person who is speaking in a one-to-one "normal" conversation. For example, when talking with a person who is speaking softly with a lower volume, the listener in turn speaks softly with a low volume. If a person is excited and expressing higher energy, the speaker should try to match it. People are attracted to voices that sound like theirs, making verbal modeling a useful way to increase engagement of the listener. Of course, this method should not be used with people who are displaying an abnormal level of suppressed speech, such as in depression, or over-heightened excitement and anger.[13]

Repeating what was just said. This communication builder is called *restating* and shows that the listener is paying attention to what is being said. Lead into the statement with "Let me know if I heard you correctly. You just said. . . ." Restating indicates good listening skills and helps keep the conversation going. But be cautious! Overuse of this technique can sound artificial and parrotlike. Paraphrasing, or restating in your own words, what the person just said is a good alternative.

Limit interruptions. There is always a tendency to identify with the speaker's recounting of an incident and interject a statement such as "I had something similar happen to me." The speaker does not want to hear about your problems. Just let them continue speaking.

Reviewing what was said and verifying understanding. This is different from repeating because rather than just repeating word-for-word what the person said, it requires analysis and synthesis of the key points and emotions of the discussion, which are then summarized in statements such as "Okay, we've been talking for a while, and it seems like you have said that you are anxious because so-and-so keeps saying to you. . . . Is that an accurate summary?"

Acknowledging what was said. Sometimes called *validating the speaker*, this communication builder makes the speaker feel that what they are saying has value and that someone cares. This technique is especially useful when the listener's perception or opinion differs from the speaker's, for example, when a patient experiencing a psychotic episode describes monsters that only they can see. Statements such as "I understand what you are saying" and "I can appreciate that you feel frightened of what you are seeing" validate the speaker. It is important to distinguish between validating the speaker and validating the content of what they are saying.

Environmental Communication Builders

Calm, nonthreatening environment. A quiet room with subdued lighting is the ideal location to help build communication. In communicating with a group, the room should be large enough to comfortably accommodate everyone with good lighting, a comfortable room temperature, and chairs for all. However, in the real world, a busy, noisy hospital room or hallway is more likely to be the environment for communication about important issues such as home medications and dressing changes. Nurses, as always, are required to do the best they can with what they have.

Blockers (Barriers) to Communication

Being able to recognize and understand blockers or barriers to good communication is a key part of being able to communicate successfully. Failures in communication in the health-care setting are not only unfortunate but can endanger the life of the patient. Communication blockers can be present in the sender of the message or the receiver of the message or both

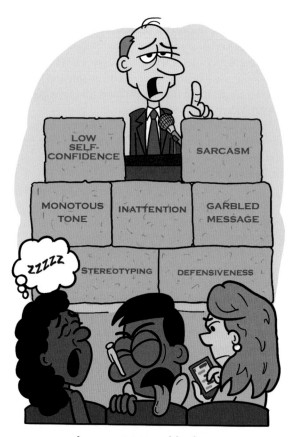

Communication blockers can ruin a presentation.

at the same time.[14] Communication blockers can exist in all three elements of communication, nonverbal, paraverbal, or verbal.

Nonverbal Communication Blockers

Eye rolling. When people roll their eyes, they are sending a message of not caring about what the other person is saying. Teens are notorious for this behavior, but adults also do it, particularly if it has become habitual.

Arm and leg crossing. This generally is interpreted as an indication of disapproval or boredom. The person listening is closed to the speaker's ideas, which are not considered very important. It sometimes can be a sign that the person whose arms or legs are crossed is feeling attacked and is trying to defend themselves.

Slouching, hunching, turning away. These nonverbal communication blockers indicate that the listener is just not interested in what is being said. It says to the speaker, "Are we done yet? I'd rather be on the other side of the room."

Fidgeting. This includes picking at fingernails, drumming the fingers, playing with buttons or jewelry, frequent shifting in the chair, rolling and unrolling hair, taking off and putting on glasses frequently, doodling extensively on a pad of paper, frequent checking of cell phone, picking at shoe laces, and so on. It delivers the message that the listener is experiencing extreme boredom and cannot wait to leave.

Deep, loud sighs. This message tells the other person that they are boring and should end the conversation quickly. What the person has to say is not worth the time it takes to say it, and there are other more productive things to be done with the time.

Multiple watch or clock checks. Like deep sighs, clock-watching indicates that the listener perceives what the person is saying is not important and that the listener is about to die from boredom.

Continuing with an activity while the other person is talking. The message is, "I'm ignoring you because you are not that important. What I'm doing is more important." Fiddling with cell phones or other electronic devices is a very common continuation of an activity. Nurses who use portable devices such as laptop computers or tablets in the patient's room to document should place the device to the side rather than right in front of the patient, blocking their view of the nurse. Documenting on these devices can be done while still facing the patient and even sharing information with them. If the computer is a permanent part of the room, it is likely located in a place where the nurse must turn their back to the patient. The nurse should let the patient know that they are going to be documenting on the computer, but if the patient needs to say something, the nurse is still listening.

Failure to make eye contact. This nonverbal technique can be used as a way to show disapproval but is often used when a person is hurt by another and is trying to hurt the person back. Again, cell phones are a major culprit in producing this blocker. Conversely, an excessively long, unblinking stare is a communication blocker that shows aggression and hostility.

Tuning out or failing to pay attention. Withholding or withdrawing attention is another way of saying, "I'm not listening—what you are saying isn't important."[6]

Verbal Communication Blockers

Differences of language. If the two people who are trying to communicate do not speak the same language, communication becomes extremely difficult if not totally blocked. Some uses of hand gestures and signals may transmit basic information, but gestures have limited effectiveness. Use of a medical translator or interpreter is essential to convey important information. Translators translate only words that are being exchanged. Interpreters also translate but add additional information about the person's mood or underlying meaning.

Automatic defensiveness. This communication blocker occurs when one person feels so threatened by the other that the first thing they say is of a defensive nature. For example, "It wasn't my fault; the thing just broke," "I really didn't want to do it, but Alexis made me," or "If you didn't push me so hard to speak, I never would have said it."

Asking closed-ended questions. These are questions that a person can answer in one or two words. For example, "Are you feeling better today?" Answer: "No." "Did you practice your responses like we discussed?" Answer: "Yes."

Accusing or blaming. This is a type of confrontational speech and sends the message that the other person is wrong even before given a chance to provide their side of the story. For example, "If you knew how to read a map, we wouldn't be lost in the middle of nowhere."

Making assumptions about meaning. Similar to accusing, confusing inferences with realities blocks the ability to convey the truth in communication. Nurses and other health-care providers have a tendency to assume, based on past experiences, that they know or understand the reasons that underlie the patient's complaint or that there is a causal relationship between certain observations and outcomes. It is important to obtain all the information possible before making a decision. After a complete assessment, and only then, should the health-care provider begin to interpret evidence. For example, a 7-year-old is examined and found to have bruising on her arms and legs. Previous examinations have never shown any type of bruising or injury, and the child is in otherwise good health. The health-care provider assumes that the child is being abused, accuses the parents of child abuse, and wants to call law enforcement. However, further testing shows that the child has an autoimmune disorder called Henoch-Schoenlein purpura, the primary symptom of which is bruising on the extremities.

Unclear message. Using abstract and overly formal language may obscure the information and message being transmitted. The use of colloquialisms, especially with nonnative speakers of English, may cause the listener to confuse the message or miss it altogether. Nurses and other health-care workers tend to use medical jargon that the listener may or may not understand.

Dysfunctional responses. Effective communication is quickly blocked when one party discounts or fails to respond to information that is being provided by the other. It makes the speaker feel irrelevant or unworthy. Similarly, responding to a speaker with a comment that does not relate to what the speaker is talking about will repress open communication. For example, if the patient reports, "When I stand up quickly, I become dizzy," the response, "Your ankles seem to be swollen," from the health-care provider would appear unrelated.

Using sarcasm. This sends the message that the other person is not respected and is untrustworthy. The statements are often said in a taunting tone with vocal overemphasis. For example, a coworker's music is audible through their ear buds. You comment, "Why don't you turn it up a little? I don't think they can hear it in Toronto!"

Constant interruptions. Over the years, some people have developed a habit of interrupting without any sort of malice or intent to hurt. However, the message is the same whether it is intentional or not—the person interrupting feels that what they have to say is more important than what the speaker is saying. Taking time-outs to answer a cell phone also interrupts the flow and meaning of the communication. It is important to allow the speaker to finish speaking before trying to interpret what they are saying; otherwise, the listener receives only part of the message. For example, a patient says to the nurse, "I started having pain in my chest three days ago when . . ."; the nurse interrupts with, "Why did you wait so long? You could be having a heart attack!"

Judging, name calling, and diagnosing. This communication blocker uses "you" messages, indicating that there is something wrong with the other person. These blockers also send the message that the person making the judgment or diagnosis is more intelligent and has a better understanding than the person with the problem. It denotes an air of superiority. It includes statements such as "You're such a perfectionist—no wonder you don't have any friends," "You don't seem to understand that we need to finish the project on time," "You know what your problem is?" "You really don't care if this issue gets resolved," "You made a mistake," "You said this about me," and "You always do this."

> *The use of colloquialisms, especially with nonnative speakers of English, may cause the listener to confuse the message or miss it altogether.*

Stating opinions as proven facts. This communication blocker prevents the other person from expressing their opinion because it discounts the importance of any evidence the person might use to support that opinion. For example, someone who lacks knowledge about the Affordable Care Act might say, "Everybody knows that the ACA created **death panels** to decide who is going to get care and who will be left to die."

Making absolute statements, being patronizing, and offering vague reassurances. Absolute statements weaken their own lucidity and reliability because nothing is absolute. When attempting to explain complex concepts or conditions, although the use of absolute statements may be easier, they do not relay accurate information. Explaining things in either black or white terms, called *polarization* or *either-or*, can reduce the complexity of the explanation but does not always provide the full picture. For example, statements such as "You always leave the break room in a mess" or "I can either change your linens now, or you can stay in the dirty ones all day" are inaccurate absolutes. In a similar way, patronization tends to oversimplify complex situations or events by reducing the accuracy of the information being conveyed. For example, "You just rest now and let us worry about the medical stuff." Vague reassurances can make the other person feel that what they have to say is not important. For example, "It always works out for the best, doesn't it?"[16]

Stereotyping. A stereotype is a form of generalization about a particular group or class of people. Stereotypes can be either positive or negative. Positive stereotypes about Americans with a Scandinavian ethnic background, for example, might be that they are generous, hardworking, fastidious about cleanliness, physically fit, friendly, outgoing, and optimistic. However, not all Scandinavian Americans have these characteristics, and some have less-desirable ones.

Negative stereotypes such as laziness, lack of intelligence, criminality, aggression, and alcohol abuse have been attributed to certain groups on the basis of their gender, race, religion, or physical traits. Research has shown that patients whom health-care workers stereotype are less likely to follow medical instructions and more likely to mistrust their doctors and other health-care providers.[17] Because of the mistrust

that has developed, they also tend to avoid accessing early or preventive care such as annual physical examinations, vaccines for preventable illnesses, and dental and eye examinations. It is important for nurses to remember that people are total and entire persons and not just a caricature of a type.

Telling people how they should feel. This invalidates the other person's feelings and shows a high degree of disrespect. These types of statements include "Don't feel like that," "Don't let that bother you," and "Getting upset is very childish."

Lacking self-confidence. Shyness, lack of assertiveness, or low self-esteem all can become communication blockers. They may hamper the speaker's ability to express their concerns and thoughts. Although health-care providers usually do not have this difficulty, patients often do. Because they are in a strange place and a dependent position, patients often feel overpowered by their environment and tend to regress to a less assertive mode of behavior and communication. Health-care providers knowledgeable in communication skills will recognize this manner in the patient and use measures to increase feelings of comfort and well-being.

Changing the subject. This can block communication by indicating that what the person is saying is not important and not worth listening to.

Expecting mind reading. Sometimes other people expect the nurse to know what they are thinking or to anticipate what they need or are going to say. People who have been very close for a long period of time sometimes get to a point in their relationship where they know the other person well enough to "mind read" (actually, anticipate) what they are going to say. However, for the vast majority of communication, telling the other person what you are thinking, feeling, or wishing them to do is the best approach.

Shaking or pointing a finger while speaking. This combines both verbal and nonverbal blockers. Much like yelling and getting too close to someone, it is an exercise of power over the other person. The message is, "You really are stupid and inferior."

Walking away. This is the ultimate communication blocker. If there is no one to talk to, there is no communication.

Paraverbal Communication Blockers

Threatening, ordering, or menacing. The message here is, "I'm angry and I don't care what you think." People often use "clenched-teeth speech" or increase the volume of their speech when being confrontational. It threatens other people and makes them keep their distance. Some people who use these blockers are deeply insecure and use these techniques to push other people away. Other individuals may resort to using threats or menacing behaviors out of frustration or pain. They also use them to make themselves feel better about themselves. It takes away the need to understand the other person.

Yelling, calling names, or hurling insults. This is a type of aggressive behavior that is immature and degrading. It shows a lack of respect for the other person and often creates deep emotional wounds. Yelling and name-calling can quickly rise to the level of physical violence such as pushing or even hitting.

Nonstop, rapid talking. When people say, "I couldn't get a word in edgewise!" it means that the other person totally dominated the conversation. Often, the speaker is attempting to avoid confrontation, stress, intimacy, uncomfortable thoughts or feelings, or a difficult situation. In some people, it can become a habit over time and shows disrespect to other people. It may also be an attempt for the speaker to hide feelings of inferiority by showing how intelligent or dominant they are.[7]

Message overload. This barrier occurs when the listener attempts to manage an excessive amount of information being put forth by the speaker. At some point, the brain of the listener has difficulty separating the unimportant from the important in what the speaker is presenting. Attempting to process excessive information produces mental fatigue and exhaustion, ultimately causing the listener to feel helpless and to give up listening altogether. The greater the feeling of being overwhelmed listeners experience, the less effort they are willing to put in to understanding the message.[14]

Different communication styles. This is a more subtle communication blocker that occurs when the speaker and listener have different styles of verbal communication. Individuals use different styles of communication often based on their ethnicity, upbringing, and geographical location.[16] Sometimes a person is so rooted in their particular way of speaking that they find it difficult to exchange information with others who use a style different from theirs. For example, some people are very direct and straightforward when they have something to say, while others use an indirect approach with small talk and talking around the topic for a while. People with a more technical or scientific orientation like to use detailed data and facts, sometimes called "getting into the weeds." Other people rely on sweeping, inclusive statements and generalities that encompass the information. Lack of specificity can cause the listener to lose interest and miss the message.

> *Sometimes a person is so rooted in their particular way of speaking that they find it difficult to exchange information with others who use a style different from theirs.*

Learning disabilities. *Learning disabilities* is a general term that is used to describe a number of more explicit disabilities. These disabilities may be genetic and/or neurobiological from injuries that modify brain operation in a way that affects one or more intellectual processes associated with learning. Individuals with learning disabilities may have difficulty speaking, reading, and/or writing. They may also have difficulties with higher-level skills such as problem-solving, organization, time planning, abstract reasoning, long- or short-term memory, and attention.[19]

Learning disabilities can affect an individual's life in many ways, including in their interpersonal relationships, work, and social settings. Many individuals with relatively mild learning disabilities may never be diagnosed and may spend their lives not knowing why they cannot keep jobs or maintain social relationships. These disabilities generally cannot be fixed or cured and are lifelong challenges for people who have them.[19] However, people with learning disabilities can achieve success in their life endeavors with proper support and interventions. Learning disabilities can range

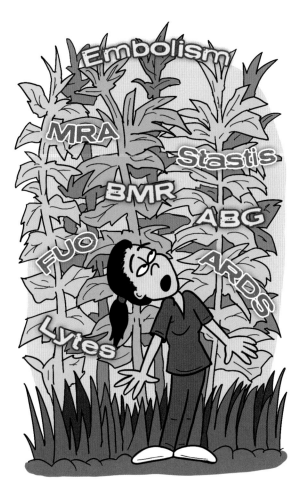

**Nurses tend to get in
the weeds with terminology.**

because of their inability to communicate verbally. Others may be unable to comprehend information that is given to them in written form or verbally. These barriers to communication can affect their health and well-being.[19]

Depending on the type of learning disability or problem a patient has, the nurse may need creativity in communicating with them. Some techniques increase the odds of success. Talking to the person one to one and face to face in a quiet space is often the preferred method, but check with them first to make sure it is acceptable to them. If communicating in writing, use black ink and large text. Try drawing a picture. Most people find it less difficult to understand objects, photos, and pictures.

Ask open-ended questions and check frequently that the person understands what you say. Confirm your understanding of what they are trying to communicate, such as "You said your head has been hurting, right?" If the patient wants you to go someplace or show you something, go with them. They may not be able to find the correct words for what they want you to see. Pay very close attention to their body language, facial expressions, eyes, and nonverbal responses. The speaker should use their own body language and facial expressions to reinforce or get a message across. Allow adequate time for communication.[20] This interaction is a learning experience on both sides. Having the same nurse care for the patient each day, if possible, allows for trust to develop and for the nurse to learn incrementally how to communicate with this person. It also alleviates the patient's stress in having to communicate effectively with multiple nurses.

Environmental (Physical) Communication Blockers

Wearing a mask. Since the COVID-19 pandemic, the wearing of masks by health-care providers has become almost universal; however, masks can be a major communication blocker. Masks muffle the voice of the speaker. Similar to what many people with hearing loss experience, masks decrease the speaker's volume, lower their pitch, and soften their tone, especially regarding consonants that often start and end words. These factors decrease the listener's understanding of words. If a person already has a hearing loss, the barriers become even worse.[18]

from dyslexia and dysgraphia to oral/written language disorder and specific reading comprehension deficit. Attention deficit-hyperactivity disorder (ADHD) and autism spectrum disorder (ASD) are not in and of themselves learning disabilities, but they can hamper classroom learning and social development.

Learning problems are different from learning difficulties and are primarily the result of visual, hearing, or motor impairments. Other learning problems are related to intellectual disability caused by emotional disorders, poor environmental background, cultural peculiarities, or economic hindrances.[19]

Some individuals with learning problems or difficulties may have difficulty expressing what they need

A normal response by a speaker to a person who has trouble hearing or understanding is to increase the voice volume, yell, or repeat the message again and again. These methods do not help in the vast majority of cases and only produce feeling of helplessness of frustration on both the speaker's and listener's parts. Several methods help increase the likelihood of success in communication when wearing a mask. Clearly enunciate and pronounce the beginnings and endings of words while speaking slowly to diminish the muffling effect of the mask. Increase voice volume a little to get past the mask's barrier. Asking the listener which part they missed or did not understand and then rephrasing that part often works well. It helps the listener focus on what was actually missed instead of listening to the whole message again. Wearing a mask with a transparent mouth window allows people with hearing disabilities to see the mouth and read facial expressions and the speaker's lips. Looking directly at the listener and giving them the speaker's complete attention lets them know that the speaker is focused on their needs.

Technology, if available, can help. Using text apps and e-tools such as *Google Live Transcribe* that write on a listener's cellphone what is being said allows for more clarity in messaging. Another useful app is the *Simply Sayin'* medical jargon app for kids. Created by Phoenix Children's Hospital, this app uses pictures, sounds, and a glossary of terms to facilitate clear conversations about conditions, treatments. and medical or health-care-related experiences. Patients with hearing aids can use the iPhone feature *Live Listen* to bring the speaker's voice literally into their ears. However, at all times, the speaker wearing a mask needs to be aware of their speech patterns and linguistics when attempting to communicate.[18]

Background noise. Effective communication is reduced when the speaker is trying to get a message across in a noisy environment. For example, on a busy hospital unit, the noise level can be very high, especially during the day shift. This background noise might cause a stressed nurse to misinterpret a physician's verbal message concerning the dosage of a medication to give to a patient. Because effective communication between the nurse and the physician was blocked by noise, the patient would receive the wrong dose of a medication, resulting in injury or possible death.[14]

Physical space. The room in which the communication occurs can serve as a communication blocker. Rooms that are too small for the number of people who are in them limit the ability to talk and alter communication. For example, "report rooms," where nurses exchange information about patients between shifts, are notoriously too small so that the nurses are packed in without enough chairs. The nurses standing or sitting on radiators or other structures in the room are physically uncomfortable and have trouble hearing the report giver and taking notes. Some facilities make nursing assignments ahead of time and then have the nurses report to each other at the doors of the patients' rooms. Small rooms combined with poor lighting and uncomfortable chairs make the listeners exasperated and annoyed. If the physical discomfort is high enough, they may just walk out.[15]

Conversely, when individuals who are trying to communicate are too far apart, they may have difficulty hearing each other. A person who intentionally maintains an excessive distance from another may transmit a sense of mistrust. However, in the age of COVID-19, maintaining what would otherwise seem to be an excessive distance has become the norm. Increasing the volume and projection of speech is a necessity to overcome the distance.

Experiencing change. Change can be a communication blocker in various ways. People may be afraid to ask questions about new procedures or policies because they fear that they might appear "stupid" in front of their colleagues. Fear of being criticized closes individuals off to positive suggestions and new ideas.[3] Others may hesitate in sharing ideas because they are afraid of being labeled as confrontational. Nurses also need to keep in mind that the communication abilities of patients experiencing change will be blocked in much the same way as those of nurses experiencing change.

> " *A normal response by a speaker to a person who has trouble hearing or understanding is to increase the voice volume, yell, or repeat the message again and again.* "

For example, a nurse is reassigned from the medical-surgical unit to the intensive care unit (ICU). This nurse will initially be somewhat fearful in the new environment with the highly trained and assertive expert unit nurses who always seem to be in control. A more positive approach would be for the new nurse to take advantage of the unit nurses' experience and learn from their examples. The new nurse needs to remember that everyone on that unit was a novice at one time. In the current health-care system, almost everyone is fearful much of the time of making mistakes and of not being able to meet the high standards of the profession.

Grief experiences. Most patients who have surgical procedures that result in major body function alterations go through the stages of the grief process: denial, anger, guilt, depression, and resolution. Communication with a patient in the anger stage who is hostile, critical of their care, and verbally abusive is very different from communication with a patient in the depression stage, who is withdrawn, reticent, and sleeps most of the time. Recognition of the communication-blocking mechanisms of each grief stage is essential to understanding why patients are acting in a particular way. A decision must then be made regarding the most effective communication technique to use when providing care (see Chapter 12 for a more detailed discussion).

Stressful situations. Stress is an environmental blocker that is produced by many factors and always affects an individual's ability to communicate. Some common causes of stress for health-care workers include institutional restructuring, group interaction and dynamics, unilateral management decisions, and personal issues and experiences. Regardless of the source, stress usually decreases people's ability to interact and communicate and increases the demands on their coping mechanisms.[8]

Policy change. Health-care reform is raising many questions about the health-care system and the delivery of care.[9] The changes produced by these transitions create a high degree of stress at all levels of the health-care system. Change and stress are major barriers to effective communication.[10] Some techniques to alleviate the stress of change include

- Active participation of the whole team in planning and implementing change.

- Open and interactive lines of communication.
- Avoiding rumors, outbursts, feelings of insecurity, and fear.

Tension and anxiety. When people are unable to successfully cope with a stressful situation, they may experience an increased state of tension or anxiety. Tense or anxious people are even more difficult to communicate with than people under stress. They may develop physiological symptoms, such as nausea, stomach cramps, diarrhea, or palpitations; in extreme cases, they may even become paranoid or psychotic. Uncontrolled high levels of stress on a nursing unit may lead to competition among the nurses that affects their teamwork, productivity, and the quality of the care given.[10]

Health-care providers who are stressed by worry about a severely ill patient or threats to their autonomy, practice, and income from changes in reimbursement policies may become tense and highly critical of or even verbally abusive toward nurses. The hospital management may also experience increased stress owing to the escalating responsibility of maintaining high-quality services with ever-shrinking revenues. Management often deals with its stress by becoming more autocratic, making increased demands on the nursing staff while reducing the control that nurses have over their practice and becoming closed off to input from nurses and physicians.

What Do You Think?

List four factors or situations that have produced high levels of stress for you in the hospital or health-care setting. Why did these incidents produce stress? How did you deal with the stress?

Stress is a major contributing factor to a variety of disorders, ranging from high blood pressure to ulcers and anxiety. In the health-care environment, stress is not experienced only by health-care providers. Stress for patients starts when they first come into contact with the health-care system; peaks when they have to undergo physical examinations, surgery, or invasive treatments; and continues throughout the recovery period. The fear that a nurse may not respond to patients' needs increases patients' stress levels, and they sometimes become more demanding of care, which in turn increases the nurse's stress levels.[21] If the nursing staff is experiencing high stress levels, patients often sense this subconsciously, and as a result, patients' stress levels also increase.

Techniques to Reduce Stress

Several techniques can be used to reduce patients' stress levels so that they can better communicate and become more receptive to teaching. Stress-reduction techniques range from very simple measures that everyone can use, such as distraction with music or simple activities, exercise, or reduction in stimuli, to more advanced techniques such as meditation, **biofeedback**, and even antianxiety medications.

Eliminate the Situation

Nurses need to be able to identify situations that produce stress, recognize the symptoms shown by someone in a stressful situation, know how to reduce stress, and be able to use appropriate communication techniques with someone under stress.

Of course, if possible, the best way to reduce stress is to eliminate the stressful situation. Consider the following case:

> The hospital management sent a memo to all the hospital units that a new patient-assessment form it has developed is to be implemented next week. This new form is in addition to the ones that the nurses already fill out each day. It is to be completed by RNs only and must be done each shift on every patient and then sent to the house supervisor so that management can track acuity. Because of recent facility restructuring and changes in staffing patterns, often there is only one RN on the 3 p.m. to 11 p.m. and 11 p.m. to 7 a.m. shifts to cover a 42-bed unit. This extra, time-consuming, and seemingly redundant paperwork increases the stress of the staff RNs to an unacceptable level.

Issues in Practice

Managing Change

The busy nonacute outpatient unit at a large hospital had become disorganized. It consistently received evaluations of "poor" when patients were asked about the care being provided. They often complained about the long waits to be evaluated and treated. The staff also recognized the problems with the care they were providing but did not have any solutions.

In an attempt to improve the evaluations, the administration replaced the director with a new director from an even larger facility across town. She was charged with the task of improving patient care and was promised that she would have whatever resources she needed.

Within 6 months, the new director completely reorganized the staffing patterns and modernized all the information systems using the latest software. She replaced old equipment with new models and bought additional equipment that the unit had never used before. She also expanded and brightened up the unit by remodeling extensively and by securing unused space from the radiology department, which occupied adjacent rooms. She increased the salaries of the nursing staff, hired new nurses, and expanded the hours of service. She implemented a "management by objectives" model for evaluation that allowed the staff nurses increased input into their working conditions and evaluations.

Patient surveys indicated an increase in overall satisfaction with the care being provided; the wait time had been decreased to a point at which there were hardly any complaints. However, approximately half the experienced nurses on the unit resigned, and the rest of the nurses began the process of organizing into a *collective bargaining unit* for the first time in the history of the nonacute outpatient unit.

Questions for Thought

1. What was the underlying issue that led to the nurses' responses to the changes?
2. What could the director have done to increase the staff's acceptance of change?

(Answers are found at the end of the chapter.)

They meet as a group with management and propose that the assessment forms they are already using be modified to include the data that management wants on the new forms. Copies of the revised form could then be downloaded by the unit clerk for each shift and given to the supervisors, thus eliminating the new form. Management notes the high stress levels of the RNs, recognizes that increased stress lowers the quality of care, and decides to follow the RNs' proposal, thus eliminating the primary source of the RNs' stress.

Although all sources of stress cannot be eliminated completely, in most situations they can be reduced to a manageable level. However, high stress levels should never be used as an excuse for destructive anger and behaviors, failure of communication, or abuse of individuals.

Anger

People who are angry almost always find it difficult, if not impossible, to successfully communicate; as such, anger is one of the environmental communication blockers, much like stress. However, because anger is also key in understanding and dealing with difficult people, is one of the stages of the grief process, and is a symptom of personal frustration, lack of control, fear of change, or feelings of hopelessness, it is discussed here in more length than other communication blockers.

Anger is one of the strong, primitive, natural emotions that help individuals protect themselves against a variety of external threats.[22] Many animals, including humans, that express anger by making loud sounds (yelling or growling), puffing themselves up to appear physically larger, or baring and gritting their teeth and staring intently are warning other possible aggressors to stop their threatening behavior. Physical violence between two people rarely occurs without a warning expression of anger by at least one of the parties. Although everyone experiences anger, how it is expressed often depends on a person's family and ethnic background, life experiences, and personal values. In some cultures, loud and physically expressive outbursts are the norm for the expression of anger, whereas in other cultures, anger is internalized and expressed only as a "controlled rage."

Positive or Negative Expression

As with most of the other factors that affect communication, anger can be either positive or negative.[22] When anger is used in a positive, productive manner, it can promote change and release tension. Anger can be used positively to increase others' attention, initiate communication, problem-solve, and energize the change process. Sensitivity to internal anger can warn individuals that something is wrong either within themselves or with someone or something in the external environment.

Many individuals have difficulty expressing and using their anger in a positive manner. Anger that is used negatively is very destructive. It hinders communication, makes coworkers fearful, and erodes relationships with others. Anger expressed by abusive behaviors, such as pounding on nursing station counters, throwing charts or surgical instruments, having verbal outbursts, or even making violent physical contact, is never acceptable and may lead to civil or criminal action against the perpetrator.

The negative expression of anger may cause the person who is the object of the anger to retaliate or seek revenge, but probably the most destructive form that negative anger can take is when it is internalized and suppressed. Long-term suppressed anger has been associated with a number of physiological and psychological problems, ranging from gastric ulcers and hypertension to myocardial infarctions, strokes, and even psychotic rage episodes.[22]

What Sets People Off

Nurses who understand what makes themselves and others angry are better able to either avoid anger-producing situations or cope effectively with their own anger or with that of others. Taking de-escalation and personal-safety training is essential for all nurses and should be offered as part of the hospital's mandatory continuing education program for employees. When dealing with an angry patient, never let the patient get between yourself and the door. Always have a safe way to exit the room. For example, even new graduate nurses soon learn that some situations will almost always evoke an angry response from hospitalized patients. These include serving meals that are cold or poorly cooked, not answering call lights in a timely manner, waking up soundly sleeping patients at midnight to give them a sleeping pill, or taking multiple attempts to start an IV line. (See Chapter 12 for more detail on angry patients.)

Similarly, unit managers and hospital administrators quickly learn that some of the things they do will almost always produce angry responses from the staff. These actions include unilateral changes in the work schedule, additional paperwork, reduction in staffing levels, and refusal of requests for vacation or time off.[22]

It is important that nurses understand that anger is a normal human emotion. Once it is recognized, it should be dealt with and then let go. Sometimes situations are not going to change, no matter how angry the person becomes, and sometimes no amount of anger will prevent changes from occurring.

What Do You Think?

Consider the health-care providers with whom you have worked in the recent past. What were their communication styles? How did those styles affect the way you communicated with them?

PROBLEM-SOLVING

Underlying the ability to problem-solve is the process of critical thinking. When an individual can mentally process conditions and analyze ideas to reach the anticipated solution, they are thinking critically. Critical thinking requires the ability to determine and evaluate a situation to find the best possible resolution to whatever issue is presented. Because they are interwoven and closely linked to each other, the primary outcome of critical thinking is problem-solving.[23] Problem-solving is the process of delving deeply into issues and questions to reach an improved and more fit resolution or answer. An accomplished problem-solver must possess good analytical skills, good reasoning aptitude, good evaluation ability, and precise decision-making ability. If a person lacks any one of these qualities, they are not going to be a good problem-solver. People who do not think before making decisions or who make quick, erroneous decisions must attempt to explain or defend them later.[23]

Problem-solving is a process that everyone uses frequently. For example, on the way to work, a tire goes flat on a person's car. That is a problem. How the person solves the problem depends on critical-thinking skills, on past experiences, and on physical abilities. If the person with the flat tire is a 250-lb, 33-year-old male construction worker in good health, he most likely has changed tires before and will probably be physically able to remove the flat tire and put on the spare without difficulty. However, if the person with the flat tire is a 90-lb, 67-year-old female church organist, her solution to the problem will likely be different. She will probably call her emergency roadside service and have someone come and change the tire for her.

One of the primary activities for nurses in the work setting is problem-solving using the nursing process. It really does not matter whether the problem is patient centered, management oriented, or an interpersonal issue; the nursing process is an excellent framework for problem resolution. It focuses on the goals of mutual interaction and communication to establish trust and respect. Using the process of assessment, analysis, planning, implementation, and evaluation helps the nurse organize and structure interpersonal interactions in a way that will produce an "I win, you win" situation.[23]

> *Sometimes situations are not going to change, no matter how angry the person becomes, and sometimes no amount of anger will prevent changes from occurring.*

The basic problem-solving steps of the nursing process also form the framework for successful conflict management. Nurses who are good problem-solvers using the nursing process also tend to be good at conflict resolution, and nurses who are good at conflict resolution tend to be excellent problem-solvers. Rather than being avoided in the work setting, conflict should be considered an opportunity to practice and grow in the use of problem-solving skills.[24]

CONFLICT RESOLUTION

Conflict resolution is the informal or formal process used to find a diplomatic solution to a disagreement or dispute between two or more parties. It is almost inevitable that conflict will arise when two or more people are working together. For example, a nurse manager may have to resolve a dispute between two nurses in the unit, or the manager may become angry at some-thing that was said about them in a meeting, or they may be required to settle a conflict between a nurse and a patient over the care being given.[24] Everyone experiences conflict at one time or another as a part of daily life. Often, people feel more comfortable address-ing the conflict that arises in their personal lives than conflicts that arise in the professional setting. Problem-solving is often perceived as less emotional and more structured, whereas conflict management is considered to be more emotionally charged, with the potential to produce hostility. However, the steps of conflict management and problem-solving are almost identical to those of the nursing process. The one additional element that must be included in conflict resolution is the ability to use assertive behaviors and communication when discussing the issues.[24]

Contributing Factors to Conflict

Many things in life con-tribute to conflicts. These can range from a differ-ence of opinion about how a job should be done to major underlying beliefs such as culture, religion, and politics. The focus here is on resolving con-flicts that affect the work environment, primarily emotional issues, insecurity, lack of skills, and diversity issues. Understanding the underlying elements of all types of conflict is a key in preventing and resolving many of the issues.[24]

Understanding what motivates the other person's behavior permits the individual to better appreciate the full scope of the conflict.[24] Conflict is often a symptom of some deeper problem, and the conflict really never gets resolved without dealing with the underlying issues. When individuals are able to sep-arate themselves from the conflict, they are less likely to take things personally and more likely to begin to focus on the underlying issues causing the problems than on the other person's behavior. The interaction becomes less judgmental and threatening to the other person. However, understanding the other person's motives never excuses unacceptable behaviors such as sarcasm, angry outbursts, and abusive language.

> *Conflict is often a symptom of some deeper problem, and the conflict really never gets resolved without dealing with the underlying issues.*

Rather, it allows for direct confrontation of the behav-ior in a more controlled and less emotional way.[23]

Emotions

Emotions and feelings are a primary contributing fac-tor to the development of conflicts. Many people are very sensitive to what others say to them or to threats to their perceived security and react aggressively to demonstrate their hurt feelings.[7]

A common situation that causes conflict is the nurse's feeling of being overworked or overwhelmed by assignments. The overloaded nurse might say, for example, "I have a huge amount of work today. Why isn't anyone helping me?" rather than ask a particular individual for help. Believing another person is, or should be, a mind reader rarely produces the results the person desires. When the person who is expected to help fails to comply with the implied request, the overworked nurse becomes angry and resentful. The other person may not understand where this anger is coming from and often avoids addressing the angry person for fear of making them angrier.[22] This type of poor commu-nication and lack of direct, respectful conflict reso-lution produces tension among workers, deterio-ration of working relationships, decreased efficiency, and, ultimately, lower-quality patient care.

Insecurity and Lack of Skills

Conflicts sometimes arise because people do not know how to deal with them or feel threatened by the thought of confronting another person. Some of the reasons people give for not resolving conflicts before they get out of hand include the following:

- Fear of retaliation
- Fear of ridicule
- Fear of alienating others
- Mistaken belief that they are unable to handle the conflict situation
- Feeling that they do not have the right to speak up
- Past negative experiences with conflict situations
- Family background and experiences
- Lack of education and skills in conflict resolution[23]

Diversity

Diversity simply means that people are different from each other. Cultural diversity is a more complex concept and denotes the cultural differences between races, ethnic groups, professions, and gender sets. Members of one culture often look on people from other cultures in terms of their own values, standards, and social traditions. Cultural diversity is a multifaceted issue that involves many areas of people's lives, including values, life experiences, instinctual responses, learned behaviors, personal strengths and weaknesses, and native abilities or skills.[17] Each time two people interact, they bring the sum total of all these elements into their communication. To communicate effectively, both parties need to first recognize that the other person is different, then understand how these differences affect the communication, and finally accept and build on these differences. (Cultural diversity is discussed in more detail in Chapter 21.)

Diversity Recognition

Conflicts based on diversity issues can be resolved by recognizing the diversity and then using it to promote teamwork, improve communication, and increase productivity. Recognizing diversity helps people better understand each other as well as themselves.[25] The ultimate goal of diversity recognition is to use each individual's strengths rather than emphasize the weaknesses, to build a stronger, more confident, and productive team. For example, consider the following scenario:

> Miguel B. is a nurse in your unit who has a reputation for being a nitpicker. He is constantly judging his peers and criticizing their actions on the basis of his own personal standards. His judgments of others are not well accepted by his coworkers, who try to avoid him as much as possible.
>
> Betty A., another nurse on the unit, always seems to be coming up with ideas for changing things in the unit but then avoids joining the committees that are formed to put the ideas into practice. When she does join a committee, she quickly gets bored and does not follow through

on her responsibilities. The other committee members become angry and frustrated by Betty's behavior. They feel that because it was her idea in the first place, she should work as hard as everyone else to make the change.

> You have been selected as the chairperson for a committee that was formed to design a new patient-care documentation tool. Both Miguel and Betty are on the committee, and the other committee members are upset by their presence. Everyone knows about Miguel's and Betty's personality quirks. As chairperson of the team, you need to draw on everyone's strengths while recognizing their diversities to develop a new, comprehensive, yet easy-to-use form. If you perform well in your chairmanship role, each team member's self-esteem should be enhanced, and the morale of the group should improve.

> *" Unfortunately, members from one culture often look on people from other cultures in relation to their own values, standards, and social traditions. "*

At first glance, these may not seem like diversity issues. However, Miguel is a detail-oriented person, whereas Betty is a visionary. Although their interests and abilities are very diverse, neither one is right or wrong. People who are preoccupied with details are left-brain dominant; creative, visionary individuals are usually right-brain dominant.[22]

Two primary tasks are required to complete the project:

Task 1. Conduct brainstorming sessions with staff members, health-care providers, and ancillary personnel to develop a general concept of what the documentation should include and how the form should look.

Task 2. Work with the print shop to design the specific layout and content of the final form.

As chairperson, you develop the following plan for the development of the new documentation tool.

Task 1. It would be most appropriate to include Betty in the group that directs the brainstorming efforts and collects different ideas. She probably had no preconceived form in mind before starting the process and will feel comfortable investigating and researching a variety of different possibilities. Miguel would have difficulty with this task. The lack of structure of the brainstorming process would make him feel out of control and would probably frustrate his urge to consider all the details of the project. Miguel would most likely already have a good idea of the form he wanted.

Task 2. Miguel would be much better at this task because of his orientation to structure and detail. Working with the print shop, he could focus his attention on each item on the form and decide where it should be placed, how much room it should be given, and how it flows in the document. He would make sure the form met all the standards and regulatory requirements of The Joint Commission and would ensure it was error free. Betty, on the other hand, would very quickly become bored with this aspect of the project. To her, all the attention given to the details would seem like a waste of time, and she would probably start recommending changes in other unit forms.

Placing people in the working environments that correspond with their strengths increases the odds for success of the project, and a successful project experience for the nurses will likely promote positive changes in peer relationships.

Resolving Conflicts

Several different strategies can be used to resolve workplace conflicts. Depending on a person's communication style and personality traits, different outcomes may occur. People who use an assertive style of communication and incorporate communication builders have much greater success in the positive resolution of conflicts.[26] Following are some strategies for conflict resolution.

Strategy 1: Ignore the Conflict
- *Submissive personality:* This person avoids bringing the issue to the other person through fear of retaliation or ridicule if they confront and express honest feelings or opinions.

- *Assertive personality:* Ignoring the conflict is never an option. This person almost always uses Strategy 2.
- *Aggressive personality:* This person has decided not to pursue the conflict because the other person is "too stupid to understand" or it would just be a "waste of my time."

Strategy 2: Confront the Conflict
- *Submissive personality:* This person does not handle the situation directly but refers the problem to a supervisor or to another person for resolution.
- *Assertive personality:* This person sets up a time and place for a one-to-one meeting. At the meeting, the two parties focus on the issues that caused the conflict and negotiate to define goals and problem-solve. If the conflict is severe, the parties may resort to negotiation or mediation.
- *Aggressive personality:* This person confronts the other loudly, in front of an audience, and attacks the other's personality rather than the issue. They either walk away before the other can speak or keep talking without stopping and do not allow the other person to respond. The communication is strictly one-sided and very negative.

> **People who use an assertive style of communication and incorporate communication builders have much greater success in the positive resolution of conflicts.**

Strategy 3: Postpone the Conflict
- *Submissive personality:* This person keeps track of the issues until they reach a critical point, then dumps all the issues at one time on the offender in a highly aggressive manner. The other person generally has no idea why they are being attacked and may respond with anger or submission.
- *Assertive personality:* This person hardly ever postpones the conflict except to allow the other person to "cool down" and become more receptive to what others have to say.
- *Aggressive personality:* This person waits until they can either use the incident as a threat or blackmail or can express the conflict in front of an audience.

Professional nurses need to be assertive and feel comfortable when handling conflict and confronting others. The conflict situations that nurses may encounter range from uncooperative patients and lazy coworkers to hostile, insecure, but influential health-care providers and administrators. Practicing the assertiveness skills needed during confrontational situations helps increase the nurse's confidence in handling daily work-related conflicts and allows the honest but respectful expression of opinions and ideas. Keep in mind that unresolved conflicts never really go away. Ignoring a conflict situation may postpone it, sometimes for a long time, but it will not resolve the issue. Unresolved conflicts often fester until they either reach a boiling point or are manifested in negative behaviors or feelings.[2] Some of the feelings and behaviors that are symptoms of unresolved conflicts include the following:

- Tension and anxiety manifested as sudden angry outbursts
- Generalized distrust among the staff members
- Gossiping and rumor spreading
- Intentional work sabotage
- Backstabbing and lack of cooperation
- Isolation of certain staff members
- Division and polarization of the staff
- Low-rated peer evaluation reports[24]

Improved Communication Skills

Often, when conflict is handled appropriately, it produces much less anxiety than was initially anticipated. An individual who prepares for a confrontational meeting by expecting the worst-case scenario may be pleasantly surprised when the meeting and discussion take place. Many conflicts turn out to be merely errors in perception, simple misunderstandings, or misquotes of something that was said. If a situation is cleared up at an early stage, this prevents the development of the symptoms of unresolved conflict (listed earlier) and improves staff relationships. Individuals feel more confident and have better self-esteem when they resolve the conflicts in an adult and productive manner.

Another advantage of good conflict management is the improvement in communication skills. As with any skill, the more that conflict management skills are practiced, the easier they become to use. A conflict situation is illustrated in the Issues in Practice at the end of the chapter.

A Focus on Strength

For many people, resolving conflicts based on diversity issues can be difficult, especially when individuals feel insecure about their skills or abilities.[25] When people feel insecure, they may revert to submissive or aggressive behavior or communication styles to hide their weaknesses or differences.

Because assertive people recognize that everyone, including themselves, has both strengths and weaknesses, they feel comfortable with diversity and are more likely to accept and support others by recognizing and using their strengths. Focusing on strengths provides them with positive feedback and helps them grow personally and professionally.[3] Focusing on weaknesses and differences tears down an individual's self-esteem, creates an uncomfortable work atmosphere, and makes people defensive and sometimes hostile.

See Box 11.5 for additional information on conflict resolution.

> *Negotiation is the process of give and take between individuals or groups with the goal of reaching an agreement acceptable to both sides.*

NEGOTIATION

There is an old saying that "everything is negotiable." Negotiation is a common method to manage conflicts. Negotiation can be between nurse and patient, nurse and nurse, nurse manager and staff, or nurse manager and administration. Negotiation is the process of give and take between individuals or groups with the goal of reaching an agreement acceptable to both sides.[24] It is a specialized two-way communication skill in which individuals or groups with differing needs or ideas settle on a middle-ground result that may not completely please either party. Negotiations may be formal or informal, hostile or friendly.[23] A cooperative atmosphere fostered by both sides that recognizes the similarity of each side's demands is the most productive in reaching a satisfactory solution.

Bargaining is a special type of negotiation that is used most often when money-related issues are being discussed. **Collective bargaining** is a formal process that is used by groups of workers represented

Box 11.5 Conflict Resolution Tips

In nursing practice, good communication and conflict management skills are essential. The following tips may help resolve communication problems:

Improve Your Conflict Management Skills
- Attend seminars.
- Read books.
- Find mentors.

Change Your Paradigm
- Focus on the positive, not the negative.
- Realize that appropriate confrontation is a risk-taking activity.

Achieve Better Communication
- Work to improve relationships.
- Encourage teamwork.
- Give and receive mentoring.

Understand Your Values
- Focus on a win-win.
- Be willing to negotiate and compromise.
- Be direct and honest.
- Focus on the issues.
- Do not attack the person.
- Do not make judgments.
- Do not become the third person; encourage peers having a conflict to communicate directly with one another.
- Do not spread rumors.

Set Personal Guidelines
- Confront in private, never in front of anyone else.
- Confront the individual; do not report them to the supervisor first.
- Do not confront when you are angry.
- Start with an "I" message.
- Express your feelings and opinions.
- Allow the other person to talk without interruption.
- Listen attentively.
- Set goals and future plans of action.
- Let it go.
- Keep it private and confidential.

and requires that the two sides designate negotiating teams that are selected by both management and employee groups. (See Bonus Chapter 30 for more details.)

Less formal negotiations found at the unit level may still have some of the elements of a formal bargaining effort. For example, if a nurse manager is negotiating with a group of staff, they may want just one or two individuals from the group to negotiate the problem. These individuals are designated as spokespersons who will be the primary representatives for the group. A formal written list of issues may be drawn up, but the exchange most likely will be informal in nature during a face-to-face meeting.[24] Informal negotiations between individual nurses can be used to resolve conflicts that, if left to fester, will eventually cause disharmony and lower morale among the staff.

Conflicting Powers

In formal contract negotiation, there is an obvious power-control conflict. Each side is reluctant to give up power or relinquish any control of key factors such as money or rights. The employees' group tries to gain some power from management and improve benefits for its members. The power tug-of-war also factors into less formal negotiations.[25] Staff negotiating with nurse managers for more staff, different length shifts, longer breaks, or fewer weekend shifts may be perceived by the nurse manager as attempting to usurp some of their power. Individual nurses negotiating a conflict may also interpret the negotiation as an attempt to reduce the other person's power.

Learn the Skills

The underlying purpose of all negotiation is to achieve a goal or objective. Negotiation is a skill that nurse managers must learn and with which all nurses should familiarize themselves. Some keys to successful negotiation include the following:

1. Do some research, particularly if negotiating with management or administration. Focusing on issues such as quality of care and patient safety is received more positively than just listing the wants or wishes of nurses.
2. Clearly identify the objectives and goals of the negotiation. The old saying, "If you don't know where you are going, how will you know when you get there?" is never so true as in negotiations.

by a union or a negotiating body to solve workplace issues such as salaries, health-care benefits, safe work environment, and hiring practices. Formal contract negotiation is a key element in collective bargaining

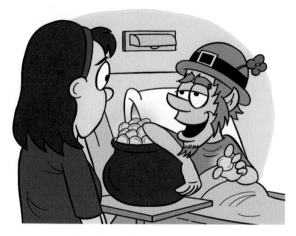

"If ye let me skip this test,
ye can have me pot o' gold!"

3. If criticized by the other person or side during the discussions, avoid taking it personally. Especially avoid becoming angry and hostile. Anger and hostility will shut down the negotiations immediately.

4. Avoid making personal attacks on the other person or group. It causes anger and hostility and shuts down the negotiations.

5. Negotiate in good faith. Effective negotiations always require give and take and a willingness to meet in the middle. Digging in one's heels and refusing to give in on any element under consideration is not negotiating in good faith.

6. Respect the other side's goals and objectives. Unless proven otherwise, assume that they are also negotiating in good faith. Trust on both sides is a key element of successful negotiation.

7. Preplan the elements of the negotiation list that can be sacrificed in order to obtain concessions from the other side.

8. Attend workshops or seminars on negotiation and bargaining. Nurse leaders in particular need to master the techniques of the negotiation process. Facilities should provide staff development in negotiating techniques for all nurses so that they can use these skills in all aspects of their professional lives.[24,25]

Mediation or Arbitration?

When the sides are unable to reach a resolution to their differences, they may resort to mediation. Mediation is a form of alternative dispute resolution that can be either formal or informal. In a formal negotiation setting such as a contract dispute, the disagreements are sometimes resolved through formal mediation in which a neutral third party provided by the Federal Mediation and Conciliation Service meets with each side.[27] The appointed mediator works with both sides to reach an agreement; however, the agreement is nonbinding, and either side can reject the settlement.

A less formal mediation process can be used to reach an agreement between two individuals who disagree.[27] Some health-care facilities select volunteers to receive training in mediation techniques. These individuals use the skills they learned to settle conflict situations between employees and colleagues. At the training sessions, the mediators learn skills such as how to identify what situations would be most appropriate for mediation, communication techniques that allow both parties to speak freely and identify their key issues, and methods of reaching a mutually acceptable resolution. The parties involved in the mediation process do so voluntarily and are not forced to participate by management. All communications during the mediation are confidential. Much like the formal mediation process, agreements developed during the informal process are also nonbinding.[27]

Arbitration is another form of dispute resolution and usually the last step before the dispute is taken to court for litigation. It can be either nonbinding or binding, in which case both parties agree ahead of time to comply with whatever decision is reached by the arbitrator. In a formal setting such as a contract negotiation or settlement for a malpractice suit, an arbitrator with binding power is appointed. This person is a neutral third party who, like the mediator, investigates the conflict, meets with both sides, and makes a recommendation for settlement.[27] Binding arbitration, by its very nature, is not appropriate for informal negotiations. Although the formal process of negotiation and arbitration is usually applied to more formal settings and situations, the skills that are involved in their practice are useful in a number of other settings and situations.

Conclusion

A person's professional and personal lives are influenced by communication styles and behavioral patterns. The ability to analyze personal strengths, weaknesses, and communication behaviors is important in everyday communication but is particularly important in negotiation and conflict resolution.

Certain specific communication qualities and skills are essential for interacting with coworkers and patients. Of primary importance is the skill of assertive communication, which allows people to express themselves openly and honestly while respecting other people's opinions and ideas. Being able to identify submissive and aggressive behavior is also essential in trying to resolve problems, as is recognizing issues of diversity, which underlie many problems in communication. Disagreements with others are ultimately resolved through the practice of conflict management. Because it is an outgrowth and extension of the problem-solving method, nurses should be able to quickly grasp its structure and master its use.

Issues in Practice

Julie H., RN, has been working the 7 p.m. to 7 a.m. shift in a busy 32-bed surgical unit of a large university hospital since her graduation from a small bachelor of science in nursing program 6 months ago. Although Julie was told by the unit director when she was hired that she would have at least a full year of training before she had to work as charge nurse, tonight the other two RNs who usually work the shift called in sick, and Julie was left in charge. The 7 p.m. to 7 a.m. shift is always busy because the unit has to discharge patients who are ready to go home after surgery and admit patients who are coming in for surgery the next day. Hospital policy requires that the RN make and sign both the discharge and admission assessments.

Although Julie is nervous about this new role as charge nurse, she feels that she can handle the responsibility if she has some additional help. Normal staffing for the unit on this shift is three RNs, three licensed practical nurse, and three unlicensed assistive personnel (UAPs). Julie calls the house supervisor to see if she can get some help. The only place in the hospital that is not busy that night is the obstetrics (OB) unit, so the supervisor sends two of the OB unit's UAPs to the surgical unit to help Julie.

It is not the help Julie really wanted, but she feels that she can handle the responsibility. However, when Julie begins to make assignments, the older of the OB unit UAPs, Hanna J., informs Julie that for the past 15 years she has worked only in the newborn nursery and does not know anything about the care of adult patients who have had surgery. In addition, Hanna states that she has a bad back and cannot lift or turn adult patients. She is also afraid that she might catch some disease from the adults that she would take back to the babies. Julie asks Hanna, "What do you feel you are qualified to do on the surgical unit?" In response, Hanna crosses her legs, folds her arms across her chest, puts her head down, and mumbles under her breath, "A lot more than a new know-it-all RN like you."

Questions for Thought

1. What messages, both verbal and nonverbal, is Hanna communicating? How should Julie respond to this comment? What should she do to rectify the situation?
2. Using what you learned in this chapter, identify the personality type of each of the persons involved in the situation.
3. How can the RN best communicate with this UAP? What were some of the communication mistakes the RN made?
4. What background, cultural, and diversity factors played a part in this situation? Develop a strategy for resolution of this conflict.

CRITICAL-THINKING EXERCISES

- Make a list of your values and where they came from. Describe how each value affects your work ethic and communication style.
- List your communication strengths and weaknesses. Rank your weaknesses on a scale of 1 to 10 (10 being the most problematic). Determine which ones you want to change, and create an improvement plan.
- Identify your primary communication style and character type.
- What methods do you use to resolve conflicts? Do these methods work for you? Identify better methods for resolving conflict situations.

ANSWERS TO QUESTIONS IN CHAPTER 11

ISSUES IN PRACTICE: MANAGING CHANGE (PAGE 312)

1. The underlying problem is that there was too much change too quickly. Even though the staff recognized that change was needed, there is always a built-in resistance to change. Sudden, unpredictable change creates the most anxiety and therefore the most resistance. It also can produce a great deal of cohesion among those being asked to change when it is viewed as a threat. This last point is borne out by the nurses seeking to organize into a collective-bargaining unit.

2. The director of the unit could have decreased resistance by garnering staff "buy-in" for the changes, allowing them to participate in decision-making from the beginning. Also, the whole process of change could have been slowed down—perhaps spread over 1 year to 18 months. A slower process would have given the nurses a chance to adjust to one change before another was implemented.

Sources: D.K. Whitehead, S.A. Weiss, R.M. Tappen, *Essentials of Nursing Leadership and Management* (6th ed.), Philadelphia, PA: F.A. Davis, 2019; E. Scott, How poor communication causes stress, Free Therapy, November 5, 2020, https://free-therapy.tumblr.com/post/685963574664953856/how-poor-communication-causes-stress.

NCLEX-STYLE QUESTIONS

1. Why is effective communication important?
   1. It is the way a sender expresses their ideas and opinions.
   2. It allows participants to share and understand one another's thoughts.
   3. It prevents misunderstanding and conflict between people.
   4. It ensures that messages are swiftly decoded by the receiver.
2. Maxine, an experienced postpartum RN, is observing as her preceptee Jan assesses a patient who is 2 days post–emergency cesarean section. The patient suddenly gasps for air and complains of chest pain. She is drenched in sweat. Maxine shouts at Jan, "Don't just stand there, dummy! Call for help!" What type of communication style is Maxine demonstrating?
   1. Assertive
   2. Nonassertive
   3. Submissive
   4. Aggressive
3. Ryan, an RN, is feeling frustrated with Ed, a CNA whom Ryan feels is lazy and not taking good care of the patients on their unit. What tools could Ryan use to address his conflict with Ed in an assertive way? **Select all that apply.**
   1. Complain about Ed's laziness to the charge nurse.
   2. Arrange to talk with Ed in a quiet, private area.

3. Tell Ed, "You do such a bad job that I always have to redo your work!"

4. Ask Ed open-ended questions about what he thinks the problem is.

5. Observe Ed's body language and note any mismatch between it and what Ed is saying verbally.

6. Be quiet and listen.

4. The process of give and take between individuals or groups with the goal of reaching an agreement acceptable to all sides is called _____.

5. The personal conflict between two employees in a busy emergency department is starting to negatively affect the morale of their coworkers as well as patient care. The two employees agree to meet with a neutral third party who will help them find a way to reach a mutually acceptable solution. What process is being described here?

1. Arbitration
2. Conflict resolution
3. Mediation
4. Litigation

6. Ryan wants to find a productive way to resolve his conflict with Ed. When the two men have their meeting, Ryan asks open-ended questions, listens closely, and pays attention to Ed's nonverbal messages. What step of the nursing process does this meeting most resemble?

1. Assessment
2. Planning
3. Implementation
4. Evaluation

7. Which statement about unresolved conflict is TRUE?

1. If you ignore an unresolved conflict, it eventually goes away.
2. Postponing a conflict gives everyone time to cool down and prevents a difficult conversation.
3. There are only minor consequences of allowing conflicts to remain unresolved.
4. Over time, unresolved conflicts can lead to significant negative behaviors or feelings.

8. Two neighbors are having a dispute over which one's property a large pecan tree is on. The neighbors have agreed to meet with a neutral third party and abide by whatever decision this person makes. What process are these neighbor's using to resolve their conflict?

1. Arbitration
2. Litigation
3. Mediation
4. Negotiation

9. At 3:30 p.m., friends of a patient who is recovering from a motor-vehicle accident ask for directions to the patient's room. Juanita, the unit clerk, tells the group that their friend has requested to have no visitors until 4:00 p.m. One of the visitors loudly demands to be taken to his friend immediately. Which response by Juanita demonstrates an assertive communication style?

1. "If you don't calm down and step away from the nurses' station, I will have to call hospital security."
2. "Well, okay, it's only thirty minutes until four o'clock, so it should be okay. His room is down the hall on the right."
3. "I understand that you are anxious to see your friend. However, hospital policy is to honor patients' requests concerning visitors. There's a waiting area you can use until four o'clock."
4. "I'm sorry. Let me see if I can get one of the nurses to explain the hospital policy to you."

10. A study group of nursing students is playing a game of charades to help them review communication builders and blockers. Each member of the group draws a card and acts out a behavior that illustrates the word on the card. Joeleen draws a card that says "Builder." Which action by Joeleen indicates she needs further study?

1. Nodding her head.
2. Making eye contact.
3. Sitting or standing in close proximity.
4. Sitting with legs crossed and picking at her shoelaces.

References

1. King P. *How to Listen With Intention: The Foundation of True Connection, Communication, and Relationships.* Publisher: Author, 2020.
2. Wilshire J. The importance of effective communication skills in healthcare. One Education September 1, 2021, https://www.oneeducation.org.uk/communication-skills-in-healthcare/
3. OptimistMinds editorial team. 5 communication styles. OptimistMinds, September 1, 2022. https://optimistminds.com/5-communication-styles/
4. Robinson M. Aggressive communication: Features and examples. Its Psychology, 2022. https://itspsychology.com/aggressive-communication/
5. Is passive aggressive communication good for you? Holistic Family Practice.com, June 13, 2022, https://www.holisticfamilypracticeva.com/is-passive-aggressive-communication-good-for-you/
6. Kelly B. Passive-aggressive communication. What you need to know. Peep Strategy, 2022. https://peepstrategy.com/passive-aggressive-communication/
7. Five steps for improving communication between your healthcare staff and patients. Ultimate Medical Academy, June 1, 2022. https://ultimatemedical.edu/blog/five-steps-for-improving-communication-between-your-healthcare-staff-and-patients/
8. Lucas S. The Gerard Egan model and SOLER. Counselling Central, 2022. https://www.counsellingcentral.com/the-egan-model-and-soler/
9. Keiling H. Nonverbal communication: 9 types and how to read and use it. Indeed Career Guide, 2022. https://www.indeed.com/career-advice/career-development/nonverbal-communication-skills
10. Paraverbal communication explained with examples. Project Practical, https://www.projectpractical.com/paraverbal-communication/
11. Evans H. Science explains why having a deep voice is critical to our success. LifeHack, February 26, 2016. https://www.lifehack.org/372669/science-explains-why-having-deep-voice-critical-our-success-2
12. Voice volume. Ifioque, 2022. https://ifioque.com/paralinguistic/voice_volume
13. Effective speaking. SkillsYouNeed, 2022. https://www.skillsyouneed.com/ips/effective-speaking.html
14. Five steps for improving communication between your healthcare staff and patients. Ultimate Medical Academy, 2022. https://www.ultimatemedical.edu/blog/five-steps-for-improving-communication-between-your-healthcare-staff-and-patients/
15. 8 physical barriers to communication and how to overcome them. Indeed Career Guide, 2022. https://www.indeed.com/career-advice/career-development/physical-barriers-to-communication
16. Business Bliss Consultants FZE. Barriers to verbal and nonverbal communication. NursingAnswers.net, February 11, 2020. https://nursinganswers.net/essays/exploring-verbal-and-non-verbal-communication-and-possible-barriers-nursing-essay.php
17. Steriotypes: What they are and why they are harmful. BetterHelp, 2023. https://www.betterhelp.com/advice/stereotypes/stereotypes-definition-and-why-they-are-wrong/
18. Cleveland Clinic. How to communicate clearly while wearing a mask. *HealthEssentials*, October 20, 2020. https://health.clevelandclinic.org/how-to-communicate-clearly-while-wearing-a-mask/
19. Types of learning disabilities. Learning Disabilities of America, n.d. https://ldaamerica.org/types-of-learning-disabilities/
20. Communicating with people with learning disabilities. Mencap, n.d. https://www.mencap.org.uk/learning-disability-explained/communicating-people-learning-disability
21. Scott E. How poor communication causes stress. Free Therapy, November 5, 2020. https://free–therapy.tumblr.com/post/685963574664953856/how-poor-communication-causes-stress
22. Webb J. Five questions to ask when you just can't bring yourself to say "I'm angry." Your Tango, 2022. https://www.yourtango.com/self/how-to-communicate-anger
23. Why are critical thinking and problem solving essential? The Black Sheep Community, 2022. https://www.theblacksheep.community/critical-thinking-and-problem-solving/
24. Shonk K. What is conflict resolution and how does it work? Harvard Law School, June 14, 2022. https://www.pon.harvard.edu/daily/conflict-resolution/what-is-conflict-resolution-and-how-does-it-work/
25. Equity, diversity, and inclusion: What is diversity? Austin Community College, 2022. https://researchguides.austincc.edu/c.php?g=522627&p=7624718
26. Structure of the brain. New Health Advisor, 2022. https://www.newhealthadvisor.org/Structure-of-the-Brain.html
27. Types of mediation. *ADR Times*, 2022. https://www.adrtimes.com/types-of-mediation/

Understanding and Dealing Successfully With Difficult Behavior

Joseph T. Catalano

12

Learning Objectives

After completing this chapter, the reader will be able to:

- Discuss the underlying issues that cause individuals to display difficult behaviors
- Develop successful strategies for communicating with persons displaying difficult behaviors
- Respond effectively to the underlying emotions that persons with difficult behaviors are communicating
- Successfully resolve problems associated with difficult behavior in both colleagues and patients
- Formulate coping strategies to adapt successfully to people with difficult behaviors

UNDERSTANDING DIFFICULT BEHAVIOR

Let's say this up front: There are no difficult people; there are, however, people who display difficult behaviors. It is important to keep in mind that behavior is a form of communication. The term *difficult people* is so often used that it has become a widely accepted way to categorize people. Labeling people as difficult is really stereotyping, which may or may not accurately reflect reality. In dealing with the group labeled as difficult, our goals are to change *our* response to the behaviors and attempt to change the behaviors they are displaying.[1] It is virtually impossible to change an individual's basic personality; however, brain injuries, extreme traumatic events, medications, and potentially lethal illnesses or injuries have been shown to significantly alter a person's personality.

The term *personality* is often misused to mean that an individual is outgoing, humorous, and generally friendly to other people. When you hear people say, "Joe has a great personality," they are usually talking about the fact that he is pleasant to be around, outgoing, and readily engages in conversations. On the other hand, you might hear someone say, "Terry has no personality at all," when they actually are talking about the fact that Terry is quiet, somewhat withdrawn, and does not easily engage in conversations.

Developing a Personality

The truth is that everyone has a personality, and although defined differently by different schools of psychology, an individual's personality is generally recognized as all those elements, both genetic and learned, that go into making that person who they are at present.[1] A personality includes strongly held beliefs, attitudes, emotions, and behaviors. Most people have identifiable personality traits soon after birth. Personality traits are the characteristic patterns that control how a person thinks, feels, and acts in response to various situations. It is a permanent pattern in a person's judgments, observations, and ability to relate to the objects and people who surround them. A personality trait is not

325

the ability to throw a baseball the fastest or hit it the farthest. Rather, it is the resolve to train the hardest and the willingness to listen to the coach. These traits are not an either-or proposition. They exist along a continuum, strong at one side and weaker at the other end. In any given individual, some traits will be more intense and dominant than others. Some of the more common personality traits include humility, kindness, extroversion or introversion, faithfulness, bravery, trustworthiness, egotism, determination, appropriate emotional expression, open mindedness, and empathy.[1] Early indicators of a personality can be seen in newborn infants. Just ask nurses who regularly work with newborn babies. Some babies are mostly quiet and seem content except when they are hungry or need to be changed, and others cry all the time and never seem to be content.

All children are genetically stamped in the womb with innate emotions that help them survive in a world that they do not understand and that is very frightening to them.[1] Feelings of anger, jealousy, selfishness, and self-centeredness, along with their behavioral expressions, help children manipulate adults, particularly the parents, and cope with what is to them a big and hostile environment. One of the primary goals parents have in raising their children is to teach them adult coping skills to deal with problems and help them outgrow the immature and childish coping mechanisms of manipulation and exploitation of others. It is evident that this outcome is not always achieved.

Some people go through their whole lives using childlike coping mechanisms and behaviors to deal with the adult world.[1] These mechanisms do not work very well, and often the people who use them get labeled as difficult people. For whatever reason, they never learned or accepted adult coping mechanisms. For example, being able to forgive is a learned adult behavior that counteracts the self-centeredness that children use as a survival mechanism. People who have never learned to forgive others, forget about insults, or let go of much of anything are sometimes afflicted, as adults, with conditions such as chronic fatigue and depression. And it is no wonder they act in these ways: they are carrying around a heavy burden of emotional baggage from a lifetime of perceived or actual events in their lives, and every day they are alive, they add another bag to the pile.

You can observe this type of behavior in a 60-year-old woman who seeks to get revenge for the way she was treated by a relative 30 years before at a wedding. She has been carrying that baggage for a long time. Often, this behavior manifests itself in activities such as hoarding. People who display hoarding behavior are not necessarily extreme hoarders, such as seen on the TV show *Hoarders*, but they tend to collect a lot of junk and pile it around the house. If you ask, for example, "Why don't we throw out these 10-year-old magazines? Everything is online now," a person with hoarding disorder will likely respond, "No, there might be something in one of them that I'll need someday." The physical hoarding of items is an outward manifestation of the person's inward hoarding of insults and emotional injuries.[2] If you look at many of the difficult behaviors discussed in this chapter from the viewpoint of what children do to get their way, you will see a great deal of similarity between the two.

> *Generally, when individuals are displaying difficult behavior, they are hard to communicate with or their behavior is such that it makes it very difficult to work with them to achieve a goal or finish a task.*

People who display difficult behaviors are everywhere. They are found at home, at work, and in the health-care setting. It is pretty obvious that communicating with them requires a special set of communication skills. Because communication is such an integral part of quality health care, it is an essential requirement that nurses be able to understand why a patient is using difficult behaviors and learn the skills that will allow them to communicate effectively with such patients.[3] The skills learned in resolving conflicts and negotiating often are used when dealing with people who have difficult behaviors. Of course, difficult behaviors are not limited to just patients in the health-care settings. They may also be the family of the patient, nurses, health-care providers, and other health-care workers. Pretty much anyone can become a difficult person to deal with under the right set of circumstances. Who knows, you might even be displaying difficult behavior.

Identifying People With Difficult Behaviors

What exactly is a person with difficult behaviors, or in common language, a difficult person? To some extent, a difficult person is one of those "you'll know them when you see them" individuals. What we are generally referring to when talking about difficult behavior is a person who is difficult to communicate with or with whom it is difficult to work. Also, it is important to recognize that identifying someone as difficult is a matter of perception. One individual's difficult person is another's "Oh, old Uncle Freddy acts that way any time there are people around."

Generally, when individuals are displaying difficult behavior, they are hard to communicate with or their behavior is such that it makes it very difficult to work with them to achieve a goal or finish a task. Difficult peoples' personalities have been described as "prickly" because if they are touched verbally, they sting back with sharp vocal barbs.[1] They often use many of the communication blockers discussed in Chapter 11 to achieve their goals. Identifying what goals difficult people are trying to achieve, whether they are a patient or a coworker, is one of the keys to understanding them and communicating with them effectively.

In the health-care setting specifically, there are two primary groups of people with difficult behaviors: coworkers and patients. Although the techniques in interacting with either group overlap to some degree, there are important differences between the two groups that need to be considered, particularly the cause for being difficult and the outcomes they are attempting to achieve. Also, although difficult coworkers can make life on the unit uncomfortable, there is no ethical or legal requirement to interact with them. However, health-care providers' relationships with patients require that nurses do everything they can to establish and maintain effective communication with them, no matter how difficult they are, to achieve the goals of quality care (Box 12.1).

Improved Understanding

All nurses recognize that obtaining a thorough history and understanding the underlying disease processes

better prepares them for the physical care of their patients. Similarly, in working with difficult people, a knowledge of their backgrounds and understanding of their needs and goals better prepares the nurse to communicate in a positive way. It would seem that nurses should be adept at handling conflict and difficult people because a large part of their education includes an understanding of the cause and effect and the intricacies of human nature. These are skills that nurses use daily in the care of patients.

Shifting the communication paradigm from instinctual, or knee-jerk, responses to one that uses the communication-building techniques discussed in Chapter 11 in combination with the nurse's relationship skills should make interacting successfully with difficult people a less imposing task. The behavior displayed by a difficult person is really a symptom of a deeper underlying problem, just as an assessment of shortness of breath is a symptom of a respiratory or cardiac disease. Identifying the cause of the problem and the outcomes the patient is attempting to achieve permits the nurse to treat the disease rather than just the symptoms.[3] The problem is never cured by merely ignoring it or dealing only with the symptoms. In the long term, the "leave it alone" approach usually only amplifies the difficult behavior.

Basic Principles

There are several basic principles to remember when attempting to work with a person displaying difficult behavior:

No change. Keep in mind that a difficult person is highly unlikely to change their behavior very much, particularly if that person is a coworker. However, one of our goals in teaching and caring for patients is to change behavior even if they are displaying difficult behaviors. The key point to remember is that we need to change our own perceptions and the way we approach a difficult person.[3] Difficult people tend to make us anxious, frustrated, and angry, but we cannot show them these feelings.

No reinforcement. It is a basic tenet in psychology that reinforcing a behavior will cause the behavior to be repeated (e.g., Pavlov's dogs). It is interesting that the reinforcement can be either positive or negative. Providing punishment for something someone is doing is often the payoff the difficult person is looking for, and they will repeat the behavior to get additional payoffs. The most powerful reinforcement is intermittent reward or punishment whereby the behavior is rewarded or punished one time and then ignored the next. It keeps the behavior going because the person is wondering when the next reinforcement will come.

No action. There is an old saying that "doing nothing is doing something." This means that when dealing with difficult people, if we do nothing, we are in reality reinforcing their behavior.

No anonymity. Identify the particular behaviors a patient is displaying as difficult and call the behaviors by name. "Letting it go" actually reinforces the behavior.

No ashes. Another old saying is "fight fire with fire"; however, the result of this approach is scorched earth and ashes. Again, this may be the outcome that the difficult person is seeking. They win when you argue with them, and in the end, nothing is left but ill feelings (i.e., ashes!).

No condemnation. The difficult people probably developed this type of behavior over a long period of time and are doing their best. Although it may not seem so, they usually are not malicious or hateful, and condemning them as such really misses the point.[4] Difficult people lack the basic communication skills to interact successfully with others and are constantly seeking to fulfill a need or achieve an outcome by their behavior.

No robbery. You must believe that you are 100 percent responsible for your own happiness, because you are.

Happiness comes from within yourself, and it is not up to others to make you happy. Similarly, it is up to you to control your unhappiness. It is the goal of some difficult people to rob you of your happiness because they are unhappy (misery loves company). Do not let them do it! Find happy people to hang out with. Find some fulfilling activity outside of the work setting.

Remembering Maslow

Maslow's hierarchy of needs is often one of the first important theories that is taught in nursing programs. It is typically introduced in the first nursing course and then reinforced in psychology courses. The primary reason it is taught is that it is one of the most effective ways of prioritizing patient care (Fig. 12.1). The needs on the bottom of the triangle, particularly the physiological and safety needs, are necessary for the patient's survival and maintenance of life. These needs must always be met first. The higher needs, such as love and belonging, self-esteem, and self-actualization, cannot be met if the person is not able to fulfill the basic needs to stay alive and remain safe.[4]

Maslow's hierarchy can also be used in understanding and interacting with people in the healthcare setting who are displaying difficult behaviors. Understanding what causes people to behave in a difficult manner is directly related to the hierarchy of

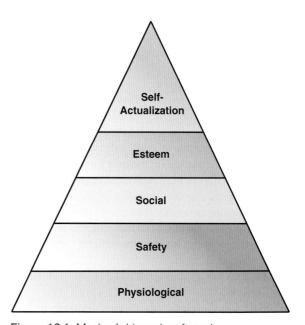

Figure 12.1 Maslow's hierarchy of needs.

needs and differentiates the causality between difficult coworkers and difficult patients. Because the causes are different for each of these groups, interacting successfully with them also requires a different approach.

It is pretty safe to believe that health-care providers, nurses, pharmacists, and other health-care workers are having their basic physiological and safety needs met. The needs that produce coworkers' difficult behaviors are generally related to the higher-level needs of love and belonging, self-esteem, and self-actualization. In the cases of difficult patients, their illnesses, injuries, or surgeries often threaten their basic needs for merely surviving physically.

Difficult Coworkers

Anyone who has been employed in or even associated with the health-care setting for any length of time soon becomes aware of a variety of personality types among the staff members. These personality types can be identified by their predominant behaviors. The behaviors vary to some degree according to how the person is attempting to meet their needs. Although there are several types of difficult personalities in the work setting, the two most common types are the persecutor and the sneak. They require different strategies for communication and for dealing with their behaviors. Keep in mind that these are stereotypes that tend to batch individuals into groups on the basis of predetermined behaviors.[5]

In reality, people may have combinations of or overlapping behaviors that may require combining strategies for communication. The various stereotypes are all interrelated and based on individual behaviors and communication styles. An increased awareness of the various identifying characteristics and communication strategies will help you develop the coping skills and communication techniques necessary for communicating with difficult people.

Also, it is possible for individuals to have true personality disorders, which are diagnosed psychological conditions. Some of these disorders, such as narcissistic personality or avoidant personality, may present with the same types of behaviors as seen with difficult people but are more pronounced and extreme.[1] If a person has a true personality disorder, it is likely beyond the floor nurse's or even the nurse manager's skill set to interact with these individuals successfully, unless the nurse specializes in psychiatric practice.

These patients are best left to the mental health professionals. However, one of the characteristics of these types of disorders is that the person does not believe they have a problem and rarely seeks help for it.

The Persecutor

Also called the *dictator*, these people generally display an attitude of being superior to others and being in control at all times. They attempt to humiliate, intimidate, threaten, or demean other individuals or groups with the goals of overcoming their own lack of confidence, feeling more powerful, and inflating their low self-esteem. They often are habitual liars and may not be able to distinguish their lies from the truth most of the time. They create their own secure world for themselves and collect a group of followers who strongly believe in their rhetoric and who reinforce the persecutor's beliefs with adulations and praise. These followers believe so strongly in the persecutor that it approaches becoming a personality cult. Persecutors often believe and express that they are the only ones who can solve a problem or do a task well; they also take sole credit for successes that they had little to do with.

They are and have been bullies for a long time and enjoy making others feel small. They like to use

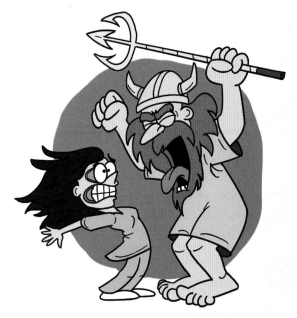

"I WANT MY PAIN PILL NOW!"

belittling terms for people to keep them in their places. This behavior is probably habitual, being used repeatedly for a long period of time, and becomes the person's primary mode of communication. The persecutor has self-esteem needs that are not being met and may also have love and belonging issues. The goal of their behavior is usually to coerce or intimidate another person into doing something they do not want to do. However, sometimes the goal is to merely humiliate a person or group due to some perceived difference or weakness because it makes them feel better about themselves.[5]

They often lash out or take outrageous actions if they feel boxed in by the truth or that things are not going the way they want. Revenge and hitting back at people who may challenge their beliefs or positions destroys their ability to establish true and long-lasting friendships.

Persecutor Tactics

Persecutors attempt to maintain control by putting others down and ruling from a command post. They often have minions working for them who are fearful of getting on their "bad side" and will help persecutors when they engage a new target. Persecutors have learned over time that being inconsistent (i.e., easy to deal with one day and demanding the next) keeps people off balance and helps them maintain power to achieve their goals. They usually are unable to accept ideas that are different from theirs and often may use loud speech and threats to keep the other person from expressing a new idea. Persecutors may attempt to provoke the other person into an angry, defensive outburst, and they enjoy the flare-up because they have achieved one of their goals. These are some of the messages they are attempting to convey by their behavior: "If you don't do what I want, I'll make your life miserable," "If you do what I want, I'll stop harassing you," and "If you give into my wants, you can become one of my minions and help me demean others."

What Do You Think?

Recall a recent exchange with someone (e.g., friend, instructor, parent, or health-care provider) in which you felt you "lost" the exchange. How did you feel? How did you respond? What could you have done differently?

If the dictator is in a superior position, such as a charge nurse or supervisor, this type of behavior is called *vertical violence*. When the dictator is a fellow employee at the same authority level, the behavior is referred to as *lateral* or *horizontal violence* (see Chapter 16 for more details). It is important to remember that the persecutor's self-image is fragile and that attempting to destroy it will be ineffective or will make the person more defensive and escalate their negative behaviors.

Taming the Persecutor

Using the basic principles discussed previously is essential in taming the behaviors of the persecutor. Communication skills can also be coping skills in interacting with these individuals. Everyone develops coping skills as they mature and uses them when confronted with complex situations. These coping skills can be used to resolve crisis situations, deal with anxiety, and resolve difficult issues of communication. This basic set of coping skills can be used as the foundation for adding to or building new coping skills to deal with difficult people.[6] Just as developing communication skills requires a willingness to change and a lot of practice, so does developing coping skills.

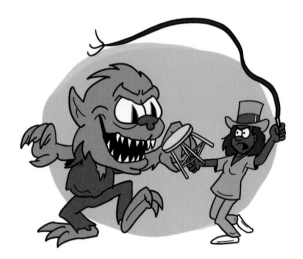

"Confronting a persecutor takes courage!"

Also, remember that perception is a significant part of dealing with the difficult behavior of people.[7] However, a lot of people really do not understand what their own perceptions are or how they affect their actions and thoughts when confronting a persecutor. When confronting a persecutor or any difficult person, it is essential to understand one's own motives, preferences, beliefs, and biases.

Dealing with difficult people requires a high level of personal confidence and inner strength: they have learned how to quickly identify weaknesses in others and to use those weaknesses in their attempt to maintain control. Confrontation is an essential element in dealing with persecutors, and courage is required to overcome their aggressiveness without becoming angry. Success in dealing with persecutors in particular also requires high degrees of self-awareness and emotional self-control. The only way to develop emotions strong enough to resist the attacks of the persecutor is through self-knowledge. Some of the particular actions that can be used in taming the persecutor include the following:

Set the stage for communication. This is an environmental communication builder. After a decision is made to deal with a difficult issue or person, it is important to set the stage for a positive experience. Because persecutors love the limelight and an audience, the location for the exchange should be private. The format of the meeting needs to be established ahead of time, including an explanation to the other person that both parties will take turns expressing their opinions and feelings without interruption.

Listen to what is really being communicated, including body language and paraverbal clues. Often, persecutors nonverbally reveal hidden messages or indications of what their real goals or needs are while giving a much different verbal message.[6] You can use the nonverbal communication builders when interacting with persecutors, but be sincere. Persecutors have learned how to quickly detect dishonesty. In some situations, merely allowing a person to vent emotions by using active listening reduces the levels of anger and animosity and sometimes even solves the conflict. Also, when intelligent people are allowed to speak openly and freely, they may be able to develop a new solution to the problem that they had not considered previously.

Use assertive but not aggressive communication. If the persecutor is in a highly animated state and speaking rapidly and loudly, your message will not penetrate the tirade. Never yell back or argue with them. Rather, say, "You are upset now; we can discuss this issue later." Then walk away.

Use a line of discussion that will get their attention and not make them defensive or lower their self-esteem, such as "Joanne, this project you have been working on shows what a hard worker you are; however, I am assigned to it also, and we need to figure out how to work together to make it the best possible"; "Liz, our relationship feels strained. I would like a good working relationship with you. What can we do to improve it?"; "Jordan, I noticed that you excluded me from meetings and communications. I feel left out. Can we talk about this?" Using the person's name eliminates a chance of misunderstanding to whom the statement was directed.

Remember that persecutors are acting the way they do because of something they lack in their lives or because of internal feelings of low self-esteem,[1] so do not take what they are saying personally. They probably say it to everyone. Also, never react emotionally in front of them by getting angry, crying, or sulking. It shows vulnerability, and that is an outcome they are seeking because it makes them feel better about themselves.

Avoid doing nothing. Persecutors want people to leave them alone so that they can continue their behavior without confrontation. After you have walked away, walk back when they calm down. Identifying their behavior to them calmly and directly is the first step in dealing with the behavior. Their behavior is not likely to change very much, but they will know that you know what they are doing. They probably will take you off their target list and seek a new target.

Avoid personal attacks. Separate the person from the behavior by focusing on the issues without attacking their personality. Having the facts about the specific behavior to be addressed makes people much more receptive to resolution of the problem than attacking their personality.[6] Remember, persecutors have fragile egos, and attacking them will only invite a more vicious counterattack. When situations are made into personal attacks, people feel defensive, responsible, or persecuted, and communication is either blocked or closed off completely. Avoid becoming personally or verbally abusive.[7]

For example,

During shift report about a particular patient, the 11:00 p.m. to 7:00 a.m. nurse forgot to tell the 7:00 a.m. to 3:00 p.m. charge nurse, Gail L., RN, that the patient had fallen out of bed during the night shift. Later in the day, the patient's physician and family confronted Gail to find out what had happened and why the patient was not placed on "fall protocols." Later, when Gail confronts the night nurse about the omission, she has two options for initiating the discussion of the incident with the responsible night nurse. Which approach would the night nurse probably take as a personal attack?

Option 1. Gail: "I was taken off guard and was ill-equipped when the family and physician asked me about this patient's fall, and I felt unprepared to explain the problem or provide a solution to them. My lack of knowledge about the fall really made me feel incompetent."

Option 2. Gail: "You failed to tell me about his fall last night. Because of you, I was not aware of the incident and was not prepared to answer questions. You always make me look like a fool!"

Avoid judging what a person is doing or what they should have done by your own standards. This type of statement becomes an arbitrary judgment call. Instead, ask the person for their ideas on how the situation could have been handled differently or what other options were available.

Ask clarifying questions that validate the person's concerns, feelings, and perceptions. Validating helps ensure that the responses address the real issues. Also, avoid reflex-type reactions to hostile or aggressive statements. It is a human instinct to become defensive when attacked and to attack back. However, this behavior only escalates the anger and tension and blocks effective communication.

Ignore trivia. Always make a conscious decision about the importance of the issue that needs to be discussed and stick with it. It is a very human tendency to become preoccupied with trivial and unimportant issues. If people spend large amounts of their energy dealing with trivia, they will have little energy left to deal with major issues when they come along. Identifying the causes and needs of people displaying

difficult behavior can sometimes be complicated and time consuming. People often try to direct the conversation away from issues they believe are painful and toward topics that are more comfortable.[3] They do not accept criticism well, even constructive criticism. By having a clear idea of the outcomes you wish to achieve, you can redirect the conversation when a person attempts to lead it in another direction.

Pathological behavior. All persecutors are bullies to some degree. The more pathological they are, the bigger the bully they become. For some individuals, the loud, aggressive, pugnacious, and vengeful behavior they display is actually a manifestation of an underlying pathological psychiatric condition such as personality disorder or bipolar disorder. These people may be very intelligent in some areas and are often highly successful. Unfortunately, their behavior usually does not rise to the level of what psychiatrists would consider a clear break from reality; and because they are not physically a danger to themselves or others, there is not much that can be done for them with counseling. They would absolutely refuse any type of counseling because they believe they are always right and everyone else is wrong. In high positions of authority, they are a nightmare, and every attempt should be made to remove them and move them to a place where they cannot do as much damage.

> *Always make a conscious decision about the importance of the issue that needs to be discussed and stick with it. It is a very human tendency to become preoccupied with trivial and unimportant issues.*

The Sneak (Manipulator, Gaslighter)

Another type of coworker with difficult behavior is called the *sneak* because of the devious, underhanded, and often malicious attacks they use to fulfill their self-esteem needs and achieve their goal to be in control. They are also called *double-crossers* or *backstabbers*. Unlike persecutors, who enjoy direct confrontation and watching others feel uncomfortable under their attacks, sneaks attack when you are not looking and get their reward by watching your discomfort and confusion in not knowing where the attack came from. Although they really do not have minions like the persecutor, they often elicit the help of others who are afraid of them and gang up on a person as a group behind their back. This process is called *gossip*, and it is a primary source of recreation and entertainment on many nursing units that should be eliminated.

The methods sneaks use are really forms of manipulation, using damaging influence over others with or without their knowledge.[8] Manipulators attack a person's mental and emotional states to get what they want and gain power over the victim. Manipulators study their future target by learning the target's genuine desires, values, and beliefs so that they can use them as weapons against the target. If a person needs something such as approval or material support, the manipulator will hold that over their head. If a person believes zealously in something, the manipulator will pretend to believe in the same thing only to betray their target at a later time when it suits their needs. Manipulators know well how to push their target's buttons and use that knowledge to set their plans in motion. Typical tactics to control a person include deception, lying, exaggeration, silent treatment, anger, and above all, fear. However, manipulators are insecure and unsure of where they belong in the work setting. Interestingly, their behavior has the same underlying causes as that of the persecutor—a need to feel in control, low self-esteem, and love and belonging issues; however, they use different methods to build up their self-esteem and sense of control.[6]

Unlike the bully who is overt in their abuse, the sneak may also be a gaslighter who uses deceptive and clandestine types of emotional abuse. Gaslighting targets a person's consciousness, their awareness and understanding of their physical environment, overt actions, and direct communication.[8] It is a form of emotional manipulation that is intended to control the way a person views themselves and their reality. (The term comes from the 1944 Alfred Hitchcock movie *Gaslight* about a husband with a secret who slowly drives his wife insane by claiming the upstairs lights are not flickering when they really are.) Gaslighters believe that they know the person they are targeting better than the person knows themself. They use methods to make a person question their own rationality and attempt to trigger a fearful or depressive state. These tactics include denial, lying, and contradiction to undermine and subvert a person's mental state. For example, the gaslighter will deny they said something, even though the person

has proof that they did say it. The gaslighter will deny that they told the person they would do some task or chore when the person knows they heard them say it. Repeated use of this tactic makes the targeted person start to question their own reality. They might start to think, "Am I going crazy? Maybe he never really said that? I must be making stuff up in my head!" Other tactics gaslighters may use include charisma and charm in the early stages of a relationship; self-pity to induce guilt in another person; explosive anger whenever rejected; and stalking in any of its forms (cyberstalking, following in a car, phone calls, or following in person).[8]

What Do You Think?

Have you ever been in a situation in which others have intentionally sabotaged your work? What was the situation? How did you feel? How did you deal with it? Did you try to retaliate?

Sneaks often have very few true friends and are generally fearful of close friendships because they do not want others to know what they are really like. Often, sneaks subconsciously feel they lack the talent, intelligence, or skills to be successful, and they use covert manipulative behavior to gain promotions and advance their position. They often behave in a way to gain attention from a superior and feel a strong sense of jealousy when the superior gives the attention or promotion they want to another person. They will work hard to bring that person down. They are very sensitive to criticism and often feel slighted and angry at people who may have unintentionally said something that hurt their feelings.

Sneak Tactics

Methods commonly used by sneaks to achieve their goals include personal digs, rumors, accusations, allegations, finger-pointing, and innuendoes. Sneaks often appear very friendly when they are communicating face to face with you, but they do not have your best interests in mind and are looking for a weakness they can exploit to lower your esteem. They will use any underhanded means to discredit a person, and by making that person appear inferior, they feel superior. They also go out of their way to avoid confrontation.

Sneaks like to keep the workplace in a state of uncertainty, tension, and disorder. One of their favorite tactics to achieve this goal is to divide and conquer. For example, the sneak knows that Bill and Cindy have a strong work alliance and friendship and rely on each other to provide high-quality care on the unit. The sneak will try to break up this alliance by first going to Bill, on Cindy's day off, and saying, "Don't repeat this, but did you hear what Cindy said about you? She said you were incompetent and shouldn't be working as an RN." Then, when Bill isn't around, the sneak would go to Cindy and say, "Don't repeat this, but did you hear what Bill is saying about you? He said you were too fat to be working on such a busy unit and provided really poor care." And the pot gets stirred!

One of the most powerful tools they use is a mixed rumor, which contains just enough truth to make it completely believable.[8] For example, Kelly is an RN on the unit who was selected by the hospital to attend an expenses-paid workshop in another state because of his interest in geriatric nursing. Taylor, who is an infamous sneak, started a rumor while Kelly was away by saying, "You know that Kelly went to that workshop paid by the hospital? Well, I heard that he skipped most of the breakout sessions and spent his time in the bar drinking with strange women!" The truth is that Kelly did go to the workshop; the rumor is what he did there. There is just enough truth in the rumor to make it credible.

Some of the messages that sneaks send out by their behavior are that no one should confront or tangle with them because, when you are out of earshot, they will put you in your place. Also, because of the covert nature of their attacks, they believe that they are unstoppable and that they are the only ones honest enough to tell the truth about other workers.

Unveiling the Sneak

The basic principles discussed previously in conjunction with some of the techniques for dealing with the persecutor will work, up to a point, with the sneak; however, there are several different techniques that must also be used to be successful. As with the persecutor, perception and self-knowledge are significant

elements in dealing with the sneak's behavior. You need to understand how and why you react the way you do when suffering the aftermath of a sneak's attack. Your reaction is a behavior that you can and need to change. Sneaks are unlikely to change their behaviors to any great degree. Understanding your own motives, preferences, beliefs, and biases can help in softening the devastation you feel after the attack.[6] Methods for revealing sneaks for who they really are include the following:

Make the decision to talk to them about their behavior. Sneaks will not change on their own and may not change anyway, but it is worth a try. Talking to them takes a high degree of courage and resolve because the exchange is going to be difficult. Do this only after you have settled down from the effects of the attack and are calm and certain of what you want to do. If you display excessive emotions while talking with them, sneaks win. They are highly manipulative and will try to make you feel bad about yourself and sorry for them.[8]

> **If you display excessive emotions while talking with them, sneaks win. They are highly manipulative and will try to make you feel bad about yourself and sorry for them.**

Let them know that you know. Catching them in the act is the best way to let sneaks know you know, but this is often difficult to accomplish. They are sneaky, after all. Pretending that you did not hear them and doing nothing is what they want you to do. You can say something such as "Taylor, you were the only one who knew that I went to that workshop. How come everyone else is talking about what I supposedly did there?" It is important that you talk with others to confirm what you heard. Make sure you have your facts straight when you do talk with the sneak, or the sneak will pick apart what you are trying to say and turn the attack on you.

Let the group know that you heard what the sneak said. Using a statement such as "Did everybody hear what Taylor said about me?" will gain you support among your peers.

Do not show your hostility toward the sneak in front of a group. Avoid being rude and aggressive. Like persecutors, sneaks have fragile egos and low self-esteem. Unlike persecutors, who will immediately attack back when confronted, sneaks will use the incident to make themselves seem like the "victim," which is another type of manipulative behavior. They revel in the "poor me" role because it garners sympathy from the other staff members and gives them more ammunition against you: "Did you see how mean Sarah was to me?"

Stay on point when you finally speak with them. Sneaks will try to turn the subject back on you to break your train of thought. Just keep saying, "We're not talking about me; we're talking about your behavior," and then continue with your train of thought. They are expert distracters, so you might want to make a list of things you want to say and take that along. Also, do not laugh at them, do not agree with them, and do not let them gain control of the conversation nor let it go.

Try to treat them with empathy and understanding, not resentment and anger. Like persecutors, sneaks have developed this type of behavior in response to something that is missing in their early lives. This has become the only way sneaks can gain attention or exercise any control in their lives. They never developed adult communication skills, and it is likely they have been using these manipulative behaviors for many years in all aspects of their lives. That is probably one of the reasons they have few friends. Sneaks tend to be negative all the time, and most people steer clear of negativity. Many people have enough negativity in their lives already and do not need any more from a coworker.

Listen carefully to their response. If you are able to complete your thoughts and finish what you are saying without them walking away, it is important to listen to how they respond. It is important to remain open-minded and to be prepared to understand what motivated them to use the behaviors they use. You might discover that you did or said something unintentionally that they took as a personal insult, which triggered their behavior. Sneaks often display paranoid tendencies. You might actually need to apologize to them. Even though you did nothing to deserve their negative behavior, be prepared to listen to what they have to say. They probably need someone to talk to, someone to confide in, and in some peculiar way, you might just be the person who is their first real

friend in many years. You might be the first person who has been prepared to really listen to them and not just turn your back on them or try to get revenge.

Plan for future interactions. After you have listened carefully to them and provided responses to questions or further explained your feelings, set the direction for your future relationship. Make them believe that their behavior must change, or you will take whatever actions are required to guarantee that they will never undermine you again. If it becomes clear that the relationship will not work, let them know that you will treat them in a civil and professional manner, but the relationship will go no further.

Forewarned is forearmed. Now that you know what types of behaviors can be expected from sneaks, you can be more cautious about leaving yourself open to future attacks. You are much less vulnerable when you can keep a close eye on them and head off covert attacks before they happen.[6]

Patients With Difficult Behaviors

Patients displaying difficult behaviors are in some ways similar to coworkers with difficult behaviors, but in other ways they are very different. The nurse is legally and ethically bound to provide the best care possible for all patients, even those who are displaying behavior that makes communication or care difficult. Although some patients may actually be persecutors or sneaks in their everyday lives or even have undiagnosed personality disorders, most patients displaying difficult behaviors are acting that way as a response to their illnesses or injuries. Their needs and goals are different from those of persecutors and sneaks.

Earlier we discussed the effects of grief on individuals. Although we usually think of grief as being associated with a loss such as the death of a loved one, patients who are severely ill or severely injured; who have had major surgeries, amputations, or loss of internal body parts; or who may be facing death also often go through the stages of grief: denial, anger, guilt, depression, and resolution. The traditional five stages of grief were first presented by Dr. Elisabeth Kübler-Ross, who had investigated grief and suffering for many years before developing her theory on grief. Some more recent theorists believe that Kübler-Ross's five-stage theory is too simplistic and have added several additional stages to the process and changed the names of the models.[9] Many sources cite seven or more phases of grief. Everyone experiences grief in their own way, and some people may not experience all the stages in order, or they may even skip some. One person may experience only one or two stages, go back to a previous stage for a while, and then advance to the next stage.[10] Others may become "stuck" in a stage and not seem to be able to move forward. Experiencing grief is a messy process that often feels like it will never end. Remind the patient that there is hope. If they can understand the process and recognize the stage they are in at any given time, they will see the light at the end of the grief tunnel.

Grief Signs and Symptoms

Just as everyone experiences grief differently, they also show different emotional, physical, and/or social symptoms of the grieving process. It is not uncommon for people in mourning to cry hard and frequently, although others may not cry at all. In either case, they may not be able to verbally express their feelings.[9] Experiencing depression is common, as it is one of the stages of grief. However, these feelings may become more intense on important days, such as the anniversary of a death or a person's birthday and particularly around holidays. Long-term unresolved depression can become a serious clinical condition.[10]

Similar to a severe traumatic event, if the source of grief is due to a sudden, unforeseen incident, the individual may experience varying degrees of posttraumatic stress disorder (PTSD). With mild PTSD, they may try to cope with the repressed anxiety through alcohol and drug abuse. In more severe cases, they may have physical symptoms, including headache, loss of appetite, nausea, vomiting, or difficulty sleeping, or psychological symptoms such as delusions and hallucinations.[10] They may express a strong desire to be alone and separate themselves from others. Routine simple daily tasks become hard to complete. Unfortunately, long-term depression suppresses the activity of the immune system and makes the person more susceptible to infections and other immune-related diseases.[9]

Despite the move to more grief stages, Kübler-Ross's five stages remain the gold standard and comprise the theory that is most often taught to nursing students.

The nurse has two primary goals in caring for patients who are working through the grief stages: (1) to provide the best care possible so that they will survive and recover from their illness (meet their physiological and safety needs) and (2) to help these patients work their way through the stages of grief until they reach resolution.[10] The ideal is to achieve both goals simultaneously, but that is not always possible. Goal 1 will always have the higher priority.

How each patient experiences grief is highly individual, and there is no right way to resolve grief. Some patients move rapidly through the stages, some skip stages, and some are unable to move on from the stage they are in. The stages of grief are guides to help determine where the patient is in the grieving and mourning process. The key to determining a patient's grief stage is to observe their behavior. It is also important to consider the effects of medications and pain on the patient's behavior. Unfortunately, our health-care system of today often sends people home well before they have had a chance to complete the grief stages. However, if the nurse is able to start the process and move it even one stage, the other stages will progress more easily at home.

As discussed earlier, coworkers with difficult behaviors have need-fulfillment issues at the upper levels of Maslow's hierarchy of needs. However, severely ill patients are often attempting to meet the needs of the lower levels of the triangle—physiological survival and safety. Maslow believed that if the lower-level needs are not met, the person is unable to move to higher-level need fulfillment. Severely ill patients, in some ways, are starting over in their needs development.[1] It is a key responsibility of nurses to aid patients in maintaining their physiological and safety needs so that they can move back up to their prior levels of adjustment.

Even more so than when working with a difficult coworker, perception on the part of the nurse plays an important part in understanding and adapting to patient behaviors. Quickly stereotyping a patient by saying, "Oh, he's just an old grouch," "She's a real whiner and complainer," or "He doesn't like nurses. He won't do anything I want him to do," completely disregards the underlying issues that are causing the patient to behave in a difficult way. Often, once a patient is labeled, the care provided to them is based on that label, and the patient's real issues are never addressed or resolved.[4]

Establishing Trust

Establishing trust is key to any successful relationship. In the nurse–patient relationship, it is the foundation upon which all nursing care is built and is particularly important when dealing with difficult behavior. In most relationships, it takes a considerable amount of time to develop trust between two people; however, in the health-care setting, time is limited, and trust has to be built quickly. Nurses have a head start in trusting relationships with patients. An annual Gallup poll surveys the nation's population asking which profession they trust most. For the past 21 years, that profession has been nursing.

Respect

Trust can be established by showing respect for the opinions and ideas of individuals and letting them know you accept their behavior even though you do not agree with it. Always be honest with patients even when it is not pleasant to do so.[11] If patients find out that you have been less than honest with them, it is almost impossible to regain their trust. Nurses sometimes are tempted to be less than 100 percent truthful because we do not want to hurt their feelings, make them angry, or upset them. By focusing on what is going well with patients rather than criticizing them or pointing out the problems in their behavior, you can soften the impact of a negative statement and show them that you are not being judgmental about them or their condition.

> *Being reliable and doing what you say you will do, even in small things, acts as a foundation for trust.*

Consistency

Another important element in building trust is being consistent in what you do and say. Patients are better able to relax if they know what is coming next. Being reliable and doing what you say you will do, even in small things, acts as a foundation for trust. If you tell the patient you will be back to check on them in 30 minutes, make sure you come back on time. If patients can trust you in the small things, they will trust you with the more critical things. Generally, nurses should not make promises to patients. Health care and health-care outcomes have too many variables to be certain about much of anything; however, if you do make a promise to a patient, make sure you keep it. Even promises about small issues, such as promising to get the patient some juice after finishing the patient next door, can have a huge impact on a person whose world is currently limited to a hospital room.

Confidentiality

In order to trust you, the patient needs to know that you will keep their confidence. Nurses are bound ethically and legally to maintain confidentiality of patient information, but nurse–patient communication is *not* considered privileged communication as exists between priest and penitent or lawyer and patient or physician and patient. (See Chapter 6 for more details.) Personal secrets that do not affect the patient's health care are easier to keep and should remain secret. Information that is important to their treatment or recovery should be revealed to the health-care provider. If a patient tells you something in confidence—for example, "Don't tell anybody, but I have seizures from time to time"—and it is not on the medical record, you need to inform the patient that the information is important to their treatment, and you are going to pass it on to the health-care provider. Sometimes patients will ask you, "I want to tell you something that I don't want anyone else to know about. Can you keep it secret?" A good response is to say, "I can keep secrets, but if what you are about to tell me is important to your care or recovery, I'll have to let the health-care provider know. If what you tell me might be harmful to yourself or someone else, then by law, I must alert other individuals who are caring for you or a legal authority such as the police. Other than in those situations, the information won't go any further than here."

Loyalty

Nurses can also foster trust in patients by showing how loyal they are to the patient and to the principles of nursing, being proficient in their health-care knowledge and nursing skills, and showing that they are ethically and morally strong. In addition, demonstrating the use of good judgment in decision making, being fair, maintaining objectivity in difficult situations, and taking responsibility for your actions also reinforce an atmosphere of trust. Once two people begin to trust each other, even if they disagree about some of the issues, they are much more likely to come to a satisfactory resolution of the problem.

Stages of Grief

This discussion of managing difficult patient behaviors is organized around the stages of grief and prioritized by the levels of Maslow's hierarchy. The behaviors most commonly associated with each grief stage are presented along with methods to respond to the behaviors. Some of the methods discussed earlier for managing coworkers with difficult behaviors also work with patients, although, because of their different needs, additional methods are also required.

Denial

Denial, sometimes called the "I'm fine syndrome," is used as a coping mechanism to give people time to adjust to sudden traumatic situations. For some people, it becomes a way of life, particularly if they have addiction issues. It is an unconscious process that protects the individual from feeling vulnerable or losing control. Because it is an unconscious process, patients often are unable to accept obvious facts, or they greatly minimize the consequences of their condition.

This stage is often very short and may take place even before the patient arrives at the hospital. Statements such as "This can't be happening," "I don't believe what you are telling me," "Are you sure about that diagnosis?" and "This treatment (surgery, medication, etc.) is a waste of time. There is nothing wrong with me" are all expressions of denial. Some patients, however, get locked into a state of denial and are unable to move from it. They may spend 2 weeks in the hospital being treated for a severe heart attack, including open heart surgery, and the day they go home, they say, "I'm glad there really wasn't anything wrong with me."

Goals

Patients in a persistent denial stage use behaviors that achieve the goal of maintaining their denial. The denial protects them from accepting the reality of their condition, which may significantly alter their body image, and precludes the need for them to make lifestyle changes, eat a restricted diet, or limit their activities after discharge.[12] There are different degrees of denial ranging from mild, which is relatively easy to overcome, to impenetrable denial, which is resistant to all rational reasoning. Common denial behaviors include refusing to take medications, refusing to go for diagnostic tests, pulling off monitor electrodes, and not following directions about activity if they decide they are not necessary because they believe they are not really sick. They might even decide to sign themselves out of the hospital against medical advice (AMA).

Autonomy

One of the important considerations in working with patients in denial is consideration of their autonomy or right to self-determination. (See Chapter 7 for more detail.) From a strictly legal and ethical point of view, they have a right to do or not do whatever they want. However, some of their autonomous actions can come into direct conflict with the nurse's obligation for beneficence, to do good for the patient.

Patients in denial pose significant challenges for nurses. Health-care providers sometimes will ask a nurse, "Did Ms. Hart take her antibiotic this morning?" The nurse answers, "No, she refused to take it because she says she doesn't need it." The health-care provider responds loudly, "When did she get her MD? She *does* need it! Get in there and make her take it!" Of course, you cannot force patients to do anything they do not want to do if they are competent. Forcing patients to take medications or undergo treatments they do not want leaves the nurse open to civil suits for assault and battery. What is the nurse to do?

Approaches

There are several approaches that can be used to achieve the goals of providing quality care and moving the patient out of denial:

Walking the tightrope. Approaching patients in denial who are refusing to take their medications or submit to prescribed treatments requires a gentle touch. Providing too much information may overwhelm them, and being too forceful in your approach may stiffen their resolve not to do what you want.[8] On the other hand, diminishing or dismissing the issue will also not accomplish your goals.

Look at the situation from the patients' point of view. They have a reason for not taking the medication or going for their treatments. Addressing that reason with compassion and rational arguments about why they should cooperate with you may work if they are in a mild denial state; however, no amount of objective reasoning will penetrate the resolve of patients in persistent denial. You must find another way to moti-vate them to take their medications. Although it is not ideal and comes very close to violating the "always tell the truth" principle, sometimes you need to use approaches that are somewhat manipulative. Follow-ing are some possible approaches that you can use:

You can trust me; I'm the nurse. You can use the trust the patient has built up in you due to your compas-sion and knowledge to change behavior. For exam-ple, "Ms. Hart, I feel like we've developed a strong relationship over the past few days. You know I have never lied to you and promise I never will. You need to believe me when I tell you that this medication is necessary for your recovery. Please take it." Be careful using this: it is right on the line of paternalism.

It can't hurt. This is sometimes called the **humor-me approach.** "Ms. Hart, I know you don't think you need this medication, but Dr. Sánchez wants you to have it. Why don't you take it anyway, since it really doesn't hurt anything, and if you really do need it, it will actually help." Or "I would really appreciate it if you would take this med-ication. I want to help you."

Let's try it and see what happens. "Ms. Hart, I know you don't believe you need this medication, but if you look at your incision site, you can see how red and tender it is. Why don't you take this medication and see if it helps with the pain? You'll probably need several doses for it to be effective."

I'll be back. "Ms. Hart, I feel like you have other things on your mind right now. I'll come back in an hour, and you can take your medication then."

Establishing a strong trusting relationship. Use the techniques discussed earlier for trusting relationships. It is particularly important in working with patients in denial.

Being consistent in your message. This approach is similar to the "walk the tightrope" approach, except now it is directed at resolving the issue of denial. You need to move slowly and let patients determine the

pace of the discussion. Agree to disagree, but do not waver in your message. Patients in denial will insist that there is nothing wrong with them, but you need to make it clear that you believe the laboratory tests, x-rays, and other objective findings that indicate that they are ill; however, do not argue with them or attempt to overwhelm them with facts and data. They will shut down completely.

Use the communication building techniques. The most important ones for patients in denial are as follows:

- Asking open-ended questions and taking the time to really listen to the responses. Try to uncover what they are afraid of losing by accepting the diagnosis: independence? lifestyle? life itself? Fear is a powerful motivator.
- Reflecting back emotions that are being expressed. Acknowledge and accept both positive and negative emotions and remember that crying is a powerful emotional release. "Ms. Bell, although you insist that there is nothing wrong with your leg, I'm getting the sense you are afraid that if the health-care provider treats it, you might not be able to clean your house or care for your grandchildren any-more. Am I mistaken?"
- Asking clarifying questions. "Ms. Bell, you said before that you are really okay, but then you just said you are afraid that the pain in your leg might lead to an amputation. I'm a little confused. Can you help me understand what you are saying?"
- Using all the nonverbal and paraverbal techniques. Eye contact, directly facing the patient, open pos-ture, quiet tone, head nodding, and light touch help to engage patients even when they prefer not to hear your message.[11]

Encourage family involvement. Families need to receive clear, timely, comprehensive, and correct information to be able to participate effectively in the patient's care. The nurse needs to make sure to include them, as appropriate, discussing patient problems and care, developing care plans, and setting outcomes

> *The anger stage may come and go quickly for some patients, whereas other patients may hang on tightly to their anger stage. Anger can be both a defense mechanism and a form of manipulative behavior.*

and goals. Two-way communication with the family is essential because they can provide the nurse with additional or missing information about the patient. If available at the hospital, a family-patient portal is an excellent method to engage family members. It will help them quickly find details and information about their loved one's care, schedule of upcoming tests and treatment, and health status updates. If the portal has a mechanism for secure messaging, the family can provide immediate information back to the nurse.[12]

However, working with the family can also be a tightrope act. You need to inform the family members of what is happening, that you need their help, and how they can be helpful. For example, "Your dad is denying that he has cancer and is refusing all treatment and medications. We are working to get him to accept his diagnosis. Denial is an unconscious protective mechanism people use to avoid the fear associated with their condition. However, we need to avoid using the 'hard sell' with him. Yelling at him and arguing with him will only make him more resistant. Letting him talk about how he is feeling is a much better approach and is more successful. Thank you for your help." Keep in mind that families sometimes go into denial, too, and reinforce the patient's denial or have a relationship that involves yelling and arguing as the usual form of communication, which only exacerbates the denial state.[12]

Provide information in small doses. Too much information at one time can overwhelm patients and increase their resistance. Leave reading materials in their room that they can consider when they are ready.

Anger

Angry behavior between coworkers was discussed earlier as one of the important communication blockers. Anger expressed by patients is also a significant communication blocker; however, it has different causes and manifestations in patients who are severely ill or injured. As patients move away from the denial stage and the protective veil of refutation and refusal falls away, patients are often unprepared for the flood of intense emotions they are experiencing. They have suddenly become vulnerable and recognize that they have lost most of their control over their lives and their future.[13] When patients accept that they are acutely ill, it means they are literally placing their lives in the hands of the health-care team.

Remember also that mild to severe episodic pain or even mild long-term chronic pain can elicit irritation and antagonism, even though the patient is not in any particular grief stage. Assessing the cause of the behavior is extremely important because the techniques used for a patient exhibiting grief-stage angry behavior will not be effective. Pain medication and distraction techniques are much more effective. However, sometimes patients displaying grief-stage anger can also be in pain.

> *Unlike patients in denial, angry patients will comply with most treatments and medications, even if they do so grudgingly, with resentment, and with some caustic comments.*

Patients' expressions of anger can range from a mild sense of frustration to declarations of injustice or raging destructive behaviors that must be stopped immediately. Patients in the anger stage often use statements that contain a small degree of recognition of their condition. Common statements that can indicate a patient is in the anger stage include "Why is this happening to me?" "This isn't right! I don't deserve this," "What has God got against me?" and "If my #%&@$ boss didn't put so much pressure on me, I wouldn't have had this heart attack!"

Other behaviors indicating the anger stage include tightened jaw; clenched fists; aggressive body language and posture; fidgeting; physiological responses such as elevated pulse rate, blood pressure, and respiratory rate; red face; raised voice; making threats; excessive demands for attention; and overt acts that express anger, such as throwing food trays or banging on bedside tables.[10] However, unlike patients in denial, angry patients will comply with most treatments and medications, even if they do so grudgingly, with resentment, and with some caustic comments. Most patients who are expressing anger believe their anger is a result of what has happened to them.

The anger stage may come and go quickly for some patients, whereas other patients may hang on tightly to their anger stage. Anger can be both a defense mechanism and a form of manipulative behavior. Anger, for those who are unwilling to let go, fulfills their needs for feeling safe and secure and meets the goal of avoiding uncomfortable feelings such as fear, particularly of pain and death, and feelings of helplessness and powerlessness resulting from loss of mobility or independence. Factors that can contribute to the anger stage are feelings of anxiety, frustration with their care, or increased feelings of stress. If they are religious, the anger may also be caused by feelings of abandonment, particularly by God or a higher power.[13] Anger is less of a threat to a patient's physical status than the behavior displayed in denial, but anger behaviors have a relatively high potential to affect the patient's safety needs, ranging from self-injury to the development of stress-related disorders.

Coping with anger is always difficult, regardless of whether it is our own anger or that being expressed by a patient. Some patients express anger easily and openly; others have little outward expression of anger and instead suppress and direct it inward. Anger turned inward is hard to assess, is very destructive, and usually is related to feelings of guilt, which is also a very destructive emotion. When patients can say, "I'm so angry at (my disease process)," the anger becomes therapeutic and part of the recovery process.

Expressions of anger always need a target, and it is usually a target of convenience and proximity. Nurses are always near their patients, so they can expect the angry behavior to be directed toward them. When patients are displaying angry behavior toward the nurse, it is a normal tendency to say, "I've had enough! They don't pay me enough to take this abuse. Put your call light on the next time you want to insult me!" and not go back in the room. This is a knee-jerk reaction and needs to be avoided.[13] By understanding that the nurse is not the real target of the patient's anger but was merely there when the patient was expressing feelings of anger at the situation can lessen the impact of the attack on the nurse, but it still hurts. It is also important to let family members, who are also often targets of a patient's anger, know that the patient is not really angry at them but is expressing feelings of loss of control and helplessness. Angry retorts from family members toward the patient can result in explosive arguments that no one wins.

Because the anger stage has fewer threats to the patient's physiological well-being than the denial stage does, the following approaches to working with a patient displaying angry behavior are focused more on moving them out of the anger stage. Many of these approaches are similar to those used for moving a patient out of the denial stage. Of course, if the patient's anger is being expressed in a self-destructive way, such as punching a glass window or throwing objects around that can bounce back and hurt them, it has become an emergency situation and action must be taken quickly to stop the behavior.

Approaches to the Angry Patient

Release anger safely. Although it is important for the patient to "get the anger out," anger should never be taken out on another person. The anger should be redirected to inanimate objects or safe activities that hurt neither the patient nor others. The ultimate goal is to have the patient redirect the anger toward the illness.[7] Throwing small plastic items such as cups or spongy stress-relief balls at a wall, scribbling hard on sheets of paper, tearing sheets of paper into small pieces, breaking pencils or tongue depressors in half, wadding paper into a ball and throwing it hard at a wall or trash can, or punching a pillow are all safe and harmless physical ways of expressing anger. Provide the patient with a stress-relief ball that they can squeeze. Be creative!

In the past, "scream therapy" was thought to be an effective way of releasing pent-up anger, but in the health-care setting, loud screaming is considered disruptive. However, depending on the unit, the number of patients, and the staffing, it may be possible to allow the patient in the anger stage to yell, scream, and stomp the feet, if able, by closing the door to the patient's room and other patients' rooms and warning the staff of what is about to happen and why. You can also include the patient in deciding on a safe expression of anger. "Mr. Pound, I appreciate how angry you are at your situation; however, yelling at me and the other staff and throwing your urinal when it is full is not appropriate. Is there something that you might want to do to express your anger that is safe and doesn't involve other people?"

Respond calmly and with respect. Although showing patients respect is an ethical requirement, when responding to angry patients, it is usually easier said than done. Patients expressing their anger are insulting, demanding, and in general, very annoying. Outside of the health-care setting, you would likely respond to this behavior by avoiding them, but as a nurse, that is not an option.[13]

Following are a few of the comments, heard over a 40-year career as an RN, made by patients who are displaying anger behaviors:

"You're not a very good RN, and you're fat too."
"Go get the pretty nurse; at least she knows what she is doing."
"Did you comb your hair with a firecracker this morning?"
"OH NO, NOT YOU AGAIN."
"If even one more person asks me how I'm doing, I'll shoot them!"
"You bring me another tray of this slop you're passing off as food, and I'll throw it at you!" (She did.)
"I want my bed bath now while I'm awake."
"You're supposed to give me my medication at 9:00 a.m.; it's almost 15 after. Where is it?"
"I've had my call light on for 2 hours. Where have you been?" (It was more like 2 minutes.)
"What do you mean you're changing my dressing-change procedure? It already hurts enough when you pull the thing off!"
"Take me for my CT scan now! I'm getting hungry."
"The care is so bad here I'm going to call my lawyer and sue you and this torture chamber for every penny it's worth."

The instinctual response to such statements is to take them personally, fire back with an even sharper verbal barb (scorched earth response), or run out of the room crying. None of these responses are therapeutic, nor do they do anything positive for the patient or you. As difficult as it might seem, the way to respond to angry behavior and speech is to remain calm, remembering that you are a professional and you are in control.[11] The statement the angry patient made was not a personal attack on you; rather, you just happened to be near when they wanted to express feelings of anger. Use acknowledgment and reflection in response to the underlying message that is in the underlying emotion being expressed.

Never respond to the actual statement. Remember, the patient is trying to achieve the goal of self-protection from the realization of the effects of his illness. However, in your best reassuring, calm, rational, professional, and "I'm in control" voice, while displaying open and accepting body language, respond by saying, "I understand how upsetting all this must be for you and how angry you are. We really need to talk about what is making you feel this way."

Sometimes the patient may actually have a legitimate complaint that needs to be addressed. If that is the case, let them know that you are doing something to fix the problem so that it does not happen again. For example, "Ms. Pesci, it appears that the food we've been bringing to you is not up to the standards you expect. I called the dietitian, and she will be here shortly to see if we can improve the selection and quality of the food you are receiving."

It is also helpful to practice by role-playing with a good friend because many people have never had another person talk to them this way. Have your friend attack you verbally with the statements presented earlier or ones that they think up, and analyze how you feel. Practice responding calmly and confidently to the emotion of the statement, not the statement itself.

Keep it cool. If the patient is in an agitated state and is hurling a nonstop barrage of insults and demands at you, step back one step, displaying accepting body language (hands off hips and no crossed arms on chest) and wait until the patient finishes. When the barrage is over and the room becomes quiet, speak calmly and softly, addressing the patient by their name. "Mr. Vance, I appreciate how scared you are. Everyone here is working hard to help you recover. All I want to do now is to listen to your lung sounds to make sure you are breathing okay." Using a calm, confident approach will help the patient relax enough to complete the rest of the physical evaluation. In some cases, the patient may even apologize for the outburst. "I'm so sorry I acted that way. I don't know what came over me." This actually may be the opening you need to address the patient's underlying feelings of fear and loss of control.

Defuse a blowup. In response to unpleasant news or some incident involving their care that they perceive as a threat, some patients with anger issues will at

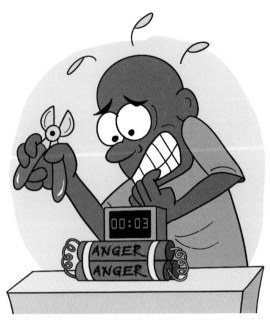

"Defusing an anger blowup can be dangerous to your health!"

times totally lose control, become irrational, and become deaf to anything you have to say. The trigger event or issue does not have to be major; patients' worlds get very small in the confines of a hospital room, and small issues can loom as giant monsters to them. The approach to a patient who has blown up emotionally is similar to the approach used to defuse the behavior of a toddler having a temper tantrum. Responding by yelling back at the patient, "Calm down," "Stop acting like a child," or "This is not acceptable behavior," will only intensify and prolong the blowup. In this situation, the patient is using the behavior to manipulate the nurse into giving them more attention or to get their way. Any type of response, either positive or negative, during the blowup just reinforces the behavior, which will be used increasingly often in the future.[13]

With toddlers who are having tantrums, the best approach, after making sure they are safe and cannot harm themselves, is to walk away. The tantrum usually stops quickly thereafter. The same approach can be used for patients, but a more therapeutic approach is to maintain eye contact with the patient in an accepting posture while they are exploding and listen

actively to the underlying emotions being expressed. Often, they will reveal what happened recently in their lives to trigger the outburst. After the patient has returned to a relatively rational state and is able to hear you again, acknowledge their feelings. If something that happened in the course of their care triggered the outburst, let them know that you regret the situation and will work to resolve it.

Involving patients in their care in general increases their sense of control and levels of compliance.[9] For patients who have blown up, asking them for their help in resolving the problem is highly effective. Use statements such as "Tell me what we need to do to resolve this issue," "Give me some suggestions on ways to deal with this," or "If you were in my shoes, how would you go about preventing this from happening again?" Try to reach an agreement with the patient on how you both can work together to find an answer. For example, "I hear what you are saying. The night nurses are very noisy and keep you from sleeping. We could approach this by having me talk to the charge nurse on the night shift about keeping the noise down. I will let her know that when you are being kept up by the noise, you will put your call light on and inform your nurse that it is getting noisy. Does that sound like a pretty good approach?" Use short, clear sentences when communicating with this type of patient.

Stop, look, and listen. As we saw with patients in denial, it is impossible to push patients off the anger stage of grief or pull them to the next stage. We can, however, facilitate their progress, but they will only move on when they are emotionally ready to do so and see some type of reward for the progress. A strong, trusting relationship is essential in making any progress and requires the use of many of the communication builders and time. The goal is to help patients understand that their expressions of anger are really a defense to accepting the realities of their illnesses or injuries.

Set aside at least a half-hour block of time and tell the patient that you will be talking with them at a predetermined time—that is, make an appointment. Make sure you show up on time and begin the communication by asking a question such as "Mr. Axelrod, I've been concerned about you for several days now. I really don't know you that well, so could you please tell me something about your background and life?" Then let him talk without interruption. Use body language that shows you are serious about the communication, including nodding, appropriate facial expressions, and eye contact. Turn off your cell phone. Listen attentively to his whole story. For many patients, this may be the first time a health-care provider has shown a real interest in them as a person and not just a disease process. "The amputation in room 234 curses at anyone who comes in the room with medications" is an example of a depersonalizing statement.

When the patient stops speaking, allow for a short pause and then begin your response by agreeing with them and showing them that you listened to what they said. For example, "I'm really glad you were willing to share that information with me about yourself, Mr. Axelrod. I can see that you have had a difficult life and appreciate the efforts you have made to improve yourself. By getting to know you better, I believe I can take better care of you." However, do not turn your reply into a lengthy monolog. Rather, see it as an opportunity to ask more questions that will help the patient attain self-realization of their behavior.

Sometimes gentle confrontation may help the patient see the issues more clearly. Statements such as "You seemed to be upset about something earlier today. Can you tell me about it?" or "You made some angry comments to the orderly who was helping you with your bath. Could you tell me what that was about?" This can open the door to deeper and more meaningful communication; however, be very cautious using any type of confrontation. The answers to these types of questions can lead to additional questions that will direct the course of the discussion.

Other techniques that help reveal the underlying causes of the patient's anger include reflection and legitimization.[10] We saw that reflective statements or questions such as "It appears to me that you became angry because you believed that I didn't think you were in pain. Is that correct?" are aimed at getting patients

> " *Use body language that shows you are serious about the communication, including nodding, appropriate facial expressions, and eye contact. Turn off your cell phone.* "

to talk about their deeper feelings. Legitimization is the acknowledgment of and agreement with the patient's perceptions. For example, you can say, "I see now why you became upset. You asked me for pain medication, and I gave you a medication different from the one you usually take without explaining what it was. I'd probably be upset also if I were in your shoes. It seems to bother you to depend on other people to meet your needs when you've been so independent all your life."

Threat of physical harm. Patients who are displaying grief-stage anger behavior usually are not physically aggressive. However, if at any time a patient threatens or attempts to harm you physically or you sincerely believe your safety is in jeopardy, contact your coworkers immediately for help and let hospital security know of the situation. Often, after they are alerted to a potentially dangerous situation with a patient, security will post a guard on the unit but will keep them out of the room and out of sight. Following are some actions by the nurse that may provoke a physical attack and should never happen when working with an angry patient, particularly one in an outburst state:

- Interrupting the patient during an outburst: "Stop yelling right now!"
- Warning a patient not to use insults, cursing, or crude language: "The hospital doesn't allow that type of speech."
- Reciprocating anger back to the patient when they make a personal insult: "You think I'm fat? Have you looked at yourself lately? You look like a pig in a mud wallow!"
- Challenging the truth of the patient's statement: "That's not true, and you know it!"
- Criticizing the patient's behavior: "You're acting like a three-year-old having a tantrum!"
- Becoming defensive: "I'm doing the best I can, but you are impossible to please."
- Using touch to try to calm down the patient.
- Blocking the patient's exit from the room.
- Getting behind the patient, out of sight, and talking to them.[12]

Documentation. It is imprinted on all nurses from the first day of nursing school that documentation is a mandatory part of the life of a health-care provider. In working with patients who display angry behaviors, or any of the grief-related difficult behaviors, documenting what was said and done becomes extremely important. Make sure to rate the level of the patient's anger, specific actions and statements by the patient that indicate anger, interventions you initiated in response to the patient's behavior, and how the patient responded to the interventions. Do not hesitate to complete an incident report if the patient in any way harms you physically. Good documentation is worth its weight in gold if the patient or family decides to initiate a lawsuit.

Bargaining

As the flames of the bonfire of the anger stage are slowly extinguished, reality again comes crashing back in, making the patient feel vulnerable. Patients begin seeking other ways to protect themselves from the things that are happening to them. It is a way for them to hang on to hope when everything seems hopeless. A general definition of bargaining is that it is a form of negotiation in which two parties attempt to reach a deal that is satisfactory to both parties over some item or issue. However, in the bargaining stage of grief, the patient has no one to bargain with except a higher power.[14]

Bargaining is an unconscious coping mechanism that seeks to fulfill the goals of avoiding the bad things that the patient anticipates will soon happen to them and regaining some degree of control over their life. It often becomes a type of "magical thinking" that is frequently seen in young children. Bargaining is also an expression of hope, often unrealistic, on the part of the patient, frequently based on irrational beliefs or incomplete information.

There is no set time limit on the bargaining stage: some patients totally skip it, and others find it very comfortable to remain in it almost indefinitely. It can become one of the most difficult stages from which to

> *There is no set time limit on the bargaining stage: some patients totally skip it, and others find it very comfortable to remain in it almost indefinitely. It can become one of the most difficult stages from which to progress.*

progress because, rather than having a large physical component that is externally disruptive, bargaining is an almost totally internal mental process.[10] The mind can have a powerful influence over beliefs and behavior. It can play all kinds of tricks on patients in this stage.

It is interesting that a bargaining stage may actually occur before the official diagnosis, when the patient merely suspects something is wrong. It serves as a means of warding off the bad news. The bargaining that occurs after diagnosis serves as a method to negotiate away the changes brought on by the disease process. As with denial and anger, the patient is seeking to meet the goals of increasing control over the situation and avoiding pain and suffering.

In all the grief stages, including bargaining, there is a relatively high level of anxiety present. Anxiety is fear of the unknown, and there are many elements of health care that always remain uncertain. Similarly, the feeling of lack of control over their own destiny causes patients to attempt to negotiate with a higher power, someone or something they believe, whether realistically or not, will help them avoid the impending changes. They often make promises to God, hoping that the pain of the illness might not occur or might at least be lessened. They look for their lives to go back to how they were before they were given the diagnosis or started the treatment.[14]

Often, patients in the bargaining stage are intensely focused on what they could have done differently in the past to prevent what is happening to them now. They also imagine all the things that could have been and how wonderful their lives could be if this bad thing had not happened to them. This type of thinking is an improvement over the denial and anger responses to their illness because it moves patients closer to accepting the changes that are occurring in their lives. They are beginning to understand and recognize the full impact their condition will have on their lives; however, it is relatively easy for excessive efforts at bargaining to produce high levels of remorse and guilt that will ultimately block their ability to successfully cope with their situation.[11]

Recognizing when patients are in the bargaining stage is fairly easy: there is a unique set of statements they often make. The following are examples of bargaining statements:

"If I do (some action), then you (God, nurse, health-care provider) will respond by (some action like taking away my disease)."

"I should have done something sooner about this."

"We should have gotten a second opinion from another physician before now."

"If only I had led a better life, this wouldn't have happened."

"I promise to stop smoking, drinking, and cheating on my wife if you (God) make this go away."

"I must have done something terribly wrong in my life to have this happen to me."

"I heard there is a doctor in Mexico who treats this type of cancer without chemotherapy or surgery (or pain)."

"I don't believe that my doctor is as smart as he thinks he is—he didn't even know about that experimental treatment I found on the Internet."

"Go ahead and fix my broken leg, arm, and pelvis. I'm still going to ride my motorcycle when I get out."

"I don't want to start chemotherapy today. Can't we wait until next week when I'm stronger? I promise to do my physical therapy every day."

"I'll give an extra-large donation to the church if you (God) can make this go away."

"You're the fifth physician I've seen about this, and none of you has given me a good answer."

People in the bargaining stage often hold tightly to irrational or illogical beliefs. However, similar to patients in anger and denial stages, understanding our own perceptions is key to maintaining a balanced approach to patients in this stage. What seems absurd and contradictory to us appears very necessary, logical, and clear to the patient. Some beliefs that bargaining patients cling to include the following:

• There should be no pain involved in this treatment.
• All problems have simple and straightforward solutions.
• Getting better shouldn't involve much time or effort.
• If I continue looking long enough and hard enough, I'll find the cure for my disease.

• Most people work out their own problems; I can too.
• All health-care providers should be smart, kind, gentle, considerate, and able to cure me.
• Health-care providers are totally responsible for solving my problem, since I don't know anything about medicine.
• I know that I am the only one who ever had this disease.
• This is my disease; I have to deal with it by myself.
• I can't burden any of my family with treating this illness.
• You must accept any problem that comes your way as a sign of your innate evil; you must accept it as the penance or retribution for your badness.
• If I get help now, the problem will go away, and I won't need any more help.[8]

Although there are relatively few immediate threats to their physiological health when patients are experiencing bargaining, one long-term effect is that they may continue the behavior indefinitely, which prevents them from moving to acceptance. The difficult behavior that nurses may encounter with patients who are in the bargaining stage occurs when patients believe that alternative and integrative treatments will work better than the ones they are currently receiving. They may stop the approved treatments and rely on alternative treatments alone or, even more dangerous, combine alternative treatments with approved treatments without notifying the health-care team. (For more detail about integrative therapies, see Chapter 25.) Also, when bargaining patients attempt to postpone treatments or attempt to seek the perfect physician with the perfect therapeutic plan, they can delay necessary interventions for a significant length of time.[14]

Because there are elements of avoidance and rejection of treatment displayed in the behaviors of patients in the bargaining stage, some of the methods used in the care of the patient with denial will also be helpful in the patient who is bargaining. However, it is important to take into consideration the differences in what these two groups of patients are attempting to avoid. Patients in denial have the goal of totally avoiding the realization that they are ill or have a severe injury, whereas patients who are bargaining have accepted their diagnosis but are now primarily attempting to avoid the discomfort that is associated with its treatment.

Providing effective care for patients in the bargaining stage requires addressing two issues: (1) the potentially dangerous situation created by their need to postpone treatments or their rejection of conventional treatments to seek alternative treatments and (2) helping them face their anxiety and fear so that they can move toward acceptance. Care for bargaining patients is made more difficult because sometimes they appear to be cooperative and compliant while they are ignoring your instructions and covertly doing what they want.[7] Resolving the emotional issues involved in bargaining can become a significant challenge. Breaking down a system of false beliefs that a patient has developed over time can be as difficult as driving a bicycle through a brick wall.

The other element to keep in mind is that when you finally get through to them and take away their false beliefs, what do they have left? Frequently, even people who are not experiencing a threat to their health and independence have difficulty dealing with the unvarnished truth. Avoid offering false hopes to patients who are in the bargaining stage. They may cling to every word, looking for a morsel of something hopeful to hang on to. You need to balance the practical things that you can offer them with their hopes; however, never offer them something that you cannot fulfill. When they are in an active bargaining state, they are often open to your support for change or new ways of believing. If you can use that moment of openness to gain their collaboration in recognizing an illogical belief, you have made a win-win deal.

Approaches

Trust, honesty, and communication approach. Trust again becomes a key to helping the patient in the bargaining stage. All the techniques for building trust and establishing open communication are required when working with these patients. They have to trust you enough and feel comfortable enough in talking with you that they will tell you if they are using alternative treatments that you do not know about.

However, if you have a sense that they are using some herbal supplements or other potentially harmful treatments without your knowledge, you may have to ask them about your suspicions. Using a quiet, calm voice, ask non-accusatory and nonconfrontational questions, such as "I noticed you have a printout of an Internet article on herbal supplements for people with cancer on your nightstand. Tell me about the ones you have tried," "Yesterday you asked me if I knew anything about using a liquid-only diet to cure cystic fibrosis. Tell me how that is supposed to work," or even a more direct question, such as "Your blood pressure has dropped quite a bit over the last two days. Tell me about what you are doing that is different from before." This can elicit honest answers if the patient trusts you.

What if the patient responds, reluctantly, "Well, okay, yes. I've been drinking this liquid that is a traditional cure for most everything. My grandmother, who is 100 percent Creek Indian, makes it. It's made from totally natural herbs and roots and other things, she says. I take it when no one is watching. Please don't tell my physician." Now what do you do with that information?

> *You are now faced with another right to confidentiality versus obligation for beneficence dilemma. Because of the real potential for harm to the patient from ingesting unknown chemical substances, you have no option but to inform the health-care provider.*

You are now faced with another right to confidentiality versus obligation for beneficence dilemma. Because of the real potential for harm to the patient from ingesting unknown chemical substances, you have no option but to inform the health-care provider. The list of substances that Native Americans have been using for centuries as home remedies that actually do have physiological effects include minerals such as lithium and selenium, which are found in the ground and in plants such as goat weed, foxglove, willow bark, and cherry bark. Sometimes substances such as ashes, which contain mercury and lead, and apple seeds or peach pits, which contain arsenic, are used. The other problem is that the dose or the concentration of the substance is unknown. Some plants taken in small doses are relatively harmless, whereas larger doses can be lethal. And the interactive effects with other medications are unknown and potentially deadly.

To soften the effect of breaching the patient's confidentiality, you can say, "I really appreciate how honest you've been with me, Ms. Crow, in telling me about the potion you are taking. As you know, we have you taking several very powerful medications here in the hospital to combat your disease. The problem is that we don't know what is in your grandmother's potion and how it affects the other medications you are taking. There may be something in it that can combine with the medications and make you very sick, or the potion may block the effectiveness of your medication. I am going to have to inform your physician about what you are taking. He will send it to the laboratory to see exactly what the ingredients are, and the pharmacist will see if any of them affect your medications. However, if they find that there is nothing harmful in your grandmother's medication, the physician may decide that you can continue taking it. Who knows, there might actually be something in it that will help your recovery."

Preempting the postponement approach. Patients in the bargaining stage are more open to logical thinking and rational arguments than patients in the denial or anger stages. Bargaining patients have already accepted that they are sick and need help; they are just trying to find the least painful way of treatment. Conversely, they are also adept at using rational arguments and logic in the attempt to postpone treatments and therapy.

Whereas a patient in the anger stage might say, "Get that #$&@ gurney out of my room; there's no way you're taking me to radiation therapy," bargaining patients are more likely say, "My back really hurts today, so let's hold off starting radiation therapy until it feels better. I don't think I can survive lying on that hard table for 45 minutes," "I've felt too nauseated and weak today to go for another chemotherapy treatment," "I'll take all the pills you want me to take if you'll stop giving me that IV medication," or "I really don't mind starting physical therapy, but I'd like to wait until the new physician I contacted consults with me."

As nurses, we have great compassion for patients we believe are trying to be cooperative and are pleasant to be around. Bargaining patients usually fit that description; however, we have to realize that we must be proactive in dealing with behaviors that may worsen their conditions. When you detect that the patient is using bargaining behavior, you need to end the behavior as quickly as possible. However, tying patients to a gurney while they are screaming that they do not want to go may leave you open to civil suits for assault and battery.

If you have built up a high level of trust with the patient, you may want to gently confront the person, identifying and pointing out the irrational beliefs that underlie the postponing behavior. For example, you can say, "I know the thought of going to radiation therapy is frightening. The machines look very imposing, and you are giving up control of your body to someone you do not know. However, all the radiation technicians are highly trained and have been certified by a national organization, so they're the best. I've seen this type of radiation decrease the size of tumors and decrease the pain it is causing. As far as your back pain goes, I have several medications that you can take to decrease it, and I'm sure the people in radiation therapy can put something on the table to make it softer."

> " *By asking questions that cause patients to consider whether their beliefs are rational, you can begin to gradually move them toward a state of reality.* "

That's a good bargain approach. Successful coping with the bargaining stage requires that patients understand the underlying causes of the behavior and acknowledge that they are using bargaining to achieve a goal. Initially, the patient needs to recognize that they are making bargains and identify what types of bargains they are making. It is essential that the patient achieve clarity on what their bargain is.[9]

By asking questions that cause patients to consider whether their beliefs are rational, you can begin to gradually move them toward a state of reality. Questions that work to achieve this goal include the following:

"Tell me why you believe that herbal substances are better than the medications we are using in the hospital when you know you have stage four cancer?"

"You've been refusing radiation therapy for almost a week, and your condition has gotten worse. Talk to me about why you feel continuing to refuse therapy will help you?"

"You seem to believe that somewhere there is a physician who can cure you without any discomfort. You've already contacted 25 physicians, and they all say basically the same thing. Does it seem logical that contacting 25 more will be any different?"

"Be honest with me—how is what you are doing now helping you?"

"You have accepted that your leg was amputated in the accident. Is it realistic to believe that nothing will be different in your future life?"

Have patients look at the bargains they have made in the past and evaluate how successful they have been. The underlying reality is not going to change.

Swapping beliefs approach. It is a well-accepted truism that when changing a behavior, we rarely stop one thing without starting something else. If we are eroding the patient's unrealistic belief system, we need to be able to replace it with a new system of realistic and rational beliefs, or the patient will be left with nothing to believe in.[10] The best method to establish the new beliefs is to have the patient actively participate in their development. Again, using reflective and thought-provoking questions is the key to the process. For example, "You've told me that seeing 25 more physicians is not going to help. What do you think would be a better way to approach how you feel about the treatments?" "Identifying that skipping treatments to avoid the discomfort is a major step forward. Talk to me about what you believe the treatments can do for you that is positive," or "Tell me what you think will change if you let go of the illogical beliefs and begin to work with your new set of beliefs."

Practice and repetition approach. Once the patient has developed a new set of behaviors to replace bargaining behaviors, the behaviors need to be practiced and

reinforced.[6] It is very easy for the patient to slip back into bargaining behaviors, and these behaviors need to be identified immediately. The patient will also likely recognize them. For example, "I'll take the medication if you let me finish my lunch first and let it digest." Nurse: "Do you recognize what you just did?" Patient: "I guess I'm bargaining again. I know that medication needs to be taken with meals."

Repetition is an essential element in learning. As the patient repeats the non-bargaining behaviors that they have developed, the behaviors soon become accepted and second nature. However, in letting go of the protective bargaining behavior, the patient may begin to experience increased anxiety, anger, and sorrow.

> *Repetition is an essential element in learning. As the patient repeats the non-bargaining behaviors that they have developed, the behaviors soon become accepted and second nature.*

Depression

As patients' stack of bargaining chips continues to dwindle and they come to fully realize the severity of the illness, the discomfort and length of the treatments, and how the illness is going to affect their future, they may slip into feelings of emptiness and sadness. It is important to keep in mind that grief depression is not a mental illness or clinical condition. Rather, it is a natural response to the loss of independence, control, self-esteem, and, to some degree, hope that patients are experiencing from their illness or injury.

Patients must experience the emotions of frustration, sadness, bitterness, self-pity, regret, pain, loss, emptiness, despair, yearning, grief, and sadness that are associated with this type of depression in order to move on to the acceptance stage. It might be helpful to think of it as anger that is being internalized. As they go through the **bereavement** and mourning process, they may cry frequently and feel emotionally out of control. They may again experience feelings of guilt and remorse that started in the bargaining stage. They take little or no pleasure in most activities of their day. There is no "normal" time span for the depression stage, but these patients are very close to resolving their grief because they are accepting the reality of their condition.[14] A depressed mood can also be caused by certain medical conditions, such as hypothyroidism, or can be a side effect of some medications, such as antihypertensives, or certain medical treatments.

Grief-stage depression symptoms can imitate the symptoms of clinical depression at times. The dividing line between the two types of depression is blurry at best, but there are several symptoms that are fairly certain indicators of clinical depression. Patients in a clinically depressed state usually experience a long-term deep state of depression that lasts more than 2 months. The depression interferes significantly with these patients' activities of daily living, and they begin expressing thoughts of suicide, hopelessness, or worthlessness. They can no longer fulfill their daily responsibilities; these patients must be referred quickly to a professional for evaluation.[9]

As with the other stages of grief, there are verbal indicators that patients are experiencing grief depression. These statements include "I just feel so sad; I don't want to do anything," "I just don't have the energy to get out of bed today," "Why bother? It's not that important," "I'll probably die soon, so what's the point?" "I can't do much of anything I want anymore, so why go on?" and "Just go away; you don't need to be wasting your time on me." The paraverbal indicators include slow, low-tone speech and long pauses after you ask them a question before they answer. Nonverbal indicators include apathy, lack of eye contact, slouched posture, and slow body movements.

One of the keys in communicating with patients in the stage of depression is to let them talk and not interrupt. Because their thinking is slowed down and they have difficulty making decisions, their speech is often slow and sometimes disjointed with long pauses. There is a tendency for the nurse to jump in and either finish the patient's sentences or respond to half of what they are trying to say. It takes practice and patience to maintain a conversation with a patient displaying depressive behaviors. Active listening for the underlying emotions the patient is expressing and reflecting those back or asking about them can help continue the conversation.[1] It is important that patients exhibiting depressed behaviors talk about their feelings as a way of resolving them. For example:

Nurse: "Ms. Daisy, are you awake? It's time for your medication."

Ms. Daisy: (Long pause) "I'm feeling so tired; I don't think I can take it."

Nurse: "It seems like today has been a hard day for you. I'd probably feel tired if I'd been through what you have. What did you find particularly tiring?"

Ms. Daisy: (Long pause) "Going for those radiation treatments always wipes me out. And my family. . . ."

Nurse: "Your family visited you today?"

Ms. Daisy: (Long pause) "I shouldn't complain; they mean well. But they sit around and yak and yak and yak and then argue about stupid things. They're always messing around with my bed and blankets and trying to get me to drink this awful-tasting water. I don't get a minute of rest. They just don't understand what I'm going through."

Nurse: "It is a lot to deal with—having cancer, being stuck in the hospital, all the uncomfortable treatments. People who haven't been through it never really appreciate how taxing it is."

Ms. Daisy: "I'm beginning to wonder if any of these treatments are really working at all."

Nurse: "When you think of that possibility, what worries you most?"

Ms. Daisy: "I guess I'm most afraid of all the pain I'm going to have to go through if the treatments don't work. And I'm not really happy about the thought of dying and leaving all the things I want to do unfinished."

Nurse: "Tell me how you feel when you think of those things."

The difficult behaviors of patients in the depression stage of grief are not as obvious as those of patients in the other stages. The primary behavior that makes communicating with patients in the depression stage difficult is their tendency to withdraw from personal relationships and to avoid interacting with others. They may refuse to see visitors and spend much of the time sleeping, crying, and grieving. These behaviors allow the patient to temporarily disconnect from the emotions of love and affection. It is an important time for grieving that must be processed before patients can move on. These patients often are preoccupied with brooding about their condition and ruminating about what they believe they will lose in the future. They hang on to memories of their past and daydream about what they might have done differently.

Depressed patients often get labeled as "good patients" because they hardly ever put on their call lights, are not demanding, and tend to be compliant with the nurses' requests. Nurses spend more time with patients who are demanding and have their lights on all the time, and patients in the depression stage are left alone except when it is time for medications or vital signs. Staying away from these patients because they are not asking for anything does not meet their needs, nor is it good nursing care.

There are few serious physiological threats to patients in the depression stage of grief. A decrease in appetite and refusal to eat due to the depression may lead to weight loss, but the nausea often associated with chemotherapy or radiation therapy may also cause weight loss. Because all depression has an anxiety component, they may experience insomnia or restlessness and may pace. Probably the most serious physiological consequence of grief-stage depression is suppression of the immune system, which increases patients' susceptibility to any number of infections, such as respiratory infections, wound infections, and urinary tract infections.[7] They have a tendency to remain immobile and can begin to experience skin breakdown. Depression can hurt physically, and it is not unusual for patients to experience muscle and joint soreness and pain, particularly if they do not get out of bed or even turn in bed frequently. They may also experience a decrease in their pulse rate and blood pressure.

The three primary goals that we have for patients in this stage are (1) preventing physiological injury of the patient, (2) allowing the patient to speak about feelings and concerns, and (3) helping the patient cope successfully with the reality of the changes brought on by the illness or injury without experiencing the accompanying sadness and grief.

Approaches

Observe and encourage. Patients in the depression stage of grief need to be observed closely for refusal to eat and weight loss, signs of infection anywhere, skin breakdown, and extremely low heart rates and blood pressures. Asking the dietitian to consult with the patient can help with selections of food that the patient may prefer to eat. Staying with the patient and using encouragement during mealtime, rather than just dropping the tray off and moving on, is also highly effective.[6] Also, bath time is an excellent time to assess patients for skin breakdown and signs of infection. Assess their lungs thoroughly for abnormal or adventitious lung sounds. A real challenge is to keep them mobile. Getting them out of bed into a chair can be a major undertaking; however, keeping them mobile is one of the best ways to prevent respiratory infection and skin breakdown.

> *Patients in the depression stage of grief need to be observed closely for refusal to eat and weight loss, signs of infection anywhere, skin breakdown, and extremely low heart rates and blood pressures.*

Although unlikely with grief depression, if the patient expresses any thoughts of suicide, a more direct approach must be used. For example, if the patient says, "My life is so worthless—I might as well end it all," the nurse can say, "How long have you been thinking about hurting yourself? How would you do it?" If the patient provides specific answers to these questions, then it is time for professional psychiatric intervention.

Prompt and suggest. One thing that makes communicating with depressed patients a little different is that they tend to be more receptive to gentle prompting and suggestions than are patients in the other stages. They often have some difficulty in making decisions, so offering them choices such as "Do you want to take your medications now or later?" does not work well for them. However, if you make a suggestion in a quiet, calm, and firm voice, the patient is very likely to be receptive to prompting. For example, after following the six rights of administering medication, the nurse says, "Ms. Daisy, it is time to take your medication. Here is a glass of water. Please take your pills now. Thank you."

What if the patient does not want to do something? Unless it is a definite refusal, as we saw in the discussion of patients in the denial or anger stage, using a prompting approach is usually effective with patients in the depression stage. For example, if the patient says, "I really feel miserable today. I don't think I can go through with chemotherapy," the nurse can say, "I can see that you are more upset today than usual and probably want to talk about it. But I also get the feeling that you realize you need the chemotherapy treatment. Let's just have you go today and do the treatment, and then when you are done, we can talk about what is bothering you."

Explain and support. Some patients who are in this stage may say, "I just feel so sad all the time and cry at the smallest thing. Why can't I seem to be happy anymore?" Although it is pretty obvious to us that the patient is in the depression stage, some of them do not realize that it is a normal part of the grief process. This is an excellent opening to do some teaching about why they feel this way and what they can do to move on to acceptance. For example, "I know that you are feeling very confused by your emotions now. You are experiencing some depression because you are beginning to accept that your life may be permanently changed by your illness. It is actually a good sign that you are feeling this way because these feelings you are having now will soon become more manageable. You are a strong person, and I can help you use your inner strengths to feel better."

However, even if the patient does not provide an opening for teaching, you need to do it anyway. A lead-in statement you can use is, "You are probably wondering why you cry so much and feel sad. You are experiencing a type of depression that most patients with your illness experience. It is due to. . . ."

Life's reality. One thing to keep in mind is that attempting to cheer up these patients or make them happier is probably not going to be successful. Statements such as "Cheer up! It's a great day outside!"

or "Stop crying so much; it isn't good for you" may only worsen the way they feel. They really do not need to interact with cheery, jolly people at this time. The nurse's goal is not to make them laugh, get them to stop crying, or take away their sadness at that moment; the real goal is to have them reconcile what has happened to them with a realistic view of their future life. To move on from the depression stage, patients must make peace with what they have lost of their past lives and look forward to what positive things their future holds for them. The important task for you is to allow them to feel your caring presence, concern for them, and willingness to help them deal with their feelings.[7]

Building coping responses. Patients in depression often are unable to summon the energy to build coping strategies on their own. It requires too much effort for them. Providing them with an opportunity to share their fears and sadness with the nurse makes patients more receptive to teaching and information to help them build their coping skills. Nurses and patients can work together toward developing an effective repertoire of coping responses. Some techniques that can be effective are slow, deep breathing; visualization exercises (thinking of a place where they feel safe and free from pain); and muscle-relaxation techniques.

The nurse can also help patients to see events and situations from a different perspective or find alternative ways of thinking about them. For example, if the patient says, "I know the radiation therapy is frying all my blood cells," the nurse can say, "It's frightening to think that it's killing off all your blood cells, but a different way to think about it is that the radiation is killing off the bad cells and making room for your new blood cells to grow."

Peel away the layers. Much like working with patients who are experiencing PTSD, patients in the stage of depression talk about their feelings to relieve the sadness, anxiety, and stress they are experiencing. They feel a sense of relief in sharing their burden with

> *To move on from the depression stage, patients must make peace with what they have lost of their past lives and look forward to what positive things their future holds for them.*

another. Depressed patients often tell you the same thing repeatedly, but each time they express these feelings, they are peeling away a layer of grief much as you peel an onion when you cook. Eventually, they get to a point where they can acknowledge how the illness or injury is going to affect their lives without the accompanying feelings of anxiety, sadness, and loss of control.

Medication maybe. The experts on treating depression disagree on whether to use antidepressants for patients with grief-stage depression. Antidepressants do not treat the underlying problems of depression; they only help relieve the symptoms. Some think that the medications may actually postpone the mourning process that patients need to go through to achieve acceptance.

Selective serotonin reuptake inhibitors (SSRIs) are one of the most widely and commonly used medications to treat mild depression. They work by increasing the serotonin levels in the synapses and have relatively few side effects as compared with the antidepressants used to treat moderate to severe clinical depression. Some patients may have been taking these medications prior to the illness and were taken off of them when they began treatment. Stopping them suddenly can have a rebound effect that causes patients to experience more depression than if they had never been on them. They need to restart taking them as soon as they can. Otherwise, generally it is best to avoid antidepressant use in patients with grief-stage depression.[11]

Acceptance

As the layers of depression fall away, patients gradually move to a mental state where they are willing to accept and to move on with their changed lives. Acceptance does not mean that patients are cured or have forgotten about what happened to them. What happened to them will be a part of their makeup for the rest of their lives, and some days they will feel it more acutely than other days. Being in the acceptance stage means that they are willing to deal with the future and to accommodate the changes wrought by the illness. Acceptance is not a period of happiness and joy but rather a state of calm and peace that comes from coming to terms with the reality they are facing. Often, patients feel a sense of strength in knowing that they have succeeded in getting past

their sense of loss of control and self-esteem and can now make sense of how their lives will be.

People in the acceptance stage may use statements such as "I'm at peace with what is happening to me," "I'm going to fight this disease with everything I've got," "It was a rough few months, but I think I'm going to be okay," and "I guess the world isn't going to end today for me." All of these statements indicate that they have decided to not let life and its experiences pass them by. Rather, they want to participate in life and the decisions that affect them and others.

Non-Grief-Stage Difficult Behaviors

Some difficult behaviors are not necessarily related to the stages of grief or Maslow's human-need stages, and they can be expressed by both coworkers and patients.

Inappropriate sexual behavior. Sexual harassment in its many forms is always toxic to the work environment because it makes people feel unsafe in the place where they work. It causes them to distrust the coworkers or supervisors they depend on to help them do their jobs and interferes with the actual care being provided to patients.[15]

Reporting and talking about inappropriate sexual behavior by celebrities and politicians have become more common in recent years. There seems to be a growing list of characters who are willing to display their indiscretions on multiple forms of social media. The origins of the #MeToo movement can be traced back to a few very courageous women who were willing to speak up about their horrific experiences with powerful and rich men. A widespread awareness of how frequently this type of unwanted behavior occurs and how to deal with it has become a national movement. In the health-care setting, inappropriate sexual behavior on the part of either coworkers or patients is harmful to the individuals who are targets of it, decreases the quality of care, and is unethical and even criminal.

Coworker behavior. Inappropriate sexual behavior or speech on the part of a coworker is a form of bullying (see Chapter 16 for more details). Individuals who engage in such conduct in the workplace are attempting to coerce or influence their coworkers using this behavior. Although this behavior contains sexual content, usually the underlying issues are the control or humiliation of others because of the perpetrator's feelings of powerlessness, inadequacy, or low self-esteem.[16] The sexual harasser has many of the same personality traits as the persecutor discussed earlier.

Workers are now legally protected from sexual harassment, and institutions are required to have written polices about it in their employee manuals. Although the definitions vary slightly from state to state, sexual harassment is generally defined as any unwelcomed sexual advances, requests for sexual favors, or any other verbal or physical behavior of a sexual nature that creates an offensive working environment.[15]

Initially, these laws were very strictly enforced, and because the decision of whether an offensive work environment existed was determined solely by the perceptions of the person being offended, some individuals had their reputations ruined by inadvertent comments or accidental incidents. In some cases, it was difficult to distinguish between "real" sexual harassment and accusations that were silly, petty, or vindictive. Sometimes accusations were made against male professors by female students who simply disliked the grade they earned. The rise in harassment claims was a response to many years of real sexual harassment, particularly on the part of male physicians toward female nurses. New graduate nurses who complained were typically dismissed with comments such as "Oh, that's the way old Dr. Smith usually refers to us. You'll get used to it." Although ethically ambiguous, in high-stress environments such as the intensive care unit or emergency department, the staff may have developed the habit of using gallows humor or dark humor (see Box 12.2) to reduce their emotional responses to life-or-death situations.

Recent legal cases of sexual harassment have taken a more commonsense approach to deciding whether statements or actions are creating an offensive work environment. However, if a nurse or anyone else employed in a health-care setting believes that a coworker is displaying inappropriate sexual behavior, they should first keep a complete record of the behavior with dates and times and what was done or said, and then contact human resources (HR). It is important to follow the facility's procedures for dealing with alleged sexual misbehavior to the letter; otherwise, the whole case may be invalidated.

Generally, these policies entail first confronting the offender with a statement that their behavior is

---

Box 12.2 Understanding "Gallows" Humor

Nurses and other health-care workers in units that experience patient tragedies on a regular basis, such as the emergency department, intensive care units, and burn units, sometimes use what is called "gallows" humor or "black" humor to reduce the emotional impact of what they are experiencing. Humor acts as a buffer to painful situations the nurse experiences that otherwise might cause them to be unable to continue providing care. In some settings, gallows humor is seen as an expression of resilience that gives people power over the heartbreaking events they are experiencing.

Newly graduated nurses and nursing students are often shocked when they first experience gallows humor in the clinical setting; however, it has probably been used as a coping mechanism since health care moved from the home to organized institutions. This does not excuse it or make it right, but gallows humor does serve its purpose on busy units where the beds literally do not cool off between patients. Nurses on these units are not afforded the luxury of time to grieve or cry for a patient to whom they have become close; rather, they must take care of the next seriously ill patient coming through the doors. Sometimes gallows humor may contain a sexual component, but unless extreme, it is not considered sexual harassment.

---

inappropriate and unwanted. For example, "Dr. Smith, I'm a professional nurse, and my primary concern is caring for our patients. I feel demeaned and belittled by the way you refer to me and my body parts and do not appreciate the jokes you tell. Please stop doing this around me." However, you need to avoid retaliating with hostile and vengeful jokes that might inflame the situation. For example, "From what I've heard, the newborn babies in the nursery have bigger ones than you!" or "You're not man enough to handle what I've got!"

The second stage in the process is a meeting with the offender, HR, and you. It is always helpful to get support from other nurses who have been harassed. It is likely that the offender has become habitual in this type of behavior and uses it with almost everyone. The third stage usually requires a meeting with the medical or hospital board. If the issue is not resolved satisfactorily by that time, then it is appropriate to seek legal resolution.

Patient behavior. Inappropriate patient sexual behavior creates a dilemma for nurses. Nurses must walk a fine line between protecting themselves and providing quality care. However, what most nurses do not know is that federal and some state laws protect them from sexual harassment by patients, and these laws should be reflected, or at least referenced, in the employee manual.[16] Unfortunately, nursing students receive little education on dealing with patients who sexually harass nurses, and there are very few continuing education programs on the topic for the working nurse.

Sexual behavior from patients may be related to a stage of grief, particularly anger, but is more typically a form of behavior that is used by patients experiencing anxiety. This behavior is disturbing, increases job-related stress for the nurse, can make the nurse feel humiliated and objectified, and can decrease the quality of care. It can also destroy the nurse–patient trust that is essential to quality care.

> *Medications that have neurological effects may lower patient inhibitions and cause them to say and do things that they would be horrified to do without the effects of the medications.*

Patients with mental illnesses, who are diagnosed with dementia, or who have brain damage or surgery may not be able to grasp the consequences of their actions or statements and therefore cannot be held legally responsible for them. Medications that have neurological effects may lower patient inhibitions and cause them to say and do things that they would be horrified to do without the effects of the medications.[10] These conditions create a unique situation for nurses because these patients may not respond to the usual approaches used for dealing with sexual harassment.

Although overt physical sexual assaults are rare from patients, the ANA reported in 2019 that more than 60 percent of nurses have experienced some type of sexual misbehavior from patients, ranging from being called "honey" or "babe" to enduring jokes with sexual content to even unwanted touching. The vast majority of this behavior is against female nurses, although male nurses also occasionally experience unwanted sexual advances. The ANA also addressed nurse sexual harassment as a part of its #EndNurseAbuseInitiative.

Nurses tend to avoid patients who are sexually abusive, entering their rooms only when absolutely necessary and skipping tasks such as physical assessments, or they may call in sick to avoid providing care for the patient. Other nurses grudgingly provide physical care, but emotional aspects of the care decline. The patient will be labeled as troublesome, and the quality of care will decrease. So, how do you effectively approach a patient with inappropriate sexual behavior without compromising care?

Approaches
Laugh and deny. Over time, some nurses build up a resistance to patients' sexual misbehavior. They often blame it on the patient's age, illness, or confused state. They may not even consider the behavior to be sexual harassment. They tend to laugh it off as another unpleasant aspect of their profession. However, this is not really the most effective approach. It may work for some nurses, but by ignoring the behavior, they have not taken any positive actions to resolve the issue.

Confront gently. There is always the temptation to respond to these patients with vengeful remarks or jokes. As with the coworker, this is not an effective method in dealing with sexual misbehavior. It is important to speak honestly to patients about what they are doing or saying and how it makes you feel. Sharp retorts such as "Knock off the jokes" or "It's really inappropriate to display yourself like that when people are around" usually only exacerbate the behavior. It does not deal with the underlying causes. The behavior may be adaptive for the patient and may have developed over a long period of time.

Confronting the patient gently but firmly may alter the behavior.[16] If nothing else, it lets the patient know you are not pleased with the sexual behavior. For example, you can say, "Mr. Blue, I appreciate that you are not feeling well; however, I feel like you are putting me down and disrespecting me every time you tell one of those jokes or pat my bottom when I'm near the bed. I would really appreciate it if you would stop when I'm in the room." This action by the nurse may make interactions with the patient tenser for a while because it creates uncomfortable feelings.

Digging deeper. As mentioned earlier, the discomfort caused by these patients' behavior often causes nurses to overlook the underlying emotional issues that may be causing the behavior. Rather than ignoring the patient or running away when they say something sexually inappropriate, the nurse can use some of the communication builders to help patients recognize why they are behaving this way.[1] The nurse can say, "Mr. Blue, I am very uncomfortable being referred to by that name; however, I realize you are concerned about your heart catheterization tomorrow. When people have high levels of anxiety, they often say things that help them relieve the tension. I'd really like to hear about what you fear most about going for the test tomorrow."

The ANA approach. The ANA has been emphatic over the years that the work setting be free from sexual harassment from either coworkers or patients. It has developed a four-step approach to dealing with patients who display sexually inappropriate behavior:[17]

Step 1: Confrontation of the offender, which is similar to the "confront gently" approach discussed earlier; however, the ANA recommends that the nurse leave no room for misinterpretation of what is being said. It insists that the nurse keep the relationship with patients professional at all times by addressing them as Mr., Mrs., or Ms. For example, "Mr. Blue, I respect you as a patient who is here to receive care, and I expect that you will treat me as the professional that I am. Please address me as Ms. Locke and not by the foul names you've been using."

In addition, the ANA believes that patients should be aware that there are potential legal consequences for their sexual harassment behaviors. Although not widely known by nurses, there are laws that permit hospitals to transfer patients who persist in sexual harassment behaviors to another facility. The ANA suggests that the nurse inform the patient of the laws associated with sexual harassment. For example, "Mr. Blue, I have asked you nicely several times to stop with the sexual jokes and crude names. The hospital has strict rules about the type of behavior you are displaying, and if you don't stop it, you will be discharged from this facility immediately." Patients in a clinic or outpatient setting are legally required to be given 30 days before they can be dismissed from care.

> *The ANA believes that patients should be aware that there are potential legal consequences for their sexual harassment behaviors. Although not widely known by nurses, there are laws that permit hospitals to transfer patients who persist in sexual harassment behaviors to another facility.*

Step 2: Notify the supervisor of the harassment. This is an important step in the process because when the employer is informed of patient sexual harassment of nurses, it becomes the employer's responsibility to do something about it. Employers have become extremely sensitized to sexual harassment issues, and they realize that if nothing is done, they can become involved in a lawsuit filed by an employee. This often spurs employers to provide continuing education programs for nurses on sexual harassment from patients and to develop policies and procedures for sexual harassment from patients if they do not already exist.

Step 3: Carefully document the harassment. It is important to keep a record of exactly what the patient said and did, what the nurse did in response, and how the patient responded to the response. The date and time also need to be documented. This is best done immediately after the incident while it is fresh in the nurse's mind.

Step 4: Involve others. Coworkers on the unit probably have similar experience with the patient because the behavior is not targeted to just one person. They can help in developing successful tactics in dealing with the patient behavior so that everyone will be consistent in the approach to the patient. Inconsistency tends to increase the inappropriate behavior. Having one or two other nurses beside you when you interact with the patient may help dampen the inappropriate speech or behavior, and they can serve as witnesses to exchanges. Make sure to include their names in the documentation. The nurse can also seek support from organizations such as the state's nursing organization or even the state board of nursing.[17]

Complaining and Whining Behaviors

One of the most common, if not most annoying, types of difficult person is the constant complainer and whiner. To complain means to verbally express unhappiness or dissatisfaction with a person, place, or thing. The strict definition of the verb *whine* is to make a high-pitched, unpleasant sound that indicates discontent, pain, or unhappiness; in colloquial usage, it means complaining, often in a high-pitched voice, about something that the person cannot or does not want to expend the effort to fix. The two words *complain* and *whine* are often used in conjunction because they mean basically the same thing.[16]

Everyone knows about the glass-half-full and the glass-half-empty division of personalities. The glass-half-full people are the optimists who see the positive aspects of life and their situation and attempt to make the best of them. The glass-half-empty people are the pessimists who see the negative aspects of their lives and situations and resign themselves to the idea that they are just going to have to tolerate it. The third type of personality are the "there's nothing at all in the glass" individuals who see their lives, work, other people, and the whole world as a black hole of existence. There is nothing good at all, and they are going to let you know about it often and convincingly. They express themselves in chronic complaining and chronic whining.

Causes of Complaining and Whining

The reality is that everyone complains at times as a way to reduce stress, lessen the impact of unpleasant news, and identify areas of concern. These types of complaints are sometimes referred to as *sporadic* because they deal with just one short-term issue or as *constructive complaining* because they are useful in focusing attention on and resolving issues the person is facing.[14] They bring difficult situations to light and allow the person to focus on the resolution of the problem and the opportunity to make right something that is wrong or unfair.

Nurses experience complainers and whiners in the health-care setting as bosses, coworkers, and patients. There are many similarities among the groups, including the reasons why bosses, coworkers, and patients complain and whine to express themselves and the approaches to dealing with them. In the discussion that follows, the groups are not separated as in previous sections because of the similarities. The differences in the care of patients are pointed out when appropriate. As with other types of difficult behavior, complaining and whining meet a need or achieve a goal that the person has. Often, this behavior is used to manipulate others, achieve some type of reward, avoid a troubling situation, or increase the complainer's sense of control.

One of the most common underlying reasons that people complain excessively is that their lives have not met the expectations they had for themselves when they were younger. The vision of the things that could have been remains in their memories, but the realities of their present lives are a constant reminder of how short they have fallen. They live in a continual state of disappointment with themselves, their circumstances, and the people around them.[8] They are truly unhappy and use complaining and whining as an expression of their unhappiness with the world.

Many people who excessively complain and whine have a pervading sense that life has not treated them justly. You will often hear from them statements such as "It's so unfair. I work my butt off every day, save every penny I can, and scrape by and have nothing while they sit back and the money rolls in." The underlying emotion leading to these feelings is a lack of control over their lives. This feeling of lack of control is often closely associated with jealousy. Although it is difficult for them to admit, they resent that someone else has something they do not. They might say, "How come Betty gets to buy a new car and I don't? She's so selfish; she probably never gives anything to charity." Complaining is a mechanism they can use to regain some feeling that they are in control.

A belief and feeling that other people do not appreciate them, understand them, or empathize with them causes some people to complain. Basically, they are expressing low self-esteem and an "I'm a born loser" self-concept. They might express this feeling by complaining: "You never do anything the right way! You should do it the way I do it because it's much quicker and better than what you are doing now." They believe that others cannot put themselves in their shoes and see things as they see them because others lack empathy for them. No one really understands or appreciates what they are thinking or the other difficulties they have to deal with in their lives. Complaining and whining, they believe, will help others appreciate them more.

They may also complain about feeling left out of important activities or being treated as a second-rate person when someone is selected over them for an important task or position. These complaints usually indicate that they are experiencing a type of anxiety similar to what children experience when they are brought to day care for the first time. Complaining makes them feel more dominant or mature when in reality they feel just the opposite.[10]

People who use complaining and whining to gain power often use these tactics much as persecutors use bullying tactics to get what they want. Often, these individuals may appear very congenial and cooperative on the outside, but when they really want something, such as a promotion or to achieve a specific personal goal, they use the complaining and whining to manipulate and harass their targets. They have no regard for how the other person feels and can make the whole work environment toxic to personnel and successful outcomes. They do not accept any excuses for someone getting in their way and often display narcissistic behavior. They are concerned only about achieving their goals and use complaining and whining to torment others until they get what they want.

> " *A belief and feeling that other people do not appreciate them, understand them, or empathize with them causes some people to complain. Basically, they are expressing low self-esteem and an "I'm a born loser" self-concept.* "

Effects of Complaining and Whining

Much like sneaks, chronic complainers love to keep the pot stirred up and boiling at work. They love to watch the drama and chaos they have created and particularly enjoy observing how their coworkers become irritated and disheartened. Unfortunately, chronic complaining is contagious, and chronic complainers may seek out other chronic complainers to commiserate with them. However, at a certain point, complainers and whiners will begin to complain and whine about other complainers and whiners. They seem to recognize the behavior in others as irritating but cannot see it in themselves.

Some studies have shown that even after just 30 minutes of listening to someone complain, the neurotransmitter levels in the brain are altered enough to cause memory loss and even permanent brain damage.[15] Even for people who are generally happy, spending too much time around chronic complainers can make it hard to remember all the good that still exists in life. A group of complainers together can make the whole workplace environment toxic. The chronic complainer infects the nursing unit by dispersing negativity and creating doubt in the minds of team members. For nurse managers and nurse team members attempting to implement a new program or policy, this annoying but effective behavior prevents the achievement of positive change.[15]

Chronic complaining destroys relationships and lowers the morale in the workplace. In the healthcare setting, it drains the energy out of the staff and decreases the overall quality of care. It creates an intense focus on only the negative issues and even reverses positive aspects of the job. Complaining makes people upset, aggravated, and generally annoyed. People who want to remain positive and provide high-quality care soon become tired of trying to ignore the negativity; it increases their stress levels way beyond what they would normally experience with their daily care activities. Nurses who try to maintain a positive attitude feel very relieved to leave work and go home at the end of the day to get away from the complaining and whining, but because they know what is coming the next day, they dread going back to work.

In facilities where there is a culture of complaining and whining, the turnover rates of nurses tend to be higher than average.[6] Nurses would rather quit and move to another facility that has a more positive atmosphere than deal with all the negativity where they are. These optimistic nurses may become depressed because no matter how hard they work, it never seems to be good enough for the chronic complainer. The awful truth is that even one person who continually complains can singlehandedly change the atmosphere of a work environment and bring a screeching halt to the productivity of an otherwise highly cohesive nursing unit.

Types of Complaining and Whining Behaviors

Most people can recognize when someone is complaining or whining about something that bothers them, but there are several varieties of this type of behavior. As with the other difficult behaviors, there is considerable overlap between the types of complaining behavior.

Duck-and-cover behavior. Some complainers have become adept at disguising their complaints by intertwining them with real problems so that it is difficult to separate the two. Because they believe they cannot fix the problem themselves, they try to place the responsibility for both the problem and its solution on another person. For example, "It's such a pain to have to document every word we say to these patients. You're the one who suggested it at the last staff meeting, so why don't you do something about it?"

Bulldozer behavior. These complainers want action and to accomplish goals. They use aggressive complaining to manipulate others to achieve their objectives. For example, "No one wants to help me get the

stuff ready for the holiday party. I guess I'll just call the whole thing off and chalk it up to your lack of interest in the unit. No wonder we have low morale around here."

Wet blanket behavior. These individuals take negativity to new lows. In their attempts to gain control and manipulate a situation, they use negative comments and complaints to dampen everyone else's attitudes. They rarely have any good ideas of their own and much prefer to sow seeds of disappointment and failure. At a meeting about a unit project, this person might say, "Jose, that's a stupid idea. We tried that in the past, and it was a miserable failure. Why should we waste our time trying it again? Sue, your idea isn't any better. I can name six reasons why it won't work! I can't believe you would even suggest that. I don't think this thing is ever going to get off the ground."

Beyond help behavior. Sometimes when people complain, it can appear that they are seeking help and support with a problem they are facing; however, they immediately reject the helping offer without even considering it. They believe the solution being offered is inappropriate or useless and that their problem is so severe or unique that there is nothing anyone could ever do to fix it.

The goal of their behavior is to gain attention and sympathy from other people, and they really do not want to solve the problem; if it does get solved, they'll find another one.[15] For example, a friend says, "That sounds like a serious problem. Something like that happened to me once, and the way I solved it was by talking to my supervisor about it. Why don't you try that as a first step?" Complainer: "Oh, that'll never work. My problem is so much worse than yours, and my supervisor is way too aloof to listen to me. I guess it's just another thing in my life that I'll have to live with."

Gossiping behavior. These people use complaining to make themselves look better, cover up their feelings of inadequacy and low self-esteem, and gain recognition

> ❝ *The awful truth is that even one person who continually complains can singlehandedly change the atmosphere of a work environment and bring a screeching halt to the productivity of an otherwise highly cohesive nursing unit.* ❞

or attention. Their tactics include interrupting others, bragging about their accomplishments, and throwing up roadblocks to progress. Some of their most effective behaviors include making unrealistic promises they cannot keep and have no intention of keeping, using others as scapegoats, and taking the credit for another nurse's work. For example, "Sorry to interrupt, but Ellen, you know that error was really your fault, not mine, and if I hadn't straightened it out as quickly and as well as I did, the whole unit would be in trouble now. No one is better at dealing with these situations than me."[16]

Needy behavior. By venting and then emotionally and/or physically withdrawing, these chronic complainers are seeking to gain the sympathy of others and develop some type of connection, even if it is dysfunctional. Often, they set up social or work situations so that they intentionally fail in order to become the victim. Being a victim is a role for which they were born, and they revel in it.[10] For example, in front of a group, this person might say, "You have put me down for just about the last time! You couldn't have hurt my feelings more if you had called me a fool! I'm going to the break room and work on my charts, and I want to be left alone."

Toxic behavior. Although all chronic complaining is destructive to a workplace environment, some complainers are so unhappy with themselves and their lives that they use their behavior to purposely manipulate or poison the environment so that everyone else will be as unhappy as they are. It can be particularly devastating if the person using this toxic complaining behavior is the boss. They sometimes have secondary goals for their behaviors, such as seeking a promotion or recognition rewards. They will attempt to falsely inflate others' perception of their skills and work hard to advance their own agenda. People who use this type of toxic behavior often retaliate and seek revenge if they are contradicted or challenged. Toxic complaining can deeply torment fellow workers and devastate their emotional state.

Underlying their behaviors may be deep-seated, long-term personality disorders, such as narcissism and even antisocial tendencies.[9] Toxic complainers seem to have no conscience or awareness of other peoples' needs or feelings and are totally focused on achieving their own goals. They have developed

manipulation into an art form and use it to control situations and people. To your face they can be very supportive of your ideas, charming, and captivating while at the same time they are creating an emotionally lethal work environment.

They may employ any of the other types of complaining discussed previously to take the focus off their own unhappiness and lack of knowledge and abilities. For example, while the nurses are still together after receiving shift report and waiting for their assignments, a toxic whiner would say, "Here we go again! Too many patients and not enough nurses. Don't they know we are all working as hard as we possibly can, and by not giving us extra help, they are killing our morale and spirit? I was so tired, and my feet hurt so bad yesterday when I went home, I got in the bathtub and fell asleep for 3 hours! It looks like today is going to be a rerun of yesterday. And these patients we have to put up with! They're old, they're grumpy, they smell bad, they can't do anything for themselves, they complain all the time, and their call lights are always on. It's like pulling teeth to get them to do anything. And all the physicians do is complain at us."

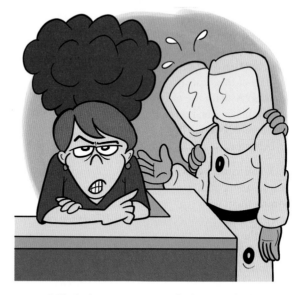

"She's having a toxic behavior day!"

Approaches

One of our goals in approaching chronic complainers is to help them recognize that their behaviors are inappropriate and that expressing their needs by complaining is harmful to themselves and the work environment. Ultimately, we are trying to get them to accept the motto "If you can't say something positive, don't say anything at all!" Of course, once they do internalize this proverb, they may not be saying much of anything for a while.

Another goal is to help them change their perspectives about why they are complaining. Often, people complain because they have little capacity for empathy. Primarily we are trying to get them to see from another person's viewpoint. If they can achieve any level of empathy at all and see other individuals more positively, they will begin to think differently, have different expectations, and find better ways than complaining to handle challenges in their lives.

A goal associated with both changing their perspective and encouraging empathy is to understand themselves better and understand why they have feelings of inadequacy. It is interesting that complainers hardly ever complain about themselves but very frequently compare themselves to others. Because they see the other person as being more intelligent, having better skills, and being more capable than they think they are, complainers are often attempting to bring the other people down to the level where they believe themselves to be.[10] If they can recognize that this is a form of jealousy and can understand that they do not have a monopoly on feelings of inadequacy, they will begin to recognize that there are many people who would like to be in their position. They can then focus more on their own lives and what makes them happy.

The chronic complaining behavior observed in patients generally has the same causes and goals as complaining behavior seen in coworkers and responds to the same approaches. However, there are several exceptions when the complainer is a patient. It is always important to listen carefully to the complaints of patients, even if they are chronic complainers. Once a patient is labeled as a chronic complainer, the tendency for busy nurses is to dismiss all their complaints as mere indications of an unhappy personality, and indeed, many of them are. However, if the complaints are different from the common complaints such as "The food is always cold," "The nurses don't talk to me much," or "Why is this room so cold (or hot)?" nurses should investigate them more closely. Although all patients' complaints about pain or discomfort need to be assessed, complaints about pain in locations where they have not complained about pain before need a more thorough assessment. It is possible for a chronically complaining patient to have a heart attack or develop a kidney stone unexpectedly while they are in the hospital.

One group that requires an approach somewhat different from coworkers is the patients who are in the depression stage of grief. They may express that grief by complaining about almost anything and everything. The approaches discussed earlier for interacting with patients in the depression stage of grief will likely be more effective than the approaches discussed next, although there are many similarities. Our primary goal for depressed patients is to move them on to the stage of acceptance.

Under the best circumstances, it is difficult to change complaining behavior. It is behavior that the person likely began using as a young child to gain recognition and attention and to manipulate the parents into giving them what they want. Because of the rewards they have received from this behavior, they will be very reluctant to give it up for more adultlike behavior. However, because it is so toxic to the work environment, it must be addressed and dealt with at some point.[6] The following approaches can be effective in altering behavior to a degree, but do not get discouraged if the chronic complainer continues to complain at times. At least it is an improvement.

The empathy approach. As it does with several of the approaches for other types of difficult behavior, active listening can also work with complainers if combined with a response that acknowledges their problems. After they finish talking, say, "Wow, that sounds really awful. I can't imagine how you handle all those problems without going crazy. I'm sure I couldn't do it." Make sure you are genuinely sympathetic and not patronizing. Many complainers are looking for someone who understands them as a person, but because of their constant complaining, people tend to avoid them. Quite frequently, they will reply, "Yes, but it's not really *that* bad and I'm handling it okay!" For this approach to work, you do need to be sincere and avoid any hint of sarcasm.

Also remember that you are not really agreeing with the complainer that their problem is worse than anyone else's or that it is so big it can never be solved.

You are just acknowledging that this is a problem for that person, which it is.

Break the vicious cycle approach. This is similar to the first approach, and like the first one, it may not completely stop the complainer from complaining. Be patient with the person and respond realistically to their complaints. For example, the complainer says, "You know, this job is really boring. I just do the same thing over and over again, and the patients are always the same." You can respond, "Getting bored with a job can be a problem. Why don't you do something about it?" Complainer (after a long pause and with a blank look): "You mean there's something I can do?" This approach will usually stop complainers from complaining to you; at the same time, you take their unhappiness seriously and offer a practical resolution. You are challenging them to take control of their situation and fix it.

Adjusting the attitude approach. Complainers often do not realize how good they actually have it and how much they can be thankful for. This approach is difficult because it requires complainers to shift their perception from one they have been hanging on to for many years. Helping adjust their perception of themselves and what they have and can do allows them to become more positive and speak of the good things in their lives.[4] They do need some degree of self-awareness, however small, for this approach to be successful.

Adjusting an attitude—whether your own or others'—can be a slow process, and the key is to get complainers to acknowledge that they have a negative attitude and that their complaining is not helping them. Continual redirection is needed when they start complaining and being negative again. For example, the complainer says, "This job is so hard. I'm always tired, and I never have any time to do what I want. They're always giving me something else to do, and I can't seem to ever say no because they'll fire me. What's wrong with me? I don't know when my life became so negative." Response: "Why don't you try

> ❝ *Adjusting an attitude—whether your own or others'—can be a slow process, and the key is to get complainers to acknowledge that they have a negative attitude and that their complaining is not helping them.* ❞

this. Tell me right now about five things that are good in your life." Complainer: "Well, I have a great husband who listens to me and encourages me and helps me with the housework. The pay I'm getting here is better than at any place else I've ever worked. I live in a nice big house with a big yard. How many is that? I've got some great friends who would do anything for me. And I love my church and the people who are there. That is five." Response: "That's great! Don't you feel better now? You have to keep looking at the positive side of things. Now I'm going to help you with this even though you'll probably get irritated with me at some point. Every time you complain about something, I want you to say something positive also, okay? It'll be hard at first, but if you forget, I'll remind you."

Complaining to the complainer approach. Unlike the first two approaches, the goal of this approach is not to alter the underlying causes of the complaining but to ameliorate the behavior to some degree. Most people who complain all the time have no self-realization of how they come across to other people and how irritating their complaining is.[3] Sometimes by hearing how they sound, they can get a sample of how other people feel about their complaining.

Step 1: Rather than trying to be empathetic and positive in responding to complainers, complain about everything, including what they are doing and how they are doing it. If they ever do a good job, complain about that. This will be tiring if you are not a born complainer, and others may look at you strangely. At some point, however, the complainer will probably start complaining about your complaining. This is a sign that your plan is working.

Step 2: Keep complaining and then, when they least expect it, tell them they are doing a great job when they do something well. Your positive words will surprise them and will likely make them ask you what you are doing. If they ask, they are showing the first signs of self-awareness, and this is your opening to have "the talk."

(text continues on page 367)

Issues in Practice

The Girl Who Cried Roach!

The incident described here really happened, but the location and some of the names have been changed to protect the innocent.

I had been pulled from the cardiac intensive care unit (ICU) to work on one of the medical-surgical units because of a low census in the ICU. My assignment that day included a 17-year-old girl who, while taking a test at school the day before, felt dizzy, had a "fluttering" in her chest accompanied by a feeling of pressure, and had difficulty breathing. The school nurse took her blood pressure and obtained a reading of 72/58 (normally 108/64) with an irregular pulse of 167 (normally 75 and regular). The nurse called the girl's parents and the ambulance. By the time the paramedics arrived, the girl's blood pressure was 104/66 with a regular pulse of 80. After being connected to the cardiac monitor, they observed normal sinus rhythm with no dysrhythmias. However, because of the potential for reoccurring cardiac abnormalities, the girl was taken to the local hospital's emergency department (ED), where she was examined by the ED physician on staff with a consult from a cardiologist. Although she had no more episodes of rapid heart rate, the cardiologist wished to monitor her in the hospital for 24 hours.

Normally, a 17-year-old child would be admitted to the pediatric unit, but that unit was experiencing a highly contagious rotavirus outbreak, and they did not want to expose the girl to the infection. She had a cardiac telemetry unit, which is a portable radio transmitter about the size of a large cell phone, only thicker and heavier, connected by wires to electrodes on her chest; the transmitter sent her heart pattern wirelessly to a room next to the ICU where monitor technicians watched it 24 hours a day for any irregularities. It allowed her complete mobility, and she was on activities as tolerated, which meant she could do pretty much anything she wanted in the hospital.

I usually was not assigned to female patients, but the charge nurse that day believed that because of my ICU experience, I was the best qualified to handle any emergency situations that might arise with the patient. Her fast, irregular heart rate was a type of supraventricular tachycardia (SVT), known as *atrial fibrillation* (A-fib or atrial fib), in which the atria of the heart becomes irritable and takes over the pacemaker function from the heart's normal pacemaker, the SA node. Many things can cause this to happen, and it is fairly common and usually transient in teenage girls and young women; however, in elderly patients, it is often chronic and an indication of an underlying cardiac pathology. Causes include increased hormone levels, as seen in teenagers; excitement; stress; and use of caffeine, tobacco, alcohol, stimulant street drugs, and a variety of prescription medications.

She was in a semiprivate room in the bed farthest away from the door, by the windows. When I went into the room, she was awake, sitting up and listening to her iPhone. I introduced myself: "Good morning, Ms. Bennett. I'm Mr. Catalano, and I'm going to be your RN today. How are—"

"Stop right there," she interrupted. "Mrs. Bennett is my mother's name. I'm just Julie."

"Okay, then," I answered. "Good morning, just Julie. I guess you can call me just Joe."

I saw her start to smile; however, it stopped suddenly when she remembered Rule Number 3 of the *Teenager's Handbook on Dealing with Adults:* Never let them know they're funny.

"How are you feeling this morning?" I asked.

"I feel great! When am I getting out of this dump?"

"Well, your cardiologist wanted to monitor you for 24 hours, and if there aren't any more episodes of what you had yesterday, you can go home, probably this afternoon or early evening. The monitor techs tell me everything has been normal since you came in. Have you felt anything like you had at school yesterday?"

(continued)

Issues in Practice (continued)

"None at all, but these things stuck on my chest are starting to itch, and I kept getting tangled up in these wires last night and pulled them off a couple of times. They won't let me use my cell phone, and this hospital phone with the wire is an antique and doesn't seem to work half the time."

"We can move the electrodes to a different spot on your chest where it isn't itchy. The cell phones send out a signal that blocks the telemetry, so we don't let anyone use them here. I realize those wires are a pain, particularly when you're trying to sleep. How did you sleep last night anyway?"

"You've got to be kidding me, right? Sleep in this place? It was noisier than our band room at break time! It sounded like someone was banging a metal garbage can top against the wall. This one over here"—she pointed to the other patient in the room—"snores like a freight train! And then there were the bugs running up and down the curtain all night."

Many teenagers are compulsive chronic complainers and use complaining like an orchestra conductor uses his baton. Complaints are a way to emphasize points, such as not being happy with a situation, and to enhance their expressions of disapproval, particularly of adults. I usually pay little attention to them, but when they sound unusual or relate to changes in physiological conditions such as pain or breathing, I tend to become curious. The bugs on the curtain complaint got my attention.

"On which curtain did you see the bugs?" I asked.

"This one here," she answered, pointing to the curtain that separated her bed from the patient in the next bed. The curtain was a heavy fabric in pastel-colored stripes and was hung from a roller track on the ceiling so that it could be pulled all the way around the bed for privacy. Usually, we just leave them pulled down to the foot of the bed.

"I think they were roaches. We had some under the sink at our new house when we moved in. My mom totally *freaked out!* She called the real estate agent who sold us the house, and a bug guy was there in 15 minutes! Roaches make kind of a clicking sound when they move around, and I thought I heard that last night."

I assessed that Julie was alert and oriented to person, place, and time and did not appear to be experiencing the side effects of any types of medications that might cause confusion. Actually, she was not on any medications at all. I pulled the curtain all the way open just to be sure and did not see any bugs of any kind.

"There don't appear to be any here now," I observed.

"Of course not. The lights are on, and the sun is out," she noted. "Don't you know anything about roaches?"

"I can't remember any nursing classes covering that topic in nursing school," I inappropriately replied. "And maintenance sprays the whole hospital for bugs about once a month. But hang on a second, I just want to check something out."

I walked around the curtain and saw that the patient in the bed by the door was a patient I had seen several times in the ICU. It was Mrs. Perry, one of our "frequent fliers" (patients who are admitted to the hospital every month or so), who was 80-something and had difficulty seeing and hearing but lived alone and was ferociously independent. She vehemently refused any kind of help with her own care or care of her living quarters. Unfortunately for her neighbors in the apartment building where she lived, she had severe self-care deficits, and her apartment was known for its cluttered and malodorous condition. I had a strong feeling that some of her admissions were related to her living conditions, because I had heard from my friends who worked in patient transport that when they returned her to her apartment after a hospitalization, it was better organized, much less cluttered, and had a lingering sent of Febreze filling the air.

"Hello, Mrs. Perry. How are you feeling today?" I asked her.

Issues in Practice (continued)

"I'm okay. Is that Joey?" (She always called me Joey because she had a son named Joe who was killed in World War II at Midway. I guess I reminded her of him.)

"Yes, Mrs. Perry," I replied. "You remembered me."

"I can't see or hear worth a flip, but my memory is like a steel trap," she replied, and then launched into the story about her Joey.

I let her talk for several minutes; then I interrupted her. "Mrs. Perry, I would like to take a look at your suitcase if you don't mind?" It was one of the old hard-side suitcases like Julie Andrews carried in *The Sound of Music* when she left the convent, except Mrs. Perry's was a faded yellow color with travel stickers on it from all over the country. It was on the floor on the curtain side of the room.

"Why would you want to look at that old thing? There's nothing in it. I put all my clothes in the closet over by the sink yesterday when I came in."

"I just want to check something out," I said.

"Well okay, go ahead."

I crouched down next to her suitcase, flipped the two worn brass latches up, and carefully opened the lid about six inches. That's all I needed to see what I was afraid I would see. There were several hundred live and healthy roaches scurrying around in the bottom. I quickly but cautiously closed the lid and latched it. I went over to the sink and got a pair of rubber gloves out of the box and then got a red biohazard plastic bag from under the sink. I carefully slid the suitcase into the bag and double tied it.

"Mrs. Perry, I'm going to need to borrow your suitcase for a little while. Is that okay?" I asked her.

"Sure, Joey, anything you want. But why don't you buy yourself one of those nice new fancy ones with the wheels on it?"

"This one will be just fine, Mrs. Perry. I promise I'll bring it back later." I wasn't sure that was a promise I could keep.

I gingerly picked it up and carried it at arm's length to the nurses' station. Never having been in this situation before, I was not quite sure what to do with it, so I set it down on the edge of the nurses' station counter. Everyone was pretty used to seeing specimens in biohazard bags that needed to be taken to the laboratory, so they did not pay much attention to my little gift. It happened that the unit manager, who was a classmate of mine from nursing school, was in the hall.

"Hi, Joe," she said. "It's good to have you back over here working with us. Did you cure all the patients in the ICU? What's in the red bag there?"

"You're probably not going to believe this," I answered. "I wasn't sure what to do with it because I've never run across this problem before. It's Mrs. Perry's suitcase, and it is full of live roaches," I said quietly.

I watched the color in her face drain away.

"Live roaches? Oh, my! I'm not sure what to do with it either," she answered. "But we need to get it out of here, now! Fern [the unit clerk], call maintenance and get them up here right now to get rid of this. Tell them it's an emergency!"

Surprisingly, three men from the maintenance department were there within about 5 minutes. We took them to an empty room and explained the situation. They said that their policy and procedure manual actually had a protocol for this. One of them put on gloves, picked up the red bag with the suitcase in it, and all three of them left. I was not sure what they were going to do with it. I was thinking incineration, but the suitcase reappeared in Mrs. Perry's room later that afternoon, a little more faded with a distinct chemical odor. I had no desire to open it again.

"We really need to get the patients out of that room," I said.

(continued)

Issues in Practice (continued)

"There is an empty private room across the hall where Julie can go, and we can put Mrs. Perry in the isolation room across the hall from the nurses' station," explained the unit manager.

I headed back to Julie's room and found her listening to her music again.

"Julie, we're going to move you to another room. Grab your makeup case and electronics and put on your shoes, okay?"

"What about my clothes?"

"I'll bring them to you later. Actually, it might be better if you call your mother and tell her to bring you some fresh clothes to go home in." We walked across the hall to the private room and got her settled in. I headed back to her old room to help with Mrs. Perry. When I got to the room, Mrs. Perry's nurse had a wheelchair next to the bed, and Mrs. Perry had a death grip with both hands on the bedrail that was still up.

"I like this room. I'm not going to go to another room!" Mrs. Perry shouted.

I walked around to the side of the bed she was facing and said, "Mrs. Perry, is there a problem here?"

"Joey, I'm glad you're back. This nurse here wants me to go to another room and won't tell me why. And she's trying to make me ride in a wheelchair. I'm not a cripple. *I can walk by myself!*" she said emphatically.

"Well, Mrs. Perry, it's like this. You've always been such a good patient for us when you come in; we wanted to put you in a nicer room. Think of it like an upgrade in a hotel when you used to travel. And you don't have to use the wheelchair. I can walk with you to your new room, you know, like we used to walk together in the ICU?" I said, bending veracity a bit.

"An upgrade? I didn't know hospitals did that. I used to love upgrades when I traveled with my husband. We were in Las Vegas one time and . . . ," she launched into her Vegas story of at least 40 years ago. I actually had not heard this one and was kind of interested in what she had to say, but I interrupted her again.

"Mrs. Perry, I really want to hear about Las Vegas, but can I hear the rest of the story after we get you to your new room?"

"Oh sure, let's go!" She was very spry for her age and walked by herself after we got her shoes on. Now, I know you are not supposed to lie to patients because it destroys the trusting relationship. However, if you rationalize it enough, I really was not lying—much. The room she was going to was actually better than her old room. She had her own TV, which she could not see anyway, and the room had some unique features, such as negative airflow and a second big sink by the door. It was larger than her old room and had a full-sized rocking recliner where she could sit comfortably. Most important, the approach her nurse was using was not working at all, and we had to get her out of that room.

A few minutes later, the three maintenance men reappeared. Two of them had Level C hazardous material (hazmat) suits on (see Chapter 26 for more detail) and were carrying a fogger and a 3-gallon spray can. The third man had on his regular blue maintenance department uniform and carried a roll of plastic sheeting and a roll of duct tape. The two with the suits and sprayers went into the room. They bagged up Julie's and Mrs. Perry's clothes in biohazard bags. They also bagged all the linens, towels, and wash cloths that were in the room in biohazard bags. Everything else was thrown away, in biohazard bags of course. A special biohazard laundry cart with a cover was brought to the unit, and all the laundry was sent for washing, no doubt in scalding hot water and undiluted chlorine bleach. I doubted Julie would ever be able to fit into that pair of jeans again.

Issues in Practice (continued)

After they were out of the room, they closed the door, and the man without the hazmat suit proceeded to tape the sheet of plastic around the doorjamb. When the other two were finished spraying, they pulled back the plastic just enough so that they could duck out and then sealed the room again. A sign was put on the plastic sheet: Do Not Enter for 48 Hours.

Julie went home later that day and had no more episodes of SVT. The nurse manager called the superintendent at Mrs. Perry's apartment and told him what we had found. When Mrs. Perry went home 2 days later, her apartment had a strong chemical odor and was cleaner than usual.

What lessons can be learned from this incident? I think there are two important ones: First, listen to your patients! When they talk to you, they usually have something to say; although it may be difficult for them to explain it and it may take some time, it is always worth listening. Second, do not totally disregard chronic complainers. If the complaint sounds strange or is about something physiological, it needs to be investigated more thoroughly.

There are also many things that do not work with complainers. These are listed here so that you do not waste your time on approaches that will only lead to more complaining or nowhere at all:[16]

1. Ignoring or avoiding complainers. They are seeking attention by complaining, and ignoring them will only make them complain more.
2. Having an aggressive confrontation. They will either hide the complaining or play the victim role.
3. Trying to fix their problems. They really do not want their problems fixed; they just want to complain about them.
4. Trying to cheer them up. Saying, "No one can have it that bad," will only make complainers try harder to convince you that, yes, their life is *that* bad or even *worse*.
5. Telling them they complain too much. They have no self-awareness of their complaining behavior and will deny it and then complain that you are being mean to them.
6. Commiserating with them. Saying to the complainer, "You know, you're right. This job is awful, and the cafeteria food stinks, and the charge nurse doesn't have a brain in her head," will make you the complainer's best buddy. You can now both face the big bad horrible world, together.
7. Using sarcasm. If you say, "Oh, you poor dear, bless your heart, it sounds like your life is just one big tragedy after another, doesn't it?" complainers may misinterpret it to mean that you really are acknowledging how big their problems are, or, if they do get the sarcasm, they will complain that you are unable to show empathy for them (and the world).[3]

Chronic complaining is bad for the work environment, bad for the people working there, and bad for the chronic complainer. No matter how difficult it is, complaining needs to be stopped somehow. A company in Germany sends employees home when they are having a "complaining day." Many employers are now including complaining behavior as a reason to avoid hiring someone. For chronic complainers, complaining is habitual, and they cannot hide it, even in an interview. However, because of the nursing shortage, HR personnel in hospitals and other health-care facilities are still using the "warm body" approach to hiring, so there tends to be a much higher number of chronic complainers in hospitals.

People can display other types of difficult behavior that were not discussed here; however, the approaches to changing those behaviors are similar to the many approaches talked about earlier. Some additional types of difficult behaviors include the following:

- Procrastination and indecision
- Nonresponsiveness and silence
- Yes people (conformist follower)

Conclusion

All professional nurses need to develop mechanisms to deal with people who are displaying difficult behavior. The very nature of the profession exposes nurses to a large number of people who are experiencing change, are under stress, and have a wide range of backgrounds and values and varying expectations. By understanding communication, using **behavior modification**, developing **assertiveness**, avoiding submissive and aggressive behaviors, and appreciating diversity, the nurse can develop the coping skills required for problem-solving, handling conflict in the work setting, and confronting the unacceptable behaviors of difficult people.[15]

Dealing with difficult people and resolving conflict are never pleasant undertakings. However, like most skills, the more they are practiced, the more comfortable you will become using the communication techniques discussed in both Chapter 11 and this chapter. The importance of handling problematic situations in a timely, honest, and caring manner is self-evident. The anxiety and fear provoked by confrontation are part of the price that nurses must pay to do their jobs well and provide high-quality patient care.

CRITICAL-THINKING EXERCISES

- Complete this statement for as many different situations as you can think of: "In a conflict situation, I have difficulty saying _____." Analyze reasons that prevent you from saying it. What is the worst thing that could have happened to you if you had said it? Create a phrase that you feel comfortable with that you could use the next time you want to say something difficult to the members of your team.
- Identify the communication and behavior characteristics of your work group or team. List areas of diversity for each member, including yourself. Identify their strengths and weaknesses. Identify methods for using the team members' diversity to enhance the team.
- Identify a person who displays difficult behaviors either at home, in the classroom, or in the clinical setting. Which of the categories discussed in the text does this person fit into? Attempt to communicate with this person using the techniques discussed in the book. Did they work? Why or why not?
- Analyze your own behavior. Are you a difficult person? Most people can have difficult behavior in some situations. What situations trigger a difficult behavior response in you? How does your behavior change when you are angry, depressed, or anxious?

NCLEX-STYLE QUESTIONS

1. Mr. Withers, a 70-year-old patient with diabetes, lived independently in his own home until he was hospitalized this week for gangrene in his foot. Since his below-the-knee amputation, he has been abusive with hospital staff, calling the nurses names and refusing to shave or wash himself or allow anyone to help him. Which response by the nurse appropriately addresses the emotions Mr. Withers is communicating?
    1. "Feeling angry doesn't give you the right to treat our staff with disrespect."
    2. "It's frightening to lose a foot. We are all working hard to help you recover and be independent again."
    3. "I think we need to call for a psychiatric consult. This could be dementia."
    4. "I'll ask the doctor to order you some medication for your anxiety."
2. How does Maslow's hierarchy of needs help to explain the difficult behavior of a patient recently diagnosed with stage 4 cancer?
    1. Stage 4 cancer threatens the patient's physiological and safety needs.
    2. Stage 4 cancer threatens the patient's need for love and belonging related to sexual intimacy.
    3. Stage 4 cancer threatens the patient's need for the respect of others related to the patient's physical appearance.

4. Stage 4 cancer threatens the patient's need for self-actualization by limiting their creativity and ability to solve problems.

3. Joleen, a new graduate nurse, is training with Mara, a senior nurse on the unit. Which of the following behaviors would support the idea that Mara is a persecutor? **Select all that apply.**
   1. Mara calls Joleen "JoJo" despite being asked not to.
   2. Mara has an answer to every question and never needs to look anything up.
   3. Mara asks critical-thinking questions to help Joleen think through problems.
   4. Mara insists that Joleen assess patients exactly the same way she does.
   5. Mara encourages Joleen to ask questions and test hypotheses.
   6. Mara compliments Joleen one day and criticizes her the next.

4. The behavior of both the sneak and the persecutor has the same underlying causes. Which of the following is NOT a cause of their behavior?
   1. Need for control
   2. Low self-esteem
   3. Desire to manipulate others
   4. Issues with love and belonging

5. Arturo, an RN in a busy ICU, decides to confront a coworker who is a sneak. Which of the following would be an effective way for Arturo to communicate with this person?
   1. "You are disgusting! I can't believe you're spreading rumors about me at work!"
   2. "I don't have time to listen to any more of your lies."
   3. "Has everyone heard what Angelica said about me?"
   4. "I never stole from the supply room, and you have no reason to say I did."

6. Tyesha is complaining again about the new charting software. "The drop-down menus aren't alphabetical, and they don't include some of the terms and diagnoses we use every day. This program runs slowly and is a pain to use. What a waste of the hospital's money!" Which response by a coworker would be most effective to counter this difficult behavior?
   1. "Just shut up, can't you!"
   2. "I know, right? And it's not intuitive at all."
   3. "I don't have time to chat now. I've got patients to take care of."
   4. "Learning new software can be challenging. Why don't you take the class?"

7. Constance is a home-health hospice nurse caring for Mrs. Alexander. Which of the following statements made by Mrs. Alexander might indicate that she is in the depression stage of the grief process?
   1. "I don't want to take any more pills. What's the point?"
   2. "If that telephone rings again, I'm going to throw it across the room."
   3. "It's so nice to see you, Constance! I enjoy visiting with you."
   4. "I read about a new type of therapy available in Mexico."

8. A patient who is in the _____ stage of the grief process may say, "I should have gotten a second opinion from another physician before now."

9. Which strategy is NOT effective in dealing with any type of difficult behavior?
   1. Ignoring the behavior
   2. Demonstrating empathy
   3. Avoiding anger or other strong emotions
   4. Listening carefully to what the person says.

10. Why do people demonstrate difficult behaviors? **Select all that apply.**
    1. It's their personality.
    2. The behavior is meeting some need for them.
    3. They are experiencing a major life change.
    4. They are in pain.
    5. They are on medication that lowers their inhibitions.
    6. They are afraid or anxious.

References

1. Ferguson S. All about human personality: Definition, disorders, and theories. PsychCentral, 2022. https://psychcentral.com/health/what-is-personality

2. Gluck S. Hording causes: Psychology of hoarding. Healthy Place, 2022. https://www.healthyplace.com/ocd-related-disorders/hoarding-disorder/hoarding-causes-psychology-of-hoarding

3. Bonlor A. 5 Things to keep in minds when dealing with difficult people. *Psychology Today*, 2022. https://www.psychologytoday.com/intl/blog/friendship-20/202206/5-things-keep-in-mind-when-dealing-difficult-people

4. How to handle a difficult coworker. Software Testing Help, 2022. https://www.softwaretestinghelp.com/how-to-handle-a-difficult-coworker/

5. What is a personality type? People Stripes, 2022. https://www.peoplestripes.org/what-is-personality-type.htm?parents&matchtype=&gclid=EAIaIQobChMIm5jc3LbC-AIVCSdMCh0yYwq0EAAYAyAAEgJFf_D_BwE

6. 8 Brilliant tips on how to handle a difficult coworker. Software Testing Help, 2022. https://www.softwaretestinghelp.com/how-to-handle-a-difficult-coworker/

7. Dean M. What are internalizing behaviors? Better Help, 2022. https://www.betterhelp.com/advice/behavior/what-are-internalizing-behaviors/

8. Bugeja M. How to disarm manipulation and gaslighting, personally and politically. Iowa Capital Dispatch, 2022. https://iowacapitaldispatch.com/2022/05/30/how-to-disarm-manipulation-and-gaslighting-personally-and-politically/

9. Gregory C. The five stages of grief. Psycom, 2022. https://www.psycom.net/stages-of-grief

10. Faubion D. The 7 stages of grief: What they are and how they affect you. ReGain, 2022. https://www.regain.us/advice/general/the-7-stages-of-grief-what-they-are-and-how-they-affect-you/

11. Cas-Alinas K. Deal with it: How to handle difficult patients. RegisteredNursing.org, 2022. https://www.registerednursing.org/articles/how-handle-difficult-patients/

12. Morrisette S. How actively involving your clients' or patients' family members can benefit your home care business. SmartCare Software, 2022. https://smartcaresoftware.com/news/involving-family-members-benefit-home-care-business/

13. How to deal with angry patients. Premier Medical Staffing Services, 2020. https://premiermedstaffing.com/blog/how-to-deal-with-an-angry-patient/

14. Gupta S. What to know about the bargaining stage of grief. Verywell Mind, 2022. https://www.verywellmind.com/the-bargaining-stage-of-grief-characteristics-and-coping-5272529

15. Inappropriate sexual behavior. Matrix neurological, n.d. https://www.matrixneurological.org/information/deficits-of-acquired-brain-injury/behavioural-emotional/inappropriate-sexual-behaviour/

16. How to deal with inappropriate patients. HealthTimes, 2021. https://healthtimes.com.au/hub/workplace-conditions/60/practice/healthinsights/how-to-deal-with-inappropriate-patients/2228/

17. Ross S, Naumann P, Hinds-Jackson DV, Stokes L. Sexual harassment in nursing: Ethical considerations and recommendations. *OJIN: Online Journal of Issues in Nursing*, 24, 2019. https://doi.org/10.3912/OJIN.Vol24No01Man01

Health-Care Delivery Systems

13

Nicole Harder | Joseph T. Catalano

Learning Objectives

After completing this chapter, the reader will be able to:

- Discuss the implications of health-care reform on the profession of nursing
- Analyze the evolution of the health-care delivery system in the United States
- Analyze the evolution of the health-care delivery system in Canada
- Evaluate the factors that influence the evolution of the health-care delivery system
- Synthesize the concerns surrounding uninsured people in the United States
- Analyze industry efforts to manage health-care costs
- Evaluate the efforts being made to ensure high-quality, cost-effective health care
- Describe and list the levels and types of health-care delivery

HEALTH CARE VERSUS HEALTH-CARE DELIVERY

Health care is often defined as the management of the resources of healing. The *delivery of health care* is the action or activities of supplying or providing services to maintain health, detect illness, and cure those who are ill or injured. In the past, these services were typically delivered in a hospital or clinic setting. A growing awareness of and interest in maintaining optimal health is resulting in a movement toward increasing preventive and primary care as a means of promoting health. This change in focus has produced substantial changes to the ways in which health-care services are delivered and the way health-care professionals interact with these systems. As professionals, nurses need to understand health-care delivery systems. Nursing practice is influenced by political, societal, and cultural realities and needs to adapt to the changing world. Today's health-care institutions are experiencing increased stress from the attempt to balance the costs of delivery, access to services, and requirements to increase the quality of care.

It has been long recognized that although individual health-care services in the United States are among the best in the world, the nation's health-care delivery system is mediocre at best. In many key health-care indicators, such as infant mortality and chronic diseases, the United States is well behind other developed countries, with a 37 out of 50 ranking. One of the goals of health-care reform is to bring the high-quality care experienced by some to those who are less fortunate or do not have employer-based insurance plans.

HEALTH-CARE REFORM

In 2010, passage of the landmark Affordable Care Act (ACA) set the stage for the largest overhaul of the U.S. health-care system in 50 years. Although the ACA got off to a somewhat rocky start, by its third year with the ongoing implementation of its provisions, many citizens were recognizing the ACA's value, particularly the 20 million or so newly insured. Nurses led the way for implementing the ACA because they saw it as a move to make the U.S. health-care system the best in the world for *all* its citizens.

However, in 2017, the Republican majority in Congress and the Trump administration attempted to repeal the ACA in its entirety. The outcry from U.S. citizens was so loud and strong that the attempt to repeal it outright failed. In response, the administration took measures to weaken the ACA. As of 2020, the ACA was still the law of the land, and although weakened, it was still providing health care for many who would not have been able to get health insurance without it. In fact, as of 2021, almost 31 million people had signed up for coverage under the ACA.[1]

With the advent of the Biden administration, many of the ACA elements that had been abolished under the previous administration were restored. These restorations and improvements include the following:

- Signing into law the American Rescue Plan (ARP), which expanded the premium tax credit (PTC) eligibility allowing Americans with income up to 150% of the federal poverty level (FPL) to obtain silver quality health plans for $0 monthly premiums
- Reducing deductible costs
- Reducing premium costs for employers
- Extending the special enrollment periods on the federal HR.gov health exchange through May 15
- Re-establishing ACA outreach efforts, such as paid advertising and promotions around the newly accessible health-care options
- Limiting association health plans and short-term, limited-duration insurance (junk insurance)
- Providing federal agencies with the authority to review regulations to identify ones that were inconsistent with ACA regulations and intent[2]

President Biden also canceled the Mexico City Policy, also known as the "global gag rule," which required foreign non-governmental organizations (NGOs) to certify that they would not perform or actively promote abortion as a method of family planning. They were forbidden to use money from any governmental source. It is yet to be seen what the effect of the 2022 Supreme Court decision that basically overturned *Roe v. Wade* will have on the abortion debate.[2]

The Biden administration put money back into the ACA that had been taken out by the previous administration, and Medicare and Medicaid were expanded in the face of the COVID-19 pandemic. The Employer Mandate, which applies to large employers (50 or more workers), remains in effect.[1]

Improving Health Care

The primary goal of the ACA is to provide affordable health care to U.S. citizens who, before its passage, were unable to pay for or obtain health insurance. Secondary goals included eliminating the insurance industry's disproportionate control of the health-care system, addressing inequities in current coverage, and helping senior citizens struggling to pay medical bills despite having Medicare. The legislative process modified or eliminated several key provisions of the ACA before it was implemented, which would have covered the almost 47 million Americans without health insurance.[3] However, more than 30 million additional citizens were added to the rolls of those with health insurance since President Obama's second term.[1] The ACA is now widely accepted as an essential part of the U.S. health-care system.

Many of the fears originally expressed by opponents of the ACA have been shown to be false or exaggerated. Because the provisions of the bill were phased in over 8 years, they proved to be less of a "culture shock" to health-care providers and citizens alike than some had imagined. Although Trump-era changes returned a substantial amount of control of the health-care system to the insurance industry, the Biden administration worked hard to reverse this trend. Biden reinstituted health-care subsidies for economically disadvantaged people, transparency requirements for insurance companies, taxes on tanning salons, and elimination of lifetime caps for insurance payouts.

Following are provisions of the ACA enacted in 2010:

- "Doughnut hole" protection for senior citizens. They received a rebate from the government to supplement the $2,700 limit on Medicare drug coverage.

> *Nurses led the way for implementing the ACA because they saw it as a move to make the U.S. health-care system the best in the world for* all *its citizens.*

One hundred percent of the doughnut hole was filled by 2020.

- Care for all children by eliminating the preexisting conditions restrictions found in most policies.
- Health-care subsidies for economically disadvantaged people.
- Access to high-risk pools for all uninsured, even adults with preexisting conditions.
- Increased age limit, to 26 years, for young adults to be covered on their parents' plans.
- Elimination of insurance companies' ability to drop coverage for someone who gets sick.
- Transparency. Insurance companies must reveal how much money is spent on overhead and administrative costs.
- A customer-appeals process to explain to customers how coverage determinations are made and claims are rejected.
- A 10 percent tax on indoor tanning services, with the money being used to fight skin cancer.
- Elimination of health-insurance **fraud** and waste with a new system of inspection and checks.
- Improved quality of information on the Web. A new Web site makes it easier for consumers and small businesses in any state to find affordable health insurance plans.
- Improved labels on food products for more accurate nutrient content to eliminate the confusing and sometimes fraudulent information provided by manufacturers.
- Less-expensive health-care plans offered to early retirees (ages 55–64 years) as part of the benefit package.

Provisions that became effective in 2011 include the following:

- Tax credits for small businesses with fewer than 50 employees to cover 50 percent of employee health-care premiums.
- Limited power of insurance companies to exploit small businesses; reduced out-of-pocket expenses for employees.
- A 2-year temporary credit (up to $1 billion) to encourage research into new therapies and procedures.

Provisions that became effective in 2014 include the following:

- Eliminating all preexisting illness limits for adults to obtain health insurance.
- Eliminating higher insurance premiums based on a person's gender or health status.
- No lifetime caps on the amount of insurance an individual can receive.
- Expanded Medicare payment to small rural hospitals and other health-care facilities that have a small number of Medicare patients.
- A minimum benefits package defined by the federal government, including certain preventive services at no cost.
- The option of coverage that can be offered through new state-run insurance marketplaces, called *exchanges*. Increased Medicare payroll taxes for high-income earners ($250,000 or more). Unearned income of $250,000 or more, now exempt from the payroll tax, would also be subject to a 3.8 percent levy.
- All new insurance plans to cover checkups and other preventive care without **copayments**.

Individuals who had health insurance plans at the time of the ACA implementation, except for those who had what professionals consider "junk policies," were allowed to keep their plans. However, by summer 2011, no health plans were able to set annual limits, drop individuals because of illness, drop children from parents' plans until they were 26 years old, or deny children coverage because of preexisting conditions.[3]

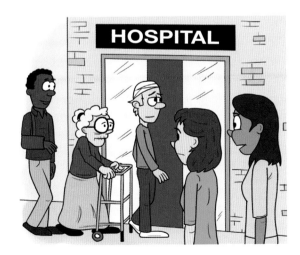

"I guess health-care reform means job security!"

Concerns About Health-Care Reform

Under the ARP, financial help for health insurance plans that meet ACA requirements is greater and more widely available than at any time in the past. However, the financial help will depend to some degree on where a person lives and what type and amount of medical care they needed during the prior year. People who wish to enroll in these types of plans do best if they shop in their own state's health insurance marketplace. It is likely they will be able to find plans for which they qualify that are free or very low cost with coverage that has strong benefits. There is no longer a federal penalty for not having minimum essential health coverage (the federal mandate); however, if a person lives in California, Rhode Island, Massachusetts, New Jersey, or the District of Columbia, there is a state penalty for not having minimum coverage. The health insurance plans people purchase in these states do not have to meet the ACA requirements for coverage (to be ACA-compliant); however, these types of plans provide the best benefits.[4]

All ACA-compliant plans are required to cover essential and basic health benefits, including almost all diagnostic and preventative care, without any caps or limits on the total amount that the plan may spend on a person's lifetime care needs. These plans offer a comprehensive safety net if a person requires substantial medical care for a long-term illness or accident recovery. Long COVID-19 recovery and medical needs are also included in all ACA-compliant plans. In addition, under the ARP, all ACA-compliant plans are required to include coverage for preexisting conditions without any waiting periods.[4]

If an individual purchases a plan that is not ACA-compliant, the insurance company will raise the cost of the premiums or reduce the amount of insurance coverage based on the person's past medical history such as preexisting conditions. These types of insurance plans all have caps on the total coverage for a lifetime and do not cover the essential and basic health benefits unless the state has its own requirements to do so.[4]

A few groups are not required to purchase health insurance. Most Native Americans can receive health care through their tribal health-care systems. Almost all federal government employees are covered by government-sponsored insurance, which is very similar to the insurance under the ACA. Also, those who have legitimate religious objections can avoid paying for insurance.[5]

Some clinicians feared that the increased number of new patients would overwhelm the health-care system, resulting in long waits at physicians' offices. However, this circumstance never developed at any time in the ACA's lifetime. Another concern was that the Medicare system would be inundated with a flood of new recipients and not have enough funding to cover everyone. This did not happen either.

Nursing and Health-Care Reform

Nurses were at the table during the planning of the ACA, and their input into the law aided lawmakers with many of its key provisions. Nurses also had a key role in its initial implementation. The initial influx of some 22 million new patients into the health-care system offered new challenges and opportunities for nurses to expand their profession and practice to the levels for which they were educated. The additional 18 million who have entered the health-care system since the initial enrollment years also have been easily accommodated into the existing health-care system.

The real test of the abilities of the health-care system to meet an influx of new and very ill patients came with the surge of COVID-19 patients in 2019. The health-care system failed miserably. Not only were traditional tactics used to handle mass casualties overwhelmed, but the very infrastructure of most acute care facilities was destroyed. The federal government's response was first to deny that there was a problem and disband the pandemic taskforce. The administration withheld the money needed to develop vaccines and purchase ventilators, fired Dr. Anthony Fauci as head of the pandemic committee, and never did develop a comprehensive plan to deal with the pandemic.[6]

With the advent of the Biden administration at the peak of the pandemic, a comprehensive COVID-19 strategy was developed and became part of the ACA. The heart of the plan revolved around an unprecedented plan for vaccinating the majority of citizens. More than 220 million Americans were fully vaccinated within the first 2 years, and over 100 million received a booster shot.[7] The plan included provisions to make the vaccinations free, generally available, and convenient for people to receive. In the first 2 years of this plan, daily COVID-19 deaths were down almost 90 percent from the start of the pandemic. Under the Biden plan, the vaccine is available for anyone above the age of 6 months.[7]

A Goal of Maintaining Health

Sometimes overlooked or discounted in discussions of the ACA is its increased emphasis on preventive care. All Americans can receive screening procedures such as prostate examinations, mammograms, annual physical examinations, and preventive care such as immunizations at no out-of-pocket costs. Almost all the preventive-care measures of the ACA have been implemented and do not require approval by Congress, as some of the other provisions do.

Opportunities and Challenges for Nurses

One commitment that has always differentiated professional nursing from medicine is the goal of maintaining health and preventing disease.[3] It makes sense, then, that the transition in health care's emphasis from illness and disease to prevention and health promotion has been easier for nurses than for physicians.

To see the effects of this transition, we have only to look at the practice of primary care. During the past decade, physician training for primary care has decreased because of low reimbursement rates from insurance companies and government programs. It is unlikely that the current crop of primary care physicians will be able to handle the increase in patients seeking preventive care. On the other hand, the education of nurse practitioners has increased by some 60 percent during the same decade. In addition, the ACA provides about $50 million per year to develop new training programs for each of the nurse practitioner roles. Also, public health finds itself on the front lines of the influx of new patients. The opportunity for nurses to lead health-care reform has been demonstrated since the ACA became law.[6]

To meet the demands of the changing health-care system, nurses must continue to do what they have always done, but to do it better. In the past, when demographic swings or governmental programs have created substantive changes in health care, nurses have been the leaders in developing new systems and models to accommodate the changes. Nurses are experts in increasing access to care while maintaining the quality of that care.

Although nurses are generally not represented at the higher decision-making levels of government and corporation boardrooms, their high-level skills and decades-long history of public trust place them in a perfect position to enter into the health-care system debate. There are any number of ways nurses can become involved in the discussion. One of the most practical and easy-to-use forums is social media. If nurses remain silent now and slip back into their pre-pandemic position of dependence, they will betray all the heroic gains that the profession made during the pandemic.[8]

The care advanced practice nurses (APRNs) provided during the pandemic cuts across diverse geographical, societal, economic, and political settings in their practice of nursing. Their type and level of knowledge is indispensable in accurately informing administrators and policymakers who are attempting to make critical decisions about health-care system reform, regulatory changes, care coordination, and health information technology. In these reforms and changes, nurses' interests and policymakers' issues run parallel. Both want the best policies to address patients' safety and health outcomes. Nurses have a unique, and perhaps one-time, opportunity to fill the vacuum created by the deep distrust the public has of politicians and policymakers.[8]

> *Nurses are experts in increasing access to care while maintaining the quality of that care.*

Policy Change via Social Media

Nurses looking for a method to engage in and impact public policy-making can find an ideal platform in social media. It has limited barriers for its use and can provide nurses a relatively simple process for getting involved with the public at large. By using social media, nurses can place before the public their real positions, values, and messages about who and what they are. They can express what they are passionate about while sidestepping the bureaucratic tangle of the hierarchy. Through social media, nurses are able to advocate for reforms in the health-care system such as safe staffing levels, care coordination, and improvements in health information technology.[8]

As nurses display their expertise, they will begin to be recognized as an authentic voice in public policy-making. Nurses can use social media to advocate for their patients and themselves. Using a written example along with a picture is the strongest way to get across a message. Remember the old saying, "A picture is worth a thousand words"? One of the best examples of the power of social media was a picture of a nurse that showed the bruises on her face caused by wearing a protective mask for a 12-hour shift. In addition to the marks produced by the mask, the picture also showed the emotional effects that providing care for COVID-19 patients had on nurses.[9]

There are risks for nurses who use social media to try to make policy change, however. During the COVID-19 pandemic, some nurses were fired for stating on social media the personal protective equipment (PPE) being provided by their hospitals did not meet the Centers for Disease Control and Prevention (CDC)'s standards, while other nurses were forbidden by their employers to talk about working conditions such as the lack of adequate masks or too few ventilators. Nurses who use social media to bring about changes in policy need to be aware of their state's licensing rules and regulations and to make sure they are not violating any part of the Code of Ethics for Nurses. One of the most basic Health Insurance Portability and Accountability Act (HIPAA) rules that is violated is sharing identifying information about patients without their consent.[8]

Other methods that can be used to influence policy decisions include phone calls to legislators, e-mails, letters to the editor of a local newspaper, and personalized notes or letters to elected officials or a face-to-face discussion with them.[9] Nurses must continue to work in the political arena to fight for the health and well-being of all U.S. citizens. They must always attempt to be at the table to help shape changes in health-care policy.

As evidence-based practice becomes the norm for health-care practice, nurses need to keep conducting the research and collecting the data that improve care. Without a solid base of research, it will be impossible to demonstrate scientifically the effectiveness of preventive care and improved patient outcomes. However, nurses cannot do research in a vacuum. It is essential that they collaborate with all health-care disciplines by understanding and acknowledging the importance of their roles in health-care reform. From collaborating with medical schools to providing training for patient care technicians, nurses can establish the trust required to work in concert with others and provide seamless, high-quality care.[9]

Health-care reform can be a double-edged sword for professional nursing. Nurses can lead the reform that will mark the success of health care for decades to come, or they can be overrun by the system and become a footnote to health-care history. Nurses who educate themselves about policy changes and who find opportunities to shape them will be the leaders health care requires now and in the future.

THE NEW FACE OF HEALTH CARE

The number of U.S. citizens not covered by any type of health insurance in 2010 was more than 49.9 million or about 16.3 percent of the population. However by 2023 (the last year for available data before publication), only 9.8 percent of American citizens, or about 28.0 million, did not have health insurance at any point during the year. In addition, 9 million children are uninsured in the United States and 73.7 percent of uninsured adults say that the cost of coverage is the reason they do not have a policy. Of those Americans who do not have health insurance, 50 percent report not having seen a physician or healthcare professional in the previous 12 months. Of those who do not have health insurance, American Indians and Alaskan Natives are the highest with 21.7 percent and Asian Americans are the lowest with 7.2 percent. The states with the highest rates of uninsured are Texas (18.4%), Oklahoma (14.3%), Georgia (13.4%), and Florida (13.2%). The states with the lowest number of uninsured are Washington DC (3.5%), Hawaii (4.3%), Minnesota (4.9%), and New York (5.2%).[10] Of the top 25 industrialized countries, the United States is the only one that does not have any type of universal health-care coverage for its citizens.[10] The ACA was a first step to developing a system that offered all U.S. residents the same type of health care distributed to members of the U.S. Congress and the president's administration. The ACA challenged politicians to develop a system that covered all citizens in the same way that the politicians are covered by their governmental health-care plan.

DEMOGRAPHICS AFFECTING HEALTH-CARE DELIVERY

Age

Between now and 2050, the number of persons 65 years or older is expected to double. By 2050, one in five people living in Canada or the United States will be elderly, and their numbers will reach an estimated 80 million.[11] Of this number, many will eventually become more dependent on the health-care delivery system as a result of chronic health problems. (See Chapter 22 for more details.)

Although an aging population constitutes a sizable number of persons who may require expensive long-term health care, their community activism and powerful influence at the ballot box can provide them with better access to health care than other less vocal and less politically savvy groups. Additional at-risk groups consist of persons residing in urban areas with limited incomes and individuals living in remote rural areas where access to care is limited.

Chronicity

Another factor influencing the climate of health-care delivery is the long-term and expensive nature of many health problems. Although significant strides have been made in treating some acute infectious diseases, many challenges still exist in the management of health concerns such as cancer, heart disease, Alzheimer's disease, diabetes, chronic obstructive pulmonary disease (COPD), and HIV.

Long COVID

Although the acute nature of COVID-19 caused major short-term disruptions in the health-care system, the extended nature of post-COVID-19 syndrome, long COVID, has added it to the list of chronic conditions. Although the exact cause of long COVID is unknown, it appears to be due to damage to the immune system, producing an autoimmune type response in many parts of the body. Long COVID symptoms persist for weeks, months, or years after the patient begins to recover from the acute disease process. Initial data shows that more than 40 percent of people infected with the COVID-19 virus show signs of long COVID, and for people who were hospitalized with COVID-19, that number increases to 57 percent. Some of the more serious of the 200 or more symptoms include speech difficulty,

> *Initial data shows that more than 40 percent of people infected with the COVID-19 virus show signs of long COVID, and for people who were hospitalized with COVID-19, that number increases to 57 percent.*

brain fog, shortness of breath, chest pain, joint inflammation, anxiety, depression, severe headaches, tachycardia, and renal insufficiency. As of publication of this text, there is no specific treatment for long COVID. Rather, treatments are directed toward the patient's symptoms. For example, if the patient is having difficulty speaking, they are referred to a speech therapist.[12] Additional concerns for chronicity include environmental and occupational safety, drug abuse, and mother and child health care.

HEALTH CARE AS AN INDUSTRY

In most developed countries, health care is one of the largest industries. Of the Organization for Economic Cooperation and Development (OECD) member countries (the 35 richest countries in the world), the United States spends the most for health care at 16.9 percent of its gross domestic product (GDP). The GDP is the total value of all the goods and services produced within a country's borders in 1 year. The United States also spends the most per person for health care at $11,072, up from $10,348 per person in 2018. The total amount that the United States spent on health care in 2018 was $16.2 billion.[13] Unfortunately, large expenditures on health care do not necessarily equal better health care. Among the wealthiest countries, the United States ranks only 11th in the quality of health services.[14]

Because the United States does not have government-supported universal health care for its citizens, Americans have increased problems paying their medical bills out of pocket. The insurance-company-run health-care system in the United States causes more people to have their insurance claims denied and a larger percentage of individuals and families forced into medical bankruptcy than in any other country.[14] Health care in the United States has been described as "lackluster" or "mediocre" when compared to other top OECD countries. Backing up these observations are the facts that the United States has the highest infant, maternal, and preventable death rates of the top 11 OECD countries. The life expectancy of a U.S. citizen at birth is 78.6 years (Canada = 82.4), which is ranked 22nd out of the 35 OECD countries. A 2018 survey of the top 11 developed countries showed the U.S. health-care system to be the worst performing, with the poorest access to care and lowest effectiveness overall. The weaknesses of the U.S. health-care system were clearly demonstrated in its handling of the COVID-19 pandemic.[14]

Health Care in the Global Context

Understanding the various approaches to health care around the globe is important in assessing the challenges to and potential of health-care delivery. How and why health-care systems differ is a function of multiple influences. These may include societal values and beliefs, sociocultural climate, the state of the economy, political ideologies, geographic density, international influences, historical realities, established practices and programs, and other factors. For health-care systems to develop, several factors must come into play at different points. This development is consistent throughout the world, as can be seen by examining the contexts in which various health-care systems were developed.

One way to think about system differences is to consider that Western countries provide for health care in several ways, all of which involve variable combinations of private or public funding of services and private or public delivery of services.[12] Table 13.1 shows the degree of public involvement in financing health services and the essential role envisioned for the health-care system.[14]

Type 1 Systems

In the type 1 health-care system, private approaches to health services predominate. Physicians, other caregivers (e.g., midwives), and patients have maximum autonomy. In this system, individuals who can afford private health insurance, or who simply can pay for their health care, choose their care providers and receive health services. Those who cannot pay do not have choice or benefit.

In its purest form, the type 1 system would not offer any option other than to pay for service. In reality, most countries have adopted a mixture of system types. For example, although the United States has a mainly private payment system of health care, some publicly funded programs assist elderly and poor people. Even with these programs, it is estimated that 30 million, or about 9.8 percent, of Americans still did not have health insurance in 2023, and therefore are limited in their ability to find treatment at health care facilities.[10]

Type 4 Systems

On the opposite end of the spectrum from type 1 is type 4. This type of health-care system focuses on keeping the general public healthy so that citizens can continue to contribute to society and the economy. Health care is considered an essential service or even a right, not necessarily involving compassionate motives. Health-care providers are considered agents of the state who work to keep others working efficiently.

In Canada, the type 4 structure is seen in such organizations as the military, hockey teams, and other sports teams. Health-care providers are hired by these organizations to ensure the players stay healthy and can do their part to achieve the goals of the group.

Type 3 Systems

Between the extremes of type 1 and type 4 health-care systems are two types—type 2 and type 3. The type 3 system is funded and operated by the government, as was seen in Great Britain some years ago. With this system, the state-operated and state-funded health

Table 13.1 Types of Health-Care Systems in the Western World

System	Type 1 Private health insurance	Type 2 National health insurance	Type 3 National health service	Type 4 Socialized health system
Primary Goal	Preserve autonomy	Egalitarian	Egalitarian	Essential service
Secondary Effect	Acceptance of social differences	Preserve autonomy	Public management	Health-care providers as state employees

services were based on an egalitarian value. Public management of each service was considered key to efficient and effective operation.

Type 2 Systems

The type 2 system is a hybrid of the type 1 and type 3 systems. Egalitarian values are given high priority, but so are practitioner and patient autonomy. The type 2 system uses tax dollars to pay for health services through health insurance available from a nonprofit agency (e.g., government).

Each health service is operated more or less autonomously by others, including municipalities, citizen groups, physicians, nurse practitioners, and physiotherapists in private offices, **group practices**, and other groups. All services rendered to patients are then paid from the central pool of health insurance funds created through taxation. This type of system is used in Canada and embodies the collective sharing of burdens and benefits while allowing a degree of autonomy in delivery.[15]

Third World Alternatives

It is important to note that the four systems just described exclude a group of third world countries that cannot afford the type of health care appreciated in most developed countries. Yet many third world countries have managed to develop primary care systems that are not as institution dependent as the systems found in Canada and the United States. In their systems, primary care includes preventive health care, first point of contact, and **continuing care**. However, in some countries, the primary and preventive systems have been undermined by the influence of Western countries promoting high technology and institutionalization.

What Do Taxes Cover?

Even in countries that finance health insurance through tax dollars, there are variations in services provided. For example, some fund home care, but others do not; some provide coverage for prescription drugs, and others do not. Regardless of the type of system, it is important to reflect on the influences that have created it and continue to maintain it.

What Do You Think?

What type of health-care system did you use the last time you accessed health care? Did you use the health-care system for preventive care or illness care?

ADMINISTRATION AND FUNDING OF HEALTH-CARE SYSTEMS

Canada's health-care system is the subject of much political controversy and debate in the United States. Those opposing universal health care question how efficient the Canadian system is at providing timely surgeries, treatments, and access to health care. Regardless of the political debate, Canada does boast one of the highest life expectancies (about 82.4 years) and lowest infant mortality rates of industrialized countries, which many attribute to Canada's universal single-payer health-care system. The Canadian system places greater emphasis on primary care and less emphasis on specialist care and on hospital-related, complex, and expensive procedures. Overall, Canada spends less per person on health care than the United States, and ordinary Canadian citizens live healthier lives than average U.S. citizens.[15]

> *Overall, Canada spends less per person on health care than the United States, and ordinary Canadian citizens live healthier lives than average U.S. citizens.*

Health Care in Canada

Financing and administering health-care systems can be an overwhelming responsibility. In Canada, health-care services are provided under the Canada Health Act. The Canadian federal government collects funds through taxes and gives the responsibility of administering health-care services to the provinces. As in the United States, the cost of financing health-care services has risen tremendously since the first Medical Care Act was introduced in 1967–1968. In Canada, medical insurance premiums became an increasing burden for the federal government as a result of the improved services promised to all Canadians.[16]

Federal Transfer Payments

In an attempt to control the costs to be paid to all provinces, the Canadian government proposed a system of block funding. In 1977, the Federal-Provincial Fiscal Arrangements and Established Programs Financing Act were established after lengthy negotiations with all provinces. The formula for federal transfer payments consisted of four components:

1. Per capita payments were made on the basis of previous expenditures and adjusted regularly in relation to the gross national product.
2. Tax points were transferred by the federal government, allowing provinces to reduce their tax contribution to the government and at the same time increase the portion of tax collected at the provincial level.
3. Equalization of tax points was distributed among poorer provinces.
4. Additional per capita payments were indexed to help pay for nursing home, residential home, and ambulatory care.[16]

This new act changed the funding formula from a 50-50 cost-sharing arrangement to one that gave taxation points to the provinces in exchange for lower cash-transfer payments. The provinces were initially very receptive, as this meant they had more taxation power in an economy that was very healthy. However, with rising costs of health care, owing in part to an aging population and the increased use of technology, some physicians and provinces struggled with reimbursement and with providing care for large numbers of patients. With extra billing or balance billing becoming prevalent, there was a heated public debate, and the new Canada Health Act was passed in 1984.

The Canada Health Act

Although the Canadian federal government has a limited constitutional basis for making health-care decisions, it has considerable economic clout to develop and shape a national health-care plan. To support its positions on health care, the federal government enacted the Canada Health Act (CHA). The purpose of the CHA is to "establish criteria and conditions in respect of insured health services and extended healthcare services provided under provincial law that must be met before a full cash contribution may be made."[16] It was last revised in 2012.

The insured health services defined by the CHA include all medically necessary hospital services and medically required physician services, as well as medically- or dentally-required surgical-dental services that need to be performed in a hospital for safety. New criteria, conditions, and provisions were formulated to eliminate extra billing and user charges.

For the provinces to qualify for full cash refunds from the federal government under the Canada Health and Social Transfer (CHST) agreement, they must meet five basic criteria and conditions. These criteria and conditions must be met for each fiscal year and must include the following:

> *The insured health services defined by the CHA include all medically necessary hospital services and medically required physician services, as well as medically- or dentally-required surgical-dental services that need to be performed in a hospital for safety.*

1. *Public administration:* The health insurance plan must be administered and operated on a nonprofit basis by a public authority, responsible to the provincial government, and subject to audit of its accounts and financial transactions.
2. *Comprehensiveness:* The plan must cover all insured health services provided by hospitals, medical practitioners, dentists, and, where permitted, services rendered by other health-care practitioners.
3. *Universality:* One hundred percent of the insured population of a province must be entitled to the insured health services provided for by the plan on uniform terms and conditions.
4. *Portability:* Residents moving to another province must continue to be covered for insured health services by the home province during any minimum waiting period, not to exceed 3 months, imposed by the new province of residence. For insured persons, insured health services must be made available while they are temporarily absent from their own provinces on the following basis:
   - Insured services received out of province but still in Canada are to be paid for by the home province at

host province rates unless another arrangement for the payment of costs exists between the provinces. Prior approval may be required for elective services.

- Out-of-country services received are to be paid, as a minimum, on the basis of the amount that would have been paid by the home province for similar services rendered in the province. Prior approval may be required for elective services.

5. *Accessibility:* The health insurance plan of a province must provide for the following:
   - Insured health services on uniform terms and conditions and reasonable access by insured persons to insured health services not precluded and unimpeded, either directly or indirectly, by charges or other means.
   - Reasonable compensation to physicians and dentists for all insured health services rendered.
   - Payments to hospitals in respect to the cost of insured health services.

Although discussion and debate continue surrounding the federal and provincial responsibilities for health-care funding and the escalating costs associated with health care, the CHA continues to be the operating model for the Canadian health-care system.[17]

Health-Care Systems in the United States

The United States' method of funding and administering health-care services is far different from that of Canada. According to the World Health Organization, the United States spends more per person on health care than does any other country; yet in overall quality, its care ranked 37th in the world before enactment of the ACA. However, there has been a marked improvement since the ACA was enacted in 2010; in 2020, the U.S. health-care system was ranked 11th against the same group. France, with its universal coverage for every citizen and its single-payer government system for health care, was ranked first in 2020.[14] Of the OECD countries, the United States has the following:

- The highest rate of death by gun violence, by a huge margin
- The highest rate of death by car accidents

- The highest chance that a child will die before age 5
- The second-highest rate of death by coronary heart disease
- The second-highest rate of death by lung cancer and COPD
- The highest teen pregnancy rate
- The highest rate of women dying due to complications of pregnancy and childbirth[17]
- The highest death rate from COVID-19[14]

This disparity is attributed in large part to the lack of access to and prohibitive cost of health-care services, not the quality of the services available.

In an attempt to contain health-care costs, **professional standards review organizations (PSROs)** were introduced to review the quality, quantity, and cost of hospital care through Medicare. The primary goal of PSROs was to review the care provided by health-care providers to determine whether the best diagnostic and treatment approaches were being used. Another measure was the introduction of utilization review committees, requiring Medicare-qualified facilities to review admission, diagnostic testing, and treatments with the goal of eliminating overuse or misuse of services.

> *In an attempt to contain health-care costs, **professional standards review organizations (PSROs)** were introduced to review the quality, quantity, and cost of hospital care through Medicare.*

What Do You Think?

Review the bill from your last hospitalization or that of a family member. Can you identify the cost of each item on the bill? What charges did you expect? Were there charges you did not expect? Is there information about how to dispute charges you disagree with anywhere on the bill statement?

Prospective Payment Systems

Although these measures have assisted with cost containment to some degree, one of the most significant factors that have influenced cost control was the **prospective payment system (PPS)** established by the U.S. Congress in 1983. This system required facilities providing services to Medicare patients to be reimbursed using a fixed-rate system and included monetary incentives to reduce the length of hospital stays. Medicare patients are classified using a **diagnosis-related group (DRG)**, and the facilities are reimbursed a predetermined amount. Patients may be classified into one of 467 DRGs, and reimbursement occurs regardless of the length of stay. DRGs may be further grouped into major diagnostic categories (MDCs).

If the patient is discharged sooner than anticipated, the facility keeps the difference. If the patient requires a lengthier hospital stay, the hospital pays the extra cost. Under the PPS, the emphasis is on the efficient delivery of services in the most cost-effective manner.

Capitated Payment Systems

Capitation, or a **capitated payment system**, was introduced to encourage cost-effectiveness in a growing health-care system. In a capitated payment system, participants pay a flat rate, usually through their employer, to belong to a managed care organization (MCO) or health maintenance organization (HMO) for a specified period of time. The health-care providers who serve the participants receive a fixed amount for each participant in the health-care plan.

Controlled Access

The goal of capitation is to have a payment plan for selected diseases or surgical procedures that provides the highest quality of care, including essential diagnostic and treatment procedures, at the lowest cost possible. Any expenses in excess of the capitated rate are the responsibility of the MCO. If the MCO spends less on the care of a patient than it is given for delivery costs, it can keep the excess as profit, providing it with a strong incentive to reduce the cost of services.

Another goal of managed care is to enhance the efficiency and effective use of health-care services. A key underlying concept of managed care is to maintain administrative control over access and provision of primary health-care services for the members of the plan. The MCO controls all aspects of care, including delivery, financing, and the purchase of health-care services for patients who are enrolled in the program. Patients are allowed to use only the services of primary care health-care providers who are approved by the organization. Any referrals to other medical specialists must be approved by the MCO. The MCO contract determines what treatments or procedures will be reimbursed.

A Spending Increase

The effectiveness of the MCO plan rests on the theory that health-care costs can be reduced by decreasing the number of hospitalizations, shortening the length of inpatient stays, providing less-expensive home-care services, and keeping people healthy through health promotion and illness-prevention services. It is logical to conclude that if people stay healthy, the cost of health-care services should decline.

Although much debate surrounds managed care and its advantages and disadvantages, the reality is that managed care has *not* reduced health-care costs nationally. Increases in spending are attributed to rising health-care wages, legislation that increased Medicare spending, increasing insurance premiums, technology, and consumer demands for less restrictive plans. Overall, managed care was deemed a failure, and many states have moved on to more efficient and effective systems.

Overview of Health-Care Plans

See Boxes 13.1 through 13.5 to compare the principal features of different health-care models.

QUALITY OF CARE

Although the primary focus of health-care delivery systems is to provide care to as many people as possible, consideration of the quality of care is also a key factor. Delivering low-quality care to large numbers of individuals is not a viable option. Health-care facilities have implemented several quality-improvement measures in an attempt to reduce the large number of injuries and deaths of hospitalized patients. (For more detailed information about quality of care, see Chapter 15.)

HEALTH-CARE LEVELS AND SETTINGS

Even though there are many methods for providing and funding health care, high-quality health-care services remain the highest priority. Consumers who have access to multiple types of health care may not always understand the differences among them.

In the past, health-care services were primarily illness or institution based and focused primarily on treating the ill or injured. The emphasis is now shifting slowly toward prevention and health promotion in the population. It is believed that a focus on wellness and a population living a healthier lifestyle will reduce

Box 13.1 Managed Care Organizations (MCOs)

Definition: Provide comprehensive preventive and treatment services to a specific group of voluntarily enrolled persons.

Managed Care Structures

Staff model: Health-care providers are salaried employees of the MCO.

Group model: MCO contracts with single group practice.

Network model: MCO contracts with multiple group practices and/or integrated organizations.

Independent practice association (IPA): MCO contracts with health-care providers who usually are not members of groups and whose practices include fee-for-service and capitated patients.

Characteristics: Focus on health maintenance and primary care. All care provided by a primary care provider. Referral needed for access to specialists and hospitalization.

Medicare MCO

Definition: Program same as MCO but designated to cover health-care costs of senior citizens.

Characteristics: Premium generally less than supplemental plans.

Box 13.2 Provider Organizations

Preferred Provider Organization (PPO)

Definition: One that limits an enrollee's choice to a list of "preferred" hospitals, physicians, and other providers. An enrollee pays more out-of-pocket expenses for using a provider not on the list.

Characteristics: Contractual agreement exists between a set of providers and one or more purchasers (self-insured employers or insurance plans). Comprehensive health services at a discount for companies under contract.

Exclusive Provider Organization (EPO)

Definition: One that limits an enrollee's choice to providers belonging to one organization. Enrollee may or may not be able to use outside providers at additional expense.

Characteristics: Limited contractual agreement; less access to specialists.

the number of people who require expensive illness-care services.

Levels of Service

Health care services are frequently categorized according to the complexity or level of the services provided. This complexity relates to the kinds, or levels, of services: primary, secondary, and tertiary.

Primary Care

In nursing, *primary care* refers to health promotion and preventive care, including programs such as immunization campaigns. Primary care focuses on health education and on early detection and treatment. Maintaining and improving optimal health is the overriding goal.

Secondary Care

In the **secondary care** level, the focus shifts toward emergency and acute care. Secondary services are frequently provided in hospitals and other acute care settings, with an emphasis on diagnosis and the treatment of complex disorders. Free-standing emergency care clinics are becoming popular to provide primary care and limited secondary care outside the hospital at a lower cost to patients.

Tertiary Care

The **tertiary care** level emphasizes rehabilitative services, long-term care, and care of the dying. Nursing services are essential in all three levels of health care, in both the hospital and community settings.

What Do You Think?

Have you ever received care in a nontraditional health-care setting? What was it? What role did nurses play in the delivery of care?

Box 13.3 **Medicare**

Definition: Federally funded national health insurance program in the United States for people older than 65 years.

Part A provides basic protection for medical, surgical, and psychiatric care costs based on diagnosis-related groups.

Part B is a voluntary medical insurance plan that covers health-care provider and certain outpatient services.

Part C is called a Medicare Advantage Plan and is a type of Medicare health plan offered by a private company that contracts with Medicare. Medicare Advantage Plans provide all of Part A (hospital insurance) and Part B (medical insurance) and usually prescription drug (Part D). Once enrolled in a Medicare Advantage Plan, most Medicare services are covered through the plan. Medicare services are not paid for by Original Medicare. Most Medicare Advantage plans may offer routine vision and dental.

Part D is an unfunded insurance for medications.

Characteristics: Payment for plan deducted from monthly Social Security check; covers services of nurse practitioners (varies by state); does not pay full costs of certain services; supplemental insurance is encouraged.

Box 13.4 **Medicaid**

Definition: Federally funded, state-operated medical assistance program for people with low incomes. Individual states determine eligibility and benefits.

Characteristics: Finances a large portion of maternal and child care for the poor; reimburses for nurse midwifery and other advanced practice nursing (varies by state); reimburses long-term care facility funding.

Health-Care Settings

While nursing care is provided in traditional settings, such as the hospital and the community, nursing services are also delivered in a growing number of

Box 13.5 **Private Insurance**

Traditional Private Insurance

Definition: Traditional fee-for-service plan. Payment, computed after services are provided, is based on the number of services used.

Characteristics: Policies typically expensive; most policies have deductibles that patients must meet before insurance pays.

Long-Term Care Insurance

Definition: Supplemental insurance for coverage of long-term care services. Policies provide a set number of dollars for an unlimited time or for as little as 2 years.

Characteristics: Very expensive; good policy has a minimum waiting period for eligibility, payment for skilled nursing, intermediate or custodial care, and home care.

nontraditional locations. One growing trend in care is seen in the outpatient departments attached to some hospitals. Outpatient services are used by patients who require a relatively high level of skilled health care but who do not need to stay in a hospital for an extended period of time. An inpatient is a person who enters a setting such as a hospital and remains for at least 24 hours. Whether patients are inpatients or outpatients, they often need assistance from the nurse to identify which services best suit their needs.

Public Health

Public health departments are government agencies that are established at the local, provincial or state, and federal levels to provide health services. The goal of early public health departments was to prevent and control communicable diseases that were rampant in the 18th and 19th centuries, producing epidemics that killed millions of people. Modern-day epidemics, such as the Ebola outbreak in western Africa and the worldwide COVID-19 pandemic, still remain a threat, and public health nurses continue their role as the first line of defense against pandemics that can potentially kill thousands of citizens. However, today, the scope of public health, while retaining its contagious disease control and prevention mission, has expanded to areas such as child health, pregnancy care, and, more recently, early detection and treatment of terrorist acts, particularly bioterrorism (see Chapter 26).

Home Health Care

Care of the ill and injured in the home is the oldest of all the health-care modalities. If you were to go back far enough, it might even be called "cave health care." The modern hospital and clinic are relatively new entities in the health-care system, having their origins in the Industrial Revolution. Before that time, the only place a person could receive care was at home, usually from a female relative.

Care in the Home Setting

Although the interest in and use of home health care have waxed and waned over time, its benefits have received new attention in the era of an aging population and health-care reform. In 2022, there were approximately 16,461 primary care home health-care agencies in the United States that provide care for approximately 9 million patients, and some of this care is at a high-acuity level.[18] Gone are the days when home health care consisted of a quick visit by a nurse or aide taking vital signs, changing a dressing, and cleaning the house. Home health care now combines the advantages of health care in a safe and familiar setting with the high-tech treatment modalities found in the most advanced hospitals.

The goal of home health care is to make it possible for patients to remain at home rather than use hospital, residential, or long-term care facilities. Most patients prefer the familiar atmosphere of their own home and neighborhood. Patients experience lower stress levels at home and have a more positive outlook, which studies have shown hastens recovery. They are active participants in their own care, increasing their independence and giving them a sense of control over the outcome. Usually, the home contains far fewer invasive and resistant pathogens than the hospital, so patients have a lower rate of infection with the medication-resistant bacteria commonly found in hospitals and extended care facilities. High-quality home care helps prevent readmissions, which benefits patients and saves money.[18] When nurses and other health-care professionals do visit the home-care patient, the patient and their health needs are the sole focus of the care provided.

The majority of home health care remains informal and is provided mostly by relatives and friends. When professionals provide care in the home, nurses are the primary group involved. Other providers include physical therapists, home health-care aides, respiratory and occupational therapists, social workers, and mental health professionals. Professional-level home health-care services can include physical and psychological assessment, wound care, medication and illness education, pain management, physical therapy, speech therapy, and occupational therapy. Assistance with activities of daily living and other daily tasks, such as meal preparation, medication reminders, laundry, light housekeeping, errands, shopping, transportation, and companionship, is sometimes referred to as *life assistance services.*[18]

Technology that was long considered the sole domain of the acute care hospital has found its way into the home. Patients who previously could receive treatment only in a hospital can now remain at home and receive the same quality of treatment. A rapidly growing industry of high-tech home care is breaking down the walls between the acute care unit and the bedroom. From IV infusions of antibiotics and parenteral nutrition to the use of ventilators, hemodialysis machines, and assistive robots, the level of high-tech home treatments continues to grow.

Automated patient records (APR) have come online in home care and reduce the number of errors caused by miscommunication with physicians and other team members. They also reduce the amount of paperwork nurses need to do. In addition, use of cloud storage services lets nurses and other health-care providers upload files to a secure server where they can be accessed through the Internet from any device with an Internet connection. Cloud services are frequently used in health care because they can be very secure and offer easy access for team members.[19]

Although it might seem logical that hospitals would resist a trend that reduces the number of patients, the opposite is true. Current funding restrictions for patients who return to the hospital too quickly with the same condition, or who have acquired a hospital-source infection, make earlier patient discharge very attractive. More continuity of care is guaranteed when patients are observed in the home. Research shows that home care reduces emergency department visits and unnecessary readmissions to the hospital. Overall, patients report an increased level of satisfaction with the care provided and the improvement of their conditions.

A Need for Skilled Care

Not just anybody can be covered to receive home health care. When a patient is referred for home health care by a physician or nurse practitioner, the provider must demonstrate that the patient requires skilled needs that can be provided only by a professional nurse or other professional, depending on the patient's diagnosis. These skilled needs fall into three categories:

- *Management of care:* For example, injections, IV lines, wound care, diabetes or its complications, urinary catheters, rehabilitation, respiratory therapies
- *Patient evaluation:* For example, unstable conditions, pain, response to medications, neurological functioning, environment
- *Patient education:* For example, medications, glucose monitoring, disease management, prevention measures, activities of daily living[20]

A Rewarding Practice

Not all nurses are attracted to home health care as a career path. Individuals who thrive on the fast pace and perpetual motion of acute care or intensive care units would find the laid-back pace of home health care boring. In addition, the mountain of paperwork that accompanies home health-care patients might deter even the most dedicated supernurse. However, many nurses find it a rewarding area of practice. The one-to-one interaction with patients and their families permits a level of care only dreamed of in the acute care setting. The ability to observe a patient over an extended period and to watch their condition improving makes all the effort seem worthwhile.

However, the nurse who provides care in the home setting must develop a number of important skill sets. Probably most important of all is ethical practice. In the home-care setting, the nurse practices with virtually no supervision. It is up to professionals to maintain their competency and provide a high level of skills. Ethical practice is at the heart of establishing trust with the patient and their family.

Flexibility is another quality that home health-care nursing requires. Things do not always go as planned. Even though appointments are scheduled well ahead of time, patients often have last-minute condition changes or conflicts that require a reschedule. Even during the visit, the nurse may find that the patient is not physically or mentally able to do the required skills or learning. Nurses are visitors in the patient's home, and the patient sets the pace for the care that is provided. It is sometimes difficult for nurses to let go of the control they had over patients in the acute care setting, but it is one of the keys to success.[20]

Nurses must also increase their **cultural competence**. Each home has its own unique cultural context. To become culturally competent, nurses must develop a high level of cultural sensitivity by respecting all cultures equally and not attempting to impose values from the nurse's culture. Using a cultural assessment such as is found in Chapter 21 can be a great help in providing culturally sensitive care. By learning about a patient's beliefs, value systems, attitudes, and customs, the nurse can enrich their own life.

Often, home health-care nurses find that the home is not a very peaceful environment but is filled with tension and conflict. The ability to apply the principles of **conflict management** (see Chapter 12) is a skill that home health-care nurses must master early in their careers. Illness is an automatic stressor, and the families of ill patients often do not know how to deal with the increased levels of stress. Family members may have widely different views of care, and patients themselves may have a variant understanding of what they can and cannot do. It is not unusual for a nurse to hear from family members, "Tell Mama she's too sick to fix supper anymore!"

The most important skill in conflict management is active listening. It is essential for the nurse to listen to patients' fears, concerns, and anger about their condition and their families' reactions and actions. The nurse must also be on the lookout for signs of elder abuse and neglect. It is not uncommon for family caregivers, either intentionally or unintentionally, to harm the patient through threats, withholding care and medications, or negative communication.

The future of home health care is full of opportunity. As the population ages, home health care will allow individuals to stay at home while receiving the same treatments and technology as they would receive in the acute care setting. Health-care reform has placed a brighter spotlight on the areas of quality and cost. Home health care allows for increased continuity of care and enhanced quality of care, while significantly reducing its cost.

School-Based Services

Nurses provide a variety of services within local school systems. These services include screenings, health promotion and illness prevention programs, and treatment of minor health problems. Emphasis is placed on physical, social, and psychological well-being. Concerns relating to self-esteem, stress, drug abuse, and adolescent pregnancy are frequently addressed by the school nurse. In addition, children and adolescents with long-term health problems often attend school, and it is not uncommon for the nurse to be consulted about such issues as seizure management, colostomy care, or gastric tube feedings.

Students who have health concerns are frequently referred to providers within the community, and an important role of the school nurse is that of community liaison. For this reason, the nurse must be knowledgeable about community resources and adept at getting patients into the system in a timely and efficient manner.

Community Health Centers

Community health centers are being more frequently used in many areas. Most centers use a team approach involving physicians, nurse practitioners, and community nurses working together to provide health services. Most centers have diagnostic and treatment facilities that provide medical, nursing, laboratory, and radiological services. Some centers may also provide outpatient minor surgical procedures that allow patients to remain at home while accessing health services as needed.

Health-Care Providers' Offices and General Clinics

The office continues to be the location where most North Americans access primary health care. The majority of health-care providers in North America continue to work either in their own offices or with other providers in a group practice. Services range from routine health screening to illness diagnosis and treatment and even some minor surgical procedures.

The responsibilities of nurses who work in offices or in general clinics include obtaining personal health information and histories of current illness and preparing the patient for examination. Nurses also assist with procedures and obtain specimens for laboratory analysis. Teaching patients basic health information

and home management of treatments and medications is also a responsibility of the clinic nurse.

Occupational Health Clinics

Maintaining the health of workers in their workplaces to increase productivity has long been recognized as an important role for nurses. In response to rising health insurance costs, today's employers are increasingly supportive of workplace health promotion, illness prevention, and safety programs. Many companies provide wellness programs and encourage or even require their employees to participate. These services range from providing exercise facilities and fitness programs to health screenings and referrals. Illness prevention focuses on topics such as smoking cessation, stress management, and nutrition. Although some companies may hire health educators to manage their clinics, community health nurses often provide these services.

In Canada, occupational health nurses are registered nurses (RNs) holding a minimum of a diploma or a bachelor of science degree in nursing. Many may also have an occupational health certification or a degree in occupational health and safety from a community college or university. Nurses who are certified in occupational health nursing must meet eligibility requirements, pass a written examination, and be recognized as having achieved a level of competency in occupational health. The certification is granted by the Canadian Nurses Association.

Hospitals

Hospitals, the traditional provider of health-care services, are still an essential part of the health-care system and still employ the majority of nurses (62 percent in 2022). Hospitals range in size from small, rural facilities with as few as 15 to 20 beds to large urban centers that may exceed a bed capacity of several thousand. However, with recent changes in health-care funding, rural hospitals are closing at an alarming rate.

Depending on the services they provide, hospitals have varying classifications. General hospitals offer a variety of services, such as medical, surgical, obstetric, pediatric, and psychiatric care. Other hospitals may offer specialized services, such as pediatric care. Hospitals can be further classified as acute care or chronic care, depending on the length of stay of the patient and the services available. Large hospitals may be designated as specific centers for treatment, such as a trauma or cardiac center, because they can offer specialized services.

Long-Term Care Facilities

The majority of senior citizens in North America continue to live in their own homes. However, a growing group of seniors have health needs that require long-term care or extended care services. Some individuals may require rehabilitation or intermediate care, whereas others require extended, long-term care. These services are provided for both elderly and younger patients who have similar needs, such as patients with spinal cord injuries.

When a person needs skilled nursing or any type of skilled therapists to treat, manage, observe, and evaluate their health care, a skilled nursing facility (SNF) is likely required. Examples of SNF care include tube feedings, intravenous injections, and physical or speech therapy. Patients usually do not stay in a SNF until they have completely recovered because Medicare covers daily required SNF care services on only a short-term basis (up to 100 days in a benefit period). Skilled nursing and therapy care is defined as care that is so intricate and complex that it can only be safely and successfully accomplished by, or under the supervision of, skilled nursing and therapy professionals. Skilled nursing and therapy professionals include registered nurses, licensed practical and vocational nurses, physical and occupational therapists, speech-language pathologists, and audiologists.

Care that can be given by nonprofessional nonlicensed staff is considered custodial care rather than skilled care. Custodial care is not covered by Medicare if it is the only kind of care a person requires. Custodial care is care that helps a person, elderly or not, with normal activities of daily living (ADLs) such as getting in and out of bed, preparing food and eating, bathing, dressing, and using the bathroom. It usually includes health-care measures that most people can handle by themselves, like using eye drops, giving self-insulin or other injections, oxygen, and changing a colostomy bag or inserting urinary catheters. Custodial care is often given in a nursing facility. These activities can also be carried out at home or in an extended care facility.[21]

The current trend in extended care facilities is to provide care in a homelike atmosphere and base programs on the needs and abilities of the patients, or residents, as they are commonly called, of the facility. Many of these residents require personal services such as bathing and assistance with activities of daily living. Because of the range of needs of patients, some facilities will admit patients with specific needs to specific areas of the facility where the appropriate services are provided. The same facility may have a place for custodial residents and another place for residents who require SNF care. Some residents may need to move back and forth between the two depending on their needs any given time.

In Canada, patients considered for admission to long-term care facilities must meet specific guidelines. Assessments of patient needs and the nursing services available must be completed before the patient is admitted to the facility. Frequently, there are waiting lists for admission to extended care facilities.

In the United States, almost all SNF long-term care facilities are **for-profit** institutions that rely heavily on the patient's **Medicaid** and **Medicare** reimbursements. When Medicare coverage is limited, the resident must use private insurance or personal resources to pay the difference in cost.[21]

Retirement and Assisted Living Centers

As the population continues to age, assisted living centers are increasing in popularity because they allow patients, or residents, to maintain the greatest amount of independence possible in a partially controlled and supervised living environment. These centers consist of separate apartments or condominiums for the residents and provide amenities such as meal preparation and laundry services.

Many centers work closely with home care and other social services to provide the resources required for residents to maintain a degree of independence. Case coordinators, often nurses, help residents navigate their way through the complex paperwork involved in obtaining required services. Some assisted living centers are attached to long-term care facilities. According to the level of care required, residents may be transferred to various facilities as their care needs change. The goal of the Gold Standards Framework program, started in the United Kingdom, is to ensure that quality of care persists up to the time of death.[22]

Issues Now

Nursing Home Fall Pays Big

An 82-year-old nursing home resident fell twice within a 6-week period. When she was admitted to the nursing home, the RN assessed that the resident had an unsteady gait from poor circulation and mild dementia and was at high risk for falls. The family also reported that she had fallen several times at home, and the falls were one of the primary reasons for her admission to the nursing home. The care plan recommended the use of seatbelt restraints and a seat alarm.

The first fall occurred in the dining room when the resident pushed her wheelchair away from the table and attempted to stand. The incident report noted that the wheelchair locks were not engaged. The second fall happened in the recreation room. The patient was left alone in her wheelchair and again the wheel locks were not engaged. She attempted to stand by herself and fell again. She did not receive serious injuries from either fall.

The patient's lawyer argued that the care plan was not followed and that the staff at the facility had neglected the protocols that called for locking wheelchair wheels when patients were left unattended. The case was settled out of court by the nursing home's insurance company. The patient and her family received $150,000 for the falls.

Source: Cebollero vs. Hebrew Home, *2009 WL 2989743 (Westchester County Court, New York, March 16, 2009).*

Rehabilitation Centers

In many acute care facilities, discharge planning and rehabilitative needs are planned at the time of admission. Rehabilitation centers or units are similar to some extended care facilities, where the patient goal is to restore health and function at an optimum level. Often, patients are admitted to rehabilitation units after recuperating from the acute stage of an injury or illness. The rehabilitation unit then provides services to complete the recovery and restore a high degree of independence. Although most post-COVID-19 syndrome (long COVID) patients manage rehabilitation at home, a small percentage require care in inpatient rehabilitation units. Their conditions can range from loss of mobility to respiratory distress to regaining mental functioning and acuity.[23]

Some common types of rehabilitation units include geriatric, chemical dependency, stroke, and spinal cord injury units. Nurses who work on these units have the responsibility of coordinating health-care services, providing skilled care when required, supervising less-qualified personnel, and ensuring patient compliance with treatment regimens.

Day-Care Centers

Day-care centers can be used by any age group. Traditionally, *day care* has referred to the care of children; however, during the past 12 years or so, adult day-care centers have become relatively common. Adult day-care centers provide services for elderly adults who cannot be left at home alone but do not require institutionalization.

Services provided by adult day-care centers include health maintenance classes, socialization and exercise programs, physical or occupational therapy, rehabilitative services, and organized recreational activities. Nurses who are employed in adult day-care centers may administer medications, give treatments, provide counseling and teaching, and coordinate services between day care and home care.

Rural Primary Care

Patients living in rural areas face some different health issues than people who live in large cities. Access to health care can be difficult for patients located in a remote area. They might not be able to get to a hospital quickly in the event of an accident or emergency and have to travel long distances for basic checkups and assessments. Rural areas often have fewer family practice physicians and often no specialists at all. Health problems in rural residents tend to be more serious because of delayed diagnoses. Chronic disease rates are notably higher in patients who live in the rural areas of the United States.

A Problem of Distance

Delivering health-care services to the rural areas of North America is a challenge because of the great distances between homes. In many rural towns, it is common to have small hospitals or other health-care facilities available to provide basic health-care services. Most of these facilities have basic laboratory and radiological services available.

In the far north of Canada, aboriginal communities have nursing stations or health centers in the community to provide basic health services. The centers are staffed by nurses. Visiting health-care providers come in occasionally to provide additional services. The nursing stations also provide emergency services to people who require stabilization before being transferred to a larger facility.

A Problem of Cost

In the United States, paying for health-care services in rural areas is a concern. Many of the residents in rural areas are farmers or employees of small businesses that do not offer health insurance. A type of group insurance called health insurance purchasing cooperatives (HIPCs) is now available to Americans who are self-employed or who do not have health insurance for other reasons.

> *In the far north of Canada, aboriginal communities have nursing stations or health centers in the community to provide basic health services. The centers are staffed by nurses.*

From the earliest beginning of public health care, cooperatives (COOPs) existed to provide low-cost insurance to farmers and others who live in rural areas. COOPs are owned by the people who use and belong to them. They serve only their owners, who determine all the elements that go into running a health insurance company, such as the cost of premiums, coverage, and governance. As not-for-profit organizations, their primary financial goal is to break even at the end of the year.

The ACA authorized and provided funds for the Centers for Medicare and Medicaid to develop a program for COOP organizations that would deliver high-quality services while reducing the cost to the people they served. However, those who resisted the ACA removed most of the money that was guaranteed for the start-up and running of the COOPs. Without these funds that were needed to support the rapid distribution of these rural health-care networks, they could no longer compete with the large insurance companies.

The service model that the COOPs focused on—low-cost premiums and low-cost out-of-pocket expenses—attracted many new members. However, the new members were sicker than the average population of their service areas, requiring the COOPs to absorb a larger-than-chance percentage of sick individuals. In order for insurance companies to balance their financial books, they need a cross section of members ranging from a fairly large group of the very healthy who need little care, a medium-sized middle group who require an average amount of care, and a smaller group who require more than average care. The larger-than-average share of sick members attracted by the low premiums strained the financial resources of the new COOPs. As a result of the decreased federal funding and overload of members who needed greater quantities of hospital time, many of the COOPs failed.[24]

Hospice Services

Hospice care originated in Great Britain and has changed the way end-of-life care is delivered. Disillusioned with health-care services that focused on technology and the preservation of life at all costs, the hospice movement gained momentum in the 1970s. Hospice care emphasizes physiological and psychological support for patients who have terminal diseases. Hospice care provides a variety of services in a caring and supportive environment to terminally ill patients, their families, and other support persons. The central concept of hospice care is not saving life but improving or maintaining the quality of life until death occurs. For example, the United Kingdom's Gold Standards Framework was developed to improve quality of life through communication, collaboration, support, and coordination of care.[22] Its principles have served as underpinnings for the National Consensus Project for Quality Palliative Care in the United States and the Framework for Palliative Care in Canada.

Telehealth and E-Health

Telehealth, or telemedicine, is the information technology (IT)–empowered delivery of health-care services without physical contact between health-care providers and patients.[25] Telehealth reduces costs by allowing a rapid and accurate answer to patients' questions and health-care needs by remote monitoring. It can act as preventative care, which allows the patient to avoid expensive emergency department and hospital admissions. Telehealth can be generally divided into three categories:

1. Telehealth visits to a provider (similar to an office visit), which use either audio-only or both audio and visual telecommunications together
2. Virtual check-ins, which are short telephone calls, video calls, secure text messages, e-mails, or communication via a patient portal
3. E-visits through an online patient portal at a health-care facility or provider office[26]

Telehealth allows health-care professionals to ask specific questions, gather essential information, triage a patient for additional health-care services, and give consultations all while the patient is at home. Telehealth visits have proven to be valuable for follow-up visits after patients have had an initial examination by a provider; for physical examination of easy-to-see areas, such as eyes or skin; for counseling and other mental health services; and for monitoring chronic conditions such as diabetes or congestive heart failure. However, telehealth visits do not work well for first visits because of the need for a complete physical examination; for clinical evaluations that require a hands-on approach, such as checking reflexes or range of motion; and of course for blood tests, x-rays, and other imaging tests.[25]

The COVID-19 pandemic imposed the need for social distancing, including in patient-to-provider interactions. Telehealth care quickly proved to be a method to improve access to care while minimizing the risk of direct transmission of the infectious agent from person to person. In answer to a unique and sudden need for virtual medical visits created by the COVID-19 pandemic, there was rapid expansion of telemedicine technologies by most health-care facilities.[25] One unanticipated outcome of this expansion of telehealth was the delivery of health-care services to populations that are traditionally underserved. Telehealth care eliminates barriers such as lack of transportation, long distances from providers, and having to take time off from work. During the COVID-19 pandemic, telehealth proved valuable for the screening of infected people based on signs and symptoms, managing the care of people who were infected but not sick enough to be hospitalized, and guaranteeing the continuity of follow-up care of patients with long COVID.[26]

At an uncertain and alarming time in history, both patients and families valued reducing the contact time with health-care providers. On the other hand, most providers exhibited positive attitudes toward the employment of telehealth visits along with an interest in continuing telehealth as a part of their practice in the future. Telehealth proved to be an effective modality during the pandemic, allowing the patient to connect in real time with health-care providers despite the need for social distancing. Because of the pandemic, health-care facilities became more flexible and accepted more technological innovation to deal with interruptions in the hospital services. Telehealth is a promising tool to help streamline traditional person-to-provider clinical practice and to inspire alternative ways of managing health care.[25] In the future, there may be total virtual hospitals built around telehealth systems and home health agencies united by telehealth-assisted visits. Telehealth is discussed in detail in Chapter 27.

E-health, or electronic health, advice takes the telephone into the computer age. The patient uses their smartphone, computer, or tablet to access any number of sites that provide health-care information. New devices that electronically record patient data, such as blood glucose levels, blood pressure, and even electrocardiograms, and then download it to a health-care provider, are becoming more widely available. Unfortunately, some of the information that patients look up online may not be completely accurate. Persons who use these resources need to evaluate the quality and accuracy of the information they find.

Parish Nurses

A parish nurse, also known as a *faith community nurse,* is a nurse who provides nursing care for members of a parish or faith community. These nurses integrate faith and nursing care in promoting health and wellness within their service community. Because of the community health component that is required for the role, the majority of parish nurses are RNs who have a bachelor's or master's degree in nursing.[27] Parish nurses must have at least 2 years of clinical work experience for certification, although it is not always required. However, certification does show that the nurse has a higher level of knowledge in faith-based nursing care and has been educated in meeting the physical, psychological, and spiritual needs of the community. The American Nurses Credentialing Center (ANCC) no longer offers faith community nursing certification; however, a number of universities do offer parish nurse certification that is available online.[28] Even if a nurse is not certified, it is advantageous for nurses who are interested in employment as a parish nurse to take additional courses that focus on the mind and spirit.

It is estimated that approximately 15,000 parish nurses throughout the United States are attempting to meet the needs of individuals who are without adequate primary care or who are experiencing escalating health-care costs.[27] Many of these nurses work part time or are volunteers, and some work in conjunction with community-based programs. Churches engage parish nurses to

• Serve as health educators and counselors.
• Do health assessments and referrals.
• Organize support groups.
• Visit parishioners who are sick or elderly.
• Serve as patient advocates or case managers.
• Organize and manage parish health clinics.

Parish nurses are in a unique position to exercise their skills as case managers. As nurses, they possess clinical knowledge and skills, understand the health-care delivery system in their communities, and know many of the key health-care providers. As members of their parish, they are intimately familiar with their communities, understand the cultural climate of their clientele, and are familiar with the services that are available. Moreover, as members of the church community they serve, they are likely to be familiar with the spiritual, psychosocial, and financial needs of their patients.[27] However, direct reimbursement is not yet available for most parish nurse services.

Voluntary Health Agencies

Since their inception in 1892, voluntary health agencies have experienced steady growth and now number

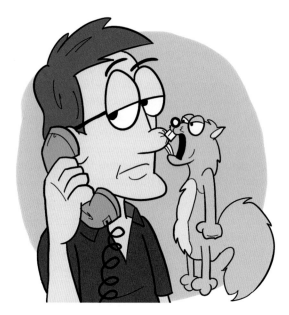

"For animal bites, please press 3."

more than 100,000. The first voluntary health agency was the Anti-Tuberculosis Society of Philadelphia. Some of the more well-known agencies that exist today include the American Cancer Society, American Heart Association, National Foundation for the March of Dimes, Easter Seals, and National Alliance on Mental Illness.

These agencies provide many valuable services, including fund-raising in support of cutting-edge research and public education. Some, such as the American Cancer Society, which has a strong emphasis on education and research, also help individuals secure special equipment, such as hospital beds for the home and wigs for chemotherapy patients. The National Alliance on Mental Illness is politically active and organizes support groups for the mentally ill and their families. These groups are **not-for-profit organizations**; all revenue in excess of cost goes toward improving services.

Independent Nurse-Run Health Centers

Similar to community health centers, nurse-run health centers tend to focus on health promotion and disease prevention. Historically, they have been service oriented rather than profit oriented and remain so today. Nurses who are interested in autonomous practice often work in these settings.

Several types of nurse-run health centers have been identified. Among these are community health and institutional outreach centers. These facilities may be freestanding or sponsored by a larger institution, such as a university or public health agency. Primary care services are generally offered to the medically underserved, and these centers are typically funded by public and private sources.[29]

Wellness and health promotion clinics are another type of nurse-run clinic and offer services at worksites, schools, churches, and homeless shelters. Many of these centers are affiliated with schools of nursing, providing health-care services while offering educational experiences for nursing students.

A final type of nursing center includes faculty practice, independent practice, and nurse entrepreneurship models. These facilities are owned and operated by nurses and may be solo or multidisciplinary practices. Services are typically reimbursed through **fee-for-service** plans, grants, and insurance. The ability of nurses in these centers to secure payments through the newly emergent and complex health-care reimbursement network will largely determine the future financial viability of these types of clinics.[29]

HEALTH-CARE COSTS AND THE NURSING SHORTAGE

Although many proposals have been put forth to solve the nursing shortage over the years, it still remains a major concern for the health-care system. The median age of nurses is 52, and over 50 percent of the nursing workforce is at or over retirement age. Nurses who are 65 years of age or older made up 19 percent (about 570,000) of working RNs in 2020, which comprised the single largest age category of nurses.[30] The Bureau of Labor Statistics projects that there will be about 194,500 openings for RNs every year between 2022 and 2030 as nurses retire and patient demand increases. That represents a 9 percent growth rate in registered nursing jobs by 2030, or approximately 276,800 new nursing jobs in the coming years.[30]

The number of people in the over-65 demographic is rapidly increasing, and many have medical and health needs that will increase the need for qualified RNs. Traditionally, as the economy grows stronger, fewer students pursue nursing as a career, further increasing the nursing shortage. However, this trend is not as pronounced currently as it was in the past.

A Cost-Cutting Measure

The managed-care model sought to lower and control the cost of health-care and health insurance by rewarding health-care companies for keeping costs down by increasing their profits. Although managed care attempted to keep costs down by cutting staff and services, in reality, the cost of health care and health insurance remained uncontrolled and unaffordable for many patients. In many areas across the country, managed care has been dropped as an effective model for delivering care, especially after the introduction of the ACA.[31] However, the implementation of managed care in the 1990s was the beginning of the RN shortage as it is known today. Not only did managed-care companies cut the number of RNs on staff in hospitals, but they also required many procedures to be performed outside the hospital, leading to patients being sicker when they did enter the hospitals.

As far back as 2002, the nursing shortage was recognized as not only a national crisis but also a global one. The pandemic with its innumerable effects on the nursing profession only worsened nursing attrition and the preexisting nursing shortage. After several years of providing care for acutely ill COVID-19 patients and watching many of them die from the virus, many nurses were suffering from anxiety, high levels of stress, differing degrees of depression, and moral distress.[31] Given this rather bleak setting, many are wondering if the profession will be able to attract enough new nurses to care for the patients of the future.

An Expensive Mistake

Health-care facilities that were attempting to cut costs hired fewer relatively expensive RNs in favor of less-expensive personnel. Nursing service at most facilities is the largest single budget item, averaging between 50 and 60 percent of the overall operating budget. At first glance, reducing the number of RNs on staff seemed like a promising way to control health-care costs, but in the long run, it turned out to be a very costly mistake. RNs who were employed in acute care settings moved in droves to the home health-care and primary care settings. At the same time, the population was aging, resulting in a need for more nurses who could deliver high-quality specialized care in the acute care facilities.

Stress on the Nurse

Even before the COVID-19 pandemic, nurses who were working in hospitals were finding working conditions to be less than ideal. Mandatory overtime, short staffing, and increased acuity of patient conditions all added to the stress these nurses experienced. As a result, they called in sick at a high rate, often for "mental health" days, or left for other facilities that had fewer demands.

As the pandemic wanes, it remains problematic to estimate the real and lasting effects on nurses because of the nursing shortages. They have experienced physical and mental exhaustion from working long shifts, lack of quality personal protective gear, practicing in poor working environments, and not being able to give the type of care that they were educated to provide. Before the pandemic, nurses already worked disruptive shift hours that had a real impact on their lives. Unknown is the number of nurses who were infected with the virus during the pandemic, but at least 2,200 have died from the disease at the time of publication.[31] Sick time, recruitment, and orientation costs for many facilities have skyrocketed as a result.

Stress on the Facility

The other area in which health-care institutions feel the cost of the RN shortage is in lawsuits and rising insurance costs. During periods when there is a shortage of RNs, the quality of health care decreases, patients become dissatisfied with the care they are receiving, and serious mistakes are made in care, resulting in injury or death of patients. It takes only a few of these cases with awards in the tens of millions of dollars to reemphasize the correlation between RN care and high-quality care.

Staffing Ratio Laws

One proposed solution to the nursing shortage problem is the passage of mandatory staffing ratio laws. Of course, hospital associations see these as increasing operating costs. However, the presumption is that more RNs will correlate to higher quality of care and ultimately reduced long-range health-care costs.[32]

Only 14 states have some type of law or regulation on nurse-to-patient ratios: California, Connecticut, Illinois, Massachusetts, Minnesota, Nevada, New Jersey, New York, Ohio, Oregon, Rhode Island, Texas, Vermont, and Washington. Seven of these states require hospitals to have staff committees that oversee nursing ratios and implement staffing policies: Connecticut, Illinois, Nevada, Ohio, Oregon, Texas, and

Washington. California is the only state that has a law requiring a specific number of nurses to patients in every unit of a hospital. For example, the California law requires hospitals to have one nurse for every two patients in intensive care and one nurse for every five patients on the medical-surgical units.[33]

Hospital association groups in several states have challenged nurse-ratio laws and effectively blocked their implementation. However, nursing groups generally support these laws and see them as a short-term solution to immediate staffing shortages. Nursing groups and other health-care entities are working on long-term, permanent solutions to the nursing shortage.

Improving Outcomes

Not everyone is convinced that fixed staff-to-patient ratios will cure an ailing health-care system, and some in the nursing profession agree. Although an ever-growing body of evidence shows improved RN-to-patient ratios also improve outcomes, still more research is required.[32] The increasing amount of research is a direct result of the Institute of Medicine's identification of a dearth of information about the quality of care being delivered in the nation's acute care facilities.

RN staffing has a direct correlation to patient outcomes and quality of care. Recent research has shown that RN staffing is essential in promoting the safety and recovery of patients. Inadequate levels of nurse staffing are related to medication errors and accidents such as falls, higher nurse stress leading to a risk for burnout, patients giving poor evaluations because they felt disregarded and ignored, poor communication and misinformation, and higher nurse turnover.[33] It has been shown that the performance of the health facility as a whole is improved and patient's outcomes are better when satisfactory nurse staffing ratios are maintained.

Similarly, better nurse staffing improves nurse-to-nurse and nurse-to-patient communication. When a unit is understaffed, nurses believe that they do not have enough time to give patients the emotional support needed during recovery or to really listen to their patient's needs.[34]

Initially, nursing leaders hoped the new staffing ratio laws would help demonstrate the important and critical part nurses play in providing high-quality care.

The American Nurses Association recognized as early as the 1990s that there is a direct correlation between the care provided by RNs and positive patient outcomes. The American Hospital Association (AHA) has formally acknowledged that RNs are critical to ensuring optimal patient care. Yet the AHA still resists the move toward mandatory staffing ratios, characterizing them as an "oversimplistic" solution to a complex problem. However, recent research has demonstrated that in hospitals with low numbers of RNs, patients are more likely to stay longer, suffer more complications, and die from complications that would be survivable if they were identified and treated sooner.[32]

Staffing ratio laws were an attempt to quickly fix a long-standing and critical problem; however, staffing ratios do not address a much wider range of problems hospitalized patients face every day. What is needed to ultimately cure the industry is a long-range plan for systemic reform on the basis of patient needs, not the needs of a profit-motivated insurance industry.[34]

Patients educated to understand what high-quality care is, and how it can best be achieved, will ultimately be the most powerful force for attaining the care they require. When all health-care facilities begin to really listen to the patients they are supposed to be serving, nurse staffing ratio laws will no longer be necessary. The facilities will meet the quality expectations by making sure that the needed number of nurses is there to provide the care the patient expects.

Although laws may not be the ultimate solution to a much deeper problem, patients in states with staffing ratio laws will be reassured to know they have a well-educated, skilled professional nurse nearby who can act as an **advocate** for their needs and monitor the care they are receiving when they are most vulnerable.

Beyond the Numbers

Some in nursing are concerned that health-care facilities will use the mandated staffing ratio as a ceiling number rather than the minimum number of nurses required to provide safe care. There is also a fear that the facilities will look only at the numbers and not at the educational, skill, and experience levels of the nurses they use to meet their quotas. Without consideration of the acuity of patient conditions on a unit and the care needs related to their illnesses, staffing ratios may actually lower the quality of care and threaten the safety of the patients. In addition, some fear that facilities in which the staffing ratio laws are unworkable will close only units where sicker patients are being treated, thus reducing access to care.[32]

A More Acute Problem

Some farseeing nursing leaders see the passage of staffing ratio laws as an important but short-term solution to a much broader problem. Unsafe nurse-to-patient ratios are just a symptom of a much more acute systemic problem in the health-care industry. The underlying problem revolves around an overly aggressive policy of cost cutting by managed care, often at the expense of the very patients who support the system with their insurance premiums.

Conclusion

Health-care delivery systems are complex and multifaceted. Nurses continue to provide the majority of health-care services to North Americans and need to understand the important role they play in the system. Changes in the health-care system are never ending. By understanding the various health-care systems and how they are related to each other, nurses put themselves at the forefront of change and can advocate for changes that benefit the health of all people.

Nursing is as complex as the health-care system itself. It occurs in a wide variety of locations, and the role of the nurse varies just as much as the health-care systems do. How a nurse functions in a hospital is different from how a nurse functions in parish nursing, but the caring and compassion that nurses bring to their roles does not vary. Nurses need to understand and develop their roles, and they will undoubtedly continue to have a significant impact on the further development of the health-care system.

CRITICAL-THINKING EXERCISES

- Select three patients you are familiar with who have different health-care needs. Describe these patients' medical histories, current problems, and future health-care needs; then determine which health-care setting and which health-care practitioners would be most appropriate for them. Identify any difficulties that might be encountered during their entry into the health-care system. How can the nurse facilitate the process?
- Skilled nursing facilities, subacute care facilities, and assisted living facilities all are forms of long-term, or extended, health care. Identify five specific problems that nurses working in such facilities encounter. What is the best way to resolve these problems?
- Identify cost-cutting measures used at a health-care facility with which you are familiar. Have these measures affected the quality of patient care? What other measures to cut costs can be implemented? How have changes within the health-care delivery system altered nursing practice?
- Identify four health-care priorities that may be initiated by the year 2030. How are these likely to affect the profession of nursing?
- Describe the advantages and disadvantages of various health-care reimbursement plans. Which ones will produce the highest-quality care? Which ones are best for the profession of nursing? Are there any payment plans that do both?
- Identify the most important elements in health-care reform. Should nurses support these changes? Why?

NCLEX-STYLE QUESTIONS

1. How has the profession of nursing in the United States affected and been affected by health-care reform? **Select all that apply.**
   1. Nurses participated in the planning of the Affordable Care Act (ACA).
   2. Nurses were vital to the initial implementation of the ACA.
   3. Thousands of new nurses have been recruited to ease the nursing shortage.
   4. Nursing's historic commitment to health maintenance and disease prevention are reflected in the preventive-care provisions of the ACA.
   5. Because of the ACA, nurse practitioners play an increasingly important role as primary care providers.
2. Of the four types of health-care systems, which is the oldest?
   1. Type 1
   2. Type 2
   3. Type 3
   4. Type 4

3. In what way do the Canadian and U.S. health-care systems differ?
   1. In the United States, health insurance must be operated on a nonprofit basis.
   2. The United States requires health-insurance coverage of all citizens; Canada does not.
   3. Canadian health care is funded by federal tax dollars and administered by the provinces.
   4. Canada is a type 4 system; the United States is a modified type 1 system.
4. Which factors will affect the evolution of health-care delivery in the United States in the future? **Select all that apply.**
   1. The elimination of contagious illnesses
   2. An aging population
   3. An increase in public wellness due to preventive care
   4. An increase in morbidity due to shorter hospital stays
   5. The increase in the number of people with chronic illnesses

5. Why is it important to reduce the number of uninsured people in the United States? **Select all that apply.**
   1. To make health care more affordable for all citizens
   2. To reduce costs passed on to hospitals and taxpayers when uninsured people receive care in the emergency department
   3. To encourage those currently uninsured to take more accountability for their health
   4. To improve public health by ensuring access to preventive care
   5. To reverse the trend of rising costs for inpatient care and pharmaceuticals

6. The insurance industry has tried to manage health-care costs in a variety of ways. What do these plans have in common?
   1. They require facilities providing services to Medicare patients to be reimbursed using a fixed-rate system and include monetary incentives to reduce the length of hospital stays.
   2. They require participants to pay a flat rate, usually through their employer, to belong to a managed care organization for a specified period of time.
   3. They seek to provide services to the maximum number of people at the lowest possible cost.
   4. They set lifetime spending caps on individuals.

7. How does Medicare encourage facilities to provide high-quality, cost-effective health care?
   1. It pays more if a patient is discharged sooner than expected.
   2. It limits the number of diagnostic tests and procedures a facility can provide.
   3. It offers facilities incentives for shorter-than-expected hospital stays and penalizes them for longer-than-expected stays.
   4. It requires patients to use physicians whose charges are below the national average.

8. What makes modern home health care a viable option for many patients with serious health concerns and medical needs?
   1. The improved training of home-health aides and other providers of life assistance services
   2. The availability for home use of technology that was once limited to hospitals
   3. The closing of small rural hospitals that would have cared for these patients in the past
   4. The greater availability of family members nowadays to care for patients at home

9. Mrs. Vazquez had hip-replacement surgery yesterday at a large hospital. Today, her case manager stops by to discuss her planned transfer to another facility for rehabilitation and physical therapy. What level of health-care delivery will the new facility provide?
   1. Primary care
   2. Secondary care
   3. Tertiary care
   4. Outpatient care

10. Mr. Nguyen takes his toddler to a facility that provides _____ care services to receive her scheduled immunizations.

References

1. Number of Affordable Care Act-related (ACA) enrollments in the Marketplace, Medicaid, and the Basic Health Program (BHP) in the U.S. from 2014 to 2021. Statista, 2022. https://www.statista.com/statistics/1280656/number-of-us-aca-related-enrollments
2. Nawaz A, Hastings D. Biden proposes expansion of the Affordable Care Act with changes to "family glitch." PBS News, April 5, 2022. https://www.pbs.org/newshour/show/bidens-proposes-expansion-of-affordable-care-act-with-changes-to-family-glitch
3. Davalon. Affordable Care Act time line. eHealth, October 13, 2022. https://www.ehealthinsurance.com/resources/affordable-care-act/history-timeline-affordable-care-act-aca#
4. Norris L. What happens if I don't buy ACA-compliant health insurance? Health Insurance.org, March 29, 2022. https://www.healthinsurance.org/faqs/what-happens-if-i-dont-buy-aca-compliant-health-insurance/
5. Health care coverage for American Indians and Alaska Natives. Healthcare.gov, 2022. https://www.healthcare.gov/american-indians-alaska-natives/coverage/
6. Greenberg J, Sherman A. How Donald Trump responded to the coronavirus pandemic. Politifact, March 20, 2020. https://www.politifact.com/article/2020/mar/20/how-donald-trump-responded-coronavirus-pandemic/
7. Fact sheet: Biden Administration announces operational plan for COVID-19 vaccinations for children under 5. The White House, June 9, 2022. https://www.whitehouse.gov/briefing-room/statements-releases/2022/06/09/fact-sheetbiden-administration-announces-operational-plan-for-covid-19-vaccinations-for-children-under-5/

8. Anders R, Engaging nurses in health policy in the era of COVID-19. *Nurse Forum,* 56(1):89–94, 2020. https//:doi.org/10.1111/nuf.12514

9. Pearce K. COVID-19 ushers I decades of change for nursing profession; HUB, October 19, 2020. https://hub.jhu.edu/2020/10/19/nursing-changes-covid-19/

10. How Many Americans Don't Have Health Insurance? Plus Over 11 Health Insurance Statistics For Apr 2023! Simply Insurance, 2023. https://www.simplyinsurance.com/how-many-americans-dont-have-health-insurance/

11. Quick Facts. U.S. Census Bureau, 2021. https://www.census.gov/quickfacts/fact/table/US/POP010220

12. Sreeniva S. What Is Long COVID? WebMD, 2022. https://www.webmd.com/lung/what-is-long-covid-pasc#1-3

13. Tina. Statistics on health care costs by country. Balancing Everything, August 11, 2022. https://balancingeverything.com/healthcare-costs-by-country/

14. Aratani L. US ranks last in healthcare among 11 wealthiest countries despite spending most. *The Guardian,* August 5, 2021. https://www.theguardian.com/us-news/2021/aug/05/us-healthcare-system-ranks-last-11-wealthiest-countries

15. Van Cauwenberghe C. Healthcare in Canada: Milestones and opportunities. Open Access Government, June 15, 2022. https://www.openaccessgovernment.org/healthcare-in-canada-system-milestones-opportunities-pandemic-covid-19/137631/

16. Health care funding in Canada. Government of Canada, 2022. https://www.canada.ca/en/health-canada/corporate/about-health-canada/funding.html

17. Canadian Health Act, RSC 1985 c C-6, December 12, 2017. https://www.canlii.org/en/ca/laws/stat/rsc-1985-c-c-6/latest/rsc-1985-c-c-6.html

18. Home health care services and statistics. AnythingResearch, 2022. https://www.anythingresearch.com/industry/Home-Health-Care-Services.htm

19. Top 3 current technological trends in home health care. Health Care Guys, June 28, 2022. https://www.healthcareguys.com/2022/06/28/top-3-current-technological-trends-in-healthcare/

20. Haupt A. How does home health care work? *Forbes,* June 11, 2022. https://www.forbes.com/health/healthy-aging/what-is-home-health-care/

21. Centers for Medicare and Medicaid Services. *Medicare Coverage of Skilled Nursing Facility Care.* U.S. Department of Health and Human Services, 2022. https://www.medicare.gov/Pubs/pdf/10153-Medicare-Skilled-Nursing-Facility-Care.pdf

22. The Gold Standard Framework network. Gold Standards Framework, 2022. https://www.goldstandardsframework.org.uk/

23. Recovery & rehabilitation after COVID-19. Alberta Health Services, December 21, 2022. https://www.albertahealthservices.ca/topics/Page17540.aspx

24. What is cooperative health insurance. Health Insurance Providers, 2022. https://www.healthinsuranceproviders.com/what-is-cooperative-health-insurance/

25. Gentry MT, Puspitasari AJ, McKean AJ, Williams MD, Breitinger S, Geske JR, Clark MM, Moore KM, Frye MA, Hilty DM. Clinician satisfaction with rapid adoption and implementation of telehealth services during the COVID-19 pandemic. *Telemedicine & E-Health,* 27(12), 2021. https://doi.org/10.1089/tmj.2020.0575

26. Cerqueira-Silva T, Carreiro R, Nunes V, Passos L, Canedo BF, Andrade S, Ramos PIP, Khouri R, Santos CBS, Nascimento JDS, . . . Boaventura A. Bridging learning in medicine and citizenship during the COVID-19 pandemic: A telehealth-based case study. *JMIR Public Health Surveillance* 7(3), 2021. https://doi.org/10.2196/24795

27. Parish nurse job description. RegisteredNurseRN.com, n.d. https://www.registerednursern.com/parish-nursing-parish-nurse-job-description/

28. What is a parish nurse? RegisteredNursing.org, November 7, 2022. https://www.registerednursing.org/specialty/parish-nurse/

29. Wilcox L. 3 benefits of nurse led clinics. *CompHealth.com,* April 11, 2014. https://comphealth.com/resources/3-benefits-of-nurse-led-clinics/#:

30. Nursing by the numbers. Carson-Newman University Online, March 30, 2022, https://onlinenursing.cn.edu/news/nursing-by-the-numbers

31. Turale S, Nantsupawat A. Clinician mental health, nursing shortages and the COVID-19 pandemic: Crises within crises. *International Nursing Review,* 68(1):12–14, 2021. https://doi.org/10.1111/inr.12674

32. Boyce H. Reducing patient to nurse ratio can save thousands of lives. *Atlantic Journal Constitution,* June 30, 2022. https://www.ajc.com/pulse/study-reducing-patient-to-nurse-ratio-can-save-thousands-of-lives/SUOJVVRCXFA5ZKHYDFTCJY4T5Q/

33. California staffing ratio law. OLR research report, 2023. https://www.cga.ct.gov/2004/rpt/2004-r-0212.htm

34. Young S. Debate over nurse-patient ratios heats up. Healthcare-brew. https://www.healthcare-brew.com/stories/2023/01/29/safe-staffing

Ensuring Quality Care

14

Viki Saidleman | Joseph T. Catalano

WHAT IS QUALITY CARE?

Like most complex concepts, *quality care* has several different definitions. The National Academies of Sciences' Health and Medicine Division (formerly the Institute of Medicine [IOM]) defines quality as "the degree to which health services for individuals and populations increase the likelihood of desired health outcomes and are consistent with current professional knowledge."[1] The three accepted elements of quality are structure, process, and outcome, and care should be safe, effective, client centered, timely, efficient, and equitable.[2]

250,000 Deaths Per Year

When the IOM published *To Err Is Human: Building a Safer Health System* in 2000, it estimated that 98,000 people die per year due to adverse events and medical errors in hospitals. Despite efforts to increase the quality of care, the number had risen to 250,000 by 2021 (the last year for which data were available), making it the third leading cause of death after cancer and heart disease.[3] COVID-19 temporarily became the third leading cause of death in 2020, but as larger numbers of persons were vaccinated, that number dropped.[4]

A medical error is a preventable adverse effect of medical care, whether or not it is evident or harmful to the client. An adverse medical incident is similar to a medical error but is defined in more detail. Generally, an adverse medical incident includes any type of medical negligence, intentional misconduct, and any other act, failure to act (negligence), or error of a health-care facility or health-care provider that caused or could have caused injury to or death of a client. The event may be caused by the unsafe use of medical devices, defects in design or manufacture of a medical device, inadequate maintenance or inapt modifications of the device by the facility, poor user instructions, lack of adequate training in use of the device, and unsuitable

- List and discuss the four concepts that underlie the Leapfrog mission
- Define and identify "quality indicators" and assess how they are used in determining quality health care
- Discuss why continuous quality improvement (CQI) is a proactive approach to quality health care
- Justify using root-cause analysis in improving the quality of health care
- Contrast and compare the Scrum framework to the nursing process
- Explain how risk reduction relates to quality
- Discuss three factors critical to quality endeavors
- Relate two educational initiatives that promote quality of care and safety

storage.[3] The three most common errors or incidents are medication errors, misidentifying clients, and surgical errors.[5] Clients often do not even know that a medical error has taken place. Not all medical errors negatively affect clients; however, a large number of medical errors are serious, causing physical and mental harm and even death. According to data from the U.S. Department of Health and Human Services, one in seven clients on Medicare in a hospital setting is the victim of a medical error.[3]

The IOM report focused on faulty systems, processes, and conditions that led to mistakes. It recommended system changes to reduce the number of errors and improve the **quality** of health care. The report recommended a four-tiered approach:

1. Establish leadership, research, tools, and protocols to enhance the safety knowledge base.
2. Develop a public mandatory national reporting system and encourage participation in voluntary reporting systems.
3. Use oversight organizations, health-care purchasers, and professional organizations to increase performance standards and expectations for safety improvements.
4. Implement safety systems at the point of care delivery in health-care organizations.

Based on the information from this report, the public became more aware of how frequently medical errors occur. Consumer demand for higher-quality care has increased dramatically. Nurses are in a pivotal position to positively influence quality and safety at local, state, and national levels.[1] Nurses can indeed make a difference in ensuring quality of health care.

The IOM's 2001 report *Crossing the Quality Chasm: A New Health System for the 21st Century* focused on developing a new health-care system that improved quality of care. It identified six aims for improvement, concluding that care should be

1. *Safe:* Avoiding injuries to clients from the care that is intended to help them
2. *Effective:* Providing services based on scientific knowledge to all who could benefit and refraining from providing services to those not likely to benefit
3. *Client-centered:* Providing care that is respectful of and responsive to individual client preferences, needs, and values, and ensuring that client values guide all clinical decisions
4. *Timely:* Reducing waits and sometimes harmful delays for both those who receive and those who give care

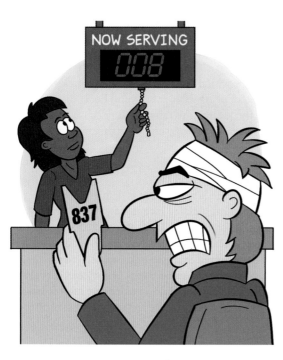

"I've already been waiting here 3 ½ hours!"

5. *Efficient:* Avoiding waste, including waste of equipment, supplies, ideas, and energy

6. *Equitable:* Providing care that does not vary in quality because of personal characteristics such as gender, ethnicity, geographic location, and socioeconomic status

Redesign priorities for health care included evidence-based decision making; safety; client as source of control; individualized client-centered care; transparency; anticipating needs; decreasing waste; and improving interdisciplinary cooperation, collaboration, and communication. Nurses are again positioned to play instrumental roles in enacting the changes necessary to overhaul the health-care system.[1]

What Do You Think?

How can nurses demonstrate their commitment to enact the required changes? Why would nurses value quality in health care? What skills should nurses have in order to provide safe and high-quality care?

Methods to Measure and Improve Quality

Quality assurance (QA) in health care attempts to guarantee that when an action is performed by a health-care professional, it is performed correctly the first time and each time thereafter. QA is evidence based and is demonstrated by best practices in identifying, assessing, improving, and monitoring all the elements of client care. In addition to improving the quality of client care, QA can improve nursing systems and reduce the number of errors or adverse events.[6] QA requires that actions and activities are continuously measured and compared to a standard of care established by a professional organization and that monitoring be in place to provide continuous feedback to prevent errors. Quality control is focused on health-care outcomes.

Quality Assurance

QA initiatives are essential when efforts are being made to cut costs and, at the same time, maintain high standards of care. To ensure high-quality care,

> *In addition to improving the quality of client care, QA can improve nursing systems and reduce the number of errors or adverse events.*

the health-care industry borrowed the philosophy of **continuous quality improvement (CQI)** from the business world. According to the CQI philosophy, there are external customers and internal customers. External customers are clients and their families; internal customers are individuals working within the health-care setting. The Joint Commission (TJC) was so impressed with CQI's potential to improve health-care delivery that in 1994 it began requiring hospitals to implement CQI strategies. These strategies target select processes to evaluate and improve. TJC has been continuously updating quality standards since its beginning, and as recently as 2021, it set standards for the use of packaged supplies and devices in response to some actions taken by facilities to reuse personal protective equipment (PPE) when shortages occurred in the early stages of the pandemic.

Exceeding Expectations

CQI, also known as **total quality management (TQM)**, is based on the belief that any organization with higher-quality services will capture a greater share of the market than competitors with lower-quality services. This approach emphasizes customer satisfaction, promotes innovation, and requires employee involvement and commitment. The goal is not only to meet but to exceed the expectations of the client. This plan uses a multidisciplinary approach in a systematic manner to design, measure, assess, and improve the performance of an organization. Standards for **benchmarking** are used to classify acceptable levels of performance. These may be written for outcomes, processes, or structures. Outcome standards focus on results of care given; process standards relate to care delivery; and structure standards relate to the organization, management, or physical environment of the organization. Different tools or indicators are used to measure performance against the set standards. Actual performance is then compared to standards and across institutions. **Dashboards** are electronic tools that act as a scorecard. They can provide retrospective or real-time data to assess quality. These informatics technologies assist the process of quality improvement.

Delivering high-quality services is valued above all else, and the goal is that every constituent—internal and external—be completely satisfied with the services provided.

Hospital Consumer Assessment of Healthcare Providers and Systems

Client satisfaction is another way to measure quality of care. The Hospital Consumer Assessment of Healthcare Providers and Systems (HCAHPS; pronounced H-CAPS) initiative began in 2008. Many hospitals at the time were using their own internal quality surveys, which made it impossible to compare one facility's quality to another's. HCAHPS developed a standardized survey to measure clients' evaluation of the quality of care they received. The HCAHPS Survey, which is also known as the CAHPS® Hospital Survey or Hospital CAHPS, has a core group of questions that can be combined with additional questions that measure the specific needs of a facility.[7] Three goals directed the survey's development: (1) produce a method to provide comparison of client satisfaction data, (2) create hospital motivation to improve care quality, and (3) increase hospital transparency in terms of quality of care. This initiative is an example of benchmarking that compares data between similar organizations in an effort to identify areas for growth (improvement) and areas of strength.

The HCAHPS Survey is composed of 29 items: 19 items cover critical aspects of the hospital experience by clients (communication with nurses, communication with doctors, responsiveness of hospital staff, communication about medicines, discharge information, care transition, cleanliness of the hospital environment, quietness of the hospital environment, overall rating of hospital, and recommendation of hospital); three items to skip clients to appropriate questions; five items adjust for the mix of clients across hospitals; and two items support congressionally mandated reports.[7]

The HCAHPS Survey reveals a client's perception of the quality of care they received. After the survey data are gathered, they are submitted to the HCAHPS data warehouse where they are analyzed by a content management system, which then calculates hospitals' HCAHPS scores and publicly reports them on the Hospital Compare website for all to see. The survey results directly impact a health-care organization's reputation.

The government provides reimbursement based on HCAHPS results; therefore, a high score on the survey helps keep the hospital financially strong. Scores, after analysis and processing, can range from a high of 100 percent to a potential low of 0 percent. In addition, readmissions to the facility sooner than 30 days after discharge lower a facility's overall average based on a complicated formula.[7] A whole new industry has grown up around helping hospitals increase their HCAHPS scores; however, the basic skills taught in every nursing program, such as communicating clearly with clients, showing that you care, and keeping the noise on the unit at a low level, are still key to client satisfaction.

There are four approved modes of administration for the HCAHPS Survey: (1) mail only, (2) telephone only, (3) mixed (mail followed by telephone), and (4) interactive voice response (IVR). The survey can be sent to clients 48 hours to 6 weeks after discharge, based on a list of diagnoses, which determine eligibility to receive the survey.[7] Because the survey does not have questions that meet the needs of pediatric or psychiatric clients, these two groups do not receive surveys (see Box 14.1). However, the criteria are broad enough to include most other hospitalized clients.

The standardized survey instrument allows health-care organizations to monitor, compare, and improve their performance. It benefits consumers by enhancing the ability to select health-care services on the basis of the institution's known and shown performance in established key areas, and it helps hospitals by providing information that can help them improve the quality of care.

The Leapfrog Group

In November 2000, **The Leapfrog Group** was officially launched to improve the safety of health care and make it more affordable. By 2017, more than 2,600 of the largest facilities in the country were monitored by the Leapfrog Group.[8] By 2022, the number of hospitals completing the Leapfrog survey exceeded 3,000. Leapfrog now serves as the gold standard for comparison of hospital performance on national standards of safety, quality, and efficiency, thereby facilitating transparency and easy access to health-care information.[8]

Leapfrog focuses solely on hospital safety as its quality measure, and participating facilities are given

Box 14.1 **Criteria for Eligibility for HCAHPS Survey**

Clients Who Are Eligible to Participate in HCAHPS Survey

- 18 years or older at the time of admission
- At least one overnight stay in the hospital as an inpatient
- Non-psychiatric MS-DRG/principal diagnosis at discharge
- Alive at the time of discharge

Clients Who Are Ineligible to Participate in HCAPHS Survey

- Clients discharged to hospice care
- Clients discharged to nursing homes and skilled nursing facilities
- Clients under court of law enforcement control (i.e., prisoners)
- Clients with a foreign home address (excluding U.S. territories—Virgin Islands, Puerto Rico, and Northern Mariana Islands)
- Clients who request not to be surveyed
- Clients excluded by state or federal rules or regulations

Source: CAHPS Hospital survey. Centers for Medicare & Medicaid Services, 2022. https://www.hcahpsonline.org

a Leapfrog Hospital Safety Grade of A, B, C, D, or F based on how they perform on the Leapfrog survey. This survey has approximately 180 questions and is completed by the facility's safety officer. A question can be skipped if it does not apply to the facility. The survey asks questions such as what the bachelor of science in nursing (BSN) nurse-to-client ratio is, how available hand washing areas are and how often they are used, and a number of questions about safe medication administration. The results from the analysis of the data provide a rapid and easy method for clients to see which facility has the safest care.[9] The Safety Grade affords consumers with all the essential information they need on how likely they are to experience accidents, injuries, errors, or harm while in the hospital. Safety Grades are updated twice per year.[8] The survey scores repeatedly gain attention from consumer media and focus attention on the client safety records of local hospitals.

The consumers who make use of the Leapfrog Hospital Safety Grade like its ease of use and straightforward letter-grade rating system. These scores are also used by numerous national and regional health insurance plans. Leapfrog's website provides additional information such as tips for effectively communicating with a physician and videos on how to stay safe while in the hospital.[8]

Performance Categories. By working with national experts in quality assurance and using the latest peer-reviewed literature, peer comparisons, and existing national standards, the Leapfrog Group establishes national standards for the comparison of all participating hospitals and ambulatory surgery centers (ASCs). The Leapfrog Standards create goalposts for which institutions can strive.[10] Leapfrog includes measures of system processes, structures, and outcomes on its biannual surveys.

Performance on each measure on the Leapfrog Hospital Survey and the Leapfrog ASC Survey is placed into easy-to-read performance categories (see Fig. 14.1).

Rewarding Performance and Quality Care. Like many quality initiatives, Leapfrog grew out of the IOM's report concerning preventable medical errors. The business leaders who founded Leapfrog were shocked by the finding that up to 98,000 Americans die every year from preventable medical errors made in hospitals alone. In fact, in 2000, there were more deaths in hospitals from preventable medical mistakes than there were from motor vehicle accidents, breast cancer, and AIDS *combined*. The report indicated that there was a need for more quality and safety in the provision of health care. Leapfrog's founders realized that they could take "leaps" forward in ensuring quality health care for their employees, retirees, and families by rewarding hospitals that implement significant improvements in quality and safety.

Inspired by the Premier/CMS Hospital Quality Incentive Demonstration project and building on the measures in the Hospital Quality Alliance initiative, the Leapfrog Hospital Rewards program measures the quality of care and the efficiency with which hospitals use resources in five clinical areas that represent the majority of hospital admissions and expenditures. Hospitals are scored and rewarded separately for each of the five areas and can participate in any of

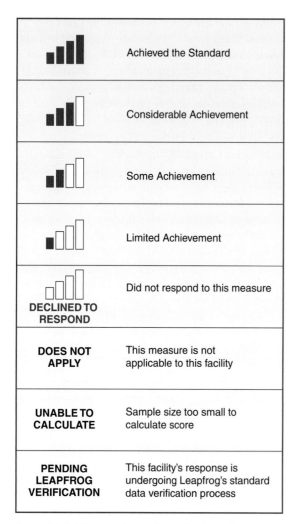

	Achieved the Standard
	Considerable Achievement
	Some Achievement
	Limited Achievement
DECLINED TO RESPOND	Did not respond to this measure
DOES NOT APPLY	This measure is not applicable to this facility
UNABLE TO CALCULATE	Sample size too small to calculate score
PENDING LEAPFROG VERIFICATION	This facility's response is undergoing Leapfrog's standard data verification process

Figure 14.1 Progress toward meeting Leapfrog standards. (*Source:* Scoring. The Leapfrog Group, 2022, https://ratings.leapfroggroup.org/scoring.)

the areas in which they provide care (see Box 14.2). If they demonstrate sustained excellence or improvement, hospitals are eligible for financial rewards and increased market share.[10]

Hospital scores can become the basis for financial incentives for consumers, such as waived copays or deductibles for choosing care at high-performing or improving hospitals. In addition, these scores can be incorporated into health plans' existing performance-based incentive and reward programs. The program is engineered by Leapfrog, with the input of a vast array of providers and health plans, but it is designed to be implemented by health plans and employers in specific markets.

A key principle of the Leapfrog program is that payers (clients) should have a say in what they are purchasing (health care). Leapfrog's pay-for-performance program for hospitals makes it easier for health-care purchasers to identify and reward those hospitals that are providing high-quality care for their employees and at the same time are helping to gain better value for health-care dollars. Facilities that meet these goals are recognized and rewarded. The Leapfrog Group is supported by the Robert Wood Johnson Foundation, Leapfrog members, and others.

Leapfrog's Mission and Goal. The Leapfrog Group's mission is to promote giant leaps forward in the safety, quality, and affordability of health care by

• Supporting informed health-care decisions by those who use and pay for health care.
• Promoting high-value health care through incentives and rewards.

Four concepts underlie the Leapfrog mission:

1. Health care in the United States is at unacceptably low levels of basic safety, quality, and overall customer value.
2. Major leaps forward in the quality of health care can be achieved if those who purchase health care recognize and reward superior safety and quality.
3. The purchasing power of America's largest employers can be used to encourage other purchasers to join and put additional pressure on health-care providers to improve quality.
4. Guided by specific innovations that present "great leaps" forward in the improvement of safety and quality of care, Leapfrog can increase media involvement and consumer support for the program.[9]

Leapfrog's goal is to promote high-quality health care through incentives and rewards. This is the first national private-sector program that responds to the urgent needs of care-service purchasers. It provides solutions for escalating health costs and substandard quality.

Box 14.2 How to Identify Quality Care and Providers

Quality Elements to Identify	YES	NO
Quality Health-Care Plan		
Is rated highly by members and on https://www.ncqa.org/report-cards/		
People who have the plan maintain their health and recover from illness		
Is accredited by a recognized organization		
The health-care providers and hospitals you use are included		
Has a list of benefits to choose from that your age and condition require		
Is affordable		
Quality Health-Care Provider(s)		
Has a certification that is appropriate to your medical requirements		
Is rated highly		
Is focused on prevention as well as treatment		
Holds admission privileges at the hospitals you use		
Is covered by your health plan		
Listens to what you have to say and encourages questions		
Explains treatments, medications, and instructions so that you understand		
Respects you as an individual		
Quality Hospital		
Is rated highly on http://www.medicare.gov/hospitalcompare/search.html or https://www.carechek.com/		
Is rated highly by your state's consumer groups		
Receives high rating post-discharge client evaluations		
Has an accreditation by The Joint Commission		
Belongs to the Hospital Rewards Program for quality care		
Holds Magnet hospital recognition		
Is included in your health plan and your health-care provider has privileges		
Has a comprehensive quality improvement and risk reduction plan		
At least 50 percent of the nursing staff are baccalaureate RNs		
Has a positive reputation for successfully treating your disease process(es)		
Uses a rapid-response team to reduce injuries to clients while in the hospital		
Bases care on scientific principles and best practices		
Provides client-centered care based on respect for the individual		
Has a low level of inpatient medication errors		
Fosters interprofessional collaboration in all aspects of client care		
Has a low number of sentinel and never events		
Fosters an environment and culture of safety throughout the facility		

What Do You Think?

What do you think about using financial rewards as a way to motivate health-care institutions to improve the quality of care? In your experience, how well do rewards work by themselves as incentives? What other things can be done to increase motivation?

It was estimated that if all U.S. hospitals implemented just the first three of Leapfrog's four "leaps," more than 57,000 lives could have been saved, more than 3 million medication errors could have been avoided, and up to $12 billion could have been saved each year.[8]

Agency for Healthcare Research and Quality

As the lead federal agency charged with improving the safety and quality of health care for all Americans, the Agency for Healthcare Research and Quality (AHRQ) helps to develop the knowledge, tools, and data needed to improve health care. These improvements include helping clients, health-care professionals, and legislators make knowledgeable and up-to-date decisions about health policies and choices.[11]

AHRQ uses **quality indicators** (QIs) as measures of health-care quality from easily accessible inpatient hospital administrative data. QIs are standardized, evidence-based measures of health-care quality that can be used to measure and track the quality of clinical performance and outcomes. Some of the benefits of using QIs include identifying areas of care that require quality improvement, tracking either improvements or declines in quality over time, and identifying areas that need additional study. Although each QI follows a rigorous process for development and a complicated process for scoring, they are relatively easy to use in the clinical setting. For example, a QI for the emergency department (ED) might be, "Clients spend fewer than 6 hours in the waiting room," or for a pediatric client in the ED treated for a urinary tract infection, "Client is reassessed for infection after 48 hours." There are QIs for all units and all types of clients with almost every condition, even clients who die during hospitalization. When a QI consistently falls short of the standardized benchmark, it is an indication that the facility or unit has potential quality concerns. If changes are made to address the QI concern, the results of the change can be tracked over time.[11]

A Proactive Approach

Continuous Quality Improvement

Unlike the AHRQ's QIs, which retroactively analyze outcomes after they have occurred, CQI is proactively oriented. Its emphasis is on *anticipating and preventing* problems rather than reacting to them. CQI requires that nurses and other health-care team members continually ask, "How are we doing?" and "Can we be doing it better right now?" With the CQI approach, the care-delivery process receives close and constant scrutiny, and everyone is encouraged to think creatively to devise and test new ideas for improving quality. New approaches based on CQI must demonstrate "meaningful use" and not just change for change's sake. CQI encourages change on the basis of systematically documented evidence and also values standardization of the process so that efficiency is maximized. For example, researchers found that using standardized processes and tools during annual wellness visits for teens with asthma significantly increased quality care provision and doubled overall adherence to the medical regimen.[12]

Nurses are in an excellent position to implement CQI strategies. On a daily basis, they assess the functioning of the health-care delivery system and the effectiveness of specific treatment approaches and care methods. For example, the unit manager (UM) in an ED noticed that an increasing number of older clients who were transgender were being admitted for a variety of conditions unrelated to their transition or their gender identity. It became evident to the UM that almost none of the staff, from the nursing assistants and volunteers to the admissions/triage nurses and the advanced practice registered nurse providers, were comfortable with caring for these clients.

> *When a QI consistently falls short of the standardized benchmark, it is an indication that the facility or unit has potential quality concerns.*

In addition, the hospital records for these clients were often incomplete or poorly documented, which indicated previous subpar care.

The UM checked the hospital's policy and procedure manual and found no policy that addressed care of transgender clients. Using the CQI process, she, in conjunction with the ED staff, selected and purchased several presentations about caring for transgender clients, to be used as part of their regular in-service training. The UM and the staff, one of whom was transgender, then developed a policy for their facility on how to appropriately address, interview, and physically assess transgender clients. After the policy was fully implemented, charting improved; scores on posthospitalization satisfaction surveys increased; and when word circulated about the care at the hospital ED, an increased number of transgender clients started coming in for care.[12]

Case Management Protocols

There is another mechanism for monitoring cost-effective, high-quality care: outcome-based case management protocols, also known as **clinical pathways**, **care pathways**, or **critical pathways**. The development of clinical pathways grew out of a need to assess, implement, and monitor cost-effective, high-quality client care in a systematic manner.[13]

Clinical pathways are an outgrowth of nursing care plans but have the advantages of streamlining the charting process, encouraging documentation across multidisciplinary teams, and systematically monitoring variances from prescribed plans of care. The ability to identify how client care and progress vary from a predetermined plan enables more accurate assessment of client-care costs and maintenance of quality-control measures. Integration of clinical pathways into practical use has been enhanced by computerization of client records and online bedside documentation.[13]

Risk Management

Risk management is a component of quality management programs. It focuses on identifying, analyzing, and evaluating risks and then reducing those risks to decrease harm to clients. When an adverse event does occur, attempts are made to minimize losses. Risk management is interdisciplinary in nature and includes aspects of detection, education, and intervention.

Nursing staff is key to any risk-management program. High-risk areas include medication errors, complications from tests and treatments, falls, refusal of treatment or refusal to sign treatment consents, and client/family dissatisfaction. Client records and occurrence/incident reports are used to track and analyze adverse events. The analysis, often called **root-cause analysis**, tracks events leading to the error, identifies faulty systems and processes, and develops a plan to prevent further errors.

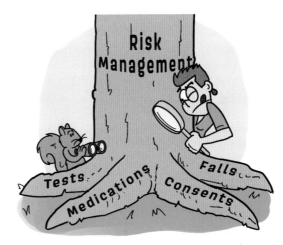

Root causes need to be examined.

TJC sets mandatory National Patient Safety Goals that address particular risks for clients. Hospitals improve quality and safety by making these goals a priority in client care:

1. Improve accuracy of client identification.
2. Improve effectiveness of communication among caregivers.
3. Improve safety of using medications.
4. Reduce risk of health-care-associated infections.
5. Identify client safety risks inherent in its client population.

TJC's central focus is to promote quality evidence-based measures to maximize health benefits. Risk management is an ongoing process that can be revised when new risks arise, when there is a change in a plan, or when risk-management documentation changes. Nurses need to closely monitor the progress of a project and make changes when needed. Risk management should be conducted before beginning a project by nurses with high levels of experience and proficiency in their specialty areas.[14]

Sentinel Events

TJC defines a **sentinel event** as an "unexpected occurrence involving death or serious physical or psychological injury, or the risk thereof. Serious injury includes loss of limb or function."[15] The Joint Commission International (JCI) definition varies slightly from the U.S. TJC. It defines a sentinel event as

> any unanticipated event in a health-care setting resulting in death or serious physical or psychological injury to a client or clients, not related to the natural course of the client's illness. These are usually the most serious events in hospitals, and include:
> Unexpected death
> Client suicide
> Wrong client, wrong side, wrong site surgery
> Infant abduction
> Sexual assault on client
> Hemolytic blood transfusion reaction resulting from incompatible blood transfusion
> Intrapartum maternal death
> Assault, homicide or other crime resulting in permanent loss of function or death[15]

Sentinel events are not always the same as errors. Not all sentinel events are due to errors, and not all errors cause sentinel events. Sentinel events indicate the need for immediate investigation and response. TJC reviews organizations' responses to sentinel events in its accreditation process. Its goal is to improve the quality of care and prevent future sentinel event occurrences.

Near-Miss versus No-Harm Incident

There are several different variations of the definition of a near miss. The World Health Organization (WHO) defines a near miss as "an error that has the potential to cause an adverse event (client harm) but fails to do so because of chance or because it is intercepted (caught before it happens)." The IOM defines a near miss as "an act of commission or omission that could have harmed the client but did not cause harm as a result of chance, prevention, or mitigation." A general definition that is often used is "an error caught before reaching the client." All these definitions focus on a type of incident

that has the potential to result in harm but, in the end, fails to cause harm.[16]

Although the variations may seem slight, they do produce some confusion as to whether a specific incident should be reported. Four factors at work in attempting to identify what a near-miss incident actually is are (1) whether the lack of harm to the client was due to a plan made by the facility to prevent it, (2) whether the lack of harm to the client was due to chance occurrences, (3) whether the incident did reach the client but was detected early and prevented by a preplanned protocol, and (4) whether the harm was prevented by accident when the incident did reach the client. Viewed from these aspects, there are actually two separate concepts to be defined: "near-miss incident" and "no-harm incident."[17]

A. Near-Miss Incident

Type 1: This is an incident that does not reach the client because of formal and planned interventions and programs that were previously developed by the hospital to specifically prevent it from happening. For example, the hospital has a policy that two RNs must check insulin doses prior to administration. A nurse draws up 20 units of regular insulin, but the second RN realizes that it should have been 10 units and prevents the overdose of insulin.

Type 2: This is an incident that does not reach the client because of interventions that occurred by mere chance or some other unplanned interventions. For example, a nurse is to hang a second unit of blood on a client with GI bleeding. When she takes down the first unit, she notices that it is O positive; the unit she was starting to hang was AB positive. She stops the procedure at that point, checks the chart, and finds that the client indeed is O positive.

B. No-Harm Incidents

Type 3: This is an incident that does reach the client but does not cause harm because of early detection, interventions, and treatment. A nurse failed to check the allergy sheet on a client with an infection on his arm. She begins to give him an IV dose of piperacillin, which is a penicillin derivative. Almost as soon as the infusion starts, the client develops a bumpy red rash and difficulty breathing. The nurse recognizes this as an allergic reaction and stops the infusion of the medication. According to a preestablished protocol, she administers IV diphenhydramine (Benadryl). The symptoms subside within a few minutes. No harm occurred to the client.

Type 4: This is an incident that does reach the client but does not cause harm because of pure chance. For example, a nurse changed an elastic (ACE) bandage dressing on a client's leg but applied the bandage too tightly, thereby restricting the flow of blood to his foot. However, when she put the bandage on, she fastened the end of it too loosely, and the bandage came loose after a short time. The blood flow restriction was not long enough to cause any damage to the client's foot, so no harm occurred because—by mere chance—the nurse did not know how to correctly apply bandages.[17]

Near misses, no-harm events, and adverse events are almost identical in their root causes; and root-cause analysis needs to be performed on all of them. Type 3 and Type 4 incidents, when they recur, carry with them a high chance of a serious adverse outcome. Such near misses fall within the scope of the definition of a sentinel event, but they are outside the scope and definition of sentinel events that are subject to review by TJC.[16]

> " *Near misses, no-harm events, and adverse events are almost identical in their root causes; and root-cause analysis needs to be performed on all of them.* "

What Do You Think?

Identify an incident that occurred during your time in health-care institutions, as either a student or an employee, that would be considered a high-risk or a sentinel event. How was the incident dealt with? What did you learn from the incident?

Hazardous Conditions

At the center of quality of care is the safety of the client and those who are responsible for their care. Anything in the environment that threatens safety can be considered a hazardous condition. Although the definition of *hazardous conditions* varies across workplace settings, the Occupational Safety & Health Administration (OSHA) defines it as "any situation or practice in a place of employment that can reasonably cause death or major physical harm."[18] In the health-care setting, particularly a hospital, it is any set of circumstances (exclusive of the disease or condition for which the client is being treated) that significantly increases the likelihood of a serious adverse outcome.

OSHA is a government watchdog organization that is responsible for making sure that all workplaces are free from hazards. However, throughout any given year, thousands of deaths and serious injuries still occur in the workplace. A portion of those accidents are due to employee gross negligence or carelessness, and the rest are caused by hazardous conditions in the workplace.[18] Almost anything can be considered a hazard if it is misused in the wrong place at the wrong time or otherwise in a state where it can cause harm. In order for a work environment to be considered hazardous or an impending danger for workers or clients, it must first meet several OHSA requirements:

1. The environment must be so bad as to provide a risk of death or serious physical harm. Serious physical harm is defined as the injury caused to a person, which will be so bad that the affected body part is no longer able to function either partially or totally (also includes the lungs and brain).

2. The environment must be toxic or filled with substances or toxic gases that expose a person to life-shortening or life-threatening properties or cause a person to experience a substantial lessening in mental or physical ability. The damage from the health hazard may be delayed for a period of time.

3. The environmental hazard must be imminent or immediate so that serious physical harm or death could result from the hazard in a short period of time or before OSHA could investigate the hazard.

4. If the environment is determined by OSHA inspectors to be an imminent danger, they must notify the workers who are potentially affected and their employer that they are invoking an OSHA intervention to immediately halt the hazardous condition.

5. Although OSHA has no law-enforcement authority itself, it does have the power to request a federal court order that the hazard be removed by the employer.[19]

Individuals who believe that their work environment is hazardous or who have suffered an injury because of a perceived hazard in the workplace should contact a personal injury lawyer for a consultation. The case may entitle the person to compensation for injuries and punitive damages, especially if the hazard had been previously reported and/or may produce long-term harm.

Most of these cases are settled out of court, and some have resulted in very large awards for the plaintiffs.

Several different types of hazardous conditions exist in the health-care setting (see Box 14.3). The COVID-19 pandemic produced a particularly hazardous condition throughout the health-care system. OSHA doubled its monitoring at workplaces with a higher potential for COVID exposures, such as hospitals, assisted living facilities, nursing homes, and other health-care and emergency response providers treating clients with COVID-19. The agency, in

---

Box 14.3 Types of Hazardous Conditions

1. **Physical hazards:** Physical hazards are factors in the environment that can cause accidental harm to a person such as pain, injuries, or death. Examples include injuries from careless coworkers; poorly placed electrical lines, panels, and power cables; loud and/or continuous noise from machines; falls from tasks that require a person to work at height or slippery floors; and prolonged exposure to extreme temperature.
2. **Chemical hazards:** A chemical hazard is a danger involved with the use of any type of potentially injurious liquid or gaseous airborne substance at home or in the workplace. Individuals exposed to dangerous chemicals in the workplace can become suddenly and acutely ill and die, or, over time, develop chronic and deadly health problems such as cancer, kidney, or liver failure. Examples of dangerous chemicals include strong acids and bases, bottled gases, solvents, dust, fumes, vapors, anesthetics, or liquids such as cleaning products.
3. **Ergonomic hazards:** Ergonomic hazards are working conditions that create wear and tear on the body and can result in physical damage to the musculoskeletal system, including the muscles or ligaments of the lower back, tendons or nerves of the hands/wrists, or structures surrounding and in the knees. These types of hazards include poor design of equipment such as workstations, desks and chairs, poorly positioned display screen equipment, repetitive strain as in typing, prolonged exposure to vibration, remaining in a prolonged awkward posture, and forceful exertion such as manual handling of heavy items such as beds or boxes and improper moving of heavy patients.
4. **Biological hazards:** Biological hazards, also known simply as *biohazards*, are organic substances or organisms that threaten a person's health. They include pathogenic micro-organisms, viruses such as COVID-19, toxins (from biological sources), spores, fungi, and bio-active substances. Biological hazards can cause various illnesses ranging from minor skin irritations to untreatable fatal diseases.
5. **Psychological hazards:** Psychological hazards are elements of the day-to-day work environment, management, or organizational practices that pose a risk to mental health and well-being by increasing the levels of stress in workers and overwhelming their normal coping mechanisms. It affects their ability to work productively and cooperate successfully with coworkers. Examples include lateral and vertical violence, understaffing, bullying, and sexual harassment.
6. **Environmental hazards:** Environmental hazards can result from chemical, biological, or physical agents produced from current industrial or health-care activity or from toxic substances not properly disposed of from previous human manufacturing that have the potential to adversely affect an individual's or community's health. Environmental hazard can also be present in the wider natural environment and include man-made disasters such as toxic chemical and oil spills, increased carbon dioxide levels in the air, pollution from natural disasters such as volcanoes that throw large amounts of pollutants into the air, or climate changes that causes prolonged droughts and temperature changes.

Source: Ubongeh, 6 Types of major hazards you should know, HSEWatch, June 28, 2022, https://hsewatch.com/types-of-hazards.

conjunction with WHO and the Centers for Disease Control and Prevention (CDC), also began developing rules and policies concerning infectious disease standards to prepare for future viral outbreaks.[20]

Between February 2020 and March 2022, OSHA issued 1,200 citations to health-care employers for hazardous conditions related to COVID-19, such as lack of PPE, inadequate staffing of areas with critical clients, and improper sterilization of invasive items. OSHA also levied fines totaling $7.2 million during the same period. More than 400 employees who filed COVID-19 retaliation claims against employers received awards exceeding $5 million.[20] Agency compliance safety and health officers (CSHOs) also interviewed employers and employees to see if there were any recorded cases or reports of active work-related COVID-19 infections that resulted in lost work time, hospitalizations, or fatalities. They determined whether unvaccinated workers were involved in tasks that required close contact with clients or other personnel. They also evaluated facilities for health hazards during their inspections, including exposure to workplace bullying and violence; slips and falls; bloodborne pathogens or other potentially infectious materials; and ergonomic hazards (devices that cause musculoskeletal problems).[20]

Six Sigma Quality Improvements

Although **Six Sigma** was developed and used initially to improve quality in the manufacturing sector in the early 1980s, it found its way into the health-care system in the mid- to late 1990s. It was seen as a way to identify problems in health-care delivery and find effective solutions.

The Tail of the Curve

The origins of Six Sigma can be traced back to the 1920s and are based on the statistical model of the bell-shaped curve. In the perfect bell curve, the mean is exactly in the center, at the highest point of the curve. Away from the mean, the curve slopes down at a predictable rate on both sides and is divided into standard deviations. Each standard deviation is designated by the Greek letter for a lowercase *s*, or σ (sigma), and given a number (e.g., plus or minus 1 sigma). Six standard deviations (six sigmas) are so far out in the tails of the bell curve that they are generally considered a total lack of error—in other words, "perfection" (statistically, 3.4 defects per million).

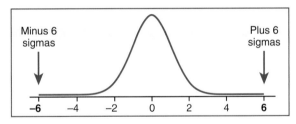

Figure 14.2 The Six Sigma bell curve.

Six Sigma's focus is a quality management program that serves as a measure, a goal, and a system of management to ensure optimal quality results (Fig. 14.2).

The Six Sigma technique was initially used by Motorola to improve the quality of its products and was then adopted by such well-known corporations as General Electric and Honeywell. This approach can be used to reduce the costs of manufacturing items or the number of steps in manufacturing, making the manufacturing process more "lean."[21]

The traditional Six Sigma process comprises five distinct phases that somewhat parallel the steps of the nursing process:

1. *Define:* The problem is identified. Why are customers dissatisfied? Why are costs excessive? Why does it take so long to complete the process?
2. *Measure:* Data are collected to pinpoint the exact issue. The whole process is reviewed in detail, and time or other elements to be measured are given numerical values.
3. *Analyze:* The root causes of the problem are identified, and the relationships of external or environmental influences are analyzed. All factors must be considered, no matter how remote (see Box 14.4).
4. *Improve:* Strategies based on the previous three phases are developed to correct the problems. Any number of techniques may be used to make the process error-proof and more efficient. Pilot projects are then established to test the effectiveness of possible solutions to the problems. Several solutions may be tested before the best one is identified.
5. *Control:* Systems are put in place to continuously monitor the changes in the process. The goal is to detect errors before they affect the whole system. A statistical process may be used to determine the level of correction and as an early-warning system for new problems.[11]

Box 14.4 Root-Cause Analysis (RCA)

In 2001, the Joint Commission on Accreditation of Healthcare Organizations (JCAHO [now The Joint Commission]) began requiring root-cause analyses for all sentinel events. Root-cause analysis is a retrospective approach to error analysis, the goal of which is to identify the original error that led to an adverse event. A root cause is the most basic causal factor or factors which, if corrected or removed, will prevent recurrence of all elements involved in the error. The purpose of root-cause analysis is to identify and remove the root cause, not assign blame for the error. A root-cause analysis should be performed as soon as possible after the error or variance occurs; otherwise, important details or information may be omitted or missed.

Sentinel events that are subject to review by The Joint Commission include the following:

- Any incident that results in unanticipated death or major permanent loss of function (unrelated to the client's underlying disease or condition)
- Inpatient suicide
- Unexpected death of a full-term infant
- Abduction
- Discharge of an infant to the wrong family
- Rape or other sexual assault
- Blood transfusion error
- Wrong-site surgery
- Foreign object retention after surgery or other medical procedure
- Severe neonatal hyperbilirubinemia
- High radiation exposure, or radiotherapy to the wrong part of the body

When developing the root-cause analysis, The Joint Commission recommends the facility incorporate the following elements:

- A determination of the human and other factors most directly associated with the sentinel event and the processes and systems related to its occurrence;
- Analysis of the underlying systems and processes through a series of questions to determine where redesign might reduce risk;
- Inquiry into all areas appropriate to the specific type of event as described in the current edition of *Minimum Scope of Review of Root Cause Analysis*;
- Identification of risk points and their potential contributions to this type of event;
- A determination of potential improvement in processes or systems that would tend to decrease the likelihood of such events in the future, or a determination, after analysis, that no such opportunities exist.

All of the personnel involved in the error must be involved in the analysis. Without all parties present, the discussion may lead to invention or speculation that will water down the facts. Asking for this level of involvement may cause staff to feel hostile, defensive, or apprehensive. Managers must explain that the purpose of the root cause analysis process is to focus on the setting of the error and the systems involved, not to identify any one individual as the causal agent.

Source: P. François, A. Lecoanet, A. Caporossi, A.-M. Dols, A. Seigneurin, B. Boussat, Experience feedback committees: A way of implementing a root cause analysis practice in hospital medical departments, *PLoS ONE*, 13(7):e0201067, 2018. https://doi.org/10.1371/journal.pone.0201067

Six Sigma in Health Care

How does the health-care system use Six Sigma to improve the quality of care? Traditionally in health care, finding and defining the specific cause of errors have been extremely difficult. Six Sigma provides a wide-reaching and more pragmatic approach to identifying and measuring the problem. By adapting and modifying the traditional Six Sigma methodology, health-care providers can develop more inclusive objectives to increase reliability and quality. The overriding goal of Six Sigma is to develop a fully reliable process or system of care. Such a system will deliver the same quality of care to all clients all the time regardless of who actually delivers the care.

The Champion

As a highly structured approach to identifying fundamental problems, the Six Sigma process uses experts or consultants to guide nurses and others through the five-phase process using highly specialized statistical tools. Specialized training is required to employ Six Sigma, and individuals can become certified as Six Sigma consultants through the Institute of Industrial and Systems Engineers or the American Society for Quality. The certification levels for Six Sigma are distinguished by "belt color": white belt, yellow belt, green belt, black belt, master black belt, and champion. Champions are upper-level managers who lead the implementation of the Lean Six Sigma plans for the institution. A person's belt level increases as they gain additional skills, knowledge, training, and expertise in the Six Sigma process. Master **black belts** serve as well-paid consultants for hospitals and other institutions that believe Six Sigma may be the answer to their QI problems.[21]

When the Six Sigma process is used to analyze a problem, it focuses on two types of statistical anomalies or variations. The primary one, usually at the root of most problems, is called *special* or *assigned variation* and shows a pattern of activity outside the patterns expected to produce high-quality care. Once this variation is detected, the five-step statistical process can be applied. The second type of anomaly is called *common* or *chance variation* and is usually attributed to environmental factors that cannot be controlled. However, in some situations, chance variations can become so significant that they affect the process and have to be addressed.

The Six Sigma process was at first used in health care on a limited basis in the Commonwealth Health Corporation in Kentucky in 2002. It was used to streamline the corporation's radiology department and increase its bottom line by reducing costs. Since that time, the use of Six Sigma has grown, as many of the original problems in using it in a health-care setting have been worked out. Six Sigma has been used successfully in many other hospitals to increase nurse satisfaction and retention by eliminating tedious factors in day-to-day operations, to reduce clients' length of stay, and to speed up the process for transferring clients from outpatient areas to inpatient rooms. Researchers have concluded that Six Sigma can assist in QI in health care as the growing evidence base demonstrates sustainability of its results.[22]

A Hybrid

A hybrid Six Sigma program called *Lean Six Sigma* focuses on identifying and eliminating waste and therefore improving the flow of processes. When Lean Six Sigma is used, more emphasis is placed on the process of delivering a product rather than on the product itself. It is similar to other agile or lean methods. Lean Six Sigma uses tools such as value stream mapping, which is a process that allows an organization to create a detailed picture of all steps involved in the product-delivery process. It is a flow chart of how resources move from the provider through the organization and to the customer.[23]

> ❝ *Champions are upper-level managers who lead the implementation of the Lean Six Sigma plans for the institution.* ❞

A research study has shown that Lean Six Sigma improved the quality of trauma care by reducing inappropriate hospital stays while reducing costs.[24] In a different study, researchers discovered that the use of Lean Six Sigma improved the collaborative efficiency of meal delivery, radiological testing, and timing of inpatient insulin administration.[25]

There are critics of Six Sigma, and several drawbacks to its use have been identified. Six Sigma is effective in modifying existing processes, but it tends to stifle creative approaches and "thinking outside the box." Although achieving perfection at the statistical 3.4 errors-per-million level might be adequate for situations such as patient satisfaction and nurse retention, it seems to fall short for activities such as administering medications and operating a ventilator. When Six Sigma is implemented in the health-care setting, it is often used as an add-on project, not connected with existing QI efforts. Nursing staff tend to resist the strange-sounding jargon and statistical emphasis and may actually attempt to sabotage implementation. Six Sigma has little regard for the interpersonal and institutional culture that is so important in the effectiveness of health-care institutions.[24]

The overall objective of Six Sigma is to increase the reliability of processes by eliminating defects and reducing system variation. Its five-phase structured approach requires high-quality discrete data that are often difficult to obtain in the health-care setting. Its orientation is more industrial than health related: it uses tools such as statistical process control and root-cause analysis to identify anomalies in the processes it is examining. Although yet to be used on a wide scale in the health-care setting, Six Sigma is gradually gaining a following, and its use in health care will probably increase in the future.[24]

Scrum

Scrum, similar to other QI processes and methodologies adopted by nursing, started its life as a business application in the software industry in 1986. Because of the rapid pace of software development, by the time an idea for a new software application was developed enough for sale to the public, it was often already outdated. Scrum allowed software companies to begin producing software incrementally in as little as 30 days rather than the usual months.[26]

Rugby enthusiasts will recognize the term *scrum* (short for *scrummage*) as the huddle-like formation that restarts play in a game. A rugby scrum involves players packed closely together in a circle with their heads down, fighting to gain possession of the ball. In the rugby scrum, the ball is passed back and forth between players on two teams in the scrum until one team is able to take control of it. In a similar process, in a software-development scrum, ideas are passed back and forth between members of a team rather than just having one person attempt to develop an idea on their own.[27]

Scrum became very attractive during the COVID-19 pandemic because of the increased use of remote work. The Scrum framework addressed the key challenges of working from home by providing increased transparency, better accountability, and more opportunities for collaboration. The overall use of the Scrum process almost tripled during the most active years of the pandemic.[27]

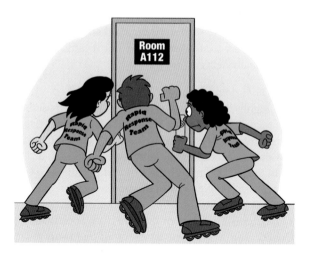

Rapid Response Team to the rescue!

There is some disagreement among the experts about whether Scrum, as it is used in the business world, is a process or a framework; however, the most accepted definition of *Scrum* is a framework within which people can address complex adaptive problems by working as an effective team through collaborating on the solutions to complex issues.[27] In business, the Scrum framework is used to identify a need (assessment), design a product (plan), list tasks needed to turn this design into a shippable product (analysis), write and complete the coding (implementation), and then test and validate that the product works (evaluation). The similarity between the Scrum framework and the nursing process is glaringly obvious. Both are grounded in observable process-control theory and employ an iterative, incremental approach to produce measurable results. As with the results of the nursing process, the results of the Scrum framework are verified through transparency, inspection, and adaptation. The major difference is that the Scrum framework is able to produce results more quickly than the nursing process.[26]

The Team Huddle

Nurses have been using a highly modified and streamlined form of Scrum in a process called a **huddle** since before 2010. It is unclear whether the informal huddle is directly linked to the formal Scrum used in business. However, the key to both processes is the interaction of the team members with each other in solving problems. The huddle in nursing is different from a regular team meeting in that it is a brief, daily discussion that focuses on the plan of action for the next shift. It encourages discussion among all workers about client safety and the goals of care rather than system problems.[28]

The huddle tends to be most effective in acute care units, where a well-planned and controllable shift can suddenly turn into pandemonium due to an event such as a client suffering a cardiac arrest or the admission of a client with complicated care needs. The workflow of the unit is forced to change, and planned, high-quality nursing care takes a back seat to the emergency. Huddles can be used to heighten awareness of an individual nurse's and client's needs so that the workload can be adjusted. An impromptu huddle can be called at any time by any nurse, even a UM or charge nurse, when they feel the unit is getting out of control. All staff members are expected to attend an emergency "stop the lunacy" huddle so that they can reevaluate plans and assignments. Scheduled huddles can also be held to deal with issues that are more long term and do not require immediate attention.[28]

EDUCATION AND A COMPETENCY FOCUS

The focus on quality care needs to begin on the first day of a health-care professional's education and continue through their whole education program and career. Certain initiatives in nursing and medical education focus on developing health-care professionals' competencies critical to providing safe, quality health care. The first of these, the Competency Outcomes Performance Assessment model, was started in the 1990s. In 2005, the Robert Wood Johnson Foundation introduced the Quality and Safety Education for Nurses (QSEN) project (see Chapter 4). In addition, the American Association of Colleges of Nursing (AACN) has developed program outcomes for baccalaureate curricula that focus on quality.

Competency Outcomes and Performance Assessment Model

The **Competency Outcomes and Performance Assessment (COPA) model**, developed in the early 1990s, has been used by medical schools and some schools of nursing to validate the skills and knowledge of their graduates. It is designed to promote competency for clinical practice at all levels. Key components in several of its eight core competencies address quality, safety, and risk reduction, aligning well with the newer QSEN competencies. One study explored the COPA model's use in two prelicensure nursing programs and in a graduate nurse internship program. Research has demonstrated the COPA model's benefits for nursing students, nursing graduates, preceptors, employers, and clients. Benefits noted for clients included increased quality and safety.[29]

Quality and Safety Education for Nurses

Driven by community and professional concerns, in 2005 the Robert Wood Johnson Foundation undertook a three-phase project to improve the quality and safety of client care by focusing nursing education on student competency. The project, QSEN, is built on five competencies initially developed by the IOM:[29]

1. Client-centered care
2. Teamwork and collaboration
3. Evidence-based practice (EBP)
4. Quality improvement[22]
5. Safety

A sixth competency, informatics, was later added as the model developed and was revised because of the important role technology now plays in health care. Subsequent research demonstrates that using the QSEN model contributed to the adoption of quality and safety competencies as core practice values.[29] (See Chapter 4 for more details.)

Essentials of Baccalaureate Education for Professional Nursing Practice

For many years, the AACN document *Essentials of Baccalaureate Education for Professional Nursing Practice* has been the gold standard for outcomes for nursing programs. AACN's *Essential II: Basic Organizational and Systems Leadership for Quality Care and Patient Safety* addresses the relationship of safety, quality improvement, and organizational and systems leadership to ensuring quality nursing care. The AACN *Essentials* have for many years defined what it means to have a high-quality nursing education program.

Skills common to both QSEN and the *Essentials* include communication and collaboration, decision making, participation in safety initiatives, QI processes, and cost-effectiveness.[30]

The New AACN Essentials

With the endorsement of the new AACN *Essentials* by the membership in April 2021, academic nursing is moving toward a new model and framework for nursing education using a competency-based education (CBE) approach. AACN is committed to providing resources, education, and guidance to bring about this transformation.[30]

The AACN *Essentials* are guidelines that define what is needed to attain high quality in nursing education. They outline the required curriculum content and anticipated competencies of graduates from baccalaureate, master's, and doctor of nursing practice programs. The new AACN *Essentials* helped academic nursing to take a major leap toward a new model and framework for nursing education using a competency-based approach.[30]

The new format has the title *The Essentials: Core Competencies for Professional Nursing Education*. Contained in the revised AACN *Essentials* is an introduction, A New Model for Nursing Education, Implementing the Essentials: Considerations for Curriculum, 10 Domains and Domain Descriptors, 10 Contextual Statements, Competencies, Entry-Level into Professional Nursing Education Sub-competencies (Level 1), and Advanced Level Nursing Sub-competencies (Level 2).[30]

With an increased emphasis on CBE, it is suggested that nursing programs begin to move to a process that guarantees that their curricula address the competencies outlined in the *Essentials*. These programs must be able to assess students' achievement of the delineated competencies. The AACN defines CBE as "a system of instruction, assessment, feedback, self-reflection, and academic reporting that is based on students demonstrating that they have learned the knowledge, attitudes, motivations, self-perceptions, and skills

> *Instead of a quick check off or "one and done demonstration" that is often now used in nursing education, students using a CBE system must be able to demonstrate that they can successfully deal with increasingly complex client situations.*

expected of them as they progress through their education."[31] CBE requires that students participate in multiple educational experiences across progressively intricate client settings and situations. The way students are assessed or evaluated with CBE measures their ability to provide care in multiple clinical settings using their learned skills and knowledge. Instead of a quick check off or "one and done demonstration" that is often used now in nursing education, students using a CBE system must be able to demonstrate that they can successfully deal with increasingly complex client situations.[31]

The AACN *Essentials* focus as they always have on baccalaureate and higher degree nursing education programs. The essentials for entry-level nursing are labeled Level 1 sub-competencies. These competencies outline a more rigorous scope of preparation for entry into practice (as compared to the previous *BSN Essentials*). These new competencies will create a much stronger generalist preparation for entry-level professional nurses who will be able to perform RN-level clinical skills upon graduation. Level 2 sub-competencies and the specialty/role competencies apply to MSN programs and/or advanced-level nursing specialties or advanced-level nursing roles.[30]

Community college–level or diploma nursing students enrolled in degree completion programs (RN to BSN) will be expected to demonstrate attainment of the entry-level 1 sub-competencies prior to graduation.[31] It would behoove associate degree nursing programs to begin adopting the competency-based elements of the *Essentials* that apply to their programs, particularly if they want their graduates to obtain a BSN.

A Difference in Opinion

Some nursing leaders believe that by conforming to QSEN-based curricula, they will transform the professional identity of nursing into something other than nursing. What about the competencies of caring, integrity, and client advocacy? What about research and scholarship? Where does prevention, a key nursing role since the time of Florence Nightingale, fit in? Those who support QSEN believe that if a nurse is providing high-quality, safe, respectful, and culturally appropriate care, caring and integrity are already included. Others contend that QSEN's inclusion of EBP as a competency addresses research concerns. QSEN's competency of QI, along with its value for updating knowledge and skills, also addresses scholarship concerns. Some argue that health promotion and disease prevention are already included in QSEN's model under client-centered care. Others believe that in order to promote nursing as a unique discipline, a seventh competency, "professional person," should be added to include those aspects of nursing that distinguish it from the medical profession.

The ANA Project

In the fall of 2010, a report by the ANA and the Constituent Member Associations (CMA) moved the discussion of QSEN-structured curricula to a new level by outlining the key messages from the IOM report *The Future of Nursing: Leading Change, Advancing Health*. This report is part of an ongoing project aimed at using EBP to advance the nursing profession so that nursing can keep pace with health-care reform activities (see Chapter 4 for more information).[29]

Federal Initiatives for Coverage of AHRQ, QIO, and CMS

The Agency for Healthcare Research and Quality (AHRQ) is 1 of 12 Department of Health and Human Services agencies that support research that improves the quality of health care and helps people make more informed health-care decisions. The agency is charged with developing partnerships that create long-term improvement in American health care. The research goal is to measure those improvements in terms of client outcomes, decreased mortality, improved quality of life, and cost-effective quality care. Its overall focus is in three areas:

- *Safety and quality:* Risk reduction by promoting quality care
- *Effectiveness:* Improved health outcomes by using evidence to make informed health-care decisions
- *Efficiency:* Translating research into practice to increase access and to decrease costs[22]

The Affordable Care Act (ACA), Section 3501, mandated that the AHRQ work through the Center for Quality Improvement and Patient Safety to conduct research on the best QI practice innovations and strategies. The center's tasks also included identifying, creating, critiquing, sharing, and giving training in these best practices. In addition, the center coordinated its activities with the Centers for Medicare and Medicaid Services (CMS) and the Centers for Medicare and Medicaid Innovation (CMI). The center was to award grants to agencies with expertise in providing assistance to health-care providers in QI activities and to the health-care providers seeking technical assistance in implementing best-practice models.[29]

The Quality Improvement Organization (QIO) is a federal program designed to review medical care, verify its necessity, and assist Medicare and Medicaid beneficiaries with complaints about quality of care. The program is also charged to implement quality of care improvements. According to the CMS, "By law, the mission of the QIO program is to improve the effectiveness, efficiency, economy, and quality of services delivered to Medicare beneficiaries."[32] The CMS identifies three core functions for QIO:

- Improving quality of care for beneficiaries
- Protecting the integrity of the Medicare Trust Fund by ensuring that Medicare pays only for services and goods that are reasonable and necessary and that are provided in the most appropriate setting
- Protecting beneficiaries by expeditiously addressing individual complaints, such as beneficiary complaints, provider-based notice appeals, violations of the Emergency Medical Treatment and Labor Act (EMTALA), and other related responsibilities as articulated in QIO-related law

How effective has the QIO been? Researchers linked reductions in both all-cause 30-day rehospitalizations and all-cause hospitalizations among Medicare beneficiaries in communities with QIO programs.[32]

What Do You Think?

What types of complaints have you made about poor care you or a loved one received while in a hospital or clinic? Did any of these complaints fall into the categories of quality-of-care items discussed earlier? If you did complain, what happened to the complaint? Were any changes made as a result?

Never Events

Starting in the fall of 2007, the CMS changed the Medicare payment program to disallow payment for reasonably preventable medical errors that occur in the hospital. These events, listed on the CMS website, are referred to as **never events**.[32] Consequently, hospitals now have to cover the costs for never events that do occur. The purpose of this change was to control Medicare costs and improve the quality of care; however, quality may come at a heavy price for institutions already financially stressed.

Never events are also considered sentinel events by TJC and must be reported to them. TJC requires that a root-cause analysis be performed after a never event. Negligent and inattentive behaviors from health-care professionals are the two primary causes of never events. Professional negligence is the very definition of malpractice, and almost all never events are followed by a lawsuit with a large payment to the plaintiff.[33]

Always Events

An always event is the opposite of a never event. An always event is what should be done in each client situation where an error could be made. In nursing, students are taught the five rights of medication administration, which improve client safety and promote better outcomes (i.e., an always event). When health-care facilities standardize processes and procedures that promote a positive, long-term culture that prioritizes client safety, they are creating always events. Always events should include the following:

- Identifying each client by more than one source for all procedures
- Being completely transparent in divulging potential adverse outcomes
- Implementing tactics for safe medication administration
- Flagging critical laboratory, pathology, and imaging results for abnormal values
- Making sure that critical client information is communicated at shift changes, in-hospital transfers, or client discharge to another facility

> *Negligent and inattentive behaviors from health-care professionals are the two primary causes of never events. Professional negligence is the very definition of malpractice, and almost all never events are followed by a lawsuit with a large payment to the plaintiff.*

The number and frequency of never events can easily be reduced through the implementation and use of always events in hospitals, outpatient facilities, and other health-care settings.[33]

Transforming Care at the Bedside

The Robert Woods Johnson Foundation and the Institute for Healthcare Improvement (IHI) joined forces in 2003 to create a framework called Transforming Care at the Bedside to institute change on medical surgical nursing units. Their goal was to improve care and staff satisfaction by addressing four main categories:

1. Safe and reliable care
2. Vitality and teamwork
3. Client-centered care
4. Value-added care processes

Ideas for change included use of **rapid response teams (RRT)**, also known as medical emergency teams (MET) or critical response teams (CRT), to "rescue" clients whose conditions were deteriorating and prevent their in-hospital deaths; specific communication models to make interdisciplinary communication clearer; a workspace that promotes efficiency and waste reduction; professional support programs; and liberalized diet plans and mealtimes.[34]

Key Factors to High-Quality Care

IOM, QSEN, and AACN *Essentials* all agree on the importance of scholarship, research, and EBP in ensuring quality and safety in health care. The developments in technology now make access to this type of information easy and immediate.

EBP/Research

For this competency, one must "integrate best current evidence with clinical expertise and client/family preferences and values for delivery of optimal health care."[35] Researchers have found multiple benefits of EBP, including cost-effectiveness, increased client safety, improved clinical outcomes, and improved client and staff satisfaction.[35]

EBP consists of three key elements:

1. *Clinical expertise:* This is the knowledge and experience of those in client care practice that provide the quality of clinical judgement and decisions in giving clients care.
2. *Best research evidence:* This refers to the highest quality and most current evidence available in clinical research that delivers the best answer for clinical problems to inform clinical decision making.
3. *Client values and preferences:* This refers to making clinical decisions about individualized client care that takes the client's values and preferences into account.[35] (For more detail on research and EBP, see Chapter 24.)

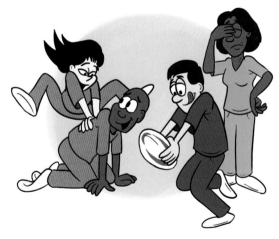

"They can't decide whether to use Leapfrog or Scrum!"

Client-Centered Care

According to QSEN, client-centered care occurs when the nurse can "recognize the client or designee as the source of control and full partner in providing compassionate and coordinated care based on respect for client's preferences, values, and needs."[29] Research about health-care institutions that utilize client and family advisors to promote client-centered care found improved client outcomes in shorter length of stay, higher client satisfaction, and improved levels of reimbursements.[33]

Teamwork and Collaboration

The IOM, the QSEN initiative, and the AACN *Essentials* all emphasize the importance of interdisciplinary teamwork, communication, and collaboration in achieving safe, quality health care. *Teamwork* is defined as the ability to "function effectively within nursing and inter-professional teams, fostering open communication, mutual respect, and shared decision-making to achieve quality client care."[36] In one study, investigators reviewed the Lewis Blackman case in which a 15-year-old boy died 4 days after routine surgical repair of a chest deformity. Researchers then devised a model to characterize the events leading to the tragic death. They proposed five strategies that nurse educators can use to promote safety and quality in nursing care. In addition to using case studies during simulation exercises, these strategies included the following:

- Use "cognitive unmooring questions" in the assessment of clients by students so that they will note subtle changes in the client's condition such as decreased urine output or low blood pressure (i.e., make them think outside the box).
- Have an awareness of and strategies for approaching authority gradients (i.e., fear of reporting something to someone in a position of authority) in interdisciplinary collaboration.
- Communication and provision of experiences that recognize client and **family** as key members of the health-care team.[36]

Informatics

IOM, QSEN, and AACN *Essentials* all agree on the importance of informatics to ensuring client safety and the quality of health care. *Informatics* is the "use of information and technology to communicate, manage knowledge, mitigate error, and support decision-making."[37] (For more details, see Chapter 17.)

Health information technology consists of the computer systems and software programs used in the health-care setting. When information technology is used to attain better client outcomes and to recognize trends and tendencies in the delivery of health care, it becomes health informatics. The two are interdependent and work together to produce better client care.[37]

Nurses who are involved in health-care informatics formulate ways to collect, evaluate, and implement solutions to client problems through the analysis of client charts, storage and retrieval of relevant information, including test results, treatments, surgeries, medications, adverse events, and all other available data sources. Their goal is to improve health-care outcomes. In addition, informatic nurses create communications procedures using the facility's electronic systems. A well-built facility informatics system enables physicians, nurses, and other professionals to have at their fingertips swift, uncomplicated, and well-organized access to all forms of client data.[37]

Lifelong Learning

Quality and safety in nursing care requires continually updating one's knowledge and skills. Because nursing has multiple levels of entry, formal education must also be viewed as a method for lifelong learning. Research studies over the past several years provide evidence of decreased client mortality with a higher proportion of baccalaureate-prepared nurses providing care in an acute care setting.[38] The AACN also supports a nursing workforce that is more highly educated.[30] In a review of the literature, researchers have discovered that through increasing nursing education levels, client outcomes and quality of care can be improved.[38]

The **Tri-Council** is composed of a group of pro-nursing organizations that represent nurses in daily practice, nurse executives, and nurse educators. It is interested in improving all aspects of nursing including the work environment, legislation dealing with health-care rules and policies, health-care outcomes and quality, nursing education, practice, research, and leadership across all sections of the health-care delivery system.[39]

The Tri-Council for Nursing issued a new Consensus Policy Statement on the Educational Advancement of Registered Nurses declaring that health-care reform requires a workforce "that integrates evidence-based clinical knowledge and research with effective communication and leadership skills. These competencies require increased education at all levels. At this tipping point for the nursing profession, action is needed now to put in place strategies to build a stronger nursing workforce. Without a more educated nursing workforce, the nation's health will be further at risk."[39] Agreeing with this stance is the Joint Statement on Academic Progression for Nursing Students and Graduates' belief "that every nursing student and nurse deserves the opportunity to pursue academic career growth and development."[40]

Environment

Nursing cultures need to make quality and safety a priority rather than focusing on what went wrong after an adverse event happens and trying to blame someone for the error. Other characteristics of blame-free or **just culture** organizations include positive working environments, commitment to safety and quality, transparency, and using errors as learning opportunities.

Blameless reporting is an important element in creating a culture of safety in health care. A blameless reporting system assists in reporting errors and near misses voluntarily and anonymously. Nurses and other health-care workers need to feel comfortable reporting adverse events and expressing their ideas for improving their work environment without being punished for past errors. Nurse managers and other management leaders should work on correcting staff actions without confronting the person individually, particularly when the error was due to procedural or system deficiency. Blameless reporting does not mean that there are no consequences; it means that an organization's culture is focused on finding solutions and learning rather than on finding culprits.[41] Without blameless reporting procedures, there is a tendency for the underreporting of negative events, which only increases the chances for the same errors to reoccur. In blameless reporting, the focus becomes an analysis of the event to identify system improvements that can positively impact quality of care and safety.[41]

However, blameless reporting has boundaries. Although it is usually imperative to work on constructive solutions for problems rather than going on

> ❝ *Research studies over the past several years provide evidence of decreased client mortality with a higher proportion of baccalaureate-prepared nurses providing care in an acute care setting.* ❞

witch hunts in order to place culpability, suspending blame is only reasonable for honest mistakes or mistakes beyond the person's control. A just culture holds staff accountable for at-risk, grossly negligent, or reckless behaviors and does not tolerate them; however, it is prepared to handle human errors justly. For example, if a nurse lacks ethical boundaries or is obviously incompetent, they should be held responsible for their actions and be reported to the state's board of nursing for punitive actions.[41]

Magnet hospitals are health-care institutions that meet or exceed the standards of excellence identified by the American Nurses Credentialing Center (ANCC).[42] The Magnet Hospital program has established 35 areas related to quality of care as its criteria for credentialing. The name "Magnet" derives from the fact that when a hospital meets the criteria, it is able to attract and retain the best qualified RNs, like a magnet attracts iron. Magnet credentialing is guided by principles in quality and expertise that ultimately advance three goals within hospitals:

1. Promoting quality in a setting that supports professional practice
2. Identifying excellence in the delivery of nursing service to clients or residents
3. Disseminating best practices in nurse services[42]

According to the ANCC, Magnet status offers these benefits to hospitals: improved ability to attract and retain the most qualified nurses, improved client care, a safe and pleasurable work environment, a collaborative culture, and an opportunity to advance nursing standards of practice and become a growing business and financial success. Only 6 percent of American hospitals have earned Magnet status.[42]

The Magnet program was started in 1983 when the American Academy of Nursing (AAN) Task Force on Nursing Practices studied work environments in hospitals that attracted and retained well-qualified nurses who promoted quality client care. Hospitals that demonstrated these qualities were designated as "magnet hospitals."[42] Building upon this study, the AAN board of directors approved a proposal for the Magnet Hospital Recognition Program for Excellence in Nursing Services. The most current Magnet Recognition Model Program has five components:

1. Transformational leadership
2. Structural empowerment
3. Exemplary professional practice
4. New knowledge, innovation, and improvements
5. Empirical quality results

Several research studies have shown a link between the Magnet hospital experience and increased client satisfaction, decreased mortality rates, decreased pressure ulcers, decreased falls, and improved client safety and quality.[42]

Conclusion

Quality can be an elusive goal for the health-care professional, the health-care institution, and the client and family. To provide the best care possible, the health-care facility must develop a culture of quality wherein quality is the central goal and not just an add-on feature to care. Quality requires commitment by multidisciplinary team members and health-care institutions to provide, monitor, assess, and evaluate the effectiveness of processes and structures to make improvements and to achieve optimal health-care outcomes. Quality challenges the nurse to be constantly vigilant; to be aware of high-risk situations; and to be dedicated to processes, structures, and policies that ensure quality.

Quality necessitates an informed health-care consumer. It is critical that the consumer is aware and informed of health-care quality and safety issues and utilizes that information to make health-care choices. The benefits of quality include efficiency, cost-effectiveness, timeliness, client and staff satisfaction, safety, and equitable client-centered care. Quality care results in positive client care outcomes. Quality care benefits the client, family, interdisciplinary health team members, and health-care institutions. In this time of health-care change, all stakeholders are poised for the challenge.

CRITICAL-THINKING EXERCISES

- Identify three quality-improvement activities that are being used in the facility where you have clinical.
- Develop a plan for quality improvement using the IOM report recommendations.
- How does the QSEN initiative improve quality and safety in health care?
- Describe what a culture of quality might look like in a hospital.
- How do client-satisfaction survey findings affect quality of care?
- Is there a clearcut advantage in using the *Essentials of Baccalaureate Education for Professional Nursing Practice* over the QSEN competencies as a curricular model, or is the best approach to integrate them?

NCLEX-STYLE QUESTIONS

1. In 2000, the Institute of Medicine's report *To Err Is Human* recommended system changes to reduce the high number of people who died each year due to adverse events and medical errors in hospitals. What has been the overall effect of these changes on client mortality?
   1. The number of deaths due to adverse events and medical errors has risen.
   2. The number of deaths due to adverse events and medical errors has decreased.
   3. The number of deaths has stayed the same, but the number of adverse events and medical errors has decreased.
   4. The number of deaths has decreased, but the number of adverse events and medical errors has increased.

2. In 2001, the Institute of Medicine (IOM) identified six aims for improving health care in the United States. Which of the following are NOT characteristics the IOM identified? **Select all that apply.**
   1. Affordable
   2. Safe
   3. Effective
   4. Local
   5. Client-centered
   6. Timely
   7. Efficient
   8. Equitable

3. Which of the following is the best definition of *quality* as it relates to health care?
   1. The extent to which clients are satisfied with their health outcomes and the care they received
   2. The provision of as much safe, effective care as the client can afford
   3. The degree to which health services increase the likelihood of desired outcomes and reflect current professional knowledge
   4. The extent to which outcomes can be quantified and compared to industry standards

4. The clinical instructor asks Darla to explain to a postoperative client the importance of using an incentive spirometer to inhale deeply. What Quality and Safety Education for Nurses (QSEN) competency is the instructor assessing?
   1. Client-centered care
   2. Teamwork and collaboration
   3. Evidence-based practice
   4. Quality improvement
   5. Safety
   6. Informatics

5. Which of the following statements about how education relates to quality and safety in nursing care is true? **Select all that apply.**
   1. Education in quality and safety begins in nursing school.
   2. Continuing education allows nurses to update their knowledge and skills to improve quality and safety.
   3. Increasing nursing education levels has been shown to improve client outcomes and quality.
   4. The type of quality and safety education a nurse receives depends on the hospital or facility in which the nurse works.
   5. Hospitals are unwilling to spend money on quality and safety education for nurses.

6. Richard, an RN, is preparing to receive Mr. Rocha, an elderly client who had a stroke 2 days ago, from the ICU. From report, Richard learns that Mr. Rocha is awake and oriented, is NPO because of swallowing problems, and is experiencing weakness on his right side. According to The Joint Commission's National Patient Safety Goals, which of the following is the most important thing Richard should do to prepare for Mr. Rocha's arrival?
   1. Wipe down the room with strong disinfecting wipes.
   2. Alert the nurse aide that Mr. Rocha is on his way.
   3. Make sure that the room is properly stocked and ready.
   4. Be sure there are signs in the room indicating that Mr. Rocha is NPO and a fall risk.

7. One system of quality improvement that has been tried in health care is _____, which was originally developed to improve quality in manufacturing but has since been used to identify problems and find effective solutions in health care.

8. Root-cause analysis, an essential part of risk management, is conducted after an adverse event. What are the components of root-case analysis? **Select all that apply.**
   1. Identifying who caused the adverse event
   2. Tracking the events that led to the error
   3. Identifying any faulty systems or processes
   4. Developing a plan to prevent further errors

9. Which of the following best describes Leapfrog Group's approach to improving the quality and safety of health care and making it more affordable?
   1. Reimbursing low-performing hospitals at a lower rate than other facilities and publishing this information to alert the public
   2. Financially rewarding hospitals that implement significant improvements in quality and safety and offering incentives for consumers who choose high-performing hospitals
   3. Requiring that consumers use only certain low-cost hospitals and submit reports on their quality
   4. Refusing to reimburse hospitals if a client is readmitted within 30 days of discharge

10. Yolanda, an RN, says that asking clients for two identifiers—name and birthdate—every time she gives them medication is a waste of time. Isn't one identifier enough? What response by the charge nurse is most appropriate?
    1. It does take a little extra time, but the safety of our clients is worth it.
    2. I agree, but that's our policy.
    3. If you don't follow the rules, I'll write you up.
    4. After the first time, you can just scan their wrist band.

References

1. Quality of Health Care in America Committee. The Institute of Medicine Report on Medical Errors: Misunderstanding can do harm. *Medscape*, September 19, 2000. https://www.medscape.com/viewarticle/418841
2. IMSS nursing essential in the comprehensive model for health and wellbeing. Archyde, May 17, 2022. https://www.archyde.com/imss-nursing-essential-in-the-comprehensive-model-for-health-and-well-being
3. Medical error statistics. MyMedicalScore, 2022. https://mymedical score.com/medical-error-statistics
4. Murez C. Covid was the third leading cause of death for 2020-2021. HealthDay, July 5, 2022. https://consumer.healthday.com/b-7-5-emb-11am-covid-was-third-leading-cause-of-death-for-2020-2021-2657592314.html
5. Schwencke M. Your right to know about adverse medical incidents. SearcyLaw.com, February 29, 2012. https://www.searcylaw.com/your-right-to-know-about-adverse-medical-incidents
6. Barry L. Why is quality assurance in health care crucial? IntelyCare, June 28, 2022. https://www.intelycare.com/blog/nursing-facilities/why-is-quality-assurance-in-healthcare-crucial
7. CAHPS Hospital survey. HCAHPS, 2022. https://hcahpsonline.org/
8. Leapfrog hospital safety grade. The Leapfrog Group, 2022. https://www.leapfroggroup.org/data-users/leapfrog-hospital-safety-grade
9. Scoring Leapfrog performance. The Leapfrog Group, 2022, https://ratings.leapfroggroup.org/scoring
10. Health care ratings and reports. The Leapfrog Group, 2022. https://www.leapfroggroup.org/ratings-reports
11. Agency for Healthcare Research and Quality: A Profile. AHRQ, 2022. https://www.ahrq.gov/cpi/about/profile/index.html
12. O'Donnell B, Gupta V. *Continuous Quality Improvement.* Treasure Island, FL: StatPearls Publishing, 2022.
13. Rosique R. Care pathways: The basics. Asian Hospital Healthcare Management, 2022. https://www.asianhhm.com/healthcare-management/care-pathways-basics
14. 5 Key elements in the risk management process. HSEWatch, 2022. https://hsewatch.com/5-key-elements-risk-management-process/
15. Recent sentinel activity. Sentinel, 2022. https://www.sentinel initiative.org/news-events/recent-sentinel-activity
16. Joint Commission sets patient safety definitions. Relias Media, January 2, 2015. https://www.reliasmedia.com/articles/67973-joint-commission-sets-patient-safety-definitions

17. Ubongeh. What is a near miss? Near miss examples. HSEWatch, 2022. https://hsewatch.com/what-is-a-near-miss/

18. OSHA Standards: A guide to health and safety compliance. SafetyCulture, 2022. https://safetyculture.com/topics/osha-standards/

19. Ubongeh. 6 Types of major hazards you should know. HSE-Watch, June 28, 2022. https://hsewatch.com/types-of-hazards/

20. Burdick G. OSHA focusing on COVID-19 inspections. *EHS Daily Advisor*, July 7, 2022. https://ehsdailyadvisor.blr.com/2022/07/osha-focusing-on-covid-19-inspections/

21. Kumar P. What is Six Sigma: Everything you need to know about it. Simplilearn, 2022. https://www.simplilearn.com/what-is-six-sigma-a-complete-overview-article

22. Scheiner M. What is Six Sigma methodology? Processes & principles guide. CRM.org, July 1, 2022. https://crm.org/news/six-sigma-methodology

23. What is value stream mapping? Benefits and implementation. Kanbanize, 2022. https://kanbanize.com/lean-management/value-waste/value-stream-mapping

24. Six Sigma belts: Definition, methodology and reasons to acquire a Six Sigma certification. Performance Institute, July 5, 2022. http://www.performanceinstitute.org/blog/six-sigma-belts

25. Brown L. Six Sigma awareness—An overview, importance, and applications. Invensis Global Learning Services, 2022. https://www.invensislearning.com/blog/six-sigma-awareness/

26. Ball K. Scrum in healthcare: Operating room process improvements lead to better outcomes for patients and more revenue for providers. Scruminc, June 22, 2020. https://www.scruminc.com/scrum-in-healthcare/

27. Iqbal M. Why teams adopted Scrum during the pandemic. Scrum.org, July 5, 2022. https://www.scrum.org/resources/blog/why-teams-adopted-scrum-during-pandemic

28. Di Vincenzo P. Team huddles: A winning strategy for safety. *Nursing*, 47(7):59–60, 2017. https://doi.org/10.1097/01.NURSE.0000520522.84449.0e.

29. Ochoa H. QSEN competencies: Set the tone of your shift. Nursing CE Central, June 10, 2022. https://nursingcecentral.com/qsen-competencies/

30. The new AACN essentials. American Association of Colleges of Nursing, 2022. https://www.aacnnursing.org/AACN-Essentials

31. Frequently asked questions. American Association of Colleges of Nursing, 2022. https://www.aacnnursing.org/essentials/tool-kit/faqs

32. Medicare quality initiative and patient assessment instruments. CMS.gov, 2021. https://www.cms.gov/Medicare/Quality-Initiatives-Patient-Assessment-Instruments/QualityImprovementOrgs

33. What are never events and why do the occur? Golden Law Office, 2022. https://goldenlawoffice.com/medical-malpractice/what-are-never-events-and-why-do-they-occur/

34. Grimes C, Thornell B, Clark A, Viney M. Developing rapid response teams: Best practices through collaboration. *Clinical Nurse Specialist*, 21(2):85–92, 2007. https://doi.org/10.1097/00002800-200703000-00007

35. Evidence based practice. Eastern Health Library, November 25, 2022. https://easternhealth.libguides.com/EBP

36. Doyle A. What are teamwork skills? The Balance, July 6, 2022. https://www.thebalancecareers.com/list-of-teamwork-skills-2063773

37. What exactly is health informatics? Healthcare Management, 2022. https://www.healthcare-management-degree.net/faq/what-exactly-is-health-informatics/

38. Androus A. Do BSN educated nurses provide better patient care? *RegisteredNursing.org*, 2022. https://www.registerednursing.org/articles/do-bsn-educated-nurses-provide-better-patient-care/

39. Tri-Council for Nursing. Homepage. n.d. https://tricouncilfornursing.org/

40. New partnership of leading organizations in nursing education and community college leadership reflects NLN's longstanding support of academic progression and lifelong learning. National League for Nursing, October 12, 2012. https://www.nln.org/detail-pages/news/2012/10/12/National-League-for-Nursing-Applauds-Landmark-Joint-Statement-on-Academic-Progression-for-Nursing-Students-and-Graduates#:

41. Stoller C. What is blameless reporting? Chirp, March 3, 2016. https://chirp.cyrusstoller.com/blameless-reporting

42. Gagnon D. What is a Magnet Hospital? Southern New Hampshire University, November 5, 2021. https://www.snhu.edu/about-us/newsroom/health/what-is-a-magnet-hospital

15

Delegation in Nursing

Joseph T. Catalano

Learning Objectives

After completing this chapter, the reader will be able to:

- Apply the principles of delegation to nursing practice
- Analyze and identify situations in which delegation is used improperly
- Discuss the legal implications of delegation in the current health-care setting
- Distinguish between delegation and assignment

AN ESSENTIAL SKILL

Delegation is an essential component of patient care and management of nursing units in today's health-care system. It allows health-care managers to maximize the use of caregivers who are educated at multiple levels in a variety of programs. Delegation, if performed properly, permits nurses to meet the requirements of high-quality care for all patients and is a basic skill that registered nurses (RNs) must learn. However, the skill set required to delegate safely is one of the most complex that nurses must master, requiring the ability to make high-level clinical judgments. The goal of delegation is to meet the increased demands for services as they intersect with the shrinking resources of the health-care system.[1]

Look to All These Things

The concept of delegation has been a part of health care since the time of Florence Nightingale, when she instructed the nurses she educated that "to look to all these things yourself does not mean to do them yourself."[2] As far back as 1991, the American Nurses Association (ANA) initially addressed and defined *delegation* when it was beginning to become more widespread in health care. The ANA further refined the definition in 1997. The National Council of State Boards of Nursing (NCSBN) addressed delegation in 1995 but made a major leap forward in development in 2016 when, in conjunction with the ANA, the NCSBN produced a Joint Statement on Delegation. The organizations recognized in this document the ever-growing demands being made on nurses from large numbers of older patients and rapidly developing technology. One essential skill that all nurses must have is the ability to delegate, assign, and supervise assistive personnel safely and effectively.[1]

DELEGATION OR ASSIGNMENT?

Although delegation and assignment are closely related concepts, they are different. **Delegation** is the process whereby a nurse (an RN) directs another health-care team member to perform specific nursing tasks, procedures, and activities that are beyond that person's traditional role and are not routinely performed by them. The NCSBN describes this process as the nurse transferring *authority* to perform the task. The ANA calls this direction a transfer of *responsibility*. Both organizations believe that an RN can direct another individual to do a task that they would not normally be allowed to do. Both organizations stress that the RN retains accountability for the delegation. This applies whether the delegate is a licensed nurse, an unlicensed assistive personnel (UAP), or another member of the health-care team, regardless of the current role of the delegatee (RN, licensed practical nurse [LPN], licensed vocational nurse [LVN], or UAP). When an RN delegates to a licensed nurse, the delegated responsibility must be within the parameters of the delegatee's authorized scope of practice under the nurse practice act (NPA) of the state where the RN is practicing.[1]

Delegation becomes a bit more confusing when one RN is delegating to another RN. The presumption is that all RNs should have the same level of knowledge and skill and be guided by the same scope of practice in the NPA. Therefore, if RN #1 can perform exactly the same tasks as RN #2, then it would appear that what RN #2 is doing when directing RN #1 to provide care for a specific patient would be assignment—not delegation—since the care being provided should be within the scope of practice of RN #1. However, in the real patient-care world, RNs may have different levels of knowledge and skill. For example, a new graduate RN, a new-hire RN, an RN pulled from a specialty unit, or even an associate's degree RN may not possess the same levels of knowledge, past experiences, skills, abilities, and competencies that the more experienced RN possesses.

The RN should delegate according to the identified skills and knowledge level for each of the staff members. The same level of patient care should not be delegated equally to a patient care technician (PCT), a certified nursing assistant (CNA), an LPN or LVN, a new graduate RN, an associate's degree RN, and a bachelor's degree RN.

For example, if an RN delegates elements of patient care to an LPN who is not trained or educated to perform the skills that are outside the scope of practice of an LPN, the RN is placing the patient in potential physical harm. In delegating to the LPN, the RN is

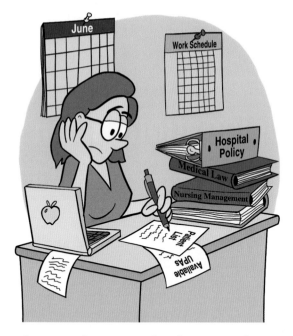

A nurse administrator's job is never done.

performing an illegal act if the LPN accepts the delegated task. If there is a bad outcome from the delegation, the RN and the LPN may be charged with malpractice or negligent homicide if the patient should die as a result of the care. (See Chapter 8.) All levels of nursing staff, including RNs, should refuse to accept any task that is outside their scope of practice or for which they do not have the expected skill or knowledge level.[3]

Responsibility can be delegated. Accountability can *never* be delegated. The nursing process cannot be delegated. The delegating RN is always accountable for all the care a patient receives, even though some of the elements of care can be, and are, delegated to other members of the health-care team. The delegating RN is also responsible for supervision and evaluation of the care being provided by the delegatee in terms of quality, appropriateness, and timeliness. The RN who has delegated patient care must ensure that the delegated activities have been carried out correctly by the delegatee.[4]

Assignment, on the other hand, is the allocation of tasks that each staff member is already authorized to perform during a given shift. For example, RN #1 assigns RN #2 to assess a newly admitted patient. RN #2 is already authorized to assess patients, which is in RN #2's skills set and scope of practice.[3]

As in the delegation process, the RN who makes assignments must guarantee that the staff member has sufficient time during the shift to complete the assignment. The RN is also responsible for monitoring and assessing the staff members' progress toward the achievement of the tasks during the shift. Ongoing monitoring, rather than end-of-shift evaluation, is essential for quality care. By the end of a shift, it is too late to correct any mistakes.[4]

Supervision is the provision of guidance and oversight of personnel to whom a nursing task was either delegated or assigned. The ANA refers to *on-site supervision*, and NCSBN refers to *direct supervision*, but both require the physical presence and ongoing direction of the supervising RN. They both also require that the supervising RN be available on site or through various means of written and verbal communication.[1]

When RNs delegate nursing tasks to both nurses and non-nurses, the RNs must always supervise those individuals to ensure that the care given meets the standards of care. However, if the facility, the state board of nursing, or some other official body has a predesignated list of tasks that non-nursing personnel may undertake in the care of patients, the RN is responsible only for ensuring that the tasks are carried out safely.

Evaluation is the assessment of the team member's ability to complete the tasks of patient care, which were delegated or assigned by the supervising RN. The art of evaluation requires that the supervising RN use direct and indirect observations of how well the staff member is providing safe, high-quality, and timely patient care. For example, the RN can directly observe if an LPN is changing a dressing properly. An example of indirect observation would be reviewing the medication sheet to make sure the LPN gave medications on time.

Most evaluation in the clinical setting should be process or ongoing evaluation; but at the end of the shift, outcome or terminal evaluation also needs to be performed. Because communication is essential for high-quality care, the supervising RN must talk with staff members during the shift and either correct any tasks that are being performed in error or inform staff that they are doing well in accomplishing their assignment.

When the shift is done, the supervising RN needs to make an outcome evaluation. The evaluation does not need to be long or detailed; it can be a simple

"You did a very good job with your care of a difficult patient" or "The majority of the care you provided today was high quality. However, although you performed adequately, we will need to review and update your technique for dressing and packing wounds." Negative evaluation should not be a harsh, unfeeling, or merciless destruction of a person's character and personality. How would the staff member feel if instead of the preceding statement, the supervising RN said, "Didn't you learn anything in nursing school? You really screwed up that dressing change. It's a wonder the patient didn't bleed to death! Go home and read about how to change a packing and dressing!" Positive reinforcement goes a long way in developing a nursing team that is high quality and functions as a unit. Negative evaluation can become toxic and destroy the unity of the health-care team. (See Chapter 11.)

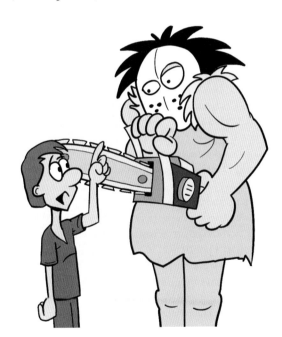

"Why don't we get someone else to remove Mrs. Lemke's sutures?"

Delegation During a Pandemic

The COVID-19 pandemic created many challenges in the delivery of health care, including a need to quickly rearrange nursing care to manage large numbers of critically ill patients. This was in addition to an existing shortage of experienced nurses. Initially, intensive care units (ICUs) required major reorganization along with structural changes such as adding bed capacity by doubling up beds in single-bed units. As COVID-19 patients overflowed into areas of the hospitals not generally accommodative to caring for critically ill patients, many facilities expanded the team nursing–care delivery model that is often used in ICUs.[3]

As nurses and support personnel were moved from their "home" units, such as labor and delivery, pediatrics, surgery, and even hospital administration, delegation became a skill in high demand.[3] Nurse managers' ability to delegate successfully was indispensable to keeping staff who were willing to stay and provide care in the midst of the health-care chaos.

One element that complicated successful delegation during the COVID-19 pandemic was the challenge of working with staff from the units that were shut down. Successful delegation requires that the delegator know the abilities and skills of the delegatee. With the arrival of personnel from other units almost every shift, nurse managers had little time to get to know the new nurses, much less time to educate them on the use of complicated life-support equipment, such as ventilators. There is nothing more terrifying for a nurse from a non-ICU area than to be thrown into the care of a critically ill patient connected to multiple IV lines, a ventilator, and a cooling apparatus.

Another factor that made pandemic delegation difficult was the lack of clarity of each person's role. Nurses tend to struggle if they do not have clearly defined roles when they are providing care, and this was particularly true while working during the confusion of a pandemic. ICU nurses did not know whether they were nurse trainers or staff nurses, and the nurses from other units did not know when they were functioning as RNs or support staff. Staff nurses need to have a clear knowledge of their role expectations. Ideally, all the "new" nurses should have been trained before being assigned to care for a COVID-19 patient. Nurses not trained in ICU care experienced the highest anxiety levels among the nurses working on COVID-19 units.[3]

Unfortunately, not every trained ICU nurse or nurse manager was interested in delegating or supervising other nurses with less training. Ineffective delegation skills on the part of nurses can produce negative outcomes for patient safety and quality of care. Due to the swift onset of the pandemic, many ICU-trained staff nurses had no prior training in delegating tasks and supervising supporting nurses.[3]

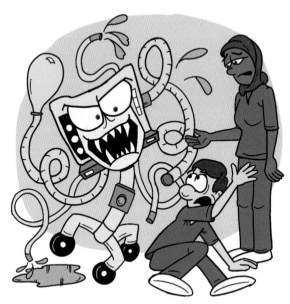

"Don't worry, ventilators don't bite."

RESPONSIBILITY AND ACCOUNTABILITY IN DELEGATING

As mentioned previously, the ANA defines *delegation* as "the transfer of responsibility for the performance of an activity from one individual to another while retaining accountability for the outcome."[5] The ANA stresses that even though the leader or manager delegates a task to another employee, the delegator remains accountable for the care that is provided. This process has become more complicated legally since advanced practice registered nurses (APRNs) are now practicing in much larger numbers. However, APRNs are held to the same standards as RNs when it comes to delegating and making assignments. Physicians follow their own practice acts and generally are not permitted to delegate to RNs or APRNs, although they may try to.[5] During the COVID-19 pandemic and its close-quarter working conditions, it became obvious that some physicians who were used to giving orders really did not understand the concept of delegation.[3]

Responsibility is the duty of a person, as a reasonable and prudent member of a particular group by training or licensure, to complete tasks and assignments that are within their power, control, and authority. For example, if a person works on a surgical unit where there are many dressing changes, it is that person's *responsibility* to learn dressing change techniques and that person's *responsibility* to perform them correctly when assigned to do so. The team member is then demonstrating the condition or actuality of being liable, or answerable, for something within their power, control, or supervision. Responsibility also includes the concept of a person being able to or authorized to take actions or make decisions by themselves, particularly when they are in charge of other individuals, by assuring that what these persons are doing is correct and safe.[1]

Accountability is an obligation or willingness to be answerable for one's own actions and/or the actions of another, particularly where there is assignment or delegation of tasks. Although the term *accountability* is related to *responsibility*, it emphasizes oversight. For example, an LPN may be responsible for checking a critically ill patient's vital signs every 15 minutes. In the event that the LPN misses several of the vital sign checks during a 12-hour shift, there may or may not be consequences, depending on the patient outcome. Accountability, on the other hand, means that the LPN and the supervising RN are held answerable for successfully completing the task and will have to at least explain why they failed to do so. Accountability can be used to identify the team member who is ultimately answerable for the correct and safe completion of the assignment as well as the one who delegated or assigned the task to the team member. It implies ethical and/or legal obligations along with the possibility of legal action or punishment.

Nurses sometimes say, "If I delegate, then that person is practicing on my license, and I don't want the responsibility." This statement implies that responsibility has legal liability attached to it. In reality, it does have liability attached, but only with the performance of duties in the specific role. When they accept a delegated task, assistive personnel accept the responsibility attached to it. **Delegatees do not practice on the RN's license.** They practice on their own license (LPNs and LVNs) or, if unlicensed, within their own level of education. Assistive personnel, when they agree to accept the delegated task, are responsible for their own actions in performance of the task.[6]

When RNs accept responsibility for delegating a task appropriately, they become accountable for the delegation process. Accountability in this situation means that the RN used their nursing knowledge, critical thinking, and clinical judgment skills in delegating a task. For example, suppose an RN delegates a task to a UAP that is appropriate for the person's educational level and skill set. The task that the UAP is assigned to perform is to give a very debilitated elderly woman a bath in the walk-in bathtub in the tub room. The UAP uses a wheelchair to transfer the patient to the tub room and places her in the tub, closes the tub door, and turns on the water. Because it takes a long time to fill the tub, the UAP tells the patient that she will be right back to help her bathe because the UAP needs to get some towels and washcloths that she forgot to bring.

When she turned on the water, the UAP determined that it was at an appropriate bath temperature by letting it run on her hand; however, while the water is running, it becomes very hot. The tub room has thick walls and is almost soundproof. The weak screams of the patient go unheard. Because of her debility, the woman is unable to adjust the water controls. While the UAP is obtaining towels and washcloths, another patient falls in the hall, and the UAP goes to help her back to her room. By the time the UAP returns to the tub room, the elderly woman is unconscious and has second- and third-degree burns over most of her body. She dies the day after the bath.

Is the RN who made the assignment accountable for the patient's death? Legally, the RN met the requirements of accountability in assigning the UAP, who by training and education was qualified to give a walk-in tub bath. The responsibility for the patient's death rests solely on the UAP, who violated several elements of

> *Delegatees do not practice on the RN's license. They practice on their own license (LPNs and LVNs) or, if unlicensed, within their own level of education.*

patient safety by not remaining with the patient and not monitoring the temperature of the bathwater.[1] On the other hand, if the RN had delegated inappropriately, such as to a first-year nursing student who is clearly *not* qualified by education or licensure, and the patient died, the RN and that person could both be held liable. So how does the RN make the decision to delegate or not to delegate? The steps outlined in the following sections are a guide to the decision-making process.

Guidelines for Delegation

Assess the Patient

Before delegating any task, RNs should carefully consider the condition of the patient and the patient's health-care needs. Assessing patients is a designated responsibility of RNs. Without a thorough assessment, it is likely that critical needs will remain unidentified by less-trained personnel, leading to potential errors in care. Patients who are relatively stable and are not likely to experience drastic changes in health-care status are the most suitable for delegation. Also, the tasks being delegated must be relatively uncomplicated and routine, must be performed without variation from policy or procedure, and should not require the use of nursing judgment while being performed. For example, the health-care provider has ordered that a patient with renal disease have his catheter outputs measured each hour to monitor hydration status. This task requires opening a drainage cap on a special collection device connected to the patient's urinary catheter every hour and measuring how much urine is present. It is a low-risk, relatively simple procedure that the RN can easily delegate to an LPN or even a UAP. Delegation of repetitive tasks to less-educated personnel produces higher efficiency because the time and skills of the RN are used more effectively.

> *The delegating nurse needs to know the availability of staff and the education and competency levels of the personnel to be delegated to.*

What Do You Think?

Is delegation used in the facility where you have clinical rotations? Who does the delegation on the unit? Does it work well?

Know Staff Availability

The delegating nurse needs to know the availability of staff and the education and competency levels of the personnel to be delegated to. These factors must be matched with the level of care required by the patient. Key information to obtain is how often the delegatee has performed the required tasks or cared for this type of patient, what units the delegatee has worked on and feels comfortable in, and their organizational abilities. It is important to keep the team informed of who is delegated which tasks and when changes are made.[1]

Know the Job Description

One large group of health-care workers to whom RNs delegate is the UAPs. This group includes individuals who have been through some type of training program ranging from a few hours to several months (Box 15.1). UAPs may receive a certificate of completion, but they do not have any type of licensure and therefore do not have legal status.

The RN needs to know the institution's official position description for the UAP as well as the individual UAP's abilities. For example, the position description may state that the UAP can care for postoperative patients who have multiple wound drains. However, when the RN assigns a specific UAP to such a postoperative patient, the nurse discovers that the UAP has worked only in the newborn nursery for the past 5 years and has no knowledge of how to care for adult postoperative patients with drainage tubes.

If the RN delegates this UAP to care for complicated postoperative patients and a major complication develops because of the UAP's lack of competence (even though the position description states that this is an appropriate function for the UAP), the RN will also be held legally liable for any injuries that the patients might suffer. When the RN determines that the patient's needs match the skills and abilities of the UAP or LPN, only then should that person be assigned.

Box 15.1 Other Names for Unlicensed Assistive Personnel (UAP)

Certified nurse assistant (CNA)

Nurse's aide

Home health aide

Registered nurse assistant (RNA)

Nurse technician (NT)

Medication technician (MT)

Nursing assistant

Patient care assistant (PCA)

Orderly

Patient attendant

Psychiatric attendant

Educate the Staff Member

RNs who assign or delegate are also responsible for educating the team member about the task to be done. If the team member is unfamiliar with the task, the RN is required to demonstrate how the task or procedure is performed and then document the training. Education also includes telling the team member what is expected in the completion of the task and what complications to watch for and report to the RN. The ANA suggests that the RN watch the team member perform the designated task at least initially, then make periodic observations throughout the shift to ensure safe and competent care for the patient.[7] Furthermore, the RN must always be available to answer questions and help the team member whenever assistance is required. Consider the following situation:

Elsie Humber, RN, is the evening charge nurse on a busy oncology unit of the county hospital. She has worked on the unit for 5 years and is usually in the charge nurse position. On one particularly busy evening, she discovers during shift report that the other scheduled RN has called in sick and no other RNs are available to take her place. Ms. Humber assigns the duties and patients that would usually be assigned to the second RN to an LPN instead. One of

the patients in the assigned group includes an elderly man on chemotherapy for colon cancer, who has a complicated tunneled wound of the abdomen that needs to be repacked and redressed each shift.

Although the LPN has worked on the unit for several months, he protests the assignment, saying he has never done one of these types of dressing changes before. Ms. Humber rebukes him, saying, "I have no one else. If you don't care for this patient, he won't get any care at all this shift, and you will be guilty of patient abandonment."

The LPN reluctantly agrees to care for the patient. During the dressing change, the LPN is fearful that the wound might bleed, so he leaves the last layer of old packing in place and puts the new sterile packing on top of it, which provides an excellent atmosphere for the growth of bacteria. In addition, he uses the sharp stick end of the long cotton swab to apply the antiseptic ointment to the edges of the wound. This process damages the newly healed tissue.

Because of the patient's suppressed immune system from chemotherapy and generally debilitated condition, he develops a serious infection of the blood (septicemia). After a protracted stay in the hospital, the patient dies. The family sues the LPN, the RN, and the hospital for malpractice. The hospital administration attempts to shift all the legal responsibility for the infection and death of the patient to Ms. Humber and the LPN.

Using the information provided, answer these questions:

- Who is legally responsible for the incident?
- Who is accountable?
- Does the patient's family's case meet the criteria for a successful lawsuit? (See Chapter 8.)

Predictable and Uncomplicated

When a nurse delegates tasks, the outcomes of tasks should be clear and predictable. For example, when a UAP is assigned the task of feeding a patient who has suffered a stroke and has hemiplegia, the predicted outcome will be that the patient will eat and not choke

Issues Now

The Professional Nurse Coach—A New Role in Practice

Although RNs regularly coach patients and other nurses informally as a part of their practice, the American Holistic Nurses Credentialing Corporation recognizes coaching as a formal role and offers certification for nurse coaches. Recently, the Interprofessional Education Collaborative Expert Panel in conjunction with the International Coach Federation identified coaching as a key element in the movement toward interprofessional education.

A professional nurse coach must be an RN who is grounded in the holistic concept of nursing care, uses evidence-based nursing theory, and has social and scientific behavioral knowledge to facilitate a process of change and development in patients and other nurses, thereby facilitating their ability to reach their maximum potential. The practice of nurse coach is grounded in the ANA *Nursing: Scope and Standards of Practice*, second edition, and the ANA Code of Ethics for Nurses. Nurse coaching is a relationship-based process and necessitates strong interpersonal relationship abilities. The skills required for a nurse coach include the ability to

- Identify individuals ready for change in their lives and then establish a therapeutic relationship with the individual. If patients or nurses are not ready for change, the process cannot go forward.
- Understand and acknowledge where patients are in their movement toward wellness. The patient may have issues and concerns that need to be identified to facilitate the coaching process.
- Work collaboratively with the patient in identifying goals and outcomes from the coaching process. If the patient does not know what they wish to achieve, then the patient will not know when they achieve it.
- Establish an agreement with the patient, either formally or informally, about how to achieve the goals. This plan should outline what the nurse's and the patient's responsibilities are in the process.
- Use communication and dialogue to motivate and help the patient work to achieve their goals. In conjunction with the patient, actions and activities are selected as interventions. Keeping the patient motivated is key in achieving established goals.
- Identify which goals the patient has achieved and which ones remain.

The nurse coach plays an important role in the development of the wellness model that is slowly but surely revitalizing the health-care system. Other nonprofessional health-care workers have embraced the coaching role, and some are seeking certification as health-care coaches. RNs, with their education in the behavioral sciences and their familiarity with research and health-care theories, are already well on the way to becoming nurse coaches. By seeking official certification as a professional nurse coach, RNs gain visibility as leaders in the emerging coach role.

Source: *Nurse health coach, RegisteredNursing.org, 2022, https://www.registerednursing.org/specialty/nurse-health-coach.*

on the food. The task should not require excessive supervision, complex decision making, or detailed assessment during its performance. If any of these elements is required, the task needs to be reassigned to an LPN or RN.

It is important to remember that when nurses delegate nursing tasks, they are *not* delegating nursing. Professional nursing practice is a science, based on a unique body of knowledge, and an art, guided by the nursing process. It is not merely a collection of tasks. Of all health-care workers, professional nurses are the most qualified to provide holistic care of the patient by promoting health and treating disease. RNs' education and experience

Box 15.2 **Five Rights of Delegation**

- Right task: Do the tasks delegated follow written policy guidelines?
- Right person: Does the person have the proper qualifications for the tasks?
- Right direction or communication: Are the instructions and outcomes clearly stated? When should the person report changes?
- Right supervision or feedback: How can the delegation process be improved? Are the patient goals for care being achieved?
- Right circumstances: Are the tasks that are being delegated possible without independent nursing judgments?

Source: S.A. Weiss, R.M. Tappen, D.K. Whitehead, *Essentials of Nursing Leadership and Management* (7th ed.), Philadelphia, PA: F.A. Davis, 2021.

provide them with the skills and knowledge to coordinate and supervise nursing care and to delegate specific tasks to others.

Although mastering delegation skills can seem like a daunting task, a nurse can take several commonsense steps to attain this skill. The Five Rights of Delegation are an easy way to remember what the RN must consider when delegating (Box 15.2). In addition, the NCSBN has developed a decision tree for delegation to nursing assistive personnel, which is very useful in making decisions about delegation (Fig. 15.1). Nursing students often have tasks delegated to them by the RNs on the units where they are having clinical rotations. It is easy to identify the RNs who have developed good delegation skills and those who still need to work on those skills.

DEVELOPING DELEGATION SKILLS

Clear Communication

In the process of developing delegation skills, students should try to emulate good delegators. Good delegators have developed good communication and interpersonal relationship skills. They make eye contact with the other person, are pleasant, and ask for suggestions. Good delegators avoid allowing the person to whom the tasks are being delegated to control the exchange by intimidation or resistance. However,

if a person sincerely believes that they lack the knowledge and skills to perform the delegated tasks, the delegator must recognize that they will have to either teach the person how to perform the task or delegate the task to another team member. (See Chapter 12 for more tips on communication.)

After a nurse delegates a task, it is a good idea to make a written list of the responsibilities that are expected from the person, if such a list does not already exist. The list will help clarify what is expected and head off possible misunderstandings. It is also important to be flexible. Patients' conditions change, new patients get admitted, and other patients get discharged. The original assignments may have to be modified in response to changes in the environment.[7]

Simulation Exercises

Both nursing education and nursing service can increase the knowledge and skills required for effective delegation through simulation scenarios that reflect daily practice. There is an increasing emphasis on simulation in nursing education, and delegation scenarios can be used alongside clinical practice ones. For students, these scenarios can be an introduction to the type of critical-thinking and decision-making skills required for effective delegation. For practicing RNs, delegation scenarios reinforce earlier learned skills and demonstrate the authority the RN has in the delegation process.

Simulations allows the student or RN to make mistakes and learn from them. Feedback is essential to the educational process and allows participants to self-evaluate their interpersonal, communication, and decision-making skills.[8]

Careful Supervision

Effective delegation and assignment of tasks requires the RN to master supervision skills, which include monitoring delegatees while they provide care and helping them when they require assistance. Are they doing what they should be doing? Do they understand the responsibilities involved in the patient's care? Effective delegation also presumes that the delegator will teach delegatees who demonstrate a lack of knowledge. Continual feedback throughout the shift allows both parties an opportunity for ongoing assessment. Most important, at the end of the shift, say,

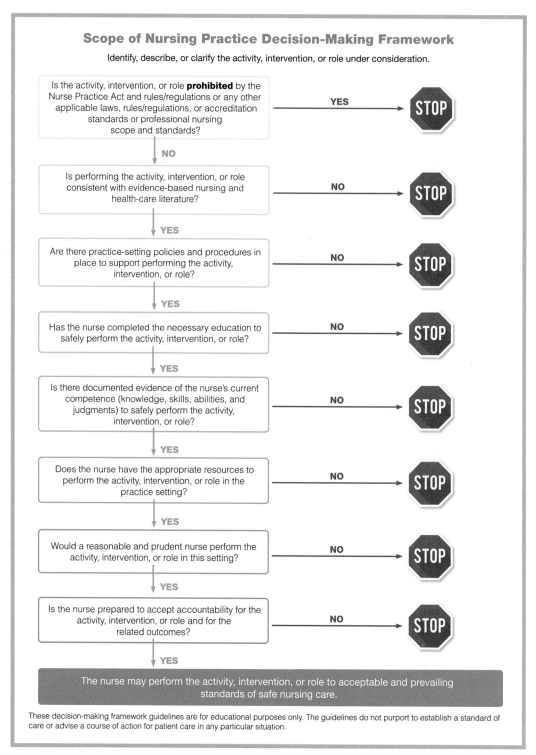

Figure 15.1 NCSBN decision tree. (*Source:* K. Ballard, D. Haagenson, L. Christiansen, et al. Scope of nursing practice decision-making framework. *Journal of Nursing Regulations*.7(3):19–21, 2016. https://doi.org/10.1016/S2155-8256(16)32316-X)

Issues in Practice

Leadership/Management Case Study: Poor Staff Performance

Angela is the emergency department (ED) nurse manager in a small rural hospital. Hiring qualified RNs for her staff became more of a challenge as the nursing shortage worsened. For 8 months, a full-time evening RN position had gone unfilled. During this time, the position was filled by cross-training nurses from other departments, paying bonus shifts and overtime, contracting with agencies, and hiring available nurses from other hospitals. These nurses were excellent, but the ED lacked the continuity of regular staffing. Angela believed this lack of continuity was negatively affecting morale and efficiency in the department.

At this hospital, the vice president of nursing services (VPNS) made all the final decisions about hiring new staff after consulting with the nurse managers. The VPNS suggested an employee who was interested in the position but did not have the experience of the nurses usually hired for the ED. Ted, who had been an LPN in a long-term care facility, had gone back to school for his BSN. After graduating, he began working in a physician's office. Although his combined health-care experience was more than 10 years, he had never worked in an acute care setting.

When Angela interviewed Ted, he appeared highly motivated, intelligent, and well groomed. Because of the nursing shortage, it had become fairly common practice to let new graduates work in specialty areas, such as EDs or intensive care units, without the traditional mandatory year of medical-surgical experience. Angela believed that Ted could, over time, learn the ED routines. He would have an experienced RN working with him for at least a year. Also, at this hospital, 90 percent of ED visits were nonurgent, office-type visits. Ted's experience of coordinating and moving patients through a busy office practice would be an asset.

Angela started by giving Ted a thorough and extended orientation to the ED. She consulted with each nurse he would be working with and asked for support in mentoring him. She encouraged the nurses to begin by letting Ted care for the more routine cases and then gradually allow him to care for patients with more acute conditions. During the orientation, Ted seemed to master the assessment and documentation aspects of the job well. Ted was also studying for advance cardiac life support (ACLS) certification. Obviously, he was unfamiliar with many of the medications routinely used in the ED. Angela encouraged him to ask questions and use the unit's medication reference books.

However, despite all the efforts at orientation, Ted made four serious medication errors during his first 2 months in the ED. Fortunately, they were discovered early enough so that no serious harm came to the patients. Ted was counseled by the hospital's nurse educator, who worked with him on a medication review. He completed the course of study successfully and passed the medication examination.

Angela began receiving feedback from the other ED staff members who had been working with Ted. They expressed insecurity about the quality of the care he was giving, and some believed he was not "carrying his load" during busy times. He would manipulate patient assignments and shift work to other nurses. A personality conflict had also arisen between Ted and some of the nurses. They had begun watching his every move and documenting what he was doing or not doing. Some observed that he would leave the ED for unscheduled long breaks without notifying anyone. Others remarked that he was not monitoring patients with cardiac problems as closely as they thought he should. Angela noted that Ted seemed to have lost the support of his coworkers and that the overall morale of the unit was deteriorating.

Angela met with Ted and suggested that he attend a certified ED nurse review course to improve his knowledge and skills in emergency nursing. He did attend the course. Angela also met with him several times to develop plans for improving his work. Each time, he would complete the requirements of the plan, and the situation would improve for a while. After a week or two, however, he would slip back into his previous behaviors.

(continued)

Issues in Practice (continued)

As the morale of the unit continued to decline, Angela began feeling depressed and under stress. She sensed that she was losing credibility and the respect of her staff. One day she overheard one of the staff nurses say, "At this hospital, any warm body can have a job," implying that the standards and quality of care were poor. On the other hand, Angela felt responsible for placing Ted in a situation in which he could not succeed.

Questions for Thought
1. Identify the erroneous assumptions used in the initial hiring of Ted.
2. What other measures could Angela have taken to help Ted in his adjustment to the ED?
3. What can Angela do now about the situation?

(Answers are found at the end of the chapter.)

"Thank you. I appreciate the hard work you've done today."

Certain delegation situations may place the RN at an increased risk for liability (Box 15.3). When delegating, try to avoid the following:

- Believing the team is not capable of completing the task as well as the nurse manager can
- Believing the team is not as dedicated to producing high-quality outcomes as the nurse manager is
- Believing the team does not have the motivation to complete the task and do it well
- Assigning tasks that are highly invasive or have the potential to cause significant physical harm to patients
- Assigning tasks that are designated under the scope of practice or standards of care as belonging exclusively to the RN (e.g., admission assessments, care plan development)
- Assigning tasks that the person is not trained for or lacks the knowledge to complete safely
- Assigning tasks when there is inadequate time to safely monitor or evaluate the practice of the person performing the tasks[7]

Delegation has the potential to be a powerful tool in improving the quality of patient care. The knowledge and judgment of the professional nurse remain essential elements in any health-care system reforms, including clinical integration, case management, outsourcing practices, total quality management (TQM), and continuous quality improvement (CQI).

Box 15.3 Barriers to Effective Delegation

A. Internal barriers (person delegating):
1. Lack of experience delegating
2. Lack of confidence in others
3. Personal insecurity
4. Demanding perfectionism
5. Poor organizational skills
6. Indecision
7. Poor communication skills
8. Lack of confidence in self
9. Fear of not being liked by everyone
10. Micromanaging management style

B. External barriers (circumstances or person being delegated to):
1. Unclear policies about delegation
2. Policies that do not tolerate mistakes
3. Management-by-crisis model for facility
4. Unclear delineation of authority and responsibilities
5. Poor staffing
6. Lack of competence
7. Overdependence on the person delegating
8. Unwillingness to accept responsibility for one's own practice
9. Immersion in trivia and gossip
10. Work overload

Source: D.K. Whitehead, S.A. Weiss, R.M. Tappen, *Essentials of Nursing Leadership and Management* (6th ed.), Philadelphia, PA: F.A. Davis, 2019.

What Do You Think?

What qualities have you observed in good delegators?
What qualities made the poor delegators ineffective?

LEGAL ISSUES IN DELEGATION

Legally, the authority or power to delegate is restricted to professionals who are licensed and governed by a statutory practice act. Because of their licensure, RNs are considered professionals with state-sanctioned powers and authority governed by an NPA and therefore are authorized to delegate independent nursing functions to other personnel. However, not all RN functions can be delegated to assistive personnel because of restrictions in the NPA or in institutional policies. For example, performing admission assessments, developing care plans, and making nursing diagnoses are activities generally restricted to RNs only.

In the everyday work setting, RNs usually make assignments and delegate tasks, often to the same individuals. Understanding delegation and assignment can be puzzling, but clarifying the difference can be helpful in reducing confusion. Understanding the concepts of supervision, authority, responsibility, and accountability are key to successful patient care.[4]

One result of managed care is the increase in nurses' liability for lawsuits in the area of supervision and delegation. In the search for cost-effective patient care, current managed-care strategies attempt to make optimal use of relatively expensive RNs by replacing them with less costly and less-educated personnel. As increasing numbers of health-care facilities restructure, the use of UAPs who have minimal education and experience will continue to increase. Although RNs have always been responsible for the delegation of some tasks and the supervision of less-qualified health-care providers, delegation is now one of the primary functions of RNs in today's health-care system.

Delegation does have some advantages. It is an RN extender that allows more care to be given to more patients than can be given by one RN. Delegation can free the RN from lower-level, time-consuming tasks so that more time can be spent planning care and performing those skills that less-prepared individuals are unable to perform. For those to whom tasks are delegated, it can serve as an incentive to learn additional skills, increase knowledge, develop a sense of initiative, and perhaps seek further formal education. Delegation, if performed properly, leaves accountability and decision-making where they belong—with the RN.

WHO CAN DELEGATE—LEGALLY?

As with most activities conducted by RNs, the legal and ethical considerations of delegation abound. The RN always must consider the probable effects and outcomes when deciding what task to delegate to which person. It is essential that RNs understand the principles of delegation and know how to delegate effectively to decrease the risk of mistakes that may cause patient injuries.

An Ethical Obligation

Most state practice acts do *not* give delegation authority to **dependent practitioners** such as LPNs, LVNs, and UAPs. In addition, professionals who delegate specific tasks retain accountability for the proper and safe completion of those tasks and take responsibility for determining whether the assigned personnel are competent to carry out the task. One exception occurs when the person who is assigned a task also has a license and the tasks fall under that person's scope of practice.[10] The RN is responsible only for supervision of the other licensed person. These situations are often seen when LPNs or LVNs are assigned to patient care.

The delegation and supervision responsibilities of RNs have been and continue to be a major concern for the nursing profession, both ethically and legally. The ANA Code of Ethics for Nurses states, "The nurse is responsible for assessing the competency of other nurses and health care personnel before transferring or assigning care duties of patients to other colleagues. The nurse is also responsible for monitoring the activities of these personnel and

> *" The delegation and supervision responsibilities of RNs have been and continue to be a major concern for the nursing profession, both ethically and legally. "*

evaluating the quality of care that is provided to the patient. RNs must not assign a task to an individual whom he/she knows is not qualified to perform it" (statement 4–4.4).[10] According to the ANA, RNs are obligated by their professional and ethical responsibilities to reject or object to any patient assignment that may put patient health or welfare at risk for a potentially catastrophic event.[10]

It is clear that RNs can, and in certain situations must, refuse assignments, but do LPNs/LVNs and UAPs also have that obligation or right to refuse an assignment they believe they are unqualified to carry out? The answer is yes, if one or more of the following conditions exist:

• There is no one to properly supervise the LPN/LVN or UAP/can.
• The LPN/LVN or UAP/CNA has not been trained to perform the assigned task.
• The LPN/LVN or UAP/CNA feels the assigned task is illegal or unethical.
• The assigned task could put the patient and/or the LPN/LVN or UAP/CNA at risk or in danger.
• The task requires that the LPN/LVN or UAP/CNA use nursing judgment.[10]

By law, an LPN/LVN or a UAP/CNA cannot delegate; however, they can ask for help with an assignment. They cannot tell or ask for another person to complete their work.[11]

When can a worker refuse an assignment? The most desirable to least desirable times are listed next.

Anticipatory. If it looks like the assignment may be in an area or with a patient the delegatee lacks the skills to provide safe care to, the worker should make an appointment with the nurse manager before the shift starts. This will put the manager on alert that there may be an issue with assignment. The worker needs to ask some questions: What are the requirements for caring for these types of patients? Does the facility have a policy manual with a competency checklist for this type of patient? Is special training required, such as Pediatric Advanced Life Support (PALS) or Advanced Cardiac Life Support (ACLS)? Is any type of orientation required before working on the unit?[12]

Report Assignments. The worker should refuse the assignment before report ends. This way the assignments can be rearranged, and another worker can be assigned to care for the patient. If the worker has received shift report and accepted an assignment, they should not refuse the assignment.[11]

Post-Report Refusal. After report is the worst time to make a patient-assignment refusal. However, if the worker really believes they cannot carry out the assignment, they need to approach the manager as soon as possible after report and say something like, "I didn't realize this patient was so critical. I am sorry, but I strongly believe that I am not safe caring for this patient, as I do not have the required skills and have never received this level of training. I believe if I care for this patient, I will put the patient at risk for injury and the hospital and myself at risk for possible legal liability. I am willing to take another assignment that I have the skills for and have been trained to carry out."[11]

Depending on the nurse manager, several outcomes are possible. The manager may decide to leave the assignment as is but assign another qualified nurse to work with the delegatee when higher level care is required. Another possibility is that the nurse manager makes a quick rearrangement of assignments on the fly with a new nurse being assigned to the difficult care patient and the original delegatee moved to the replacement nurse's assignment. Or if the nurse manager is really poor at their job, they may just leave the worker with the assigned patient and say something like, "Do your best. I know you are qualified to do it." Of course, this leaves both the nurse manager and the worker responsible for any injury that may occur to the patient. Also, if the nurse manager is completely unprofessional, they may just tell the worker to go home and not come back.

There may or may not be consequences for the change in assignment. The nurse manager may require that a protest of assignment (POA) be filled out by the worker who refused the assignment. Additional paperwork, as required by the facility, may need to be completed as well. In some facilities, the refusal of an assignment may be grounds for dismissal.[12] Under no circumstances can the worker merely deny the patient care and leave them alone. Leaving the assignment may be considered patient abandonment, which carries severe professional and legal penalties.

Direct and Indirect Delegation

The legal side of the delegation issue has also been addressed by the ANA in its Principles for Delegation by Registered Nurses to Unlicensed Assistive Personnel (UAP). This document makes a distinction between direct delegation, which is a specific decision made by the RN about who can perform what tasks, and indirect delegation, which is a list of tasks that certain health-care personnel can perform that is produced by the health-care facility.[5]

The consensus among many experts is that *indirect* delegation is really a form of covert institutional licensure. Lists of activities from the facility that allow nonnursing personnel, who do not have the education of the RN, to carry out professional nursing functions is de facto permission to practice nursing without a license. Indirect delegation places not only the person performing the tasks but also the RNs at the facility in a precarious legal position.

Basically, indirect delegation takes away almost all of the RN's authority to delegate personnel tasks, yet the RN remains accountable for the safe completion of the tasks under the doctrines of *respondeat superior* and **vicarious liability**. Although some states have addressed the UAP and delegation issues in their NPAs, many states either have no official standards for UAP delegation or include UAP standards under the medical practice acts that often allow physicians to assign UAPs tasks and duties that are far beyond their education.[13]

Delegation and the NCLEX

Because delegation is such an important issue in today's health-care system and because decisions about delegation require considerable critical-thinking skill, the number of questions about delegation on the NCLEX has been increasing steadily. It is not unusual for 10 to 25 percent of questions to deal with delegation issues. One problem nursing graduates may encounter with these questions is that the NCLEX uses strict parameters for determining delegation. In the real world of health care, LPNs, LVNs, and UAPs often perform functions beyond their legal scope of practice (see Fig. 15.2). The following lists may be helpful in answering NCLEX questions about delegation.

Although LPNs and LVNs can do most skills, for the NCLEX they *cannot*

- Do admission assessments.
- Give IV push medications.
- Write nursing diagnoses.
- Do most teaching.
- Do complex skills.
- Take care of patients with acute conditions.
- Take care of unstable patients.

For questions concerning UAPs, CNAs, and aides on the NCLEX,

- Look for the *lowest level of skill* required for the task.
- Look for the *least-complicated* task.
- Look for the *most stable* patient.
- Look for the patient with the *chronic illness*.

Conclusion

With the increased use of less-educated and unlicensed personnel in today's health-care system, it is essential that the nurse develop effective delegation and supervision skills. The nurse needs to be mindful that delegated tasks can change on the basis of work setting, patient needs, position descriptions, institutional training of personnel, and the everchanging requirements of NPAs and professional standards. Nurses also need to know when delegation is inappropriate.

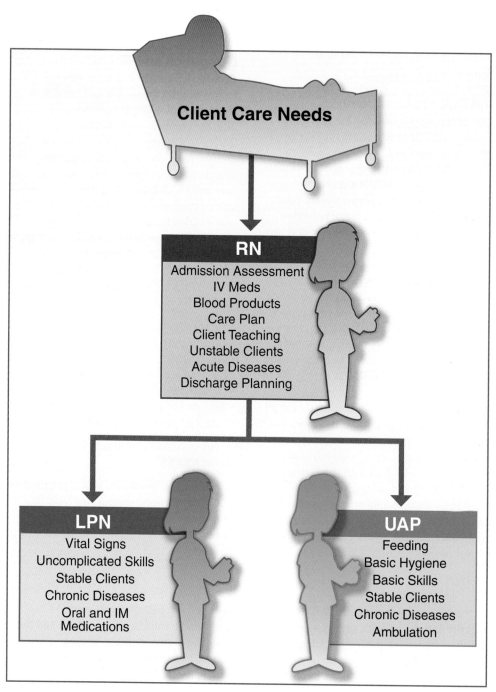

Figure 15.2 Delegation of responsibilities.

CRITICAL-THINKING EXERCISES

- Obtain a copy of your state's nurse practice act. Review the section that deals with delegation. Apply those criteria to the case study starting on page 435.
- As a nursing student, you have had tasks delegated to you. Identify how delegation has changed as you have progressed through your program.

- Obtain a copy of the policy on delegation from at least two of the clinical sites where you have practiced. How do these policies differ? How are they similar? What are the reasons for the similarities and differences?

ANSWERS TO QUESTIONS IN CHAPTER 15

ISSUES IN PRACTICE: LEADERSHIP/ MANAGEMENT CASE STUDY (P. 435)

1. The first erroneous assumption was that a nurse with no acute care hospital experience could be taught to provide safe care in a specialty area with only minimal orientation. The second assumption was that the other nurses would be enthusiastic about spending extra time and effort in orienting and teaching a new nurse. This group seemed to resent the imposition. The third assumption was that, because most of the care in the ED was "routine," a person with only limited experience could work there.
2. When Angela first discovered that Ted was having problems adjusting, she could have suggested that he work on a medical-surgical unit and cross-train for the ED. This approach would have given him a range of learning experiences that he could later apply to his work in the ED. After Ted had received 6 to 8 months of medical-surgical experience and cross-training, Angela and the other unit managers would have been able to better evaluate his skills and knowledge.
3. Because of the declining morale and the loss of trust in Angela by the staff, Ted needs to be removed from the ED. If his performance so indicates, he may be terminated. However, in this age of nursing shortages, a better option would be to place him on another unit and evaluate him there. Not everyone is destined to be an ED nurse, and Ted may find another unit with a more relaxed pace to be better suited to his personality and skills.

NCLEX-STYLE QUESTIONS

1. Which action is most appropriate for the nurse to delegate to an unlicensed assistive personnel (UAP)?
   1. Assisting a patient with a prosthetic leg to ambulate to the bathroom
   2. Teaching a patient with diabetes about the importance of eating an entire meal
   3. Helping a patient to drink contrast media that was poured into a cup by a nurse
   4. Asking a patient who recently had surgery about the intensity of pain being experienced

2. A nurse is in charge of a team consisting of a registered nurse (RN), a licensed practical nurse (LPN), and a nurse aide (NA). Which tasks should the nurse delegate to the LPN for the most effective use of the expertise of staff members? **Select all that apply.**
   1. Take vital signs on a postoperative patient one day after surgery.
   2. Perform a bed bath for a patient on contact precautions.

3. Obtain a blood glucose level on a patient with diabetes.
4. Provide patient education regarding a dressing change.
5. Discontinue tubing used to administer blood.

3. A charge nurse is making assignments to staff members working on a surgical unit. Which patient should be assigned to a recently registered nurse rather than to an experienced registered nurse?
1. A woman with an elevated temperature after surgery for an ectopic pregnancy
2. A middle-aged patient who had elective surgery for repair of an abdominal hernia
3. A young adult who had a fractured femur as well as multiple soft tissue injuries from an automobile accident
4. An older adult male who had a transurethral resection of the prostate who has cherry red drainage from the continuous bladder irrigation

4. A nurse in charge of a patient care unit is considering staff member assignments. What criterion is most significant for the nurse to consider when delegating a task to another member of the nursing team?
1. Who will ultimately be responsible for the patient's care?
2. Is the activity within the person's job description?
3. How much experience does the person have?
4. What is the acuity level of the patient?

5. _____ is the transfer of responsibility for the performance of an activity from one individual to another while retaining accountability for the outcome.

6. The nurse is managing care of a school-age child with new-onset insulin-dependent diabetes. Which tasks must be performed only by the RN and cannot be delegated to an LPN/LVN or a UAP? **Select all that apply.**
1. Teaching parents how to give subcutaneous injections of insulin
2. Performing blood glucose monitoring before meals and at bedtime
3. Evaluating the child's response to insulin doses
4. Determining the educational goals for the day
5. Teaching the child signs for hypoglycemia and hyperglycemia

7. Assigning the right task to the right person is a principle of nursing delegation and assignment. Which of the following scenarios meets this principle?
1. A 4-month-old with Down syndrome is assigned to a nurse whose own child died of heart disease due to Down syndrome 6 months ago.
2. A child with a central IV line that occluded on the previous shift is assigned to a new LPN.
3. A child newly diagnosed with acute leukemia is assigned to an experienced pediatric oncology nurse who floated to the general pediatric unit.
4. A child with new-onset insulin-dependent diabetes is assigned to an RN who has four other complex-care patients.

8. The RN is assigning tasks for the care of a patient after surgery for colon cancer. Which of the following assignments should the RN reconsider?
1. The UAP is to check the patient's new stoma for redness when assisting the patient with a bed bath.
2. The LVN is to report blood glucose readings that are outside a given range.
3. The UAP is to assist the patient in ambulating twice per shift.
4. The LVN is to administer medications as ordered by the health-care provider.

9. When caring for a patient in pain, which activity is appropriate to delegate to unlicensed nursing personnel?
1. Coaching the patient during painful procedures
2. Assessment using a self-report pain scale
3. Evaluating pain after giving medication
4. Bathing the patient and performing hygiene measures

10. When making assignments for the oncoming shift, the charge nurse assigns a float RN from another unit to care for a patient with complex needs. What is the legal responsibility of the charge nurse in this situation?
1. Assurance of scope of practice
2. Duty to orient, educate, and evaluate
3. Patient's rights and responsibilities
4. Determination of nurse/patient ratios

References

1. Barrow J, Sharma S. Five Rights of Nursing Delegation. In *Stat-Pearls*. Treasure Island, FL: StatPearls Publishing, 2021. https://www.ncbi.nlm.nih.gov/books/NBK519519/

2. Nightingale F. *Notes on Nursing: What It Is and What It Is Not*. London: Harrison & Sons, 1859, p. 17.

3. Geltmeyer K, Denoit N, Hilde-Goedertier M, Duprez, V. Implementing mixed nursing care teams in intensive care units during COVID-19: A rapid qualitative descriptive study. *Journal of Advanced Nursing*, 78(10):3345–3357, 2022. https://doi.org/10.1111/jan.15334

4. Delegation skills in nursing. University of Texas at Arlington Academic Partnerships, 2021. https://academicpartnerships.uta.edu/articles/healthcare/delegation-skills-in-nursing.aspx

5. Position statement: Registered nurse utilization of unlicensed assistive personnel in all settings. American Nurses Association, July 13, 2007. https://www.nursingworld.org/practice-policy/nursing-excellence/official-position-statements/id/RN-utilization-of-nursing-assistive-personnel-in-all-settings

6. Faubion D. 10 Ways to demonstrate accountability in nursing practice. Nursing Process.org, 2022. https://www.nursingprocess.org/accountability-in-nursing.html

7. Vardhan H. Delegation at work: Everyday mistakes, and how to avoid them. Hiver, 2022. https://hiverhq.com/blog/delegation-skills-avoid-mistakes

8. Weydt A. Developing delegation skills. *OJIN*, 15(2), May 31, 2010. https://doi.org/10.3912/OJIN.Vol15No02Man01

9. Nurse case study: Wrongful delegation of patient care to unlicensed assistive personnel. National Service Organization, n.d. https://www.nso.com/Learning/Artifacts/Legal-Cases/Wrongful-delegation-of-patient-care-to-unlicensed

10. Samuel. A nurse's right to refuse a patient care assignment. Excel Medical, January 16, 2022. https://www.excel-medical.com/a-nurse-s-right-to-refuse-a-patient-care-assignment/

11. CNA responsibilities: The five rights of delegation for certified nursing assistants. 4CNAs, n.d. http://www.4cnas.com/cnaresponsibilitiesthefiverightsofdelegationforcertifiednursingassistants.html

12. Should a nurse refuse a patient assignment? Critical Cover-up, 2022. https://criticalcoverup.com/should-a-nurse-refuse-a-patient-assignment/

13. Delegation types and skills for delegation: Examples. Indeed, 2020. https://www.indeed.com/career-advice/career-development/delegation-examples

Incivility: The Antithesis of Caring

16

Cheryl Taylor | Sharon Bator | Edna Hull | Jacqueline J. Hill | Wanda Spurlock | Joseph T. Catalano

Learning Objectives

After completing this chapter, the reader will be able to:

- Define *caring* in the context of civility: the importance of caring relationships
- Define *incivility* and related concepts in academia (among faculty and students) and in the workplace
- Discuss the ethical codes violated by incivility in the profession
- Describe behaviors that are considered uncivil and civil in the academic and clinical settings
- Define and discuss the similarities and differences between bullying and lateral violence

CIVILITY VERSUS INCIVILITY

Concepts and ideas can be either-or propositions, where one idea excludes the other, or they may exist on a continuum that identifies a range. Civility and **incivility** are the second type, and it can sometimes be difficult to identify when an action is civil or uncivil. The context of a situation, the culture of an organization, and the power difference between the participants can all affect perceived civility or incivility.

Current newspaper, television, and Internet reports indicate that incivility is escalating in the world. Some experts believe that the news media's continual reporting of violence between people has desensitized them and caused them to accept this type of behavior as the norm. Incivility in the form of bullying and intimidation is often exploited in the media on reality television programs that use it for entertainment.

What Is Civility?

Although almost everyone has a basic understanding of what civility is and is not, it is more difficult to actually define. The word *civility* is derived from the Latin word for *citizen*. It appears that to be a good Roman citizen, a person had to be polite and helpful to their fellow citizens. In a global context, civility is often thought of as good manners; however, its meaning is much broader. Civility is based on recognizing that all human beings have value. A simple definition of civility is for people to treat others as they would wish to be treated (the Golden Rule). Empathy is key to recognizing how others might want to be treated and what they may perceive as unpleasant actions by others. A more activist view of civility sees it as taking positive actions that fight injustice and oppression while at the same time respecting the rights of others. For example, the Civil Rights Act of 1964 requires that all individuals have equal protection under the law, regardless of race, color, religion, gender, national origin, or disability.[1]

An analysis of existing research shows that even perceived discrimination as a form of incivility can produce negative mental and physical health outcomes such as elevated stress levels and self-destructive behaviors. Protection from the incivility caused by discrimination can be found in social support, active coping styles, and group identification.[2]

Civility in Nursing

In nursing, civility is one of the underpinnings of caring and can even be considered a moral imperative (i.e., a rule or principle originating in a person's mind that forces the person to act in a certain manner).[3] For most people entering the profession, the motivation to be a nurse stems from the moral values of helping and caring coupled with a deep desire to make a positive impact in the lives of individuals.

Civility in the profession enables nurses to make caring the focal point of their practice. Being civil to each other, to students, to colleagues, and to clients promotes emotional health and creates a positive environment for learning and for the promotion of healing. It also develops emotional intelligence and empathy in nurses.[1] Emotional intelligence, the ability to be aware of feelings and thoughts of others by using behavioral cues, promotes the nurse's personal growth. It also transforms negative actions and attitudes into positive responses to health-care issues and is considered critical to the foundation of nursing practice. A workplace culture of civility necessitates cultivating a compassionate, kind atmosphere where respect and skillful communication are encouraged and modeled throughout the institution. In a culture of civility, racism, bullying, and harassment cannot exist because such deviant behavior is neither excused nor tolerated.[3]

Communication and Civility

In Watson's model of human caring (Chapter 3), caring can be demonstrated and practiced through interpersonal interactions (Box 16.1). Similarly, the consideration of others within interpersonal relationships is a fundamental part of being civil.[3] Incivility in nursing today contradicts the primary requirement that nurses be caring professionals. The reasons for incivility can be uncovered by a closer examination of the interpersonal relationships found in toxic work and learning environments.[4]

Box 16.1 Watson Model of Human Caring

"Caring Science is the starting point for nursing (in) relational ontology that honors the fact that we are all connected and belong to Source."

Source: J. Watson, *Nursing: The philosophy and science of caring* (rev. ed.), Boulder: University Press of Colorado, 2011.

Toxic work and learning environments can be identified by recurring exposure to overt and/or covert insults and hostile remarks from nurse managers or coworkers. Unfortunately, most people do not recognize that their place of employment is toxic until it has produced excessive stress and enough anxiety that it affects their mental and even physical health. Some things an employee might observe that indicate a toxic work environment include physical and mental stress from working long hours, continual negative comments from the supervisor or other employees, lack of signs of appreciation for the work being done, one-way communication from the top down, and inability of the workers to express themselves due to fear and intimidation.[4]

The health and well-being of clients are predicated on excellence in communication and a culture of civility in the workplace. The Institute of Medicine's 2001 report *Crossing the Quality Chasm: A New Health System for the 21st Century* notes that finding new strategies to improve communication is critical in promoting a culture of civility. Furthermore, intimidation, even when subtle, results in harmful outcomes of psychological abuse, horizontal and lateral violence, bullying, relationship aggression, workplace incivility, and mobbing when a group is involved. Ethical codes and values in society affirm civility as the antidote to incivility.

What Is Incivility?

This conversation between two experienced nurses was overheard at a major state nursing conference:

Nurse 1: "I can't believe how impolite people are now. No one ever seems to say *please* or *thank you* or *you're welcome* anymore."

Nurse 2: "I know! I had my arms full of packages when I arrived yesterday, and not even one of the three or four people standing by the door offered to help."

Nurse 1: "I was almost hit in the hotel parking lot by some guy who tried to muscle into a space I was already pulling into!"

Nurse 2: "I guess our society has just gotten a lot ruder over the years."

Society in general and the nursing profession in particular seem to be filled with complaints about "incivility," both in academia and in the workplace. The simplest definition of incivility is the lack of civility. The American Nursing Association (ANA) defines incivility in nursing as "one or more rude, discourteous, or disrespectful actions that may or may not have a negative intent behind them."[5] However, *incivility* is a very broad term that includes a wide range of what is considered unacceptable behavior in a civilized society. Incivility can be viewed as a continuum of impolite behaviors with a lot of overlap between them. Each stage typically begins with some type of covert, subtle psychological behavior. However, incivility can lead to physical violence if taken to its extreme. As shown in Figure 16.1, on the right end of the scale are overt violent actions such as vandalism, physical assault, and battery. On the left end of the scale are more surreptitious and psychologically based behaviors such as discrimination, rudeness, verbal bullying, and psychological abuse. The continuum of incivility moves from relatively minor behaviors, such as eye rolling and sarcastic comments, to bullying and racial or ethnic slurs to more aggressive and potentially violent behaviors like intimidation and physical violence. Between the extremes is a range of behaviors that are either more or less overtly violent with a great deal of overlap.[5]

In the academic or classroom setting, incivility is any type of human activity or interaction that creates an unpleasant or negative learning atmosphere. Examples of classroom incivility engaged in by students include inattentiveness (e.g., texting, side conversations), coming unprepared for class, not listening, interrupting others who are speaking, and tardiness. Examples of faculty incivility include not addressing students by their preferred name, belittling or demeaning students because of questions they ask or answers they give, and not keeping scheduled office hours. Classroom incivility can also arise due to grading procedures, faculty evaluations, and cheating or attempting to cheat. The end result is that students do not learn, and the stress levels of both students and faculty increase. In the health-care work setting, incivility takes on many forms, but they all produce a threatening and polarized work environment that reduces the quality of client care. Subsequently, nurses feel dissatisfied, angry, anxious, and unhappy. Stress levels are unnecessarily high, and turnover rates increase.

Generally, incivility is a societal problem. Many professional psychologists, educators, and health-care providers agree that civility has declined in society, but they are hopeful that behavior and relationship education will result in more harmonious discourse while elevating expectations for appropriate behavior. People under stress can potentially lose their sense of civility, which can escalate, turning into outright violence if left unchecked (Box 16.2).

What Do You Think?

Is incivility present in your nursing classes? What types of things are other students doing that you consider to be uncivil? Are offenders reprimanded for their behavior?

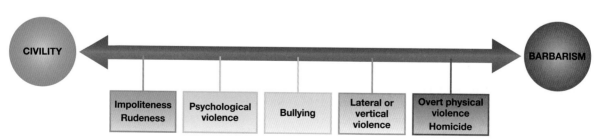

Figure 16.1 Incivility continuum.

Box 16.2 Common Examples of Incivility in the Workplace

- Acting temperamental and yelling at others
- Showing up late repeatedly to meetings
- Being disrespectful to other employees
- Blackmailing or talking about other employees behind their backs
- Sabotaging someone's project or assignment
- Trying to ruin an employee's reputation
- Failing to pay attention during meetings
- Refusing to respond to e-mails or calls or purposely responding late
- Interrupting employees during meetings, presentations, or conversations
- Ignoring employees as they talk
- Keeping important client or company information from an employee.

Source: P. Ogbuagu, Learning to manage incivility in nursing, Nursing CE Central, June 28, 2022. https://nursingcecentral.com/incivility-in-nursing/

Toxic Technology

Incivility and intimidation in academic and workplace environments are not new. However, technological developments have made them even more toxic, more widely distributed, and more damaging. Research indicates that cyber-harassment, vicious anonymous e-mails, hate text messages, harmful social media posts, acts of rudeness, and social rejection are on the rise. Often, students targeted in this way experience more fear, anxiety, and avoidant behaviors than if they were victims of an actual theft or physical assault.[6]

Incivility in the health-care setting is by no means an original problem. Over the years, it has been called by several names: *nurses eating their young, the doctor–nurse game, assertive versus aggressive, passive-aggressive behavior, lateral violence,* and *workplace violence,* to mention a few. The ultimate consequence of incivility in this setting is that it jeopardizes quality of care and client safety.[7] Researchers have found that incivility in health care is a problem nurses have experienced in all health-care settings and that it can be dangerous not only to nurses but also to clients. Up to 88 percent of nurses have witnessed physician incivility toward nurses. According to a review of the literature, incivility in nursing was discussed as early as 1980; however, it became a more widely researched topic in early 2000s, and both violence and research on it have steadily increased since then.[7] Research has shown that more than 7 out of 10 nurses have experienced episodes of incivility from other nurses and physicians during their careers.[7]

The COVID-19 pandemic increased the number of nurses who experienced incivility while working. With its sudden and total rearrangement of the workplace setting, the pandemic exposed nurses to situations with which they had no familiarity. In addition to a shortage of experienced bedside nurses, nurses also experienced extreme work demands, severely high patient acuity, poor delegation of tasks from nurse managers, and lack of teamwork among nurses who did not know each other. All of these conditions added to nurses' increased anxiety and stress levels, conflicts with coworkers, and depression.[7]

Incivility has been linked to increased medical errors and the creation of hostile academic and workplace environments. Such negative environments can create situations that end in decline of health or even loss of life. For example, a newly licensed nurse asks his preceptor how to properly place sequential compression devices (SCDs) on a postoperative client's legs. The experienced nurse "hazes" the trainee by telling him to "just figure it out." The trainee does his best, but the client later develops a deep vein thrombosis (DVT). What about a licensed practical nurse (LPN) in a nursing home who routinely treats her nurse aides and unlicensed assistive personnel (UAP) badly, telling them how stupid and lazy they are? The aides and UAPs respond to the LPN's incivility by not repositioning bedbound residents as frequently as ordered. These residents soon develop pressure injuries that require wound care. Could these incidents have been prevented by early recognition of the signs of severe incivility?

Bullying

Bullying is a type of incivility that is one step beyond impoliteness. The ANA defines bullying as "repeated, unwanted harmful actions intended to humiliate, offend and cause distress in the recipient."[7] It can also be defined as any behavior that could reasonably be considered humiliating, intimidating, threatening, or demeaning to an individual or group of individuals. Bullying can occur anywhere and at times becomes habitual, being repeated over and over.[8]

Although almost everyone has experienced some type of bullying during their lives, bullying is a complex concept that includes several elements.

Bullying can be classified into three general types: verbal bullying, social bullying, and physical bullying. Verbal bullying, the most common, is saying, writing, or otherwise communicating unkind, cruel, and/or false information about a person that causes them emotional distress. These communications can include teasing, insults, unbecoming sexual remarks (sexual harassment), mocking, and threats of physical harm. Almost as common as verbal bullying is social bullying, sometimes call relational bullying, which attacks a person's good reputation or personal relationships. Actually, it is hard to have social bullying without the verbal component, and cyberbullying has added a whole new dimension to bullying with the addition of pictures and videos. Social bullying occurs through gossip and rumor spreading, saying something embarrassing about someone in public (assault), organizing a group activity and leaving someone out on purpose, or texting someone untoward or graphic photos. Although physical bullying is not usually seen in the health-care setting, it consists of unwanted physical contact, which may or may not cause harm to a person's body or their possessions (battery).[9]

Physical bullying can take the form of throwing something that hits another person, pushing a person out of the way, breaking a person's possessions, making rude or nasty hand gestures, and such direct physical attacks as slapping, punching, kicking, and pinching.[9]

In the U.S. legal system, physical abuse, emotional abuse, verbal abuse, or any combination of the three are considered bullying and may be punished by fines in the civil system or jail time in the criminal system (see Chapter 8). The goal of bullying is usually to coerce or intimidate another person or group of people into doing something that they do not want to do. However, sometimes the goal is to merely humiliate a person or group because of some perceived difference or weakness. Hazing and initiation rites are also a form of bullying. Most people who bully others have low self-esteem along with a poor self-image and a lack of empathy, and they use bullying to make themselves feel more powerful.[6]

Although not often discussed, *workplace mobbing* or *mob bullying* can be a serious problem in the health-care work setting. It is also fairly common.

Surveys show that during their careers, at least one out of three workers has experienced it. Mobbing is a type of bullying in the workplace that occurs when one person (a known bully) enlists coworkers to pester and damage the reputation of another worker. Another definition is the repeated psychological and health-harming maltreatment of one person by one or more coworkers. It is most often verbal and social in nature. Once mob bullying begins, there is a tendency for additional people to join the mob (mob mentality). These mob actions create a toxic and unfriendly work environment, which may ultimately cause the targeted person to resign. Similar to individual bullying, mob bullying includes offensive actions such as disruption of the person's work, personal insults, intimidation, embarrassment, and threats of physical harm.[10]

Some psychologists believe that bullies are born and not made (i.e., the tendencies to be a bully are genetic). People who display bullying behaviors have more than double the number of depressive and acute anxiety episodes as others and are likely to have attention deficit hyperactivity disorder (ADHD). They also have a much higher rate of suicide than the general public. Although not commonly evaluated for psychological disorders, bullies who were evaluated were six times more likely than others to be diagnosed with oppositional defiant disorder (ODD). Persons with ODD show symptoms of frequent and persistent patterns of anger, irritability, arguing, and defiance or vindictiveness toward authority figures, such as parents, teachers, or other adults.[8] Treatments such as medications and therapy that are started in childhood or the teenage years may not cure ODD or bullying, but they can give the person some control over the disorder and control the expression of the symptoms. Despite the treatments for ODD, in reality it is difficult to change people's basic personalities.[7]

Targets

The victim of bullying, or any level of incivility, is often called the *target*. Typical targets are discussed next.

Vulnerable Individuals. These people are bullies' favorite target. Vulnerable individuals usually feel powerless. The powerlessness of these individuals feeds into the bully's need to feel powerful by putting them down. People who are vulnerable are unlikely to retaliate against the bully or to report the behavior.

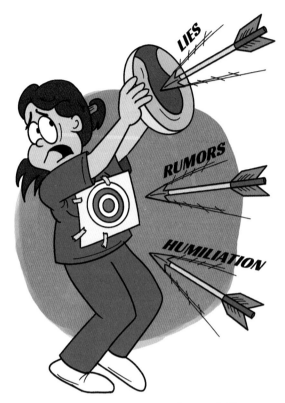

Bullies target anyone who is different.

Threatening Individuals. This group includes individuals who demonstrate intelligence and competence in their job performance, who possess a high level of skills, and who are working toward career advancement. Threatening individuals are more dangerous for the bully to attack because of their knowledge levels and probable awareness of what the bully is trying to do. However, because the bully fears that the target's abilities make them (the bully) appear inadequate and negligent or because of strong feelings of jealousy, the bully may resort to sabotage, spreading lies, and belittling to bring the target down to their level. Cyberbullying is a favorite tool because of its anonymity.

Caring Individuals. People who have workplace support networks and strong friendships will often make the bully jealous because the bully lacks a meaningful social support system. The bully will try to destroy the target's social support system by telling lies about the target's friends, starting negative rumors about the target, and using cyberbullying techniques.

Ethical Individuals. People who treat others fairly and ethically may be targeted because bullies see these individuals' characteristics in opposition to their own deficits. Also, ethical individuals often believe in giving another person a second chance and may not recognize that the actions the bully is taking are on purpose.

The Newbie. The new kid on the block, or new employee, makes a tantalizing target for bullies because the bully sees them as timid and weak. New employees are also common targets of both lateral and vertical violence (discussed shortly). The new person usually has a low level of self-confidence, similar to the vulnerable person, and has not developed any strong or meaningful relationships this early in their job life. Bullies know that these people have a feeling of powerlessness and are easy prey for intimidation, teasing, and personal threats. The new employee will be fearful of reporting the bully and may not even know they are being bullied if the bully is a sneak.

Anyone Who Is Different.
- *Racial identity:* If the person is of a different racial or ethnic background than the bully, they are likelier to become a target than individuals who are of the same racial or ethnic background as the bully. Hispanic workers are targeted the most frequently at 26 percent. African Americans are targeted 21 percent of the time, and Asian workers are targets in 7 percent of bullying cases.[11]
- *Physical appearance:* Anyone with a physical characteristic that is not "normal" may become a target for the bully. This includes individuals with physical or mental disabilities, people who are unusually short or tall, people who are very slender or obese, people with unusual facial features, and people with obvious scars or unusual tattoos. Although some of these individuals, like vulnerable individuals, may feel powerless, bullies may target them just to ridicule and make fun of them as a form of self-entertainment.[11]
- *Gender:* In a workplace that is predominantly male, women are more likely to be the target of male bullies than men are. Interestingly, women bullies who work in a primarily male work setting are also more likely to bully other women. In the health-care setting, particularly in nursing where women make

up 95 percent of the employees, women-on-women bulling is the norm.[11]

• *Sexual orientation, religion, speech patterns:* Although diverse sexual orientations and gender identities are becoming more accepted, in a predominantly male workplace, nonbinary men are often targeted by bullies. In a predominantly female workplace, sexual orientation and gender identity do not appear to make a person a target. Bullies tend to leave people who have a different religion alone because of the laws against religious discrimination. However, individuals who wear different garments, such as a turban (Sikh), yarmulke (Jewish), or hijab (Muslim) for religious reasons, may become targets. Regional or foreign accents may also attract a bully's attention. Speech patterns can easily become the butt of jokes when the bully tries to imitate them.[11]

Bullying also involves making intimidating comments on social media (cyberbullying), ostracizing a person from the group, or making a person the butt of practical jokes. One-on-one bullying from peers is sometimes called *peer abuse* or *lateral violence*, but in groups, the primary bully may have co-conspirators who contribute to or prolong the bullying activities. Sometimes a bullying culture can develop in the workplace or educational setting, to the point that it becomes the normal environment, no matter how toxic it is.[10]

Lateral Violence

Lateral violence, also known as *horizontal violence*, has many of the same characteristics as bullying except that it takes place almost exclusively in the work setting. Applying to interactions between professional colleagues at the same organizational level, such as staff nurse to staff nurse, lateral violence is usually limited to psychological harassment. Some of the forms it can take include verbal abuse, intimidation, exclusion from unit activities, unfair assignments, denial of access to opportunities to advance, and withholding of information.[12]

Lateral violence has been recognized by the National Institute for Occupational Safety and Health (NIOSH) as one of the leading causes of poor staff morale, excessive sick days, turnover of staff, nurses leaving the profession, poor quality of care, and physical symptoms such as insomnia, hypertension, depression, and gastrointestinal upset. Over the past

several years, the ANA has produced many position papers that discuss lateral violence as a major problem for practicing nurses.[12]

Lateral violence can be either covert or overt. Overt lateral violence can include name calling; threatening body language; physical hazing; bickering; fault finding; negative criticism; intimidation; gossip; shouting; blaming; put-downs; raised eyebrows; rolling of the eyes; verbally abusive sarcasm; or physical acts such as pounding on a table, throwing objects, or shoving a chair against a wall. Covert lateral violence is initially more difficult to identify and includes marginalizing a person, refusing to help someone, ignoring someone, making faces behind someone's back, refusing to work with certain people, whining, sabotage, exclusion, and fabrication.

Lateral violence is a well-known phenomenon in nursing. It has been part of the health-care culture almost since the beginning of the profession. Those experiencing lateral violence also include nursing students, pharmacists, unit secretaries, and others. Oppression theory notes that marginalization is a key contributing factor to lateral violence. Nurses sometimes use horizontal violence to attack one another as

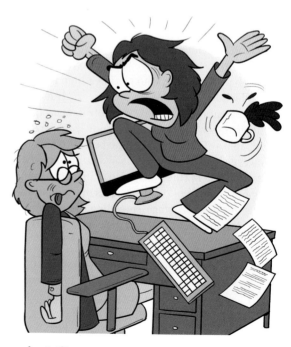

Incivility can create a toxic atmosphere.

a means of venting their frustration with and anger against a supervisor or institution they feel helpless to change. When lateral violence occurs among health-care providers, it leads to decreased communication and, ultimately, poor care and reduced safety of clients.[12]

Vertical Violence

Bullying from a superior, or vertical violence, is a type of harassment that can permeate the entire organization and have a detrimental effect on its effectiveness. The ANA's 2019–2020 Healthy Nurse, Healthy Nation (HNHN) survey showed that 23 percent of nurses said they have experienced bullying from those in authority.[13] The concept of inappropriate use of coercive power becomes a key element in vertical violence. When bullies are in a position of power or are perceived to have power, they can do a lot of damage to the organization and the people who work for them. The people they supervise are in a constant state of fear and work in a defensive mode, avoiding contact with the bully or anything that may bring attention from the bully. They feel anger toward the bully and have lower self-esteem; because of the bully's position of power, they do not know what to do about the bullying.

Vertical violence can also be covert or overt. Covert actions include withholding information needed for client care, exclusion from unit activities, difficult assignments, sighs and making faces when the person speaks, annoyed glances, and condescending remarks. Overt actions may include insulting or rude responses to a person's statements or ideas, name-calling, yelling and swearing when a mistake is made, openly criticizing and purposely embarrassing the subject in front of their peers, blaming them for things they did not do, and even making ethnic jokes or using slurs. These types of actions are a major issue in health care today because they destroy effective communication and teamwork and lead to poor quality care and unsafe conditions for clients.[13] As a result of this type of atmosphere, productivity and innovation decrease, morale suffers, and the best workers seek employment elsewhere.

Vertical violence can move in both directions, however, and superiors themselves may become the targets of bottom-up vertical violence. Although subordinates may seem to be powerless in the face of a bullying superior, they actually do have considerable power both as a collective and as individuals (see Chapter 1). The superior's position is often dependent on the productivity of the people being supervised. Some extremely disgruntled employees may devise subtle, passive-aggressive ways to decrease productivity, sabotaging the boss and the organization. When workers lower productivity enough, the boss is going to be confronted by their superior to see what the problem is and may get fired as a result. In the extreme, bottom-up vertical violence may result in the employee "going postal" and causing physical injury or even death to those they hold responsible for causing distress. (See "Workplace Violence" later in the chapter.)

Vicious Circle

Another negative outcome of vertical violence is the "bullying vicious circle" that is perpetuated in the organization. This phenomenon is particularly evident in organizations such as health-care facilities and educational settings, where the persons who are bullied when they first start are likely to move into positions of power later. An example is when a new faculty member who was bullied when they first started now has several years of experience and bullies newly hired faculty. The same cycle often occurs on nursing units in a hospital, where new nurses who were bullied become the charge nurses and bully other new nurses. Bullying may become part of the culture to the point that it is not even recognized as bullying. Often, there is an attitude of "I went through it, so now it's time for you to pay your dues."

INCIVILITY IN NURSING EDUCATION

In its broadest sense, academic incivility is any speech or action that disrupts the harmony of the teaching or learning environment.[14] Incivility in nursing education can take the form of lateral violence, vertical violence, bullying, and eating the young. Incivility endangers the physical and emotional well-being of both faculty and students. It exists at all levels in higher education: student–student, student–faculty, faculty–student, and faculty–faculty. Incivility is damaging to the relationships between professionals and impedes the exchange of information, research findings, and evidence in the academic setting. In higher education, acts of incivility can range from impolite body language or nonverbal expressions and displays of arrogance or rebuffing remarks to overt bullying, xenophobic and damaging comments, and even intimidation. Incivility is an ongoing problem in nursing education that leads to detrimental learning on the part of students and the disillusionment of nursing faculty leading to resignations and a worsening nursing faculty shortage.[14]

Incivility in nursing education takes the form of lateral violence when faculty, students, and staff are demeaning to their peers. It becomes vertical violence when department chairs, deans, and other administrators bully those who have less power than they do. Vertical violence also exists in faculty–student relationships that become unprofessional. Incivility is destructive to the emotional and physical well-being of those affected.[14] Significant financial costs result from a fear-based environment due to missed work, legal fees for lawsuits, rehiring, and decreased work output. Although data about the costs of bullying in higher education are limited, it is estimated that it may cost large educational institutions more than $96,595 to replace each faculty member who has left due to lateral violence. This figure includes the cost to recruit, hire, and train a new nursing faculty member but not the overtime costs for other faculty while the position remains open.[14]

The classroom reflects the larger society, with inequities as well as humanitarian qualities such as caring. Academic incivility is an interactive and dynamic process in which individuals or groups make the choice to behave uncivilly. Within nursing education, the three parties or groups who need to take primary responsibility for incivility are administrators, faculty, and students.[14]

An Escalating Problem

Administrators

The term *administrator* includes several levels of persons who are responsible for the running of an organization or a unit of that organization. The role of administrators is to oversee the operations within their organization, to coordinate with other managers in the organization, to initiate planning for the organization, and to provide guidance for employees. The administration sets the tone and creates the atmosphere for the entire organization. The efficiency and success of an organization are directly linked to the administrator's skills in communicating well,

promoting staff development, finding solutions to problems, and creating a positive work environment. However, administrators are human and are sometimes responsible for incivility in their organization.

Some administrators can be uncivil and can even be bullies. The very characteristics that helped them rise to a position of power may also contribute to a personality that tends to be uncivil. Administrators who are uncivil are likely to be self-centered and to have difficulty feeling empathy with others. They may have little concern about the consequences of their actions, and they seem to feel good about themselves most of the time. However, they have a brittle ego and retaliate against negative comments by belittling others. This behavior trickles down and promotes a culture of incivility throughout the organization. When employees complain of bullying from other employees or supervisors, their complaints often are dismissed outright or placed in the system where they become lost.[14]

Faculty

Differences of opinion and academic conflicts are common within groups of highly educated and extremely motivated individuals such as are found in nursing faculty. These conflicts generally occur as collegial differences and intellectual debates and are a natural phenomenon within intellectual communities. These types of purely academic differences, if expressed in a positive way, can contribute to a constructive learning environment. However, if the differences get out of hand or are ignored, they can, over time, lead to incivility or even become full-blown battles.

Faculty-to-faculty incivility is not uncommon in higher education and is frequently left unaddressed and unresolved. Administrators may actually encourage this type of activity to promote "survival of the fittest" among the ranks. Friction among faculty can stem from personality conflicts, extreme self-interest, a high need for control or power, jealousy, spite, or even revenge. In some cases, faculty may be oblivious to how their behaviors affect others. Faculty incivility increases in the presence of heavy workloads, unclear role expectations, pressure to publish, evolving technological demands, and the lack of skills to manage conflicts with other faculty. Higher education often places a lot of pressure on faculty to move up through the ranks. "Publish or perish" (meaning if you do not publish, you are not getting promoted and may even be let go) is the mantra in many institutions. Because slots for promotion are limited, a faculty member who does not get promoted or granted tenure may have feelings of envy and jealousy of the achievements of others, which can be triggers for incivility.

An uncivil culture or environment in the nursing program can lead to psychological and physical stress conditions such as sleep disorders and depression among faculty. Faculty incivility also affects the students in the program who are sensitive to the ongoing stress or strife. Faculty members will sometimes complain to students about other faculty, which puts the students in an uncomfortable position. It is essential that there be increased awareness by faculty and administrators about the variety and frequency of faculty-to-faculty incivility and how it impacts everyone in the nursing program. Faculty must be educated in how to treat one another with civility and respect and how to recognize incivility when it is in its early stages so that it can be stopped.[14]

Some faculty report being the target of negative remarks, insinuations, and harassment from their faculty peers, all of which are counterproductive to their work and their credibility. Some faculty dismiss this type of lateral violence as "part of the job" and look the other way. Others note the rise in incivility and report feelings of anger, disappointment, and embarrassment as the result of colleagues' actions.[14]

Expressed in many different forms, workplace incivility can include a toxic work environment, workplace violence, and bullying. Faculty themselves experience psychological pain as well as anger, fear, anxiety, feelings of being devalued, and decreased self-esteem. These emotions may prompt competent teachers to resign rather than confront the incivility.[10] But avoiding confrontation is not a suitable response for a professional educator. In the words of Dr. Martin Luther King Jr., "Our lives begin to end the day we become silent about things that matter."[14]

Cause and Effect

The increase in incivility among nursing faculty has several causes. The academic culture is often controlling and driven by faculty insecurities and competitiveness. It is historically based on a rather inflexible hierarchical management structure (see Box 16.3). Many nursing faculty, who may have been excellent clinical practitioners, entered the teaching profession with little preparation in the basics of higher education. On-the-job training became the norm as nursing faculty adapted to the academic setting with its triple requirements of teaching, research (publication), and service. Being unprepared, they often found themselves victims of lateral violence through unequal relationships or discrepancies in faculty status and rank.[15]

Normally, nursing faculty work in a highly interactive social system. Most of the day-to-day operations of classes and committees require working closely with other nursing faculty. In some cases, when faculty disagree strongly with policies, procedures, or lines of authority, they may develop feelings of exclusion or alienation. Although nursing educators

Box 16.3 Traditional Faculty Ranks in Higher Education (From Lowest to Highest)

Higher Educational Faculty Hierarchy	Degree Required
Adjunct instructor, clinical instructor, special instructor	MSN—BSN for AD
Instructor, lecturers	MSN—non-tenure track
Assistant professor	PhD/EdD—tenure track
Associate professor	PhD/EdD—tenured
Professor	PhD/EdD—tenured
Distinguished professor, endowed professor	PhD/EdD—tenured
Professor emeritus (retired)	PhD/EdD—tenured

Note: Rankings may vary somewhat among institutions.

recognize that challenging the status quo is essential for the growth of the profession, it is still often resisted. Faculty members who challenge the system can be silenced and sometimes even shunned by colleagues when they attempt to take a contradictory stance on an important decision.[15] This is most noticeable when a new faculty member with many years of experience in the clinical setting, but none in education, is hired and then is expected to blend seamlessly into the academic realm.

Mentoring

Mentoring is a relationship between two people, one a mentor with considerable experience and the other a new employee (mentee) with limited experience in the role. The goal of mentoring is the professional and personal development of the mentee.[16] When mentoring is successful, it can also become a long-term relationship between two people who share knowledge, experience, and advice with each other. After a career as an expert clinician and/or nurse administrator, new faculty members are often surprised by the demands of their new role. The new faculty member may be shocked by the complexity and requirements of the nurse educator's role and the challenges of being a novice educator.

The mentoring relationship can be formal and planned or may be informal and just occur by accident. In the nursing higher education setting, mentoring should be planned and formal, with one person assigned to mentor the new faculty member. The procedure manual should list specific items that the mentor needs to cover with the mentee, such as university policies on vacation and sick days, where to get office keys and a parking permit, how to advise students, and how to log on to the computer network. While the mentor is covering the formal items, a relationship may develop with the mentee, and informal mentoring can take place. Informal mentoring may include what the janitor's name is and how to get them to vacuum your office carpet, when the best time is to go to lunch to avoid the crowd, or which faculty member keeps a bowl of candy on their desk. When a faculty member lacks a formal mentor, mentoring usually occurs informally through professional and social interactions such as faculty meetings or new faculty picnics. The experienced faculty member will take the new person under their wing. In nursing education, typically the mentor is an experienced faculty member or even the administrator of the program.[16]

A positive mentoring process requires an appropriate match between the mentor and the mentee. The mentor needs to be committed to the mentoring process with a sincere desire to help with development of the mentee. The mentor must also be willing and able to commit considerable time and energy to the process. The mentor must support the empowerment of the mentee as they advance and must know when the mentoring process is over.[16]

For a program to become accredited by the ACEN, mentoring is mandatory for the nurse administrator as well as for full- and part-time faculty.[16] Because of the ongoing scarcity of qualified nursing faculty, nursing programs are required to actively find and retain individuals who will be able to educate the next generation of nurses. High-quality mentoring for new faculty members helps to build healthy faculty relationships. Constructive mentor relationships require respectful listening, focused thinking, maturity, wisdom, and positive energy, all of which help those being mentored correct mistakes and accomplish goals.[16]

Students

Some nursing faculty are too embarrassed to admit that incivility exists in higher education, particularly in their own classrooms, despite a documented increase in student hostility, insubordination, and even intimidation.[14] Although students are often considered subordinates in the classroom setting, they wield a considerable amount of power derived from their numbers and the policies of the institution. Students can exercise this type of bottom-up vertical violence in undeservedly poor teacher evaluations, low levels of attention, inadequate note-taking, and poor grades. Examples of student-to-faculty incivility typically include the following:[5]

- Harassing and threatening behaviors by students toward certain instructors over grades
- Filing false complaints about inappropriate sexual behavior
- Cutting classes because students consider them boring or the instructor stupid
- Cheating on tests and homework assignments to get better grades

- Refusing to participate in class activities
- Being unprepared for classes by not doing reading assignments or written work
- Distracting teachers and other students by asking irrelevant or confrontational questions
- Complaining behind the teacher's back to the teacher's superiors
- Complaining behind the teacher's back to other instructors

The impact on nursing students experiencing horizontal violence from their peers is both psychological and physical. Psychological issues include low self-confidence, insecurity in classes, trouble forming relationships with peers, and appearances of physical illnesses. In severe cases of horizontal violence, students may feel isolated, helpless, and unappreciated. Physical complaints of students who are victims of horizontal violence can include minor to severe headaches, higher than normal levels of stress, apprehension, insomnia, and fatigue. In the worst cases, horizontal violence can cause depression and inability to concentrate leading to falling grades.[17]

Often students do not recognize what is causing their distress. Because they lack self-confidence and may not be able to express their apprehensions, they will sometimes turn to experienced instructors for appropriate direction to deal with their issues. Without a solid advisor or mentor, nursing students may continue to try to solve the situation themselves or turn to other students for help, which may lead to more difficulties in the long run. Nursing students who are victims of horizontal violence almost always have low self-esteem and feel ignored and unwanted by faculty or other nursing students.[17]

Examples of student-to-student incivility include the following:

- Obtaining study notes from the previous year's classes and using them as bargaining chips with their classmates
- Ridiculing (bullying) students who are considered outcasts because they do not fit the model of the majority in terms of weight, clothing, hairstyle, and disposable income
- Two-faced behavior, where students act nice to a classmate's face but are nasty behind their back
- Intentionally excluding a student from study groups or group social activities

What Do You Think?

Are any of the previously listed behaviors present in any of your classes? What are some other uncivil things students do in class?

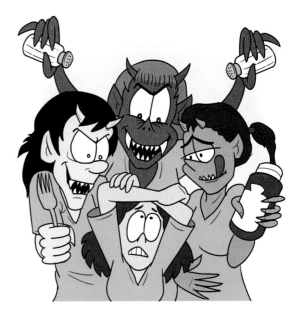

Nurses are known for eating their young.

These uncivil behaviors are found throughout higher education. It is critical for nursing faculty to deal constructively with disgruntled students in a timely manner. When students' rude and disruptive behavior is not addressed, it may turn into physical violence. Most nursing students recognize the importance of treating others respectfully, studying diligently, disagreeing graciously, and listening attentively. However, when stress levels are high, they may struggle to remain civil.[12] Studies show a correlation between increased student stress and increased student incivility, resulting in some faculty doubting their abilities as educators or even having concerns for their personal safety. The key to effective education lies in the quality of the interpersonal relationship between student and teacher.[17]

What can nursing educators do to promote positive interpersonal relationships that encourage civility?

The National League for Nursing (NLN) faculty development program includes strategies to manage incivility and offers a program of co-sponsorship for those interested. (See NLN Incivility, Bullying and Workplace Violence 2015, https://www.nursing world.org/~49d6e3/globalassets/practiceandpolicy/nursing-excellence/incivility-bullying-and-workplace-violence–ana-position-statement.pdf.)

Although many schools of nursing actively engage in curriculum- and program-improvement measures, few examine the impact of incivility on student learning. Examples of incivility in nursing education range from minor insults, delivered either electronically or face to face, to full-blown acts of physical violence.[17] Regarding the rise of incivility in nursing education, two questions have dominated the literature in recent years: (1) What factors contribute to it? (2) What measures can be taken to minimize its impact on student learning?

Being a Nursing Student in a Pandemic

During the best of times, nursing students experience high levels of stress as they attempt to earn a degree in one of the most difficult majors on campus. During the worst of times, such as a worldwide pandemic, even the most unflappable student experiences catastrophically high levels of stress. Stress in this setting is a specific relationship between the nursing student and the environment that is judged by the student as highly demanding to a point where it surpasses their abilities to cope and which may also imperil the student's health and well-being.[18] Due to the transactional relationship between the person and their immediate environment, stress develops because of elements and situations beyond the person's control. Stress situations affect the nursing student and, in turn, impact the student's reaction to each situation. For example, many nursing students experienced highly stressful situations when, in the spring of 2019, their nursing programs shut down a few months before graduation due to the onset of the COVID-19 pandemic.[19]

Some hospitals attempted to compensate for the sudden loss of nurses by enlisting nursing students to join the fight against COVID-19. The hasty move to shore up the workforce was sometimes called *rushed labor insertion*.[19] While the experience provided nursing students the opportunity to practice their clinical skills, replace some of their required clinical practice hours, and help in the care of those suffering from COVID-19, it also increased their stress and anxiety levels.[18]

During the pandemic, nursing students experienced added stress factors such as the fear of being infected and of infecting their close family members. Lack of adequate PPE, safety, and disease control measures, as well as a general lack of knowledge of the disease, increased their fears. Other causes of stress were fear and uncertainty of what was going to happen (daily changes were not unusual), fear of making medication errors, working with new and complicated equipment, and lack of time to apply nursing theory learned in the classroom.[19] Nursing students' stress levels increased because they believed that they were not prepared to care for COVID-19 patients or to use safety protocols and PPE that they had never used before in the clinical setting. The most stressful clinical settings cited by nursing students in rank order were the intensive care unit, the emergency department, and the surgical unit. The least stressful setting was the general medical unit, at least until that unit started receiving COVID-19 patients. Many hospitals relied heavily on in-house classroom simulation for training nursing students along with additional online assignments at home to maintain their skills advancements, and the stressful learning environment hindered student success.[18]

When classes suddenly were suspended, uncertainty about the students' academic future also produced stress. Students had many questions, including the following:

- Will I have to retake all the skills tests, quizzes, and exams I've already taken to this point?
- Will I need to redo all of the assignments I've already done?
- What does this mean for my scholarships and financial aid?
- I was supposed to graduate this May. How is the school shutdown going to affect my graduation date?
- What am I supposed to do about the NCLEX? I already have a date.
- Am I going to get any refund on my tuition if I drop out?
- Are there going to be classes in the fall? When should I register?

- Do I have to repeat all the classes from this semester?
- The hospital where I usually do my clinicals isn't letting students in. Can I do clinicals at another hospital?
- If the hospitals reopen to students, can I complete my clinical hours over the summer?
- My nursing school has some great simulation manikins and programs. Can I complete my clinical hours with simulation?
- My nursing instructor resigned. What do I do now?

A lot of these questions had no answers at the time everything closed down. All answers were dependent on the particular nursing program, college or university, and the individual instructor. Overall, nursing programs and colleges worked diligently with students to make sure they could graduate and get the best educational experience possible.[20] However, high levels of student anxiety and stress continued. This type and level of stress increased student self-doubts and contributed to poor academic performance for some students. Stress also led to some students withdrawing from their nursing program and to others experiencing a deterioration in mental and physical health.[18]

Contributing Factors

It is common knowledge that attending nursing school increases students' stress levels. Identified stressors include juggling multiple roles, such as meeting the demands of work, study, and family responsibilities; financial pressures; time management; lack of family support; demanding faculty; and students' own emotional issues.[20] Students automatically find themselves in a dependent and relatively powerless position compared to the instructor or institution.

Even in a non-pandemic setting, the clinical setting is vulnerable to incivility due to rapid technological changes, staff shortages, and poor staff-to-staff interpersonal communication and relationships. There is a need for ongoing research into the negative consequences of the clinical environment on students and faculty.[21]

One study reported that other factors contributing to incivility include student developmental issues caused by isolation from high-quality professional role models and reduced exposure to the faculty's

decision-making process. Other nursing students did not believe in the hierarchical social structure of nursing school but rather felt that everyone was a peer. For these students, the chain of command did not exist, and there were no boundaries in the lines of communication between students and faculty.[5,20]

Ignoring incivility does not make it go away. Rather, disregarding incivility sends the message that uncivil behavior is the norm and something to be tolerated. Denial of problems often leads to bigger and more severe problems down the road. It is far better to take measures to prevent incivility and to stop it as soon as it starts. Once incivility becomes a common occurrence, it is almost impossible to stop without radical intervention.[17]

Solutions to Academic Incivility

Once incivility is identified and acknowledged in the academic and clinical settings, effective measures can be taken to either decrease it or totally eliminate it. All the most effective measures to deal with lateral incivility are based on effective communication skills.

Don't Eat Your Young

The ritual of "eating the young" is seen in both the classroom and clinical settings. It is a form of vertical violence because it is based on an inequality of power between the experienced nurse or faculty member and the new nurse or nursing student. There has long been a practice of having the new members of a profession undergo a rite of initiation, or "hazing." These initiation rites often involve intimidating and belittling the student or the new nurse to help them "learn their place" in the organizational chain. Common eating-the-young activities include punishing, shaming, or ridiculing students or new nurses for their lack of knowledge. Using caustic humor or sarcasm or setting up victims by placing them in a situation in which they will likely fail also serve to demoralize students and new nurses. Although this initiation process has diminished to some degree in recent years, it still exists in many institutions.[13]

As an alternative to on-the-job training for nurses interested in nursing education, universities are now offering master's degrees in nursing education; these programs teach students how to teach and explore the political ins and outs of the academic setting. Graduates of nursing education programs enter their teaching careers with an understanding of curriculum development, evaluation, testing, course preparation, and many other aspects of surviving in higher education, such as yearly evaluations, the rank and promotion system, and the need to publish. They are taught to be more assertive and to express their opinions without trepidation. Nowadays, senior nursing educators are much more sensitive to the needs of new faculty and have a strong incentive to nurture them and help them develop into high-quality educators.[20] They realize that this new generation of instructors will replace them as they retire in large numbers over the next few years.

Preceptor and mentoring programs for new nurses have been developed in clinical facilities as a result of the IOM's report *The Future of Nursing: Leading Change and Advancing Health Care*.[13] Box 16.4 provides examples of classroom and clinical behavioral norms for nursing students. These have been co-created with colleagues and clinical-setting partners so that everyone clearly understands the expectations for appropriate behavior.[21]

Alternatives to Incivility

It is a well-known psychological principle that all behavior has meaning. (See Chapter 12 for more detail.) An individual's behavior also expresses their intrinsic values, including whether or not they treat others with respect and dignity or in a way that disrespects them and drags down their self-esteem. An individual who helps in a soup kitchen, provides pro bono nursing care at a free clinic, or drops a few coins in a homeless person's cup is displaying behavior that indicates a fundamental belief that all human beings are valuable and deserve basic respect.[21] As noted in the later discussion of the ANA Code of Ethics and civility, disrespectful and poor treatment of others, whether they be coworkers, clients, family members, or strangers, is inconsistent with the basic tenets of nursing.

Because every action toward others, whether conscious or reflexive, contributes to a culture of either civility or incivility, it is essential that every individual be committed to eliminating negative, uncivil thoughts and behaviors. For example, simple negative actions that should be eliminated include groaning out loud when a classmate in the front row asks another a complicated question, gossiping about a classmate during break times, disparaging the instructor's clothing, making cynical comments about a classmate's presentation, and so forth. Instead, it is much more productive to use positive actions such as saying "good morning," "please," and "thank you" to everyone, even individuals who are not well liked; opening doors for people; putting your phone away when someone is talking to you; complimenting people when they do a good job; asking people if they need help; and so forth. A culture of civility is based on respecting everyone's dignity all the time.[15]

Box 16.4 Civility in the Classroom and Clinical Settings

Dr. Clark's Classroom Norms	Dr. Clark's Clinical Norms
• Practice proper door etiquette. • Assume goodwill. • Listen to and respect others. • Be flexible and open-minded. • Keep cell phones on silent and use proper cell phone etiquette. • Use laptops for class work only. • Do not have side conversations. • Give notice of change in advance (faculty). • Be present and on time. • Have fun!	• Assume goodwill. • Respect and celebrate differences. • Communicate respectfully. • Listen carefully. • Come to clinical prepared and on time. • Share work equally among group members. • Resolve conflicts directly and with respect. • Have fun!

Source: Clark, C. M. (2017). *Creating & Sustaining Civility in Nursing Education.* United States: Sigma Theta Tau International.

Over time and with the accumulation of life experiences, many people become cynical. Cynicism develops when people have been hurt, no longer trust the motives of others, and try to keep people from hurting them again. This distrust is just the opposite of what is required for civility. The ability to assume that the intentions of others are positive and good (or at least neutral) is key to establishing a culture of civility.

Another method to decrease incivility is to avoid escalating uncivil behavior. It is a natural tendency that when someone is uncivil to us, we respond with similar behavior. This creates a cycle of incivility that escalates until the cycle is broken by one of the individuals. Would it not be better to break the cycle at the beginning? However, breaking the cycle does not mean ignoring another person's inappropriate words or actions. Dealing with conflict and the difficult behavior of individuals is a skill that all nurses must master.[21] For a more detailed discussion of dealing with difficult behavior, see Chapter 12.

A Model for Civility
Administrators in colleges and universities have an important role in building a proper workplace environment. This begins with the first interview of the hiring process. Applicants need to be asked specific questions about civility. Following are some samples of these questions:

- What things about the people you are working with really irk you?
- What do you do when you become angry or irritated with another employee or supervisor?

- On a scale of 1 to 10, with 10 being the best possible, how would you rate your abilities in the areas of collaboration, collegiality, and civility? Explain your answers.[15]

The positive or negative attitudes of administrators can determine whether uncivil behaviors are addressed or ignored. Unaddressed, the culture of incivility permeates all aspects of the organization, but when constructive problem-solving and respectful encounters are the norm, a culture of civility can prevail. A civil climate enhances both teaching and learning.

A recently developed model allows faculty and students to promote civility in the academic setting. Although the model does not include administrators, their responsibilities, or their perceptions about incivility, it emphasizes the critical importance of the climate and infrastructure established by administrators. It is called the *conceptual model for fostering civility in nursing education* (Fig. 16.2). The model depicts how, as stress levels increase for both students and faculty, student attitudes of entitlement and faculty attitudes of condescending superiority can lead to incivility.

The conceptual model provides a basis for creating a culture of civility by focusing on the levels of stress for nursing faculty and students. Possible research questions include the following:

1. What do you perceive to be the biggest stressors for nursing students?
2. What uncivil behaviors do you see nursing students displaying?

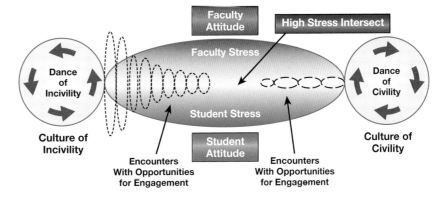

Figure 16.2 Conceptual model for fostering civility in nursing education. (Reprinted with permission from SLACK Incorporated: C.M. Clark, P.J. Springer, Academic nurse leaders' role in fostering a culture of civility in nursing education, *Journal of Nursing Education*, 49(6):319–325, 2010, https://doi.org/10.3928/01484834-20100224-01.)

3. What do you perceive to be the biggest stressors for nursing faculty?
4. What uncivil behaviors do you see nursing faculty displaying?
5. What should be the nursing administration's role in addressing incivility?[20]

There are some methods faculty can use to overcome academic incivility. Becoming a catalyst and a change agent in one's own nursing program will set an example that others can follow. Make civility and cooperation a key element in the vision, mission statement, and outcomes of the program. Revise the curriculum so that shared values, collegiality, and collaboration are threads that guide students and faculty in the learning process.

ETHICAL PROHIBITIONS TO INCIVILITY

As of now, there are no federal standards to regulate workplace violence; however, several states have attempted to develop laws to control it. In most cases, these laws are confusing and difficult to enforce. To help fill this void, in 2016 The Joint Commission developed guidelines under its Leadership standard to deal with behaviors that are interpreted as lateral violence. These include the following:

> *A caring attitude is not transmitted from generation to generation by genes—it is transmitted by the culture of a society.*

- Requiring hospitals and other organizations to develop their own codes of conduct defining behaviors that are considered lateral violence
- Requiring hospital administration to develop and implement a process for managing individuals who are displaying disruptive and inappropriate behaviors
- Requiring additional standards for medical staff to follow for the credentialing process, including demonstrating interpersonal skills and recognizing interprofessionalism[22]

A Guide for Caring

The Joint Commission notes:

Intimidating and disruptive behaviors can foster medical errors, contribute to poor patient satisfaction and to preventable adverse outcomes, increase the cost of care, and cause qualified clinicians, administrators, and managers to seek new positions in more professional environments. Safety and quality of patient care is dependent on teamwork, communication, and a collaborative work environment. To assure quality and to promote a culture of safety, health-care organizations must address the problem of behaviors that threaten the performance of the health-care team.[22]

The ANA Code of Ethics also has principles that support ethical, civil, and caring relationships. (For more information on the code, see Chapter 6.) The code was developed as a guide for carrying out nursing responsibilities in a manner consistent with quality in nursing care and the ethical obligations of the profession. The NLN website gives high priority to the Code of Ethics and to faculty responsibility as a way of dealing with student behavioral problems. The specific parts of the ANA Code of Ethics (2015) that relate to incivility are as follows:

1.0 "The nurse, in all professional relationships, practices with compassion and respect for the inherent dignity, worth, and uniqueness of every individual. . . ."

1.5 Principles of respect extend to all encounters, including colleagues. "This standard of conduct precludes any and all prejudicial actions, any form of harassment or threatening behavior, or disregard for the effect of one's actions on others."

3.5 "Nurse educators have a responsibility to . . . promote a commitment to professional practice prior to entry of an individual into practice."[23]

The Joint Commission, the ANA, and the NLN make it clear that underlying attitudes of caring and respect are essential expectations of those who enter the profession of nursing. It is essential for nurses to learn and internalize these attitudes. A caring attitude is *not* transmitted from generation to generation by genes—it is transmitted by the culture of a society.[7] The ANA's Task Force on Workplace Violence maintains a Web site that assists nurses in understanding more about this problem.

Professional Standards

Ethical behaviors in nursing school correlate with ethical behaviors in professional practice.[21] The American Association of Colleges of Nursing (AACN) notes the importance of professional standards, including the development and acquisition of an appropriate set of values and an ethical framework. It stresses that incivility is unethical and notes that nursing faculty have a "moral imperative" to deter incivility.[15] Early identification of incivility in a culture of violence is very important in preventing severe physical harm (see Fig. 16.3). The AACN strongly suggests that educators try to determine the presence of incivility before students enter a program.[21]

Honor Codes (Codes of Conduct)

Some universities and colleges have instituted honor codes or codes of conduct. An honor code is a type of social contract between a student and the educational institution that systematically describes the basis for conduct that is deemed honest and ethical for the student while at the institution. Traditionally, honor codes include the requirement that the student sign a written pledge affirming that assignments are their own work (anti-plagiarism); that the student affirm that they will complete un-proctored exams without help (anti-cheating); that the student participate in university judicial bodies (community service); and that the student report violations that they observe (honesty). Honor, in general, is a commitment to excel in the achievement of virtue, to adhere to core values, and to do what is right. Honor codes are designed to motivate students to demonstrate personal integrity and support their peers and to create and maintain an environment that is supportive of the growth of virtues and excellences.

Studies have shown that academic settings with an honor code have less cheating. One type of honor

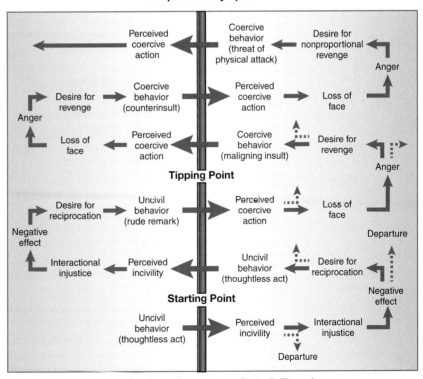

Figure 16.3 The incivility spiral. (From L.M. Andersson, C.M. Pearson, Tit for tat? The spiraling effect of incivility in the workplace, *Academy of Management Review*, 24(3):453–471, 1999, https://doi.org/10.5465/AMR.1999.2202131; with permission.)

code for students and faculty is called **HIRRE**, which stands for **honesty, integrity, respect, responsibility, and ethics**. In HIRRE, students sign a pledge promising not to cheat or plagiarize. Faculty and students can use a reporting system to identify violations of the honor code. Enforcement by faculty, directors, or the dean can include expulsion for honor code infractions.[24]

WORKPLACE INCIVILITY

Workplace incivility is a broad term that includes workplace hostility, bullying, lateral violence, vertical violence, and workplace violence. It is the threat of violence or the actual causing of physical harm to workers either inside or outside the workplace. Workplace incivility spans a continuum, ranging from verbal abuse to physical violence and homicide.

Workplace Violence Is Epidemic

More than 2 million workers are targets of workplace abuse each year, and workplace violence is blamed for the deaths of more than 1,000 people a year in the United States. When uncivil behavior causes someone bodily harm, it becomes workplace violence. The cost of violence in the United States each year ranges between 250 and 330 billion dollars with almost 400,000 violent assault cases per year. A recent study revealed that as many as 25 percent of nurses are physically assaulted on the job, with 69 percent of physical workplace violence assaults and 71 percent of nonphysical workplace violence assaults reported in the health-care and social service professions. Violence against health-care workers is 12 times higher than that directed at the rest of the U.S. workforce; and overall, 75 percent of all workplace violence incidents that happen each year in the United States involve health-care professionals.

According to the Occupational Safety and Health Administration (OSHA), hospitals are one of the most dangerous places to work in the United States. Hospitals recorded more than 221,000 work-related injuries in 2019 (the last year that data were available), according to OSHA. Due to the high number of incidents, workplace violence remains a primary concern for the roughly 4 million nurses in the United States, according to a study by the Government Accountability Office. Data show that these numbers are largely due to workers'

close contact with the public, inadequate staffing levels, and poor workplace protection policies.[25] Still, it is estimated that as many as 25 percent of incidents of workplace violence go unreported, often because of the multiple requirements and reams of paperwork that go into reporting incidents.[26]

Hospitals and health-care providers spend a tremendous amount of money in planning for and reacting to violent events. The cost includes paying for uninsured care, enhanced security measures, and injuries to hospital personnel. The health-care professionals at highest risk for workplace violence are nurses. Whether in the form of workplace incivility or full-blown workplace physical violence resulting in injuries, these behaviors result in negative outcomes for clients as well as employees, administrators, and facilities.[26]

Along with the COVID-19 pandemic came an increase in hospital workplace violence. In addition to the stress placed on the entire health-care system, the pandemic also raised the level of anxiety and stress in clients, visitors, and family members. There have been many reports of health-care staff being attacked and placed in physical jeopardy while attempting to provide care. Approximately 44 percent of nurses reported experiencing some form of physical violence from clients and visitors, and 68 percent reported experiencing verbal abuse during the COVID-19 pandemic.[26]

Not only does violence cause physical and psychological injury for health-care workers, workplace violence and intimidation make it more difficult for nurses, physicians, and other clinical staff to provide high-quality client care. Nurses and physicians cannot provide the best care possible when they are afraid for their personal safety, distracted by disruptive clients and family members, or traumatized from prior violent interactions. Violent exchanges at health-care facilities reduce both client satisfaction and employee productivity, and they increase the potential for adverse medical events and costly malpractice suits.[26] It is not completely clear whether client or visitor violence against health-care professions is horizontal or vertical violence.

Even before the COVID-19 pandemic, workplace violence in the health-care setting was a growing problem. It is important to be able to recognize characteristics that may indicate escalating cycles of violence in nurses, health-care providers, clients, family members, visitors, or others. The following actions can occur in an environment of horizontal hostility, leading to the compromise of client safety and quality of care:

- Failing to clarify an unreadable order because of fear of the health-care provider
- Lifting or ambulating heavy or debilitated clients without assistance rather than asking for help
- Using an unfamiliar piece of equipment without asking for instructions first
- Carrying out orders that the nurse did not believe were correct[26]

Institutions need a comprehensive plan to deal with violence, including client violence toward health-care workers. Without appropriate interventions, disrespect and unresolved conflict can quickly spiral out of control and eventually lead to physical violence. OSHA has developed a set of guidelines for limiting workplace violence and stopping it once it gets started. This document is an appropriate place to start developing an institutional plan. It is comprehensive yet flexible and can be modified to fit almost any workplace environment.

> *To break the cycle, it is necessary to be proactive about incivility incidents and to see them as signs of potentially more dangerous problems.*

Stop the Spiral

The incivility spiral (Fig. 16.3) depicts uncivil behavior between two people or two groups. The behavior can escalate into violence, or those involved can let go of their resentment and stop the incivility from progressing. The path chosen depends largely on communication, both at the beginning of the conflict and during its progression. Conflict resolution interventions are essential to the process.

The higher up the spiral the uncivil behavior advances, the more coercive behavior is displayed and the greater is the desire for violent revenge. The victim of the incivility experiences loss of face, increased anger, and a desire to fight back against the one creating the hostile environment. Once the tipping point is passed (i.e., the point in the spiral where neither party can back down), the potential for physical violence increases dramatically. Interrupting the spiral with positive interventions and communication before the tipping point is reached is essential in defusing the anger.

What Do You Think?

How is workplace violence similar to child abuse or elder abuse? Are the measures to overcome child or elder abuse similar to those required to overcome workplace violence? Should there be a mandatory reporting requirement for workplace violence?

Solutions to Horizontal Violence in Nursing

Nurses must try to prevent a situation from reaching the tipping point where incivility turns into violent actions. The importance of providing safety in practice needs to be continually reinforced to prevent negative outcomes from an unsafe work environment. The Quality and Safety Education for Nurse (QSEN) competencies developed by the AACN can be successful in reducing educational and workplace incivility when they are efficiently implemented into a facility or nursing program. The six QSEN areas for prelicensure and graduate nursing programs include client-centered care, teamwork and collaboration, evidence-based practice (EBP), quality improvement (QI), safety, and informatics.[27] Although these areas are being addressed in the clinical setting, there is still a need to promote these competencies in education (see Chapter 4).

Creating a Positive Work Environment

Alertness is essential to defuse incivility in the work setting. Listening to fellow workers' accounts of incivility is a first step and should be followed by reflection and development of an action plan. Ignoring the problem never solves it and often escalates the frequency and intensity of the incivility. To break the cycle, it is necessary to be proactive about incivility incidents and to see them as signs of potentially more dangerous problems.

The Nursing Organizations Alliance (NOA) recommends eight actions to help create a positive workplace environment and overcome incivility:

1. Build a collaborative culture that includes respectful communication and behavior.
2. Establish a communication-rich culture that emphasizes trust and respect.
3. Make accountability central to the culture with clearly defined role expectations.
4. Maintain adequate staffing.
5. Train leaders competent in cooperation and communication.
6. Share decision-making with all those it will affect.
7. Continuously develop employee skills and clinical knowledge.
8. Recognize and reward employees' contributions.[28]

Other identified methods that help reverse horizontal violence include the following:

1. Recognize and acknowledge that horizontal violence exists in the workplace.
2. Adopt a continuous, consistent, integrated approach to promote a culture of cooperation and address instances of horizontal violence.
3. Provide regular education for all staff on the subject of horizontal violence; for example, what it is, how to address it, and so on.
4. Institute mechanisms that enable and allow staff members to safely address issues of horizontal violence.
5. Talk to all staff members about the phenomenon, breaking the silence.[28]

Nurses can break the cycle of incivility by looking at their own acceptance of or participation in the negative behavior and using organizational structures and personal influence to change the organization's culture of horizontal violence. Some important actions nurses need to take individually to reduce the effects of both vertical and lateral violence on their own careers and lives include the following:

1. Document, document, document! Keep a detailed record of horizontal and vertical violence episodes including dates, times, witnesses, and so on. These will be useful in making a solid case that there has been a breach of the culture of safety.

2. Establish unit-level programs to create awareness about and provide tools to address workplace violence.
3. Establish a zero-tolerance policy against workplace violence, with clear boundaries and early enforcement.
4. Compliment at least one nurse colleague each day.
5. Assign qualified and willing nurses to mentor students and new nurses.
6. Name the problem—refer to the situation as *horizontal violence*.
7. Raise the issue of workplace violence at staff meetings—bring the light of day to the problem.
8. Learn from experience—keeping a journal about personal values, beliefs, attitudes, and behavior, raises self-awareness.
9. Pursue a path of personal growth—finding those things that create happiness and satisfaction and developing them goes a long way to counteract incivility.
10. Ensure that you are part of the solution, not part of the problem.
11. Maintain self-care behaviors—peer support, good nutrition, adequate sleep, time-outs, meditation, and exercise.
12. Speak up when workplace violence toward others is witnessed.
13. Provide team members with tools to help them navigate uncivil relationships, such as team building skills, interdisciplinary teamwork, and conflict resolution skills.[29]

Although both vertical and horizontal violence are endemic in the workplace, they can be decreased and, at some point in the future, may even be eliminated. It requires that all employees of every workplace work together to eliminate oppression and unhealthy behaviors from the environment. Nurses must be vigilant for acts of incivility that are less obvious but affect the work of nurses in all settings.

Leadership for Job Satisfaction

Healthy workplace environments that empower nurses are critical to the success of the profession. A healthy workplace decreases absenteeism, increases productivity, and dramatically reduces turnover rates.[28] Mentoring has been shown to lower incivility in the workplace. Mentoring partnerships, along with updated educational models, increase cultural competence and enhance job satisfaction for both the new person and the mentor.[29] Mentoring eases the new nurse's transition into their new role and helps the mentor to better understand the problems the new nurse is having in completing the role transition. Mentoring also helps make the new person a genuine member of the group much more quickly than if they were learning by trial and error.

Transformational leadership (TL) is a key element in reversing incivility in the academic or workplace environment. TL acts as a lens through which leaders can see themselves and the workplace inequalities that need to be changed. *Transformational leadership* can be defined as a style of management or control that emphasizes ethical principles, teamwork, and shared values that work

> *Healthy workplace environments that empower nurses are critical to the success of the profession.*

together to provide high-quality outcomes. It has a goal of empowering workers to produce at a higher-than-expected level. Because workers have a positive emotional orientation toward their work, they also have high levels of job satisfaction. Consequently, patient satisfaction increases with the end result of higher quality of care, improved client outcomes, and fewer medical errors.[30]

As an intervention, TL requires a leader to have an extraordinary capacity for self-restraint and self-reflection and deep consciousness of the inner sense of responsibility. In addition, TL plays an important role in implementing needed changes in present and future practices.[30] Box 16.5 lists 13 transformational leadership qualities that can work toward increasing civility in the workplace.

Box 16.5 Thirteen Qualities of Transformational Leaders

1. You hold a vision for the organization that is intellectually rich, stimulating, and rings true.
2. You are honest and empathic. People feel emotionally safe and trust that you have their interests at heart.
3. Your character is well developed, without the prominent dark side of ego power.
4. You set aside your own interests in looking good and getting strokes, instead making others look good and giving others power and credit.
5. You evince a concern for the whole (not just your own organization), reflected in your passionate and ethical voice being heard when necessary.
6. Your natural tendency is to help others engage, deepen their perspectives, and be effective.
7. You can share power with others—you believe sharing power is the best way to tap talent, engage others, and get work done in optimal fashion.
8. You risk, experiment, and learn. Information is never complete.
9. You have a true passion for work and the vision. It shows in your time commitment, attention to detail, and ability to renew your energy.
10. You communicate effectively both in listening and in speaking.
11. You understand and appreciate management and administration. They appreciate that you move toward shared success without sacrifice.
12. You celebrate the now. At meetings or anywhere else, you sincerely acknowledge accomplishment, staying in the moment before moving on.
13. You persist in hard times. That means you have the courage to move ahead when you are tired, conflicted, and getting mixed signals.

Source: Schuster, J. (1994). Transforming your leadership style. *Association Management*, L39-43. This article originally appeared in *Association Management*. Reprinted with permission. Copyright ASAE: The Center for Association Leadership (January 1994), Washington, DC.

Conclusion

Incivility violates trust and undermines the nurse's obligation to care. It creates insecurity and hostility; and it degrades learning, collaboration, and performance in all institutions where it is found. In all settings, relationships are adversely affected by incivility. Research and active efforts to deal with the problem will help to ensure better client care. TL qualities can be used to transform uncivil environments into civil and caring ones. TL can stop upward-spiraling incivility and help with spotting, intervening in, and overcoming incivility. Constructive mentor–mentee rather than tormentor–tormentee relationships promote professional growth in nurses and improve both the academic environment and the health-care setting. Emotional intelligence arising from the practice of civility is essential and basic to the practice of nursing.

Issues Now

It's the Simple Things

There are several rather simple strategies that you, as a nursing student, can use to reduce incivility in nursing education. Initially, you need to think about your own behaviors, identify any that are uncivil or could be perceived as such, and then work to change the behaviors or rid yourself of them. Although this is the first step in the process, it may be the hardest. Identifying your own faults is not something anyone wants to do. Look over the section in the chapter that describes the characteristics of a bully or uncivil actions and honestly attempt to see which ones you have.

Whenever you encounter incivility in the classroom or clinical setting or anywhere, carefully consider and attempt to determine the purpose and contextual background of what is going on. Are you contributing to the incivility by gossiping or laughing at an uncivil joke? Is the incivility directed at you? The next step also takes some courage. If after careful consideration you decide that the disrespectful remarks are about you, you need to elucidate what the interaction actually meant with the person. If you are feeling too uneasy to approach the person in a face-to-face meeting, sending a polite e-mail asking for clarification about the incident is a productive substitute. Although the e-mail message may help get the discussion started, following up with an in-person meeting is more powerful. As Margaret Wheatley so beautifully reminds us, "We can change the world if we start listening to one another again, [because] it is the simple art of conversation that may ultimately save the world."

You, as a nursing student, have a responsibility to be a model for civility. Some actions you can take to fulfill your role as a model of civility include encouraging respectful social discussion and taking a leadership role, in conjunction with your student nurses association's faculty representative, to develop classroom and clinical standards that will provide a safe and open environment to express conflicting views.

It is important to co-create class civility norms. On the first day of class and clinical sessions, you, your fellow students, and the faculty representative need to work together to establish civility behavioral norms based on the vision and mission of the university, the college, and the department of nursing. The following are some examples of possible norms for the semester:

- Be prepared, attend class, and pay attention
- Be on time
- Greet each other before class starts
- Treat each other with dignity and respect at all times
- If late, enter quietly and inconspicuously
- If leaving early, inform the professor and sit near the door

Issues Now (continued)

- Avoid side conversations when the professor is speaking
- Raise your hand if you have a question or wish to speak
- Stay on topic and avoid monopolizing class discussion
- No sleeping, talking, checking social media during class
- No working on assignments for another class
- Share positive comments when appropriate
- Avoid negative comments at all times
- Engage in meaningful dialogue at all times
- Offer positive suggestions and solutions to problems
- Assume the best intentions with all classmates and faculty
- Listen with attention before speaking
- Be respectful when communicating; avoid grunting and under-the-breath comments
- Use computers in class for class-related content only
- Keep cell phones off or on vibrate during classes and clinicals
- Make every effort to minimize classroom distractions
- Revisit your civility norms several times during the semester and use them as a guide for class discussions and activities
- Conduct solution-focused open forums that include faculty, where action plans can be developed to prevent and address incivility in a safe environment
- Take civility reminders into the clinical setting
- Discourage or interrupt group gossip
- Speak openly about the need for change when things aren't working
- Hold one another accountable for incivility issues as they develop
- Deal with incivility issues before they become impossible to resolve

If someone tells you that another person is saying something negative about you, you have at least two options: (1) Assume goodwill about the person and say, "Interesting. That doesn't sound like something so-and-so would say." (2) If you suspect it might be true, check it out by going to that person and asking if the report is accurate. If so, discuss the issues and, if possible, come to a mutual understanding. Taking a direct and honest route is clearly the best strategy. Constructive dialogue improves the quality of human interaction and thus enhances civility.

Ultimately, however, it's the simple things that matter most.

Source: *Clark C, Cardoni C, What students can do to promote civility, Nursing Centered, November 16, 2020, https://nursingcentered.sigmanursing.org/features/more-features/Vol36_2_what-students-can-do-to-promote-civility#:.*

CRITICAL-THINKING EXERCISES

- Obtain the policy and procedure manual for your nursing program. Try to find the policy on lateral violence or bullying. Does it include the guidelines to stop bullying discussed in this chapter? What should be added? If your nursing program does not have a policy, ask the dean if you can develop one.

- Obtain the policy and procedure manual for your primary clinical site. Try to find the policy on lateral violence or bullying. Does it include the guidelines to stop bullying discussed in this chapter? What should be added? How does the facility's policy compare to the policy from your nursing program?

If your clinical site does not have a policy, ask the CEO if you can develop one.
- Ask your fellow nursing students about their experiences with lateral violence. Take notes and see if there is a common thread that runs through the stories.

- Ask your fellow students and/or faculty how they feel about honor codes. Are they for them or against them? How would they feel about adding an honor code to your policy and procedure manual if the manual does not already have one? What about updating the current honor code?

NCLEX-STYLE QUESTIONS

1. Which statement best describes the relationship between caring and civility in nursing?
   1. Giving care that exactly follows facility policies and procedures is how nurses show civility.
   2. It is easier to assess a nurse's caring than it is to assess their civility.
   3. Engaging in civil behavior is a way to demonstrate caring for clients, coworkers, and others.
   4. Focusing on civility takes time and attention away from caring in nursing practice.
2. A nurse manager is concerned about incivility on her unit. The nurses on day shift gossip about the night nurses; unlicensed assistive personnel complain that the nurses refuse to help them turn morbidly obese clients; and during staff meetings, everyone looks at their phones. When the nurse manager shares her concerns with her supervisor, she identifies the specific problem as _____.
3. Which statement about incivility in the educational setting is true? **Select all that apply.**
   1. Incivility in the educational setting may involve administrators, faculty, and students.
   2. In the nursing classroom, instructors are responsible for policing uncivil behavior.
   3. Incivility among nursing educators is sometimes related to differences in educational backgrounds and professional preparation.
   4. Students are typically uncivil to one another, not to instructors.
   5. There is a correlation between increased student stress and increased student incivility.
4. Students in Dr. Reynolds's nursing fundamentals class routinely leave scathing reviews of him on a professor-rating Web site, refuse to participate in class activities, and complain to the dean about how strict Dr. Reynolds is. What activity are these students engaged in?
   1. Academic incivility
   2. Bullying
   3. Vertical violence
   4. Lateral violence
5. Rodney, a new RN, just started training on a busy medical-surgical unit. He has been warned that the experienced nurses on the unit will probably expect him to "pay his dues" just as they had to. This type of initiation practice is commonly referred to as _____.
6. Mara is reviewing her class notes on incivility and nursing ethics. Which of the following notes should she request clarification about?
   1. In 2016, The Joint Commission developed guidelines to address lateral violence.
   2. The Joint Commission noted that lateral violence contributes to medical errors, patient dissatisfaction, and adverse outcomes.
   3. The ANA Code of Ethics has principles that support civility.
   4. The ANA Code of Ethics mentions extending respect to all encounters, except for colleagues.
7. Which of the following behaviors would be considered civil in both the classroom and the clinical setting? **Select all that apply.**
   1. Assume goodwill.
   2. Listen to and respect others.
   3. Be on time.
   4. Do not ask questions.
   5. Do not share information.

8. Carol is listing examples of civil classroom behavior for the nursing students in her study group. Which example should the other members of the study group question?
    1. Play computer games quietly so as not to disturb others.
    2. Turn cell phones on silent.
    3. Do not allow the door to slam shut.
    4. Be present and on time.

9. Which of the following behaviors are characteristic of both bullying and lateral violence? **Select all that apply.**
    1. Can escalate to physical actions
    2. Intimidation
    3. Name calling
    4. Verbal sarcasm
    5. Use of social media to attack target

10. What is the main difference between bullying and lateral violence?
    1. Bullying can result in physical violence; lateral violence does not.
    2. Lateral violence is a response to vertical violence; bullying is not.
    3. Lateral violence occurs primarily in the work setting.
    4. Targets of bullying are chosen because they have attributes that are foreign to the bullies; targets of lateral violence are chosen because the bullies see their own despised attributes in the target.

References

1. Dinkin S. Toward becoming an antiracist: The journey continues. *San Diego Union Tribune*, June 19, 2020. https://www.pressreader.com/usa/san-diego-union-tribune-sunday/20220619/282329683608625

2. Snook A. Discrimination in the workplace: What it is and how to avoid it. i-Sight, July 7, 2022. https://www.i-sight.com/resources/discrimination-in-the-workplace-guide/

3. Carlson K. Investing in the future: Positive workplace culture in healthcare. NursesUSA, n.d. https://nursesusa.org/article_positive_workplace_culture_in_healthcare.asp

4. Agape C. How to cope with anxiety in a toxic work environment. Wellahealth, August 16, 2022. https://www.wellahealth.com/blog/how-to-cope-with-anxiety-in-a-toxic-work-environment/#:

5. Ogbuagu P. Learning to manage incivility in nursing. Nursing CE Central, June 28, 2022. https://nursingcecentral.com/incivility-in-nursing/

6. Top 7 impacts of social media: Advantages and disadvantages. Simplilearn, 2022. https://www.simplilearn.com/real-impact-social-media-article

7. Nurses unite to end incivility and bullying. *OR Today Magazine*, July 1, 2022. https://ortoday.com/nurses-unite-ending-incivility-and-bullying/

8. Oppositional defiant disorder: Diagnosis and treatment. Mayo Clinic, 2022. https://www.mayoclinic.org/diseases-conditions/oppositional-defiant-disorder/diagnosis-treatment/drc-20375837

9. What is bullying? Stopbullying.gov, June 30, 2022. https://www.stopbullying.gov/bullying/what-is-bullying

10. What is workplace mobbing? Regain.us, 2022. https://www.regain.us/advice/psychology/what-is-workplace-mobbing/

11. Who could be a target in workplace bullying? Swartz Swidler LLC, 2022. https://swartz-legal.com/target-workplace-bullying/

12. Morse K. Lateral violence in nursing. *Nursing Critical Care*, 3(2):4, 2008. https://doi.org/10.1097/01.CCN.0000313323.72329.8e

13. Vertical violence and workplace bullying. *OR Today Magazine*, October 31, 2020. https://ortoday.com/vertical-violence-workplace-bullying/

14. Clark C, Landis T, Barbosa-Leiker C. National study on faculty and administrators' perceptions of civility and incivility in nursing education. *Nurse Educator*, 46(5):276–283, 2021. https://doi.org/10.1097/NNE.0000000000000948

15. Reed J. Reducing lateral violence: A humanistic educational approach. *RN Journal*, 2022. https://rn-journal.com/journal-of-nursing/reducing-lateral-violence-a-humanistic-educational-approach

16. Ard N, Beasley S. Mentoring: A key element in succession planning. *Teaching and Learning in Nursing*, 17(2):159–162, 2022. https://doi.org/10.1016/j.teln.2022.01.003

17. Burda M. Student nurse perceptions of horizontal violence during clinical hospital rotations [dissertation]. Walden University, 2021. https://scholarworks.waldenu.edu/cgi/viewcontent.cgi?article=10812&context=dissertations

18. The COVID-19 impact on nursing students. Palomar College, 2022. https://www.palomar.edu/nursing/covid-19-impact-on-nursing-students-faqs/

19. Barret D. The impact of COVID-19 on nursing students. What does the evidence tell us? *Evidence-Based Nursing*, 25(2):37–38, 2022. https://doi.org/10.1136/ebnurs-2022-103533

20. Hamadi H, Zakari N, Jibreel E, Nami F, Smida J, Haddad H. Stress and coping strategies among nursing students in clinical practice during COVID-19. *Nursing Reports*, 11(3):629–639, 2021. https://doi.org/10.3390/nursrep11030060

21. Dillon S. Workplace bullying in nursing: Why it happens and how to confront it. Bravado Health, 2021. https://www.bravadohealth.com/2021/01/07/confronting-nurse-bullying/

22. Arnetz J. The Joint Commission's new and revised workplace violence prevention standards for hospitals: A major step forward toward improved quality and safety. National Library of Medicine, 2022. https://www.ncbi.nlm.nih.gov/pmc/articles/PMC8816837/

23. American Nurses Association (ANA). *Code of ethics for nurses with interpretive statements.* Silver Springs, MD: ANA, 2015.

24. Academic and professional ethics. John Hopkins School of Nursing, 2021. https://nursing.jhu.edu/information/current-student/student-affairs/academic-professional-ethics.html

25. Boskamp E. 29 Startling workplace violence statistics [2022]. Zippia, 2022. https://www.zippia.com/advice/workplace-violence-statistics/

26. Fact sheet: Workplace violence and intimidation and need for federal legislation. American Hospital Association, June 2022. https://www.aha.org/fact-sheets/2022-06-07-fact-sheet-workplace-violence-and-intimidation-and-need-federal-legislative

27. Alemar D. Utilizing the QSEN framework to redesign nursing orientation competencies. QSEN.org, October 6, 2021, https://qsen.org/utilizing-the-qsen-framework-to-redesign-nursing-orientation-competencies/

28. Anti-discrimination policy. Nursing Organizations Alliance, 2022. https://www.nursing-alliance.org/anti-discrimination-policy

29. Ackerman-Barger K, Dickinson J, Louisa M. Promoting a culture of civility in nursing learning environments. *Nurse Educator*, 46(4):234–238, 2022. https://doi.org/10.1097/NNE.0000000000000929

30. Wijayanti K, Aini Q. The influence of transformational leadership style to nurse job satisfaction and performance in the hospital. *Journal of World Science*, 1(7):485–499, 2022. https://doi.org/10.36418/jws.v1i7.69

17

Nursing Informatics

Kay Lenhart | Joseph T. Catalano

Learning Objectives

After completing this chapter, the reader will be able to:

- Analyze the relationship of nursing informatics to the other health-care sciences
- Justify why nursing informatics is not a monolithic career
- List and describe the four common roles that an informatics nurse assumes
- Appraise the relationship of computer, information, and cognitive science to nursing informatics
- Summarize the key points in the history of nursing informatics
- Defend the importance of nursing informatics to nursing practice
- Evaluate the importance of human factors on equipment design
- Extrapolate the relationship of nursing informatics, artificial intelligence, and interoperability
- Describe the legislative changes that have fostered the role of informatics nurse
- Critique the changes in the HIPAA law and their effect on nursing informatics
- Discuss the steps in becoming a nursing informatics specialist

WHAT IS NURSING INFORMATICS?

Most nurses recognize that health care is becoming increasingly computerized. Home automation, or the "internet of things," where everything that runs on electricity is assigned an Internet Protocol (IP) address, has become common in new home construction. Home-owners are able to control heating and cooling, outlets, light switches, and almost any appliance from a computer or a smartphone. Many of these devices are now voice activated. Can the same technology be very far behind for health-care facilities?

Informatics is simply defined as the science of processing data for storage and retrieval. It uses computer calculations as a universal means of solving problems in any discipline whose data can be organized as 0s and 1s; it is also used to communicate information and to express ideas related to organization and management. Health informatics (HI) is an interdisciplinary field that narrows the focus of informatics to the health-care industry. HI integrates health-care science with information technology (IT), business and management technology, and computer science. The goal of informatics in health-care is to develop technology-based software (computer programs) and hardware (computers that run the software) to improve the quality of health-care and patient outcomes.[1]

Nursing informatics (sometimes abbreviated NI) is a subdivision of HI that focuses on the practice of nursing. It integrates nursing science, knowledge, practice, and information with technology to better manage all aspects of patient care. Nursing informatics uses many types of health-care information to better manage and support nursing practices.[1] Using information and communication technology, nursing informatics enables nurses to recognize, delineate, control, and communicate statistics, information, comprehension, and insight in nursing practice.

Informatics nurses were on the cutting edge when computer technology first started being used in health care. These nurses helped to develop user-friendly software and systems and to educate other nurses in their use. As technology has expanded, the nursing informatics role has also grown to meet the needs of patients, families, health-care providers, hospital staff, insurers, and government agencies. In fact, so many informatics competencies now exist that a new nurse entering the informatics field would be totally overwhelmed attempting to learn them all at once.

Like nursing science, informatics has a unique language that sounds rather strange to a newcomer in the specialty. Because informatics is also interwoven with computers and IT language, it uses many abbreviations in describing its process and systems. To help the reader better understand the terminology, the major nursing informatics abbreviations and their meanings are listed in Box 17.1.

Many disciplines are related to nursing informatics, including, but not limited to, the following:

- Evidence-based practice (EBP)
- Project planning/management
- Population health
- Genomics
- Nanotechnology
- Organizational theory
- Systems theory
- Educational theory
- Game theory
- Change management

Nursing informatics also relies on four sciences: nursing science, information science, computer science, and cognitive science. Nurses who specialize in informatics are nurses first and foremost and apply their nursing knowledge and skills to patient care while integrating technology. More important, all nurses use informatics simply by doing what nurses do every single day.

Nursing informatics integrates nursing science with multiple information management and analytical sciences to identify, define, manage, and communicate data, information, knowledge, and wisdom in nursing practice. Another definition of *nursing informatics* is the meaningful use of data by health-care professionals to improve patient safety and quality-care outcomes, advance decision making, and optimize human work processes using technology for and by all. More simply, nursing informatics is the use of nursing skills in tandem with information and technology to improve health-care outcomes.

It supports nurses, consumers, patients, the interprofessional health-care team, administrators, and other stakeholders in their decision making in all roles and settings to achieve desired outcomes.[2] This support is accomplished through the use of information structures, processes, and technology.

Every day, nurses use the nursing process to organize, classify, and analyze data. While gathering data, nurses assess the situation, diagnose its cause or causes, plan what to do on the basis of evidence and experience, intervene with steps that should improve outcomes, and evaluate the outcomes to make sure they meet the preset standards. Nurses continually analyze and communicate data; therefore, in their daily practice, all nurses function as informaticists.

WHAT DO INFORMATICS NURSES DO?

The informatics nurse role is not monolithic. Many specialty areas in informatics are available to nurses, such as trainer, project manager, project design analyst, application and project architect, application consultant, and even programmer, among many others. Nursing informatics positions include the following:

- Informatics nurse specialist (entry-level)
- Nurse informaticist (mid-level)
- Nursing informatics director (senior-level)[2]

Some of the other common roles an informatics nurse might have in a health-care facility are discussed next.

Software Developer

Software developers typically analyze users' needs and then design, test, and develop software to meet those needs. They also either design or recommend software upgrades for customers' existing programs and systems. The nursing informatics developer can guide end-user nurses to select the program that best meets their needs and has the fewest negatives. For example, nurses might want to keep track of the total time a team member spends providing specific care to a patient across different departments; however, one of the electronic medical record (EMR) or electronic health record (EHR) systems they were considering for purchase might not have the capacity to perform this task. The software development role of the informatics nurse involves developing a solution to

Box 17.1 **Abbreviations and Their Expansions**

ADT	admission, discharge, transfer
AHMI	American Healthcare Information Management Association
AI	artificial intelligence
AMIA	American Medical Information Association
ANCC	American Nurses Credentialing Center
ANI	Alliance for Nursing Informatics
ANIA	American Nurses Informatics Association
ARPA	Advanced Research Projects Agency
ARPANet	Advanced Research Projects Agency Network
ARRA	American Recovery and Reinvestment Act of 2009
BCMA	barcode medication administration
CARING	Capital Area Roundtable on Informatics in Nursing Group
CCC	Clinical Care Classification
CDSS	clinical decision support system
CHIP	Child Health Insurance Plan
CINAHL	Cumulative Index for Nursing and Allied Health Literature
CIS	clinical information system
CMS	Centers for Medicare and Medicaid Services
CPOE	computerized provider order entry
DSS	document security system
EBP	evidence-based practice
ENIAC	Electronic Numerical Integrator and Computer (the first general-purpose computer)
GIGO	garbage in, garbage out
HF	human factor
HIPAA	Health Insurance Portability and Accountability Act of 1996
HITEC	Technology for Economic and Clinical Health Act
HL7	Health Level 7
ICNP	International Classification for Nursing Practice
IMIA	International Medical Informatics Association
MACURA	Medicare Access and Reauthorization Act of 2015
MeSH	Medical Subject Headings
MIPS	Merit-based Incentive Payment System
MIS	medical information system
MU	meaningful use
NLM	National Library of Medicine
NANDA	North American Nursing Diagnoses Association

(continued)

Box 17.1 **Abbreviations and Their Expansions** (continued)

NDNQI	National Database of Nursing Quality Indicators
NIC	Nursing Intervention Classifications
NMDS	Nursing Minimum Data Set
NOC	Nursing Outcome Classifications
ONC	Office of the National Coordinator for Health Information Technology
OS	operating system
PCS	patient care system
PDA	personal data assistant
PoCT	point-of-care technology
PrOMIS	problem-oriented medical information system
QPP	Quality Payment Program
QM	quality metrics
ROI	return on investment
SNOMED-CT	Systematized Nomenclature of Medicine–Clinical Terms
SCAMC	Symposium on Computer Applications in Medical Care
TIGER	Technology in Informatics Guiding Education Reform
UMLS	Unified Medical Language System
URL	uniform resource locator (Web address)
WINI	Weekend Immersion in Nursing Informatics

the problem, either by contacting the vendor of the software system with an enhancement request (which might take months if not years) or by devising an alternative workaround to solve the issue.

Coordinator

In a coordinator role, the informatics nurse may organize and lead meetings in which nurses provide information that the informatics nurse uses to analyze and change the system design to make it more useful. During these meetings, the informatics nurse may ask nurses about their daily work to understand how the department functions. This information is known as the *workflow* of the unit or department. Once the informatics nurse understands the workflow of the department, they will make recommendations to the vender of the program about how to best reconfigure the program to meet the needs of the nurses. After the program is reconfigured, the floor nurses give additional input on whether the proposed revision

will work. This process might take weeks. The willingness of vendors to reconfigure programs varies; some respond quickly, while others are slow to respond or may refuse to change their programs at all.

Tester

Once a module of the program is reconfigured and approved by the floor nurses, the informatics nurse tests it to see if the module works as advertised. Often, several modules may be tested at the same time. After each module has been tested individually, integration testing takes place. For example, a patient is registered in the registration module, then the patient is scheduled by importing data from the registration module into the scheduling module. Finally, the patient appears in a tracking board indicating they have been admitted. It is important that the informatics nurse ensure that each module *and* the overall program work together to promote a smooth transition from one module to the next.

Issues Now

There's an App for . . . Diseases?

Health-related apps for wireless devices are wildly popular. Currently, there are more than 350,000 of these apps. Many of these apps deal with exercise, diet, and healthy living, but some are specific to medical care, and the number of disease-management apps is increasing. Apps that emphasize managing specific diseases or health conditions now make up 47 percent of health-care apps as compared with 28 percent in 2015. Mental health–, diabetes-, and cardiovascular disease–related apps make up almost half of condition-specific apps.

The COVID-19 pandemic forced patients and health-care providers to implement digital health tools as care moved from face-to-face to electronic media. More than 90,000 new apps came online between 2019 and 2021, the two peak years of the pandemic. One commonly downloaded app during that time was the telehealth app Doximity, whose use increased by 38 times in 2020. This app is directed at health-care providers. Doximity aims to decrease miscommunication and patient handoff errors by creating a platform that enables quick and easy communication between physicians, HIPAA-compatible document transfer, and a streamlined service to securely contact patients and colleagues. Other apps whose use increased during the pandemic included exercise apps, mental health apps, and blood pressure apps. COVID-19 also increased the market for wearable devices that could measure oxygen blood saturation in patients who had survived COVID-19 or were being treated at home.

People who are about to undergo surgery often have high anxiety levels due to fear of the unknown. What's going to happen? Is it going to hurt? How long is it going to take? Well, there's an app to help with that. Touch Surgery is an app that allows patients who are preparing for operations to download videos of their actual surgery or computer-based simulations of it. Health-care facilities use apps like this to educate patients about procedures and also to build trust and confidence in anxious patients. Some of the surgeries that can be viewed include removal of the gallbladder (cholecystectomy), removal of the appendix (appendectomy), and common orthopedic surgeries such as hip and knee replacement and shoulder reconstruction. Because many of these surgeries are done in one-day surgery units, nurses have little time to educate patients about postoperative care. The app provides patients with instructions about deep-breathing exercises, activity limitations, and the use of medications. The app has the potential to increase patient satisfaction and improve outcomes.

Feeling stressed? There are apps that can help with that! Stress-reduction apps monitor your daily stress by using sensors built into mobile devices that measure physiological changes. Devices built into some smartphones can measure environmental noise level; social activity, such as the number and frequency of texts and calls; temperature; and even the user's posture. Biometric measuring watches can track moods and emotions by analyzing pulse and heart-rate data and relay it to a provider if so desired. The app can make people more aware of their internal stress levels, which may be helpful for patients with cardiovascular disease or anxiety disorders.

Although not an app, there is a Web site where patients can find out if the hospital they are being admitted to has had any patient-care violations. By logging on to www.hospitalinspections.org, the patient can find information about deficiencies cited during complaint inspections at acute care and critical access hospitals throughout the United States. The site is run by the Association of Health Care Journalists (AHCJ) in conjunction with the U.S. Centers for Medicare and Medicaid Services (CMS). The goal of the site is to make federal hospital inspections easier to access, search, and analyze. However, inspections of psychiatric or long-term care facilities are not included in the database. Previously, this information could be accessed only by hardcopy written request through the Freedom of Information Act. The AHJC continually updates and fills in missing information.

Sources: *E. Olsen, Digital health apps balloon,* mobihealthnews, *August 4, 2021, https://www.mobihealthnews.com/news/digital-health-apps-balloon-more -350000-available-market-according-iqvia-report; DigiPrima Technologies, How mobile apps are transforming healthcare, LinkedIn, July 25, 2022. https://www.linkedin.com/pulse/how-mobile-apps-transforming-healthcare-digiprima-technologies.*

Trainer

After the informatics nurse decides that all the modules and the total program are working as they should, staff needs to be trained. The informatics nurse may also be the staff trainer, or there may be a separate education nurse who is responsible for staff training. Whatever the situation, one person should be in charge of developing educational materials to train the team members on using the program and teaching the new program. Often, vendors have educational materials and demonstration programs that can be modified or used as is. The goal of the training is to ensure that the majority of end users successfully master the program and feel comfortable in its use.

When a new system or a system update is ready to "go live," the launch is coordinated by the informatics nurse and other members of the project team, such as a vendor representative, IT personnel, and the facility's nurse educator. The informatics nurse is responsible for planning every aspect of the rollout months before the actual go-live date. Often, the vendor provides a small support team that can address glitches that may occur during the rollout. Their role is to quickly solve any technical issues that may occur with the new program. Although for some team members, this is the exciting part of the project, for the informatics nurse, it is usually the most stressful part of the job.

WHERE DO INFORMATICS NURSES WORK?

Informatics nurses' work is not limited to hospitals or clinics. Informatics nurses are also hired by program vendors as analysts or consultants.[1] Nurse analysts work with program developers, who know technology well but know little or nothing about nursing, to make sure the programs they are developing are user friendly. Consultants work to design solutions either for one facility or for many facilities within a network. Being a consultant often involves significant travel.

HOW DOES INFORMATICS FIT WITH NURSING?

Nursing informatics as a discipline did not spring up overnight. In fact, its origins actually precede the

work of Florence Nightingale.[2] Milestone achievements in nursing informatics are noted on the timeline shown in Figure 17.1. As you read through the timeline, try to organize the major events into categories and analyze why those classifications are meaningful or useful. This analysis can be done using the nursing process, which informs the data-to-wisdom model in nursing informatics.

Data-to-Wisdom Model

Data to wisdom is the model that nurse informaticists use to transform basic data into innovations that augment safe, quality health care. It is the primary connection between informatics and EBP. The four steps in the model include data, information, knowledge, and wisdom; each piece of data can become wisdom when analyzed accurately. Let's look at an example.

Raw Data

If given the number 2010, the year when artificial intelligence (AI) became a reality, many people would not automatically associate it with a milestone on the nursing informatics timeline. The number 2010 by itself is just raw data and holds no value or meaning; it is only a group of four numbers in a row and could mean anything. It could be the number of people attending a conference, the number of feet a person walked during a day, a locker combination, the name of a movie, an AM radio station, or a version of a software program.

Information

A good way of thinking about information is data + meaning. To construct information, a person must be able to combine diverse raw data points into a meaningful picture within a specified context. In this way, information becomes a continuum of progressively emerging and grouped data that can answer the basic questions such as who, what, where, and when.[3] If, from the raw data point of 2010, the nursing informatics milestone comes to mind, it is only because the person thinking about the number remembers the timeline. If additional data, the fact that the number appears on the nursing informatics timeline, is

> *Wisdom results only from the most profound analysis and combining of data, information, and knowledge.*

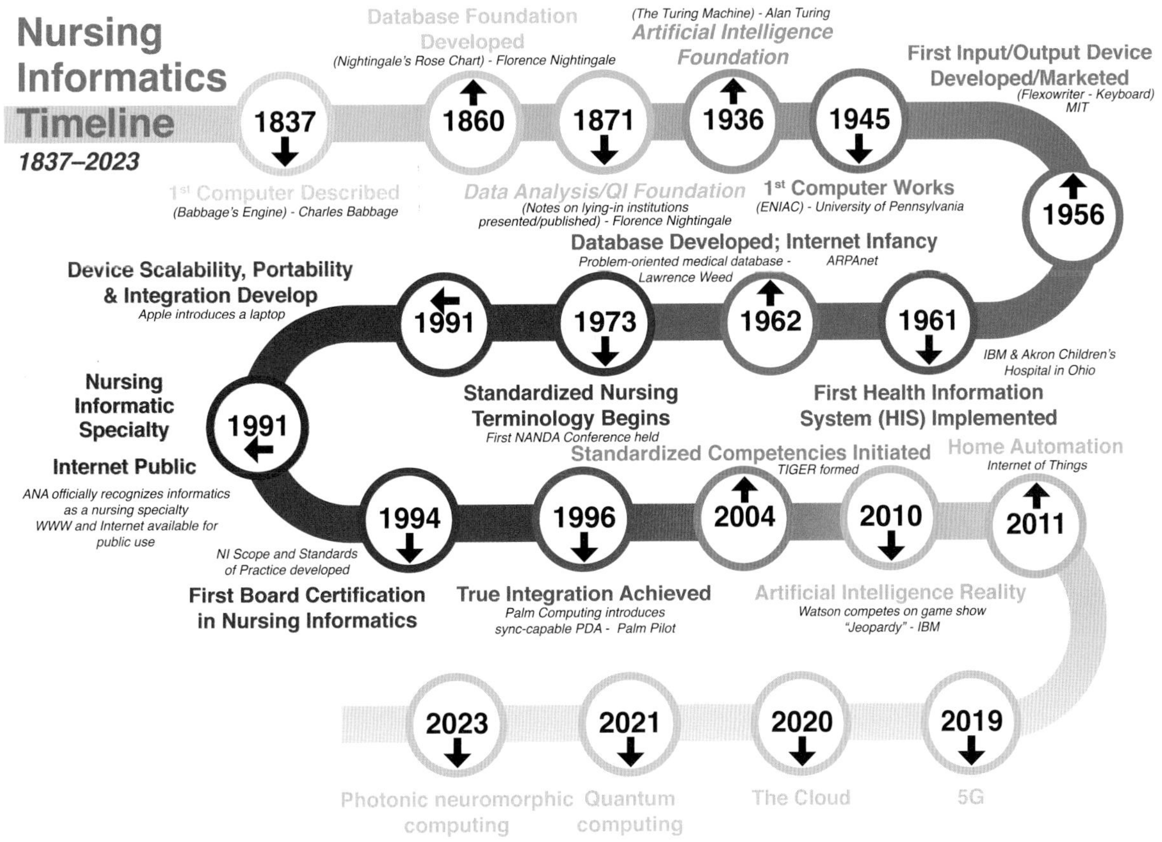

Nursing Informatics Timeline
1837–2023

Nursing Informatics Timeline

1837	**1860**	**1871**	**1936**	**1945**		

Database Foundation Developed
(Nightingale's Rose Chart) - Florence Nightingale

(The Turing Machine) - Alan Turing
Artificial Intelligence Foundation

First Input/Output Device Developed/Marketed
(Flexowriter - Keyboard) MIT

1st Computer Described
(Babbage's Engine) - Charles Babbage

Data Analysis/QI Foundation
(Notes on lying-in institutions presented/published) - Florence Nightingale

1st Computer Works
(ENIAC) - University of Pennsylvania

1956

Database Developed; Internet Infancy
Problem-oriented medical database - Lawrence Weed   ARPAnet

Device Scalability, Portability & Integration Develop
Apple introduces a laptop

1991	**1973**	**1962**	**1961**

IBM & Akron Children's Hospital in Ohio

Nursing Informatic Specialty

1991

Standardized Nursing Terminology Begins
First NANDA Conference held

First Health Information System (HIS) Implemented

Internet Public

ANA officially recognizes informatics as a nursing specialty WWW and Internet available for public use

Standardized Competencies Initiated
TIGER formed

Home Automation
Internet of Things

1994	**1996**	**2004**	**2010**	**2011**

NI Scope and Standards of Practice developed

First Board Certification in Nursing Informatics

True Integration Achieved
Palm Computing introduces sync-capable PDA - Palm Pilot

Artificial Intelligence Reality
Watson competes on game show "Jeopardy" - IBM

2023	**2021**	**2020**	**2019**

Photonic neuromorphic computing   Quantum computing   The Cloud   5G

Figure 17.1 Nursing informatics timeline.

provided, that data adds value and makes it easier to interpret the data 2010 as a year in a sequence of years.

Knowledge

Knowledge is defined as information that has been analyzed and synthesized so that the relationship and interactions between data points are defined and formalized. Knowledge can be thought of as the building up of meaningful information created from discrete data points. Knowledge is often affected by the expectations and central theories of a scientific discipline and is originated by learning the patterns of relationships between different collections of information. Knowledge answers questions of why or how.[3] The process of combining the raw data, 2010, with the information from the timeline produces knowledge. Knowledge consists of data that have been given form and have been interpreted. In this case, knowledge is recognizing that AI became a reality in 2010.

Wisdom

The American Nurses Association (ANA) in 2008 defined *wisdom* as the appropriate use of knowledge to manage and solve human problems. Ethical behavior informs wisdom so that the nurse knows why certain actions or procedures should or should not be employed in nursing practice. Wisdom, when applied to nursing science and practice, guides the nurse in identifying the evolving issue, illness, or condition based on the patients' values and the nurse's experience, knowledge, and skills. The nurse must combine all these elements, decide on a nursing intervention, and then act accordingly. Wisdom is how a nurse makes an effective and safe clinical judgment.[3] Wisdom results only from the most profound analysis and combining of data, information, and knowledge. Starting with the number 2010, the resulting wisdom could be a portion of the mixture of sciences that created nursing informatics.[4]

What Do You Think?

Describe your feelings about using an EHR during your clinical experiences. What was the most difficult part of using the system?

ANALYZING NURSING INFORMATICS

Data points on the nursing informatics timeline can be sorted into three categories of knowledge: (1) computer hardware and software, (2) data organization and integration, and (3) AI.

In addition, each data point can be classified as a science. In general, each meaningful achievement on the timeline is mapped to a science. Computer hardware and software information becomes computer science knowledge. Data organization and integration information becomes information science knowledge. And AI, or logistical process, information becomes cognitive science knowledge.[4] There is no wisdom, only knowledge about the pieces that make up nursing informatics.

Computer, Information, and Cognitive Science

The founders of nursing informatics are considered to be Charles Babbage, Florence Nightingale, and Alan Turing, even though Babbage's and Turing's work was unrelated to nursing. Because of the innovative and persistent work by these three prominent pioneers, nursing informatics is possible. Each science included within informatics is represented by one of these trailblazers: computer science, information science, and cognitive science.[3]

During the Industrial Revolution in the early 19th century, Charles Babbage, a mathematician and statistician who was friends with the Nightingale family, introduced the world to concepts that would later become computer science and information science. In 1837, Babbage published meticulous instructions for what he termed the *Babbage Engine*, a type of early computing machine. Following Babbage's instructions, modern engineers actually built the engine in 1991.[1] Once built, it worked exactly as he had described.

As a child, Florence Nightingale began organizing, classifying, and analyzing every type of data she could find using statistical principles she learned from Babbage. Her statistical fascination led her to develop the Nightingale rose diagram, a type of early pie chart that presented data about health conditions during the Crimean War in a standardized, accurate format in order to improve care.[5] Nightingale did not like the term *rose* or *coxcomb* (the red top of a roster's head) but preferred simply *diagram*. Nightingale's diagram in Figure 17.2 shows two circles divided into 12 wedges whose size illustrates the number of soldier deaths that occurred per month per year at Scutari Hospital in Turkey from April 1854 to March 1856. A modern pie chart would likely include the actual numbers of deaths to compare with each other rather than just the size of the wedge. The wedges are color-coded: blue represents deaths by disease; red indicates deaths from battle injuries; black shows other causes of death. The two "roses" (diagrams) show the months from April to March illustrating what was happening before and after Nightingale instituted the hand washing and other sanitary measures in March 1865. Comparing the two diagrams, two differences become obvious: first, how much larger the blue wedges (death by disease) are than the red wedges (death from battle wounds) in both diagrams; and, as a result of the use of sanitary interventions, how the total size of the chart (representing the total number of deaths) is vastly reduced from April 1885 to March 1886 compared to the previous year without sanitary measures.[5]

Nightingale was the first nurse to use information science—data, data presentation, and data analysis—in showing a cause-and-effect relationship between a nursing action and a health-care outcome. The overall death rate among soldiers from disease and infection fell from a high of 40 percent to 2 percent.[5] Nightingale's use of information science provided the foundation of nursing informatics and quality improvement, which was most evident in her 1871 publication "Notes on Lying-in Institutions."[4]

Before and during World War II, Alan Turing, the father of AI, studied Babbage's analytical writings. Turing described his own computer, which he called the Turing machine, in 1936 and proposed the Turing test in 1950.[5] Turing's work, based on Babbage's initial reflections a century earlier, became the classic text on AI because it showed how machines can emulate human thought processes via logical analysis.

The pace of technological advancement increased after World War II, when computer science,

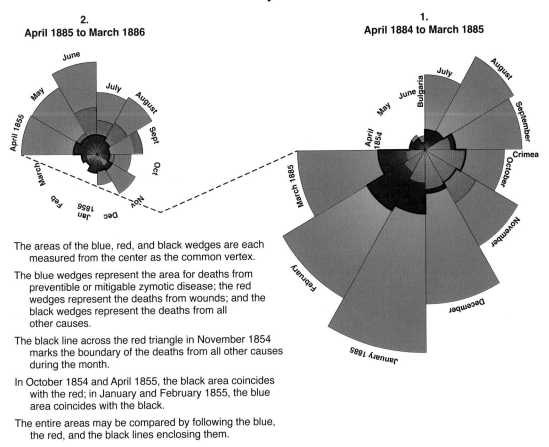

**Diagram of the Causes of Mortality
in the Army of the East**

The areas of the blue, red, and black wedges are each
measured from the center as the common vertex.

The blue wedges represent the area for deaths from
preventible or mitigable zymotic disease; the red
wedges represent the deaths from wounds; and the
black wedges represent the deaths from all
other causes.

The black line across the red triangle in November 1854
marks the boundary of the deaths from all other causes
during the month.

In October 1854 and April 1855, the black area coincides
with the red; in January and February 1855, the blue
area coincides with the black.

The entire areas may be compared by following the blue,
the red, and the black lines enclosing them.

Figure 17.2 Nightingale rose chart.

information science, and cognitive science thrived
and began to meld into what became known as
informatics.

Development of Computer Hardware and Software

In 1945, engineers at the University of Pennsylvania
built the first working electronic computer named
the Electronic Numerical Integrator and Computer
(ENIAC).[6] The development of the ENIAC ignited
research and innovation in the field of computer
science. A mere 11 years later, in 1956, the Flexowriter was introduced by computer scientists at
Massachusetts Institute of Technology (MIT).[6]

The Flexowriter allowed the user to input information from a keyboard rather than using a tape or
punch cards. Modern input/output (I/O) devices,
such as mice, pens, printers, voice, and video-
capture hardware, began with the Flexowriter. The
new hardware and software capabilities could be
combined to process data using heuristics, shortcuts
that allow for rapid decision making or the quick
resolution of problems. In the world of computers,
heuristics take the form of algorithms, or logical-
order problem-solving, to create results with greater
efficiency and accuracy than humans are capable of
achieving. In other words, I/O devices such as the
keyboard forced the integration of computer science

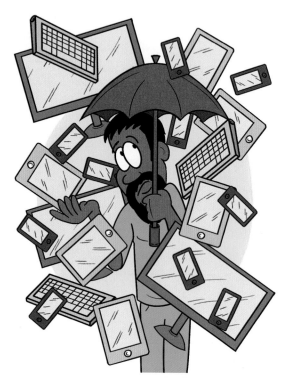

Technology can be overwhelming.

and cognitive science so that the computer hardware could manipulate rational and coherent input data in order to produce usable output results. The reverse of this idea is the familiar saying "garbage in, garbage out," which means if the data that are entered in the system are of poor quality, then the results of the data analysis will be trash.

Development of Information Systems

The International Business Machine (IBM) Corporation, in conjunction with Akron Children's Hospital, pioneered the first health information system (HIS). This task required the use of all three sciences—computer, information, and cognitive—in order to be successful. Furthermore, because this information system was implemented in a health-care setting, it became the genesis of nursing and health-care informatics. In 1961, a working HIS was demonstrating process integration, decreasing paperwork, and improving quality and safety.[8] Review the multitude of information systems available today in Box 17.2.

While the HIS at Akron Children's Hospital eventually led to a nation filled with information systems, similar foundational design began just one year later on the largest information system in the world. The Advanced Research Projects Agency (ARPA) formed the network basis for the Internet, known at that time as the ARPANet. The ARPANet increased Internet hosts, network numbers, and technological advances over the next three decades, ultimately evolving into the World Wide Web (WWW), which was made public in 1992.[7] The instantaneous and global I/O processes and responses of today are possible because of the foundational work of ARPA.

EHR or EMR?

What is the difference between an EHR and an EMR? The EHR is classified as a clinical information system (CIS), whereas the EMR is classified as a standalone system. The difference has to do with the ability of a system to work with various other computers and different computer programs.

Integration means that several systems or electronic entities all work together. A wireless smartphone exemplifies hardware integration because the small computer processor in the phone works as a computer, phone, and camera, among many other things. Software integration is best exemplified by an operating system, which is one large collection of computer programs that work together. Similarly, "bundled" software, the kind that comes with a new computer, is an integrated system that includes an operating system, a database program, a number of different software applications, and a presentation program. In those types of software bundles, the data entered into one program can often be used in a different program. For example, the software in the database program works with the software in the presentation program, and so forth. This type of programming is integrated.

An EHR is integrated because it is able to communicate with other systems, such as administrative systems, financial billing systems, laboratory systems, and even systems outside the facility, such as health insurance systems. By contrast, an EMR is not integrated because it is located on a single computer system and is unable to network with computer systems outside its designated sphere, although it may be located on several computers. For example, EHRs are usually used in a large health-care facility with many

Box 17.2 Classification of Information Systems

Classification	Key Points/Examples

Bibliographic retrieval system	• Online library search (or catalog) systems using standardized terminologies:
	  • Medical Subject Headings (MeSH)
	  • Unified Medical Language System (UMLS)
	  • NLM (National Library of Medicine) Vocabulary
	• Can combine Boolean or advanced search for further retrieval
	• Examples: PubMed, Medline

Clinical information system (CIS)	• Also known as patient care systems (PCS)
	• Integrated system that provides all patient care and administrative information at the point of care
	• Benefits:
	  • Shared data between multiple information systems to improve quality and safety of care
	  • Increased financial responsibility and return on investment (ROI) for facilities, as costs are captured
	• Example: Electronic health record (EHR) system

Communication system	• Systems that are increasingly integrated with CIS • Used for spoken, written, and nonverbal messages • Examples: Nurse tracking system, wireless nurse call system, patient educational messaging system

Decision support system (DSS)	• Based on algorithms, a database that aids human decision making through a series of input/output, or questions and answers
	• Specific type: Clinical decision support system (CDSS)
	  • Algorithmic-based decision-making tool
	  • CDSS used every day
	  • In terms of informatics, DSS and CDSS are computer based
	  • Any scale used to rate a patient is an algorithm, or decision support
	• Simplistic example: Glasgow Coma Scale score
	• Complex example: Computerized provider order entry (CPOE) drug warnings—the provider enters a medication that may interact with another medication and immediately receives an alert

Health information system (HIS)	• Also known as *core business system* • Similar to CIS but with focus on administration rather than on patients • Includes admission, discharge, transfer (ADT) system • May integrate with finance/billing, MIS, acuity, payroll, and scheduling
Management information system (MIS)	• Used to create reports for administration • Reports used for increased quality decision making • Can be linked with quality measures
Natural language system	• Database search inquiries using cognitive science (artificial intelligence) to understand written requests • Used as an alternative search technique in most online library catalogs, such as Cumulative Index for Nursing and Allied Health Literature and ProQuest • Also used for voice recognition, such as dictation • Largest example: Google search systems

(continued)

Box 17.2 **Classification of Information Systems** (continued)

Classification	Key Points/Examples
Point-of-care technology (PoCT) system (or PoC system)	• Devices that may or may not integrate with other systems • Provides ability to document and deliver testing at the bedside • Simplistic (nonautomated) example: Urine dipstick • Automated examples: EHR tablets, glucose meters, barcode medication administration (BCMA) devices
Standalone system	• Also known as a *dedicated system* or a *turnkey system* • Overriding classification of systems • System will not share data, or communicate, with other computers or computer programs • Example: Electronic medical record (EMR) system
Transaction processing system	• Financial system that includes accounting and billing • Examples: Patient billing and payroll

different services or departments, such as laboratory, radiology, medical records, admitting, and so forth. An EMR is more likely be used by a health-care provider's office as a patient record on the office's computer system, which does not communicate or share data with any other system outside the office except for functions such as e-mail.

Integrated Devices Everywhere!

The late 20th century brought major advances in computer, information, and cognitive science. Hardware became more affordable, portable, and accessible. A number of technology companies made landmark achievements advancing portability, scalability, and integration, and each achievement created more devices.

Portability and Scalability

Portability is the ability to move a device easily from one place to another. Compare ENIAC's weight of more than 30 tons with the first laptop, which weighed a mere 5.1 pounds.[2] *Scalability* is a forward-thinking property of a hardware/software/network system's ability to scale, or grow, to accommodate anticipated needs. For example, the first laptop had a *million times* more computing power than the ENIAC, in a much smaller size. And compare the function of a desktop computer from the year 2000 with the computing abilities of a smartphone today. The smartphone has more memory and much faster computing power. The smartphone demonstrates scalability by having more functionality in a smaller size.[6]

Integration and Interoperability

Integration and *interoperability* are often misused or mistakenly used interchangeably. They do not mean the same thing. *Integration* refers to one or more electronic devices sharing data with another device, regardless of whether data sharing was the original goal of the device. For example, if a smartphone of one brand can synchronize with a desktop or laptop computer of another brand in order to use some of the computer's data, then integration exists. Neither the computer nor the smartphone was originally designed to share data with the other device; however, a program was developed that allowed the devices to communicate, or share, data with each other.

Interoperability is the ability to use, or share, data among any number of devices, regardless of the type or brand of device. A common example of interoperability is televisions. Regardless of brand, all televisions will correctly receive the signal sent by the station or signal provider. A corollary is that it does not matter what television provider is chosen by any given household; the signal is still displayed appropriately on the television. The television signal data and the multitude of brand-name televisions, or television providers, are interoperable.[7]

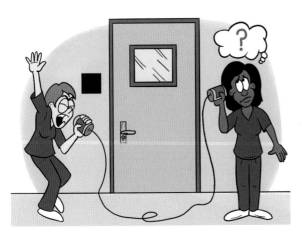

"I don't think our system has interoperability!"

Still in Development

Unfortunately, true interoperability does not yet exist in health care or informatics. The interoperability goal in health care is for all information systems to share data, regardless of the brand of hardware or software used or the facility using it. The nursing informatics timeline shows that Palm Computing attempted to create interoperability in 1996 but achieved only true integration instead. The Palm Pilot could synchronize with desktop computers, regardless of operating system, via a desktop software program.[7] Full interoperability has yet to be achieved.

Creating Standards

After World War II, the need to categorize and label information so that it could be accurately and efficiently retrieved and used by end users grew dramatically. The work of Lawrence Weed, Norma Lang, and Virginia Saba standardized nomenclature, database design, and retrieval. Their work on early EBP principles, terminology standardization, and interoperability contributed greatly to informatics as a science. These efforts optimized nurses' workflow and contributed to safer and higher-quality care for patients.

Weed chaired the formation of the patient-reported outcome measurements information system (PrOMIS) in 1962 at Cleveland Metropolitan General Hospital.[8] It is a set of person-centered measures that evaluates and monitors physical, mental, and social health in adults and children. PrOMIS can be used with individuals living with chronic conditions.

Weed did not believe that all medical knowledge should, or could, be memorized but rather that safe, high-quality care would result when information could be easily retrieved and used. Weed developed a database of usable data, information, and standardized medical terminologies, comprising nearly 5,000 problem-oriented categories that could be used for patient care and research.[8]

NANDA

The development and use of the term *diagnosis* in nursing was a long and hard-fought battle. The most universal and general definition of diagnosis is "the collection and analysis of data in order to identify and name problems of various kinds." Using this general definition as a starting point and adapting it to the type of work nurses perform on a daily basis, such as caring for individuals with various illnesses and injuries, *nursing diagnosis* can be defined as identifying the elements and characteristics of altered human responses to a health problem. The international North American Nursing Diagnoses Association (NANDA) has further refined the definition of nursing diagnosis as "the clinical judgment that nurses formulate about the responses of the individual, the family, or the community to the vital conditions or processes." Nursing responsibilities that arise from the nurse's use of clinical judgment include monitoring the patient's responses to various treatments and medications and developing a care plan for the implementation of interventions that include nursing actions, interdisciplinary therapies, and transfers if judged necessary.[9]

NANDA began categorizing nursing diagnoses in St. Louis, Missouri, in 1973.[10] Lang pushed for standardized nursing terminology. Saba,* another well-known informatics nurse, supported the need for standardized terminology as well. Saba, however, focused on the need for terminology integration to promote HIS interoperability. To meet this goal, Saba released the Clinical Care Classification (CCC) system in 1994. The CCC integration list includes

- Cumulative Index for Nursing and Allied Health Literature (CINAHL).
- Unified Medical Language System (UMLS).
- Systematized Nomenclature of Medicine–Clinical Terms (SNOMED-CT).
- Health Level 7 (HL7).[11]

*Dr. Virginia Saba, RN, passed away on November 24, 2021.

Each clinical term, procedure, medication, or diagnosis in the CCC automatically links to a similar term, procedure, medication, or diagnosis in any of the preceding systems and indices. Because of the automatic links in databases and the communication between different systems, the foundation for true interoperability has been formed. This process of mapping one health-care language, or standardized terminology, to another is similar to the database design and retrieval that occurs within AI systems.

ARTIFICIAL INTELLIGENCE

To some, the term *artificial intelligence* conjures images of out-of-control home appliances and robots that want to kill humans and take over the world. Because of these unfounded fears regarding artificial intelligence, some people working in technological fields of study now recommend using the alternative terms *knowledge engineering, machine learning, neural networks,* or *expert systems*. None of these alternative terms has caught on for general use, and AI remains the dominant term. Realistically, there is little reason to fear AI independently taking over all computer systems because the systems are only as intelligent as the people programming them.

Hello, Watson

Electronic automation in homes and industry ignited the quest for interoperability in the beginning of the 21st century. The first steps toward interoperability were the development of advanced AI systems. IBM developed high-level artificial intelligence with natural language skills with a computer named Watson. Watson was composed of five large computers that that took up the space of a good-sized bedroom. In 2011, Watson competed on the game show *Jeopardy* and eventually beat the show's top human champion! But Watson was not perfect; sometimes, the computer answered incorrectly because it did not understand the question. These incorrect answers demonstrated the limitations of database design, data analysis, natural language heuristics, and database retrieval capabilities.

Home-automation systems use algorithms, not artificial thought processes, to benefit humans. In 2011, Nest Labs released the Nest Learning Thermostat to benefit both humans and the environment. The thermostat "learns" what temperature the house occupants like and then builds a schedule around the times the temperature is adjusted. The Nest can save both money and natural resources by turning the temperature either up or down when no one is at home. This device expedited development of a form of integration that approaches comprehensive interoperability. From the Nest thermostat, additional home-automation devices, such as the Amazon Echo, Apple HomeKit, and Google Home, were developed.[12]

AI in Health Care

Although AI use has been rapidly gaining ground in commercial and industrial applications, in health care, by comparison, it is growing at a snail's place. However, where AI has been used in health care, it has had a substantial impact on patient-related processes. It has even greater potential. For example, from the time a patient decides to engage a health-care provider, the patient can register for an appointment at home from a device that has fingerprint or retina identifying technology or, in the facility or office, at a kiosk using the same type of technology. They then can add the reason for the visit with voice-recognition technology. All their data that have been collected so far during previous visits at any facility are electronically recovered along with their method of payment. Having health-care information linked to the insurance information allows the patient to know whether there is a copayment and, if so, how much it is. It also eliminates the tedious in-person insurance information–gathering process. After the patient has electronically checked in, the provider has all their medical information in hand without the patient ever having encountered an employee.[12]

AI can also help the patients take greater responsibility for their own care with wearable monitoring device technology that is electronically linked to a provider's office. An example of the current use of a wearable device is the continuous blood glucose monitor. These medical monitoring devices track the patient's health information and alert the patient and provider of changes in data that could be a cause for concern. A new device that holds great promise is the blood pressure (BP) tattoo. It is a noninvasive method for continuous BP monitoring in the home. Currently, many individuals with hypertension have home BP devices called *sphygmomanometers,* or *blood pressure cuffs*. Most are the automatic type that require the user to put the cuff on the person' arm or wrist, press a button, and in a minute or two read their BP. Unfortunately, even though the reading is highly accurate, it is just one reading. Health-care providers know that a person's BP varies throughout the day, especially in people who have labile, or unstable, hypertension. Their BP swings from very high to low over short periods of time.

The BP tattoo is a thin, sticker-like wearable electronic device that can provide continuous and accurate BP monitoring. The tattoo is composed of thin layers of graphene, a single sheet of carbon atoms arranged in a crystal lattice similar to a honeycomb pattern. Graphene is also the core element in the development of nanotechnology. The graphene layers conduct electrical impulses from the skin, which are captured as raw data. The data are then transferred by a tiny electronic machine embedded in the tattoo to a learning algorithm. The learning algorithm then analyzes and interprets the information, the results of which are translated into mmHg, the units used for measuring blood pressure.[13] The tattoo is temporary and similar to the stick-on tattoos that children like to wear. This new technology allows providers to understand how a patient's blood pressure fluctuates during the day in response to certain activities and to adjust the treatment accordingly. When AI is used in this manner, it is called predictive analytics, and it allows for early interventions that reduce morbidity and save lives.[12] It is only a matter of time before other monitoring tattoos are developed for a variety of diseases that would benefit from continual monitoring.

INFORMATICS ORGANIZATIONS AND THE PEOPLE BEHIND THEM

In 1981, Saba presented at the Symposium on Computer Applications in Medical Care (SCAMC), which was a conference for nurses that finally showed acceptance of informatics as a legitimate field for nursing.[2] One year later, Susan Newbold founded the Capital Area Roundtable on Informatics in Nursing Group (CARING), the first informatics organization for nurses on the East Coast.[2] The major health-care informatics organizations with their Web addresses are listed in Box 17.3.

Box 17.3 **Nursing Informatics Organizations**

Full Name	Informal Name	Exists Today?	Web Site
American Health Information Management Association	AHIMA	Yes	http://www.ahima.org
American Medical Informatics Association	AMIA	Yes	https://amia.org
Alliance for Nursing Informatics	ANI	Yes	https://www.allianceni.org
American Nurses Informatics Association	ANIA	Yes	https://www.ania.org
Capital Area Roundtable on Informatics in Nursing Group	CARING	Merged with ANIA	https://www.ania.org/about-us
Health Information and Management Systems Society	HIMSS	Yes	https://www.himss.org
International Medical Informatics Association	IMIA	Yes	https://imia-medinfo.org/wp
Symposium on Computer Applications in Medical Care	SCAMC	Renamed American Medical Informatics Association (AMIA)	https://amia.org
Technology in Informatics Guiding Education Reform	TIGER	Merged with HIMSS	https://www.himss.org/professionaldevelopment/tiger-initiative

Nursing Informatics Gets Recognized

By 1992, the American Nurses Association recognized nursing informatics as a specialty practice. That year, Pat Schwirian became the editor of *Computers Informatics Nursing*, the first official journal for the specialty, which remains in publication today.[3] Also in 1992, the University of Maryland in Baltimore graduated the first class of nursing informatics doctoral students, which included Nancy Staggers.[2] In 1994, Staggers, along with Carol Bickford, drove the publication of *Scope and Standards of Practice for Nursing Informatics*; Staggers also chaired the second edition in 2001.[3]

The American Nurses Credentialing Center (ANCC) offered the first nursing informatics board certification in 1994. Newbold passed the first certification offering and went on to create the Weekend Immersion in Nursing Informatics (WINI) classes in 1995; to date, these classes have aided hundreds of individuals studying for the nursing informatics certification examination.[3] Finally, June Kaminski and Staggers were instrumental in developing competencies for nursing informatics, which is crucial for advancement of the field. Just as terminology must be standardized, so must aptitude expectations. A list of nursing informatics pioneers with their critical contributions can be reviewed in Box 17.4.

THE LAWS THAT MADE IT HAPPEN

Nursing informatics is the meaningful use of data by health-care professionals to improve patient safety and quality-care outcomes, to advance decision making, and to optimize human work processes using technology. However, the evolution of computer, cognitive, and information sciences did not create the need or desire for informatics in health care. Rather, the impetus of the federal government made informatics a specialty in health care, specifically in nursing. Let's take a closer look at how legislation made it happen.

The Health Insurance Portability and Accountability Act

In 1996, the Health Insurance Portability and Accountability Act (HIPAA) was signed by President Bill Clinton as legislative law. Its primary purpose was to allow patient records to be transferred from one provider or institution to another provider or institution. Because these records were starting to be computerized and digitized, the law also provided

---

Box 17.4 Nursing Informatics Pioneers

Pioneer Name	Contribution
Carol Bickford	Drove creation of first *Scope and Standards of Practice for Nursing Informatics*
June Kaminski	Nursing informatics standardized competencies
Norma Lang	Standardized terminology: ICNP, NANDA, NIC, NOC, NMDS, NDNQI
Susan Newbold	CARING founder Passed first ANCC Nursing Informatics board certification WINI creator
Virginia Saba	Standardized terminology: CCC development with integration to CINAHL, UMLS, SNOMED, HL7
Patricia Schwirian	First Cumulative Index for Nursing and Allied Health Literature editor Early informatics theorist (Schwirian's Cube)
Nancy Staggers	First doctoral graduate in nursing informatics, University of Maryland Drove creation of first *Scope and Standards of Practice for Nursing Informatics* Chaired publication of second edition of *Scope and Standards*

regulations for the privacy and security of the records during the transfer process. The privacy and security part of the law became the main focus of health-care providers. In fact, if asked, most nurses would say HIPAA was about privacy of patient information. The law also includes more protections than most health-care professionals realize. Five titles comprise this law, but *Title II: Preventing Health Care Fraud and Abuse, Administrative Simplification, and Medical Liability Reform* affects nursing informatics the most. The main HIPAA components in Title II and their subsequent effect on informatics are defined in Box 17.5.

The initial HIPAA legislation required health-care facilities and providers to ensure that patients understood the care provided. It also required that the care provided remained confidential and private. The provision for administrative simplification forecasted the need for protection of electronic data and information. HIPAA, therefore, marked the start of database design in health care.

- Data had to be protected, anonymous, confidential, and collectible, but without individually identifiable features.
- Data had to be able to be placed in groups so that patterns within that data could be identified during collection.

- Data had to be meaningful.
- Data had to be inaccessible to anyone who should *not* have access to it.

All of these requirements created a whole new world for databases within the field of health care. If HIPAA's criteria could not be met, consequences could be enforced under civil law.

What Do You Think?

Have you witnessed any HIPAA violations in your clinical experiences or in your interaction with the health-care system? If so, how could they have been prevented?

SECURITY ISSUES

Most people assume that all physician–patient communications are strictly confidential. However, in the new electronic world, confidential information has become a commodity that is bought and sold in the electronic marketplace. Although the HIPAA laws have tried to deal with this issue, people who use the Internet quickly realize that their personal information is no longer so personal. For example, health-care providers often look up information on friends and family members who are not under their care, thereby violating HIPAA regulations and hospital policies.

Box 17.5 HIPAA's Effects on Informatics

HIPAA Provision	Date of Effect	Effect on Informatics
Administrative Simplification Provision	1996	• Subsection 2 of Title II in the law, which contains the rules adopted for electronic standards, safety, and security, inclusive of coding requirements and unique health identifiers • Requires notices and paperwork for patients to be understandable
Privacy Rule	2003	• Personally identifiable information must stay confidential or be removed if information is to be shared or studied • Only those who need to know should know
Security Rule	2005	• Information must be confidential and safe • Logins or other electronic methods must protect electronic information
Enforcement Rule	2006	• Defines penalties for breaking any part of the HIPAA law • Denotes prosecution will be under civil law

Confusing Laws

Unfortunately, no one comprehensive federal law governs data privacy in the United States. There have been many proposals over the years for such a law, but for a variety of reasons, they keep being rejected. Rather, the United States now has a complex and confusing patchwork of federal and state laws, including laws and regulations that address telecommunications, health information, credit information, financial institutions, and marketing. The Federal Trade Commission (FTC) is one of the major players in enforcing privacy laws. Its authority to regulate on behalf of consumer protections comes from the Federal Trade Commission Act (FTC Act), which has broad jurisdiction over commercial entities under its authority to prevent unfair or "deceptive trade practices." In 2021, a proposal to grant the FTC an additional $500 million was rejected by the U.S. Senate, but the Biden administration continued working to get the FTC the money, resources, and personnel it needs to become the country's primary privacy regulator.[14] Currently, the Federal Bureau of Investigation (FBI) is the primary enforcement and investigative arm of the Department of Justice that deals with breaches of privacy laws.

> *Attacks on health systems, including hacking into patient databases and facility shutdowns due to ransomware attacks, were up 66 percent over 2020.*

Information for Sale

Examples of violations of patient confidentiality abound. Early in 2022, the University of North Carolina (UNC) Lenoir Health Care and business partner Medical College of Georgia (MCG) Health had an incident involving unauthorized access to patient information. MCG Health was contacted by a hacker who claimed to have obtained protected health information from MCG patients. The hacker then demanded payment in exchange for returning patient files to MCG. An investigation by the FBI and computer forensic investigators found that patient health records had been listed for sale on the dark web. While these records all belonged to MCG patients, hospital administrators believed that the hacker may also have gained access to UNC Lenoir's patient records as well. Therefore, the personal, financial, and medical information of several thousand patients was in jeopardy.[15]

One of the most egregious violations of privacy occurred in 1996. A convicted child rapist working as a technician in a Boston, Massachusetts, hospital rifled through 1,000 computerized records looking for potential victims. He was caught when the father of a 9-year-old girl whom the rapist was harassing used caller ID to trace a call back to the hospital.

In 2010, a family member of a patient in the Charleston Area Medical Center in West Virginia discovered how to access the facility's patient information database while trying to find information on the Internet about the quality of the hospital. The database contained thousands of patients' names and Social Security numbers as well as medical and demographic information. The breach resulted in a lawsuit, *Tabata v. Charleston Area Medical Center*, based on the lack of security of the system.

In 2011, a class-action lawsuit was filed by patients of the University of California–Los Angeles (UCLA) health system. An external hard drive was removed from the home of a former UCLA physician with information pertaining to more than 16,000 patients. Although the hard drive was encrypted, a piece of paper with the password was also taken. In the class-action suit against UCLA, lawyers sought $1,000 for each patient as well as attorneys' fees and other costs, exceeding $16 million.

In another case, a banker on Maryland's State Health Commission pulled up a list of patients with cancer from the state's medical records, cross-checked it against the names of his bank's customers, and revoked the loans of the patients diagnosed with cancer. In addition, at least one-third of all Fortune 500 companies regularly review health information of applicants before making hiring decisions.

In Washington State in 2017 at a large medical center, a health-care employee was terminated for inappropriately accessing more than 600 confidential patient health records. The employee accessed private patient information including addresses, phone numbers, diagnoses, and Social Security numbers;

but there was no evidence that the information was misused. The breach in confidentiality was uncovered during a routine file audit.[15]

Cyberattacks on health systems mushroomed during the COVID-19 pandemic, and 2022 was their worst year on record. Attacks on health systems, including hacking into patient databases and facility shutdowns due to ransomware attacks, were up 66 percent over 2020.[16] The unrelenting increase in attacks on health-care facilities places patient safety in jeopardy and adds both emotional and financial strains on providers who are just now recovering from the pandemic.

How do hackers do it? Here's an example. Provider #1 receives a legitimate-looking e-mail from Provider #2, a person she knows, asking her to log into a hospital's portal to obtain a copy of one of a patient's past medical records to aid in the patient's care. However, Provider #2's e-mail is counterfeit, mocked up by hackers to look real. When Provider #1 logs into the portal, she has just unknowingly given her login password and credentials to a hacker who now can access the patient information portal and thousands of patient records.[16] This login access also allows the hacker to upload any kind of virus, such as a ransomware, into the hospital's computer system.

The cost of these attacks to hospitals and other health-care facilities is tremendous. On average, hospitals and health-care systems spend $7 million per year for a cyberattack. A small, nonprofit hospital, Sky Lakes Medical Center in Oregon, decided not to pay the ransom the attacker was demanding. Rather, they chose to rebuild their information system by replacing its 2,500 computers. They also had to completely clean their network before they could again access the Internet. Even after the hospital hired extra staff, it took six months to re-input all the paper records into the system. The total cost for the reactivation of their information services was $10 million.[16] However, with the upgrades in security that they incorporated during the revamping of their system, the hospital believes it will be able to stop new cyberattacks before they do any damage.

ETHICAL ISSUES

As discussed in Chapter 6, the study and science of ethics are concerned with placing value on people and situations that are encountered in everyday life. Ethics help people to determine whether what they are doing is good or bad, right or wrong. Although personal ethics are not usually written down, professional ethics are, and they aid in guiding the professionals in the group to make sound decisions. Some ethical precepts are so important that they are written into laws that can be enforced. The data management and information computing professions are no exception and have their own guidelines and laws that govern the conduct of their professionals.[17]

Computers and information technology burst so suddenly on to the scene that computer use initially had no regulations at all. Its rapid growth caused both ethical and legal problems, and guidelines had to be quickly formulated, often *post facto*, to deal with them. With the freedom of the Internet, new issues emerge all the time, and computer ethics attempts to address these threats.

Some of the more common threats include the following:

- Computer crimes
- Cybercrimes committed with the intent to harm an individual's reputation
- Malware insertion, uploading a computer virus or a Trojan horse that harms data stored in the computer by corrupting it
- Identity theft that allows a criminal to obtain personal information and use it as their own (credit card theft)
- Cyberstalking, a form of harassment using electronic communication devices

It is evident that all computers are vulnerable to some type of electronic wrongdoing. These crimes can be committed through the Internet, a computer network, or even a person's own personal communication device. Being ethical helps an individual avoid committing inadvertent computer crimes; it is equally important to use computer protection measures to reduce your susceptibility to a computer crime.[17] Box 17.6 lists a number of unethical, and in some instances illegal, actions from the Computer Ethics Institute.

A Question of Ownership

One of the key ethical questions in nursing informatics is, Who owns the patient's health-care data? Does the health-care information belong exclusively to the

Box 17.6 Computer Ethics Guidelines From the Computer Ethics Institute

- It is unethical to write a program with wrong motives such as harming users.
- It is unethical to access and destroy other people's files.
- It is unethical to generate and spread computer viruses.
- It is unethical to read other individuals' information without their permission because it violates their right to privacy.
- It is both unethical and illegal to use an electronic device to steal money, property or anything of value because it is deemed computer fraud and there are laws against it.
- It is unethical to use an electronic device to spread lies (slander).
- It is unethical and illegal to violate software, books or other written sources that are guarded by intellectual property rights (copyright).
- It is unethical to use any software or products that are not legally acquired.
- It is unethical and illegal in most cases to hack into a computer or information system for which the person has no legal authorization. *Hacking* is generally defined as the illegal bypassing of passwords or other authorization measures that allow access to a system.
- It is unethical and illegal to "pirate" the intellectual property of another.
- It is unethical to copy another person's work without authorization.
- It is unethical and illegal to write a computer program that is harmful to society (terrorism).
- It is unethical to use an electronic device that will show disrespect and a lack of consideration toward other individuals (cyberbullying).
- It is unethical and illegal to use a computer in any aspect of a crime, and the user will become one of the targets of the investigation and prosecution.

Source: Ethical issues in an age of information and communication technology. Ivy Panda, July 27, 2022. https://ivypanda.com/essays/ethical-issues-in-an-age-of-information-and-communication-technology.

patient? Does it belong to the organization that is storing the data or to the organization (e.g., insurance company, preferred provider organization) that paid for the care? Should it belong to the health-care provider who directed and ordered the care? What about the facility in which the care was given? Can it claim some ownership of the information, particularly if it is stored there? Do all these groups and individuals own a part of the information? No one really knows the answer.

Should Society Benefit?

Those who argue for individual rights believe that each person should have total and exclusive control over the disclosure of information concerning their health and the care rendered. Those who take a utilitarian, or "social good," position believe that society as a whole benefits from shared information about disease occurrence, treatment, and outcomes. Therefore, information should be available to all interested parties. As with most ethical dilemmas, a single definitive answer does not exist regarding who owns health-care data.

However, the number of public-policy debates concerning the collection of health-care information is increasing, especially regarding the use of aggregate databases to underpin health-care planning. Still, many consumers are concerned about the confidentiality of future physician–patient relationships. Driving the development of data-collection policy is the public's fear of the damage that may result from excessive and uncontrolled disclosures through automated health-care information systems.

The Implications of Consent

When patients enter the health-care system, they are generally asked to sign consent forms so that other organizations, such as insurance companies, can obtain information about their health status and the care that they receive. Patients are usually unaware that this information can also be supplied to many other organizations or institutions.

For example, facilities report injuries resulting from accidents to the trauma registry. The tumor registry collects information about benign and malignant tumors, and the public health department collects infectious disease reports. Currently, health-care information is shared to develop payment systems, examine access to care, identify cost differences in treatment modalities, research disease trends and epidemiological implications, and expand consumer information.

Threats to Security

Unauthorized Access

Unauthorized sharing of health-care information is both unethical and illegal. The codes of ethics for most health-care professions prohibit unauthorized or unnecessary access to patient information. In addition, most health-care institutions have policies prohibiting unauthorized access to confidential information. Individuals can lose their jobs, and nurses can lose their licenses for unauthorized access or sharing of patient information; and under HIPAA laws, they may be convicted of a crime.

As with all laws, there are limits to the security of patient information. After more than 20 years, many of the provisions of the Patriot Act remain on the books and in effect despite bipartisan congressional recognition that this act violated a number of information privacy rights by allowing the use of mass spying on U.S. civilians. Without further congressional action, much of the Patriot Act will remain permanent.[18] Under the Patriot Act, some federal agencies, such as the FBI, Immigration and Customs Enforcement (ICE), and the National Security Administration (NSA) have the authority to wiretap or access, without court approval, any electronic information they believe may be associated with a terrorist threat. This information includes physicians' and nurses' records, laboratory information such as DNA profiles and blood type, and financial information. Although some people believe this unrestricted access is necessary to prevent future terrorist attacks against the United States, others believe that it is a major violation of U.S. citizens' right to privacy.[18] It certainly seems to violate the regulations set forth in HIPAA.

Unauthorized access to or sharing of information is not a new problem. It was just as easy to gain unauthorized access to a paper record as it is to access the electronic record. The professional codes of ethics that stress confidentiality have *always* been the primary protector of patient information.

In some ways, the automated electronic record provides greater privacy than paper did. Access to the automated record is generally restricted to employees who have been issued a password. Also, most organizations have periodic **audits** that track each person who has accessed a record, and some systems can even detect unauthorized access at the time of entry into the system.

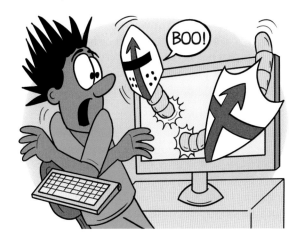

"I think it has WORMs!"

Accidents

Threats to information security can be either accidental or intentional and can affect both paper and electronic systems. Accidental threats involve events such as floods, fires, earthquakes, electrical surges, and power outages.

The paper record has little security against natural events. Typically, paper records are secured in a locked file cabinet or medical records room. Although current safety regulations require fire detection and suppression systems in these areas, even a small fire can destroy a large number of paper records very quickly. Little can be done to protect paper records against major flooding either. Once the charts are destroyed, they cannot be reproduced.

Facilities with automated systems usually have well-developed natural-disaster plans built into the system design. These plans include the automatic production and storage of backup data to a remote server at a protected location some distance from the health-care facility. The frequency of data backup varies with the organization's requirements. Most systems automatically save all the data in the system every 24 hours, although this time interval can be shortened or increased to meet the facility's needs.

Although these backup measures provide a high degree of protection from major natural events such as floods and fires, power surges and outages create problems for electronic systems but leave paper systems unaffected. Anyone who works with computerized equipment recognizes the major disruptions in service and work that occur when the system goes down. Again, some safeguards can be built into the system so that not all of the most recent information is lost when the power goes out, and power surges can be controlled with surge-protection devices.

Intentional Acts

Intentional threats to the security of information involve the actions of an individual or group who wishes to damage, destroy, or alter the records. In most cases, protecting paper records from intentional tampering is difficult. A determined individual can gain access to paper records and erase, add to, or rewrite sections of the chart. These changes are often very difficult to detect. In addition, a person could simply remove the chart and destroy it. Although automated electronic records are vulnerable to several kinds of intentional threats, they are, overall, more secure than paper records. All current automated systems have computer malware–checking programs that protect the electronic record from both intentional and accidental introduction of destructive computer viruses and other malicious programs.

Once data have been entered into the automated system, they are difficult to alter. Modern automated systems are designed with write once, read many (WORM) programs. If a legitimate change in the electronic record needs to be made, it must be an addendum. Any changes made in the electronic record are logged by the date, time, and the person who made them and can always be tracked to the point of origin.

A determined and gifted hacker can still obtain unauthorized access to almost any electronic database. However, after each hack, electronic security systems are made increasingly difficult to breach. Terrorist acts, ranging from detonation of bombs in key locations to development of "superviruses" to destroy electronic records, are more difficult to defend against.

Although criminal and civil penalties may result for those found guilty of data breaches, the consequences do not appear to deter hackers from attempting to break into secure databases. Health-care data are routinely hacked, as are other data sources in the United States. Because of the Breach Notification Act of 2009, all known data breaches involving more than 500 records are public record. The enforcement provisions of HIPAA detail the criminal and civil penalties attached to data breaches, and entities who receive these penalties are also a matter of public record.[19]

After the peak number of HIPAA health-care-related violations during 2019 through 2021, the number of breaches decreased during 2022. During the peak period, 80 percent of the electronic breaches were due to hacking and IT incidents. Unsanctioned access or disclosure accounted for 15 percent; and loss, theft, or improper disposal of records accounted for 5 percent of the breaches.[20] However, AI technology is a powerful deterrent to these types of breaches. Where it has been used in health-care facilities, AI and automated detection systems caught and halted information breaches 27 percent faster than facilities without the technology.[20]

HIPAA 2.0

To manage the regulations and requirements set forth in HIPAA, the Office of the National Coordinator for Health Information Technology (ONC) was officially established in 2009 by legislative law.[20] Title XIII of the American Recovery and Reinvestment Act of 2009 (ARRA) created the Health Information Technology for Economic and Clinical Health Act (HITECH), which mandated the use of informatics in health care.[21] For highlights of legislative and administrative mandates contributing to the rise of nursing informatics, see Box 17.7.

Some of the most important elements of this legislation for nurse informaticists pertain to electronic protection of health information. Penalties for breaches—or security and privacy violations—now include criminal as well as civil punishments. In addition, HIPAA underwent a revision in 2013 that refined and clarified all previous provisions and rules. This revision also created the meaningful use (MU) designation, officially titled the Medicare Electronic Health Records Incentive Program.[22]

Box 17.7 Important Legislative Effects on Informatics

Legislation	Date of Effect	Effect on Informatics
ARRA	2009	• An omnibus act including major provisions for health care • Only those who need to know should know
HITECH Act	2009	• Title XIII of ARRA • Officially created the Office of the National Coordinator for Health Information Technology • Allowed for processes—and money—to adopt and expand health information technology • Initial goal to create a national network of EHR systems
Breach Notification Act	2009	• Part of the HITECH Act • Outlines what to do if protected health information (PHI) is inadvertently, accidently, or purposely distributed in any form • Requires media notification • Criminal penalties now apply
ACA	2010	• Changed Medicare from a fee-for-service to a bundled payment system • Created/allowed accountable care organizations that could continue billing as a fee for service with a bonus/penalty system for quality • Required EHRs be adopted for meaningful use
HIPAA Omnibus	2013	• Final rule consolidating all previous HIPAA/HITECH rules • *Breach* defined more clearly • Enforcement rules more stringent
MACRA	2015	• Established a value-based system for Centers for Medicare and Medicaid Services payments • Transitions MU to one of four parts of the Merit-based Incentive Payment System • Established Quality Payment Program (QPP)

Sources: R. Smith, A. Coustasse, The HITECH Act and financial challenges of health information technologies in the United States with bottom up approach, *Insights to a Changing World Journal*, 2014(2):39–53, 2014; *HIPAA Administrative Simplification: Regulation Text*, 45 C.F.R. §162., 45 C.F.R. §§ 160, 162, 164, U.S. Department of Health and Human Services, 2013, https://www.hhs.gov/sites/default/files/hipaa-simplification-201303 .pdf; MACRA RFI posting: RFI on physician payment reform [CMS-3321-NC]: External FAQ, Centers for Medicare and Medicaid Services, 2016, https://innovation.cms.gov/Files/x/macra-faq.pdf; EHR incentives and certification: Meaningful use definition and objectives, Office of the National Coordinator for Health IT, https://www.healthit.gov/providers-professionals/meaningful-use-definition-objectives; Here are the degree options available to become a nurse informaticist. All Nursing Schools, 2018, https://www.allnursingschools.com/nursing-informatics/degrees.

Meaningful Use

Meaningful use refers to the use of certified EHR technology in a meaningful manner, for example, using electronic nursing records or electronic laboratory results to guide patient care. MU provides for the electronic exchange of health information (interoperability) with a goal of improving the quality of patient care. The MU program was phased in gradually in three stages: (1) data capture and sharing in 2011, (2) advanced clinical processes in 2013, and (3) improved outcomes in 2015. As of 2022, the majority of facilities that opted into MU were either in the latter phases of Stage 1 or in the early phases of Stage 2. A small percentage were beginning Stage 3.[22] To encourage adoption of EHR technology that would improve efficiency and outcomes, the federal government offered providers monetary incentives. Improved outcomes are linked to incentive payments of up to $44,000 over 5 years for Medicare providers and up to $63,750 over 6 years for Medicaid providers. Participation in the incentive program is totally voluntary; however, if eligible providers or hospitals failed to join by 2015, they experienced negative adjustments to their Medicare/Medicaid fees starting at 1 percent reduction and escalating to 3 percent reduction by 2017 and beyond.[22]

MU is built upon five health-care priorities:

1. Improving quality, safety, and efficiency and reducing health disparities
2. Engaging patients and families in their health
3. Improving care coordination with other health-care team members
4. Improving population and public health
5. Ensuring adequate privacy and security protection for personal health information[22]

The Challenges of Implementing Meaningful Use

One of the major challenges the MU system faced was the requirement for rapid implementation. The MU program initially required facilities to implement an EHR that met all the requirements within a short 2-year period. Despite the mandate and heroic attempts by health-care facilities, the goal could not be achieved, and the quality of care suffered.[22] Most facilities at the time had only paper systems for storing and moving data from one information point to another. A classic example is the patient chart, which had paper notes, laboratory data, the patient's history, a list of medications, and so forth. In some facilities, it was possible to use a computer to enter laboratory or dietary orders. Some facilities used computers for calculating staffing ratios or identifying patient acuity. However, laboratory results, dietitians' notes, and providers' notes came back in paper form and were pasted into the chart, the central database for that patient. The computers could not communicate with each other or with the chart.

Another challenge to implementing MU was that the infrastructure for integration within systems and interoperability among systems did not yet exist. Health-care facilities rushed to buy EHR systems, often without clinician or informaticist input. The EHR systems purchased may have been demonstrated to only a small number of available personnel. Often, the decision-makers were from non-nursing departments such as purchasing, finance, and administration; and many of the decision-makers had no idea how the technology would be used in everyday patient care. Even so, if the price was right, facilities purchased the system with the hope that it would meet the MU requirements.[22]

Another challenge to implementation was a lack of trainers and nursing informatics experts. Many early EHR systems advertised support for training and implementation. This promise of support made facilities feel secure with their decision to buy systems without seeking input from the people who were going to be using them daily. The plan usually was to train "superusers" who would then train and assist the other nurses and team members within their assigned units. Ideally, there would be a trained informatics person to assist the trainers and superusers. However, even if facilities had wanted to hire dedicated informatics personnel, qualified clinical informaticists were few and far between.[22]

> *MIPS seeks improved health-care outcomes through a quality- and value-based payment system that benefits the provider.*

A recent outgrowth of MU technology is the MyChart patient portal. The MyChart tool can provide all the laboratory data and various other pieces of information to providers and patients. It can also be focused to better manage a particular population of patients, such as those with diabetes. In large institutions that serve very diverse health-care populations, many of whom may never return to the facility for care, MyChart can be used to electronically share patient data with primary care providers in distant states.[22]

Despite the ANA declaring nursing informatics a specialty in 1992 and offering board certification in 1994, fewer than 1,000 board-certified nurse informaticists existed in the United States in 2010. To implement MU, it was projected that 20,000 to 100,000 nurse informaticists were needed. Those facilities that did hire additional staff usually hired information technologists, who knew a lot about computer systems but had no clinical background. This created additional problems with communication between the floor nurses and nonclinical computer technicians.[22] Informatics nurses were needed to bridge the gap.

Merit-Based Incentive Payment System

The attempt to implement the MU program demonstrated both its flaws and its strengths. Subsequently, its strengths became one of four components of the Merit-based Incentive Payment System (MIPS) introduced in 2019. MIPS seeks improved health-care outcomes through a quality- and value-based payment system that benefits the provider. This is different from MU, which benefited the payer.[23]

More than 200 quality measures exist on which a MIPS-eligible provider, provider group, or virtual group can report. To meet the MIPS's quality performance category requirements, data on 6 of the 200 quality measures (including at least one outcome measure or one high-priority measure if no outcome measure is selected) need to be collected and submitted for each quality measure during the 12-month performance period. The current data-completeness requirement is that 70 percent of the patients who are eligible for inclusion in the group's measurements must meet the quality measures.[23]

MIPS allows technological improvements to occur at the organizational level rather than via governmental mandate. The focus of MIPS, like MU, is on safe, high-quality patient outcomes. The difference is that with MIPS, organizations focus on improved patient care and outcomes rather than on mere technology implementation mandated by the government. The technology to achieve MIPS already exists and is being modified to meet its goals. In addition, a new structure of rewards and penalties for institutions, based on patient outcome data, has been developed for MIPS.[23]

WHAT IT TAKES TO BE AN INFORMATICS NURSE SPECIALIST

Early in the development of nursing informatics, any nurse who displayed minimal computer ability would often be pulled off their floor nurse duties and be unceremoniously designated as the informatics nurse. Usually, there were no written job descriptions or standards, and the nurse would literally have to write their own. There were no requirements for entry education level. However, a nurse who was truly dedicated to the role would seek additional nursing informatics training through seminars and workshops. Although the early technology was not that difficult to master, nurses' lack of knowledge of computers and hesitation to use them made nursing informatics training very difficult.

Today, the informatics nurse position is usually classified as a specialist.[24] A bachelor of science in nursing (BSN) degree is generally the entry-level degree required for informatics nurse specialists, although the masters of science in nursing (MSN) or doctor of nursing practice (DNP) is now preferred.[24]

Career prospects for nurses with advanced degrees in nursing informatics are growing exponentially because of the rapidly increasing use of EMRs and the general growth in the complexity of information technology. Informatics nurses work in a variety of areas; most commonly they work for large health-care organizations or technology companies. As the role of the informatics nurse grows and technology expands, so will the number and variety of professional positions.[24] (See Box 17.8.)

An informatics nursing degree can be earned through a specialized master or doctoral program. Coursework educates nurses to adapt technology to facilitate health-care goals and standards set by various organizations and the government.[24] Nurses study database management, computer systems analysis, and software design. They learn to use technology to support clinical decisions, maintain the quality and security standards of patient records, and manage government regulatory requirements. They become experts in communication and teaching skills and train new hires in the use of the facility's computer system. They also learn how to coordinate with vendors of informatics systems so that they can offer suggestions to improve systems and manage updates from the vendor.

The Bureau of Labor Statistics (BLS) projects that by 2030 an additional 276,800 informatic nurses will be needed, which is an expected increase of 9 percent over current levels. However, this number may be even higher because of the growth of large health-care

Box 17.8 Nursing Informatics: Positions and Settings

Some of the places informatics nurses can work:

- Academic setting
- Ambulatory care center
- Consulting firm
- Counseling center
- Electronic medical record company
- Government or military
- Health-care product company
- Hospital or health system
- International organization
- Private contractor
- Research facility
- Technology company
- Urgent care clinic
- Utility company

Career titles for nursing informaticists:

- Chief information officer
- Chief nursing officer
- Clinical analyst
- Clinical informatics nurse
- Clinical specialist
- Health informatics officer
- Informatics nurse
- Nursing informatics specialist

Source: Nursing informatics, *Nurse.org*, 2022, https://nurse.org/resources/nursing-informatics.

systems using complex data and information technology, the aging nurse population, nurse burnout related to the COVID-19 pandemic, and the increasing number of nurses leaving bedside nursing due to stress and workplace violence. In addition, the implementation of HITECH and the Patient Protection and Accountable Care Act (PPACA) have both led to the increasing need for technology savvy nurses. The American Medical Informatics Association (AMIA) believes that there will be a need for an estimated 70,000 new nursing informatics nurses per year just because of the rapid technological advancements that are occurring in health care.[24]

The ANCC offers an informatics certification that signifies a high level of competency in nursing informatics and is valid for 5 years. To be eligible to take the ANCC certification test, RNs must hold at least a BSN and complete 2 years of nursing practice. Continuing education credits in informatics must be earned. Nurses must also hold a graduate degree in informatics or have completed at least 2,000 hours of practice as informatics nurses. According to the 2022 data from PayScale.com, informatics nurses earned a median annual salary of $79,272 per year or $35.73 per hour. However, depending on years of experience, where the nurse lives, and additional education such as a PhD or DNP, salaries can range from just over $70,000 per year to as much as $107,000 per year.[24]

User Issues

Nurses are resourceful by nature and problem-solvers by vocation and education. Early health-information systems were primitive by today's standards; they were not user friendly and frequently did not work as advertised. Often, if a program did not perform a task the way it was supposed to, nurses would figure out a way to make the system do what they wanted it to do. Nurses, in general, did not attempt to alter their own daily routine to carry out the intended technological processes. This ability to make the computer perform tasks it was not initially intended to perform or using one of its features to defeat another feature became known as a *workaround.*

Workarounds can be either negative or positive. They are negative when they take the nurse's time away from patient care to fix a computer glitch or when they create errors in data or place patient safety at risk.[25] Positive workarounds can lead to new and innovative ways to complete tasks and increase the quality of patient care. Analyzing workarounds calls attention to design or programming inadequacies of the system being used. When these inadequacies are addressed, nurses' routines can actually become quicker and safer, and quality can be improved.[25] This improved process is called *workflow optimization.*

Although current EHR and other systems used to manage health-care data are much improved over the early ones, a number of workarounds still persist. There are two primary types of workarounds: in-system workarounds that occur when the user is working within the EHR system and out-system workarounds that occur when the user takes actions outside the EHR to supplement or bypass the system's practices. Some of these workarounds are discussed next.

Ignoring Pop-ups

Ignoring pop-ups is an in-system workaround. Pop-ups are part of the EHR's warning system to ensure tasks are implemented. However, in actual use, EHRs seem to open pop-ups way too often. Pop-up warnings, such as allergy warnings, that reoccur frequently can be very annoying to a provider or staff nurse. When pop-ups appear on a screen, it means the nurse has to stop what they are doing to answer the pop-up question. Instead, they just close it. Habitual ignoring of pop-ups can produce a false sense of safety, which could jeopardize patient well-being.

Pre-Starting a Patient's Visit

Pre-starting a patient visit is a an in-system workaround that uses the information in the EHR to pre-order treatments such as blood tests and x-rays to save time during the visit even before the patient physically arrives for the appointment. This process is done by clicking the "start patient visit" button that opens a new window through which orders can be placed whether or not the patient has arrived. However, if the patient does not show up for their appointment, this workaround will lead to an invoice for the patient because the tests have been registered as part of their care.

Copy-Pasting

Copy-pasting is an in-system workaround that involves using the "copy and paste" feature of the device to move data from one part of the system or record to another part. Ideally, all data should be recorded or entered individually and separately into the system. Although this workaround may save some time, it produces problems when developing statistical data with the information in the EHR.

Using Separate Text Fields

Using separate text or note fields is an in-system workaround that a nurse or provider can use that adds a separate note field called a *specialty comment* to the main chart. Use of specialty comments sometimes occurs because the EHR has only a fixed number of words or characters that can be entered in a particular field, leading the user to use a separate note

for the additional information. This workaround also affects the ability to do research on the data generated. It produces a separate piece of plain text that can lead to an unfinished overview of the data.

Leaving Data Fields Empty

Deliberately leaving data fields empty is an in-system workaround that occurs when certain patient-specific information is not entered into the EHR. A reason for this workaround is that users feel that the EHR restricts their autonomy and discretion to enter the data they wish to enter. Although not entering data cuts down on the amount of time needed for charting, this workaround damages the information quality that the EHR can provide. Moreover, not registering data potentially leads to errors in prescribing medications and other treatments where end dates are not entered. Incomplete vital sign data or neurological evaluations can be used in lawsuits when a patient injury occurred during the time period of the empty data entries. "If it's not written down, it wasn't done" is the legal precept.

Sharing Login Details

Sharing login details with other nurses or providers is an in-system workaround and a clear violation of hospital policies and HIPAA regulations. This workaround is done either because of a lack of time or a lack of a computer at hand. Once login details are shared, there is no control over potential abuse of this information.

Entering Incorrect or False Data

This in-system workaround involves entering data that does not represent reality. It can be used to intentionally bypass restrictions placed in the system to control the work process, such as avoiding delays in ordering medicines. It can also be used to avoid an inaccurate picture of the current day to improve the workflow of the next day.

Using Paper

This is a very common out-system workaround where information is first written down on paper and then later transferred to the EHR. Nurses will write notes on anything that is available, including their hands, paper towels, napkins, and meal menus. The nurse may feel that first writing down information on paper and later recording it in the EHR helps to produce better written information. This action may also indicate a lack of trust in the nurse's ability to enter the data correctly the first time. Sometimes the presence of a computer in the room may interfere with the nurse's ability to observe how the patient responds to questions. Although using paper notes allows the nurse to review information provided by the patient before entering it, it adds extra work and time. There is also the risk that the notes may get lost. However, during a power outage or computer failure, nurses and others will need to fall back on using pen-and-paper methods of documentation.

Using Shadow Systems

Another out-system workaround is the use of a data-processing system other than the one dedicated for EHR. These are called *shadow systems* and are used either as a substitute for or as a complement to the EHR. For example, a provider may open a Word document in a window next to the EHR and create a file as a continuous record instead of the piecemeal one on the EHR. Some providers dislike the layout in the EHR and prefer to use one they are more comfortable with, such as Word. Shadow systems place the completeness and timeliness of data in the EHR at risk due to the chance of the provider forgetting to register data in the EHR alongside the shadow system.[25]

Imagine the time involved in training staff to use new technology. Now imagine the time involved in fixing the technology because it did not work properly for the staff after implementation. Finally, imagine the time needed to retrain staff when the technology is fixed or upgraded. You can easily see why it is important that working staff nurses *must* be involved in evaluating and selecting new technology as well as planning for its implementation. The end users, in this case the floor health-care team, are the only people who really know how the technology will impact the day-to-day workflow. Involving the end user from the beginning can decrease costs, increase efficiency, and improve staff morale.

The Human Factor

All humans commit errors from time to time, and health-care providers are only human. Unfortunately, medical errors can cause the injury or death of a patient. As of 2021 (the last year complete data was available at the time of publication), medical errors had been the third-leading cause of death in

the United States for 4 consecutive years. According to a Johns Hopkins study conducted by Dr. Martin Makary, medical errors result in more than 250,000 preventable deaths per year. Because of the way medical errors are reported, some studies estimate the number may be as high as 440,000 per year.[26] Informatics, when well designed and optimally used, has the potential to reduce the number of hospital-related deaths and injuries. Nurses should be on the forefront of using informatics technology to reduce patient-care errors.

The human factor (HF) is a term used in nursing informatics and refers to the interaction of the human with a technology or an automated process. (See Box 17.9.)

HIGH-QUALITY DATA AS THE BASIS OF NURSING INFORMATICS

Data are the cornerstone of nursing informatics. Without data, knowledge and wisdom cannot occur. Without high-quality data, safe, quality care cannot be delivered.

The Five Rights of Informatics

Nursing students are taught early in their programs that safe medication administration requires nurses to use certain safety checks, called the Six Rights, to prevent errors. Some of these same rights can be applied to the use of data. If the rights of (1) time, (2) person, and (3) route are applied to data, nursing informatics can promote a safer health-care environment with the use of high-quality data.[27] In addition, the rights of integrity and confidentiality coupled with right documentation virtually guarantee clean data (that is, data that are accurate, retrievable, confidential, meaningful, and usable).[26] The Rights of Informatics are reviewed in Box 17.10.

Additional rights that apply both to data-handling and medication administration include right documentation, right action, right form, and right response, discussed next.

Right Documentation. After nurses administer a medication, they must sign the medication sheet or make the appropriate entry in the EHR. The nurse's signature is legal evidence that the patient received the medication. Students are taught never to sign the medication chart before administering the medication. Doing so is illegal and endangers the patient.

Box 17.9 **The Human Factor**

Factor	To Human or Computer?	Key Points

Ergonomics	Human	• *Problem:* The human body wears out
		  • Repetitive motion
		  • Muscle strain
		  • Extensive reach
		• *Workarounds:* If technology not within reach, transcription errors—double documentation—may occur
		• *Fix:* New technology should match workflow and be optimized and adjustable for height/body type. Voice-activated systems eliminate the need to type data into the computer.

Alarm/alert fatigue	Human	• *Problem:* Multiple notices given by the computer or monitoring devices
		  • Results in critical notices being ignored
		  • Medical error or death may occur
		• *Workarounds:* Notices are clicked before being read; alarms are turned off
		• *Fix:* New technology—and existing clinical information system (CIS)—should review alerts/alarms
		  • Only critical alerts/alarms should be set
		  • Alerts/alarms should generate reports to monitor frequent nuisance warnings
		  • Create policies, procedures, and education

Garbage in, garbage out (GIGO) principle	Both	• *Problem:* Data entry issue
		  • Inaccurate data-entry results in inaccurate data output
		  • Aggregate data used to make decisions will be wrong
		  • Document security system (DSS) can lead the human to an incorrect solution
		  • Medical errors can result
		• *Workarounds:* None—individuals are unaware that data entered was incorrect
		• *Fix:* Ensure individual entries are correct
		  • Enter information at point of care
		  • Do not use the copy-and-paste function
		  • Do not use narrative charting unless absolutely necessary (narrative charting does not translate to data-entry output)
		  • Avoid checkbox charting or charting by exception

Evidence-based practice (EBP)	Both	• *Problem:* Current research is not placed into practice for approximately 15 to 20 years
		  • Computer might provide best procedure
		  • Computer might not have the most up-to-date information and provide an alarm/alert
		• *Workarounds:* The way it has always been done
		• *Fix:* Culture of EBP
		  • Create EBP committee—update CIS
		  • Subscribe to EBP databases that communicate with CIS
		  • Journal clubs for increased EBP awareness
		  • Dissemination of knowledge

Source: HIPAA, HITECH, and Omnibus Rule: What are they? TotalHIPAA, n.d. https://www.totalhipaa.com/hipaa-hitech-omnibus-rule.

Box 17.10 The Five Rights for Handling Data

Right	Key Points
Time	• Data should be entered at the time it is received. • Data should be available in real time. • Disaster planning should be practiced and perfected.
Person	• Only those with a need to know should know. • Data needs to be entered on the correct person. • Levels of security need to be implemented to ensure data is secure.
Route	• Data should never leave the system. • Data should be available to anyone who needs it and has a right to it. • Security needs to be in place to ensure the route traveled by the data is right.
Integrity	• Data should be protected so that it is not breached. • One datum compromised leads to all data compromised—GIGO.
Confidentiality	• Multilevel system security ensures only safe data are entered. • An entire chart is not needed for one laboratory order. • Security measures must be in place (password, antivirus, firewall, etc.).

What if the patient refuses the medication or the nurse forgets to administer it? A more dangerous scenario is failing to sign when a medication *has* been administered. Another nurse may conclude that it has not been administered, and the patient will receive a double dose. For prn medication, it is essential to document the reason for administering the medication and what effect it had on the patient.

Given these legal requirements, how does a nurse "sign" a record that is totally electronic? The answer is to use an **electronic signature**, or e-signature. This type of signature provides the same legal standing as a handwritten signature if it adheres to the requirements of the National Institute of Standards and Technology–Digital Signature Standard (NIST-DSS) regulations in the United States.[28] There are several different types of electronic signatures. Some are as simple as a nurse's name entered in an electronic document. The basic requirements for an electronic signature are as follows:

1. The person who signs can be uniquely identified and linked to the signature.
2. The person who signs must have sole control of the private key that was used to create the electronic signature.

3. The person who signs must be able to identify data that are attached to it and also identify if any data have been changed.
4. In the event that the attached data have been tampered with, the signature must be invalidated.[28]

Right Action (Right Integrity). For many years now, the legal defense "I was just following the physician's orders" has not been available to nurses. Nurses need to know why the patient is receiving a medication and how the medication works. They need to know if the prescribed medication and its dose are appropriate for the patient. Administering an antihyperglycemic agent to a patient who does not have diabetes but does have an infection is a medication error, even if the medication was prescribed. Nurses also need to be aware of laboratory values associated with certain medications. Administering a daily dose of potassium to a patient whose morning laboratory work shows a blood potassium of 7 mEq/mL could lead to cardiac arrest.

In data-handling, right action is similar to right integrity. Nurses are sometimes told by providers to chart untruths. Legally, one false statement in charting invalidates all the data entered in that section of the chart.

Right Form. Right form data, or data form validation, helps nurses and other users to fill out forms in the correct format, guaranteeing that the data presented will work successfully with the base application. When the user enters data into the computer, the Web application verifies that the data are entered correctly. If the data are correct, the application allows the information to move to the server where it is saved in a database.[27] For example, a nurse is about to enter the time of a just-administered medication, and the EHR asks for the nurse's password. If they make a mistake and do not enter a valid password, the application sends back an error message explaining what corrections need to be made.

Right form data is similar to the right route of medication administration. It is possible to administer various medications by different routes. For example, a licensed practical nurse (LPN) in a long-term acute care facility became confused about how to administer a bag of enteral nutrition. The nurse on the shift before had mistakenly put IV tubing on the bag of enteral nutrition and had hung it at the bedside to save the next nurse time in hooking it up. When the LPN heard the pump alarm that the bag was empty, he came in and hooked the new enteral nutrition line to the IV. The patient died about an hour later. In another case, a pharmacist drew up an oral medication in a syringe to obtain a more accurate measurement. The nurse was not familiar with the medication and, because it was in a syringe, gave it by IV.

In entering data into the system, the nurse must follow the instructions for data entry, or else the data may be compromised and even removed when the system goes through its "cleaning" process. *Cleaning* is the process of detecting and correcting (or removing) corrupt or inaccurate data points. Data corruption occurs when the data code is changed or changes by itself into an incorrect form that cannot be processed. Data cleaning also includes identifying incomplete, incorrect, inaccurate, or irrelevant parts of the data set and then replacing them with accurate information. Once data are in the system, the nurse as well as others who have access to the information must make sure that it is retrieved following the technological and legal guidelines established by the facility.

> *Cleaning is the process of detecting and correcting (or removing) corrupt or inaccurate data points.*

Right Response. This could also be called *right assessment* or *right observation*. Right response or assessment of data quality is determining whether the data meet the goals or stated purposes. Elements of the data such as their precision, comprehensiveness, trustworthiness, relevance, and timeliness all feed into the evaluation of data quality. The end measurement is when patients are receiving the level of care they deserve.[28] As data are increasingly coupled with the functions of health-care organizations, the emphasis on the assessment of data quality will gain greater consideration.

In nursing care, right response is key in determining if the nursing action was successful and if the standard of quality was met. For example, after a medication is administered, the nurse must go back to evaluate whether the medication is doing what it is supposed to do. Most nurses know this is mandatory for pain medications and recognize the need to chart whether or not the pain level was reduced. However, it is also important for almost all other medications. If the patient was given an antacid for ulcer pain, the nurse needs to note whether or not it helped. Right response is particularly important for dangerous medications such as insulin, anticoagulants, and cardiac medications. The nurse must respond quickly if a patient on anticoagulants begins to have blood in their urine or is oozing blood from the IV site. This may indicate that the patient is receiving too high a dose of the medication. And of course, it is essential to check for allergic reactions to antibiotics and other medications. (See Box 17.10.)

What Is Quality?

Health care is increasing its focus on quality initiatives as it moves toward a value-based payment system. However, many health-care organizations are still being thwarted in their ability to identify, monitor, and use appropriate quality metrics. One of the major sources of this problem is that there is no standard definition of "quality." Perhaps people know it when they see it, but they cannot define it. However, to be able to accurately measure the quality of health care, it is necessary to describe what is being measured. An IOM study found more than 100 different definitions of quality used in health care. The IOM itself defines *health-care quality* as "the degree to which health services for individuals and populations increase the likelihood of desired health outcomes and are consistent with current professional knowledge."[29]

Not knowing the definition of quality health care has not stopped or even slowed down the development of quality measures. There may be as many as a thousand different quality measures in use. Quality measures are the yardstick for measuring the ability of health-care providers to care for patients and populations. However, each quality measure focuses on a different aspect of how patient care is delivered.[29]

OUTCOME DATA AND QUALITY METRICS

Outcome data (OD) and quality metrics (QM) are the products of evaluation systems for electronic data used in health care and similar industries to assess data quality. OD are now required by the government, insurance companies, and providers to demonstrate the quality of care provided at the facility. If high-quality care is not demonstrated, the facility will lose federal government funds. The process of gathering outcome data, tracking changes over time, and determining the quality goals to be measured is known as *quality metrics*. QM are data collection tools ranging from questionnaires to electronic patient checklists that help quantify health-care processes, outcomes, patient perceptions, and organizational structure and/or systems. These data relate to one or more quality goals for health care: effective, safe, efficient, patient-centered, equitable, and timely provision of care. Some of the more commonly used quality measures include the following:

- Mortality rates
- Hospital readmission rates under 30 days

- Timeliness (how long patients had to wait)
- Effectiveness of care (using best practices and meeting outcomes)
- Patient safety of care (accidents, wrong medication incidents, falls, etc.)
- Care coordination (team members know what they are supposed to do)
- Patient engagement in their own care
- Patient perceptions of their care (e.g., patient complaints or satisfaction)[29]

QM are stored in and retrieved from central databases. The OD is compared to predetermined standards. If the OD meet the standards, then the institution is presumed to be providing high-quality care. These standards can also be used to improve patient care.[28] The gathered data are analyzed so that all providers can be compared with each other.

The experience of the patient has become an important data point for QM and has driven *patient-centered care*. In addition, the ANA's National Database of Nursing Quality Indicators (NDNQI), which collects yearly data from nearly one-third of the nation's hospitals, confirms that employee satisfaction, along with shorter work shifts, better staffing, and increased patient communication all positively affect the patient health-care experience. As a result, employee satisfaction is also being measured as a QM.[28] For several years, the Triple Aim in health care was to improve population health while satisfying the patient and decreasing costs. However, the Quadruple Aim added a new goal—staff outcomes. These outcomes include staff retention, satisfaction, autonomy, and empowerment.[29] These data points have been added to the quality metrics now being collected at most facilities.

Conclusion

In health care and nursing, informatics can truly help to provide new care-delivery methods and make safe, quality care a reality. The history of informatics is a story of innovation to improve workflow and make better decisions that can ultimately save lives.

The nursing informaticist represents the end user (i.e., the floor nurse) and advocates for technology that helps the end user deliver safe and high-quality care. To connect the world of technology to patient

care, specialists in informatics educate other nurses, identify and report workarounds, and demonstrate flexibility and being open to innovation. The competent nurse informaticist knows that not all technology is good and that only some of it should be implemented for use in patient care. Finally, the nurse informaticist should be able to assess and evaluate new technologies to choose technology that is user friendly and meets the needs of the nursing unit.

Informatics includes the ability to store, retrieve, and analyze data. EBP brings recent best research data into clinical practice to make the best clinical judgements possible. The integration of informatics and EBP increases the quality of care by providing data and information to assist in accurate and appropriate decision making to improve patient care quality and safety. The process of applying technology to nursing knowledge helps the nurse recognize potential problems earlier and develop plans of care to successfully resolve them. Informatics and computer skills are the essential mechanisms and underlying framework that supports and reinforces EBP in nursing.

CRITICAL-THINKING EXERCISES

- Debate the ethical issues of personal privacy and the greater social good in relation to access to health-care information.
- Discuss how the design of equipment increases or decreases error rates.
- Write a vision paper describing your view of new technology in health care in the year 2030.

- List all the pieces of data you had to give at your last visit to a provider or hospital. Was all of the information necessary for your care? Who needed the information? How was the information recorded or transmitted? How many times did you have to write the same information on different forms? How could that duplication have been prevented?

NCLEX-STYLE QUESTIONS

1. Which statement BEST describes the effect of HIPAA on nursing informatics?
   1. HIPAA accelerated the development of electronic safeguards for transmitting and storing patients' medical data.
   2. HIPAA made previously public medical information confidential.
   3. The first generation of HIPAA required that paper medical records be turned into electronic files.
   4. HIPAA recognized the valuable contribution of informatics nurses to nursing knowledge.
2. To become a nursing informatics specialist, what credentials and/or experience does a person need to have? **Select all that apply.**
   1. A bachelor of science in nursing (BSN) degree
   2. A master or doctoral degree in nursing informatics
   3. Informatics certification through the ANCC
   4. A bachelor of science in computer science degree
   5. At least 5 years' experience working as an informatics nurse

3. Luís, a nursing informatics specialist, is interviewing nurses and support staff who work in the hospital's emergency department to find out if the facility's electronic health record system adequately meets its needs. What nursing informatics role is Luís performing?
   1. Software developer
   2. Coordinator
   3. Tester
   4. Trainer
4. Ming and Christy, two newly graduated RNs, are discussing the role of an informatics nurse. Christy says, "Our generation is really technology savvy. I don't see the need for a separate informatics nurse." Which statement by Ming is the most appropriate response?
   1. "Yes, the need for informatics specialists is decreasing every year."
   2. "Well, somebody has to be able to analyze and interpret all those statistics!"
   3. "Technology is changing so fast that full-time floor nurses aren't able to keep up with the latest innovations."
   4. "Nurses take care of people. The information technology folks take care of the machines."

5. Alan Turing is considered one of the founders of nursing informatics. What area of nursing informatics did Turing contribute to?
   1. Computer science
   2. Information science
   3. Cognitive science
   4. Nursing science

6. Rachel is a family nurse practitioner in private practice. She is concerned that her office's electronic medical records (EMR) system does not share information easily with the computer systems at the laboratory service her practice uses or the insurers it seeks payment from. Rachel's EMR system lacks _____.

7. An informatics nurse notices that a large number of data-entry errors occur on a surgical unit because nurses must type in the names of their patients' surgical procedures, such as *cholecystectomy*, the surgical removal of the gallbladder. What solution would the informatics nurse most likely suggest?
   1. Require nurses to attend a medical terminology spelling class.
   2. Reprogram the system to recognize common terms for procedures, such as "gallbladder removal."
   3. Buy a voice-recognition system that turns nurses' speech into typed words.
   4. Change the system so that nurses can select the names of the procedures from a drop-down menu.

8. How did the meaningful use program encourage providers and facilities to switch from paper to electronic health records (EHRs)?
   1. It required providers and facilities to enroll in the Medicare Electronic Health Records Incentive Program.
   2. It offered providers and facilities that participated in the program incentive payments for improved outcomes.
   3. It withheld payment to providers and facilities that refused to switch from paper to EHRs.
   4. It published a list of providers and facilities that refused to switch from paper to EHRs in newspapers around the country.

9. Which of the following is an example of a quality metric (QM)?
   1. Employee satisfaction
   2. Year-end profits
   3. Winning a best-in-city award
   4. Low staff turnover rates

10. Who benefits from the data gathered, analyzed, and disseminated by nursing informatics specialists? **Select all that apply.**
    1. Health-care providers
    2. Creators of public health policy
    3. Insurance companies
    4. Patients
    5. Nursing educators and students

References

1. Holly P. Deep dive: What is health informatics? HIT. Academy, July 8, 2022. https://healthit.academy/blog/what-is-health-informatics/

2. Naghiloo S. Nursing informatics history and evolution [online course lecture]. In *Nursing 301: Nursing Informatics*, July 22, 2022. https://study.com/learn/lesson/nursing-informatics-history-evolution.html

3. Panda T, Sojor B. History of informatics. Nursing Informatics, 2022. https://sites.google.com/site/ni100bsummer/products-services/history-of-informatics

4. Kiel J, Linkov F. The role of artificial intelligence in enhancing the delivery of healthcare. *Journal of AHMIHA*, July 11, 2022. https://journal.ahima.org/page/the-role-of-artificial-intelligence-in-enhancing-the-delivery-of-healthcare

5. Sherlock A. Florence Nightingale's "rose" diagram. Maharam, n.d. https://www.maharam.com/stories/sherlock_florence-nightingales-rose-diagram

6. Statler T. History of computers with timeline. Comp Sci Central, n.d. https://compscicentral.com/history-of-computers/

7. Interoperability in health care. HIMSS, n.d. https://www.himss.org/resources/interoperability-healthcare

8. PrOMIS. HealthMeasures, 2022. https://www.healthmeasures.net/explore-measurement-systems/promis

9. Nursing diagnosis: A comprehensive guide and list. NANDA Diagnosis, 2023. https://nandadiagnoses.com/

10. Nursing diagnosis guide for 2023. Nurse Labs, 2023. https://nurseslabs.com/nursing-diagnosis/

11. Coding for nurses. HCA Healthcare, 2022. https://careclassification.org/

12. Kiel J, Linkov R. The role of artificial intelligence in enhancing the delivery of healthcare. *Journal of AHMIA*, July 11, 2022. https://journal.ahima.org/page/the-role-of-artificial-intelligence-in-enhancing-the-delivery-of-healthcare

13. Sabin N. The next blood pressure breakthrough: Temporary tattoos. Medscape, July 25, 2022. https://www.medscape.com/viewarticle/977914?reg=1

14. Data privacy laws: What you need to know. Osano, December 14, 2022. https://www.osano.com/articles/data-privacy-laws

15. Data breaches in healthcare companies. American Medical Compliance, July 12, 2022. https://americanmedicalcompliance.com/hipaa-violation/data-breaches-in-healthcare-companies/

16. Reader R. Healthcare systems want government to help with hackers. Politico, June 22, 2022. https://www.politico.com/news/2022/06/22/health-systems-government-help-hackers-00041084

17. Ethical issues in an age of information and communication technology. Ivy Panda, July 27, 2022. https://ivypanda.com/essays/ethical-issues-in-an-age-of-information-and-communication-technology/

18. Bennett M. Is the Patriot Act still in effect? *Straight Arrow News*, February 16, 2022. https://straightarrownews.com/cc/is-the-patriot-act-still-in-effect-jim-jordans-tweet-triggers-discussion/

19. What is a HIPAA violation in the workplace? What to Become, July 18, 2022. https://whattobecome.com/blog/what-is-a-hipaa-violation-in-workplace/

20. Mensik H. Health data breaches slowing from 2021's record high, report suggests. Healthcare Dive, July 19, 2022. https://www.healthcaredive.com/news/cyberattack-hacking-IT-breach-healthcare-providers-plans-targets/627511/

21. HIPAA, HITECH and Omnibus Rule: What are they? TotalHIPAA, n.d. https://www.totalhipaa.com/hipaa-hitech-omnibus-rule/

22. Larsen K, Wilson M. Using meaningful use to improve quality of care. Medscape CME and Education, August 7, 2014. https://www.medscape.org/viewarticle/829169_2

23. MIPS quality reporting requirements. Polaris, n.d. https://polaris.figmd.com/weightage-requirements/

24. Gaines K. Nursing informatics. Nurse.org Career Guide Series, July 18, 2022. https://nurse.org/resources/nursing-informatics

25. Boonstra A, Jonker T, van Offenbeek M, Vos J. Persisting workarounds in electronic health record system use: Types, risks and benefits. *BMC Medical Informatics and Decision Making*, 21, June 8, 2021. https://doi.org/10.1186/s12911-021-01548-0

26. Knapp C. How many deaths are caused by medical errors? Knapp and Roberts, December 14, 2021. https://www.knappandroberts.com/how-many-deaths-are-caused-by-medical-errors/

27. Nursing informatics in the healthcare professions. Scribd, n.d. https://www.scribd.com/presentation/299284467/Nursing-Informatics-in-the-Health-Care-Professions

28. Paula. Then vs now: The evolution of digital signatures in healthcare. eSignly, n.d. https://www.esignly.com/electronic-signature/technology/then-vs-now-the-evolution-of-digital-signatures-in-healthcare.html

29. Orand J. Most important metrics for a healthcare quality management dashboard. Symplr, January 21, 2022. https://www.symplr.com/blog/most-important-metrics-healthcare-quality-dashboard

The Politically Active Nurse

Joseph T. Catalano

A NUTS-AND-BOLTS APPROACH

Politics, and the consequences of political action, touch people's lives at the national, state, and local government levels. It has famously been said that "all politics are local." This statement means that whatever happens in the political arena at any level eventually affects all citizens no matter their societal status.

Nurses need to understand how politics work because they have the potential to influence policy decisions that could ensure both better health care for patients and improved work environments for themselves. Moreover, it is important for nurses to be able to critically analyze proposed policies for any unintended consequences. With their understanding of both the health-care system and human experiences as well as their leadership and negotiation skills, nurses are well prepared to become active in the political system.

This chapter provides a foundation for understanding the political basics with the intention of motivating nurses to become active in the political world. Politics is examined both within the profession of nursing and within society at large. In addition, this chapter discusses the forces that drive politics and the three concepts it comprises: partisanship, self-interest, and ideology.

THE INTERSECTION OF NURSING AND POLITICS

Policy that most influences nursing is instituted at both the state and federal levels and sometimes overlaps. States are responsible for licensure and nurse practice acts, so any legislation that regulates the criteria for licensure and certification or defines the scope of practice is determined by individual states. Nurses who aspire to influence their work environment or practice need to become active at the state level, preferably through state professional organizations.

The American Nurses Association (ANA) has been involved in politics at the federal level for many years and has the ANA Political Action Committee (ANA-PAC), which is now the second-largest federal PAC in Washington, DC, engaged in political activities

- Discuss how a bill becomes a law
- Identify the major committees at the federal level that influence health policy
- Identify four points at which nurses can influence a bill
- Give examples of how nurses may become politically involved

exclusively at the federal level. The ANA focuses on influencing policy to ensure high standards of nursing practice, promoting the rights of nurses in the workplace, projecting a positive and realistic view of nursing, and lobbying Congress and regulatory agencies on health-care issues affecting nurses and the public.[1] Provision 9 of the ANA Code of Ethics for Nurses calls for nurses to be active in social policy and politics. (See Chapter 6 for more detail on ethics.)

Sometimes conflict arises between the federal and state governments about what constitutes a legitimate course of action for the federal government and what constitutes the same for the state government.

The 10th Amendment to the Constitution says that any powers not expressly identified as being under federal control should be delegated to the states, unless the states are willing to give control to the federal government. This amendment is part of the current debate about whether the states should be responsible for administering certain elements of the Affordable Care Act (ACA), particularly where they pertain to Medicaid and Medicare. This becomes an issue because, unlike the federal government, state governments are required by law to balance their budgets.[2] When the federal government passes unfunded mandates on to the states, such as with Medicaid, the governors are left to struggle with funding and possibly administering programs they cannot afford.

Federal Issues

Federal concerns that directly involve nursing include the nursing shortage, burdensome tuition debts, and patient safety. Indirectly, legislation such as the ACA significantly affects nursing services, in particular, by potentially expanding the demand for nurse practitioners (NPs) and altering the way nurses work within health care.

The Nursing Shortage

In 2022, the last year data were available before publication, there were approximately 3.9 million registered nurses (RNs) in the United States. The U.S. Bureau of Labor Statistics (BLS) projects that more than 500,000 RNs will retire by the end of 2022 and that 1.1 million new RNs will be needed to prevent a shortage.[3] By 2030, the shortfall is expected to be more than twice as large as any nurse shortage experienced since the introduction of Medicare and Medicaid in the mid-1960s.

The COVID-19 pandemic has also accelerated the need for new RN graduate nurses. When the pandemic started and as it peaked, nurses were heralded

as heroes on the front line of the health-care battle, facing difficult conditions and inadequate staffing. Since the waning of the pandemic, many nurses are experiencing decreases in salaries, loss of bonuses, increased numbers of shifts due to loss of personnel, and again inadequate personal protective equipment (PPE) as problems with the distribution system continue. The enormous pressure during the peak of the pandemic for frontline nurses to conform to the requirements of the institution led many nurses to decide that their passion for the profession did not offset the negative effects on their mental and emotional well-being.[2] The aging nurse workforce and the stressful working conditions produced burnout, and nurse turnover rates are now as high as 37 percent, depending on geographic area and specialty.

Both the federal and state governments are searching for solutions. The U.S. Senate created a 12-member Senate nursing caucus to provide a forum to address these issues. It was followed quickly by the development of a House of Representatives nursing caucus.

A bill introduced by Senator Jeff Merley [D-OR], called the Future Advancement of Academic Nursing Act, or the FAAN Act (S. 246), authorizes the Health Resources and Services Administration (HRSA) to award grants to nursing schools to increase the number of nursing students who can respond to public health emergencies and pandemics and otherwise enhance nursing education programs. The bill calls on HRSA to prioritize giving grants to historically Black colleges and universities and other minority-serving institutions, schools located in medically underserved communities, and schools in areas with shortages of health professionals. The bill has been read twice and referred to the Committee on Health, Education, Labor, and Pensions. Although it has not yet passed, it is still alive, and nurses and nurse educators should

Issues in Practice

How Do Politics Affect You and Your Family?

Why should nurses be involved in politics? Does it really make a difference who is elected and who makes the laws? Take a minute to answer the questions that follow and check the items you think may be affected by politics.

Between the time you wake up and the time you leave the house, you have already interacted with the world outside your home. Do you think any of the following subjects are affected by politics?

- The water with which you wash your face and brush your teeth
- The electricity that lights the room
- The price and quality of food you have for breakfast
- The safety of the products you buy

As the average person's life span grows longer and the retirement age is increased, these later years become more meaningful. Are any of the following affected by our political systems?

- The age at which you can retire
- The income that you get during retirement
- The quality and cost of health care
- Your life expectancy

We value our leisure time and the chance to "get away from it all." Are any of the following areas affected by politics?

- The parks and lakes where vacationers fish and swim
- The air you breathe and the water you drink
- The radio and television programs that entertain you

Take some time to think about these questions. The answers will make you think some more.

---

contact Senator Merley, chairman of the Senate nursing caucus, and express their support.[2]

Nurses can contact members of this caucus to offer suggestions and help work toward effective solutions. In addition, the American Association of Colleges of Nursing (AACN) has a position statement on the nursing shortage and is working with policymakers at both the state and national levels to bring attention to this healthcare concern and develop plans to resolve the shortage.

Tuition Debt

Like other college students, nursing students often leave college with large amounts of debt. The amount of debt a nursing student takes on to earn their nursing degree varies widely, however. On average, associate degree nurses (ADNs) take on close to $20,000 in debt; those with a bachelor of science in nursing (BSN), nearly $24,000; and those with a master of science in nursing (MSN), more than $47,000.[4]

In fulfillment of one of President Biden's campaign promises, in August 2022, the administration officially launched its plan to cancel as much as $10,000 in federal student loan debt for single people earning less than $125,000 a year or less than $250,000 for married couples. Students who received Pell Grants, a federal program to provide aid for lower-income students, could receive up to $20,000 in loan forgiveness. Most individuals with federal student loans are already below the income threshold for forgiveness and qualify for Biden's cancellation plan. Undergraduate loans, graduate loans, and Parent Plus loans held by the Department of Education are also all eligible for cancellation.

Although Biden's plan will increase the amount of money for loan forgiveness, there remain a number of other ways that many of the 43 million federal student loan borrowers may qualify for some student loan forgiveness. The federal government already has a number of programs that offer student debt forgiveness. Some of these programs have been temporarily expanded by the Biden administration, reducing the difficulty for some borrowers to qualify for student debt forgiveness. So far, in excess of $26 billion in targeted debt cancellation for more than 1.3 million borrowers has been approved by the administration—more than under any other president.[4]

The federal government assists nursing students with education costs through programs such as the Nursing Education Loan Repayment Program administered by the Department of Health and Human Services. A loan repayment plan through Titles VII and VIII of the Health Resources and Service Administration (HRSA) awards several different types of loans to nursing students and also has loan repayments in exchange for working with underserved populations and in rural areas. These programs need to be funded biannually by Congress; nurses can contact their representatives to ensure they understand the importance of funding these programs.

Patient Safety

Patient safety is the protection, security, and well-being of individuals who entrust their care to the supervision of health care professionals in a variety of settings. Patient safety revolves around the prevention of injuries, harm, or death due to errors in diagnosing diseases and conditions, errors in medical treatments or surgeries, medication errors, or other preventable mistakes that a patient may experience while receiving care in a hospital or other health-care facility. It also involves the lessening of the risk of accidental injury or harm associated with health care.[5]

What the government's role in patient safety should be has been discussed for many years in the United States. However, since the 1999 Institute of Medicines (IOM) report on the number of deaths caused by medication errors, U.S. hospitals have gradually become safer places for patients. According to federal government data, medical errors and adverse events such as medication errors, hospital-acquired infections, surgery-related adverse events, pressure injuries from inactivity, and serious falls that cause injury, have declined meaningfully across the nation. It is acknowledged that some of the decline is likely due to advances in technology and medical procedures. For example, patients undergoing laparoscopic surgery are at much lower risk of complications than patients who used to require large open incisions for the same surgery.[5]

However, the improvement in patient safety is also due in large part to safety improvement programs developed by hospitals to reduce detrimental events such as medication errors and hospital acquired infections. Hospitals have been focusing on improving the quality and safety of care for many years. There has been an acceleration of efforts to rigorously evaluate care inside hospitals and to identify methods of improving it.[5] Outcome data (OD) and quality metrics (QM) have helped identify behaviors and processes in which a hospital may be falling short in providing a safe environment for patients. Applying these data to the actual care of patients has led to better staffing and increased patient satisfaction. (For more details, see Chapter 17.)

What Do You Think?

What experiences have you encountered, either as a patient or as a health-care worker, related to the nursing shortage? How might the political system help solve the shortage? How might the political system worsen the shortage?

States Issues

States, through their state boards of nursing and nurse practice acts, are the primary regulators of nursing licensure and certification. The states are ultimately responsible for patient safety, so they have the capacity to pass any legislation and to set the requirements for who is qualified to practice and how and where they may practice. The mandate for nursing is to help legislators understand how nursing standards are established and then to help develop legislation with an achievable agenda for political action by nurses at the state level through the state boards of nursing.

Like the federal government, states are searching for solutions for the nursing shortage. Some states are opting for a short-term solution of recruiting foreign nurses. The National Council of State Boards of Nursing (NCSBN) requires that all nurses who work in the United States must hold a license to practice in the state where they work. The federal government has the authority to provide the required visas to allow foreign nationals to work in the United States, but states have the authority to ensure that these foreign nurses obtain a license to practice. Many boards require a CGFNS (Commission on Graduates of Foreign Nursing Schools) certificate before they will issue a license.

Prior to the COVID-19 pandemic, foreign educated nurses (FEN) comprised approximately 8 percent of nurses now practicing in the United States, and the licensing and credentialing barriers were very strict.[6] As the pandemic surged, five states—Colorado, Massachusetts, Nevada, New Jersey, and New York—modified their licensing guidelines to ease the requirements for FENs to work in hospitals overwhelmed by pandemic-induced staffing shortages. The normal requirements for FENs to work in U.S. health-care facilities included the following:

1. Meet the educational requirements (4-year BSN or equivalent)
2. Complete a FEN course
3. Take and pass an English language proficiency test
4. Pass the National Council Licensing Examination-Registered Nurse (NCLEX–RN)
5. Obtain credential evaluation
6. Find a nursing recruiting agency or U.S.-based employer
7. Apply and obtain an RN immigrant visa/green card
8. Accept an RN position[6]

FENs who are *not* eligible to work in the United States include the following:

1. Nurses with less than 2 years' experience
2. Nurses lacking a 4-year nursing degree
3. Nurses who have committed a crime either before or after becoming a nurse
4. Nurses who lack sponsorship from a reputable nursing agency

The five states created temporary licenses for FENs who required supervision from a licensed professional RN. They also relaxed the scope-of-practice rules for nurses, allowing them to perform any task their supervisors assigned to them. The temporary licenses were valid only as long as the state governor's public health emergency declaration remained in effect, generally to the end of the emergency. Most of these temporary licenses expired in 2022.[7]

There were several unforeseen difficulties with this attempt to employ more FENs. First, for any individual to enter the United States, they first must have a visa from their home country and obtain the proper visa applications and paperwork from the U.S. Citizenship and Immigration Services department. When the pandemic first started, almost all countries, including the United States, shut down all their governmental facilities due to fear of the infection. In most countries, these shutdowns lasted a year or longer, creating a huge backlog of people desiring to enter the United States. When the offices did open, it was only for a few hours per day, and visa applications were processed in a first-come, first-served order. By the time the FENs had completed all the educational and other requirements for entry, they were far down on the application lists.[7]

A second problem was the way the new temporary license laws were written. FENs with temporary work visas would be practicing nursing on the licenses of their supervising RNs. Few RNs were willing to allow this to take place. In the past, some RNs believed that nursing students practiced on their licenses. This is not true. Nursing students practice on an exemption in the nurse practice act that allows students to perform certain nursing actions at their level of education under the supervision of a nursing education instructor.

> *All nursing organizations and state boards of nursing believe that allowing unlicensed individuals to practice as RNs has the potential to risk patient safety and quality of care.*

By the time the pandemic was resolving, only one FEN was being employed by a Colorado hospital. However, even after the pandemic, some health-care facilities held on to the idea that employing FENs was a way to deal with the nursing shortage (and to reduce costs). To avoid delay in allowing foreign nurses to practice, some institutions continued to support legislation to allow FENs to practice either with a temporary license or without a license altogether until they legally obtained a license. This type of employment would actually be a type of hospital licensure, where the facilities would determine the nursing actions that the FENs could perform. All nursing organizations and state boards of nursing believe that allowing unlicensed individuals to practice as RNs has the potential to risk patient safety and quality of care.[7] Nurses can contact their state legislators to lobby for upholding nursing licensure so that the same standards apply to foreign nurses as to U.S. citizens. (See Chapter 5 for more detail.)

Advanced Practice Nursing

State regulations also vary on advanced nursing practice. Currently, 26 states have full practice authority laws that allow advanced practice nurses (APRNs) to evaluate patients, diagnose, order and interpret diagnostic tests, and initiate and manage treatments, including prescribing medications without any physician supervision.[8] This is the model recommended by the NCSBN and eliminates unnecessary, outdated regulatory barriers that prevent patients from accessing vital care services directly from APRNs.[9]

In 13 states, APRNs have what is called *reduced practice*, in which state practice and licensure laws reduce the ability of APRNs to engage in at least one element of full APRN practice. APRNs in these states are required to have some type of collaborative agreement with a physician in order for the APRN to provide patient care. Reduced practice may limit the ability of the APRN to practice in one area, usually in prescribing medications.[8]

In the remaining 11 states, APRNs are governed by restricted practice acts in which patient care must be done under the *supervision, delegation,* or *team management* of another health discipline.[8]

In the states that have granted full practice authority, APRNs are practicing more in rural communities and underserved areas. The states that do not allow full practice authority to APRNs are noted to have higher levels of health disparities among minority groups and primary care shortages in rural areas of their states. Decades of research show that states with full practice authority improve patient access to care, increase their workforces, and work toward reducing health-care disparities.[9] APRNs deliver high-quality health care in more than 1 billion patient visits each year. As of 2022, more than 355,000 licensed NPs in the United States were providing care in communities of all sizes across the nation.[10]

Many of the states that do not yet give APRNs full practice authority have bills before their legislatures to do so. Nurses can work with their professional organizations and directly contact their representatives to help enact legislation to ensure all APRNs can practice to the full extent of their education.

Professional Organizations

Professional organizations provide another way to influence policy change and legislation at both the state and federal levels. As previously mentioned, the ANA has a large PAC that focuses on influencing federal legislation. In addition, because the ANA establishes the standards for nursing, it can influence how nurses deliver care.

Magnet Hospitals

In 1980, the American Academy of Nurses conducted a study to identify the elements present in hospitals that attracted and retained nurses. Retaining nurses is cost-effective for hospitals because recruiting and training new staff is very expensive. Several key factors were identified in hospitals that seemed to fulfill the Magnet status, including a participative management style, allowing the nurses a relatively high degree of autonomy in practice and decision making; high-quality leadership at the unit level; a horizontal organizational structure, allowing nurses to practice as full professionals; opportunities for career development; and high-quality patient care. Nurses employed at Magnet hospitals have a high degree of job satisfaction and a much lower average turnover rate than nurses in other hospitals of similar size.[11]

The Magnet hospital program has grown markedly since the original study. The American Nurses' Credentialing Center (ANCC) has established rigorous standards for hospitals to meet to obtain the

Magnet designation. Most hospitals have found achieving Magnet status to be very challenging, and only a small percentage are able to achieve it on the first try. Only 475 facilities in the United States have Magnet designation at the time of publication.[11] However, hospitals that do acquire Magnet status have achieved a well-deserved level of prestige among their peers. Nurses working at these hospitals have more control over their practice, and the result is that higher-quality care is provided to patients.[11] Magnet designation of a hospital is now considered to be the gold standard for nursing practice and innovation. Magnet hospitals are considered to be institutions where nurses are empowered not only to be leaders in patient care but also to be the force behind the transformation and innovation in their facility. Empowering nurses to improve patient care is a primary focus of the Magnet Recognition Program. This program is now available to countries throughout the world. The program creates an environment where nurses, in collaboration with the facility's interprofessional team, establish the standards for excellence through management, scientific research, and use of new knowledge.[11]

> *In most health-care settings, nurses stimulate and lead change through research and their involvement in interprofessional teams.*

Although many in the general public measure the quality of a hospital by its physicians, it is usually the nurses who play the primary role in producing high-quality patient outcomes. In most health-care settings, nurses stimulate and lead change through research and their involvement in interprofessional teams. The Magnet program for improving health outcomes revolves around reducing medical incidents and complications, shortening the length of hospitalizations, improving patient and employee satisfaction levels, and reducing the costs of care.[11]

Nursing Education Organizations

In the past, most nursing students entered the profession right after graduating from high school, and recruiting sufficient students was not a huge issue. Before the 1960s, nursing was one of the few occupational opportunities for women. Society has changed markedly since that time, and now women have opportunities to pursue fields that were traditionally male dominated. Today, it is not unusual for students seeking nursing school admission to be in their late 20s and early 30s. Some are non-nursing associate or non-nursing baccalaureate graduates looking for a second career, possibly motivated by the well-publicized nursing shortage and the promise of a well-paying career with lots of job security. So far, recruiting these "nontraditional" students has not reduced the nursing shortage or its projections for the future. Increasing the supply of nurses by any means remains a high priority for alleviating the worsening nursing shortage.[2]

One reason for the nursing shortage is the acute shortage of nursing school faculty, which forces nursing schools to turn away qualified students. Although there has been some movement to resolve this issue, the AACN reports that 80,407 qualified applicants were turned away from nursing programs in 2019 (the last available statistics), primarily because of a faculty shortage and lack of resources such as clinical sites.[12] The same survey identified 1,637 faculty vacancies in 892 nursing schools with baccalaureate and/or graduate programs across the country. Besides the faculty vacancies, schools cited the need to create an additional 134 faculty positions to accommodate increased numbers of students. Most of the vacancies (89.7 percent) were faculty positions requiring or preferring a doctoral degree.[12]

For those who do choose to enter the nursing profession and manage to get into nursing school, the future looks bright. There are many opportunities, and health-care facilities are beginning to appreciate and reward nurses at the level they deserve. Funding to increase educational resources is essential to help resolve the nursing shortage. Nurses, nursing students, and their friends and families can contact their representatives and encourage them to place funding for nursing education in the federal budget.[11]

Another factor contributing to the nursing shortage is the aging workforce. As experienced nurses retire or approach retirement age, there simply are not enough new young nurses of the same quality to replace them.

Also contributing to the shortage is the huge population of baby boomers (people born between 1946 and 1964), whose health-care needs have increased as they near or reach retirement age. More nurses are needed to care for this rapidly growing number of patients. A third factor is greater career opportunities for women, whose career options in the past were limited to nursing, teaching, or secretarial positions. Women can now pursue all types of careers, which reduces the percentage of women who become nurses. Finally, one factor that contributes both to a high nursing turnover and to the lack of interest in the profession by young people is working conditions. Nurses are expected to work long shifts, often caring for more patients than is safe; to keep medically complex patients alive; to educate patients about their health; to anticipate physician's needs; to mentor new nurses and nursing students; and to remain calm and compassionate with overwrought patients and their families.

POLITICS AND POLITICAL ACTION

Politics can be seen as the complex interaction between public policy and various public and constituent interests. Politics is directly and indirectly influenced by the self-interest of political officials, both elected and appointed. The mass media also have both a direct and indirect impact on the political process through political commentators, commercials, and investigations into the backgrounds of selected political figures.

Political action is a set of activities, methods, tactics, and behaviors that affect or potentially affect governmental and legislative processes and outcomes. One example of political action is grassroots efforts to change policies or deal with issues such as voters' rights. *Grassroots* refers to political movements that are started at the local level by volunteers in the community who give their time to support an issue that is important to them. Grassroots movements are typically spontaneous in nature, unlike movements that are organized and supported by money from traditional political organizations.

Another example of political action is the activities of lobbyists to change elected officials' opinions or votes and support the give and take of political compromise within legislative bodies. A **lobbyist** is anyone who talks to a legislator to express the lobbyist's opinion about an issue that interests them. Paid lobbyists have to be registered with the political institution they are working in and follow a set of rules and guidelines governing what they can and cannot do. Paid lobbyists usually represent large organizations or businesses and must be registered as professional lobbyists. The goal of the lobbyist is to provide information about issues that legislators may know little or nothing about. For example, nurses who speak with legislators about health-care or nursing issues they wish them to support are acting as lobbyists. Most legislators come from a legal or business background and often are very appreciative of health-care information from nurses.

The image of lobbyists has been tainted in recent years because of the excessive amounts of money provided by large corporations and interest groups to change legislators' positions on issues. Although there are regulations to control this type of activity, some savvy lobbyists have found loopholes and ways around them.

> *A lobbyist is anyone who talks to a legislator to express the lobbyist's opinion about an issue that interests them.*

A Series of Processes

Government is often thought of as a series of processes used to maintain society. As both an element of and a result of politics, government is also influenced by the forces that drive politics. The three concepts that constitute politics include partisanship, self-interest, and ideology.

Partisanship

Partisanship refers to membership in a political party or supporting a political party's position. Numerous political parties exist; however, because of its limited scope, this chapter focuses on three: Democrats (who tend to be progressive or liberal and are considered to be on the "left" side of the political spectrum); Republicans (who tend to be conservative and are considered to be on the "right" side of the political spectrum); and to a lesser extent, Independents (who tend to be populists and incorporate positions from both the left and right).

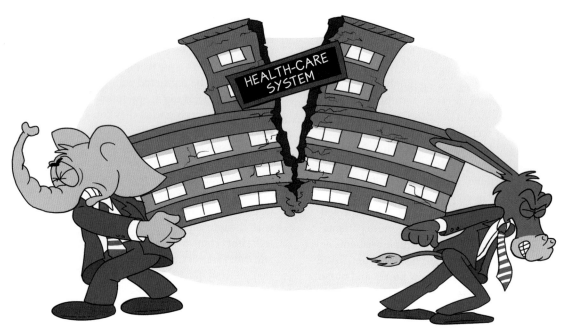

Political rivalries threaten the health of the U.S. health-care system.

Self-Interest

Self-interest is almost always the most important factor in politics. It dictates the kind of issues that legislators become involved in and present to their constituencies (the public members of their party) as the key issues. For instance, a congressperson who resides in a blue-collar industrialized district that has a majority of constituents who support unionization will most likely be pro-union. The legislative structure in the United States was designed so that elected officials represent the people in their districts rather than the whole population of the country. If a candidate does not represent the beliefs of the district, it is unlikely that they will succeed in that district.

In the larger world of electoral politics, the principle of self-interest often means that an elected official will not make legislative or political decisions that could lead to their professional demise, namely loss of an election. There have been exceptions to this rule where elected officials were so ideologically committed to an issue that they defied conventional wisdom and made decisions that went against their self-interest. Politicians whose ideology does not represent that of their constituents often are not re-elected. Generally, to be effective in politics, a person needs to understand and accept the self-interest of their constituents and use it as the driving force in political decision making.

Ideology

Ideology is a broad concept that embodies the beliefs and principles of an individual or group. However, within each group, not every member shares the same opinion on every issue. For instance, persons can be conservative on fiscal issues and liberal on social ones. Conservatives, ultraconservatives, liberals, populists, libertarians, and radicals represent six examples of ideologies. Ultimately, all groups have their own vision for American safety and prosperity. The groups disagree mostly on who should be responsible for making that vision a reality and how it should be done. These opposing ideologies usually act as counterbalances for each other and prevent one ideology from taking over the government and moving the country in just one direction.

UNDERSTANDING THE POLITICAL PLAYING FIELD

Government

Government can be defined in multiple ways. In general, government is a group of people (political system) by which a country, community, or any relatively large group of individuals is managed, regulated, or controlled. Through government action, organizational policies and rules are developed, and means for enforcement of the rules are established. Government also sets the direction or goals for the country, prioritizes the goals for its citizens, and establishes a means of providing safety and protection for its citizens from enemies foreign and domestic.

Types of Governmental Systems

Authoritarian. This type of government, whether it be an individual or group of powerful individuals, has total control over the leadership of the country. An authoritarian leader usually has gained their position of power by armed revolution or military force. Some of these regimes may, on the surface, look like other forms of government such as a democracy, but the regime controls who wins the elections and all the other elements of the government, including making and enforcing the laws. The only way the government changes is if a stronger group or individual takes over by armed force.

Monarchy. In the past, monarchies were the most common forms of government. In an absolute monarchy, the king or ruler is in total control of all governmental functions. Only one family rules the country. Government changes hands when the ruler either dies or abdicates their position and the title and power of the ruler are passed down to the next generation of their bloodline. In the monarchy system, transfer of governmental power is usually peaceful; however, when the successors disagree about who is next in line, bloody battles over succession have occurred, including the murder of the king and siblings.

> *One of the hallmarks of a democracy that differentiates it from other forms of government is the peaceful transfer of power from one governing body to the next through the peoples' vote in an election.*

Oligarchy. This type of governmental structure places the political power with a few powerful individuals or families. Unlike the monarchy, continuation of leadership is not dependent on birth into a particular family. Types of oligarchies include plutocracy (rule by the wealthy), stratocracy (rule by the military), and theocracy (rule by one dominant religion or religious leader). Transfer of power usually involves some type of armed conflict among the top groups or leaders.

Totalitarian. This type of government can be viewed as an authoritarian government on steroids. It can also be called an autocracy. Not only does the ruler (sovereign, king, general, dictator, etc.) have absolute power over all the functions of government, they also exercise control over the personal lives of their subjects. They use force and punishment to ensure the cooperation of the people to stay completely in charge. Governmental leadership changes only by the overthrow of the ruler by armed force.

Democracy. This is a form of government in which the people of the country hold the power to govern through their right to select new leaders by their vote.[21] The U.S. Constitution states that the government is "of the people, by the people and for the people." Democracy is a type of government that is limited in its powers, which is different from the authoritarian or totalitarian governments where there are no limits on the powers of the government. One of the hallmarks of a democracy that differentiates it from other forms of government is the peaceful transfer of power from one governing body to the next through the peoples' vote in an election.[21] The saying "ballots not bullets" applies to a democracy.

Democratic government can be thought of as a three-legged stool. One leg is the right of people to vote in free and open elections. The second leg is the rule of law, which states that if anyone, regardless of rank or wealth, violates a law, they are to be held liable for the violation and punished according to their crimes.[21] The third leg is truth, honesty, and commitment to a democratic form of government that is exhibited by the politicians who make up the governing body and leadership. If any of the three legs is missing or damaged, the democracy will fall.

Early in the development of the United States, confusion arose over the terms *democracy* and *republic*. They had been used interchangeably for some time, and the founders of the country were not sure of their meanings. James Madison attempted to untangle the confusion when he published the following definitions: "a pure democracy is a society consisting of a small number of citizens, who assemble and administer the government in person, and a republic is a government in which the people vote for individuals to represent their values and needs in a legislative assembly."[22] According to his definition, the United States is a republic.

However, John Marshall, the first chief justice of the U.S. Supreme Court, declared that the "Constitution provided for 'a well-regulated democracy' where no king, or president, could undermine representative government."[22] Marshall's designation of the form of government for the new nation as a democracy stuck, and the United States has since identified itself as a such.

There are several types of democracy. The United States is representative democracy (republic) in which the people vote for representatives (senators and representatives) who will support their values and ideals when decisions need to be made. In addition, the United States can be considered a federal republic with a democratic government and a capitalistic economy. It also can be designated as a presidential democracy, which has an elected president as one of the three branches of government (executive, legislative, judicial).[22]

Threats to Democracy

Because human nature has a built-in drive to gain and increase power over others, democracies tend to be fragile. Many past attempts at democratic forms of government have failed, primarily due to takeover by an authoritarian leader. The minimum condition for the survival of a democracy is that a large proportion of both the people and the leadership believe that a democracy is better than any other type of government.[23]

Threat 1: *Apathy*. Because democracy is a form of government in which the power to govern rests in the people, when the people lose interest in governing the country by not participating in the political process, not paying attention to what is going on, and particularly by not voting, they give up their power. This leaves a power vacuum that savvy and unscrupulous individuals can fill by getting themselves elected through manipulation of a small percentage of the voting public.

Threat 2: *Factionalism*. A political faction can be defined as a group whose interests are in conflict with the goals and purposes of the people and democracy. A faction can be either a majority or a minority of the whole group, who are united and activated by an individual with a cult personality or some common passion, cause, belief, or motive that is antagonistic, hostile, or contrary to the rights of other citizens.[23] The existence of factions in a democracy or republic tends to destabilize the government. Factions introduce dishonesty, injustice, prejudice, bias, inequality, and confusion into the workings of the legislative bodies. Factions are considered a mortal disease that causes the "people's" government to perish. Factions are most dangerous when they deny the rule of law and the basic principles of a democracy.

Factions differ from political parties, which are essential in a democracy. Political parties mobilize voters and increase their interest in the political process. They stabilize the legislative bodies and enable the majority to prevail over the opposition of a minority.[22]

Threat 3: *Restrictions on the right to vote*. The right to vote is the most basic principle of a democracy. When restrictions are placed on the right to vote, particularly when the restrictions disproportionately affect the voters of one party, they undermine the fundamental democratic principle of a voting population.[23]

One common type of voter restriction is gerrymandering, which is a process of dividing or arranging a region of a state into election districts in a way that gives one political party an unfair advantage in elections. The term is named after Elbridge Gerry, governor of Massachusetts in 1812. He signed a bill that formed a district in Boston that looked like the mythological fire salamander.[23] The mythological salamander is believed to have hibernated on logs, which when thrown in the fireplace, snuffed out the fire due to the salamander's presence. (See Figs. 18.1 and 18.2.) A disastrous result of voter restriction is that

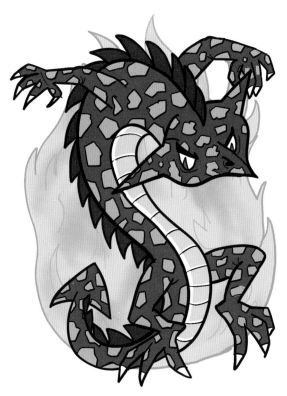

Figure 18.1 The mythological (fire) salamander.

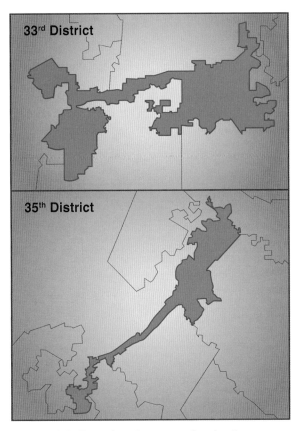

Figure 18.2 Examples of gerrymandered voting districts.

one party, through the manipulation of the electoral college, could consistently win elections while lacking a popular majority of votes nationwide. This practice would be a violation of the core democratic principle that elections should be won by a majority of the people's votes. It gives rise to the idea that some people's votes are worth less than other people's votes.

Threat 4: *Cult of Personality*. A cult of personality, sometimes referred to as a personality cult, is defined as "exaggerated devotion to a charismatic political, religious, or other leader."[23] These types of leaders are one of the primary reasons past democracies failed. The founding fathers of the United States were particularly afraid of this type of individual. After the Revolutionary War, some in the country's early leadership wanted to make George Washington king of the United States. To avoid this outcome, the founding fathers built into the Constitution a system of checks and balances among the three branches of government so that no one branch could exert unilateral

control over the other two branches. Although some individuals in the past have had strong personalities and have met the definition of a cult leader, the system of checks and balances has worked in keeping them from exerting excessive power over the government.

Leaders of cults of personality use their charisma to present themselves as bigger-than-life figures, the only ones capable of solving all the country's problems.[23] They may burst on the scene as a new figure, or they may take many years to develop a loyal following before exerting a major political influence. Although they will complain that the mass media treats them unfairly, they will use it to inflate their image and manipulate it to produce an exalted, even heroic, version of their persona in the minds of their followers. Dishonesty is one of a cult leader's foremost and deadliest weapons.[24]

There is great power in the frequent telling of big lies to manipulate at least part of the public's opinion. "Alternative facts" is a comparable modern-day equal to the big lie process that has become popular with some political figures. That is why a free and unencumbered press is necessary to the life of a democracy.[24] The press are the ones who can unearth the big lie and shine the withering spotlight of truth on it.

Cult leaders are particularly dangerous to a democracy when their antidemocratic message resonates with even a portion of the electorate. This group becomes fanatic followers who accept the cult leader's façade and bravado as authority and knowledge. These followers will believe whatever the leader says as the truth and have an almost religious devotion to the leader making their ideology their mission.[23]

One of the primary goals of the cult leader is to interrupt the established order, such as the balance of power of the three branches of government. The more followers who buy into the idea that the current government is in crisis and that society is on the eve of destruction, the better the cult leader can make their case that they are the only hope for survival. To maintain the interest of their followers, the cult leader speaks the same language as their followers, even to the point of using hate messages and vulgarity in public speeches.[23] This will guarantee that the followers comprehend and agree with what the leader is feeding them.

Followers also must feel that they are members of a special in-group. As members of the in-group, they will have their own beliefs and rituals, such as chanting at rallies, wearing special clothing, or displaying large signs and pictures that strengthen their dedication to the leader. To maintain and display their status in the group, followers will often increase their radical (and sometimes violent) behaviors, especially when the leader stirs prejudice against out-groups who have little or no possibility of ever belonging in the in-group. In this setting, laws, established values, and even ties to their own family take a back seat to the loyalty to the in-group and obedience to the leader.[23]

Creating and maintaining cults of personality has become easier in the modern era. Cult leaders have become masters of using the increasingly sophisticated and accessible mass media, often designating one or more media outlets solely for their support. This allows leaders of cults of personality to more easily spread and control their messages. This is an unprecedented threat to the survival of democracy.[22]

Structures of Democracy

The three branches of the U.S. government are the executive, judicial, and legislative branches. These branches exist simultaneously at the federal, state, and local government levels.

The Executive Branch

At the federal level, the executive branch consists of the president, vice president, cabinet, and various executive administrative bodies. Only the president and vice president are elected by the people. The others are appointed by the president and accountable to them. These appointees take the same oath to uphold the Constitution of the United States as the military and other elected officials and, therefore, are working for the people of the country and not the president. The executive of a state is the governor, who is elected by the people. Boards and commissions are also part of the executive branch because they are appointees of the chief executive. In county or parish government, one or more elected county commissioners function as executives. Larger cities usually have an elected mayor. Smaller cities and townships sometimes also elect mayors. (See Fig. 18.3 and Box 18.1.)

The Judicial Branch

The judicial branch is the court system. It is important to note the distinction between federal court, state court, and local court; appeals and supreme courts are found at both levels. At the federal level are the U.S. Supreme Court and district, or circuit, courts. At the state level are supreme courts, appeals courts, and the lower courts. Many cities and counties also have a local court system. Justices in the federal system, including Supreme Court justices, court of appeals

> " *There is great power in the frequent telling of big lies to manipulate at least part of the public's opinion.* "

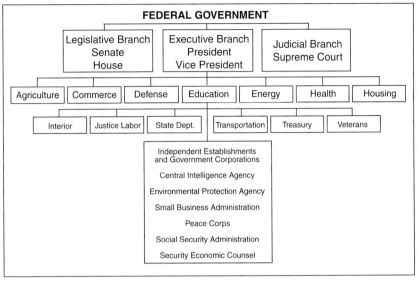

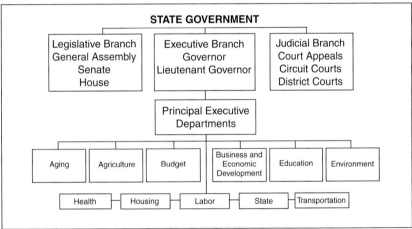

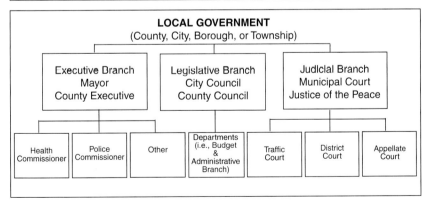

Figure 18.3 The organizational structure of the U.S. government.

Box 18.1 Know the Structure to Play the Game

One of the keys to creating power is understanding the organizational structure of the government. The Constitution of the United States establishes three separate branches of the federal government: legislative, judicial, and executive. Unless specifically granted to the federal government by the Constitution, the powers are supposed to go to the individual states. However, since the Constitution was signed, the federal government has taken on more power than was originally intended by the framers. It is the role of the state governments to serve their citizens within these parameters and to delegate discrete areas of activity to local governments.

Beneath the federal and state levels of government, there exist five layers of local government identified by the U.S. Census Bureau: county, municipal, township, school district, and special district governments (which include various utility, construction, and facility authorities). The qualifications for the classification of these local government structures are generally determined by the parent state governments. State governments are defined by their individual state constitutions and in turn delineate responsibility for the local governments.

Nurses must understand that there are three branches in each level of government: legislative, judicial, and executive. These distinctions are important and are the most common source of confusion for nurses.

judges, and district court judges, are nominated by the president and confirmed by the U.S. Senate, as stated in the Constitution. They hold their positions for life or until they retire. Appointed judges are supposed to be *nonpartisan*, that is, not strongly affiliated with any particular political party or ideology, and are supposed to base their decisions solely on the law. Although the U.S. Supreme Court is and has been since its beginning composed of nine members, the Constitution does not specify any particular number of justices. State court judges are selected in a variety of ways. Some are elected; some are appointed for a

given number of years or for life; and others are chosen by a combination of these methods (e.g., appointment followed by election). Local court judges are usually elected.

The judicial branch of government should not be discounted or perceived as unimportant to nurses. Over the years, both federal and state courts have decided several important issues that have an effect on the practice of nursing. These include the U.S. Supreme Court's decision regarding the right of nurses to organize into collective bargaining units, the requirement of health-care providers to report potentially violent patients to the police, the obligation of nurses to refuse to carry out physician orders they deem dangerous, and the establishment of criteria permitting nurses to withdraw life-support measures. Because of the influence courts can have on nursing practice, it is important to be aware of judicial decisions and keep them in mind when electing judges to office.

The Legislative Branch

At the federal level, the legislative branch of government consists of the House of Representatives and the Senate. Each state also has a legislative branch of government. All states except Nebraska have a bicameral legislature with both a house of representatives and a senate. The primary function of the legislative branch of government is the formation of policy by making laws.

Key Players in the Legislative Process

Members of the legislative branch of government have a wide range of influence. It is important to remember that legislators are human and respond to the same forces that all people respond to, including interpersonal dynamics, peer pressure, and both internal and external factors. All members of the legislative branch are elected by the people to represent their interests. It is the people's responsibility to make sure their officials do that rather than promote their own self-interest, party affiliations, or ideologies.

The Majority Leader

The majority leader in the House of Representatives is the person who generally supervises and directs the activities on the House floor. Some consider this position to be the most powerful job in politics. The majority leader has control over the legislative calendar, which ultimately determines when many of the House session activities take place and even when, or if, bills are introduced for consideration. The majority leader is also the central figure in crafting the budget, which is the most important activity the legislature performs on an annual basis. The majority leader of the House of Representatives is the third person in line for the presidency should something happen to the president and vice president preventing them from governing.

The Majority Whip

The majority whip is responsible for collecting votes when legislators may be leaning toward voting against their party. At the same time the majority leader is supporting a bill, the whip is negotiating on the House floor for the votes necessary to pass the bill. The whip is responsible for collecting support and votes for various issues both during the legislative session and when it is in recess. They "whip-up" their party members to vote for the bill.

The Minority Leader

The minority leader represents the party that does not have a numerical majority in the House and helps organize support against bills introduced by the majority leader. The minority leader presents an alternative point of view. There is an expression in the legislature: "The majority will have their way, and the minority will have their say."

In most cases, the majority party can pass almost any bill it supports over the objections of the minority. The minority leader usually can only speak against it. However, there are some issues that legislators will almost never vote against: "mom," "pop," and "the little guy." Depending on the area of the country, mom and pop and the little guy may represent older citizens, family farmers and ranchers, or local small business owners. When these issues are included in a bill, most legislators will support the bill, even if they must vote against their party. To ensure representatives vote the will of the people, they need to hear the opinions of their constituents.

The Conference Committee

The conference committee attempts to reconcile differences in bills, where one is passed by the House and another by the Senate on the same issue. The rules governing the structure, composition, and function of the conference committee vary from state to state. Generally, they consist of an equal number of appointed members from both the House and the Senate. Often, a specified combination of votes, such as two votes from the House and two votes from the Senate, is necessary to approve a compromise bill and move it out of committee.

What Do You Think?

Whom do you know in the legislature of your state government? Who is your representative or congressperson? Make a list of the things you would want that person to know about or do for health care and the nursing profession.

Caucuses

Caucuses are formed when the legislature divides into groups consisting of people with mutual interests. These groups operate as a unit rather than as individual voters, trading on their capacity to bring a block of votes for or against an issue or bill. Examples are the Senate Nursing Caucus, the Women's Caucus, the Black Caucus, the Hispanic Caucus, and the Business Community Caucus.

Although caucuses may be bipartisan, many are partisan. For example, the largest caucus groups are the Democratic Caucus and the Republican Caucus. Each caucus develops its own internal governance structure and leadership, including a speaker who leads the caucus and speaks for the group. After a group member achieves a leadership role, they must try to balance the wishes of the group against their own political survival in the caucus and the political pressures exerted by the larger world.

THE POWER OF THE MEDIA

The media and the voters exert external forces on policymakers. In recent years, the media have become a powerful influence on government, often driving and shaping public opinion that eventually evolves into a legislative agenda. In the 2020 election cycle, social media shaped the opinions of many voters. Advanced technology targeted specific groups of voters and sometimes even individual voters to deliver political messages tailored to the voters' beliefs and viewpoints, even when the messages were untrue.

Evidence that social media was and continues to be manipulated by foreign powers also was discovered. Outside forces invest vast sums of money under false corporate names to flood social media with false or misleading information in support of the candidate who supports their position.

When Is It News?

Because of limited time and resources, major news outlets must choose which stories are most important to report on; that is, they must decide what is and what is not news. These outlets can focus on certain elements of the news, thereby making them seem to be more important than others. To form a more complete and well-rounded understanding of current events, it is helpful to get news from reputable national and international sources with a range of perspectives.

In recent years, the Internet has become a major source of information for people. Those interested can, and should, inform themselves about all sides of the issues. Just as when doing research in nursing, it is advisable to locate and read the original sources rather than rely on the explanation of an issue by a news agency that may present only positions that support its viewpoint. (For more on Web site credibility, see Chapter 24.)

Politicians well versed in electronic media have learned to use it as a tool both to get their message out and to raise funds for their campaign. Younger voters no longer rely on the national networks' nightly newscasts to get their information about politics and other issues; instead, they use the Internet and a variety of apps and newsfeeds to access information. Most legislators now have weekly newsletters and updates by e-mail and social media that they send out to anyone who wishes to sign up for them. When viewing these sites, keep in mind the ideological position of the creator. It is always best to consider multiple reputable sources of information before accepting an observation or conclusion as true.

Well-funded fringe groups are able to put sophisticated and professional-looking political advertisements on the Internet and social media that attack a candidate in a personal way or falsely attribute a radical viewpoint to that candidate. In other cases, partisan elements create *memes*—humorous images, videos, or pieces of text that are copied and spread rapidly by Internet users—containing unsubstantiated or even blatantly false charges against a candidate. These memes are then picked up by the network or mainstream media, and candidates have to spend time and money refuting false claims or allegations. However, once these stories are out in the media, they often are perceived as true, regardless of any denial or evidence a candidate may offer.

Election by Media

Before media campaigns became the norm, with millions of dollars being spent on television and radio advertising, the printed news media used to publish what the candidate said and often printed whole speeches. This approach allowed the public to read the speeches and make up their minds about which issues the candidate supported. Today, the trend is to give a 30-second soundbite of a candidate's speech, then have 10 minutes of political analysis by a well-known commentator who tells the public their opinion of what the candidate said.

Some members of the print media have adopted a similar approach to political issues. In newspapers, it is not unusual to see a lengthy editorial comment positioned next to a brief statement made by a candidate. In some ways, media has come full circle. With the advent of the Internet, interested citizens can watch, listen to, or read the text of important speeches in their entirety at their own convenience.

Unfortunately, in recent elections, huge sums of money from foreign countries with business interests in the United States have been illegally funneled through political organizations and PACs in an effort to influence election outcomes. The U.S. Constitution makes any contributions from foreign sources illegal.[13] Because the laws that required the tracking of these sources of money were repealed by the U.S.

> *To form a more complete and well-rounded understanding of current events, it is helpful to get news from reputable national and international sources with a range of perspectives.*

Supreme Court, it left large loopholes in the law, and now no one really knows where the money comes from. The result has been a blizzard of negative political attack ads that can influence the outcome of both state and national elections.[14]

Legislator Beware

Legislators, while recognizing and using the power of the media to promote their messages, have also become wary of it. Statements can be taken out of context and used to undermine the real intent of their message by news organizations and Web sites that oppose their views. So, while it is important for legislators to use the media to promote their position, media exposure also puts them at risk for potentially unfair criticism. Political organizations that support candidates for election have become highly sensitized to attacks and generally try to post rebuttal ads within 24 hours of the airing of attack ads. This helps prevent the attack ad from going viral. But it remains important for the informed voter to beware: always check the original source to make sure a soundbite or opinion attributed to a speaker has not been taken out of context.

> *... while it is important for legislators to use the media to promote their position, media exposure also puts them at risk for potentially unfair criticism.*

A Story With Legs

As an example, suppose a legislator has a large population of senior citizens in his district who have supported him for many years. The legislator publicly supports senior-citizen issues and believes that the senior support will always be there. However, during an election campaign, a political opponent's investigation uncovers information that the legislator voted against several bills that would have increased senior citizens' benefits. Keep in mind that amendments are routinely added to unrelated bills, so the legislator may have voted against a bill they viewed as detrimental to their constituents but that had an amendment that was beneficial to them. Although the legislator may agree with the amendment, they elected not to vote for the entire bill. Still, an opponent can take that fact out of context and use it to harm the legislator's reputation.

Scandals involving moral issues, such as sexual misconduct, have overshadowed almost all other issues in past years. If a legislator's opponent found something that was questionable and posted this information on some obscure Web site or social media platforms, the story could be picked up by the network media, immediately reported on television news programs, and make the front page of the local newspaper the next day. Eventually, the major networks would perform investigative reporting on the issue, which will either support or disprove the allegations. But by then, people have often already made up their minds about the candidate's guilt or innocence. However, in recent elections, moral issues have not been seen as important as in the past. Candidates who have been divorced several times, admitted to cheating on their spouses, and even admitted on tape to harassing women have managed to win elections. They believe that their celebrity and wealth will protect them from suffering any consequences.

A normal news cycle is about 24 hours, which means that a story will be reported for one day, then dropped for the next new thing. If the story develops "legs," meaning it takes on a life of its own and continues to grow without further information from the opponent, it will be on other Internet sites, all the television news programs, and in the major national newspapers. Stories with legs can stay in the news for days or even weeks.

The Internet has contributed to the "legs" phenomenon. Today, almost everything a person in a public position has ever said or done is recorded somewhere, and political Web sites show these recorded clips. If they are entertaining enough, the clips are often picked up by the network media and shown repeatedly, giving the information a much wider audience than it might otherwise have had. Internet-savvy people are proficient at "data mining" and can obtain private records and information on individuals running for office. This information can become a potent tool in the hands of a political rival. Unfortunately, in some instances, the actual story may be untrue, but because it gets so much exposure by respected news sources, it becomes accepted as true.

At this point, the legislator who is the subject of that story is in political jeopardy. There is little that a politician fears more than being the subject of this type of negative story. Constituents need to be wary of stories such as these. Consider who may benefit from such a story before accepting it as fact. Get to know your representative by keeping abreast of the work they are doing and how they vote. Doing so can help you discern the authenticity of a story about that representative.

THE POLITICAL PROCESS

Laws maintain order in a complicated society and regulate the interactions of its citizens. As a society becomes more complex, existing laws are revised or new ones are passed to ensure they are still relevant for the survival and smooth functioning of that society.

Who Introduces Legislation?

Where Laws Begin

Federal laws are legislative, meaning they are passed by Congress and signed by the president. For example, just a few years ago, there were no laws that dealt with hacking, computer fraud, computer theft of bank funds, or online pornography. Today, there is an ever-growing body of law that focuses on computers; whole sections of police agencies, such as the Federal Bureau of Investigation's Computer Crime Unit, are dedicated to enforcing these laws. Where do ideas for laws and policies come from, and how do these ideas become laws?

Elected Officials

Any elected official, including governors, mayors, county commissioners, and city council members, can propose a program or an initiative that requires passage by the legislature. This initiative is called a *bill*, and once a bill is passed, it becomes a *legislative law*. The elected official goes to the legislative leadership in the parties and asks them either to submit the bill or to help move the bill through the legislative process.

Lobbyists, the constituency, and advocate groups are a major source of proposed legislation. These groups represent various interests ranging from public interest groups to corporate lobbyists. Lobbyists frequently craft legislation and then pass it on to a friendly legislator. Consumer groups are often visible at the legislature through demonstrations and lobbying.

Constituency groups are groups of individuals and networks of people who share common interests and concerns with a major organization. They work collaboratively with the primary organization on specific issues to support and develop policies and provide additional voices to influence legislators' opinions. For example, the ANA is composed of individual nurse members who are interested in advancing an agenda that promotes a range of issues based on quality health care and the nursing profession. The state nursing associations and other organizations, such as the National Organization of Nurse Practitioner Faculties and the American Association of Critical-Care Nurses (AACN), are constituency groups to the ANA.

> *Advocacy groups are sometimes known as pressure groups, campaign groups, or special-interest groups and are different from constituency groups in that their main focus is to change the way the public views an issue.*

Advocacy groups are sometimes known as *pressure groups, campaign groups,* or *special-interest groups* and are different from constituency groups in that their main focus is to change the way the *public* views an issue. Advocacy groups can range from very small to very large, and they freely use the media to increase their power and influence. They can be motivated by a current hot political issue or a long-term issue that affects society. Examples of these groups include organizations such as the National Rifle Association (NRA), which acts as a lobbying group for gun manufacturers and enthusiasts, and the American Association of Retired Persons (AARP), which is concerned about the long-term effects of legislation on older Americans.

Government Agencies

Legislation is also generated from government agencies. When agencies seek fee increases or another type of policy reform, they can introduce legislation.

For example, policy reforms in the Internal Revenue Service are a type of agency-initiated legislation. Frequently, the employees of the agency draft the legislation and then direct it toward a supportive legislator.

These agencies can also create regulations referred to as administrative law. Bureaucratic agencies, such as the U.S. Department of Health and Human Services (DHHS), create the regulations of issues under their authority. These regulations that have the force of law can be problematic because they are written by unelected administrators, so elected representatives are not accountable for the consequences of imposing these regulations on their constituents. This process is one of the criticisms of the ACA. The bill, as passed, defines outcome goals and provides the DHHS with wide authority to write the rules. That places the responsibility for the effects of the ACA on unelected administrators and provides some cover for elected officials who then do not need to take responsibility for any problems.[15]

What Drives Legislation?

Funding. Because almost all government agencies depend on legislative funding to sustain their operations, they become actively engaged, overtly or covertly, in seeking the passage of a budget that will sustain their survival.

Public Demand. Legislators are very careful to listen to the demands of their voters and typically vote for an issue that the majority of their constituents supports. A classic example of this process was seen in New Jersey, where a child was sexually molested and murdered by a known convicted sex offender who moved into the child's neighborhood. The tragedy prompted a public outcry: How could this happen? Something needed to be done! Ultimately, the outcry produced the now famous Megan's Law, which requires public disclosure of a known sex offender's residence. The power of individual constituents to demand laws or changes to laws should not be underestimated. Legislators listen and will conform to the will of the people if they hear from enough of them.

Program Issues. These issues recur periodically and require legislative attention. Requests for increases in television cable rates constitute an example of a programmatic issue. The cable industry will be very interested in the outcome of legislation that may affect what cable companies can charge for their services.

Both cable and consumer group lobbyists actively seek the opportunity to influence key legislators on these and similar issues.

Constituent-Specific Issues. Groups of voters may have specific interests that can lead to introduction of a bill. For example, in legislative districts where a large population of senior citizens resides, escalating costs of prescriptions or decreased access to health care may be an important issue. Legislation specific to that constituency will be introduced at a greater rate than in areas with fewer senior citizens. Issues related to nursing practice regulations fall into this category.

How Bills Become Law

The Tracking Number

Legislators in both the House and the Senate can introduce a bill from any source into their respective chambers. Additional legislators can sign on as the bill's cosponsors. A bill is considered to be strong if it has strong sponsorship, including a number of powerful cosponsors, a high degree of bipartisanship, and the interest of powerful individuals, both political and nonpolitical. After the bill is introduced, it is taken to the chief clerk, who assigns it a number that permits it to be tracked throughout the process.

What Do You Think?

Visit your state legislature's Web site and identify two bills that deal with health care. How do you feel about these bills? How should your representative vote on this issue? How can nurses influence these bills to ensure effective health-care policy?

The Committee

After a bill is assigned a number, it is referred to a **committee**. Most congressional committees deal with passing laws. Thousands of bills are proposed in both chambers of Congress, but only a small percentage ever gets considered for passage. A bill that is favored usually goes to a committee that focuses on the issues that the bill would address, but House and Senate leaders decide which committee considers the bill. This decision, greatly influenced by politics, is critical to the survival and ultimate passage of a bill.

In committee, members consider written comments on the measure, hold hearings in which witnesses testify and answer questions, make any needed changes based on the information gathered, and then send the bill to the full chamber for debate. Conference committees, usually composed of standing committee members from the House and Senate who originally considered the legislation, help reconcile one chamber's version of a bill with the other chamber's version.

It is no coincidence that most bills die in committee. Invariably, the leadership discusses its expectation for the bill with the committee chairs. If the leadership wants a bill to fail, it is referred to a committee that will never vote on it or will not pass it on to the House.

In the U.S. Congress, the committees with greatest jurisdiction over health matters and their subcommittees are the following:

- *House Ways and Means Committee:* Social Security and Medicare (health-care subcommittees)
- *House Commerce Committee:* Health legislation, including Medicaid (subcommittees on health and the environment)
- *Senate Finance Committee:* Medicare and Medicaid (health subcommittees)
- *Senate Labor and Human Resources Committee:* Health legislation in general; also works cooperatively with the Senate Finance Committee in considering issues involving Medicare and Medicaid
- *House and Senate Appropriations Committee:* Authorizes all money necessary to implement action proposed in a bill (subcommittees for labor, education, and health and human services)

The Next Step

As a result of full committee hearings, several things may happen to a bill. It may be

- Reported out of committee favorably and be scheduled for debate by the full House or Senate.
- Reported out favorably, but with amendments.
- Reported out unfavorably.
- Killed outright.

For example, a bill reforming the way judges are elected ideally would go to the judiciary committee. However, there is no legal requirement that the Speaker of the House or the Senate president pro tempore to send the bill to any particular committee. For political reasons, the speaker may refer the bill to the committee on intergovernmental affairs, where it will languish and die.

Can the Bill Survive?

For a bill to survive, its sponsor must have the knowledge and the political standing to move the bill out of committee. If sponsors are truly committed, they will trade on their political capital. **Political capital** generally refers to some type of favor or action that a politician can exchange for something they want. It is an extremely important element in the legislative process and consists of, but is not limited to, votes, amendments to bills, appointments, and support from constituency groups. Political capital often consists of an "if you vote for my bill, I'll vote for your bill" type of exchange. Legislators can be motivated to consider a bill if they get feedback from enough of their constituents.

> **If the leadership wants a bill to fail, it is referred to a committee that will never vote on it or will not pass it on to the House or Senate.**

A Scheduled Debate

After a bill has been reported out of a House committee (with the exception of the ways and means and appropriations committees), it goes to the rules committee, which schedules bills and determines how much time will be spent on debate and whether or not amendments will be allowed. In the Senate, bills go on the Senate calendar, after which the majority leadership determines when or if a bill will be debated.

After a bill is debated, possibly amended, and passed by one chamber, it is sent to the other chamber, where it goes through the same procedure. If the bill passes both the House and the Senate without any changes, it is sent to the president for signature.

Opposing Versions

However, if the House and Senate pass different versions of a bill, the two bills are sent to a conference committee, which consists of members appointed by both the House and the Senate. This committee seeks to resolve the differences between the two bills; if the differences cannot be resolved, the bill dies in committee. When the conference committee reaches agreement on a bill, it goes back to the House and

Senate for passage. At this juncture, the bill must be voted up or down, because no further amendments are accepted.

Passage or Veto?

If the bill is approved in both houses, it then goes to the chief executive—at the federal level, the president, or at the state level, the governor—who makes determinations about the bill. Governors can do one of two things: sign the bill into law or actively **veto** it. At the federal level, the president has the same options, with the addition of the pocket veto. Pocket vetoes, found only at the federal level, occur when the president, rather than actively vetoing a bill, simply does not sign it so that it does not become law. If vetoed, the bill is sent back to the House and Senate. To override the veto, a two-thirds vote by both chambers is required.

The Fiscal Note

Clearly, the passage of a law can be a long and difficult process. This is often quite frustrating for action-oriented nurses who are used to seeing immediate outcomes—forming plans and making things happen quickly.

All bills that are passed need a fiscal note attached to them. Therefore, the appropriations committee is operationally very powerful. A piece of legislation that is passed without a fiscal note attached will never become a law. Over the years, many pieces of legislation have been passed by the legislature but have been starved to death financially. These are called *unfunded mandates*.

Housekeeping Bills

A *housekeeping bill* is used to update a law by clarifying obscure language, eliminating obsolete sections, or modernizing sections to keep in step with changes in technology or society. However, some housekeeping bills go beyond a simple cleaning up of the law. Major regulatory changes can be put forth in laws in the form of housekeeping bills. Legislators can use this tactic to move a piece of legislation through the process, especially when the bill is more significant than the leadership acknowledges it to be. Although regulatory reform and change may seem tedious, they are important to the legislative process and have the capacity to benefit the public immensely or do irrevocable harm.

Executive Orders

Executive orders provide the chief executive, the governor or the president, a means for moving an agenda item forward. Executive orders are in many cases a convenient way to formulate policy with minimal involvement of the legislature. They also allow the executive to make a statement about an issue that can be entered on the public record.

The legislature can leave executive orders uncontested or challenge them by characterizing them as beyond the scope of the executive branch. This may involve turning to the third branch of government, the judiciary.

> *Pocket vetoes, found only at the federal level, occur when the president, rather than actively vetoing a bill, simply does not sign it so that it does not become law.*

HOW TO BE A POLITICALLY ACTIVE NURSE

The first step in becoming a politically active nurse is to identify the specific goals that nurses, as a group, want to accomplish.

Why Be Active?

Nurses recognize many important issues in today's health-care system:

- Increasingly acute conditions of hospitalized patients who require higher levels of care and more complex levels of support than ever before
- Increasing responsibilities for nurses in supervision of rising numbers of unlicensed health-care personnel
- Loss of control of the work environment caused by managed care organizations
- Ever-shortening hospitalizations resulting in patients being sent home "quicker and sicker"
- Attempts by non-nursing groups to alter nurse practice acts and change the nature of state boards of nursing
- Expanding the scope of practice for APRNs

Any one of these issues can become a target at which nurses can aim their considerable political power.

For example, most nurses are concerned that RNs, who have traditionally been at patients' bedsides, are being replaced by individuals who are less prepared and less able to deal with high-acuity patients. Nurses believe that when they are replaced in large numbers by unlicensed assistive personnel, including nursing assistants, and by personnel who provide specific services, such as technicians who sit in front of cardiac monitors, the quality of patient care decreases. Nurses know that these technicians often take on responsibilities for which they have had little training. Rarely are there established national standards that require these assistive personnel to demonstrate their ability to provide a specific level of care or even standards that protect public safety.[1]

Feeling Powerless

Nurses are usually employees at will and can be fired for any reason. Although some efforts have been made in this direction, whistleblower protection is generally not available to protect nurses who wish to speak out against unsafe staffing levels or employment practices. Nurses are, at times, torn between their obligations to maintain high standards of safe, ethical care and their obligations to their families to remain employed.

Although nurses often feel powerless against a monolithic health-care bureaucracy, in reality they have the potential to be a potent political force. Nationally, with almost 4 million nurses licensed to practice, the nursing profession constitutes the largest single body of health-care providers in the country.[2]

Finding a Voice

Nurses in all health-care settings are saying, "Somebody's got to do something about this situation." The reality of the situation is that nurses themselves are the best group to do that something. Once nurses identify exactly what it is that needs to be accomplished and understand what is possible within the

> *Although nurses often feel powerless against a monolithic health-care bureaucracy, in reality they have the potential to be a potent political force.*

political framework, they can use their significant political power to make changes that will benefit both the patients and the profession.

Three Groups of Constituents

Although most nurses understand the problems they face as a profession, not all will be motivated to take the steps to make changes via the political process. Some are more comfortable taking leadership roles in political encounters, while others prefer to follow and provide needed support. Others may want to get involved but need to weigh family responsibilities and their perception of their ability to make a difference. As situations change, they may choose to become more active. Generally, however, they can be grouped by their state of involvement and beliefs.

Group 1: Have a Little

One problem that nurses in this group encounter is the ongoing conflict between the status quo and progress. They want to obtain more power and control, gain more benefits, earn more money, and have more respect as professionals. However, the strong desire to advance is counterbalanced by fear of jeopardizing their current jobs and/or their professional standing. Their motivation to be something more, to do something new, or to believe in something bigger is held back and pulled in another direction by their fear of change or the demands of their personal life. The result of this internal tug-of-war is an attitude of inertia and ambivalence that has traditionally prevented nurses from organizing politically and effectively using their numerical power.

Group 2: Want More

Despite the inertia and ambivalence of individuals in the have-a-little category, some of the most notable revolutionaries in history have come from this group, including Thomas Jefferson, Dr. Martin Luther King Jr., and Loretta Ford, who founded the nurse practitioner movement. Each of these individuals came from the working middle class with a belief that it could be made better and that they could "want more." Nurses who overcome their fear of change and risk their comfortable status quo position can make great strides in the profession. They can use their actions as examples of what individuals can accomplish to raise their own motivation levels to a point at which they overwhelm their trepidation.

Group 3: Sit Back and Watch

A third group of people, who share the inertia found among the have-a-little and want-more groups, are the "do-nothings." These individuals can be heard making comments such as "I agree with what you are saying; I just don't agree with your means," "I'm not going to get involved in this," and "I'm too busy to belong to the organization." The do-nothings tend to watch the activities of others, and if their efforts are successful, then they will join in as beneficiaries because they feel they have supported the effort from an ideological standpoint. However, they avoid any active involvement in politics. The 18th-century British politician Edmund Burke recognized the danger of the do-nothings. He said, "The only thing necessary for the triumph of evil is for good men [and women] to do nothing."

What Can One Nurse Do?

It is important to remember that politics is a free-market enterprise open to anyone who is willing to become involved and play the game. Success in the political arena is contingent on three elements:

1. Knowledge and understanding of the process
2. The ability to offer something of value to the political figure
3. The capacity to identify what will be necessary to accomplish the objective

Anyone who is interested in becoming politically active must recognize that all candidates and elected officials need three things: resources to run their political operation (money and volunteers), votes, and a means to shape public opinion. Learning about politics through the mentoring process is often a successful strategy for nurses who have had little past **political involvement** but are interested in advancing a health policy.

Resources

Money

Sufficient resources are essential to running a political campaign. The first and most necessary resource is always money. Would-be candidates soon discover that a lack of money to fund a campaign will inevitably lead to political failure. An unfunded candidate cannot travel, send mailings, produce radio and television commercials, post signs, or organize a telephone bank.

Voters often fail to realize that political candidates are only as available as finances permit. Frequently, promising candidates lose because they fail to garner the financial resources necessary to run an effective campaign.

Nurses can gain a candidate's support for issues by donating to their campaign chest. Many nurses feel that they are just struggling to make ends meet and do not have a lot of extra money to spend on candidates. The reality is that everybody can afford something, even 5 or 10 dollars. Although the small sum may not seem like much when compared to the millions and millions donated by big business and foreign donors, because of the large numbers of nurses, the small amounts will quickly add up. The nurse's name will show up on the candidates' donor list, and the candidate will be more likely to consider the nurse's opinion when the nurse calls or writes about an issue.

Nurses can also contribute to PACs such as ANA or state-level organizations that collectively can have a greater voice than one individual.

Volunteers

A second important resource in an election campaign is volunteers. Volunteers work in campaigns by staffing telephone banks, making literature drops, placing

> *Anyone who is interested in becoming politically active must recognize that all candidates and elected officials need three things: resources to run their political operation (money and volunteers), votes, and a means to shape public opinion.*

signs, conducting voter registration drives, and distributing issues electronically to garner more interest in a position. Usually, political candidates are very glad to have free help for their campaigns, and many movements gain significant traction at the local level.

Although nurses may not be able to make large monetary contributions to a candidate's campaign, they can always volunteer some time. Working closely with a candidate on a volunteer basis allows individuals to discuss important issues and helps candidates who support issues important to nurses. Most candidates need a considerable amount of education on health-related issues because of their lack of knowledge about medical and nursing concerns.

Votes

The 14th and 15th Amendments emphasize that the right to vote is the most fundamental act in a democracy. Obviously, votes are essential to any candidate. If a candidate does not have votes, they will not be elected. One of the most significant activities nurses can become involved in is to join and support a political party and then vote in elections for the candidates who most closely reflect the nurse's value system and fundamental beliefs.

Requirements to Vote

The first step in being able to vote is to meet the established requirements for voting. These are established by the individual states but are very similar in many states. They include being a U.S. citizen, establishing residency in a particular location, not being a convicted felon (some states), and being 18 years of age or older. If people meet these requirements, they next go to a location where they register to vote. In some states, this can be done by mail or even at the voting polls the same day as people vote. In other states, it is much more restrictive, and the locations may be at state offices. Also, some states require voters to present a government-issued photo ID, birth certificate, written proof of residency, or passport to register. In 23 states, voting rights have been restricted by the addition of more than 100 highly selective voting requirements, including purging voter registration lists without notification of the voters; closing voting sites where underrepresented groups are concentrated; eliminating ballot drop boxes; restricting the use of mail-in ballots; and shortening voting times, which produces long lines and discourages people from voting. These measures were aimed at certain groups such as college students and various racial and ethnic minorities who tended to vote for Democratic candidates. These restrictions came about as a result of the 2014 Supreme Court decision to repeal several requirements in the Voting Rights Act that prevented certain states from enacting regulations that would restrict minority voting.[16]

> *In 23 states, voting rights have been restricted by the addition of more than 100 highly selective voting requirements, including purging voter registration lists without notification of the voters; closing voting sites where underrepresented groups are concentrated; eliminating ballot drop boxes; restricting the use of mail-in ballots; and shortening voting times, which produces long lines and discourages people from voting.*

There are several different types of elections in which people can vote. Local elections are for the election of local officials such as councilpersons, mayors, and various other local officials. Special elections occur when there is a specific issue that needs consideration or when a state is attempting to replace a legislator who was removed or who quit, retired, or died before the end of their normal term in office. The governor of a state has particular power over special elections and may hold off having them until the climate is more favorable for their party's candidate. State elections are for the election of state officials such as governors, state senators, and state representatives. "Off-year" elections are held every two years primarily to elect members of Congress. General elections are for the election of national officials such as the president and vice president and are held every 4 years on the first Tuesday in November. Sometimes local, state, and general elections all occur at the same time, or they may be held at different times throughout the year.

Primary elections are for the selection of candidates for the various levels of office. These are held at times selected by the governors of the individual states. For primary elections, most states require that voters must vote within their own party (i.e., if they are Democrats, they must vote for a Democratic primary candidate; if they are Republicans, they must vote for a Republican primary candidate), but several states have open primary elections in which the person voting can vote for any primary candidate regardless of party affiliation.

Keep in mind that people almost never find a perfect fit with any political party. Almost everyone who belongs to a political party will disagree at some point with some element of the party's platform. However, differing opinions and beliefs should not be a barrier to membership in a political party. The only way to change a view or opinion is by active participation from within the party.

The ultimate political power is the vote. Nurses must be registered to vote and must go to the polls. They can make the difference for a candidate who supports legislation that empowers nurses and who recognizes what is needed for beneficial health-care reform.

Shaping Public Opinion

Candidates need endorsements from their constituents (voters) so that they can build their support base. They generally consider endorsements from nurses as one of the most valuable assets to their campaign.

Public Trust in Nurses

Supporting nursing organizations such as the ANA or the American Academy of Nurse Practitioners that lobby for the concerns of nurses is essential because this is exactly the type of organizational endorsement that candidates try to get. By careful selection of candidates who support legislation favorable to nursing and health care, endorsements can give nurses the capacity to shape public opinion. Large organizations have people whose job it is to study the candidate's position on issues important to the profession. Why are endorsements from nurses so valuable? Periodic polls conducted by national news magazines, asking readers to rank various professions by how much they are trusted, have consistently shown that the public views nurses very highly, in the same category

as police officers, firefighters, and teachers. For the past 20 years, nurses have ranked number one on the Gallup Poll list of the most ethical, honest, and trusted professionals, outranking the second-place finisher, pharmacists, by 12 points.[17]

Why the Governor Matters

Nurses should endorse candidates in campaigns that have an impact on important issues. Often, the campaign for governor falls into this category because governors, as chief executives, have a great deal of political power within a state and can appoint people to a number of boards, committees, and other positions. Nurses need to recognize that the members of the board of nursing in their state, as well as important appointed positions in health departments and other regulatory agencies, may be appointed by the governor and that this board has the final decision on the way that nurses practice.

When nurses establish a working political relationship with the governor either individually or via their state nursing organization, the governor is more likely to look favorably on them as those who have sustained them, provided financial support, and given endorsements during the political campaign. They will be the people the governor is likely to appoint to board positions.

Grassroots Effort

A model for individual political development encourages grassroots involvement in local issues. This model is based on the belief that grassroots efforts may be more fulfilling than involvement in partisan politics.[18] This model is an activity-oriented ladder, including activities at four distinct levels:

- *Rung 1: Civic involvement.* Children's sports, Parent Teacher Association (PTA), neighborhood improvement group
- *Rung 2: Advocacy.* Writing letters to public officials and newspapers and making organized visits to officials to discuss local issues
- *Rung 3: Organizing.* Independent organizing on local issues, incorporation of single-issue citizens' groups, and networking with similarly situated citizens' groups
- *Rung 4: Long-term power wielding.* Campaigning for oneself or another, local government planning, and agenda setting

Sometimes grassroots movements are not so grassroots. How can you tell the difference? The key is the funding source, which some movements attempt to hide. If the source of money for the movement is from a large corporation, a politically slanted cable news channel, a political party, or other organization that has strong leanings toward one particular position, it is not a true grassroots organization. If large groups of people are bussed in for rallies from a great distance away and their signs are professionally printed, this may be a tip-off that they are being funded by a politically motivated enterprise.

True grassroots movements tend to be more spontaneous and less well organized. They have little funding from large organizations and come from a locally developed movement. A good example of this is the high school student protests that arose after the 2018 shooting event that took place in Parkland, Florida. Another one that helped boost the image of nursing was the Show Me Your Stethoscope movement that was initiated completely through a group of nurses on Facebook. These movements tend to focus on one particular issue, and the life cycle of their organization is relatively short, lasting until the issue is resolved. This may be for only a few weeks or months at most, although some may spin off a better-organized group that can have considerable political power.[18]

> *"True grassroots movements tend to be more spontaneous and less well organized. They have little funding from large organizations and come from a locally developed movement."*

Nurses in Office

Most nurses prefer not to run for political office. However, some do and achieve high status in public office. One way that nurses can become more politically involved is to become knowledgeable about key issues that have an effect on health care and the profession. Often, issues that may not seem at first glance to be associated with health care or nursing, such as tax cuts, have a profound influence on how a state can care for those most in need. Almost always, the first items cut from a budget are social safety net and health-care programs such as school nurses.

Another way to become politically involved is to develop a political relationship with an elected official at the state or local level or a political operative who can mentor and guide you in finding a route through the political maze. As discussed earlier, the principle of self-interest is one of the most critical elements in politics, and to establish a relationship with a political figure, nurses must demonstrate that the issues they support have value to both themselves and to the politician.

Making Alliances

There are several ways that a nurse can decide whom to support when becoming involved in the political process. A first step is to identify those legislators interested in issues related to health care and nursing. Editorial opinion pieces in newspapers can give nurses a sense of the issues of concern, and representatives' Web sites can reveal their positions on issues.

It is a good idea to begin with local legislators and candidates, such as the state representative, state senator, or councilperson serving the neighborhood. Call their offices and find out when and where they are scheduled to speak, then go and listen to the speech to get a sense of who they are and what issues they support. Their speeches and the way they answer questions will reveal their ideology and partisanship. Also, during question-and-answer periods, ask elected officials what they think about issues important to you.

Attending some of the partisan events that occur during an election season or volunteering at election headquarters will help with getting exposure to prominent political figures. An advantageous way to visualize the local political landscape is by observing who is talking to whom at the event. Nurses can make their own assessments of political candidates by observing the candidates in action, calling their offices for information, reading published literature, checking their positions on their Web site, and talking to people who know the candidates.

Beginning the process may seem difficult, but once you decide to become politically active, you'll become more confident, and your interest in the process will grow.

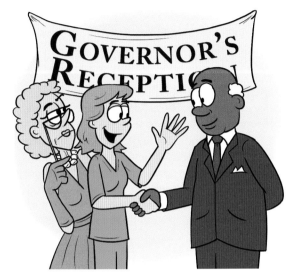

Nurses make alliances with politicians through direct contact.

Know the Issues

For nurses to be successful in the political process, they must know and understand the issues. At times, an issue may be readily apparent in a nurse's community—for example, an increased number of homeless people. Other issues are easily identified by reading newspapers and a variety of Web sites that focus on current issues. Issues are generally presented in the editorial section; most newspapers also have a political watch section, which reports the results of any significant votes at the state and federal levels. Keep in mind, however, that most media outlets have a political view that influences the way they present their news and opinions. It is best to research an opposing view to get a full understanding of the issues.

The ANA newspaper, *American Nurse*, is an excellent source of information on issues of concern to the profession. In addition, the *American Journal of Nursing* Newsline feature and *Nursing and Health Care*'s Washington Focus are excellent, easily readable sources of information in journals. *Capitol Beat*, the ANA legislative newsletter for nurses, reports on the activities of its nurse lobbyists and on significant issues in Congress and regulatory agencies. This publication requires a subscription but is available in most nursing school and hospital libraries. Most state legislatures now have online access to their proceedings so that bills of interest to nurses can be tracked as they progress through the legislative process.

State nurses' associations and many specialty nursing groups also publish newsletters or legislative bulletins. Many of these are free to members but may be sent only when requested. Most state nurses' associations have Web sites where members can find information on important bills that will affect their practice or the health of their states. Tracking these bills is very important. The best way to influence a bill that will adversely affect nursing practice or health care is to present an opposing view *when the bill is in committee*. Writing or calling committee members is key to the success of this tactic. The practice in the past was to have public hearings when a bill was in committee. This allowed for thoughtful discussion about the effects of the bill on the various constituencies. However, in recent years in some state legislatures where one party has an overwhelming majority, house speakers have adopted the practice of not permitting public debate in committee. They cite "streamlining the process" as the reason but use the practice to quickly move their partisan agendas to approval. Constituents often have less than 24 hours to do anything while the bill is in committee.[17]

Action alerts may also be sent by e-mail or phone to inform members of vital issues that come to the table. It is critical that nurses take action and make their positions known. Often, as few as 20 phone calls to a legislator can make a difference in the way they vote. Remember, a legislator is not a health-care practitioner and probably knows little about the issue. A nurse's opinion provides a valuable level of expertise.

Tactics

Tactics, essential tools for those who desire to be politically active, are the conscious and deliberate acts that people use to live and deal with each other and the world around them. In a political sense, *tactics* usually means the use of whatever resources are available to achieve a desired goal.

Nurses, with their long history of accomplishing much with few resources, are natural tacticians.

As nurses learn how to organize themselves for political purposes, they can use their well-developed tactical skills to achieve important political goals. Listed next are some easy-to-use tactics for political action.

Engage in Bipartisan Tactics

All nurses need to be politically active to achieve unified goals. Political action across the spectrum of issues and across partisan lines is necessary to pass legislation that is in the best interest of all citizens, regardless of party affiliation. Nurses should understand that only by supporting candidates who advocate for nursing, regardless of political party, can the profession make changes that will advance its agenda. The most important thing, always, is the issue being addressed, not the personality or party of the candidate.

Lobbying

Sometimes communication with legislators takes the form of lobbying. *Lobbying* may be defined as attempting to persuade someone (usually a legislator or legislative aide) of the significance of one's cause or as an attempt to influence legislation. Lobbying methods include letter writing, face-to-face communication or telephone calls, e-mails, letters to the editor, and written or verbal testimony. In addition, legislators have a place on their Web site to invite comments on issues.

To lobby effectively, you should be both persuasive and able to negotiate. Lobbying is truly an art of communication, an area in which nurses can become skilled. Before beginning any lobbying effort, it is vital to gather all pertinent facts. If the legislator asks you a question you do not know the answer to, be honest and reply that you will get that information. Then get back to the legislator as soon as you can.

If the plan is to visit the legislator's office, an appointment should be set up in advance. Usually, the meeting will actually be with the legislative aide, particularly at the federal level. This should not be discouraging because this individual is often responsible for assisting in the development of position statements and offering committee amendments for the legislator.

To ensure that legislators and support staff listen to your concerns, it is important not only to be well prepared but also to show that others support your position. When one person speaks, legislators may listen; but when many people voice the same concern, legislators are much more likely to pay attention. Always leave a business card, contact sheet, or both with your personal information so that the legislator can contact you. Send a thank-you note expressing your gratitude for the meeting.

Collaborate With Constituency Groups

Nurses can increase their political power by making alliances with other powerful constituency groups that support similar issues, such as the American Hospital Association, the American Medical Association, and other organizations interested in healthcare issues. Nurses who are organized into collective bargaining units can use an alliance with powerful unions. Unions are traditionally concerned with issues such as working conditions, including staffing patterns in hospitals, wages, job security, and benefits. Nurses are concerned about the same issues.

Be a Political Organizer

"Know thy enemy" is one of the most fundamental rules that tacticians must follow, whether in war or politics. Napoleon was successful as a tactician and general because, before he fought any battle, he walked the battlefield. He knew what the terrain was like and where the rocks and crevices were. He knew what to anticipate when he arrived on the battlefield. Nurses who want to be successful in a political battle must first learn the hills, valleys, rocks, and crevices of the primary political battlefield, their own state demographics.

Comparing numbers helps define the political landscape of a state. Important demographics for organizing nurses at the state level include the following:

- Total population of the state. This provides a demographic overview of the political arena.
- Total number of registered voters.
- Total number of registered voters by political party.
- Total number of likely voters in any given election cycle. To determine this number, the difference between an on-year and an off-year election cycle should be understood. An on-year election cycle occurs when there is a major race in the state,

Issues in Practice

How to Effectively Lobby Your Legislators

The first time you communicate with a legislator can be intimidating. The key element to remember is that legislators are people, just like you. They work for you because you put them in office. The other thing to remember is that they really do not know much about nursing and health care, but you do. You are an excellent source of information for them.

The hierarchy of communicating with legislators is listed here in order from the most effective to the least effective:

1. **Personal contact.** This is the best way to make your opinion known, but it is unlikely you will be able to do so very often. During legislative sessions, lawmakers are very busy and have little time for personal interaction with constituents. The next best option is to meet with their staffers. Ask for the one who deals with the specific issue. During times when Congress is not in session, you might reach legislators when they are home in their districts.
2. **Phone calls.** During legislative sessions, phone calls are a powerful method of communication. It is timely if you are attempting to influence a vote on a particular bill that is being considered. It is unlikely that you will talk to the legislator directly. Rather, you will get an office staff member. Make sure you give the number of the bill you are either supporting or opposing and make it clear as to which position you are taking. What happens is that the staff person has a sheet of paper with the bill number at the top that is divided in half with pros in one column and cons on the other. Your phone call will get a check mark in one or the other of these two columns. This may not sound important, but decisions about how to vote have been decided by as few as 20 phone calls.
3. **Written letters.** Letters are effective but tend to have a time-lag problem. If a bill is being pushed through a committee in 24 hours, the letter may arrive a day or two too late. If you know the bill is coming up in a week or so for a floor vote, a timely letter can be effective. Make sure you identify the bill number and whether you are for or against it in the first paragraph. Keep the letter short—one page is best—and sign it with your name, credentials (e.g., LVN/LPN, RN, APRN), and address. Make sure you clearly indicate if you are for or against the bill. The legislator will probably not read your letter, but the staff will place it in one of two piles—a pro pile or a con pile. At the time of the vote, the number in each pile is counted.
4. **E-mails.** All legislators' Web sites have a place for constituents to comment on issues. Some legislators pay little attention to e-mails and may never read them. Some are more involved with e-mails and may actually respond to yours. Most of the time, a staff person is assigned to read them and make, again, a pro or con list for various bills.

No matter how you communicate with your legislators, consider following these practical suggestions to maximize the success of your message:

• **Know your legislators.** You will be most effective by getting to know the senator and representative from *your* district on a personal basis. Find out which committees and subcommittees your legislators serve on and their voting records. They have much more influence over legislation within their committees' and subcommittees' jurisdiction. This information is available on your state's legislative Web site.

(continued)

Issues in Practice (continued)

- **Know the legislation.** Just as your time is very limited, so is a legislator's. Know the bill number and the issues. Have your facts ready when you approach a legislator. State your position clearly and then be available to either answer any questions the legislator may have or offer to find out the answer to any question you do not know. All bills are listed on the legislative Web site by number and have a reference to the full text.
- **Know the legislative process.** Understand the steps that a bill goes through to become law. Review the steps in this chapter.
- **Be firm but friendly.** Do not try to force a commitment on how your legislator is going to vote. However, when your legislator is aware of the issue and your position, it is then time to begin asking for a position. Remember to be courteous.
- **Keep in touch throughout the year.** Legislators do not like it when the only time you contact them is when you are upset about something. Send them a Christmas card—you will get one back!
- **Concentrate on the issue, not the person.** Doing your homework and preparing for your conversation with your legislator will allow you to concentrate on the issue. Even though it is not always possible to remain in harmony with your legislators, remember that with rare exceptions, they are honest, intelligent public servants trying to represent *all* of their constituents.
- **Lobby like you run your unit/floor/hospital/business.** Be cooperative. Be realistic. Be practical. Never break your word. If you tell a legislator that you will do something, keep your promise. Continue to educate yourself regarding the legislative issues that are of concern to you. Bills change during the process. Sometimes you may find yourself supporting a bill and the next week opposing it because it was changed. Know where your bill is and what it looks like at all times. Despite popular perception, things sometimes happen fast with legislation.
- **Don't threaten the legislator.** Comments such as "If you don't support this bill, I'm not going to vote for you next election" and "I'm not going to give any more money to your campaign" are counterproductive. Think about how you respond to threats.
- **Don't try to do it by yourself.** Work with your fellow nurses in your community and your state. Work with and through your place of employment, your local chamber of commerce, state chamber of commerce, and of course your state nurses' association.

Source: *Student Guide to Legislative Day, 2022, Governmental Activities Committee, Oklahoma Nurses Association.*

usually during a presidential or gubernatorial race. An off-year cycle occurs when a major race is not being run. Lower levels of political activity are seen in an off-year election cycle.
- Total number of registered nurses. This information can be obtained from the state board of nursing. Comparing the number of actual voters with the number of nurses in a state provides an indication of the potential power of nurses voting as a block. For example, if there are 800,000 people who regularly vote in a state and there are 100,000 nurses in the state who are organized into a voting block about a particular issue, that group of nurses represents a

significant percentage of voters, and candidates running for statewide office will be interested in having nurses' support. Nurses must be encouraged to register and vote to increase the power of the block.[18]

Important Characteristics of an Organizer

Many of the characteristics of an organizer (see Box 18.2) are the same characteristics that are required of nurses on a daily basis in the practice of their profession. Although these characteristics may have varying degrees of value for the organizer, the one critical element a political organizer has to have

Box 18.2 **Characteristics of an Organizer**

- Curiosity
- Motivation
- Reverence
- Realism
- Flair for the dramatic
- Sense of humor
- Charisma
- Self-confidence
- Communication skills
- Clear vision of the future
- Capacity to change
- Persistence
- Ability to organize
- Imagination

is the capacity to communicate in an honest and factual manner. Although nurses usually have a well-developed ability to communicate at the bedside, they may lack the confidence to communicate in the larger public and political arenas. Nurses need to recognize that the communication skills they use on a daily basis, as when explaining complicated medical jargon to patients, are the same skills they can use in translating health-care issues into language that the public and elected officials can understand.

One way to gain the public's interest and elected officials' support is to personalize health-care issues by stressing the fact that nurses are the professionals who provide the bulk of direct care for their mothers, fathers, siblings, and children. Communication of issues that touch people personally is usually the most effective method.

WHAT FOLLOWS ORGANIZATION?

Drafting Legislation and Creating Change

Certain critical questions must be asked. The first question always must be, Who is the decision maker? For example, if an issue needs to be resolved in the state board of nursing, the first step is to identify who makes the decisions at the board. Although the board members make decisions, it is important to remember that the people who sit on the board are appointed.

Who appoints them, and what is the basis of those appointments? If they are political appointees, they usually have some sort of political benefactor or a political relationship with someone in power.

Understanding these types of relationships makes it easier to determine the appointees' ideological and partisan positions on many issues.[19] For example, if a nursing board is newly appointed by a recently elected Republican governor, there is a chance that most of the board members are Republicans who agree with the governor on many key issues.

The second question to address is, How accessible is the appointee's benefactor? Sometimes board members are appointed by the legislative leadership, not the governor. It is important to discover who appointed the board and whether or not individual voters have access to them. Generally, access by individual voters to the power figures who make these types of appointments is very limited. Organized groups, such as the ANA, provide the best avenue of access at the federal level, whereas state nursing organizations focus their efforts on states issues.

Also consider which organizations have opposing views. Understanding their positions provides the opportunity to research data to refute their position.

Questions About Health Care

Other questions that need to be answered include the following:

- How successful have nurses been in the past in achieving specific goals?
- What positions do nurses hold in government?
- What does the state board look like politically?
- Which legislators have supported nursing issues in the past?
- Which legislators traditionally oppose nursing and health-care issues?
- What is their voting record on similar bills? Do they have a record of support?

Failure to ask and answer these questions has led numerous pieces of pro-nursing legislation to die in committee or to lack sponsors to move the bill through the process. In states where nurses are in tune with the political issues and powers, they have more success moving bills through the legislative process than in states where nurses are apathetic about the political process.

If a Bill Is Not Filed or Does Not Pass

Even if a bill favorable for nurses or health care does not pass the first time, the fact that it was brought to a vote is important for several reasons. First, it has brought an issue to the attention of the whole legislature that they might otherwise have dismissed as unimportant. Also, it can expose those entities that support or oppose the issues and provide important information about planning future efforts.

Second, the legislative process brings to light the proponents and opponents of the issue and allows nurses to specifically target legislators who voted against the bill. One of two approaches can be used at this point. Nurses can either communicate with the legislators to explain why the bill is important in hopes of changing their minds, or they can organize as a voting block and attempt to vote the opposing legislators out of office.

Third, after a bill has gone through the process the first time, it becomes much easier to identify the obstacles and sticking points in the language of the bill. Before the bill is reintroduced in a later session of the legislature, it can be modified and amended to eliminate those parts that may have caused ideological problems for specific legislators.[20]

The Nurse as Political Ally

Historically, very few nurses have ever served in local or state governments or in the U.S. House of Representatives or the Senate. However, some have. Nurses who are elected to political office should identify with the nursing profession and have the courage to support legislation that promotes health care and the nurses; however, after they are elected, for whatever reason, some former nurses decide to support legislation that is contrary to the profession's best interests.[20] These officials need to be reminded by their constituents of the values that make nurses the most trustworthy professionals.

Conclusion

There is nothing magical about nurses becoming involved in politics. It is simply a matter of hard work and use of the critical thinking, decision making, and persuasion skills that nurses already possess. It is clear, however, that nurses can and do make a difference in the political arena. Nurses must ask themselves how and where they can make a difference and how they can become involved in the process. Not every nurse will choose to run for political office, but each nurse can make a contribution. The willingness of nurses to become involved in politics is the key to developing legislative respect for the profession and improving health care.

CRITICAL-THINKING EXERCISES

- Go online and find out who the state and national senators and representatives are for your district. Ask your classmates and professors who their state and national representatives and senators are. Are you surprised by the results?
- Are you a registered voter? If not, investigate the voter registration process in your state. Was it easy or difficult? If it was difficult, what factors contributed to the difficulty? How can you change the voter registration process?
- What political issues do you feel strongly about? Look up the location of the local party headquarters that supports your position on an issue and go there to see what type of volunteer work you can do.
- Find a bill online at your state government bill-tracking site that deals with an issue important to nursing or health care (e.g., tobacco related, Medicare or Medicaid issues, or changes in the nurse practice act). Track the bill as it goes through the bill-making process. What legislators are key in its passage? Contact them by phone or letter to let them know that you either support or disagree with the bill. Did the bill pass?

NCLEX-STYLE QUESTIONS

1. To help his students review for a quiz, an instructor asks his class to name causes of the nursing shortage. Which answer given by a student indicates a need for clarification?
   1. Historically low wages for nurses
   2. Stressful working conditions
   3. Increased career opportunities for women
   4. Lack of nursing faculty to teach students
2. What are the MAIN reasons nurses become politically active? **Select all that apply.**
   1. To improve their working environments
   2. To advocate for their patients and for public health
   3. To assume high government office
   4. To express their dissatisfaction with nursing as a career
   5. To influence legislation that affects their ability to practice
3. A group of representatives supports a bill to allow APRNs to practice independently nationwide. What process must be followed for this bill become a law? Place the steps in the correct order.
   _____ 1. The chief clerk assigns the bill a number.
   _____ 2. A representative introduces the bill.
   _____ 3. The bill is debated by the full House and passed.
   _____ 4. The bill is referred to a committee where hearings are held and revisions are made.
   _____ 5. The bill is sent to the Senate for debate and approval.
   _____ 6. The president signs the bill.
   _____ 7. The approved bill is sent to the president for signature.
4. What do housekeeping bills and executive orders have in common?
   1. They shape policy with minimal involvement from the legislature.
   2. They involve revising and updating existing policies.
   3. They are both initiated by the chief executive.
   4. They can both be used to move forward a policy that faces strong legislative opposition.

5. Mara has organized a meeting between a group of hospice nurses and their representative at the state capital. The group wants to persuade the representative to vote for legislation to expand Medicaid coverage of hospice care to pediatric patients who qualify for it. Mara and her group are engaged in _____.
6. Omar and Joleen, two nursing students, are arguing about the effects of the media on the legislative process. Omar points to the negative effects of soundbites and social media memes that oversimplify or, even worse, misrepresent candidates' positions. What positive examples of media's effects might Joleen respond with? **Select all that apply.**
   1. Media shape public opinion.
   2. Transcripts of candidates' speeches are available online.
   3. News media focus on sensational or "click-bait" stories.
   4. Audio or video files of speeches may be watched or listened to any time.
   5. Candidates can use social media to communicate in real time directly with their constituents.
7. Malia, an RN, educates herself about upcoming legislative initiatives, writes and calls her representatives to share her opinions, and votes in every election. However, she feels as though she is not making much of a difference. What simple action would give Malia more political clout as a nurse?
   1. Organizing a nurses' union at her hospital
   2. Joining the American Nurses Association
   3. Running for government office
   4. Encouraging coworkers on her unit to share their opinions on health-care legislation with their representative
8. Zavyon, an RN in the cath lab, has decided to become more politically active. What can Zavyon do to convince his senator to take him and his agenda seriously? **Select all that apply.**
   1. Write the senator a letter presenting his agenda.
   2. Donate to the senator's election campaign.
   3. Volunteer to phone bank for the senator.
   4. Organize a block of voters to support the senator.
   5. Offer to endorse the senator in campaign ads.

9. How does the American Nurses Association (ANA) influence politics in the United States?
   1. The ANA provides financial support for nurses who run for political office.
   2. The ANA crafts health-policy legislation that the House and Senate then vote on.
   3. The ANA lobbies Congress and regulatory agencies on health-care issues affecting nurses and the public.
   4. The ANA uses social media to manipulate public opinion.

10. What are state governments responsible for regarding nursing and health care? **Select all that apply.**
    1. The Medicare program
    2. Nursing licensure and certification
    3. How Medicaid funds are used
    4. Nurse practice acts
    5. The Affordable Care Act (ACA)

References

1. Carlson K. Politics and nursing: Strange bedfellows? NursesUSA, 2022. https://nursesusa.org/article_politics_and_nursing.asp
2. Edmonson C. The pandemic's consequences. AMN Healthcare, 2023. https://www.amnhealthcare.com/siteassets/amn-insights/surveys/amn-rnsurvey-2023-final.pdf
3. Martinovich M. The nursing shortage is a national problem. how we can solve it. Science of Caring, January 18, 2022. https://nursing.ucsf.edu/scienceofcaring/news/nursing-shortage-national-problem-how-we-can-solve-it
4. Lobosco K. What to know about these 5 student loan forgiveness programs—and how Biden has expanded them. CNN Politics, August 4, 2022. https://www.cnn.com/2022/08/04/politics/biden-student-loan-forgiveness-programs/index.html
5. Study: Medical errors declined: Safety increases in U.S. hospitals. Newsmax, July 20, 2022. https://www.newsmax.com/health/health-news/hospital-safety-study/2022/07/20/id/1079592/
6. Gaines K. How to work in the US as a foreign educated nurse. Nurse.org, 2022. https://nurse.org/articles/work-in-us-as-foreign-educated-nurse
7. Hawryluk M. Amid Covid health worker shortage, foreign-trained professionals sit on sidelines. KFF Health News, January 25, 2021. https://khn.org/news/article/amid-covid-health-worker-shortage-foreign-trained-professionals-sit-on-sidelines/
8. State practice environments. American Association of Nurse Practitioners, 2022. https://www.aanp.org/advocacy/state/state-practice-environment
9. State of New York grants full and direct access to nurse practitioners. American Association of Nurse Practitioners, April 11, 2022. https://www.aanp.org/news-feed/state-of-new-york-grants-full-and-direct-access-to-nurse-practitioners
10. Fernandez A. Looking back and moving forward: Reflecting on the nurse practitioner role. American Association of Nurse Practitioners, August 3, 2022. https://www.aanp.org/news-feed/looking-back-and-moving-forward-reflecting-on-the-nurse-practitioner-role-in-2022
11. Gagnon D. What is a Magnet hospital? Southern New Hampshire, 2021. https://www.snhu.edu/about-us/newsroom/health/what-is-a-magnet-hospital
12. Nursing shortage factsheet. American Association of Colleges of Nursing, 2022. https://www.aacnnursing.org/Portals/42/News/Factsheets/Nursing-Shortage-Factsheet.pdf
13. Crabtree S. Will Congress close the foreign-donor loophole? Real Clear Politics, August 1, 2022. https://www.realclearpolitics.com/articles/2022/08/01/will_congress_close_the_foreign-donor_loophole__147975.html#!
14. 52 U.S. Code § 30121 - Contributions and donations by foreign nationals. Cornell Law School, 2022. https://www.law.cornell.edu/uscode/text/52/30121
15. Blumenthal D, Collins S, Fowler R. The Affordable Care Act at 10 years: What's the effect on health care coverage and access? Commonwealth Fund, February 26, 2020. https://www.commonwealthfund.org/publications/journal-article/2020/feb/aca-at-10-years-effect-health-care-coverage-access
16. Timm J. 19 States enacted voting restrictions in 2021. NBC News, December 21, 2021. https://www.nbcnews.com/politics/elections/19-states-enacted-voting-restrictions-2021-rcna8342
17. Registered nurses top Gallup Poll for 20th year. National Nurses United, January 13, 2022. https://www.nationalnursesunited.org/press/registered-nurses-top-gallup-poll-for-20th-year-row
18. Lampert L. How grassroots efforts can change the nursing profession. Daily Nurse, August 30, 2016. https://dailynurse.com/how-grassroots-efforts-can-change-the-nursing-profession/
19. Gattozzi K. Who are the decision makers? What politics teaches us about diversity. TalVista, January 21, 2021. https://www.talvista.com/who-are-the-decision-makers-what-politics-teaches-us-about-diversity/
20. Cato D, Costello D. Advocacy: From the patient to the profession. *Nurse Leader*, 20(5)490–493, 2022. https://doi.org/10.1016/j.mnl.2022.06.005
21. The Theory of Democracy. Britannica.com, 2022. Retrieved from: https://www.britannica.com/topic/democracy/The-theory-of-democracy
22. American democracy is under threat. Vox.com, 2022. Retrieved from: https://www.vox.com/22798975/democracy-threats-peril-trump-voting-rights
23. Vinney C. What Is a Cult of Personality? Very Well Mind.com, 2022. Retrieved from: https://www.verywellmind.com/what-is-a-cult-of-personality-5191337
24. Buckenmaier C. If you tell a big enough lie and tell it frequently enough, it will be believed. U.S. Medicine.com, 2018. Retrieved from: https://www.usmedicine.com/editor-in-chief/if-you-tell-a-big-enough-lie-and-tell-it-frequently-enough-it-will-be-believed/

4

Delivering High-Quality Care

The Health-Care Debate: Best Allocation of Resources for the Best Outcomes

19

Linda Newcomer | Rob E. Newcomer | Joseph T. Catalano

Learning Objectives

After completing this chapter, the reader will be able to:

- Briefly discuss the history of past attempts at health-care reform
- Identify the position of the American Nurses Association on health-care reform
- Explain how legislative changes affect health-care reform
- List future challenges to health-care reform
- Explain why nurses and prospective nurses need to know about health-care reform

100 YEARS OF CONTROVERSY

In the United States, the conversation concerning health-care reform started more than 100 years ago and is likely to continue as long as the quality of health care is less than ideal, the cost is more than expected, and the access to care remains less than 100 percent. More recently, health-care reform and one of its key legislative outcomes, the Affordable Care Act (ACA), have been the subject of much public debate. Unfortunately, much of the conversation has continued to revolve around the political talking points, misinformation, and the trepidation of the people the ACA affects.[1] The debate is likely to continue as long as there are disparate and strongly held ideologies on the role of government in the lives of U.S. citizens.

WHAT NURSES NEED TO KNOW

With the rapidly increasing volume of information addressing improvements in patient care, new medical technology, and ever-evolving regulatory changes, a legitimate question that many nurses would ask before starting to read a chapter on health-care reform is *Why?* Although a case could be made that every concerned citizen should be spending more time learning about the scope and implications of health-care reform, there are many important reasons this argument applies particularly to nurses.

The Institute of Medicine's (IOM) report *The Future of Nursing: Leading Change, Advancing Health* (see Chapter 14) recommended that nurses "should be full partners, with physicians and other health care professionals, in redesigning health care in the U.S."[2] It is impossible to be a full partner in this process without some knowledge of the history, scope, cause, and potential solutions to the issues.

More Than a Job

Some nurses say they just want to do their job, take care of their patients, and go home at the end of the day without being involved in the political process. These nurses need to understand that health-care policy affects patients, families, communities, and nurses every day. Health-care policy is about people, and nurses often care for the most vulnerable people every day—the very young, the old, and the severely ill. The decisions made in health-care policy decide which providers people can see, which patients can afford medications, which patients can receive preventive care or early diagnosis and treatment, and ultimately, who lives and who dies. (See Chapter 18 for more details about the political process.) The decisions in the health-care policy arena determine where nurses practice, what they are allowed to do, and their ability to be reimbursed for the services they provide at individual and collective levels.

Eliminating Waste

Many hospitals and providers already use value-based purchasing, ensuring that health-care providers are held accountable for both cost and quality of care. Value-based purchasing is a method of obtaining products and services at a lower price and has been used by private industry and the federal government for many years. By using mass purchasing power, they can negotiate lower prices and better quality of services, including health care. According to one report, value-based purchasing attempts to reduce inappropriate or ineffective care by identifying and rewarding the providers who perform best, possibly by using the National Database of Nursing Quality Indicators (NDNQI), along with other well-developed indicators as measurement tools. It has been suggested that nursing-sensitive measures, those that promote optimal staffing and practice environment, could demonstrate what floor nurses already know: adverse events and mortality are highly dependent on the quality and number of nursing staff.[3]

Nursing-sensitive value-based purchasing is tied directly to the fourth message identified in *The Future of Nursing*: "Effective workforce planning and policy making require better data collection and an improved information infrastructure."[2] The information infrastructure will be developed and implemented *whether or not nurses participate in the process*. Therefore, it is important for staff nurses to be a part of the conversation that chooses the data-collection tools that will determine adequate and appropriate nurse staffing levels.

THE NEED FOR HEALTH-CARE REFORM

Four broad categories—economic, societal, ethical/moral, and health outcome—delineate the need for health-care reform. Another noteworthy issue is the inconsistent state policies for consumer protection. For example, in the mid-2000s a congressional committee conducted investigations that revealed some insurance companies carrying out bad-faith and unethical practices such as canceling or denying claims after a policy had been issued because of a client's costly disease, denying all claims for a period of time and then paying only those that were formally challenged by clients, and failing to pay claims for nonexistent "preexisting conditions."[4] The data collected across the nation demonstrated a lack of self-regulation by the insurance industry and a lack of federal oversight and enforcement because the individual states are responsible for regulating insurance companies within their boundaries. Although some insurance companies' negative practices are blatantly unethical, other insurance companies claim that their bad-faith negative practices were a result of the regulations imposed on them by state and federal governments.

> ❝ *Repeated studies have shown that nurse practitioners can safely provide 80 percent of the care provided by family practice physicians without any decrease in quality or health outcomes and with an increase in patient satisfaction.* ❞

More Patients, Increased Demands

After the full implementation of the ACA, more than 30 million new patients have health insurance. According to the Department of Health and Human Services (DHHS), the number of uninsured Americans fell from 10.3 percent in 2020 to 8.9 percent during the third quarter of 2021. In 2022, a record 14.5 million Americans purchased health insurance under the ACA.[3]

Repeated studies have shown that nurse practitioners (NPs) can safely provide 80 percent of the care provided by family practice physicians without any decrease in quality or health outcomes and with an increase in patient satisfaction. Even with the current numbers of nurse practitioners and family practice physicians, a shortage of primary care providers still exists. Regulatory barriers in many states prevent advanced practice nurses from functioning to the full extent of their education and from being fairly compensated for their work.[4] Legislative decisions made at both the state and federal levels will either reduce or increase these barriers and compensation for NPs.

Registered nurses (RNs) are the largest single group of health-care providers in the United States. Nursing as a profession has not historically participated collectively in full partnership with other players in the health-care industry in determining health-care policy. Nurses need to be heard as advocates for health-care decisions that have the most positive impact on the patients for whom they care. To lend informed opinions to the conversation and process of finding solutions to the current health-care problems,

nurses—current and future—need to educate themselves on the economic, political, ethical/moral, and health-outcome issues that drive health-care policy.

A BRIEF HISTORY OF HEALTH-CARE REFORM IN THE UNITED STATES

It is easy to think of health-care reform as just the latest in a series of political topics that provide a framework for political parties to air their differences. Health-care reform as a political issue in the United States actually surfaced in 1912 and has resurfaced periodically since that time. Although everyone wants good health care that is easily available and affordable, there is little consensus on how to accomplish it. The debates about health-care policy revolve around some of the most fundamental issues in a democratic government: the roles of government and individuals, regulation versus the free market, rights versus privileges, and federal versus state responsibility and control. Added to this mixture are powerful special interests, such as large pharmaceutical companies, insurance providers, and physician associations, which are all concerned with financial outcomes.

Issues in Practice

Resolving the Health-Care Reform Debate Using Critical Thinking

Although critical thinking is used in all aspects of decision making, it is particularly important in resolving issues such as the health-care reform debate. As a way of looking at the world, critical thinking allows the nurse to consider new ideas and then evaluate those ideas in light of reliable information and the nurse's own value systems. Nurses are constantly making important decisions in both their professional and personal lives. By viewing critical thinking as a purposeful mental activity in which ideas are evaluated and decisions reached, nurses can make ethical, creative, rational, and independent decisions related to patient care.

Critical thinking, when applied to the health-care reform debate, is a powerful problem-solving tool. When used purposefully, it becomes a gestalt that allows the nurse to sort through the multiple variables that exist in the reform debate. Effective use of critical thinking is evident when nurses successfully apply their knowledge about the issue and come to a creative solution to a complex and multifaceted debate.

Questions for Thought

1. How much do you know about the ACA of 2010? Putting aside your ideological perspective and thinking about it critically, is the law helping or hurting people who formerly lacked health insurance? What evidence supports your answer?
2. What additional information about the ACA would clarify its effects on health care? Where can you find additional information about it?
3. Have there been other recent issues in health care that you can apply critical thinking to?
4. How have the changes made to the ACA since 2016 affected the ability of this health-care legislation to achieve its stated goals?

Presidents Get Involved

As a presidential candidate of the Bull Moose Party in 1912, Theodore Roosevelt became the first national political figure to call for some type of reform for national health coverage. This call started the century-long quest for universal health care. It is reported that President Franklin Delano Roosevelt (FDR), after starting a conversation about the establishment of national health insurance, retreated from including it in what became the Social Security Act of 1935, in large part due to the opposition from the American Medical Association (AMA). FDR instructed aides to begin working on national health insurance legislation, but he died before any bill was introduced.[5] One of the primary reasons health insurance became a benefit offered by employers at this time was that FDR implemented wage controls that capped how much employees could earn. Employers used health benefits to attract employees because benefits were exempt from wage controls. Offering health care as a benefit was the first time the person who uses health care was separated from the one who pays for health care (third-party payer), a practice that is the norm today.

President Harry Truman pressed Congress on multiple occasions to enact into law a plan known as the Truman-FDR plan. This plan proposed a single-payer public health insurance plan similar to the Canadian health-care plan. Again, powerful interests applied enough pressure that Truman scaled back his original plan until it was reduced to providing health coverage only to older adults.

In 1961, President John F. Kennedy began his vigorous advocacy of a plan to provide health benefits to older adults. This became the framework for the Medicare program. Kennedy was assassinated before he could see these new laws enacted. His successor, Lyndon Baines Johnson, presided over passage of the Medicare and Medicaid Act in 1965, considered the most ambitious health insurance advance in U.S. history until the enactment of the ACA.

Richard Nixon is credited by many as the first president to attempt to hold down the rising cost of health care and health insurance through health-care reform.

In 1973, he signed a law to encourage development of health maintenance organizations (HMOs) that were the first manifestations of managed care. A Republican, Nixon demonstrated that universal health insurance was not a goal of just the Democratic Party when he proposed private coverage for citizens through a federal mandate on employers and individuals. Nixon believed a nationwide mandate that would require all citizens to have and pay for health insurance was necessary to reduce the cost of health insurance, but it was not popular with most Americans. Nixon's proposed underlying structure for comprehensive health-care reform became the basis for the plan Governor Mitt Romney would implement in Massachusetts and the framework that President Barack Obama would pursue three decades later in developing the ACA. The Watergate scandal and subsequent resignation of Nixon stopped any further progress in health-care reform by his administration. The increasing costs of health care and health insurance were to become a continuing concern in politics from this point forward, regardless of any plans or attempts to provide universal coverage.

President Jimmy Carter introduced a health reform plan similar to Nixon's, including coverage for catastrophic illnesses or injuries. It had an employer's mandate and a replacement for Medicare and Medicaid to cover older adults, persons with disabilities, and people living in poverty.[7] This plan was united with a cost containment package directed at hospital and physician costs. The cost containment legislation passed the Senate in 1979 but was defeated in the House of Representatives.

A call for universal health coverage did not re-emerge in presidential politics until the presidency of Bill Clinton. In 1993, his wife and future presidential candidate, Hillary Rodham Clinton, took charge of a task force to reform health care and developed the Health Security Act of 1993. However, this initiative failed to yield any significant health reform. The backlash and the divisiveness from this very public failure, in addition to other factors, helped the Republicans to reclaim control of the House and Senate in the midterm elections, ending any presidential conversation on universal health coverage

> *Based on the belief that health care is a right of U.S. citizens and not just a privilege, the ACA immediately began enrolling large numbers of citizens who had never before had health insurance into affordable plans.*

until the election of Barack Obama as president in November 2008.

After almost two years of negotiation, the Democratic Congress under the leadership of President Barack Obama managed to get the Affordable Care Act passed in 2010. Based on the belief that health care is a right of U.S. citizens and not just a privilege, the ACA immediately began enrolling large numbers of citizens who had never before had health insurance into affordable plans. The number of enrollees in the ACA plans continued to increase, and the coverage of the plans broadened to include more conditions until the election of President Donald Trump in 2016.

The Republican Trump administration almost immediately tried to rescind the ACA. His attempt failed by one vote in the Senate, so the ACA remained in effect as the law of the land. However, Trump's commitment to rescinding the law seemed only strengthened by this failure. Through executive actions that did not require approval by the Congress, he chipped away at coverage and to suppress enrollment. Congress contributed to these efforts by refusing to fund or by underfunding some of the provisions of the ACA that required money. Nonetheless, people continued to enroll in the program.

Under President Joe Biden, the ACA was revived. This was important because Biden was elected just as the COVID-19 pandemic was starting in 2020. Many people lost their jobs and, along with their jobs, their employer-based health insurance. People who were without insurance who became sick from the virus were covered by a governmental program that paid for their health care. As the pandemic waned and was declared to be endemic by Dr. Anthony Fauci in 2022, the Biden administration worked to pass bills that would expand many of the elements of the ACA. One of these bills that became law was the American Rescue Plan (ARP). Under the ARP, affordable health insurance coverage became available to more people than ever before.[4]

Historical Factors Related to Health Insurance

The first country to provide a form of national insurance coverage was Germany under Chancellor Otto von Bismarck in 1883. Other countries in Europe soon followed. Anti-German sentiment in the United States was strong at the time. Theodore Roosevelt introduced the idea of national insurance coverage in the United States in 1912. However, anti-German sentiment has been cited as one of the reasons Roosevelt's idea did not make progress at that time.[5] The original purpose of health insurance was to share financial risk across a large group so that health care could be provided when needed. Providers could get paid without depending on the current financial ability of the person needing health care. With no government initiatives being considered, hospitals and physicians began to offer nonprofit private insurance plans in the 1920s and 1930s. This type of insurance required that the individual be treated only by a physician in the hospital with whom the patient was insured.

In response to declining hospital occupancy during the Great Depression, the American Hospital Association established statewide Blue Cross insurance plans that provided hospital coverage at a choice of any hospital in the state. Soon, state medical societies began to provide Blue Shield insurance to cover physician services.[6] Because of wage and price controls during World War II, employers discovered they could legally use employer-paid health insurance to compete for scarce employees. After World War II, unions began to negotiate for health benefits in their contracts. These factors encouraged the growth of private for-profit commercial insurance plans.

Community Rating Versus Experience Rating

The original Blue Cross/Blue Shield insurance set premiums by what was called **community rating**, where rates were set by medical costs across a geographic area, region, or even across the whole nation. The commercial profit-based insurance companies introduced the concept of experience rating. An **experience rating** system is used to estimate how much a specific individual or group will have to spend on medical care within a very limited setting, such as an industry. This rating is based on how much the person has already spent, what health conditions are already present, and what risk factors a person has compared to what would be considered a "normal" expenditure. Experience rating tailors health insurance policies to the specific group or individual rather than to a geographic area, and these policies tend to have lower rates because the people using them tend to be healthier and younger.

Experience rating was used as a competitive tool because it set low premiums for special organizations that had primarily young, healthy employees. However, this scheme left other insurance companies and the government paying increasingly higher insurance rates for older people and those with chronic diseases. Older Americans, who tend to have more age-related illnesses, were one of the groups hardest hit by use of experience rating. Community rating was unable to survive in an insurance market that was using experience rating. In 1945, the Blue Cross/Blue Shield providers outnumbered commercial insurance providers two to one. By 1955, commercial insurance providers outnumbered the "Blues." Legislation, including the exemption from taxes of employer-paid health insurance, was signed into law by President Dwight Eisenhower in 1954, making the private for-profit insurance business once and forever part of the American health-care landscape.[6]

Because of the high cost of experience-rated insurance, by the late 1950s, less than 15 percent of people over the age of 65 had any type of insurance.[6] The federal and state governments' first attempts to fill in large gaps in the availability of health insurance for select groups in the population started with the Medicare and Medicaid legislation of 1965. First was the coverage of persons over age 65, people with disabilities, and children in poverty. In 1997, the Children's Health Insurance Program (CHIP) was created to extend Medicaid coverage to many uninsured children and their parents.[6]

Government Gets Involved

Although the entry of the government into the health insurance industry assisted those people left behind by the private insurance companies, it also created a guaranteed source of income to the health-care industry. Health-care costs rose rapidly when large sums of government dollars began to be funneled into a system that rewarded health-care providers for increasing the number of services rather than for producing positive health outcomes. Combined with the unrestrained use of new and increasingly complicated technology, health-care costs exploded, exceeding the inflation rate tenfold.[6]

The biggest expansion of Medicare since its initial enactment occurred under Republican president George W. Bush, who signed into law an unfunded prescription-drug benefit bill. The bill increased senior citizens' access to prescription medications through the Medicare Part D program. The bill also provided subsidies to private companies to compete with Medicare, such as the Medicare Advantage program. Proponents hailed the bill as the answer to seniors' financial problems with purchasing needed medications; however, opponents called the bill a giveaway to drug companies because it prevented Medicare from negotiating for discounts with drug companies or purchasing medications from other nations. Although providing additional services for seniors, the Medicare Part D bill was an unfunded mandate that increased the cost of providing these Medicare services and included no cost-saving measures.[6]

Rising Costs Spur Reform

After the failed attempt at health-care reform in 1993, serious political discussion did not re-emerge until the presidential campaigns for the 2008 elections. During this interval, many organizations interested in health-care costs and outcomes, such as the IOM, the Kaiser Family Foundation (KFF), and the World Health Organization (WHO), began to release reports about the rising cost of health care and the declining state of U.S. health care compared with other countries. Many of the recommendations produced by these reports become part of the ACA.

In 2008, a large group of bipartisan veterans of the 1993–94 national health-care reform campaign met to discuss the future of health-care reform.[7] All three leading Democratic presidential candidates had presented similar plans for comprehensive health-care reform. The Republican nominee, John McCain, produced a markedly different plan for reform. Most of the attendees at the meeting believed that a Democratic president in 2008 would make a concerted effort to achieve comprehensive health-care reform. The group was less confident about *actually* achieving comprehensive reform unless there were a Democratic congress.[1]

> *The biggest expansion of Medicare since its initial enactment occurred under Republican president George W. Bush, who signed into law an unfunded prescription-drug benefit bill.*

After a long discussion with expert advisors from both political parties and many health providers, a "10 commandments" for presidential leadership on health-care reform was produced with the goal of assisting the president-elect to avoid the pitfalls of previous attempts to bring about health-care reform:

1. Clearly communicating the vision and goals to the public
2. Keeping all the stakeholders at the table
3. Tasking Congress to work out the details of the plan
4. Involving the states
5. Reducing partisanship
6. Moving the legislation to a speedy completion
7. Being politically forceful while moving the legislation forward
8. Selecting advisors and spokespersons who the public trusts
9. Limiting the scope of the reform legislation to a manageable size
10. Getting the congressional leadership onboard early in the process

President Obama was successful at achieving most of the commandments except for managing the partisanship of a recalcitrant Congress.[1]

Economic Issues

The Organization for Economic Co-operation and Development (OECD) is an international organization, representing 35 industrialized countries, that compiles and analyzes international health-care data.[8] (See Figure 19.1.)

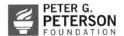

U.S. per capita health-care spending is over twice the average of other wealthy countries

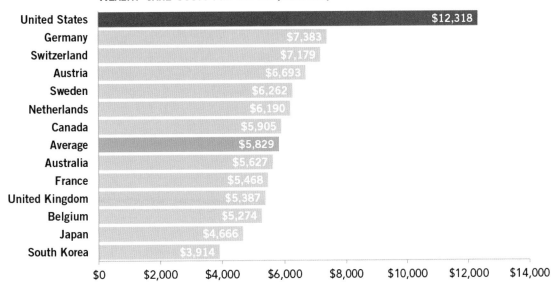

SOURCE: Organisation for Economic Co-operation and Development, *OECD Health Statistics 2022*, July 2022.
NOTES: Data are latest available, which was 2019, 2020, or 2021. Average does not include the United States. The five countries with the largest economies and those with both an above median GDP and GDP per capita, relative to all OECD countries, were included. Chart uses purchasing power parities to convert data into U.S. dollars.
© 2022 Peter G. Peterson Foundation   PGPF.ORG

Figure 19.1 The U.S. spends on average double the amount of money per person on health care than the 12 other richest nations. (*Source:* How does the U.S. healthcare system compare to other countries? Peter G. Peterson Foundation, July 19, 2022, https://www.pgpf.org/blog/2022/07/how-does-the-us-healthcare-system -compare-to-other-countries.)

According to the OECD's recent reports, the United States spends two-and-a-half times more than the OECD average health expenditure per person; however, the life expectancy in the United States is below the average for the 35 countries evaluated. These figures can be misleading, however, because health-care expenditures include administrative costs, costs such as paying for treatments not always available in other countries, cost of research that is funded in the United States in greater amounts than in other countries, and the cost of self-medication and treatment. U.S. health-care costs per person are twice as much as those in France, for example—a country that is generally accepted as having a high-quality health-care system.[8]

Health-care costs have grown more rapidly than most other sectors of the economy, and health care's share of the national economy has increased disproportionally. Some critics suggest that the costs began to escalate once the Medicare act was passed, and more government funds were available to provide health care without restrictions. To get a balanced picture of health-care cost comparisons across nations, it is important to look at both expenditure as a percentage of gross national product (GNP) and expenditure per capita. The United States leads other countries in both measures. In 1970, total health-care costs in the United States were approximately $75 billion, or $356 per person. With the increase in spending to $12,318 per person for health care in 2021 and $3.9 trillion for total health-care costs, the industry's share of the overall U.S. economy has risen from 7.2 percent in 1970 to 17.2 percent in 2017 and 18.8 percent in 2021.[8] Projections suggest that by 2025, health care's share of the GNP will be more than 20 percent.[9] Predictions see marked increases in health-care costs due to the increased numbers of aging baby boomers and the elimination of tax-related provisions, such as the individual mandate in the ACA and the passage of new laws that expanded Medicare such as the Inflation Reduction Act (IRA) of 2022.

The large percentage of U.S. GNP that is spent on health care limits the amount of money that is available for education, transportation infrastructure, and many other needed programs. These excessive health-care costs create a competitive disadvantage for American companies in the international market.

Impact of Ever-Increasing Costs

Health-care costs impact not only the national economy but also personal finances. The average American's salary increased 31.7 percent from 2010 to 2020. During this same period, the cost of health insurance premiums rose 30 percent.[10] One study found that in the United States, almost 17 percent of the population, or 59.5 million, experienced bankruptcy in 2021 because of excessive medical bills; many of these people with high medical bills were well educated, owned homes, and earned a middle-class income.[11] More than 75 percent of people filing for medical bankruptcy had health insurance at the beginning of their illness. After the enactment of the ACA, the number of bankruptcies due to medical bills dropped to 770,000 in 2016; however, the bankruptcy rate has leveled off since then.[10] The truth is that just about anyone who does not have good-quality health insurance is one bad diagnosis or one serious accident away from financial ruin.[11]

> **Young adults often find themselves staring down the barrel of medical debt that prevents them from building savings, finishing their education, or getting a job.**

Societal Issues

Issues other than economics and politics can interfere with access to health care and affect the quality of care. Health status can also be affected in part by social and economic conditions and the resources and support systems that exist in our neighborhoods, schools, and homes.

Socioeconomic Disparity

Recent studies support the findings of research conducted by the IOM in 1999 at the request of Congress. Researchers found that the extent of health-care disparities in the United States required strategies for intervention. They looked into racial and ethnic minority health outcomes, the percentages of racial/ethnic minorities who were uninsured, and the perceptions by minority populations of their access to health care and its quality. Although rising health-care costs cause many people to have difficulty paying their medical bills and to put off needed health care because of cost, the percentages are noticeably higher for those with lower incomes and even higher for those without any insurance (public or private). Nationwide, Black adults are 50 percent more likely than Whites to owe money for past medical care. Hispanic adults are 35 percent more likely. Young adults often find themselves staring down the barrel of medical debt that prevents them from building savings, finishing their education, or getting a job.[11]

In 2010, a study by the KFF showed that only 10 to 11 percent of the nonelderly adult population with insurance or Medicaid had no regular source of health care. The rate among uninsured people was 55 percent. Under the ACA, this rate had dropped to 8.6 percent by 2022 (last year of available data).[12]

The data concerning insured and uninsured children is even more revealing. Children with no insurance are over seven times more likely to have no regular care provider than are those with Medicaid and almost 10 times more likely than those with private insurance. In 2022, the percentage of uninsured children in the United States dropped from 13 percent in 2010 to 2 percent in 2022 due to the ACA.[13]

What Do You Think?

Do you or does someone you know lack health insurance? Do you or they avoid seeking health care for illnesses or injuries?

Pervasive Disparity

The socioeconomic conditions that created traditional health disparities are further causing the same groups to experience an ever-increasing loss of health insurance. According to the U.S. Census Bureau in 2020, individuals at or below the poverty level had lower health insurance rates than those who were above the poverty income level.[13] Health-care disparities among minority groups undermine health-care outcomes for all aspects of care, including access to care, quality of care, and efficiency of delivery of care, which leads to missed opportunities to help ensure long, healthy, and productive lives.[13]

The COVID-19 pandemic highlighted the health-care disparities among minority groups. Data from the time of the pandemic demonstrate that the hospitalization rates during the pandemic for African Americans, Alaska Natives, Hispanic/Latino, and American Indian populations were five times those of non-Hispanic White persons.[14] Rates of COVID-19-related deaths were notably higher in African Americans and Hispanic/Latino populations.

Biological, social, and structural elements all contributed to the disparities seen during the COVID-19 pandemic.[14] Comorbidities such as diabetes, obesity, coronary artery disease, and hypertension were more likely to be present in minority populations, biologically worsening the effect of the virus. Socially, even with the ACA, minority groups tend to be less likely to have access to high-quality health care and are more impacted by their environment. African Americans and Latinos/Hispanics were more likely to work in jobs that were categorized as "essential jobs" or "frontline" occupations and to work during stay-at-home orders. This job designation increased their exposure to the virus. Essential workers were defined as those who performed a range of services that are typically essential to maintain critical infrastructure processes. *Critical infrastructure* is as umbrella term that encompasses energy production, national defense, agriculture and food production, child care, critical retail (such as grocery stores, hardware stores, transportation), critical trades (construction workers, electricians, plumbers, etc.), health-care workers, law enforcement, and nonprofits and social service organizations.[15] Many of these workers belonged to minority groups. The social determinants of health created an ideal environment in which COVID-19 could thrive.

Although some people deny it exists and others rally against the concept, structural racism contributed to COVID-19 health disparities. The situation is better today than in the past, but there is still an unwillingness among many to confront the issue of structural racism in health care. Without dealing with the issue directly, it will remain a stumbling block to achieving true health equity.[14]

Cost Shifting

Health-care costs increase for everybody when people without insurance receive no preventive care. Without preventive care and early treatment interventions, individuals with chronic health problems and late-stage serious diseases end up being treated in a more

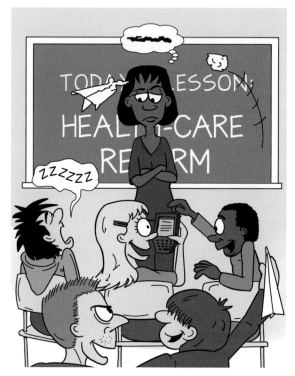

Student motivation is key to learning.

expensive hospital setting rather than in a less expensive physician's office or clinic. Those costs accrue regardless of the person's ability to pay, and uncompensated costs are shifted to hospitals and health-care providers and eventually to those with insurance.

The costs for people who lack health insurance end up falling on taxpayers for government-supported programs or private insurers in the form of increased taxes and premiums. It is often referred to as the *hidden health-care tax*. In essence, those with health insurance end up paying twice—once for themselves and once for their uninsured counterparts.[15]

According to DHHS, in 2022 (the last year for available data before publication), the number of American citizens without health insurance coverage hit an all-time low of 8 percent. The downward slide in uninsured Americans began in 2021, when Congress and President Biden agreed on a $1.9 trillion COVID-19 relief bill. This agreement allowed lower premiums and out-of-pocket costs for new or returning customers who were purchasing plans through the ACA's private health insurance markets.

However, a 9 percent uninsured rate translates into approximately 26 million people who still do not have health insurance in the United States. And about 2 percent of children are still uninsured.[16]

Health Outcome Issues

Despite spending significantly more for private pay and out-of-pocket costs for health care, the United States does not always have the best health outcomes in the world for some health concerns.[17] These failures are not always due to the way in which health care is delivered. Societal issues such as drug use, obesity, poor lifestyle choices, and gun violence play a significant role and do affect the measures. However, the single major differentiating factor between other developed countries and the United States is access to health care. Following are some of the key health-care measures in which the United States lags among 37 wealthy countries:

- Mortality rates: The United States ranks 30th.
- Mortality rates from preventable diseases and illnesses: The United States ranks 19.
- Long-term kidney transplant failure was highest in the United States when compared to other wealthy countries.
- Number of hospital beds per 1,000 citizens: The United States ranks 23rd.[17]
- Infant mortality: The United States ranks 19th (although this was an improvement since the advent of the ACA—the United States ranked 23rd in 2008).[17]
- Overall quality of health care: The United States ranks 10th.
- Preparedness for the COVID-19 pandemic: The United States ranked 17th
- Health-care spending: The United States ranks number one, spending per person $12,318, whereas Switzerland with its socialized system of health care spends $7,919 per person and is ranked number one in quality of health care.[17]

Moral/Ethical Issues

The idea that access to health care is a basic human right is supported by WHO, the AMA Code of Ethics, the ANA Code of Ethics, the Democratic Party, and many social and religious groups.

Although almost everyone agrees that health care should be available to everyone without risking bankruptcy, the ethical issues focus on the most equitable way to make that possible. Should those who have more economic advantages bear the bulk of the costs? Should those who choose a less risky lifestyle pay less than those who do not? Should people pay for services they do not need because others need them? Do those who pay for the insurance or administer insurance programs get to create regulations to force those who make poor lifestyle choices to modify their behaviors? If a single-payer option is instituted, does the government get to force healthy lifestyles on individuals? Can the government force people who have health insurance coverage to actually receive health care when they need it? Who gets to determine appropriate treatments, and how much should they cost?

These questions and many others come with consequences, regardless of the health-care model selected. Nurses need to understand these issues if they are to be prepared to deal with them in the future.

What Do You Think?

Select one of the ethical questions posed in the preceding section. Do you agree or disagree with its proposition? Why? What are the ethical issues involved in the dilemma?

Questionable Insurance Practices

Several of the OECD countries use private insurance companies to pay for part or all of their health-care costs. However, the United States, in addition to being the only wealthy industrialized nation not to provide basic health care to all citizens, is the only OECD country to allow private companies to profit from providing *basic* health care. The insurance companies in other OECD countries make profits only on non-basic, or sophisticated, services that go beyond the basic care required by the government.[18]

All companies are run by humans; as a result, unethical business leaders can overlook or even encourage unethical business practices. Regulations need to be in place to prevent unscrupulous insurance companies from trying to increase profits by selling **junk policies**, also called *short-term policies* or *limited policies*. These policies became illegal under the ACA; however, changes made by President Trump's administration allowed these policies back on the market again. Under the Biden administration in 2020, the ACA restrictions on junk policies were reinstated.

Other ways insurance companies increase profits is by selectively withholding services and delaying or denying services that are included in the policies. Because insurance companies receive tax subsidies from the government, regulating their practices should fall under government control; however, in early 2018, many of these controls were lifted.

Separate from the issue of whether tax dollars should subsidize insurance companies are the ethics of increasing profit by limiting financial losses for covered services. These limits are usually spelled out in the policy, but persons purchasing the policies may have little understanding of the cost of a chronic or traumatic event or do not think it will apply to them. As most people understand it, the purpose of insurance is to spread the risk across the largest pool of people. It is accepted that some people will receive more care than others due largely to unforeseen medical needs.

In some cases, insurance companies have suddenly added policy-limit caps to policies held by employees who have worked for the same company for many years and have had the same insurance plan. These employees have paid into the company-sponsored insurance for themselves and their families all during their employment. After years of paying their health insurance premiums regularly, they or their family could be left without sufficient insurance coverage if they exceed the cap. Subsequently, they may be unable to get new insurance that they can afford due to a preexisting condition. For people with high-cost chronic disorders such as hemophilia, lifetime caps pose a serious threat that affects health care, career choices, and financial stability.

Another practice of unethical insurance companies is **rescission**. *Rescission* is a legal term for when a health insurance policy is canceled unilaterally by an insurance company without the knowledge of the owner of the policy. Under the ACA, an insurance company can cancel a policy only if the patient has committed fraud or if the patient lied deliberately about a material fact in a way prohibited in the terms of the health insurance plan. The practice of rescission was all but eliminated by the ACA when it removed cost caps and made it illegal for companies to deny health insurance for preexisting conditions.

However, some companies have mechanisms or even whole departments in place whose sole job it is to try to find technicalities or errors that would justify the unilateral cancellation of medical insurance policies for holders who develop new illnesses that require expensive treatment and care while the policy is in effect.

Congress Investigates

A 2008 congressional investigation into the problem of rescission found that insurance was being canceled retroactively "over minor and/or unintentional discrepancies and omissions in a person's application materials or medical records when high-cost healthcare claims were submitted."[19] Chief executives of three of the largest health insurance companies in the nation were called before this congressional committee. Lawmakers were appalled and outraged as they listened to case after case of actual rescissions by these three companies. For a brief list of Congress's findings, see Box 19.1.

Horror Stories

After being diagnosed with an aggressive form of breast cancer, a nurse from Texas recounted losing her health insurance coverage. The reason she was given for the policy cancellation was that she had not disclosed a visit to a dermatologist for acne many years before, which the insurance company considered a preexisting condition for cancer. A sister of an Illinois man told Congress that he died of lymphoma after the insurer canceled his coverage. At the time, he had already been approved for a lifesaving bone marrow transplant. The rationale for the policy cancellation was failing to report gallstones and the possibility of an aneurysm that were on his chart after an x-ray many years before. This x-ray was never discussed with the patient, and even the insurance company was never able to find any evidence that indicated intentional deception on the part of the patient.[20]

When the executives of these three major insurance providers were each asked separately by the chairman of the committee if they were willing to limit the cancellation of policies to only cases in

> *Lawmakers were appalled and outraged as they listened to case after case of actual rescissions by these three companies.*

which they could prove "intentional fraudulent misrepresentation," all three said they would not stop the practice. They noted that there were no state laws that prevented the practice of canceling the policies of patients with high-cost diagnoses and illnesses.[20]

Insurance Regulatory Issues

In the individual health insurance market, regulation is still provided through a mix of state and federal rules and laws. Although insurance regulation is primarily delegated to the states, the federal government often writes federal policies or protections that are supposed to be incorporated into the state regulations and enforced. An example of a federal attempt at consumer protections was the Health Insurance Portability and Accountability Act (HIPAA) of 1996.[21] Two of HIPAA's key purposes were to allow employees to bring with them their health insurance policy when they changed jobs and to prevent cancellation of polices due to preexisting conditions.

The Pandemic Sheds Light on Reform

The COVID-19 pandemic focused attention on the need for health-care reforms, particularly ones that promote universal access to affordable care. All facets of the U.S. health-care system faced challenges during the peak months of the pandemic, and the patchwork system of governing and paying for health care started to unravel. Millions of people were left jobless and without health insurance, requiring a rapid, coordinated political response to guarantee meeting their care needs.[22]

Meeting the needs of patients with COVID-19 required Congress to quickly pass two significant pieces of legislation. The Families First Coronavirus Response Act (FFCRA) required all private insurers, Medicare, Medicare Advantage, and Medicaid to cover COVID-19 testing during the pandemic. It also eliminated all cost sharing (copayments, deductibles, and coinsurance payments) associated with testing services while the pandemic was still a public health emergency. To cover the cost of testing for uninsured individuals under state Medicaid plans, $1 billion was

Box 19.1 Selected Findings of the 2008 Congressional Investigation of Health Insurance Rescissions

- Rescinding coverage on the basis of typos in the application form
- Rescinding coverage on the basis that individuals failed to disclose conditions they were unaware they had
- Rescinding coverage for family members incurring high-cost claims, even if they were not involved in the omission or discrepancy
- Investigating the medical histories of all enrollees diagnosed with certain high-cost illnesses or conditions
- Evaluating employees on the basis of how much money they save the company by retroactively canceling policies
- Using a computer algorithm to identify women recently diagnosed with breast cancer to trigger an investigation into their records to find a pretext to rescind coverage

Sources: Howell A, What is insurance rescission, and what do I need to know about it? *Good RX Health,* 2021. https://www.goodrx.com/insurance/health-insurance/insurance-rescission; Prohibiting rescissions fact sheet, National Partnership for Women and Families, 2012, http://www.nationalpartnership.org/site/DocServer/HCR_Prohibiting_Rescissions.pdf.

appropriated for the Public Health and Social Services Emergency declared by President Trump.[22]

The second legislation passed was the Coronavirus Aid, Relief, and Economic Security (CARES) Act that provided $2.2 trillion in pandemic-relief. It required that all private health insurance plans cover COVID-19 testing and future vaccines, but it stopped short of eliminating copayments for COVID-19 treatment. Most private insurers, including Humana, Cigna, UnitedHealth Group, and Blue Cross Blue Shield, agreed to waive copayments for insurance plan members treated for COVID-19. The CARES Act also appropriated $100 billion for hospitals and health-care providers to cover the costs of providing care for pandemic patients. Uninsured patients were not to be billed at all for COVID-19 treatment because the federal government reimbursed providers at Medicare rates for treating uninsured patients. The CARES Act also provided substantial tax credits, emergency grants,

and loans to help businesses keep employees on the payroll or on furloughs while extending and increasing unemployment benefits for those who lost their jobs. These types of laws provide a framework that universal health-care coverage could be built upon.[22]

In 2022, the U.S. House and Senate passed the Inflation Reduction Act of 2022 (IRA), which was signed into law by President Biden. Although not primarily a health-care bill, the IRA includes provisions dealing with health care. The health-care provisions in the bill include important reforms that will directly impact patients and health-care providers. The key provisions of the bill include the following:

Reducing medication prices by permitting medication price negotiation. This provision reverses a requirement introduced by President George W. Bush, which prevented the government and health-care institutions from negotiation for lower medication prices.[23]

Rebates for prescription medication inflation. Although a bit complicated, this newly introduced provision requires drug manufacturers to issue rebates to the Center for Medicare and Medicaid Services (CMS) for brand-name medications without generic equivalents under Medicare that cost $100 or more per year per individual when prices increase faster than inflation. Medications will be re-evaluated every calendar year on or after January 1. This provision also requires the CMS to calculate the inflation-adjusted payment amount with a reduction or waiver for medication shortages and severe supply-chain disruption. Manufacturers that fail to comply will be subject to civil monetary penalties.[23]

Medicare beneficiaries will receive Part D improvements and maximum out-of-pocket caps. Also somewhat complicated, starting in 2026, a benefit structure goes into effect that modifies the payments for applicable medications to 20 percent of the insurance cost of the medication. For nonapplicable medications, the payment amount is 40 percent of the cost. In 2025, the secretary of Health and Human Services (HHS) can make agreements with medication manufacturers that participate in Medicare Part D to provide additional discounts for medication prices. A medication manufacturer that fails to provide discounted prices for applicable medications will be subject to a civil monetary penalty for each failure.[23]

Prescription drug rebate rule delayed. This rule was inserted by the previous Congress into one of its anti-ACA bills. It allowed for rebates to states and other entities for medication purchases. The IRA put off the implementation of this rule until January 1, 2032.

Full cost coverage for adult vaccines. These are the vaccines that are recommended by the Advisory Committee on Immunization Practices under Medicare Part D.[23]

Expanded eligibility for low-income children. It increases subsidies under Part D and improves access to adult and child vaccines under Medicaid and the Children's Health Insurance Program.

A $35 monthly cap on out-of-pocket spending on insulin for Medicare beneficiaries only. The cap does not apply to private payers.[23]

Extension of the value of ACA subsidies to certain consumers who receive subsidies for health insurance through the ACA marketplace through 2025.[23]

Although health care for all U.S. citizens remains unfinished, the ACA along with the passage of the above types of laws push the country closer a little at a time. However, it is obvious that there remains a need for health insurance reform and an increase in regulation by outside entities. The question, of course, becomes *how* to go about fixing this large and unwieldy system.

What Do You Think?

How much did you know about health-care reform before reading this chapter? How much do your parents or older relatives know?

THE DEBATE

Even though the ACA has been in effect for more than a decade, there remains a fundamental disagreement about whether the United States should have universal health care or keep its patchwork system that covers some individuals but not others. Both sides agree on several issues:

- Health-care reform should not take big slices out of the GNP.
- Successful reform of health care begins with the realization that all health-care systems have problems.

- Reform needs to be accomplished within a reasonable amount of time.
- Different approaches to reform meet different needs and set different priorities.

All solutions will have both positive and negative aspects. The goal needs to be to find those actions, solutions, and measures that improve the system, have the fewest drawbacks, and address the priorities of cost, quality, and coverage.[23]

ANA POSITION ON HEALTH-CARE REFORM

The ANA's 1991 document *Nursing's Agenda for Health Care Reform* was endorsed by more than 60 nursing and other health organizations. This document has since undergone two significant updates. The ongoing shortage of both nurses and other health professionals as well as the rapidly growing body of scientific research reinforced the critical need for reform. The ANA continues its strong commitment to its belief that health care is a human right. The ANA believes that all persons should have access to affordable, high-quality health-care services when they need them. The health of individuals, the strength of society, national well-being, and the overall productivity of the United States will be positively impacted when all citizens have accessible, affordable, and high-quality health care. The updates made to the initial ANA document include the following:

- The ANA reaffirms its support for a restructured health-care system that ensures universal access to a standard package of essential health-care services for all citizens and residents.
- The ANA believes that the development and implementation of health policies that reflect the six IOM aims (safe, effective, patient-centered, timely, efficient, and equitable provision of care) are based on outcomes research and will ultimately save money.
- The current system must be reshaped and redirected away from the overuse of expensive, technology-driven, acute, hospital-based services to a model that strikes a balance between high-tech treatment and community-based and preventive services, with emphasis on the latter. The solution is to invert the pyramid of priorities and focus more on primary care, thus ultimately requiring less costly secondary and tertiary care.

- Ultimately, the ANA supports a single-payer mechanism as the most desirable option for financing a reformed health-care system.[24]

The ANA believes that new reforms should be designed to move the country from a system that provides illness care to one that provides patient-centered, preventive health care. This type of care is provided best by nurses. The ACA addressed most of the ANA Reform Agenda. However, the ACA does not explicitly declare health care a human right and does not provide for a single-payer system. The American Association of Retired Persons (AARP) agrees with the ANA concerning nurses, the amount and type of funding provided, and the administrative division responsible for the provisions.[25]

Since its first involvement in designing the ACA, the ANA has been a strong proponent of its success. The ANA was a powerful political voice fighting for the survival of the ACA when attempts were made to repeal or dismember it. Millions of people are still enrolling in the ACA during the enrollment periods, and its provisions to improve the quality of care remain in place.[22]

Evaluating Health-Care Reform

With all the state-of-the-art diagnostic tests and treatments available, highly respected and innovative doctors, and many of the world's best hospitals, the United States produces many of the significant advances in medical technology and biomedical research. However, with a health-care delivery system that in many cases is fragmented, wasteful, inefficient, irrational, and unsustainably expensive, the United States continues to lag in many categories that define a healthy country.[26]

According to the Centers for Disease Control and Prevention (CDC), health performance indicators showed only some improvement between 2016 and 2018 (last year for available data). These indicators included insurance costs and access to care, affordable care, primary and preventive care, hospitalizations from nursing homes, and rehospitalizations. However, additional indicators of concern are opiate abuse; infant mortality; childhood obesity; safe care;

> *" The ANA was a powerful political voice fighting for the survival of the ACA when attempts were made to repeal or dismember it. "*

patient-centered, timely, coordinated care; and racial and ethnic disparities. In addition, suicide rates increased among all categories (men, women, teens), and life expectancy from birth dropped 0.2 years between 2014 and 2018.[27]

Cost Effectiveness

Along with identifying health-care delivery issues that need to be improved, cost effectiveness needs to be addressed. There is no question that health-care costs are rising. One of the main reasons for this problem has been anticipated since the late 1940s, when the birth rate escalated after World War II. Baby boomers (born between 1946 and 1964) have significantly influenced societal costs throughout their lives, beginning with increasing the need for more schools and eventually, as they enter their older years, creating a huge demand for health-care services.

During the COVID-19 pandemic, health-care costs escalated. Many people lost their health insurance when they lost their jobs and had insufficient income to purchase insurance privately, which cost more because of their age and preexisting conditions. If the government had not stepped in and passed the FFCRA and CARES acts, many individuals would have been left homeless and penniless.[12]

However, the money for these pieces of legislation had to come from somewhere. For taxpayers and government budgets, programs such as Medicare, Medicaid, and the pandemic bills increased the share of financial coverage of health care more than ever before. This meant a larger share of government budgets was absorbed by increased health-care costs.

Since the pandemic, the U.S. economy has turned around, with job growth at an all-time high and unemployment at historic lows. Many individuals who had lost their jobs are again employed and receiving health insurance from employers. In addition, the ACA provided millions more people with health insurance.

Another cost-saving feature of the ACA was offering federal incentives to facilitate the adoption of meaningful use of health information technology (HIT). HIT advances can decrease health-care expenses through lowering administrative costs related to recordkeeping and provision of data to compare effectiveness, helping identify root causes of problems, and identifying ideal staffing ratios. This same information technology can increase safety by enabling portable electronic health records (EHRs) that prevent duplicate or inappropriate treatment because of a lack of complete information, potentially reducing medical errors. HIT can increase the use of latest research and evidence by clinicians and allow patients to compare treatments, facilities, and providers. This technology developed so rapidly that it is already entrenched in the health-care system.[1]

ACA POLITICAL BATTLE CONTINUES

The passage of the ACA was a significant achievement, but it was just the beginning of health-care reform in the United States. Initially, many states attempted to overturn or not comply with the law because of the impact they feared it might have on their budgets. However, over the years it has been in effect, these states have quietly adopted ACA measures through backdoor means. With its renewal and expansion under President Biden, the ACA could someday form the foundation for universal health care in the United States.[27]

Electronic Enrollment

Exchanges allow consumers to apply for and enroll in coverage online, in person, by phone, by fax, or by mail. They provide culturally appropriate assistance in a variety of languages. Call centers and a Web site with information about insurance options and application assistance still exist. Funding for the navigator program has been reinstated so that there is plenty of help available to aid individuals in selecting the best plan for their needs. The computerized system determines eligibility for public programs, premium tax credits, and cost-sharing subsidies for those purchasing insurance through the exchange.

Improving Health-Care Outcomes

The ACA was a major reform of the health-care system, and it also tackled health-care financing and outcome measures. As it is now implemented, the ACA impacts federal revenues, direct or mandatory spending, and discretionary spending. Some of these changes in spending are directly related to quality of care and health-care outcomes. The ACA links

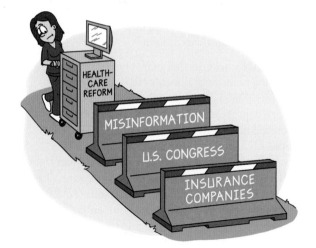

There are many obstacles to health-care reform.

certain types of payments, especially to hospitals, to their ability to demonstrate successful outcomes. The use of the ACA's complicated formula, which hospitals initially complained about, has led to an overall improvement in care quality and increases in patient satisfaction levels. Hospitals now advertise their high-quality care as a reason to seek medical services there.[25]

CHALLENGES FOR THE FUTURE

Controlling the Costs of Medical Care

Many people are concerned that the changes in the ACA will cause costs to go out of control for the average American citizen. The ACA was meant to address three key components of health care—cost, access, and quality—ensuring better, more affordable, and more equitable health care for all people. As provisions are removed from this landmark legislation, what will be the effect on the three key components of health care? Will only those who can afford the cost receive the access and quality?

The political realities of bipartisan negotiating, compromising, and consensus building often require politicians to accept less than what their constituents want. Many economists believe that the market control exerted by insurance companies, medical providers, and pharmaceutical companies is the primary driver of increasing costs. Numerous reports show that procedures and medical products cost far more in this country than they do elsewhere.[24]

Increased Health Literacy

The National Patient Safety Foundation (NPSF) produced a fact sheet in 2018 called "Health Literacy: Statistics at a Glance." It reported that 36 percent of adults in the United States are at risk due to limited health literacy, and higher rates of health illiteracy are found among lower-income individuals who qualify for Medicaid.[28]

Lack of health literacy is present in all demographic groups but is more common in the same demographic groups that determine eligibility for Medicaid (i.e., lower socioeconomic status, limited education, and people with mental or physical disabilities). People with health literacy deficits have difficulty navigating the health insurance market in several ways. It is difficult for them to understand the multiple types of coverage offered by the ACA and which one is best for them. They find it difficult to make an informed choice and to complete the complicated forms for eligibility.[28] This group typically also has problems in initiating their own care and in interacting with health-care providers to make their health-care needs known. Their problems will only increase with the elimination of the navigator program caused by cuts in the ACA.

Public Opinion

There is a reciprocal relationship between public opinion and politics: public opinion helps drive political decisions, and politics helps form public opinion. In the midst of formulating comprehensive health-care legislation affecting everyone's lives, some people focus on what they might lose rather than on understanding what benefits their family or the nation would gain. Change requires letting go of the familiar and accepting something that is new. Change is on the health-care horizon again. Many people have gotten used to the benefits of the ACA and look forward to the increased coverage elements found in the IRA of 2022.[2]

Lessons From Other Countries

Why does the United States not look to other countries to find solutions to its health-care problems? The reality is that many wealthy, technologically advanced countries have found ways to provide all their citizens with basic health care, spend less money, have better health outcomes, and increase patient satisfaction with their care. By analyzing both positive and negative outcomes of health-care payment systems in other nations, the United States could design a system that ensures personal freedom while supporting those most in need.

Reforming American health care does not mean that the United States could or should copy any other country's institutions exactly. Americans cannot *adopt* another country's health-care structure, but they could *adapt* those approaches to America's inherited conditions.

OPPORTUNITIES FOR NURSING IN HEALTH REFORM

The old question asks: "How do you know you are there if you don't know where you are going?" All nurses know that after you assess a problem, you need to establish goals for its solution. It is no different for health-care reform. To develop any type of meaningful and useful strategy, the process must have well-defined goals. The primary goal for health-care reform from the viewpoint of health-care professionals is to improve health outcomes for patients while making the system more efficient and not increasing expenses or compromising results. The three objectives of health-care reform are (1) decreasing the number of uninsured people, (2) decreasing the cost of health care to the public, and (3) improving the quality of care. The goal of health-care reform from the political viewpoint is to have universal health care that includes all citizens of the country and a single-payer system that reduces the high administrative costs of a patchwork insurance system.[29]

The ACA, as a first step in U.S. health-care reform, partially achieved several of the key objectives. It was also welcomed by most health-care professionals and citizens who realized that there was a desperate need for reform. After the ACA passed, many Americans were able to access health care who had never had it before. This was good news for those needing primary care, health care at home, and urgent care; but it led to a shortage of qualified nurses to meet these additional patients' needs. The more educated nurses were to fill the numerous nursing vacancies created under the ACA, the higher the quality of health care became for the general public.[26]

The COVID-19 pandemic reinforced the obvious need not only more nurses but also for nurses who were able to demonstrate leadership in the health-care system. As the health-care system transforms ever so slowly from a fee-for-service, provider-based model to a model that focuses on quality, affordability, and seamless care, nurses must be a part of the transformative change.[22] Nurses, who have always been agents of change, need to step up and reassume this role as its primary catalysts. In the age of reform, the role of nurse leaders is evolving and expanding.

Reshaping Knowledge

These new nurse leaders are required to reshape their knowledge base, focusing on personal professionalism, knowledgeable leadership, informed communication, and up-to-date business skills. Additional knowledge that nurse reform leaders must attain to be successful includes mastery of quality and safety improvement techniques, an understanding of theories of innovation, internalization of the basic tenets of ethical care, familiarity with ways to enhance collaborating with other professionals, and knowledge of care delivery systems. Health-care reform requires nurse leaders and managers to bridge the gap between administration and the clinical setting.[1]

In the age of health-care reform, the new nurse manager must be able to use a style of leadership that interweaves collaboration and mutual respect of personnel with the coordination of care and complex care systems. This type of manager will experience increased respect along with lower staff turnover, fewer medical errors, and reduced numbers of patient complaints. High-quality nurse leadership can be promoted by educating nurses on change theory so that they can better implement new changes introduced by reform. For example, a new responsibility for the nurse leader (and the team) will be finding and introducing ways to reduce or prevent early patient readmissions. This is one outcome that all reform models have as an indicator of quality of care. To successfully meet this goal, it is necessary that nurses understand the economics of how payments are made under different payment models. Communicating what changes are going to be made and how they will be made effectively requires that the nurse leader also understand and use the skills necessary for producing change.[24]

Meeting the goal of delivering efficient and safe care in health reform requires nurse leaders to help build and promote a high-quality health-care system. By working with other health professionals, the team will be able to deliver high-quality and patient-centered care. When nurses are directly involved in patient-centered care, they can aid in averting nursing workforce shortages, increasing access to care, improving quality, and reducing errors.

Need for Advanced Practice Registered Nurses

Since the passage of the ACA and its recent expansion in scope, more patients are seeking primary health care. Studies have shown that advanced practice registered nurses (APRNs) can meet the primary care needs of large segments of the population, ranging from well-child evaluations for pediatric patients to screening for chronic diseases found in older adults.[15] There are additional demands for qualified nurses in any number of health-care fields, such as nursing informatics, case management, and nurse navigation.

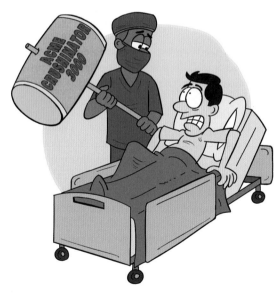

"This is the only procedure your junk insurance policy allows for breaking up kidney stones."

Remaining Vigilant

Nurses need to remain vigilant and involved in the politics and legislation of nursing, particularly at the state level. It is important that APRNs, as key providers in the health-care system, be included in any discussions of state revisions of nurse practice acts. APRNs must be allowed to practice to the full extent of their education and capabilities and receive appropriate reimbursement. As decisions are made on how to contain costs, nurses working every day with patients must participate in the decision-making process to ensure that nursing activities are identified and measured.[19]

RNs are the largest group of providers of care who directly impact patient outcomes. It is part of the professional responsibility of nurses to educate themselves about the health-care debate. If more nurses joined their primary professional organization, the ANA, it would give nursing one of the largest and most powerful political voices in the country. Nurses can work with their local or state representatives on issues important to health care, identifying misinformation or distortion of facts, and providing opinions based on their expert knowledge and experience. The American public trusts nurses to advocate for their best interests. Nurses have been rated number one for over 10 years on the Gallup polls for most trusted and honored professions.[2]

Conclusion

The debate about the best way to pay for health care and improve patient outcomes will continue well into the future. With a law as extensive as the ACA, it would be expected that provisions will be modified or eliminated as unforeseen problems and unintended consequences become evident. There is also no doubt that ongoing efforts to repeal, replace, or change key provisions of the health-care law will occur.

It is important that nurses have input into all phases of the implementation and outcome analysis of health-care changes. They were at the table when the ACA was initially designed, and they should be there as it is revised and reconfigured. Nurses have a wide range of knowledge and first-hand experiences in the health-care system at all levels, knowledge and experiences that are very useful and highly sought after by many policymakers. The most effective way for individual nurses to make their voices heard is by joining a professional organization. Groups that represent large numbers of voters have lobbying power.

CRITICAL-THINKING EXERCISES

- Find one of your classmates whose opinion of the ACA differs from yours. Have a thoughtful discussion with them about health-care reform. Try to formulate a middle-ground approach to reforming the health-care system.
- Research "myths about health-care reform." Make a list of at least 10 myths. Without stating that they are myths, read the list to several friends or relatives and ask them which ones they agree with. Are you surprised by their answers?
- Do a Web search for groups who may lack adequate health insurance (e.g., women, children, older persons). How does the lack or inadequacy of insurance affect their health and well-being?

NCLEX-STYLE QUESTIONS

1. What are the main issues that health-care reform has traditionally targeted? **Select all that apply.**
   1. Access to care
   2. Cost of care
   3. Patient satisfaction
   4. Retention of nurses
   5. Quality of care

2. Marla, a newly graduated RN, says she has no interest in understanding health-care policy and reform. What is the BEST reason for Marla to change her mind?
   1. Nurses must pass a continuing education examination on changes in health-care policy.
   2. Marla will be better prepared to debate health-care reform if she understands it.

3. Health-care policy affects the patients Marla cares for, Marla herself and the staff she works with, and the facility she works in.
4. Marla's patients and their families may have questions for her related to health-care policy and reform.

3. Which of the following statements best summarizes the American Nurses Association's overall position on health-care reform?
   1. Health care is a human right, so universal access should be our goal.
   2. Health-care costs are increasing rapidly, so cost containment is essential.
   3. Reform should include a greater emphasis on high-tech medical and nursing care for chronic illness.
   4. Encouraging competition among payers is the best way to finance a reformed health-care system.

4. In 1965, President Johnson signed the _____, which was the most ambitious health insurance advance in U.S. history at that time.

5. Which American president first supported a nationwide mandate requiring all citizens to have and pay for health insurance?
   1. John F. Kennedy
   2. Richard Nixon
   3. Bill Clinton
   4. Barack Obama

6. A nursing instructor asks the class to name some of the arguments made against the Affordable Care Act (ACA). Which answer given by a student indicates the need for further instruction?
   1. Health insurance, like car insurance, should be bought and sold in a competitive free market.
   2. The ACA suppresses wages because companies will reduce employees' work hours to avoid the mandated employer-provided health insurance.
   3. The ACA invades workers' privacy because employers need detailed household information to supply mandated health insurance.
   4. The ACA eliminates cost shifting in which higher premiums and taxes are used to pay for uninsured people's health care.

7. A 2019 tax bill removes the individual mandate, the requirement that all citizens must purchase some type of health insurance, from the ACA. What is a likely effect of this change? **Select all that apply.**
   1. Healthy young people will opt out of buying health insurance.
   2. The cost of health insurance premiums will go up.
   3. The number of citizens who have health insurance will go down.
   4. The quality of health care provided will decrease.
   5. People will engage in more unhealthy behaviors.

8. Miguel, an RN with 5 years' experience on a medical-surgical unit, is considering going to graduate school to become a family nurse practitioner (FNP). What effect is the ACA likely have on Miguel's career opportunities as an FNP?
   1. Miguel likely will not be allowed to practice to the full extent of his education and abilities.
   2. Miguel will probably have a long job search ahead of him.
   3. Miguel should plan to pursue a degree in nursing education as well so that he can teach.
   4. Miguel should easily be able to find a job as a primary care provider.

9. Since 2017, changes were made to the ACA that shortened and reduced funding for the open-enrollment period and reduced funding for the navigator program that helps people select the right policy. Which aspect of health-care reform has been primarily affected by these changes?
   1. Accessibility to care
   2. Affordability of care
   3. Quality care
   4. Satisfaction with care

10. Which benefit of the ACA is most likely to endure?
    1. Improved access to health care
    2. More affordable health care
    3. Widespread use of health information technology (HIT)
    4. Coverage for citizens with preexisting conditions

References

1. Archer D. Health care reform in 2021: What you need to know. Just Care, November 25, 2020. https://justcareusa.org/health-care-reform-in-2021-what-you-need-to-know/

2. Stringer H. IOM Future of Nursing report card: Progress after 10 years. Nurse.com, July 1, 2019. https://www.nurse.com/blog/2019/07/01/iom-future-of-nursing-report-card-progress-after-10-years/

3. What is NDNQI? Well and Empowered, February 1, 2021. https://wellandempowered.com/what-is-ndnqi

4. Trattner C. U.S. Uninsured rate drops as 14.5 million sign up for 2022 Obamacare coverage. *Newsweek*, January 27, 2022. https://www.newsweek.com/us-uninsured-rate-drops-145-million-sign-2022-obamacare-coverage-1673745

5. Kelly M. Overview of Roosevelt's Bull Moose Party beliefs. ThoughtCo, September 5, 2019. https://www.thoughtco.com/bull-moose-party-104836

6. Miller W. History of health insurance. *Mendocino Voice*, July 18, 2022. https://mendovoice.com/2022/07/miller-report-for-july-18-22-history-of-health-insurance/

7. Horstman C, Bryan A, Lewis C. How the CMS Innovation Center's payment and delivery reform models seek to address the drivers of health. The Commonwealth Fund, August 8, 2022, https://www.commonwealthfund.org/publications/issue-briefs/2022/aug/how-cmmi-payment-delivery-reforms-address-drivers-health

8. How does the U.S. healthcare system compare to other countries? Peter G. Peterson Foundation, July 19, 2022. https://www.pgpf.org/blog/2022/07/how-does-the-us-healthcare-system-compare-to-other-countries

9. U.S. healthcare coverage and spending: Statistics. Congressional Research Services, 2022. https://crsreports.congress.gov/product/pdf/IF/IF10830

10. American Wage Index (AWI). Social Security Administration, 2022. https://www.ssa.gov/oact/cola/awidevelop.html

11. Levey N. 100 Million people in America are saddled with health care debt. *Idaho Capital Sun*, June 20, 2022. https://idahocapitalsun.com/2022/06/20/100-million-people-in-america-are-saddled-with-health-care-debt/

12. Uninsured and underinsured. Consumer health Ratings, 2022. https://consumerhealthratings.com/healthcare_category/uninsured-under-insured/#:~

13. Seitz A. Number of uninsured Americans drops to record low. AP News, August 2, 2022. https://apnews.com/article/biden-health-us-department-of-and-human-services-government-politics-24684188cb67c576ed00d01b2f53c09c

14. Wilder J. The disproportionate impact of COVID-19 on racial and ethnic minorities in the United States. *Clinical Infectious Diseases*, 72(4):707–709, 2021. https://doi.org/10.1093/cid%2Fciaa959

15. COVID-19: Essential workers in the states. National Conference of State Legislatures, 2021. https://www.ncsl.org/research/labor-and-employment/covid-19-essential-workers-in-the-states.aspx

16. Study: Medical errors declined: Safety increases in U.S. hospitals. Newsmax, July 20, 2022. https://www.newsmax.com/health/health-news/hospital-safety-study/2022/07/20/id/1079592/

17. U.S. healthcare system ranks sixth worldwide: Innovative but fiscally unsustainable. Peter G. Peterson Foundation, February 3, 2022. https://www.pgpf.org/blog/2022/01/us-healthcare-system-ranks-sixth-worldwide-innovative-but-fiscally-unsustainable

18. The history of healthcare insurance in the United States. Healthcare Information Network, n.d. http://healthncare.info/history-healthcare-insurance-united-states/

19. Fraud alert: 10 ways to stay away from health insurance false promises. Care Health Insurance, August 5, 2021. https://www.careinsurance.com/blog/health-insurance-articles/fraud-alert-10-ways-to-stay-away-from-health-insurance-false-promises

20. Quigley F. American healthcare horror stories: An incomplete inventory. Truthout, April 28, 2019. https://truthout.org/articles/american-health-care-horror-stories-an-incomplete-inventory/

21. Godard R. Which matters more? HIPAA or state law? I.S. Partners, August 11, 2022. https://www.ispartnersllc.com/blog/hipaa-or-state-law-health-info/

22. King J. Covid-19 and the need for health care reform. *New England Journal of Medicine*, 382, e104, 2020. https://www.nejm.org/doi/full/10.1056/NEJMp2000821

23. Taylor N, Meyer T. Inflation Reduction Act of 2022: Key health-care provisions. *National Law Review*, 2022. https://www.natlawreview.com/article/inflation-reduction-act-2022-key-health-care-provisions

24. Healthcare system transformation. American Nurses Association, 2022. https://ana.aristotle.com/SitePages/healthcarereform.aspx

25. Healthcare service delivery reform. *Policy Book AARP 2021-2022*, 2022. https://policybook.aarp.org/policy-book/health/health-care-service-delivery-reform

26. What you need to know about the Affordable Care Act (Obamacare). WebMD, 2020. https://www.webmd.com/health-insurance/affordable-care-act-provisions

27. Arispe IE, Gindi RM, Madans JH. *Health, the United States, 2019*. National Center for Health Statistics, 2021. https://www.cdc.gov/nchs/data/hus/hus19-508.pdf

28. Health literacy interventions. County Health Rankings and Road Maps, 2017. http://www.countyhealthrankings.org/take-action-to-improve-health/what-works-for-health/policies/health-literacy-interventions

29. Kumar U. Healthcare reform: The strategy. TechBullion, July 27, 2022. https://techbullion.com/health-care-reform-the-strategy/

Spirituality and Health Care

20

Roberta Mowdy | Joseph T. Catalano

ROUGH SPOTS ALONG THE TRAIL

The road of life often is filled with twists and turns, ups and downs, and precipitous waysides. People who are facing potentially long-term or debilitating illnesses, confronting acute health crises, or suffering from loss and grief may find themselves re-examining the foundational beliefs they have held since childhood. Seldom is a person so focused on evaluating the spiritual self than during such crises. Yet the times when patients are most vulnerable also can be opportunities for personal and spiritual growth.

Nurses have the unique task of working with patients at various points throughout their life journeys. Often, nurses encounter patients during the "rough parts of the trail." The holistic nursing perspective requires nurses to view each person as a biopsychosocial being with a spiritual core. Each component of the self (physical, mental, social, cultural, and spiritual) is integral to and influences the others (Fig. 20.1). Nurses spend more time with their patients than do other health-care workers. Therefore, the spiritual needs of patients must be recognized as a domain of nursing care. Holism cannot exist without consideration of the spiritual aspects that create individuality and give meaning to people's lives.[1] Thus, nurses must be sure to address the spirit along with the other dimensions to provide holistic care.

NURSING AT LIFE'S JUNCTURES

The human life cycle is marked by a rhythm of transitions: birth, the entry of a child into society, puberty, sexual awakening, entry into adulthood, marriage, parenthood, illness, loss, old age, and death. In all cultures, there are other rhythms that people honor, such as the solar and lunar cycles, the agricultural cycle, and the reproductive cycles. These cycles constitute the rhythm of human life.

Developmental Crisis

All people recognize the importance of transitions and in some way have ritualized them through their religions or through custom.

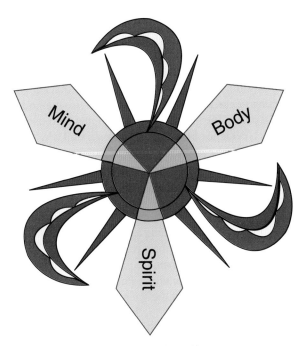

Figure 20.1 Components of the self.

People learn from their own cultural groups how to behave during each transition, and each cultural group has conceptualized an understanding of these human experiences. Their importance is universally recognized.

Nurses have contact with patients in the health-care setting primarily within the context of these transitions. Developmental crisis theory holds that transitions are times of anxiety and vulnerability for families. Therefore, nurses are required to treat people who are going through transitions with great tenderness and care. It is a sacred trust for nurses to be allowed into a family system in transition. Patients and families may seek spiritual support or may feel spiritual abandonment. Ideally, nurses can help people identify and find the spiritual support they require.

SOCIAL AND SCIENTIFIC EFFECTS ON SPIRITUALITY

Science as Magic

The term *magic* is sometimes used when events occur that people do not understand. In the past, these occurrences were attributed to a supernatural source of power. Early in the history of health care, there was little understanding of the causes of illness, such as viruses and bacteria, and many people thought that illness was caused by bad magic. Of course, the way to treat an illness caused by bad magic was to use a stronger good magic.

Over a long period of time, from the Enlightenment of the 17th century to the dawn of the 21st century, political leaders and educated people in Western cultures came to believe that the answers to human suffering could be found in science and technology. In a sense, science became the new magic for the general population. For example, early in the 20th century, antibiotics were thought of as "magic bullets" that cured diseases and reduced suffering. People were eager to believe that science and technology would soon be able to cure any disease. This belief still exists among a large segment of the population today.[1]

It was in this context that the nursing profession embraced the Western scientific method as the measure for defining itself. Many in the nursing profession believed, and still do believe, that rigorous research involving the testing of hypotheses provides the soundest theoretical base for the practice of professional nursing.

More recently, pandemics, terrorism, climate change, major natural disasters, space exploration, and the mapping of the human genome have given urgency to reconsideration of the question, What does it mean to be fully human in the universe as it is now understood? It is evident that science and technology cannot offer the solutions to all human problems; in fact, they have contributed to them.

What Do You Think?

Make two lists: a list of the problems that science and technology have caused during the last 20 years and a list of the problems that have been solved by technology and science. Which list is longer? Why do you think that is?

To Be Fully Human

Science, electronic communications, and the great social experiments of the past two centuries are among the influences directing humans to a consciousness that individuals are connected to all peoples and to the whole of creation. There is a growing belief that all people share a common basic sense of existence that encompasses everyone and everything. This sense of oneness with the universe that is often associated with severe illness or injury and near-death experiences has the potential to produce profound changes in the way that people view themselves and the world around them. Some people who have had these experiences take life events less personally and tend to see the similarities in all people as if they were members of their family regardless of how different their external appearances may be. They may also experience a heightened compassion for the suffering of others, become involved in altruistic acts, or forgive others more easily. These actions often correspond to finding more meaning, richness, and joy in their lives. Many spiritual leaders believe this type of change is the essence of becoming more human.

In the realm of health care, the increasing awareness that true healing occurs only when there is a reintegration of the physical with the spiritual and the mental gives testimony to the need for increased emphasis on the spiritual aspect of care. Health-care providers need to recognize that spiritual traditions other than their own contain valuable insights into the nature of human beings and the oneness of creation.

Phenomenology

Phenomenology is a branch or type of philosophy that studies the relationship of our experiences to our consciousness. Rather than viewing the world as sets of objects that bump into or interact with each other, phenomenology believes that the experiences of persons should be explored through the gathering of conscious experience rather than just objective data. As a feature of postmodernism, phenomenology suggests that truth is relative, allowing for an appreciation of diverse perspectives on what is true.

Since the mid-1980s, science, including nursing science, has expanded its ways of discerning truth not only by using traditional hypothetico-deductive, quantitative, "fact"-driven research but also by widening research discovery using less-restrictive research methods. (*Hypothetico-* means using a hypothesis as the basis of research; when *deductive* is added to it, the term refers to using deductive reasoning to either support or disprove the hypothesis with

quantitative data.) The hypothetico-deductive quantitative method is the foundation of scientific research, regarded by some as the only true scientific research method. (See Chapter 24.)

Phenomenology is one major influence that has led nursing researchers to appreciate qualitative methods of discovery. The objectivity of developing hard data through evidence-based research works well when dealing with the physical aspects of patient care. However, phenomenological research approaches are much better suited when attempting to develop information about the nonphysical elements of patient care, such as emotions and spirituality.

In the health-care setting, a phenomenological approach to understanding a patient's spirituality recognizes that that person's experiences may be more "true" than those of the nurse. Phenomenological research does not reject the scientific method but rather sees it as an aid to understanding individuals and their needs through their reflections upon their lived experiences. The patient's past experiences and knowledge include rich information about the person's being as they progress through life transitions. In nursing, intuition, perception, memory, and internal awareness can all be better understood through a phenomenological research approach. This change in viewpoint coincides with increased interest in complementary and alternative medicine (CAM) therapies and with the importance of spirituality in healing and wellness. (See Chapter 25 for more details on CAM.)

> **As a feature of postmodernism, phenomenology suggests that truth is relative, allowing for an appreciation of diverse perspectives on what is true.**

THE NATURE OF SPIRITUALITY

Spirituality is a broad and somewhat nebulous concept that has to do with the search for answers to certain questions and issues (Box 20.1). In fact, answers to these large questions are sought across cultures. In research on the development of spirituality, children of various cultural backgrounds express similar issues and questions.

A Diverse Heritage

A rich heritage of spiritual practices is found in all the major religions of the world. The roots of the great

Box 20.1 Spiritual Questions

Why are we here?

How do we fit into the cosmos?

What power or intelligence created and orders the universe?

What is the nature and meaning of divine or mystical experiences?

How are we to make meaning of suffering?

How are we to behave toward other people?

How are we to deal with our own shortcomings and failures?

What happens to us when we die, and where were we before we were born?

traditions, including each religion's prayer practices, can be traced to the shift in human consciousness that occurred around 500 BCE. During this period, many great teachers and spiritual leaders emerged, including Confucius; Lao-tzu; Siddhartha Gautama, who became the Buddha; Zoroaster; the Greek philosophers Socrates, Plato, and Aristotle; and the Hebrew prophets Amos, Hosea, and Isaiah.

St. Augustine, a Roman Catholic bishop who lived in North Africa during the fifth century CE, is credited with first identifying the relationships among contemplation, action, and wisdom within the Christian tradition. For Augustine, the contemplative life was properly focused on the discernment of truth and was open to all people. Augustine equated truth with God.

Hope Through Compassion

Spirituality is often defined as integrative energy, capable of producing internal human harmony, or *holism*. Other definitions refer to spirituality as a sense of coherence. Spirituality also entails a sense of transcendent reality, which draws strength from inner resources, living fully for the present, and having a sense of inner knowing. Solitude, compassion, and empathy are important components of spirituality for many individuals.

The concept of hope is central to spirituality. Spirituality may be regarded as the driving force that pervades all aspects of and gives meaning to an individual's life. It creates a set of beliefs and values that influence the way people conduct their lives. Spiritual activity involves introspection, reflection, and a sense of connectedness to others or to the universe. For many people, this connectedness focuses ultimately on a supreme being who is sometimes called God.

When providing spiritual care to their patients, nurses must base their actions on compassion, or sensitivity to the suffering of others. Compassion is a way of living that is born out of an awareness of one's relationship to all living creatures, a sensitivity to the pain and brokenness of others. The Greek word for compassion, σπλαγχνίζομαι, means "to feel movement in one's viscera" (heart and other internal organs). The Greeks believed that the internal organs, particularly the heart, were the seat of human emotions. When the Greek word was later translated into Latin, an ecclesiastical translation was used, *compassionem*, which is what most people accept as its present meaning: "suffering with" or "sharing of affliction or suffering of another." Given this definition, you can easily see how compassion is part of spirituality and the life journey.

A Sense of Meaning

Traditionally, *spirituality* has been defined as a sense of meaning in life associated with a sense of an inner spirit. However, it is difficult to identify what such a spirit is like and how it can be observed. Spirituality can be defined from both religious and secular perspectives. A person with spiritual needs does not necessarily participate in religious rituals and practices.

Despite the lack of consensus regarding the definition of spirituality, several themes emerge from an interdisciplinary review of the literature:

- All human beings have the potential for spirituality and spiritual growth.
- Spirituality is relational.
- There is a necessary link among religion, moral norms, and spirituality.
- Spirituality involves lived experience; it is a way of life.

In some ways, spirituality is a mystery. Although human beings can experience spirituality, appreciate it, and grow in it, there is much about spirituality that cannot be explained or reduced to human language.

Based on these themes, spirituality is defined as a way of life, usually informed by the moral norms of one or more religious traditions through which a person relates to other persons, the universe, and the transcendent in ways that promote human fulfillment (of self and others) and universal harmony.

The Religious Perspective

From a religious perspective, spirituality can be defined as encompassing the ideology of the *imago dei* (image of God), or soul, that exists in everyone. The soul makes the person a thinking, feeling, moral, creative being, able to relate meaningfully to a supreme being and to others. This being or force may be called God, Allah, the divine creator and sustainer of the universe, the divine mystery, or other names that convey a profound sense of transcendence and awe. A religious perspective often entails a set of beliefs, or a *creed*, that helps explain the meaning of life, suffering, health, and illness. Most religions also incorporate and promote a set of positive values, such as charity to others, faith in a supreme being, and a requirement for a lifestyle that involves honesty, truth, and virtuous living. Persons who accept and follow the beliefs and tenets of their religion should be able to develop a deep spirituality that will ultimately lead to their self-actualization. These beliefs can be crucial to a believer's physical well-being.

Spirituality is often mistakenly understood to mean just religious practice; however, it should be considered in the broader sense of the term. Religion can be an approach to or expression of spirituality, and spirituality is a component of religion, but the two concepts are different.

> *Each of the world's religions is different because it has evolved to respond to unique histories and different cultural developments.*

Religious Practice Gone Astray

It is quite possible for a member of a religion to be limited in their spirituality. Most people have known individuals who dutifully follow the rules of their religious tradition. They strongly believe that if they adhere to the rules correctly, God will reward them with blessings such as health, success, affluence, social status, and power. For these individuals, adverse events such as disease, death of a loved one, or loss of investments can be devastating because these events are perceived as a failure in religious practice or punishments from God. On the other hand, there are many deeply spiritual persons who do not belong to any organized religion but who may be profoundly reflective about the meaning of their life and experiences.

Specific Values and Beliefs

Some religious leaders attempt to help a diverse population appreciate religious traditions other than their own. They point out that all the world's major religions seek to answer the same questions: Why are we here? What does it all mean? and What, if anything, are we supposed to be doing with our lives? All religions taken together can be perceived like a stained-glass window that refracts the light in different colors and offers reflections of different shapes. Each of the world's religions is different because it has evolved to respond to unique histories and different cultural developments.

Definitions of *religion* usually identify a specific system of values and beliefs and a framework for ethical behavior that the members must follow. Religion can be thought of as a social construct that reflects its cultural context and specific philosophical influences. Religion, as an institutionally based, organized system of beliefs, represents only one specific means of spiritual expression. Participation in a religion generally entails formal education for membership, an initiation ceremony, participation in worship gatherings, adherence to set rules of behavior, participation in prescribed rituals, a particular mode of prayer, and the study of that group's sacred texts. Religious groups vary widely in their tolerance of intragroup diversity of beliefs and behaviors as well as their respect for the belief systems of others. In addition, a specific religious group may encompass a wide range of understanding of what its practices represent.

Occasionally, health-care professionals may encounter individuals whose spiritual practices are highly questionable or discomfiting to witness, such as worshippers of Satan or those who seek to cause harm to others through their prayers and rituals.

The Secular Perspective

Although some people believe that secularism or humanism are synonymous with nonspirituality or even antispirituality, these philosophies try to separate organized formal religion from government. The principle of secularism is centered on humans and looks to science and rational thought to understand the world. Secularism endorses the right of people to be free from governance by organized religious creeds and teachings and asserts the right to freedom from governmental imposition of one particular religion upon the citizens of a country. Secularism in the United States also acts to protect all organized religions and the people who belong to them from interference by the government.

Although the secular perspective separates religion from government, it is not necessarily nonspiritual. Secular spirituality is seen as a set of positive values, such as love, honesty, and truth, chosen by the individual to ultimately become that person's supreme focus of life and organizing framework. It is a type of spiritual ideology without an external religious structure or organization that emphasizes the search for an inner peace rather than a relationship with a divine being. People who seek a secular spirituality are often motivated by the wish to live a happy existence, which may or may not involve the need to help others. They believe in a human life that goes beyond the materialistic, yet often they do not believe in a supreme being. For the individual who subscribes to secular spirituality, living a good life involves nurturing positive thoughts, emotions, words, and actions and believing that everything in the universe is mutually dependent.

> *Some say Nightingale was a modern prophet of God and saw herself as a liberated human being.*

Manifestation of Spirituality

The religious and secular perspectives can exist together in the totality of a person's life. A person's spirituality may be nourished by the ability to give and receive touch, caring, love, and trust. Spirituality may also entail an appreciation of physical experiences such as listening to music, enjoying art or literature, eating delicious food, laughing, venting emotional tension, or participating in sexual expression. In the context of a person's spiritual growth and development, a series of

four developmental stages have been proposed for human spirituality:

- Stage 1: The chaotic (antisocial) stage, with its superficial belief system
- Stage 2: The formal (institutional) stage, with its adherence to the law
- Stage 3: The skeptic (individual) stage, with its emphasis on rationality, materialism, and humaneness
- Stage 4: The mystical (communal) stage, with its "unseen order of things"[2]

A SPIRITUAL TRADITION IN NURSING

Modern nursing has a rich legacy of the appreciation of spirituality in health and illness. Florence Nightingale's views of nursing practice were based on a spiritual philosophy that she set forth in *Suggestions for Thought*. She was the daughter of Unitarian and Anglican parents, and among her ancestors were famous dissenters against the Church of England.

The skepticism fostered by her Unitarian upbringing may have influenced her to question and critique established religious doctrine. Her search for religious truth caused her to become familiar with the writings of Christian mystics (e.g., St. Francis of Assisi, St. John of the Cross) and with various Eastern mystical writings, including the *Bhagavad Gita*.

What Do You Think?

How would you define your spirituality—religious or secular?

The Lady of the Lamp

Most modern nurses consider Florence Nightingale (1820–1910) to be the mother of the nursing profession (see Chapter 2). Most know her as "the lady of the lamp," who almost single-handedly brought about sweeping changes in British medicine, care delivered on battlefields, and public health. Nightingale realized a call to care early in her life. She was a sickly child, and as the recipient of care from family members, she began to reciprocate in kind by nursing other sick relatives.

A Modern Prophet?

Nightingale sought places where she could learn to care for the sick and dying in a way that distinguished what she did from the work of common chambermaids. She attended the Institution of Deaconesses at Kaiserwerth in Dusseldorf, Germany. This was a Protestant training hospital that taught something akin to nursing as a call from God. Through her time at Kaiserwerth and her contacts there, she came to believe that all persons on a mission or quest to become Christlike are given certain gifts and talents. Some say Nightingale was a modern prophet of God and saw herself as a liberated human being.

For Nightingale, spirituality involved a sense of a divine intelligence that creates and sustains the cosmos, and she had an awareness of her own inner connection with this higher reality. She regarded the universe as the embodiment of a transcendent God. She came to believe that all aspects of creation are interconnected and share the same inner divinity. She believed that all humans have the capacity to realize and perceive this divinity. Nightingale's God can be described as perfection or as the "essence of benevolence."[3]

The Thoughts of God

Nightingale saw no conflict between science and religion. To her, the laws of nature and science were merely the "thoughts of God." Spirituality for Nightingale entailed the development of courage, compassion, inner peace, creative insight, and other "Godlike" qualities. Based on this belief, Nightingale's convictions commanded her to lifelong service in the care of the sick and helpless.[4]

Nightingale endorsed the tradition of contemplative prayer, or attunement to the inner presence of God. All phenomena, Nightingale believed, are manifestations of God. A spiritual life entails wise stewardship of all the earth's resources, including human beings. She saw physical healing as a natural process regulated by natural laws, and as she stated in her *Notes on Nursing*, "What nursing has to do . . . is to put the patient in the best condition for nature to act upon him."[3]

> ❝ *Paying attention to the spiritual domain in providing holistic care depends on the beliefs and values of both the nurse and the patient.* ❞

Spirituality and Religion in Nursing Theory

As nursing sought to establish itself as a profession with a legitimate knowledge base, the concern with human spirituality was downplayed and even consciously ignored until the early 1980s. Typically, the spiritual domain is assigned to the art rather than to the science of nursing because its seemingly subjective nature is mistakenly equated with esthetics and intuition. Paying attention to the spiritual domain in providing holistic care depends on the beliefs and values of both the nurse and the patient.

More than 26 major nursing theories and conceptual frameworks have been developed since the 1960s. Although 14 of them recognized the spiritual domain of health somewhere in their assumptions, only two theories mention it by name.

Energy Fields

Martha Rogers's science of unitary human beings theory is an example of a profoundly spiritual view of humanity that does not directly name the concept of spirituality. Rogers's framework suggests that there are unbounded human energy fields in interaction with the environmental energy field. Her spiritual definitions can also apply to the concept of the soul (discussed later). Rogers, who grew up in Tennessee amid fundamentalist Christians, was loath to be interpreted in that light; moreover, she had to establish her credibility at New York University during the 1950s, before nursing was accepted as a scientific discipline.

An Aspect of Holistic Health

Betty Neuman, in the later development of her theory, and Jean Watson are the only theorists who clearly acknowledged the impact of spirituality in the development of their theories (see Chapter 3). Watson alone defined and explained the spiritual terminology she used to discuss the spiritual aspect of holistic health.

Watson specifically identifies the awareness of the patients' and families' spiritual and religious beliefs as a responsibility of a nurse.[5] She advocates that nurses should appreciate and respect the spiritual meaning in a person's life, no matter how unusual that person's belief system may be. Watson states that nurses have an obligation to identify religious and spiritual influences in their patients' lives at home and to help patients meet their religious requirements in inpatient settings. For example, nurses can facilitate patients' use of religious measures, such as the lighting of candles (real or electric), putting flowers and personal objects in the room, ensuring privacy, and playing music to promote increased comfort and relieve anguish.

Spiritual Distress

Since 1978, the NANDA-I has recognized the nursing diagnosis of spiritual distress. In reality, any disruption in the life principle that pervades a person's entire being and that integrates and transcends one's biological and psychosocial nature can be considered spiritual distress.[6]

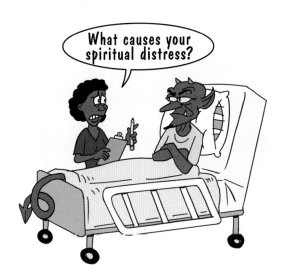

Defining characteristics of spiritual distress include concerns with and questions about the meaning of life and death, anger toward God, concerns about the meaning of suffering, concerns about the person's relationship to God, the inability to participate in preferred religious practices, seeking spiritual help, concerns about the ethics of prescribed medical regimens, preoccupation with illness and death, expressing displaced anger toward clergy, sleep disturbances, and altered mood or behavior. Spiritual distress may occur in relation to separation from religious or cultural supports, challenges to beliefs and values, or intense suffering.

At first glance, *religiosity* might seem to be something spiritually good or desired. Why, then, do the nursing diagnoses that are directed toward it seem to be negative? For both Christians and non-Christians, *religiosity* refers to extreme religious activities. Religiosity is an excessive devotion to the conduct of the rituals and traditions of a particular religion.[7] Because some people find it easier to observe the rules, rituals, and traditions of a religion than to maintain a personal and fervent relationship with the Creator, they become excessively or sentimentally religious. They also often practice their religiosity in an intrusive and pushy way toward others by speaking excessively about their beliefs. They display an extreme passion for rituals outside of and beyond the norms of faith. People who are afflicted with religiosity often appear to serve God to earn God's love and salvation or to be seen and admired by other people rather than serving God and neighbor because they love God and are expressing gratitude for God's love for us and the gifts of salvation and eternal life.[7]

Illness as Punishment

Nurses should be aware that some individuals have been seriously harmed by their religious communities. Examples of harm might include being shunned or excommunicated, being told that they are evil, being forced into a rigidly controlled lifestyle by a cult, or being physically or sexually assaulted by members of the religious community. For these people, illness may be seen as punishment for some sinful action, and they may perceive any offer of spiritual support from the religious community as profoundly threatening. They may believe that God has abandoned them or that the idea of God is foolish or even destructive.

Given the rapid turnover of patients in most health systems, there may be little that the nurse can do other than to acknowledge a patient's spiritual pain and accept them with the assurance that "I am here for you now." If there is more time for contact, the nurse may be able to refer a patient or family to appropriate support groups or clergy.

Going Against Traditions

At times, patients make health-care decisions that conflict with the beliefs of their religious communities. These decisions often produce high levels of spiritual distress that may affect both the mental and physical well-being of the patient. Patients also make choices that are difficult for nurses to accept. For instance, because of religious beliefs, patients may refuse commonplace treatments, such as blood transfusions, medications, and even minor surgeries.

End-of-life decisions are often made by family members guided by their spiritual beliefs. Such decisions can be controversial among the health-care personnel who are involved. In some acute-care settings, chaplains and psychiatrists conduct regular group sessions with staff nurses to assist them in understanding and accepting controversial patient decisions.

The Human Energy System and the Soul

Most religious traditions include a concept called the "soul." Religious traditions usually offer explanations of what the soul is, how and when human beings acquire a soul, and what happens to the soul after death; but soul need not be a religious concept.

Images of the Soul

Thomas Moore, a psychotherapist who has written extensively about spiritual development, describes the soul "not as a thing, but a quality or a dimension of experiencing life and ourselves. It has to do with depth, value, relatedness, heart, and personal substance . . . [not necessarily] an object of religious belief or . . . something to do with immortality." Yet Moore observes that the soul must be nurtured, and religious practices can provide that nurturance.[8] For Moore, spirituality is the effort a person makes to identify the soul's worldview, values, and sense of relatedness to the whole of the person and of creation. The work of the soul is the quest for understanding or insight about major life questions.[8]

Some people may depict the soul as an image of the person that extends several feet beyond the physical self or characterize it by color and energetic movement. Many people believe that the soul enters the body at some point during gestation and leaves the body at approximately the moment of death. Reincarnation, or the return of a soul for many earthly lifetimes, is a concept encountered in numerous religious frameworks, including certain mystical traditions within Judaism and Christianity, although not all denominations subscribe to it. The reason for the soul's return to earthly life is to learn, to develop, and to be purified. Some traditions express this process in terms of earning an improved position in the spiritual world to become closer to God after the final judgment.

The soul would seem to be an exquisitely precise and vast center for communication. Souls have the capacity to communicate with one another, with all living things, and with the divine source of all energy. Their capacity is not limited by the laws of physical matter. Some alternative modalities of healing rely on energy movement through the soul.

Examples of therapies that capitalize on knowledge of the soul and the movement of a divinely generated energy, life force, or grace (*chi* in Chinese, *ki* in Japanese, *prana* in Indian traditions) include therapeutic touch, Reiki, and shiatsu. Energy can move in many directions. When a person needs it, energy can be drawn from its divine source into the person. Excess energy can be moved from one person to another, and the flow of energy throughout the person's energy field can be balanced to achieve a state of health.

Human Energy Centers

Some alternative healing practices that use colors, herbs, aromas, and crystals can be regarded as consistent with a paradigm of repatterning the human energy field or altering the flow of energy throughout the person's body. The circulation of divine energy may be thought of as coming from God and circulating through all living things, the Earth, and all the celestial bodies, thus interconnecting all creation.

Religious traditions of India and other Eastern cultures teach that the human energy system contains seven energy centers, or *chakras*. These can be considered the primary openings in the human energy system through which energy flows. Each center has or controls a unique type of energy and spirituality that it allows to enter or leave the body. The root chakra is located at the base of the torso or the perineum, and its energy has to do with the material world. The crown chakra, the highest level of energy at the top of the head, relates to spirituality (see Fig. 20.2).

Issues in Practice

The Terri Schiavo case in Florida demonstrates how well-meaning people with strong religious beliefs can be diametrically opposed when it comes to end-of-life decisions. This is what happened:

In 1990, 25-year-old Terri Schiavo suffered a cardiac arrest and, after heroic measures, was revived. However, because of the length of time her brain was deprived of oxygen, she fell into a persistent vegetative state, or coma. She remained in this condition until she was 41, being sustained by tube feedings and IV hydration. Michael Schiavo, her husband, began requesting in 1995 that she legally be allowed to die by removing the feeding tube and IVs. Terri's family vociferously objected, and thus began a highly publicized legal battle between Terri's family and her husband that roused debate across the United States and around the world.

At the heart of that case, Michael believed, as did every physician who examined Terri, that she would never emerge from her comatose state. He did not want her to merely exist in a permanent vegetative state, unconscious, unresponsive, and unable to interact with the world. His personal knowledge of her as his wife and her wishes to him while they were married led him to believe that she would not want to remain in that condition indefinitely. He believed that the feeding tube and hydration were just prolonging her death.

Terri's family bitterly disagreed. They still believe to this day that she would have wanted to live even if it was in a coma, that her husband did not have her interests at heart, and that they were unfairly pushed aside in their effort to save her life. They believe that a miracle could have happened or that medical science might have come up with a cure and she would have awakened.

The underlying issue is an ethical question: What does it mean to be alive? If a person has a beating heart and working lungs, but no ability to sustain themselves, interact with others, or respond to the world, are they alive? Does the right to life always supersede quality of life concerns?

What began as a private dispute in a hospital room between Michael Schiavo and Terri's family ended up in a local court. From there it moved to a Florida circuit court, then to district courts and to state and federal courts, to Congress, and eventually to the U.S. Supreme Court. President George W. Bush, a strong state's right proponent and believer in limiting the reach of the federal government, almost created a constitutional crisis between the courts and the executive branch when he tried to override with an executive order the Florida courts' decision to allow Michael Schiavo's wish to permit his wife to die naturally. During his tenure as Florida governor, Jeb Bush, President Bush's brother, decided to fight his own state courts in trying to override their decision to let her die.

Eventually, the Vatican got involved. It challenged U.S. law that, in general, allows the stopping of artificial food and water, under certain circumstances, to allow for a natural death. The Vatican said food and water could not be stopped; however, within the Church there was disagreement over the definitions of active and passive euthanasia, extraordinary measures, and the right to die (for more information, see Chapter 7). The result was that the Vatican's decision created a great deal of confusion and left many Catholic health-care institutions and Catholics unsure about what they should do when requests were made to let patients die by removing a feeding tube, a common practice carried out by most hospitals when requested by family. These results made a strong case for the Church's earlier belief that these types of decisions should be made at the bedside, perhaps with the help of a clergy person, and that the legal system and courts were poorly prepared to deal with such issues.

Although Terri Schiavo's parents believed that she was *not* in a permanent coma and could one day "wake up," an autopsy found that her brain was severely atrophied, weighing less than half of what it should have. No treatment then or now could have reversed the brain damage she suffered.

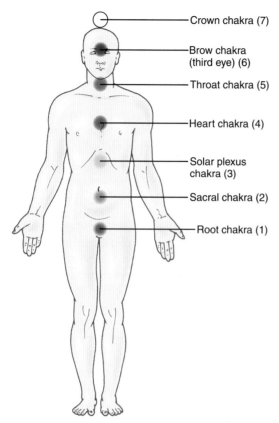

Crown chakra (7)

Brow chakra
(third eye) (6)

Throat chakra (5)

Heart chakra (4)

Solar plexus
chakra (3)

Sacral chakra (2)

Root chakra (1)

Figure 20.2 Chakras are energy wheels located throughout the body.

Examining the religious art of many cultures over many centuries, artists depict these areas of their subjects' bodies in similar ways. For instance, holy people are depicted with vivid, large, or colorful hearts, and their heads are surrounded by halos. At the very least, the chakras represent a paradigm for ordering the archetypal issues of human life.

What Do You Think?

What sources of religious energy do you have? When and how do you use them?

Communication Between Worlds

Some individuals seem to be more aware of the nonphysical or spiritual realms than others. Many people have had a precognition or déjà vu experience during their lives. However, nurses may have more opportunities to glimpse a different reality than laypeople. Nurses have been involved in research on the near-death experience for more than 20 years.

The Near-Death Experience (NDE)

Across religious and cultural traditions and throughout history, a common NDE has been documented, but only since the early 1980s has it gained credence among Western health professionals.

Many patients describe the experience of near death as a sensation of floating in the air while visualizing their body lying below on a hospital bed, at the scene of an accident, or where the near death occurred. They often watch health-care personnel who are working to resuscitate the body. The person then experiences being drawn into a tunnel, perhaps accompanied by other forms or spiritual beings, and moving toward a bright light that exudes great energy or love. They also describe a communication with the light being, generally identified as God, about whether they are to remain there or return to the earthly body.

The COVID-19 pandemic yielded a new crop of NDE stories. Although many patients are reluctant to talk about their experiences, a number have related them. A man living in Braselton, Georgia, who contracted the virus and was hospitalized for 4 months, described his NDE as feeling like being submerged in thick mud. He explained that while in the mud, he could not hear or see anything except people floating by him.[9]

Another man went into the hospital diagnosed with COVID-19. Shortly after he was admitted, he developed severe pneumonia that was quickly worsening. Because his organs were beginning to shut down, he was placed in a medically induced coma and connected to a ventilator. He described his experience as passing through a brightly lit tunnel. The light was beautiful, warm, and loving. He looked over his shoulder and saw a big, beautiful white staircase rising up and disappearing into the sky. The thought came to him that if he could get onto that staircase, maybe somebody would find him. He made his way to the staircase and began crawling up it. He made it partway up but was unsure how far when he heard somebody yelling, "There he is!

There he is!" Then it felt like they grabbed him by his shirt collar and just pulled him off the steps, returning him to his black, small, murky, sedated hospital bed.[10] There are many other COVID-19 NDE stories, and their number will likely increase as the pandemic ends and more survivors are willing to talk about their experience.

Obviously, in cases of near death, the person makes the decision to return. Individuals who have experienced near death often report that they have developed a great inner peace, that they no longer fear death, and that their lives have been transformed by what they experienced. They feel more loving and open toward their families and even strangers.[10]

Nurses who spend much of their time working with patients who are near death, such as hospice nurses, are most likely to have witnessed the experience of deathbed visions and gained a glimpse of a different realm of reality. Dying patients who are having a deathbed vision are often aware of multiple realities: the tangible here and now that family members and caretakers can observe and "the other side," where they see loved ones who have died and are waiting for their arrival.

Some medical researchers attribute near-death and deathbed experiences to progressive hypoxia in specific brain centers. However, others give the experiences a spiritual interpretation. Could a deceased husband, for example, really come to meet his wife of many years? A vast amount of literature on angels and spiritual guides emphasizes that people need not feel alone or frightened by future situations or crises. Angels and other spiritual guides are available to comfort them just for the asking.

Spirituality in Children

Some authorities believe that children are more open than adults to communication from the spiritual world because they have not yet been contaminated by the laws of natural science that are generally accepted by Western society. Nurses can watch for and nurture spirituality in children. When a nurse is open to such an occasion and acts on it, an opportunity for transcendent and reciprocal spiritual growth is available to both the child and the nurse. Children may be conscious or unconscious participants in a spiritual life.

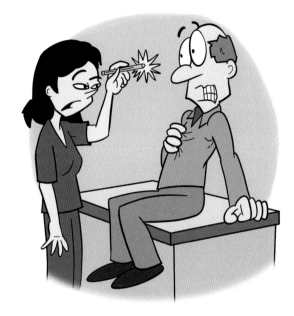

"Sir, the bright light you see is my penlight, not the afterlife."

By their mere presence, their demonstrations of love, their ability to draw love from their family and friends, and their expression of awe of the natural world, children provide strong aspects of spirituality to the world. Children express their spirituality primarily through behaviors. They imitate ritual and use symbols in imaginative play. They question with innocence and intent. Children express values and make value judgments. They use art, dance, song, and movement to express joy, despair, awe, and wonder; to deal with suffering; and to question meaning in their experiences. Children who have developed and are supported in spiritual and religious expression or practices develop a framework for the understanding of social relations and the natural world.[11]

Mysticism

Mystics are people believed to have a different relationship to time, space, matter, and energy than most of the population. It seems that they can understand the real nature and full capability of their souls and can apply that knowledge and ability to the physical world, producing changes that science has difficulty explaining and that some call miracles. For example, in India, a Hindu holy man named Sai Baba, who died in 2011, generated ash in his hands that brought miraculous healing to some people who touched it. Although some discredited it as just sleight-of-hand tricks, he had many devoted followers and established houses for the poor all over the Far East and Africa. Far from India, many healing miracles were documented by physicians and scientists during the lifetime of the Italian Franciscan priest St. Padre Pio before his death in 1968.

The common message of mystics from around the world is that people are to live lives of love and compassion for all. The extraordinary love and compassion that most mark the early life of the Dalai Lama, a Buddhist holy man, is depicted in the historical films *Seven Years in Tibet* and *Kundun*.

SPIRITUAL PRACTICES IN HEALTH AND ILLNESS

The way that nurses care for and nurture themselves influences their ability to function effectively in a healing role with another person or patient. Spirituality is an important component of a life's journey. Tending to matters of the soul aids a person in living a healthy lifestyle and is fundamental to integrating spirituality into clinical practice.

Nurturing the Spirit

Caring for their spirits or souls requires nurses to pause, reflect, and take in what is happening within and around them; to take time for themselves and their spiritual or religious practice, for relationships, and for other things that animate them. Maintaining and nourishing one's spiritual disposition can be achieved in a variety of ways, and nurses can give the same suggestions that they themselves use to heal internally.

Issues in Practice

Religion Versus Care

Angie and Edward are a couple with two teenage children. They are a close and loving family who have a large network of family and friends. The entire family is active in their church, school, and other community groups.

Angie and Edward's 15-year-old son, Alan, has just been severely injured in a motor vehicle accident. Angie and Edward are summoned to the hospital where they are told that Alan has multiple fractured bones and possible internal injuries. While they are waiting for the surgical team to arrive, the couple keeps vigil at their son's bedside in the pediatric intensive care unit (PICU). The surgeon informs the distressed parents that there is evidence that Alan's injuries are more serious than previously diagnosed. Alan has active internal bleeding and will need a blood transfusion to survive. Although genuinely devastated, the parents adamantly refuse to sign consent for the lifesaving blood transfusion, stating that they are Jehovah's Witnesses and that receipt of blood is against their religion. The surgeon asks you, Alan's nurse, to get the parents to change their minds. You talk with the couple, but they continue to refuse to sign the surgical consent form.

Questions for Thought

1. What are the primary underlying spiritual principles involved in this dilemma?
2. Do Alan's parents have the right to refuse their consent for a blood transfusion on the basis of religious beliefs?
3. Do you think that Alan's being a minor (under 18 years old) makes a difference in this situation?
4. What actions do you think the charge nurse should take?
5. How would you resolve this dilemma?

Spiritual Assessment Questions

Nurses may have difficulty assessing the spiritual status of a patient. Following are some questions that facilitate gathering this information:

- What is strength for you?
- Where can you get your strength?
- Who gives you strength?
- How can you increase your inner strength?
- What does peace mean to you?
- Where do you feel at peace?
- Who makes you feel more peaceful?
- What situations will increase your sense of peace?
- When do you feel most secure?
- Where do you get your security from?
- Who makes you feel secure?
- How can you increase your security?[1]

To support the "whole" person, health-care providers should be willing and able to address their patients' spiritual needs. How do you feel about discussing such matters with your patients? If you feel uncomfortable about addressing the issue of spirituality, is there someone with whom you can discuss these matters and perhaps alleviate your discomfort so that you can better serve your patients?

A Professional Responsibility

Care of the spirit is a professional nursing responsibility and an intrinsic part of holistic nursing. Nurses must become confident and competent with spiritual caregiving, expanding their skills in assessing the spiritual domain and in developing and implementing appropriate interventions. A caring relationship with a patient is necessary to show the person that they are significant. Effective spiritual care requires self-awareness, communication, trust building, and the ability to give hope.[12]

The nursing profession must understand and support holistic care. Therefore, spirituality and the delivery of spiritual care become fundamental content areas for nursing students.[12] What the nurse needs is a set of social, psychological, and personal skills combined with sensitivity, open-mindedness, and tolerance. These skills include such things as listening, responding appropriately, correctly identifying emotional states, showing accurate empathy, and so forth. Sensitivity enables nurses to detect the sometimes-subtle cues given by the patient; open-mindedness prevents nurses from automatically interpreting what they see and hear in terms of their own worldview and beliefs; and tolerance enables nurses to accept beliefs expressed and requests made that may not accord with their own sentiments. Guidelines and policies must be developed to fully support nurse educators in their endeavors.

A persistent barrier to the incorporation of spirituality into clinical practice is the fear of imposing religious beliefs and values on others. Nurses who integrate spirituality into their care of others need to recognize that, although each person acts out of and is informed by their own spiritual perspective, acting from this foundation is not the same as imposing these beliefs and values on others. In fact, many practitioners believe that the more grounded they are in their own spiritual understandings, the less likely they are to impose their values and beliefs on others.

Several organizations and agencies encourage the incorporation of spiritual practices into health care. The American Holistic Nurses Association (AHNA) was founded in 1980 by a group of nurses dedicated to bringing the concept of holism to every arena of nursing practice. They define *holism* as wellness—that state of harmony between body, mind, emotions, and spirit—in an ever-changing environment. The AHNA offers certification in holistic nursing and has endorsed programs in aromatherapy, interactive imagery, and healing touch.

Parish (congregational) nursing is a movement of the past two decades in which churches, synagogues, mosques, and other faith communities designate nurses to serve their membership. Parish nursing is viewed as a healing ministry, and parish nurses are attuned to spiritual issues raised by health transitions and the healing nature of spiritual practice. They may assist people to remain in their own homes, connect them with other health services for which they are eligible, or provide needed health teaching and support. At times, their role is simply to be present with people.

The David B. Larson Fellowship in Health and Spirituality offers funding to those interested in researching religiousness and spirituality, and physical, mental, and social health. For more information visit https://www.loc.gov/programs/john-w-kluge-center/chairs-fellowships/fellowships/larson-fellowship-in-health-and-spirituality/.

Prayer and Meditation

Prayer and meditation are spiritual disciplines practiced in many traditions, both cultural and religious. Appreciating the personal nature of these disciplines, the nurse, with respect and sensitivity, can help patients remember or explore ways in which they reach out to and listen for God or the absolute. Recalling the place and meaning of prayer and the ways in which they experience the presence of and communion with God or the absolute provides patients with a rich resource.

In the clinical setting, both the nurse's and the patient's understanding of prayer will determine its role. Clarifying the patient's understanding of and need for prayer is part of holistic nursing. Some patients want others to pray with or for them, whereas others do not believe in prayer. Nurses should support each patient's request and need for prayer, which may mean inviting others to take part in various forms of prayer with and for the patient or simply praying with the patient themselves if prayer is part of the nurse's spiritual practice. Facilitating the appreciation and practice of prayer in a patient's life is an important aspect of caring for the spirit.

Does Prayer Help Healing?

The literature is well populated with accounts of individuals who were miraculously healed when people prayed for them. These are individual cases and personal accounts of the effectiveness of prayer. However, hypothetico-deductive quantitative research has been difficult to carry out on the causal relationship between prayer and healing because of the many variables involved in the studies.

Studies of the effectiveness of prayers on health generally have focused on one of three separate categories of prayer: the effects of the patients praying for themselves (first-person effects), the effects of a close friend or relative praying for the patient (second-person effects), and the effects of a person or group of persons not known by the patient who are praying for them (third-party effects). Second-person and third-party praying are also identified as *intercessory prayer*, which is a type of prayer also used by those who pray to saints to intercede with God on their behalf.

One of the largest attempts at a scientific study of the causal relationship between prayer and healing was the Study of the Therapeutic Effects of Intercessory Prayer (STEP). The researchers studied 1,802 patients who had undergone coronary bypass surgery in six different hospitals. The patients were randomly divided into three groups, with groups 1 and 2 told that they may or may not be prayed for, while group 3 was told they would receive prayers for healing. Congregations at three different Christian churches in the area were then told to pray for 30 days for the full recovery of patients in groups 2 and 3, while group 1 did not receive any prayers from the congregations. At the end of the study, there were no noticeable differences in the 30-day recovery or mortality rates among the three groups. The conclusion drawn was that prayer had no significant effect on the recovery or mortality of the patients in the two groups who did receive prayer.

Follow-up investigation of the STEP demonstrated several variables that had not been considered in the original research design. Group 3, who knew they were being prayed for, noted a higher level of stress than the other two groups, a sort of "performance anxiety." They felt that because they were receiving prayers, they should have a better recovery. Some of the individuals who were praying commented that they had been required by the research design to use the scripted prayer: "For a successful surgery with a quick, healthy recovery, and no complications." These participants noted that this was not the way they usually prayed, and it felt abnormal. For this reason, they said that their prayers lacked the power or weight that they would normally have had. The researchers also did not account for a placebo effect among group 3 from their knowledge of having prayers said for them. Finally, even though groups 1 and 2 did not know if they were being prayed for by the three congregations, some of them had other individuals or even groups praying for them that were unknown to the researchers.

The results of a much smaller study by Duke University researchers seem to reinforce the positive results of prayer in treating illness. Similar to the STEP, Duke researchers used the third-party, or intercessory, prayer of off-site prayer sessions of seven prayer groups of various denominations around the world. The prayer groups included Buddhists, Catholics, Moravians, Jews, fundamentalist Christians, Baptists, and the Unity School of Christianity. A group of 150 patients was divided into two random groups of 75, one that received prayers and one that did not. Being a double-blind study, none of the 150 patients knew if they were or were not receiving prayers. However, the age and illness of each patient assigned to prayer therapy groups was sent to each prayer group. The patients in the study had prayers from all over the world said on their behalf for healing and recovery. All the patients in the study suffered from similar heart disease conditions and were to undergo stent placement in one or more coronary arteries to keep the artery open.

The results of the study showed that the patients who received prayers had better outcomes and fewer adverse results than the patients who did not receive prayers. Researchers are still unsure of the mechanism of causality—that is, why the prayer intervention helped. They believe that the prayers may have helped calm the patients, which aided their recoveries. Researchers were so pleased with the results that the study added a Phase II on a much larger sample of patients. However, Phase II seemed to indicate that there was no significant difference between the control group and the study group.

Whether or not prayer can promote healing is a topic that has been studied for many years and is still the focus of much research. Although difficult to study because of the large numbers of variables ranging from the patient's own personal beliefs in a higher power to the sincerity of those praying for healing, several studies seem to show that intercessory prayer can work to help patients heal. On the other hand, there are just as many studies that seem to confirm that there is no connection between prayer and healing.[13]

Should prayer be categorized as an alternative integrative health practice? Any nurse who has spent much time with patients and families who have a strong belief in a higher power has seen the real-life effect of praying together. It lowers anxiety levels, reduces stress, and overall lessens the fear associated with illness and dying.

Relief Through Imagery

When a person is physically confined to a hospital room, the practice of imagery may enable them to experience another space. Imagery can take a person to a temple, an ocean, a place of religious worship, a breakfast nook, or any "sacred space"—that is, a life-giving and healing place for the patient. In this other space, the patient may feel more comfortable in spirit and more able to engage in prayer or meditation. Family and friends, as well as other patients and other staff, may be resources in this practice of imagery.

Exploring as many aspects of the prayer experience as possible enriches both the nurse's and the patient's understanding of the nature and place of invocation. Sacred or inspirational readings, music, drumming, movement, light or darkness, aromas, and time of day are among the many factors that may be important considerations in meditation.

The patient's method of reflection, in all its fullness and meaning, nurtures the spirit, and the nurse may be able to support the patient's prayer or meditation needs by facilitating changes in the environment or schedule. It is wise to remember that merely the process of listening to and appreciating self-reflection of another person nurtures the spirit and acknowledges the spiritual dimension of that person.

> *" When a person is physically confined to a hospital room, the practice of imagery may enable them to experience another space. "*

Relaxation Response

The relaxation response and prayer have been demonstrated to affect illnesses. The ability of people to participate in their own healing through prayer or meditation may rely on a source of healing power called *remembered wellness*, sometimes also called the *placebo effect*. Remembered wellness is the belief that all people have the capacity to "remember" the calm and confidence associated with emotional and physical health and happiness. As a source of energy that can be tapped into, remembered wellness should not be regarded suspiciously but instead should be used for healing. However, its effectiveness depends on the individual's belief system.

Remembered Wellness

Remembered wellness depends on three components: belief and expectation of the patient, belief and expectation of the caregiver, and belief and expectation generated by a caring relationship between the patient and the caregiver. A warm and trusting relationship seems to enhance the effectiveness of the care provided.

Everyone involved in providing health care is able to use remembered wellness as an energy source to enhance the healing process. One thing health-care providers can do to promote healing is to speak positively of treatments and medications being used. For example, positive reinforcement occurs when the nurse refers to the patient's medication as the "drug your doctor prescribed to help your heart" or the food tray as "nutrition to help your body fight your infection."

The Nocebo Effect

In contrast to the placebo effect, the "nocebo" (negative placebo) effect is the fulfillment of an expectation of harm. If a patient is told something bad is going to happen to them and believes it, the likelihood of it happening increases. It is also an effect that health professionals can cause. Examples of the nocebo effect include advising patients that a medicine will probably make them sick, telling them that chemotherapy will drain their energy and cause more of their hair to fall out, or informing them that a certain percentage of people die from a given procedure. Such warnings can bring about the complications. Any teaching about the side effects of medications has the potential to produce a nocebo effect, and there really is no way to prevent it. It creates a difficult ethical dilemma for the nurse, who is caught between the obligation of beneficence (do no harm) and the obligation of informed consent (see Chapter 6 for more details).

Some have proposed a middle ground called *contextual informed consent*, where the information given to patients is adapted to their specific levels of knowledge and anxiety. Basically, the patient is not told about *all* the potential side effects in detail, particularly those that commonly have a psychological component such as headaches, back pain, and shortness of breath. Other experts believe that the contextual informed consent approach may invalidate consent forms and destroy the nurse–patient relationship, which is built on trust.

What Do You Think?

Is the practice of contextual informed consent ethical? Under which system of ethical thinking is it more likely to be considered ethical: utilitarianism or deontology? (See Chapter 6.) How would you approach a patient who was anxious about the side effects of a medication or a surgical procedure?

A Quiet Focus

Sometimes called *transcendental meditation* (TM) or *mantra meditation*, the relaxation response entails 20 minutes, twice each day, of quiet meditation with the eyes closed, focusing on a word or image that is spiritually meaningful to the person. When an intrusive thought enters the person's consciousness, the person should lightly dismiss it, as if gently blowing a feather away, and return to the meditation word or image. Over time, individuals who use this method have lowered blood pressure, decreased incidents of dysmenorrhea, and reduced chronic pain; this practice has brought about improvement in several illnesses.[14]

Peace Through Awareness

Relaxation, meditation, visualization, and hypnosis can help seriously ill patients, including many with cancer. Meditation is a way of focusing the mind in a state of relaxed awareness to pay attention to deeper thoughts and feelings, to the products of the unconscious mind, to the peace of pure consciousness, and to deeper spiritual awareness.

Some teachers of meditation suggest that the person select a spiritually symbolic word (e.g., God, love, beauty, peace, Mary, Jesus) on which to focus, whereas others suggest watching a candle flame. Still others teach practitioners to focus on their breathing. All these methods are intended to bring the person to a deeply restful state that frees the mind from its usual chatter. This is the experience of being centered. People may experience spiritual insights, but more often they experience a gradual enhancement of well-being.

Visualizing an Outcome

Visualization is the practice of meditating with an image of a desired outcome or the process of attaining it. It is preferable that the image be selected by the person using it rather than by someone else. For example, a person with a tumor might visualize miniature miners mining the unhealthy tissue and carting it away. Hypnosis is the process of suggesting an image of a desired reality to someone. Both these techniques have been demonstrated to stimulate the immune system.

Researchers have also observed that some seriously ill people believe that they deserve their illness as a punishment for something they did in the past. Helping them forgive themselves often brings about dramatic improvements in their conditions. Releasing fear and hate has a similar effect. This process reflects Nightingale's belief that nurses need to help patients get out of the way of their own healing.

It might seem logical to conclude that patients who do not recover from illness, or who die, have failed to help themselves or did not adequately use their spiritual powers. That is not the case. Spiritual modes of healing do not always lead to cure. Spiritual healing takes a much broader view and includes enhanced comfort and an inner peace with disability or death.

Therapeutic Touch

Therapeutic touch (TT) is an active alternative healing modality that involves redirecting the human energy system. In recent years, TT has been retrieved from ancient traditions, studied, and refined.

Altered Wave Patterns

As a healing practice, TT is consistent with the science of unitary human beings developed by Martha Rogers. The science of unitary human beings defines people as energy fields interacting with the larger environmental energy field. The energy fields are characterized by patterns of waves. One way of altering the wave patterns of the human energy field is to use TT to move energy into and through it in deliberate ways.

The TT practitioner acts with the intent of relaxing the recipient, reducing pain and discomfort, and accelerating healing when appropriate. Early controlled studies showed that the hemoglobin levels of a group of patients who received TT increased significantly more than the levels in a control group who did not receive TT.[11]

The TT practitioner should approach the patient with compassion and the intent to heal, and the recipient of care ideally approaches the healing encounter with receptivity and openness to change. The practitioner of TT first centers and then assesses the state of the recipient's energy field, noting energy levels and movement around the chakras. Cues may be determined through physical sensations in the practitioner's hands, direct visualization, inner awareness, or other intuitive modes of insight.

After assessing the recipient, the TT practitioner, working from the center of the patient's energy field to the periphery, directs energy from the environment into the patient's field as needed, then stimulates energy flow through the patient's field, clears congested areas in the energy field, dampens excess energetic activity, and synchronizes the rhythmic waves of the energy flow, depending on the patient's needs. The practitioner is not diverting their own energy into the patient because it would be detrimental to the practitioner. Rather, the TT practitioner redirects the patient's energy field or directs energy from the environment outside the patient. (CAM therapies such as TM and TT are discussed in more detail in Chapter 25.)

An Expression of Care

Families and friends may need encouragement to share physical expressions of care and concern in the sometimes-intimidating hospital environment. Nurses may encourage them with statements such as the following:

> *At times when words cannot be found, or in circumstances in which people are more comfortable with physical expression than with words, touch is a powerful expression of spirit and an instrument of healing.*

"It's okay to hold her hand; you won't interfere with the tubes."
"He mentioned that you give a wonderful back rub; would you like to give him one today?"
"She seems to know when you are in here holding her hand."
"I can show you how to massage her feet."
"Would you like to brush her hair?"

Persons vary in their degree of comfort with touch and the conditions in which they may want to share touch. The nurse's own feelings about and comfort with touch help in assessing the place and potential use of touch in the patient's situation. At times when words cannot be found, or in circumstances in which people are more comfortable with physical expression than with words, touch is a powerful expression of spirit and an instrument of healing.

NURSING AS A PROFESSION OR VOCATION

Although the nursing profession is deeply rooted in religious traditions, modern nursing has spent considerable energy attempting to distance itself from this aspect of its history. Nursing as vocation has given way to nursing as profession (see Chapter 1). The current health-care system has required nurses to shift their identity from vocation to profession to achieve appropriate value in a system that is increasingly economically oriented.

Nursing as Spiritual Calling

Nursing is much more than the mere secular enterprise the modern world perceives it to be. Perhaps it is time that nurses re-evaluate the work they do and consider it a vocation—that is, a life calling in the spiritual sense of that word. The world's religions consistently allude to the symbolic and deep meaning of the work that nurses do. Nursing practice has the capacity to be richly imaginative and to speak to the soul on many levels. It can be carried out mindfully and artistically, or it can be done routinely and unconsciously, like any other job. When nursing is practiced with deep consciousness and purpose, it nurtures the nurse as well as the patient.[9]

Some experts perceive that nursing is directly connected to the nurse's fantasy life, family myths, ideals, and traditions. The profession of nursing may be one way nurses sort out their major life issues. Although the choice of nursing as a career may often seem to have been serendipitous, in the spiritual context it is reasonable to question whether anything really happens by accident. As nurses practice nursing, they craft themselves, undertaking the soul's lifetime work of self-definition and self-identification.

When the Well Runs Dry

As with most professions, at times it may become difficult, even impossible perhaps, to feel good about the work that one is doing. Negative attitudes about work are detrimental to a person's self-development and often cause people to become overly invested in the surface trappings of work, such as money, power, and success. The phenomenon of burnout among nurses has been identified and studied for many years (see Chapter 9). The COVID-19 pandemic with its large numbers of severely ill and dying patients raised both the number of nurses with burnout and interest in how to prevent it. Burnout can be viewed from a spiritual perspective as the well running dry, energy fields becoming unbalanced, or the nurse experiencing a prolonged "dark night of the soul" or even feeling that their life work is devoid of meaning.[15]

Wounds to the Soul

At the peak of the COVID-19 pandemic, nurses caring for patients with the disease encountered extreme working conditions that compromised the quality of the care they were providing. When nurses believed that the nursing actions they were forced to take or had to witness violated their deeply held ethical beliefs, a condition called **moral injury** (nursing diagnosis: *moral distress*) developed. Unlike burnout that develops from long-term workplace stress, moral injury results from a type of cognitive dissonance in which nurses know the quality of care their patients need but are unable to provide it because of elements they cannot control. One of the most serious results of moral distress is a type of deep wound to the nurse's soul that produces symptoms similar to the post-traumatic stress disorder (PTSD) seen in soldiers after they have experienced a prolonged, intense, and bloody battle. The disconnect between the values that directed people to become nurses in the first place and the compromises they had to make while providing care during the pandemic produced a deep emotional impact on some nurses' psyches.[15]

Although some symptoms of burnout and moral injury can be similar, moral injury can also produce feelings of shame, inadequacy, distress, guilt, and remorse. Long-term effects of moral injury can include the development of mental health conditions and decreased sense of worth. Similar to the long-term effects of PTSD, nurses can experience negative changes in behavior such as sudden angry outbursts or social withdrawal, decreased motivation, deteriorated senses of empathy and compassion for others, obsessive-compulsive behaviors, inability to sleep, and increased use of alcohol or drugs.[15]

Sometimes the aftereffects of burnout can be long term and difficult to treat, but people who experience it usually have enough internal resilience to overcome it after a period of rest and anxiety reduction without much help from others. Because of the deeper type of damage caused by those experiencing moral injury, a longer and often professional type of treatment may be needed. It is necessary for the nurse to have a strong support system. It is especially important for those who experience a moral injury to have a support team who also experienced the same painful work conditions. This team will help diminish their feelings of isolation and despair.[15]

Issues in Practice

The Pin

I received my basic RN education in a Catholic diploma nursing school in Upstate New York. Our nursing pin is inscribed with the Latin words *caritas benigna est*, which is most often translated "love is kind." It is part of St. Paul's Hymn to Love that is found in 1 Corinthians. At the time I graduated, I thought, "That's a nice saying," and rarely thought about it anymore, although I wore the pin every day for the next 40 years.

Over the past few years, I have begun to think about it again. I was honored as the alumnus of the year and invited to give a keynote presentation at my nursing class's 30th reunion. I based my talk on what the pin means. In English, *kind* is one of those words we use as an automatic response, such as *fine, okay*, and *nice*. But as I started to wonder why such a trite word would be on an item that is the miniature battle shield and identifying logo of my nursing school, I started to believe that there must be more to *benigna* than being merely kind, especially when it is equated to as powerful a word as *love*. Translated another way, it says, "Kindness is the same thing as love," which puts a whole different slant on it.

Of course, the word "love" also has become well-worn in the English language. Love—we hear that word so often that it starts to lose its meaning to us. It appears 317 times in the Old Testament and 221 times in the New Testament. More than 1,200 songs in English contain the word *love* in their titles. Despite its familiarity to us, we must never forget that LOVE is the substance, the essence, and the very being of God. If you could physically touch God, you would be touching love. If you experience Jesus, you are experiencing love. When you hold your spouse or children, you are holding love. When you help your friend, enemy, or patient, you are helping love.

Love is an all-pervasive force that pulls us toward one another and toward God, a type of celestial magnetism. It demands that we create and live in relationships with others. The more we love someone or something, the closer we want to be to that person or thing. We become all absorbed by the thing we love and forget about ourselves. We do things and make sacrifices we would otherwise consider ridiculous. We love what the other loves. Witness a mother holding her new infant or a young couple pressed tightly against each other holding hands.

Now if love is the same as kindness, then what really is kindness? When we think of kindness, we often think of warm, fuzzy acts that make us feel good all over when we perform them. Good examples would be buying a present for a needy child at Christmas, visiting an elderly relative—even one we do not much like—in a nursing home, or bringing a tuna casserole to someone who has had a hip replacement. But I believe that kindness involves more. It involves relationships with and service to others.

A classic example of kindness can be found in the Catholic story of a woman named Veronica. Veronica's act of kindness took a supreme effort of courage and persistence. The story takes place while Jesus was being led through the streets of Jerusalem to his crucifixion on Golgotha. Jewish law of the time required that women stay separate and apart from men, yet Veronica, an ordinary Jewish woman from Jerusalem, pushed through a crowd of men and soldiers to get to Jesus. Jewish law required that women cover their heads at all times when they were in public, yet Veronica took off her veil in the middle of a crowd and, bareheaded, gave it to Jesus. Jewish law strictly forbade women from touching men they were not married to, yet Veronica wiped Jesus' face. For her reward, she was roughly dragged away and physically thrown out of the crowd. Initially, Veronica saw only a bleeding, beaten, and pain-filled person who needed help. Yet her seemingly minor act of kindness established a relationship and provided a service that impressed the true image of Jesus both on her veil and on her heart.

In the nursing profession, we call this type of kindness *caring*. Perhaps Veronica was one of the first to demonstrate true nursing care merely by wiping the face of a man in need.

(continued)

Issues in Practice (continued)

But what is the nature of care? What does it mean to those of us who are supposed to be caregivers? Do we give care to others generously or is it a list of tasks to squeeze into our shift?

Is there a difference between "care for" and "care about"? Is what we do as nurses just a job, or is it a profession based on our ability to build relationships and provide service?

Maybe it is all of the above. Care and caring are complex concepts, and no two patients or situations are identical. Most basically, to care, to be kind, is to enter into the experiences of someone whose life has been invaded by illness, injury, suffering, and feelings of powerlessness and depression. As nurses, we need to recognize not only others' need for the care we provide but also our need to provide that care.

Increasing numbers of our patients are aging and elderly. We recognize that better health care means more people need care not only at the end of life but also while they make their developmental transitions through minor and serious illnesses and injuries, age-related changes in health and activity, and hidden mental health conditions that become evident only when they are extreme. As nurses, we need to set examples, for those around us, that demonstrate true caring and true kindness. We need to show what it means to give care that is not merely a list of tasks to check off on our shift-report sheets.

Maybe a better translation for *caritas benigna est* is *love is caring*. The act of caring in this sense means establishing relationships with others, some of whom we do not know very well and some of whom are not very pleasant and may be irritating and demanding. As nurses, we can touch these individuals not only through listening, teaching, and encouragement but also through actual physical touch. This is a great power and privilege we are given when we become members of our profession. It might even be considered a type of consecration or knighting.

Pope Francis, in a talk with thousands of Italian nurses in March 2018, told of his experiences with nurses when he was a young man of 20 and almost died. He called nurses "promoters of the life and dignity of the person," "truly irreplaceable," and "experts in humanity." He believes that the profession of nursing is a "mission" or "calling," wherein a joyful word, a smile, a simple touch, makes all the difference in the world to the one who is sick. It makes the person feel closer to someone who really cares and closer to being healed. The patient feels like a real person and not just the hip in Room 315. Pope Francis told the nurses that their care was particularly important in a society that often leaves the weak and poor on the margins, a society that places value only on people who are wealthy or famous.[*]

I believe that what the Pope is talking about is the type of kindness that St. Paul meant in his Hymn to Love. It seems that the good sisters of St. Francis who taught me at my diploma school had understood the real meaning of the saying long before I did!

Joseph T. Catalano

[*] A. Gibson, Pope Francis calls nurses "experts in humanity"—Thanks nurse who saved his life, Nurse.org, 2018, retrieved from https://nurse.org/articles/pope-francis-thanks-nurses-remembers-nun

People working in the helping professions, the work of which is rooted in compassion and concern for others, are prone to burnout and moral injury. A concerted effort at spiritual development, or the nourishment of the soul, is essential to nurses' overall mental and physical well-being.

Maintaining Balance

As discussed earlier, the integration of the mind, body, and soul is required for a balanced, productive, and fulfilled life. Because of the close interconnection of the three elements, any time one becomes imbalanced, the other two are affected. For example, high levels of anxiety or emotional stress of the mind increases the pulse and blood pressure and has been linked to peptic ulcers and chest pain in a person with an otherwise healthy body. Similarly, a physical illness or injury can cause anxiety and depression in a person with a usually healthy mind.

Self-Restoration

To maintain an internal state of balance, the first thing nurses need to do is take time to feed their spirit. Daily prayer or meditation is an important source of insight and energy. Belonging to a group or community that actively pursues spiritual growth is also a powerful source of spiritual nourishment. Many individuals find that their spirits are nourished within the setting of a formal religion, although not necessarily the one in which they were reared. It is not uncommon for people to seek a faith community in midlife or later life, perhaps after being away from one for many years. The experience of trying various religions and modes of worship is by itself a broadening, nurturing experience.

A Sense of Sacredness

Periodic retreat from the hustle and bustle of modern living can be highly restorative to the spirit. A retreat may be for a few hours, a half-day, a weekend, a week, or longer. For some people, keeping a journal is a retreatlike experience. For others, it may be a stroll through a beautiful park, a few hours watching waves on a beach, or a trip to the woods. Retreat is most effective when time is consistently set aside for introspection and reflection rather than for tasks.

A sense of sacredness can infuse everyday life with meaning and zest if nurses open themselves to it. It is a part of normal human activity to celebrate seasonal and family holidays with specific rituals, music, decorations, group gatherings, and foods. These types of activities honor life cycles that are greater than the individual and nurture important relationships that serve as a **support system**.

Enjoy Special Moments

Many people have routines for their weekends or days off that allow time for self-restoration. These special activities may include making a large country breakfast while listening to favorite music; baking cookies, bread, or a pie; sitting for an extended period in a favorite easy chair; or even playing a physically demanding sport such as basketball. Many people have favorite coffee mugs or dishes or special objects in their homes that are not only beautiful but may also remind them of loved ones, wonderful trips, religious experiences, or other events that nourish them each time they view the object.

One of the most spiritual aspects of a person's life is the enjoyment of beauty. It costs little or nothing to plant or cut flowers or to listen to music. It is in these moments that a person's creativity and insight are most evident.

Regaining the Center

The hectic modern world continually urges people to enhance their capacity for dealing with multiple concerns at the same time. Some people even define success by looking at how many tasks they can juggle simultaneously. *Multitasking* is the buzzword for the health-care environment of the 21st century. Nurses are required to be able to talk on the telephone, send faxes and e-mails, look up EBP, and use a word processor for entering patient data while they are developing care plans, evaluating patients, answering call lights, supervising unlicensed assistive personnel, and providing physicians with information. However, recent neuroscience studies have demonstrated that it is *impossible* to do two or more things at the same time that require cognitive thinking. Scientists now refer to this process as **rapid task switching**, whereby the person cognitively switches quickly from one task to another and then back again.[16]

In the past, multitasking was viewed as a highly productive method of working; however, recent studies have shown that forcing the brain to switch rapidly between cognitive tasks is highly unproductive. It can reduce productivity by as much as 40 percent; that is, it can take up to 40 percent longer to complete two tasks by multitasking (rapid task switching) than it would have taken to complete first one task and then the other. One of the big problems in using rapid task switching is that nurses have difficulty filtering out irrelevant information. This not only slows down the task completion process but is a major obstacle in making sound nursing judgments.[16]

Rapid task switching is also spiritually unhealthy. The more nurses multitask, the more disconnected they become from the elements that center them. Multitasking can be thought of as the antithesis of spiritual nurturance, or as a type of spiritual centrifugal force that scatters a person's focus. Spirituality is about personal wholeness, whereas multitasking is about fragmentation. When nurses slow down and center their energy fields, they have the capacity to be fully present and the ability to attend with complete consciousness to their loved ones, colleagues, and patients.[15]

Conclusion

Spirituality in the nursing context needs to be seen as a broad concept encompassing religion but not equated with it. Fundamental to this concept is a search for meaning in life and its events, such as ill health. Nursing students need to be aware of the many forms that spiritual distress may take.[14]

Nurses are in an ideal position to provide spiritual care that positively affects the mental and physical health of their patients. To be able to focus clearly on patients' spiritual needs, nurses must first consider their own spirituality as a starting point for self-knowledge. The means of supporting patients with spiritual problems must be explored. Teaching methods should be participatory and student centered. The means of assessing and meeting spiritual needs hinges on effective communication skills and determines whether the nurse is "being with" the patient as opposed to merely "being there." The meaning of the holistic moment emerges through the synergistic interaction among its elements (Fig. 20.3). Just as a person is greater than the sum of their parts, so too the holistic moment is greater than the sum of its parts, namely spirituality, presence, and relationship to others.

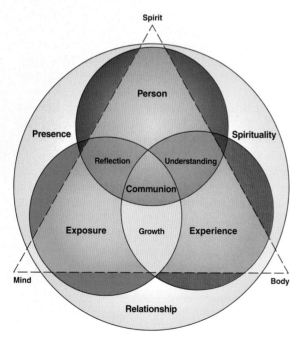

Figure 20.3 Elements involved in experiencing spirituality and presence in the nurse–patient relationship.

CRITICAL-THINKING EXERCISES

Mrs. Jan Steiner, 73 years old, has outlived two husbands. Ted, her second husband, died 20 years ago. Reared in the Roman Catholic faith, Mrs. Steiner converted to Judaism when she married Ted. Her two daughters by her first husband were also reared in the Roman Catholic tradition. One of them, Kathy, continues to practice her religion. The other daughter, Judith, is Unitarian.

Mrs. Steiner experienced a stroke 2 years ago that left her moderately disabled. At that time, she moved into a long-term care facility. She was still able to read and to enjoy visits with friends and family, but a second stroke 3 months ago left her incontinent and aphasic.

Mrs. Steiner has just had a major heart attack. Although bypass surgery could extend her life, she has never articulated any end-of-life desires. Her daughters are in conflict over how Mrs. Steiner's medical management should proceed. Kathy strongly believes that as long as Mrs. Steiner is alive, life should be actively supported. It would be morally wrong to do less than that. Judith, on the other hand, believes that what has been the "life" of Mrs. Steiner is essentially over and it is a waste of resources to merely delay the inevitable. The nursing staff, as they attempt to facilitate communication between the family and the medical staff, feel caught in the middle.

- What are your own spiritual beliefs about the proper approach to Mrs. Steiner's medical management?

- Analyze the positions of Kathy and Judith from the perspectives of both their ethical and spiritual contexts.
- What resources are likely to be available in the hospital or the community to help the daughters come to a decision?

Bypass surgery is not performed, and Mrs. Steiner returns to her long-term care facility. Her overall condition continues to deteriorate, and within 3 months she is very near death. She seems to have little awareness of her surroundings and does not consistently recognize or respond to her daughters.

- Knowing the religious divergence in Mrs. Steiner's family, how might the nursing staff facilitate their preparation for the death of their mother and her funeral?
- What would happen in Mrs. Steiner's circle of family and friends if any "side"—Catholic, Jewish, or Unitarian—"won" in planning her end-of-life care?
- Have you seen blending of religious traditions in rituals of marriage or burial? What are the advantages and disadvantages of such an approach?
- What might be the outcomes of handling their mother's death in a strictly secular or nonsectarian way and allowing all relatives and friends to mourn privately in accordance with their own spiritual traditions?

NCLEX-STYLE QUESTIONS

1. Mr. Mason, a 54-year-old evangelical Christian, is in the cardiac ICU after experiencing a massive myocardial infarction. Mr. Mason angrily questions why God allowed him to have a heart attack, since he has followed his church's teachings and has never smoked tobacco or drunk alcohol. Which of the following is an appropriate nursing diagnosis for Mr. Mason's anger?
   1. Risk for spiritual distress
   2. Impaired religiosity
   3. Spiritual distress
   4. Readiness for enhanced religiosity

2. Nursing students are making a list of the health benefits of spiritual practice to hospitalized patients. Which items belong on the list? **Select all that apply.**
   1. Reduced pain
   2. Increased response to medication
   3. Reduced anxiety
   4. Improved orientation in patients with dementia
   5. Lower blood pressure
   6. Faster wound healing

3. _____ is the consciousness that all individuals are connected to one another and to the whole of creation.

4. What distinguishes spirituality from religion?
   1. Spirituality identifies a supreme being or life force in the universe.
   2. Religion emphasizes the interconnectedness of all life.
   3. Spirituality does not necessarily have a religious component.
   4. Religion does not necessarily have a spiritual component.
5. A component of some alternative healing modalities is spirituality. What best describes the relationship between spirituality and therapeutic touch (TT)?
   1. An individual's energy field and that of their environment are mobilized through touch to bring about relief or healing.
   2. The TT practitioner prays over the patient to bring about relief or healing.
   3. Through touch, the patient receives energy from the TT practitioner that brings about relief or healing.
   4. Therapeutic touch is consistent with Martha Rogers's spiritual nursing theory, the science of unitary human beings.
6. Which of the following would you expect to observe in a patient diagnosed with spiritual distress?
   1. Statements indicating belief in a secular morality and science
   2. Statements indicating the patient feels abandoned by their God
   3. Weeping over the recent death of a loved one
   4. An angry outburst directed at the cancer growing inside them
7. Modes of prayer, sacred texts, an initiation ceremony, and an organized system of beliefs are essential elements of _____.

8. Which area of research supports the idea that spirituality may be a universal human experience?
   1. Therapeutic touch
   2. Meditation
   3. The nocebo (negative placebo) effect
   4. Near-death experiences
9. What is the relationship between spirituality and the nocebo (negative placebo) effect?
   1. Having patients visualize a negative response causes that response to manifest.
   2. Negative spirituality can cause unintended negative reactions to medications or treatments.
   3. The power of belief can lead to negative effects if patients believe strongly that these effects will happen.
   4. Telling patients about possible negative side effects of treatment causes them to have spiritual distress.
10. Richard, a nursing student, thinks the nursing diagnosis "spiritual distress" applies to a patient he saw in clinical practice today. What evidence would support Richard's diagnosis? **Select all that apply.**
    1. The patient's religion teaches that disease is caused by evil spirits.
    2. The patient tearfully states that he is "going to Hell" when he dies.
    3. The patient is the only local practitioner of his faith.
    4. The patient states that he fears God is punishing him for his sins.
    5. The patient requests that he be allowed to fast for a day as his religion dictates.

References

1. Helming M. *Dossey and Keegan's Holistic Nursing: A Handbook for Practice.* Burlington, MA: Jones & Bartlett Learning, 2022.
2. Cherry K. Kohlberg's theory of moral development. Verywell Mind, 2021. https://www.verywellmind.com/kohlbergs-theory -of-moral-development-2795071
3. Florence Nightingale Biography. Biography.com, 2014. https:// www.biography.com/people/florence-nightingale-9423539
4. Nightingale F. *Notes on Nursing.* New York, NY: Dover, 1969. First published 1859 by Harrison (London).
5. Watson J. *Nursing: Human Science and Human Theory of Care: A Theory of Nursing.* New York, NY: National League for Nursing, 1988.
6. NANDA Diagnoses: A Comprehensive Guide and List. NANDA Diagnoses, 2022. https://www.nandadiagnoses.com/
7. What is religiosity? Got Questions, 2022. https://www.gotquestions .org/religiosity.html
8. Moore T. *Thomas Moore Care of the Soul* (25th anniversary edition). New York: Harper Collins, 2022.
9. Georgiou A. Man who got COVID-19 describes near-death experience: "Like you are in mud. You can't hear. You can't see." *Newsweek*, August 5, 2020. https://www.newsweek.com/ covid-19-survivor-near-death-symptoms-1522932
10. One man recounts his near-death COVID story. National Public Radio, July 14, 2022. https://www.npr.org/2022/07/ 14/1111473823/one-man-recounts-his-near-death-covid-story

11. Mata J. *Spiritual Experiences in Early Childhood Education: Four Kindergarteners, One Classroom.* Hoboken, NJ: Taylor and Francis, 2022.

12. Spirituality in nursing. BrainMass, n.d. https://brainmass.com/health-sciences/spirituality-in-nursing

13. A scientific study of prayer. Subtle Energy Science, n.d. https://subtle.energy/a-scientific-study-of-prayer/

14. Welch A. 7 Types of meditation. Everyday Health, August 6, 2022. https://www.everydayhealth.com/meditation/types/

15. Cornell A. Understanding nurses experiencing moral injury. Nurse.com, August 22, 2022. https://www.nurse.com/blog/nurses-experiencing-moral-injury/

16. Hill B. Ethics in action: Multitasking during a pandemic. *Financial Management*, February 4, 2021. https://www.fm-magazine.com/news/2021/feb/cima-ethics-professional-competence-due-care.html

Diversity, Equity, and Inclusion

21

Joseph T. Catalano

TRANSCULTURAL NURSING

Culture is a powerful influence on how nurses and patients interpret and respond to health care and to each other. Both nurses and patients expect to be treated with respect and understanding for their individuality regardless of their cultural origins. Nurses who understand essential characteristics of transcultural nursing can provide competent and culturally sensitive care for patients from all cultural backgrounds.

WHAT IS CULTURE?

Culture is defined and understood in several ways. Culture may be seen as a group's acceptance of a set of attitudes, ideologies, values, beliefs, and behaviors that influence the way the members of the group express themselves.[1] It is a collective way of thinking that distinguishes one relatively large group from another over generations. For example, members of a political party, although diverse in other ways, may be viewed as belonging to a particular culture because of their beliefs and ideologies. Cultural practices are often handed down from parents to children over generations. Culture adapts and changes through time, learning, and societal events. For example, older people in a family may be more "traditional"; younger family members, while still a part of that culture, may not want to speak the language or may reject other parts of their culture in order to assimilate in the larger group.

Cultural expression assumes many forms, including language; spirituality; works of art; group customs and traditions; food preferences; response to illness, stress, pain, **bereavement**, anger, and sorrow; decision making; and even world philosophy.[1]

A Powerful Influence

An individual's cultural orientation is the result of a learning process that literally starts at birth and continues throughout the life span. Behaviors, beliefs, and attitudes are transmitted from one generation to the next. Although expressions of culture are primarily unconscious, they have a profound effect on an individual's interactions with and response to the health-care system—for better or worse.

Concepts of Culture

Culture is not a monolithic concept. Each individual probably belongs to several subcultures within their major culture. Subcultures develop when members of the group accept outside values in addition to those of their dominant culture. Even within a given culture, many variations may exist.[1] For example, it is logical to conclude that people who live in the United States belong to the American culture; this commonality is a part of every citizen's identity. However, teenagers living in the rural areas of Oklahoma may find it difficult to relate to teenagers raised in Philadelphia. Even though they may speak the same language and share a cultural perspective based on their ages, their life experiences are so different that it may be difficult for them to relate to each other.

Issues Now

When Cultural Traditions Are a Barrier to Care

Mrs. Sung, who is 74 years old, is brought into the emergency department (ED) by her family because of "very bad indigestion that won't go away." Three family members (a middle-aged man and woman and a younger woman) accompany her. They are discussing her condition in a mixture of English and another language the nurse does not recognize. Because the patient does not seem to understand any English, the nurse attempts to address the family. The younger woman speaks some English and manages to explain that the patient is her grandmother and that she is accompanied by her mother and father, who speak even less English than she does. The granddaughter explains that her grandmother arrived in the United States for a visit only 2 days ago from a small mountain village in Korea where she has lived all her life. She had been having periodic episodes of indigestion for several weeks before the visit and used traditional herbal teas prescribed by the local healer to treat her condition. On the basis of further assessment and a diagnostic test, it is determined that Mrs. Sung had an extensive myocardial infarction at least 1 week before her trip and is currently in a mild state of congestive heart failure (CHF).

She is given medications for the chest pain and CHF and is started on anticoagulant medications in the ED. She is then transferred to the coronary care unit (CCU), where she is scheduled to have a coronary angiography the next day. The angiogram shows multiple blockages in her coronary arteries and extensive myocardial damage. Because of her age and the extensive damage to her heart, the physician thinks it would be too risky to attempt bypass surgery and decides to monitor her closely and treat her medically until she is stable enough to have a balloon angioplasty.

When the CCU nurse assigned to Mrs. Sung enters the room at the beginning of her shift the day after the angiogram, she finds the patient covered with four heavy blankets and a bedspread and sweating profusely. When the nurse attempts to remove the excessive bedcovers, the patient's daughter protests vehemently and puts the blankets back on as soon as the nurse leaves the room. The daughter seems to think that her mother is sick because she is too cold and gives the elderly woman hot herbal drinks from a Thermos bottle she has brought from home.

Using a telephone medical-interpreting service, the nurse explains to the patient and her daughter why excessive heat is harmful to the patient's cardiac status and why she needs to follow the diet restrictions prescribed by the physician. The ingredients of the herbal drinks are unknown, and there may be some serious interactions with the numerous medications the patient is receiving. Although the patient's daughter outwardly seems to comply with the restrictions, she continues the traditional folk treatments in secret, believing the Western hospital food is bad for her mother's health.

(continued)

Issues Now (continued)

Mrs. Sung's condition gradually deteriorates during her hospitalization, despite all the medical treatment.

Questions for Thought

1. What factors should the nurse have noted during a cultural assessment of Mrs. Sung?
2. Besides the communication barrier, what cultural issues are involved in the care of Mrs. Sung?
3. Is there any way the nurses could have worked with the patient's belief system to aid in her care?
4. Are there any other measures the nurses could have taken in order to communicate better with the patient and her family?
5. The situation presented here is fictitious, but situations like it occur regularly in health-care facilities. How can nurses use transcultural nursing to avoid assuming that patients from other cultures are uncooperative and/or superstitious?

Culture can be envisioned as a flawed photocopy machine that makes duplicates of the original document with minor modifications. As a society attempts to preserve itself by passing down its values, beliefs, and customs to the next generation, slight variations in the practices inevitably occur. For the most part, the key elements of the culture remain intact. However, other elements change greatly due to influences from both within and outside the group.

Diversity

Diversity is a term used to explain the differences between cultures. The characteristics that define diversity can be divided into two groups: primary and secondary.

1. Primary characteristics tend to be more obvious, such as race, skin color, age, and possibly religious beliefs.
2. Secondary characteristics include socioeconomic status, education, occupation, length of time away from the country of origin, residential status, and sexual orientation. Secondary characteristics may be more difficult to identify, yet they may have an even more profound effect than the primary characteristics on the person's cultural identity.[2]

When individuals make generalizations about others based on the obvious primary characteristics or less evident secondary characteristics, they are stereotyping. A **stereotype** is an oversimplified belief, conception, or opinion about another person (or group) based on a limited amount of information.

MELTING POT VERSUS SALAD BOWL

The United States has traditionally been considered a melting pot of world cultures. Early in the history of the United States, most people who came from distant lands assimilated into American culture. Many people Americanized their names, shed their traditional dress, learned American manners and customs as quickly as possible, and learned English often without the benefit of formal schooling—all so that they could "fit in" with their new homeland. This practice of acculturation, altering one's cultural practices in an attempt to become more like members of the new culture, resulted in a blending, or melting pot, of cultures.[3] In the past, immigrants felt compelled to acculturate, and doing so was stressful. *Acculturative stress* occurs whenever a person from a minority or marginalized group adopts the ways of the dominant culture.

The Multicultural Salad

At present, individuals who migrate to the United States from other countries may maintain many of their traditional cultural practices and languages while learning American culture, resulting in a phenomenon called **multiculturalism**.[3] Rather than "melting" into the bigger pot as former immigrants did, many modern immigrants maintain their own unique cultural flavors and textures, much like the ingredients in a large tossed salad. As a growing phenomenon, multiculturalism is something that health-care providers need to be aware of; they must learn ways of adapting their health practices to allow for these diversities.[2]

Cultural Relativism

The current salad-bowl approach to acculturation has the advantage of allowing individuals in the dominant culture to gain an appreciation of other cultures for their unique contributions to society. A possible drawback of the salad bowl is that it can create pockets of culturally different individuals who have only minimal interaction with other parts of American society. If these individuals do not learn English or decide not to participate in the customs of the dominant culture, it can be challenging for them to gain an education, access health care or social services, find employment, or advance their socioeconomic status.

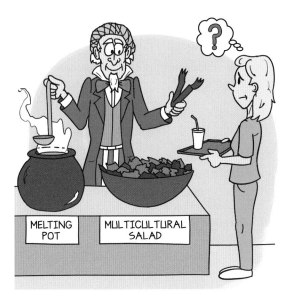

MELTING POT   MULTICULTURAL SALAD

The concept of cultural relativism can help people avoid having a knee-jerk negative reaction to cultural practices that are different from their own. Cultural relativism refers to not judging a culture according to one's own standards of what is right or wrong, strange or normal. Instead, it is trying to understand the cultural practices of the other group *in that group's own cultural context*. For example, let's say you hear that a new restaurant in town is serving fried crickets. If you are not familiar with this food, your first thought might be, "That's disgusting!" But take a moment to think like an anthropologist and ask, "Why do some cultures eat fried insects?" With a little research, you will learn that fried crickets or grasshoppers are full of protein and are crunchy and tasty. In Mexico, this food is part of Oaxacan regional cuisine. In fact, cultures around the world have used insects as a healthy food source for thousands of years. In cities on the east and west coasts of the United States, one of the hot "new" food trends is fried insects.

Cultural relativism is the opposite of ethnocentrism, which judges another culture's values and standards from the viewpoint of one's own culture. Ethnocentrism is the belief that one's own culture is better than that of others, not just different.

What Do You Think?

Identify and rank by priority at least five of your own health-care values (e.g., exercise, immunizations). Identify five health-care values of a culture different from yours with which you are familiar. How do these values compare with your own?

The salad-bowl approach to acculturation has the advantages of allowing immigrants to fit in and advance within the larger culture, while retaining many of the cultural elements that feel like home, which provides a sense of stability in their lives. In some individuals, however, it may create a type of cultural confusion that may lead to increased tension and anxiety.

A Population Shift

According to the U.S. Census Bureau in 2021 (the last year of available data before publication), approximately 130 million, or 42.2 percent, of the entire U.S. population was composed of underrepresented groups, up from 36.3 percent in 2010.[6] Between 2010 and 2021, the Hispanic/Latino population increased by 11.9 million, from 50.7 million in 2010 to 62.6 million in 2021. The White (non-Hispanic) population had the largest decrease, dropping 5.9 percentage points between 2010 and 2020.

If current trends continue, it is projected that by 2045, the White population will be a minority group, constituting 49 percent of the total U.S. population. In states such as California, the White population may be a minority as early as 2030. These shifts will require a redefinition or rethinking of the term *minority*, as it is currently defined as a racial or ethnic group that composes less than 50 percent of the population.[5]

The Need for Transcultural Nursing

Thanks to efforts on the part of the National League for Nursing (NLN), the American Association of Colleges of Nursing (AACN), and other organizations concerned with nursing education, the number of minority nurses has risen markedly from 10.7 percent in 2007 to 25.6 percent of the registered nurses (RNs) practicing in the United States in 2020 (the last year for available data). During the same time, the percentage of men who are RNs has risen from 5.4 percent to 9.4 percent.[6] The latest reported statistics from the AACN in 2020 demonstrate a marked increase in the number of minority students enrolled in basic nursing programs, from 29 percent in 2017 to 35 percent in 2020. To reflect American demographics accurately, the percentage of RNs from various minority groups should be approximately 33 percent and should mirror the percentage from each minority group.[7]

Culturally Competent Care

Cultural competence is the ability to successfully interrelate with individuals who belong to different cultures. In nursing, the goal of cultural competence is to focus on equality of care through the lens of patient-centered care that requires viewing each patient as a unique and individual person.[5]

Nurses from one culture should be able to give culturally competent care to individuals from any other culture. Health care is considered culturally competent when health-care providers and institutions provide care that meet patients' cultural needs. Ultimately, individuals and institutions with cultural competency provide high-quality care to every patient, regardless of language, race, or ethnic background.

Being on the front lines of health care, nurses are continually confronted with cultural changes that result from ethnic shifts in the population. Nurses lead the way in promoting an understanding of individuals from other cultures and in improving the overall quality of health care for everyone.

The Effects of Medicare and Medicaid

Medicare and Medicaid laws evolved out of the social programs of the 1960s. Because of increasing enrollment in these programs, there has been a corresponding increase in the number of economically and culturally diverse patients with whom nurses come in contact.

Before the Affordable Care Act (ACA) was enacted, the poorest segments of the population had the lowest percentage of insurance coverage. Before Medicare and Medicaid legislation, economically disadvantaged people of all racial and ethnic groups were unable to afford health care and were seen in the health-care setting only when severely ill. People with limited financial resources and those over age 65 are now covered by Medicaid and Medicare, respectively, and their presence in all levels and areas of health care has prompted nurses to become more sensitive to the transcultural aspects of their work. The ACA of 2010 also increased insurance coverage for citizens from the working-poor class so that they are now being seen more regularly in the health-care system.[8]

Since the 1970s, transcultural nursing has been an important subject in most nursing programs. However, nursing education lagged behind in taking steps to integrate cultural competence into daily practice. Nursing education programs, with incentives from accrediting entities, are now moving to incorporate cultural competency into their curricula. As technological and transportation advances bring increasing numbers of people from different cultures closer together, there will be an increased demand for nurses who can practice effectively in a culturally diverse society.[7]

> " *In nursing, the goal of cultural competence is to focus on equality of care through the lens of patient-centered care that requires viewing each patient as a unique and individual person.* "

DEVELOPING CULTURAL AWARENESS

Developing cultural awareness is the first step in becoming a culturally competent nurse. One of the main challenges for nurses who practice in a culturally diverse environment is to understand the patient's perspective of what is happening in the health-care setting. The patient's understanding may be very different from what the nurse believes is occurring.[9]

Awareness Begins at Home

Cultural awareness begins with an understanding of one's own cultural values and health-care beliefs and an exploration of one's own potentially prejudiced and biased views of others. Nurses need to become aware of their own biases and how they respond to people whose upbringings and cultural experiences differ from their own. For example, a nurse may realize that they think of all Hispanic immigrants as "illegal aliens." This nurse is beginning to develop an awareness of a cultural bias toward a particular group of people. A nurse develops cultural awareness only when they recognize and value a patient's culture, including beliefs, customs, responses, methods of expression, language, and social structure. However, merely learning about another person's culture does not guarantee that the nurse will have cultural awareness.

Beliefs about health care are based in part on knowledge and are often related to religious beliefs. To those unfamiliar with a particular culture's health-care beliefs, some of the health-care practices may appear meaningless, strange, or even dangerous. For example, if a particular group has no knowledge of bacteria as a cause of infection, antibiotics may seem useless in achieving a cure for the disease. With that in mind, if a society believes the illness is caused by evil spirits entering the body as the result of curses by witches or medicine men, practices such as incantations; use of ritualistic objects like bones, feathers, or incense; and even bloodletting and purgatives to release the spirit from the body are acceptable approaches to achieving a cure.

Cultural Belief Systems

Cultural belief systems are highly complex. Some beliefs and practices are kept as closely guarded secrets among the group's members, and there may even be some type of sanction or punishment for members who reveal the belief. Many cultural beliefs develop over time from a trial-and-error process that has both benefits and drawbacks. Some cultural beliefs have a primary purpose of explaining unusual or unpredictable events.

Cultural Values

Sources of cultural values include religious beliefs, worldviews and philosophies, and group customs. The values that underlie any culture are powerful forces that affect all aspects of a person's life, ranging from individual actions and decision making to health-care behaviors and life-goal setting. Values, which are discussed in Chapter 6, are the ideals or concepts that give meaning to an individual's life. They are deeply ingrained, and most individuals will strongly resist any attempt to change their value structure.[5]

Recognizing Health-Care Practices

Although nurses strive to provide the highest quality health care possible, a report by the Institute of Medicine (IOM), now called the National Academy of Medicine (NAM), indicates that multicultural health care often falls short of the mark.[10] In addition to patients who belong to racial or ethnic minorities, patients who are lesbian, gay, bisexual, transgender, queer/questioning, intersex, or asexual (LGBTQIA) also experience discrimination and worry about their ability to get equitable care.

Most nurses are conditioned to address problems that are obvious and within their line of sight, but sometimes it is necessary to take a step back and look at the bigger picture. Interprofessional collaboration provides a wider view and higher-quality culturally competent care.[8]

Motivating Patients to Change

It is important to recognize that one of the primary functions of nurses is to motivate patients to change ineffective health-care behaviors to ones that promote health. It is not an easy task. The first step, always, is to recognize that the nurse comes from a particular culture that has its own set of health-care values. Like all values, these have developed over time and are dependent on the nurse's education, upbringing, religious beliefs, and cultural background.

The next step is to identify the culture of the patient and recognize specific health-care beliefs and practices that are both similar to and different from those of the nurse. The nurse must then make a decision about whether it would be constructive or even possible to change the patient's belief on a specific matter and if the end result would be beneficial enough to put forth the necessary effort.[10] The nurse seeking to change a patient's ineffective health-care behaviors should look for ways to motivate the patient that are congruent with the patient's belief system.

> *To those unfamiliar with a particular culture's health-care beliefs, some of the health-care practices may appear meaningless, strange, or even dangerous.*

Issues Now

More Diversity Needed for the Future of Nursing

The nursing literature contains numerous studies showing the benefits to patients of having health-care providers who are "congruent" with them—that is, providers who are of the same race, cultural group, or gender as the patients. Yet despite these findings, the health-care workforce remains predominately white, and most nurses are women. Recruiting and retaining increased numbers of nurses from under-represented groups has been a primary goal of the health-care industry for almost a decade. Initiatives have been implemented by both the private sector and governmental agencies to increase the numbers of nurses from underrepresented groups to meet the needs of ever-shifting patient demographics.

A comprehensive report of all RNs in 2022 shows a moderate increase in the number of nurses from underrepresented groups since 2010. In 2010, there were 2.8 million RNs in the United States, and 24.6 percent were from underrepresented groups. In 2020 there were 4.9 million RNs with 32.3 percent in underrepresented groups. The following data is from 2022 and based on an estimated 4.2 million RNs. Numbers in parentheses indicate data since 2017.

80.6% (3,385,200) White/Caucasian (down from 80.8%)

11.4% (478,800) men of all ethnic groups (up from 9.1%)

7.2% (302,400) Asian (down from 7.5%)

6.7% (281,400) Black/African American (up from 6.2%)

2.3% (96,600) Other (down from 2.9%)

2.1% (88,200) More than one race category selected (up from 1.7%)

0.5% (21,000) American Indian or Alaska Native (up from 0.4%)

0.4% (16,800) Native Hawaiian or other Pacific Islander (down from 0.5%)

0.2% (8,400) Middle Eastern/North African (2020 was the first survey with this category)

In addition, 5.6% (235,200) of RN respondents self-identified as Hispanic/Latino/Latina, up from 5.3% in 2017.

Hospitals have been the primary employer of nurses of color and recognize that their employment is a matter of survival. In the competition to attract patients, hospitals cannot afford to have patients feel uncomfortable because of cultural diversity issues. Having a health-care workforce that is more reflective of the community it serves is essential because diversity in the nursing staff increases the quality of care for minority patients.[9] To help recruit nurses of color and retain those who are already practicing, several organizations have been established that nurses can contact. The National Coalition of Ethnic Minority Nurse Associations and the Tennessee Hospital Association's Council on Diversity are available for assistance.

Sources: *By the numbers: Nursing statistics 2023.* Carson-Newman University Online, *2023. https://onlinenursing.cn.edu/news/nursing-by-the-numbers*

Racial/ethnic composition of the RN workforce in the U.S. Campaign for Action, 2022. https://campaignforaction.org/resource/racialethnic-composition-rn-workforce-us/

When Is Persuasion Appropriate?

Many cultures have strong values concerning pregnancy and the birth of children. In some cultures, for example, the birth process is valued as an event strictly involving women, and the father is usually not present to either witness or assist in the delivery.[9] However, midwives and obstetric nurses from the mainstream American culture place a high value on the father's participation in the birth as a way of promoting stronger family ties and starting the bonding

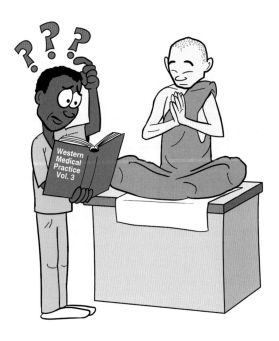

process as soon as possible. The nurse who takes care of a family that does not want the father involved in the birth can invite the father to stay in the delivery room during the delivery but must understand, if he refuses, that it is not due to his unwillingness to be there but to the cultural norms of the group.

Members of some cultures believe in the effectiveness of "medicine bags" and special leather or beaded necklaces in protecting infants from harm and promoting their growth. A medicine bag is a spiritual container used by some Native Americans, which takes the shape of a small pouch made of leather often decorated with beads. It can be filled with just one or several sacred objects and is worn around the person's neck to keep the bag close to the wearer's heart. The object placed in the bag is usually something the person feels a close affinity to. For example, if a person believes that bears are their animal spirit, they may place a bear tooth in the bag. However, they may also place items such the ashes of a beloved family member who was cremated or dirt from a sacred prayer location. These types of items cause nurses to have concerns about hygiene and sterility of procedures.

It is not unusual to observe infants wearing these types of necklace bags when they come to medical clinics for care.[11] The main concern of providers in these clinics is the possibility of the infant choking if the necklace should become entangled. But the cultural importance of the necklace is so strong that parents may refuse to remove the necklace, or they may remove it for the clinic visit and then put it back on after.[11] Because of the ethical principal of autonomy or self-determination, the most health-care providers can do is teach the parents about the potential dangers of the necklaces and hope they will reconsider the risk.

Assessing Culture

Obtaining accurate cultural assessments can be time consuming and difficult. However, such assessments help nurses to avoid imposing their own cultural values and practices on others and to develop plans of care based on their knowledge about others' beliefs and customs.

Beginning the Assessment

The following key questions can serve as a starting point for a cultural assessment:

- Why do you think you are ill? What was the cause of the illness?
- What was going on at the time the illness started?
- How does the illness affect your body and health?
- Do you consider this to be a serious illness?
- If you were at home, what type of treatments or medications would you use? How would these treatments help?
- What type of treatment do you expect from the health-care system?
- How has your illness affected your ability to live normally?
- If you do not get better, what do you think will happen?

Because patients from different cultures may feel uncomfortable revealing information about cultural beliefs, values, and practices to strangers, it is a good idea to begin your assessment by asking some general questions. A patient is more likely to trust a nurse who demonstrates interest in that person as an individual. Only after a warm and trusting environment has been established will a patient be willing to reveal the more personal aspects of their culture to the nurse.

Understanding Physical Variations

Physical assessments made on individuals from other cultures also require a certain level of cultural awareness and competence. Before the assessment begins, health-care workers need to be aware that certain garments are worn for a variety of religious, cultural, or other deeply personal reasons. Sensitivity is needed, for example, when asking a Sikh patient to remove his turban, a Muslim patient to remove her hijab, or a transgender man to remove his chest binder. Although the assessment techniques used for different individuals may be identical, the nurse also needs to know the basic biological and physical variations among ethnic groups.[12] The interpretation of assessment findings may be affected by ethnic variations in anatomical structure or characteristics (e.g., children from some Asian and Central American cultures may fall below the normal growth level on a standardized North American growth chart because of their genetically smaller stature).

> *Only after a warm and trusting environment has been established will a patient be willing to reveal the more personal aspects of their culture to the nurse.*

Changes in skin color may also affect the interpretation of assessment findings (e.g., cyanosis in people with a light versus a dark complexion). To determine whether the patient's skin color is normal or abnormal, the nurse must know what constitutes the normal color for a particular complexion. In assessing for cyanosis, the nurse may need to examine the patient's oral mucosa and may also need to measure capillary refill times to determine whether the patient has cyanosis.

As with all assessments, the ultimate goal of cultural assessment is to provide the best care possible for the patient.[12] A fundamental nursing principle is that all patients have a right to self-determination, including the customs, practices, and values that emanate from their culture. By considering cultural variables of each patient, nurses will avoid practice that is ethnocentric and conducted strictly from the nurse's cultural viewpoint.

Issues in Practice

Cultural Aspects of Organ Donation

"Sarah, are you going to ask them?" The tall, haggard third-year trauma resident stood across the desk from me and eyed me with apprehension.

"Well," I sighed, "he's medically suitable and has been declared brain dead. So, yes, I'm going to ask them." I had been coordinator of the New Mexico Organ Procurement Organization for more than 2 years and had asked families for permission to obtain organs for transplantation literally hundreds of times.

"But they're Navajo," he said.

"Organ donation is an option for them," I replied. "They deserve to be offered the option at the very least."

"Can I come in with you?" he asked. "There are a lot of people in there."

"Sure," I said.

So, after reviewing the patient's case file to identify the legal next of kin, the resident and I went into the ICU conference room to approach a traditional Navajo family for consent for organ donation.

As I entered the room, 13 pairs of eyes looked up at me. I took a deep breath, let the resident introduce me, and we began our conversation.

The family was young, and the patient had never married, so the oldest daughter was making the decisions. She had a lot of good questions for me, as did the rest of the family, and I talked with them for a long time.

Issues in Practice (continued)

"You know we're Navajo?" one of her brothers asked me. "Organ donation is against our beliefs."

"I realize that," I said, "but you have the option to save a life, possibly as many as three lives, and I wanted to let you know."

"Our uncle got a kidney transplant last year," the oldest daughter said while looking at her brother. "I think we owe something back. Can we have some time to talk about this?"

I thanked them for their time, expressed my condolences again, and left the room with the resident. Once we were back on the unit, the resident got excited.

"Oh, man. I think they're going to say yes," he said, shifting from one foot to another.

Just then, the doors to the ICU swung open and a pair of elderly Navajo women walked into the unit and right up to the desk where I was sitting. They inquired which room my patient was in and went in after I told them. They hovered at the patient's bedside for several minutes, regarding the medication pumps, the monitors, and the ventilator with disdain.

Silently, the pair left the unit through the doors they had just entered.

"Who are they?" the resident asked.

"I believe those were the tribal elders," I said.

He looked at me with disbelief. "What do we do now?"

"Now we wait," I said.

Minutes later, the oldest daughter appeared around the corner. I could tell she had been crying.

"Can we see the doctor in our room?" she asked.

"Sure. Wait here and I'll go get him," I said.

I went around the corner where he was lounging with his feet propped up on the desk. He was chatting with the unit clerk. "I really think they're going to do it," he said.

"The family wants to see you," I interrupted.

When he looked at me, I saw a question mark on his face. I returned the look with one of my own. Having been in this situation a couple of times before, I had a feeling I knew what the outcome would be.

We walked around the corner, and he went into the conference room with the family, and I returned to my desk to wait.

Two minutes later he was back. He slumped into the chair beside me. "They declined," he sighed disappointedly. "What do I do now?"

"You," I said, "are done. Thank you very much for all your time and hard work. I've got to do some paperwork and call in the decline, and then I'm going home."

He sighed again. "Well, good effort."

Questions for Thought

1. Was it ethical to ask the family about organ donation when their beliefs generally prohibit it?
2. Was there another possible approach to seeking permission from the family?

Source: *Sarah T. Catalano, coordinator, New Mexico Organ Procurement Organization.*

Transcultural Understanding

Cultural competence has become a buzzword in the health-care system. It describes the skill to successfully interact with people who belong to dissimilar cultures and the preparedness to comprehend and interact with individuals of different races, ethnicities, gender identities, and sexual orientations. Even when the patient's beliefs, health-care practices, and values directly conflict with orthodox medical and nursing practices, using cultural competence skills allows the nurse to gain the patient's trust, be empathetic to their needs, and be successful in treating them. Cultural competence as it relates to nursing can be regarded as the provision of effective care for patients who belong to diverse cultures, based on the nurse's knowledge and understanding of the values, customs, beliefs, and practices of the culture.[9]

Providing culturally competent care requires the development of certain interpersonal skills that allow nurses to work with individuals and groups in the community. The primary skills required for cultural competence include communication, understanding, and sensitivity. Although the basic types of cultural skills are similar, their application within and between cultural groups may differ greatly. The development

of cultural competence is not a one-time skill to check off on a skills checklist; rather, it is an ongoing process that continues throughout the nurse's career.[9]

Transcultural Communication

The ability to communicate is the foundation on which culturally competent care is built. The most obvious barrier to culturally competent care for the non-English-speaking patient is the lack of a common language (Box 21.1). Be aware that patients who are deaf or hard of hearing also face a communication barrier. It is recommended that all communication between a patient who does not use the same language as the care providers should be carried out through an approved medical interpreter. In the case

---

Box 21.1 Guidelines for Communicating With Non-English-Speaking Patients

1. Avoid using relatives as interpreters; they may distort information or not be objective.
2. Avoid using children as interpreters, especially with sensitive topics.
3. Maintain eye contact with both the patient and the interpreter to elicit feedback and read nonverbal clues.
4. Remember that patients can usually understand more than they express; thus, they need time to think in their own language. They are alert to the health-care provider's body language and may forget some or all of their English in times of stress.
5. Speak slowly without exaggerated mouthing, allow time for translation, use active-voice verbs rather than passive voice (e.g., say "Take the medicine every 4 hours" instead of "The medicine should be taken every 4 hours"), wait for feedback, and restate the message. Do not rush; do not speak loudly. Use a reference book with common phrases, such as *Roget's International Thesaurus* or *Taber's Cyclopedic Medical Dictionary*.
6. Use as many words as possible in the patient's language and use nonverbal communication when unable to understand the language.
7. Use same-age and same-gender interpreters whenever possible. However, patients from cultures who have a high regard for elders may prefer an older interpreter.
8. Use interpreters rather than translators. Translators restate the words from one language to another, whereas interpreters decode the words and provide the meaning behind the message.
9. Use dialect-specific interpreters whenever possible.
10. Use medical interpreters if at all possible.
11. Give the interpreter time alone with the patient.
12. Provide time for translation and interpretation.
13. Be aware that interpreters may affect the reporting of symptoms, insert their own ideas, or omit information.
14. Note that social class differences between the interpreter and the patient may result in the interpreter's not reporting information that they perceive as superstitious or unimportant.
15. If an interpreter is unavailable, the use of a translator may be acceptable. The difficulty with translation is omission of parts of the message; distortion of the message, including transmission of information not given by the speaker; and messages not being fully understood.

Source: S. Groenwald, *Designing and creating a culture of care for students and faculty: The Chamberlain University College of Nursing model*, Washington, DC: National League for Nursing, 2017.

of patients who are deaf or hard of hearing, a medical interpreter proficient in American Sign Language (ASL) is needed. If an interpreter is not available, a translator can be used; however, the two are not the same. The key skills of the translator include the ability to understand the source language of the patient and then to repeat those words clearly and accurately in the second language. In other words, the most important mark of a good translator is the ability to translate the source language word for word into the second language.[13] For some cultural groups, having a translator who is of the same generation and the same gender as the patient is also a consideration.

An interpreter, on the other hand, must be able to translate in both directions on the spot. Interpreters must have extraordinary listening abilities, especially for simultaneous interpreting. Simultaneous interpreters need to process and memorize the words of the source language while the patient is speaking, then translate into the second language the words that the speaker said 5 to 10 seconds ago. This process allows interpreters to instantly transform emotions, idioms, colloquialisms, and other culturally specific references into analogous statements enabling the second-language care provider to understand. Medical interpreters must be fluent in the medical terminology of both languages. They must also able be to "read" the emotional context of the translation source and relay that to the secondary hearer.[13] Hospitals refer to the U.S. Department of Health and Human Services standards for Culturally and Linguistically Appropriate Services (CLAS) when providing language services for patients (Box 21.2).

Box 21.2 U.S. Department of Health and Human Services' Culturally and Linguistically Appropriate Services (CLAS) Standards

Principal Standard

Standard 1: Health-care organizations should provide effective, equitable, understandable, and respectful quality care and services that are responsive to diverse cultural health beliefs and practices, preferred languages, health literacy, and other communication needs.

Governance, Leadership, and Workforce

Standard 2: Health-care organizations should advance and sustain organizational governance and leadership that promotes CLAS and health equity through policy, practices, and allocated resources.

Standard 3: Health-care organizations should recruit, promote, and support a culturally and linguistically diverse governance, leadership, and workforce that are responsive to the population in the service area.

Standard 4: Health-care organizations should educate and train governance, leadership, and workforce in culturally and linguistically appropriate policies and practices on an ongoing basis.

Communication and Language Assistance

Standard 5: Health-care organizations must offer language assistance to individuals who have limited English proficiency and/or other communication needs, at no cost to them, to facilitate timely access to all health care and services.

Standard 6: Health-care organizations must inform all individuals of the availability of language assistance services clearly and in their preferred language, verbally and in writing.

Standard 7: Health-care organizations must ensure the competence of individuals providing language assistance, recognizing that the use of untrained individuals and/or minors as interpreters should be avoided.

Standard 8: Health-care organizations must provide easy-to-understand print and multimedia materials and signage in the languages commonly used by the populations in the service area.

(continued)

Box 21.2 U.S. Department of Health and Human Services' Culturally and Linguistically Appropriate Services (CLAS) Standards (continued)

Engagement, Continuous Improvement, and Accountability

Standard 9: Health-care organizations should establish culturally and linguistically appropriate goals, policies, and management accountability and infuse them throughout the organizations' planning and operations.

Standard 10: Health-care organizations should conduct ongoing assessments of the organization's CLAS-related activities and integrate CLAS-related measures into assessment measurement and continuous quality improvement activities.

Standard 11: Health-care organizations should collect and maintain accurate and reliable demographic data to monitor and evaluate the impact of CLAS on health equity and outcomes and to inform service delivery.

Standard 12: Health-care organizations should conduct regular assessments of community health assets and needs and use the results to plan and implement services that respond to the cultural and linguistic diversity of populations in the service area.

Standard 13: Health-care organizations should partner with the community to design, implement, and evaluate policies, practices, and services to ensure cultural and linguistic appropriateness.

Standard 14: Health-care organizations should create conflict- and grievance-resolution processes that are culturally and linguistically appropriate to identify, prevent, and resolve conflicts or complaints.

Standard 15: Health-care organizations are encouraged to communicate the organization's progress in implementing and sustaining CLAS to all stakeholders, constituents, and the general public.

Source: National standards on culturally and linguistically appropriate services (CLAS) in health and health care, U.S. Department of Health and Human Services, Office of Minority Health, https://thinkculturalhealth.hhs.gov/assets/pdfs/EnhancedNationalCLASStandards.pdf

---

Communication is a highly complex process that requires both verbal and nonverbal exchanges. Nonverbal communication includes (but is not limited to) body language, facial expressions, eye contact, personal space, touch and body contact, formality of names, and time awareness. Other factors that affect communication are volume of voice, tone, and acceptable greetings. Often, patients communicate differently with family and friends than they do with health-care personnel. Nurses should be aware that in some cultures (e.g., those with a strong caste system or class structure), communication between those in the upper and lower classes may be affected by tradition. For example, some cultures hold the role of women in health care in high esteem, whereas other cultures may consider women in health care as the bottom rung on the social ladder.

Nonverbal Responses

Nurses who work with non-English-speaking patients need to develop alternative ways to measure a patient's understanding rather than depending only on a verbal response. Nurses must be cautious when interpreting the nonverbal responses from some cultural groups, which may respond to all questions with a yes, a nod, or a smile. In the American culture, this response usually indicates understanding and **compliance**. However, in some cultures, nodding and smiling can be signs of respect for the nurse's position or an attempt to avoid confrontation. For example, see the Issues Now box at the beginning of this chapter.

Speech Patterns

The use of silence by some cultural groups has led to misunderstandings in the health-care setting. For example, some cultures may consider silence to be a sign of respect, particularly for elders, whereas individuals of other cultures use silence to gain privacy or to indicate agreement.[12]

Variations in communication styles also account for misunderstandings and miscommunications. Factors such as loudness, intonation, rhythm, and speed of speech all are important in communication. Some nurses may speak at a rapid rate and use medical jargon. Others may increase the volume of their voices when communicating with patients who do not speak English, as if talking more loudly will increase understanding.[12]

On the other hand, members of some cultural groups often speak more softly and may be difficult to hear even when the nurse is standing at the bedside. These individuals may misinterpret the louder, more forceful tone of the nurse as an indication of anger. To prevent misunderstandings, nurses need to analyze their own speech patterns and consciously modify their tone and pace when working with different cultural groups.

Personal Matters

Nurses also need to recognize that some people are much less willing than others to disclose private matters or personal feelings. Members of some cultures tend to be less secretive about almost all issues because the practice of sharing has been encouraged from an early age, but members of other cultures may be highly reluctant to discuss personal topics at all. Other groups may discuss personal issues openly with friends and family members but may be reluctant to do so with healthcare providers whom they do not know well.[10] There can also be wide variations within cultural groups.

Open-Ended Language

It can be productive to start the communication process with small talk and general, nonthreatening questions to establish a trustworthy rapport. Often, the use of open-ended questions and statements allows the patient to express beliefs and opinions that would be difficult to discover through closed-ended questions that the patient can answer with a simple yes or no.

As the level of trust increases, the patient will be more likely to reveal important information in the more sensitive areas of the assessment. In addition, sensitivity to the nonverbal aspects of the communication process allows nurses to use behaviors that increase trust and to avoid gestures, facial expressions, or eye contact that the patient may interpret as superiority, hostility, anger, or disapproval.

Touch Misinterpreted

A leading cause of miscommunication in the healthcare setting is touching patients in ways that they consider inappropriate.[10] In the United States, nurses are taught early in their first nursing classes, usually in physical assessment or basic skill courses, that it is necessary to "lay on hands" in order to provide quality care. Students who are reluctant to palpate the femoral pulses of their laboratory partner or remove a patient's shirt for **auscultation** of anterior heart and breath sounds may receive a failing grade for the course.

However, touching can convey a number of alternative meanings, ranging from power, anger, and sexual arousal to affirmation, empathy, and cordiality, and the meaning of touch varies across cultures. As a standard practice, do not ask a patient to take off any clothes and do not touch any part of their body that is not directly related to the presenting problem. It is extremely important for the nurse to ask permission and to explain, *before the particular physical contact occurs*, what they are going to do and why it should be done. The nurse should also avoid any unnecessary contact, such as palpation of femoral pulses when the patient has pneumonia.

> **When a person's personal space is violated, it often creates a generalized feeling of discomfort or threat, which causes the person to move away from the offending individual.**

Personal Space

Closely related to the issue of touch is the concept of personal space. Personal space is a zone that individuals maintain around themselves in most casual social situations. When a person's personal space is violated, it often creates a generalized feeling of discomfort or threat, which causes the person to move away from the offending individual. Nurses routinely violate patients' personal space when performing physical assessments or providing basic care.

The distance required to maintain a comfortable personal space varies widely from one culture to another. Members of some cultures prefer close contact, standing face to face, and maintaining eye contact throughout an entire conversation. Members of other cultures may prefer between 18 and 22 inches of space and intermittent eye contact for comfort.[2]

It is easy to understand why misinterpretations in communication might arise. A patient from one culture might judge a nurse from another culture to be cold and aloof, although the nurse is merely maintaining what for them is a comfortable personal space from the patient. Likewise, the same nurse may feel physically threatened by the close communication style of a patient and continually back away from the patient in an attempt to reestablish a comfortable personal space.[2]

Eye Contact

Similarly, the use of eye contact differs among groups and between individuals and can lead to miscommunication. People on the autism spectrum may avoid eye contact because it makes them uncomfortable. In the United States, frequency of eye contact differs between people who identify as men and those who identify as women. Among some cultures, making periodic eye contact during conversations indicates

Issues Now

Informed Consent Requires Understanding

Sinwan Ho, an elderly woman who spoke very little English, was admitted to the Gastromed Health Care Center for a routine colonoscopy and polypectomy, which was performed on May 20, 2003, by Lawrence Kluger, MD. During the procedure, the bowel was perforated. The next day, Ms. Ho underwent a laparotomy with removal of the damaged part of the colon and the formation of a colostomy.

Ms. Ho was readmitted on September 2, 2003, to have the colostomy closed and the colon reconnected. She recovered well, but several years later, she began experiencing abdominal pain and gastrointestinal symptoms. It was determined that lesions had formed in the reconnected bowel and were closing the bowel. On April 20, 2006, Ms. Ho was readmitted, and another colostomy was performed. Later that year, on September 6, 2006, the colostomy was again closed with reconnection of the bowel. The patient had a total of five surgeries related to the first routine procedure.

Dr. Kluger was initially sued for malpractice, but the court could not find conclusive evidence that he had committed any medical errors, and the case was dismissed as a "bad outcome."

Later, a suit was filed on behalf of Ms. Ho. According to her testimony and that of a friend, Kenneth Lee, she had not been properly informed of the possible complications of the procedure in language that she could understand. She did sign the informed consent form when it was handed to her. The court determined that lack of clear communication of the possible complications was a deviation in the standard of care.

In further testimony, Dr. Kluger admitted that he knew the patient did not speak much English and that he had made no attempt to find an interpreter to help explain the procedure and the possible complications, such as bowel perforation and colostomy. However, his lawyer argued that because the possibility of an intestinal perforation with a resulting colostomy is so low, revealing that information did not meet the state's requirement as a "reasonable degree of medical probability."

The court ruled that Dr. Kluger's failure to adequately communicate the complications of the procedure did not meet the requirement for malpractice. However, it did rule that there was a case for medical negligence based on the premise that failure to disclose what a reasonable and prudent patient would want to know is a deviation from a standard of care.

In 2010, the hospital's insurance company settled the case for an undisclosed sum, imposing a gag order on all parties and without acknowledging wrongdoing by the hospital or the physician.

Source: Ho v. Kluger, A.2d, 2009 WL2431591 (N.J. App., August 11, 2009), http://www.leagle.com/decision/In%20NJCO%2020090811191.

attentiveness to the communication and is a means of measuring the person's sincerity. Common sayings such as "Look me in the eye when you say that" and admonitions for public speakers to make eye contact with the audience emphasize the underlying positive value these cultures place on eye contact. Lack of eye contact may be interpreted as inattention, insincerity, or disregard.

In contrast, other cultures believe that the eyes are the windows of the soul and that direct eye contact by another may be interpreted as an attempt to "steal the soul" from the body. In other cultures, direct eye contact is a sign of challenge and aggression and may precipitate a violent physical confrontation.[12] Sustained eye contact can also be seen as sign of disrespect, and eye contact with a child is believed by members of some cultures to convey the *mal de ojo*, or "evil eye." Many childhood and adult illnesses among these cultures are attributed to the effects of the evil eye, and practices such as tying red cloths or strings around children's wrists may be used to ward off illnesses.[2]

> *Nurses may label patients from other cultures as noncompliant, when in reality the nurse has an incomplete understanding of the patient's culture or unrealistic expectations for behavior.*

The complexity and importance of communication should never be underestimated when working with patients from diverse cultures. Merely speaking a language does not encompass the entirety of communication. Awareness of the meanings of gestures, body positions, facial expressions, and eye movements is essential in culturally competent communication.

LOOKING DEEPER

Several other elements must be considered for effective transcultural nursing, including passive obedience, cultural synergy, building on similarities, and conflict resolution. *Passive obedience* refers to a type of behavior that develops when patients from a different culture believe that the nurse is an authority figure or expert in health-care matters.[15] Members of these cultures may try to cope with the uncertainty of their health status and the threat of an authority figure by becoming passively obedient. Rather than asking questions they think will reveal their lack of

knowledge or confusion about some health issue or that they believe may challenge the authority of the nurse, they become compliant.

Cultural Conflicts

It is inevitable that conflicts will arise from time to time when a nurse cares for patients of different cultures. Nurses may label patients from other cultures as noncompliant, when in reality the nurse has an incomplete understanding of the patient's culture or unrealistic expectations for behavior. Common reasons for noncompliance among culturally diverse patients include the lack of external symptoms of disease, inconvenient or painful treatments, and lack of external support from family members or close friends. However, it is the nurse's responsibility to dig deeper to understand the reason for the patient's resistance to a particular treatment. For example, some patients may not be taking their prescribed medication because they cannot afford it, not because of their cultural beliefs.

What Do You Think?

Think of the last patient for whom you provided care. What were the cultural differences that affected the care you gave? What measures did you use to overcome these differences? What might you have done differently to improve care?

Respect for Healing Traditions

The nurse first needs to ask the patient what, if any, traditional treatments they use in dealing with this disease. In cases in which the traditional treatments are similar to the ones used by the health-care facility, the nurse may be able to demonstrate this similarity to the patient.

In other cases, the treatments may be very different. However, if culturally based alternative treatments do not interfere with the prescribed treatment plan or threaten the patient's health, they can be used simultaneously with the standard medical treatments.

Cultural Synergy

Cultural synergy is an attempt to bring two or more cultures together to form an organization or environment that is based on combined strengths, concepts, and skills. Cultural differences are used to encourage mutual growth by cooperation.[2] Developing cultural synergy implies that health-care providers make a commitment to learn about other cultures and to immerse themselves in those cultures. Nurses who work actively to develop cultural synergy tend to be more successful in the delivery of competent transcultural care. Nurses achieve cultural synergy when they begin to selectively include values, customs, and beliefs of other cultures in their own worldviews. The first step in building cultural synergy is the desire to know everything about another culture and to purposely establish relationships with individuals from other cultures.[2]

More Alike Than Different

Closely related to cultural synergy is the recognition that most cultures are alike in many respects. Many books and publications written about cultural diversity present only the differences between cultures and not the similarities. Although recognition of cultural differences is important, it should be just one step toward the ultimate realization that there are more similarities than differences among diverse cultures.

INFORMATION SOURCES FOR TRANSCULTURAL NURSING

Like all practice areas in the profession, transcultural nursing is also striving to increase the quality of care by using best practices based on evidence-based practice (EBP). Through the rapid growth of research and information sources on transcultural nursing, new models and theories have been developed. However, these new theories and models may lead some individuals to assume that patients can be categorized by race, culture, and ethnicity. The reality is that individual patients cannot be put into culturally specific boxes or labeled by virtue of their culture or skin color. People are individuals, and the common beliefs or behaviors of a particular cultural group do not accurately describe every patient who belongs to that racial, ethnic, or cultural group.

> *People are individuals, and the common beliefs or behaviors of a particular cultural group do not accurately describe every patient who belongs to that racial, ethnic, or cultural group.*

From a Conference . . .

With the rapidly increasing diversity in the United States, there is a growing need for nurses who can practice transcultural nursing. The origins of the current transcultural movement can be traced back to 1974, when a transcultural conference on communication and culture was held at the University of Hawaii School of Nursing. Following the success of this conference, a series of transcultural conferences was planned over the next year to bring together nurses, sociologists, anthropologists, and other social scientists to discuss issues that would eventually form the basis for transcultural nursing.

Not long after the Hawaii conference, the Transcultural Nursing Society was organized. It was incorporated in 1981 and began publishing its semiannual *Journal of Transcultural Nursing* in 1989. The publication is now a peer-reviewed quarterly journal that provides information on all aspects of culture and nursing both in print and online. In 1976, the American Nurses Association (ANA) recommended that multicultural content be included in nursing curricula. Since then, the ANA, in conjunction with the Expert Panel on Global Nursing and Health, developed Standards of Practice for Culturally Competent Nursing Care in 2010 and revised them in 2014.

. . . to a Specialty

Since the 1980s, increasing numbers of universities and colleges have started offering graduate degrees in transcultural, cross-cultural, and international nursing. Graduates are now able to become certified transcultural nurses (CTNs) by completing oral and written examinations offered by the Transcultural Nursing Society. Nurses do not need to be from underrepresented groups to obtain the CTN qualification.

Society has not remained stagnant during this period of development and organization. Growing numbers of immigrants, changing governmental regulations, and grassroots movements all have contributed to the pressure placed on nursing to recognize and effectively care for patients from different cultures.

Issues in Practice

Case Study: Cultural Conflict Within a Family

Jose Bisigan, age 87 years, and his wife Carmen, age 85, sold their small restaurant and immigrated to Los Angeles from a small town in the Visayan region of the Philippines. They came to join their firstborn daughter, a nurse named Felicia, age 54; her husband; and their three children, ages 10, 13, and 18. Mr. Bisigan speaks limited English and is in a poststroke rehabilitation unit. Since the stroke, he has had mild aphasia, mild confusion, and bladder and bowel continence problems. His hypertension and long-standing diabetes are controlled with medication and diet. His wife, daughter, and grandchildren have been supportive of him during this first hospitalization experience. Mr. Bisigan's family has cooperated with the health team, often agreeing with minimal resistance to the prescribed treatment management. The rehabilitation team recommended subacute rehabilitation treatment as part of the discharge plan.

As a businessman and the elder in the family household, Mr. Bisigan is looked to for counsel by the immediate and extended family. Mr. Bisigan's status, however, has caused friction between Felicia and her husband, Nestor, an American-born Filipino who works as a machinist. Nestor has accused Felicia of giving excessive attention to her mother and father. Felicia's worries about her parents' health have made Nestor very resentful. He has increased his already daily "outings with the boys." Felicia maintains a full-time position in acute care and a part-time night-shift position in a nursing home.

Mr. Bisigan's discharge is pending, and a decision must be made before Medicare coverage runs out. Felicia has to consider the possible choices available to her father and the family's circumstances and expectations. Mrs. Bisigan, who is being treated for hypertension, has always deferred decisions to her husband and is looking to Felicia to make the decisions. Because of her work schedule, the absence of a responsible person at home, her mother's health problems, and intergenerational friction, Felicia considers nursing home placement. She is, however, reluctant to broach the subject with her father, who expects to be cared for at home. Mrs. Bisigan disagrees with putting her husband in a nursing home and is adamant that she will care for her husband at home.

Felicia delayed talking to her father until the rehabilitation team requested a meeting. At the meeting, Felicia indicated that she could not bring herself to present her plan to put her father in a nursing home because of her mother's objection and her own fear that her father will feel rejected. Feeling very much alone in resolving the issue about nursing home placement, she requested the team to act as intermediary for her and her family.

Questions for Thought

1. Identify cultural family values that contribute to the conflicts experienced by each family member.
2. Identify a culturally competent approach the team can use when discussing nursing home placement with the Bisigans.
3. How might the rehabilitation program be presented to Mrs. Bisigan and still allow her to maintain her spousal role?
4. Discuss at least three communication issues in the family that are culture-bound and suggest possible interventions.
5. Identify psychocultural assessments that should be done by the rehabilitation team to have a greater understanding of the dynamics specific to this family.
6. Identify health promotion counseling that might be discussed with the Bisigans' grandchildren.
7. Identify and explain major sources of stress for each member of this household.

Source: *S. Groenwald,* Designing and Creating a Culture of Care for Students and Faculty, *Washington, DC: National League for Nursing, 2017.*

Diversity and Sexuality

Sexuality is the way humans experience and express themselves through sex, which involves biological, erotic, physical, emotional, social, and even spiritual feelings and behaviors. *Sexuality* is an expansive term and does not have a precise definition. Many factors can influence a person's sexual interest in and attraction for another person. Profound feelings of trust, love, or care combined with physical and erotic aspects of sexuality establish strong bonds between individuals.[14]

Sexuality can be thought of as a spectrum of behaviors and orientations. For example, people may be heterosexual, homosexual, bisexual, or asexual; or they may choose not to label their sexuality at all. The majority of the world's population is heterosexual, or straight; that is, they are sexually attracted only to members of the opposite sex. But, as is true with virtually everything related to patients, health-care providers should not make assumptions about sexuality but rather should ask, sensitively and professionally, and only when appropriate.

Sexual orientation refers to where a person's sexual attraction is directed. Terms related to sexual orientation include the following:

- *Asexual (also "ace")* refers to someone who has no sexual attraction toward others but who may experience emotional or romantic attraction.
- *Bisexual* (also *polysexual, heteroflexible, homoflexible*) refers to a person who has sexual feelings toward both cisgender men and cisgender women. Bisexual individuals commonly have a distinct, but not exclusive, sexual preference for one gender over the other.
- *Heterosexual* refers to sexual attraction to members of the opposite gender, whether they are cisgender or transgender.
- *Homosexual* refers to sexual attraction to members of the same gender.
- *Gay* refers to sexual attraction between people who identify as men, but the term can be used by women also.
- *Lesbian* refers to sexual attraction between people who identify as women.
- *Pansexual* (also *omnisexual*) refers to sexual attraction to persons including cisgender men and women, transgender men and women, and people who identify as nonbinary.

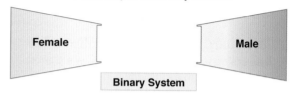

Female only or male only normal?

Figure 21.1 Binary system. A system of identification that divides its members into one of two sets of identities based on the appearance of the genitalia at birth.

Gender identity is an individual's experience of their gender. Gender identity can correlate with the sexual assignment at birth (cisgender), or it can differ from it (Fig. 21.1). In most societies, the dominant culture has a set of beliefs about "appropriate" masculine and feminine behavior based on sexual designation. Behavior that differs from cultural expectations can create problems for individuals in all aspects of their lives. Terms related to gender identity include the following:

- *Cisgender (cis)* refers to individuals whose gender identity aligns with their sex assigned at birth.
- *Gender neutral* refers to individuals who do not feel or a have strong personal connection to either gender role despite their sex assignment at birth. At times, they may display actions of either gender or assume gender-neutral clothes, hairstyle, behaviors, and actions. They may adopt and use gender-neutral first names and prefer the use of the plural pronouns *they, them, their,* and *theirs.*
- *Gender nonconforming* refers to a person whose behavior or gender expression does not match masculine or feminine gender behavioral norms of the society. These individuals are also sometimes referred to as *gender variant, gender diverse, gender atypical,* or *genderqueer.*
- *Genderfluid* refers to individuals who do not identify themselves as having a fixed gender.
- *Intersex* is a general term used for a variety of congenital conditions in which a person is born with a reproductive or sexual anatomy that does not fit the typical definitions of female or male. For example, a person might be born with the external genitalia of a female and be assigned the female sex while having components of male-typical genitalia internally. However, the term *intersex* is sometimes incorrectly

used to identify individuals with ambiguous genitalia or atypical genitalia. Some experts believe that in order to be truly intersex, the brain of the person has to be exposed to an unusual mix of hormones in utero so that even if a person is born with atypical external genitalia, they may not actually be intersex.[14] *Intersex* has replaced the offensive term *hermaphrodite.*

- *Nonbinary (enby,* also *agender, genderqueer)* refers to someone who doesn't identify with any gender.
- *Transgender (trans)* refers to individuals whose gender identity does not correspond with their sex assigned at birth.

People have sex, so it is important for nurses and health-care providers to be able to have knowledgeable, nonjudgmental conversations with their patients about this topic. Asking patients about their sexual partners and the kinds of sex they are having helps health-care personnel assess for sexually transmitted illnesses and secondary conditions related to certain types of sexual acts, to make effective differential diagnoses, and to provide teaching customized to the patient's needs.

Nurses should not assume that everyone they care for is cisgender or straight; neither should they make assumptions about a patient's sexual behavior without asking. For example, men who have sex with men (MSM) may or may not identify as exclusively homosexual or gay. Anal sex is usually associated with MSM; however, many MSM do not engage in anal sex and may engage in oral sex or mutual masturbation instead.[14]

Gay men typically have about the same number of unprotected sexual partners annually as straight men and women. However, human immunodeficiency virus (HIV) is transmitted by anal sex more frequently than by any other transmission route because of the difference in the anal and vaginal mucosa. A worrisome statistic is the rise in the incidence of syphilis among MSM in the United States. Contracting syphilis increases the likelihood of HIV transmission. In addition, anal warts are significantly more common among men who recently had sex with men than among men who recently had sex only with women (MSW). On the other hand, genital herpes is less common among MSM than among MSW. Chlamydia, human papillomavirus (HPV), gonorrhea, and genital lice saw no significant difference between MSM and heterosexual groups.

Infectious disease specialists in 2022 noted that anyone can be infected with monkeypox, and the disease is not limited to gay men; however, gay men did have the highest incidence of the infection at that time. Monkeypox is not officially classified as a sexually transmitted infection but rather as a contact infection. It can spread not only through oral, anal, and vaginal sex but also through close personal contact; contact with fluid from a skin lesion; touching objects, fabrics, and surfaces used by someone with the virus; and contact with respiratory secretions. Monkeypox can also infect a fetus through the mother's placenta.[15]

Women who have sex with women (WSW) may or may not identify as exclusively homosexual or lesbian. Like all sexually active women, WSW are at risk of acquiring sexually transmitted infections (STIs) such as genital herpes, genital warts, or other pathogenic infections. When sexual activity is nonpenetrative, the risk of WSW exchanging bodily fluids is generally lower, and therefore the likelihood of transmitting STIs is also relatively low. Although the risk for HIV transmission from exclusively lesbian sexual activity is significantly lower than it is for male–female and male–male sexual activity, it still can occur. HIV can be spread through bodily fluids, such as blood including menstrual blood, vaginal fluid, and breast milk. It can also be transmitted by oral sex if the person has cuts or sores in the mouth or poor oral hygiene. Pathogens such as metronidazole-resistant trichomoniasis; genotype-concordant HIV; HPV, which has been linked to nearly all cases of cervical cancer; and syphilis can be spread through sexual contact between women.[15]

TRANS-AFFIRMATIVE NURSING CARE

As discussed earlier, nursing education places an emphasis on teaching students to provide culturally competent, patient-sensitive care. Over the past few decades, another group—the transgender community—has joined the diverse patients whom nurses care for. Information about trans-affirmative care, much like culturally competent care, should be infused throughout the nurse's whole education program and not just as a one-hour unit during the junior year.[16]

Not All the Same

Gender identity is self-determined and based on many factors and life experiences, including in utero hormone exposure, home life, social experiences, personal relationships, and cultural environments. (See Fig. 21.2.) Gender identity cannot be assigned by someone else based only on the appearance of a person's genitalia. Defining some terms will help to clarify the discussion that follows:

• *Gender-affirmation treatments and procedures* (also called *medical transitioning*) describes the hormone treatment and/or surgery a transgender individual may undergo to attain the physical characteristics that conform to their gender identity.
• *Social transitioning* occurs when a transgender person assumes a name, appearance, and clothing that correspond to their gender identity.
• A *cross-dresser* is a person who wears items of clothing and other accessories associated with the opposite sex within a particular society. Cross-dressing has been used for purposes of sexual gratification, disguise, comfort, and gender identity self-discovery. Also called *transvestic fetishism*, it is most often practiced by heterosexual men and is not related to being transgender.
• In *drag*, a person, typically male, cross-dresses as a form of performance art or theater. Often, drag involves exaggeration or parody of gender differences through dress and behavior as a means of provoking an audience reaction.

• *Disorders of sexual development (DSD)* (also *disorders of sex differentiation* or *differences of sex development*) are medical conditions that involve the reproductive system. Although the use of the terms is controversial and somewhat nonspecific, they are similar to intersex conditions. The terms are often used with older children who have abnormally developing genitalia.
• *Sex assignment* is the male or female designation given to an infant either before birth by use of ultrasound examination or at the time of birth based on the appearance of the external genitalia. Sex assignment can be very difficult to legally change on official documents such as birth certificates, hospital records, and passports.
• *Misgendering* is wrongly identifying the gender identity of a person either intentionally or by mistake. Misgendering is insulting, insensitive, demeaning, or even abusive. A common form of misgendering is *deadnaming*, using the transgender person's former, opposite-gender name.
• *Gender dysphoria (GD)* (or *gender identity disorder [GID]*) is the emotional or mental distress individuals experience because the gender they were assigned at birth does not match their gender identity. GD, although a psychiatric diagnosis, by itself is *not* categorized as a mental disorder or disease. However, if the person with GD displays clinically significant distress or symptoms such as eating disorders, depression, stress, isolation, anxiety, poor self-esteem, and suicidal behavior, then psychotherapy or counseling is recommended to support the individual's identified gender.[16]

Respectful and Sensitive Care

Each person is an individual, and part of any good nursing assessment is obtaining as much pertinent information possible about a patient's health, history, and culture. One element to remember in providing respectful and sensitive care to transgender patients is that they likely have known and possibly struggled with their gender identity for most of their lives, starting as early as 4 or 5 years of age. Older transgender patients who grew up at a time when their identity was considered a mental disability, mental or physical illness, moral transgression, or even a crime may require special sensitivity on the part of the nurse. Despite improvements, discrimination still exists against transgender elders in nursing homes

Gender identity is:

• Usually established by age 3 but may take into adulthood
• Deeply felt sense of a woman being a man, a man being a woman, or a person being both man and woman or being in a state of uncertainty or being neither woman nor man

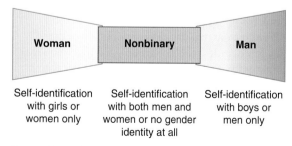

| Woman | Nonbinary | Man |

| Self-identification with girls or women only | Self-identification with both men and women or no gender identity at all | Self-identification with boys or men only |

Figure 21.2 Gender identity.

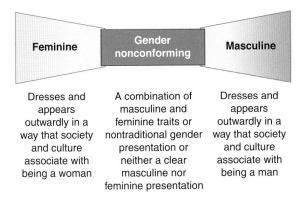

Figure 21.3 Gender expression: Outward physical ways for a person to display their inner beliefs about their real gender identity through appearance, clothing, behavior, mannerisms, adopted roles, and outward signs.

and long-term care facilities.[17] And discrimination against transgender people of all ages is still relatively common.

Although mainstream American culture is becoming more accepting of the spectrum of sexual orientations and gender identities, a significant percentage of the population still clings to the biases and stereotypes of prior generations. (See Fig. 21.3.) Recent legislative decisions restricting transgender people's use of public restrooms, military changes in recruiting and deploying transgender service members, and court decisions allowing businesses to refuse service to gay or transgender people display the deep-rooted and ongoing cultural bias against these groups.[16]

Some health insurance companies deny payment for gender-affirming treatments and surgery for transgender patients because companies code these procedures with the patient's gender marker used when the insurance policy was initiated. Some insurers will deny payment for routine screening tests, such as a Pap smear, if the patient is designated a male on insurance documents, despite the fact that a transgender man may still have a cervix.[16]

NANDA Approved

LGBTQIA patients, when they come into a provider's office or a facility for physical health care, will likely have a history of discrimination and bias due to their sexuality or gender identity in addition to a presenting physical complaint. For this reason, a variety of NANDA-I diagnoses may be appropriate, depending on the patient's experiences, behaviors, and presence or absence of social support.

Advancing Equity

It is important to assess and monitor transgender patients for symptoms of depression, anxiety, or particularly suicidal ideation. Many transgender patients experience changes in their relationships with families, friends, and coworkers during their transition that may include intimate partner violence or workplace abuse. Transgender patients also are frequent targets of street violence, which disproportionately affects transgender women of color. The social stigma that these patients may have experienced can take a toll on their emotional state, and they may display societal phobias. Some transgender individuals are fearful because many have experienced bullying and violence and have been targeted for hate crimes in their past.[17]

In 2022, the Biden administration issued an executive order aimed at advancing LGBTQIA health equity. The order was based on the recognition that health equity for the transgender patient population has historically been marginalized by the health-care system. Research shows that transgender individuals experience much higher rates of chronic health conditions as compared with the cisgender population. Prior discrimination and social stigma influence their physical and mental health. The Biden administration's efforts in advancing equity for transgender individuals was in response to new legislation by some states that attempted to limit the rights of LGBTQIA individuals. These new state laws were based on biased misinformation that spread across the nation focusing on reducing transgender health-care rights.

Taking time to establish a nonjudgmental, trusting nurse–patient relationship is critical. Doing so can be challenging because many transgender people have experienced negative interactions with past health-care providers who may have been uninformed, insensitive, or openly negative to them about their status. Some individuals are very sensitive about their body and may have fragile body images. If physical care is required that involves the genital area, such as inserting a urinary catheter or giving an enema, make sure to ask, if possible, what gender nurse the patient would prefer to perform the procedure.[18]

An important fact to remember is that the nurse is caring for the transgender person at one point in time for one particular health issue. The process of transitioning, however, occurs over a long period of time, sometimes with stops and starts along the way, and is a deeply personal decision. The needs of a person at the end of the process are very different from those of a person who is just beginning to transition.

Sensitive Care Begins at the Door

A transgender patient's first contact with the health-care setting, whether it is the waiting room, clinic receptionist, admissions personnel, or ward clerk, may set the tone for the entire visit. When the patient is standing at the admissions desk for a regular office visit, they have taken a hugely courageous step that will involve disclosure of some of their most personal information.[16]

Health-care environments can be made more accepting of transgender patients by simply having signs for gender-neutral bathrooms. Physicians, nurses, as well as intake personnel should be trained to ask *every* patient what name they prefer to be called and what pronouns the person prefers. This practice allows all patients, including transgender and nonbinary ones, to relax and feel accepted.[16] Not all transgender persons use the pronouns listed in Box 21.3, but some do, so it is important to be familiar with them.

Although basic standards of care have been developed for use with transgender patients (discussed

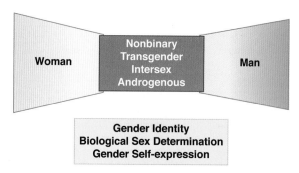

Figure 21.4 Elements in gender formation.

shortly), providing respectful and sensitive care for this population is an ongoing process with a rather steep learning curve for many nurses.[16] Terminology and the words used to describe gender identity and sexual orientation are evolving. Because of the diversity of experiences among individuals, when a patient tells you they are transgender, never assume that you understand the entire story for that person. (See Fig. 21.4.) Everyone's journey is different.

What Nurses Can Do

Nurses can do what they have always been good at doing. They can create a warm and trusting environment where *all* patients can feel safe in divulging highly personal information about themselves. In order to obtain the information required for high-quality nursing care, the nurse must be sensitive to patients' emotions and open to their information without any appearance of judgment, bias, or rejection.

The best and simplest way to find out what title to use with a transgender patient is to ask the patient how they wish to be addressed.[16] If you make a mistake, apologize sincerely. Also, listening carefully to patients and how they speak about themselves and others can be helpful in determining what particular titles and pronouns to use.[12]

Using good communication skills is essential with *all* patients. Review the section in Chapter 11 on therapeutic communication, keeping in mind how these techniques might best be used in communicating with transgender patients. One of the best methods to obtain information is to use open-ended questions or statements. For example, "How can I help you today?" or "Tell me what your major concern is." Be careful

---

Box 21.3 **Respectful and Sensitive Care**

Using Gender-Neutral Pronouns

- Ze (pronounced *zee*) instead of she. "Ze bought a new dress."
- Xe (pronounced *zshee*) instead of he. "Xe went to the potluck for dinner."
- Hir (pronounced *here*) instead of her. "Hir new dress was too big."
- Zir (pronounced *zhere*) instead of him. "They welcomed zir at the dinner"
- Hirs (pronounced *heres*) instead of hers. "The last dress on the rack was hirs."
- Zirs (pronounced *zheres*) instead of his. "Zirs ate a lot at the dinner."

about how you address visitors in the patient's room. Rather than asking the visitor, "Are you Lee's wife?" it is better to ask the patient, "Who is with you today?"

Transgender patients have a variety of health-care needs that are not related to their transition. Patients who are undergoing gender-affirmation treatment or surgery have their own expert provider who is supervising the hormone and/or surgical treatments; these patients will go to that provider for transition-related health care. However, like any other person, transgender patients can have gallbladder attacks, fractures, infections such as flu or cystitis, cardiac issues, and so forth.[12]

It is not always necessary to ask about a patient's sexual history or gender history (if their gender differs from the sex assigned at birth). However, if this part of a patient's history does need to be evaluated, it may be best to lead into the topic with a statement such as "So that I can provide you with the best care possible, I need to ask some questions related to your sexual activities and/or your transition" or "It is our standard practice here to take a sexual history for every patient we serve." If the health issue is related to the patient's transgender status, the nurse should ask about how the patient defines their identity, where the patient is in the transition process, and what their transition goals are.[16]

Transgender patients may also be hesitant to provide information for a spiritual assessment. (See Chapter 20.) Many transgender individuals have had strong negative experiences with organized religion, ranging from intensive religious-related psychiatric counseling and medications and physical abuse to outright banishment during a church service.[19] Sometimes transgender persons may feel that God made a mistake when He created them or that they are terrible sinners with no hope of redemption. On the other hand, many transgender individuals are very spiritual.[19] Some may attend church and be an active part of the church community if it is accepting of them.

Because transgender individuals are also at relatively high risk for intimate-partner violence, the nurse may wish to carefully investigate if there are any obvious indications of abuse.[18] Nurses who feel particularly uncomfortable communicating with transgender patients should try role-playing responses with other nurses who are more skilled in communication. However, the bottom line is that patients have the ethical right to self-determination and can choose not to answer questions they do not wish to answer.

As with all patients, confidentiality is of utmost importance. Transgender individuals, particularly those in the early stages of transition, may not have revealed the information to anyone. When they reveal the information to the nurse during the admission assessment, it is best for the nurse to ask, "Have you told anyone else about your status?" If they say no, then that should be noted so that other nurses will not accidently "out" the patient to family or friends.

The Health Insurance Portability and Accountability Act (HIPAA) can be violated easily by sharing this type of information with anyone who is not directly involved in the care of the patient. It is both an ethical and a legal violation that may result in employment termination, lawsuits, and heavy fines for the nurse and the facility. Nurses often do not realize how much patients are able to hear of what is being discussed at the nurses' station. Unbecoming or demeaning comments made between nurses or other care providers at the nurses' station about a transgender patient are a sure way to erase a caring atmosphere, destroy trust, and shut down future communication. Jokes about a patient's, visitor's, or coworker's sexual orientation or gender identity are on the same level of incivility as racist jokes. Such comments or jokes about a transgender patient carry the same penalty as any other violation of protected health information.

Education Tips

Health education for transgender patients is key for their health and well-being in the future.[20] Unless they have been under the care of a provider who specializes in gender affirmation or transgender issues, they may require help "unlearning" false information and letting go of false beliefs before learning new information. Transgender patients who are unable to find a provider near them who can or will prescribe hormones may self-medicate with nonprescribed hormone medications obtained online, on the black market, or in unregulated countries. Stressing the dangers of taking these medications without the supervision of a knowledgeable provider is essential.

Of course, nurses need to be well grounded in accurate information before they attempt to educate transgender patients. The *Standards of Care* published by the World Professional Association for Transgender Health is a highly useful source of information for providers. It uses a comprehensive approach to transgender-specific health care, including changes in gender role, hormone use, and feminizing or masculinizing surgical procedures. A number of other high-quality sources of information are listed at the end of this section.

When teaching transgender patients, it is important to stress the need for regular screenings and physical examinations. If the patient feels comfortable with a particular provider in a clinic, have the patient ask for that person. Screenings and examinations should include the full range of tests. For example, a transgender woman who has had bottom surgery needs to have regular prostate examinations because that gland is not usually removed during gender-affirmation surgery.[16]

Transgender men who choose to pursue surgical transition may have male chest reconstructive surgery ("top surgery") and/or removal of the uterus, fallopian tubes, and ovaries ("bottom surgery"). If the internal organs are left intact, a regular Pap smear is recommended, as is routine breast examination, even if the patient has had top surgery.

Patient education should also include the information that smoking increases risks for blood clots and breast cancer among transgender women taking estrogen. Transgender patients should be made aware that they are at higher risk for alcohol abuse, drug misuse, higher rates of anxiety and depression, and greater risk of STIs (including HIV) than the cisgender population.[20] These patients may also need additional information on resolving gender-identity issues and how to respond to individuals who are ignorant or insensitive about transgender issues.

Developing a Trans-Affirmative Climate

Being a patient advocate is one the nurse's primary roles. For many years, LGBTQIA patients have experienced the same type of health-care disparities that other cultural minorities did and still do. To change the way transgender patients are treated, facilities must create an atmosphere of transgender inclusiveness.[20]

> ❝ *When teaching transgender patients, it is important to stress the need for regular screenings and physical examinations.* ❞

Nurse advocacy can begin with individual nurses who are personally or professionally motivated to learn as much as they can about transgender patients and then informally educate their colleagues in key aspects of communication and care. It may also involve speaking out to interrupt jokes about transgender patients or correcting other providers who are displaying unprofessional behavior.

If the nurse believes that there is an institution-wide deficit of knowledge about the care of transgender patients, advocacy should be expanded to the development and adoption of transgender-inclusive policies. Most nurses currently in active practice were educated when the box at the top of the chart admission sheet was checked either "M" or "F" and all of the rest of the care that was provided was based on that dichotomy.

In today's health-care system, nurses are finding that the binary sexual designation on the chart is not always accurate. Over the past few generations, Western understanding of gender identity, including gender expression, has evolved from an either-or designation to a continuum of internalized identities. On any given day, nurses work with patients who express their gender in various ways and patients who are at different places along the continuum in their gender transformations.

Admission forms should be modified so that patients can fill in their sex assigned at birth and their current gender identity. Alternatively, checkboxes for sex assigned at birth (male, female), transgender woman, transgender man, gender queer, or other could be included. When the provider or staff member sees that the patient's birth-gender designation is different from the gender identity they listed, the nurse will know immediately that this person is transgender.

Some transgender and nonbinary patients may not want any gender at all noted on the medical record, which would require a "none" or "not given" box. Many hospitals have no mechanisms for dealing with requests for no gender designation.

Advocating for a facility-wide trans-affirmative atmosphere includes ongoing education in the care needs of transgender patients.[20] If the facility does not have routine in-service training on the care of transgender patients, these modules need to be developed or purchased and added to the nurses' regular in-service education program. There should be a section in the policy manual that deals with transgender patient care and issues. If there is not, the nurse should ask the policy and procedure committee to develop one or should develop a policy and submit it for approval.

Nurses as Life Savers

For transgender patients, positive experiences with health-care providers have sometimes been an important element in saving their lives. These patients report that nurses have cared for them through difficult issues, such as when they came out to their families and friends, or helped them to strengthen their identities, build self-esteem, and overcome depression. When nurses demonstrate genuine interest, patience, and a willingness to spend time and listen to patients, the transgender patients will begin to feel that they are in a safe environment where their most personal and guarded information will not be ridiculed by uninformed or biased people.

Sources of Information on Transgender Issues

- National Resource Center on LGBT+ Aging, https://www.lgbtagingcenter.org
- World Professional Association for Transgender Health Standards of Care, https://www.wpath.org
- SAGE, https://www.sageusa.org
- National Coalition for LGBT Health, https://www.jointcommission.org/lgbt
- Center of Excellence for Transgender Health at the University of California, www.transhealth.ucsf.edu/trans/page=program=care
- Facts on LGBTQ aging. *SAGE & National Resource Center on LGBT Aging*, 2021. https://www.sageusa.org/wp-content/uploads/2021/05/sage-lgbt-aging-final-2021.pdf
- *More Than Pink: LGBTQ Breast Health*, http://komenpugetsound.org/wp-content/uploads/2016/11/More-Than-Pink-LGBTQ-Breast-Health_web.pdf

Source: Resources for LGBTQI+ Students, U.S. Department of Education Office of Civil Rights, 2022, https://www2.ed.gov/about/offices/list/ocr/lgbt.html.

Conclusion

The major changes in U.S. demographics that began in the 1980s—and have been accelerating ever since—require nurses to provide culturally sensitive care to an ever-growing number of individuals. Although not yet highly likely, there is a chance nurses will find themselves caring for a transgender patient from a different culture who may not even speak English. A fundamental belief of professional nursing holds that *all* individuals are to be cared for with respect and dignity regardless of sexual orientation, race, culture, beliefs, gender identity, or disease process. Therefore, nurses must actively seek to educate themselves about the diversity of human experience in order to practice at the top of their license.

However, nurses need to keep in mind that assessments of and decisions about care of their transgender patients are relative to the nurse's own personal experiences, beliefs, and culture. There is a natural tendency among people to unconsciously stereotype, on the basis of their own internal value system, individuals who come from other cultures or whose gender expression differs from expectations. There is also a tendency to generalize about individuals from one culture or group when in reality there may be wide variations within that group.

Nurses who have a high level of cultural knowledge and sensitivity maximize their nursing interventions when they become coparticipants and patient advocates for individuals who might otherwise be lost or mistreated in the health-care system. When nurses understand the patient's perspective, develop an open style of communication, become receptive to learning from diverse patients, and accept and work with the ambiguities inherent in the care of these individuals, they become truly competent health-care providers for all patients.

CRITICAL-THINKING EXERCISES

- Look up the census data for your city or town for the years 2010 and 2020. Did the percentage of culturally different individuals change? What changes do you anticipate seeing in the 2030 census or in the 2040 census if the same trends continue?
- What cultural group(s) do you belong to? Identify and list five traditions or cultural practices that you and your family follow.
- Is it possible for people from a different culture to use both the salad bowl and melting pot approaches to acculturation at the same time? Provide an example of how this might occur.
- List the elements of culturally competent care that you have developed so far in your career. What other skills do you need to work on to become fully culturally competent?
- Find the policy and procedure manuals for your nursing school and the primary facility you attend for clinical experiences. See if there are policies on the care or treatment of transgender individuals. Is the policy up to date? Does it include the information presented in this chapter? If there is no policy, try developing one with the help of your fellow students or nursing professor.
- Have you or any of your classmates taken care of transgender patients during your clinical experiences? If you have, how did you deal with the various issues outlined in the chapter?

NCLEX-STYLE QUESTIONS

1. Which of the following statements about the melting pot and salad bowl theories of acculturation is TRUE?
    1. In the melting pot, immigrants must give up their cultural practices.
    2. In the salad bowl, members of different immigrant groups live separately from each other and from members of the dominant culture.
    3. The salad bowl allows members of different groups the opportunity to learn about one another's unique contributions to society.
    4. The melting pot helps prevent people from judging other cultures according to their own standards of what is normal.
2. Raquel, a nursing student, just learned about secondary cultural characteristics and is making a list of hers. Which of the following should she include on this list? **Select all that apply.**
    1. Olive complexion
    2. Woman
    3. Middle class
    4. Lesbian
    5. 20 years old

3. Marcus, an RN, is assessing his new patient, Mr. Hassan, a 68-year-old Syrian immigrant admitted to the hospital with pneumonia. Marcus asks Mr. Hassan, "What do you think caused this illness?" What is Marcus trying to elicit from Mr. Hassan?
    1. Mr. Hassan's cultural health beliefs
    2. Mr. Hassan's medical opinion
    3. The underlying cause of Mr. Hassan's pneumonia
    4. An assessment of Mr. Hassan's ability to speak English
4. Thalia, a nurse at a community health clinic, needs to teach a patient who speaks only Spanish about the medication he has been prescribed, which must be taken with food every 6 hours. Thalia took 2 years of Spanish in high school. What should Thalia do to ensure her teaching is as effective as it can be?
    1. Give the patient a Spanish-language pharmaceutical pamphlet about the medication.
    2. Speak loudly and slowly, using as much Spanish as she can remember.
    3. Ask the patient's young son to translate for her.
    4. Use a medical interpreter to communicate her teaching and relay questions from the patient.

5. In a report, Sue, a new-graduate RN, learns that one of the patients she and her nurse-trainer will care for today is an elderly man from South Korea. Sue has never met anyone from Korea, and she is eager to do so. Sue and her trainer enter the man's room to conduct their start-of-shift assessment. Which action by Sue indicates the need for more training in culturally competent care?
   1. Sue clearly introduces herself and her trainer and asks the patient what he prefers to be called.
   2. Sue quickly explains that they are there to assess the patient and begins to untie his gown.
   3. When the patient smiles and nods in response to a question about pain, Sue follows up to verify that he understands the question.
   4. Sue listens carefully when the patient answers questions and gives him plenty of time to answer.

6. A community clinic wants to show that it welcomes all patients. Which of the following actions can the clinic take to show that it is inclusive and welcoming? **Select all that apply.**
   1. Posting stickers of the rainbow flag, the human rights flag, and/or the transgender flag in its window
   2. Asking patients what they prefer to be called
   3. Using patients' preferred pronouns
   4. Not assuming that a transgender patient's visit relates to his or her transition
   5. Having gender-neutral restrooms

7. Tayesha, a triage nurse in the emergency department, is assessing a patient who presents with a fever of 101°F, nausea, sharp pain in the right lower quadrant of the abdomen, and abdominal swelling. The patient is a transgender man who is scheduled to have bottom surgery in 2 months. What priority nursing action should Tayesha take?
   1. Contact the surgeon who will be performing the patient's bottom surgery.
   2. Get a complete history of the patient's transition so far.

3. Report the patient's symptoms to the physician on duty.
4. Place a damp washcloth on the patient's forehead to lower their temperature.

8. Dr. Ochoa asks the nursing students in his class to list elements that should be included in a teaching plan for a patient who is a transgender woman. Which element named by a student indicates the need for further instruction?
   1. Smoking increases the risk of blood clots among transgender women taking estrogen.
   2. Regular mammograms are recommended.
   3. Having annual wellness examinations and getting scheduled immunizations are important to maintain health.
   4. After bottom surgery, there is no need to have regular prostate examinations.

9. Jordan, a new patient who identifies as nonbinary, is checking in at the doctor's office for a wellness examination. Which response from the front-desk administrator demonstrates culturally competent care?
   1. "Do you go by 'Jordan,' or is there another name you would prefer we use?"
   2. "Hi, Jordan! I need to know if you're a man or a woman in order to file with your insurance company for today's visit."
   3. "I hear you are nonbinary. That's so cool!"
   4. "Will you be needing a Pap smear today?"

10. When is it appropriate for a health-care provider to ask a patient about their sexual partners, the kind(s) of sex the patient is having, and their gender history (if the patient's gender is not the same as the sex assigned at birth)? **Select all that apply.**
   1. To assess the patient's risk for sexually transmitted illnesses (STIs)
   2. To provide teaching about safe sex practices
   3. To determine if the patient requires additional health screenings (e.g., prostate examination)
   4. To assess the patient's need or desire for contraception
   5. To demonstrate interest in the patient as a person

References

1. Deering M. Cultural competence in nursing. *NurseJournal*, November 29, 2022. https://nursejournal.org/resources/cultural-competence-in-nursing/

2. Why is cultural diversity important in patient care? Excel Medical, January 30, 2022. https://www.excel-medical.com/why-is-culturally-diversity-important-in-patient-care/

3. The Diversity Digest: Spring 2023 Edition. *AACN*, 2023. https://www.aacnnursing.org/news-data/all-news/article/diversity-digest-spring-2023-edition

4. Our changing population. USA Facts.org, 2022. https://usafacts.org/data/topics/people-society/population-and-demographics/our-changing-population

5. Frey W, The US will become "Minority White" in 2045, census projects. *Brookings*, 2018. https://www.brookings.edu/blog/the-avenue/2018/03/14/the-us-will-become-minority-white-in-2045-census-projects/

6. 2020 U.S. population more racially and ethnically diverse than measured in 2010. United States Census Bureau, 2021, https://www.census.gov/library/stories/2021/08/2020-united-states-population-more-racially-ethnically-diverse-than-2010.html

7. Diversity in nursing begins at the student level. *ONS Voice*, March 1, 2022. https://voice.ons.org/news-and-views/diversity-in-nursing-begins-at-the-student-level

8. McKnight G. How did the ACA increase healthcare coverage? Very Good Coverage, n.d. https://www.verygoodcoverage.com/post/how-did-the-aca-increase-access-to-health-insurance

9. How to practice cultural competence in nursing. *St. Catherine University*, 2021. https://www.stkate.edu/academics/healthcare-degrees/cultural-competence-in-nursing

10. Diversity and inclusion at IOM. IOM.int, 2022. https://www.iom.int/diversity-and-inclusion-iom

11. What is a medicine bag? Thunder Wolf Medicine Lodge, 2022. https://thunderwolfmedicinelodge.weebly.com/what-is-a-medicine-bag.html

12. Cultural physical assessments: What they are and how to conduct one. Indeed, 2021. https://www.indeed.com/career-advice/career-development/cultural-assessment

13. How to become a certified medical interpreter. Medical Interpreting Training School, March 2, 2022. https://medicalinterpretingtrainingschool.com/how-to-become-a-certified-medical-interpreter/

14. Lockwood J. Getting gender identity and sexual orientation right. TheHRDirector, August 25, 2022. https://www.thehrdirector.com/business-news/diversity-and-equality-inclusion/getting-gender-identity-sexual-orientation-right/

15. Kochi S. Fact check: Monkeypox can spread to anyone through close contact. *Austin American-Statesman*, August 17, 2022. https://www.statesman.com/story/news/factcheck/2022/08/17/fact-check-monkeypox-can-spread-anyone-through-close-contact/10262679002/

16. Eight tips for creating a trans-affirming health care environment. Center for Community Practice, 2022. https://www.urccp.org/article.cfm?ArticleNumber=31

17. United States: Transgender people at risk for violence. Human Rights Watch, November 18, 2021. https://www.hrw.org/news/2021/11/18/united-states-transgender-people-risk-violence

18. Fatal violence against the transgender and gender non-conforming community in 2022. Human Rights Campaign, n.d. https://www.hrc.org/resources/fatal-violence-against-the-transgender-and-gender-non-conforming-community-in-2022

19. Weitzman C. Religion vs. transgender mental well-being. Religion can present itself as a cultural foundation that is challenging to overcome. Gender Wellness of LA, n.d. https://genwell.org/complications-religion-transgender-mental-well-being/

20. Siwicki B. How health IT can advance health equity for transgender and nonbinary patients. *Healthcare IT News*, August 3, 2022. https://www.healthcareitnews.com/news/how-health-it-can-advance-health-equity-transgender-and-nonbinary-patients

Impact of the Aging Population on Health-Care Delivery

22

Joseph Molinatti | Joseph Catalano

THE SILVER TSUNAMI

The U.S. health-care system was designed primarily to treat acute illness and injury. But today, the health-care system is evolving to provide high-quality care for chronic illnesses and to address behaviors and personal issues of an aging population. This rapid growth in the older population has been coined the "silver tsunami," the "gray tsunami," or the "silver/gray wave." Like a huge wave flooding the land, the large numbers of baby boomers are increasing the demand for health services focused on chronic disease, comorbidity, and the unique health promotion needs of older adults. However, most older adults are relatively healthy and manage their chronic conditions at home. Although older Americans' concept of what it means to be healthy is different from the expectations of younger people, as long as they can continue to live independently, they consider themselves to be in good health.[1]

Nurses are dealing with a rapidly aging population as the baby boomers (adults born between 1946 and 1964) become 65 and older. More than 49.2 million people in this group will have one or more chronic illnesses by 2030. Older adults have an increased risk for chronic illness, which includes diseases and conditions such as obesity, diabetes, coronary artery disease (CAD), chronic obstructive pulmonary disease (COPD), dementia, cardiovascular disease (CVD), cancer, osteoarthritis, and depression. Even though the majority remain in their homes, the older population has more hospitalizations, more admissions to nursing homes, and a higher likelihood of losing the freedom of living in their own homes; therefore, the possibility of experiencing low-quality care increases for older adults simply because they are participating in the health-care system more frequently.[1]

What Do You Think?

Have you ever taken care of an older patient in a hospital setting? How was the experience different from providing care for younger patients?

- Critique the elements in disaster preparation for the elderly and generate an effective evacuation plan
- Discuss older adults' view of spirituality and how it impacts their health status
- Identify the key elements in the transitioning of care of the older adult and discuss the nurse's role in promoting a safe transition for the patient

Ageism

Ageism is a type of discrimination that includes prejudice against people based on their age and comprises holding negative stereotypes about people of different ages, both younger and older.[1] Age discrimination can be seen in a wide variety of settings and situations, including the workplace and in health care. The impact of ageism can be serious and can lead to pay disparities, forced retirement, or difficulty finding employment.[2]

Following are several signs of ageism:

- Exclusion from a group, such as at school or at work
- Being passed over for promotions or raises
- Being laid off or forced to retire
- Negative comments about a person's age
- Having the older person's input or ideas ignored or dismissed
- Losing out on benefits such as paid time off
- Not having access to new learning opportunities[1]

Stereotypes such as the following frequently develop among the younger population because of their expectations of how older people should behave:

Succession: Younger people often assume that older individuals have "had their turn" and should get out of the way for the younger generations.

Consumption: Younger people may feel that older individuals have used their share of limited resources, which now should be used on themselves.

Identity: Younger people often feel that the older generation tries to act younger than they really are by, for example, using contemporary jargon or wearing progressive fashions.[3]

Ageism is a commonplace occurrence. As many as one out of every two people may hold moderately or highly ageist attitudes. Ageism also has a damaging impact on both the physical and mental health of the individuals who are targeted. It can lead to isolation, deterioration of overall health, and reduced life expectancy.[1]

A Major Killer

Because the older population is living longer, chronic disease has become a major problem and a leading cause of death, although falls and the resultant injuries remain one of the top causes of death. The healthcare system is continually increasing its focus on the chronic disease process. Nearly half of Americans ages 20 to 74 have some type of chronic condition.[2] Each year, 7 out of 10 Americans die from chronic diseases, with strokes accounting for more than 50 percent of all the deaths. Chronic disease accounts for more than 36 million deaths per year globally.[2]

All the major health organizations have identified obesity and diabetes as major health concerns. More than 25 percent of people with chronic conditions are limited in one or more activities. Arthritis is the most common cause of restricted activity, and diabetes continues to be the leading cause of kidney failure and blindness among adults. The reality is that chronic diseases have no measurable cures. The best that can be hoped for is to treat the symptoms and slow the disease's progress.

❝ Being in a familiar environment makes the older adult more apt to remain independent and have a sense of comfort and belonging. ❞

Individuals who have multimorbidity problems require longer hospital stays. Although *morbidity* can have different meanings in different contexts, here it refers to the condition of being in a disease state or poor health. Although each disease in a multimorbid presentation may not be acute or fatal in itself, together they contribute to factors that ultimately cause death.

Chronic-disease management has changed over the years, enabling an improved treatment approach for those with chronic illness. In line with the approach advocated by the Affordable Care Act (ACA), the newer management programs emphasize prevention and wellness throughout the health-care system, particularly in community care.[2]

Self-Care

In Dorothea Orem's model of nursing, individuals are responsible for their own health.[3] Callista Roy's model focuses on how the choices people make help them adapt to illness and maintain wellness. Several mid-range nursing theories also address the process of maintaining health and managing chronic illness with health-promoting practices such as self-care maintenance, self-care monitoring, and self-care management (see Chapter 3).[3] As people age, their ability to perform activities of daily living often decreases if any type of illness occurs that impinges on their physical and/or mental function. It is evident that most adults would prefer to reside in their own community and home as long as possible. Being in a familiar environment makes the older adult more apt to remain independent and have a sense of comfort and belonging. Often, when independence is removed from older adults, they do not have a family support system to help them. States that invest in home support services for elders have reduced the number of patients receiving long-term institutional care and lowered overall spending in their Medicare programs.

Aging in Place

Many older adults wish to "age in place"; that is, stay in their own homes as they get older. The truth is that in today's culture, an elderly person can get almost any type of help they want right in their home—but for a cost, which may be covered by Medicare or supplemental plans.[1] Information on the available services in any particular area can be obtained online or from the local Area Agency on Aging, local and state offices on aging or social services, tribal organization, or nearby senior center. Some of the major concerns for older adults who wish to remain in their homes as they age include the following:

- Personal care
- Household chores
- Food and meals
- Money management
- Medications and health care
- Getting around—at home and in town

- Social isolation
- Safety concerns in and outside the home
- Housing costs such as maintenance and insurance[4]

Resources for older adults who wish to age in place include the following:

1. *Family, friends, and neighbors.* Older adults need to communicate with relatives and friends about what they need and the best way to go about obtaining it. If the older person is physically able, they might want to consider trading services with a friend or neighbor. For example, one person who is more mobile could do the grocery shopping, and the other, who has difficulty getting around, could cook the meals.[5]
2. *Community and local governments.* A number of government resources can be accessed by older adults. They can learn about the services in their community from health-care providers and social workers. The state or local Area Agency on Aging, local and state offices on aging or social services, and tribal organizations will have lists of services that can be contacted. Churches and religious groups often offer senior services such as help with utility bills, free meals, and spiritual support.
3. *Case managers or geriatric care managers.* These specially trained professionals can help older adults and their families find essential resources. They will help with transitions between health-care facilities and home, help form a long-term care plan, and find the services needed to help sustain the person. Geriatric care managers can be helpful when family members live far apart by coordinating communications and sharing important health information.
4. *Federal government.* With the revival of the ACA, the federal government has expanded its resources for aid to older individuals. LongTermCare.gov at the Administration for Community Living is a good place to start the search for federal resources.[6]

Health-Care Costs and Coverage

Health-care expenditure in the United States neared 4.3 trillion in 2021, more than 17 times the $256 billion spent in 1989, with $12,914 being spent for each U.S. citizen. Between 2008 and 2016, the growth rate in health-care expenditures declined slightly as compared to the late 1990s and early 2000s, as the provisions of the ACA were phased in. Total health-care spending accounts for almost 18.3 percent of the nation's gross domestic product (GDP).[4]

Medicare and Medicaid account for a large portion of this expenditure. Medicare is a federal government–sponsored health-care program developed primarily for citizens over the age of 65, those with end-stage kidney disease, and disabled persons who are eligible to receive Social Security benefits. To maintain consistent and uniform coverage across the country, the program is run and maintained by the federal government and is divided into Part A, which covers hospital care; Part B, which covers medical insurance; and Part D, which covers prescription drugs. Participants in the program may be required to pay a deductible and a relatively small copay for medical services.

Medicaid differs from Medicare in that it is primarily for low-income families and individuals. There is much variability in who qualifies for Medicaid and the benefits that are available because it is administered and managed by the individual states, which receive matching funds from the federal government. Some states are very restrictive in who can receive benefits and may require that patients have virtually no income and meet other criteria such as passing drug screening tests and demonstrating the inability to find a job. In states with more progressive Medicaid programs, patients can receive services such as hospitalization, x-rays, laboratory services, midwifery services, clinic treatment, pediatric care, family planning, nursing services, in-home nursing facilities for patients over age 21, and medical and surgical dental care. A large percentage of Medicaid expenditures go for nursing home care and children.

Employers faced with increasing expenditures in premiums for family health insurance coverage for their employees tend to hire more part-time employees, who are not required to be covered. From 2008 to the present, unemployment rates have dropped drastically; however, many of these jobs are still at the lower end of the pay scale, which leads to an overall lower income for middle-class Americans. As a result, there is greater government health-care spending through the Medicaid program, which covers low-income families.[4]

Medicare covers not only older adults but also people with disabilities. Both state and federal budgets are affected by these increased costs.[4] Medicare covers some costs for those who need a skilled nursing facility, require rehabilitation, and receive service from a Centers for Medicare and Medicaid Services (CMS) nursing home after a qualifying hospital stay. To qualify for such coverage, the patient must have spent a certain amount of time in a hospital prior to admission to a skilled nursing facility. Conversely, only Medicaid patients who are in a facility that is certified by the government are eligible for Medicaid coverage.[4]

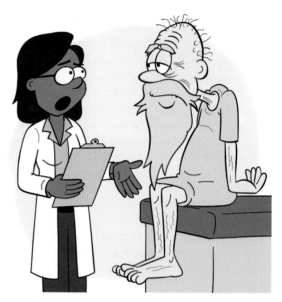

"Your chart indicates you're 34 years old. We need to talk about wellness and prevention."

Health-Care Ruling

When the Supreme Court issued its ruling upholding the ACA in 2013, it had a favorable effect for seniors on Medicare. A large segment of the older population expressed a sense of relief regarding their health-care options. When the ACA was passed by Congress in 2010, the changes in coverage were spread out over several years. If the bill had not been reaffirmed by the Supreme Court as being constitutional, none of the provisions would have been implemented, leading to a marked decrease in coverage for seniors and a pullback on coverage for previously uninsured people.

The National Committee to Preserve Social Security and Medicare believes that because of the ACA, the average Medicare beneficiary will continue to save an average of $650 a year, a significant sum, especially for seniors on fixed incomes without supplemental insurance. The ACA also expanded Medicaid to anyone who earns up to 133 percent of the federal poverty level, or $14,856 for a single person. According to projections by the Congressional Budget Office, approximately 40 million people are expected to sign on to Medicaid by 2025.[5]

One key provision of the ACA still in effect at the time of publication is assisting low-income couples to save more of their assets in qualifying for Medicaid. In the past, couples often had to decrease their assets or become unemployed in order to qualify for Medicaid. Such people comprise the "working poor."

The Gerontological Society of America (GSA) believes that older adults should have a high quality of life and receive patient-centered care. It also believes that for this vision to be realized, federal and state policies must expand the health-care options available to older adults to include in-home and other care that enables them to live independently as long as possible. Members of the GSA have been informing policymakers about the growing health-care needs of the older population of adults.[6]

> " *Although Healthy People 2020 began to include specific objectives for the care of older adults, Healthy People 2030 recognized the growth in this population and the need for more attention to its needs.* "

Older adults and their caregivers need support and resources to better understand their needs and to make the most of Medicare and other benefit programs.

What Do You Think?

Has the Affordable Care Act improved or hurt health care in the United States? Since the implementation of the ACA, have you experienced any advantages or disadvantages in the health-care system? Have you experienced any changes in health-care provision since the attempts to repeal the ACA began?

In 2022, the U.S. House and Senate passed the Inflation Reduction Act of 2022 (IRA), which was signed into law by President Joe Biden. Although not primarily a health-care bill, the IRA includes provisions dealing with health care that affected older adults. The health-care provisions in the bill include important reforms that will directly impact patients and health-care providers. Key provisions include the following:

- Reducing medication prices by permitting medication price negotiation
- Rebates for prescription medication inflation
- Part D improvements and maximum out-of-pocket caps for Medicare beneficiaries
- Full-cost coverage for adult vaccines
- A $35 monthly cap on out-of-pocket spending on insulin for Medicare beneficiaries only
- Extension of the value of ACA subsidies to certain consumers who receive subsidies for health[6]

Healthy People 2030

Healthy People 2030 builds on information accumulated over the past 40 years and addresses the latest public health priorities and challenges. The mission of *Healthy People 2030* is to "promote, strengthen, and evaluate the nation's efforts to improve the health and well-being of all people."

The framework for *Healthy People 2030* incorporates the essential ideas and purpose of the project and is the primary plan of action. It was based on recommendations made by the Secretary's Advisory Committee on National Health Promotion and Disease Prevention Objectives for 2030 (Committee).[7]

The objectives for *Healthy People 2030* underwent a multiyear development process that included input from a varied group of experts, different health-care organizations, and a group of public contributors. The Department of Health and Human Services (DHHS) reviewed and finalized the list of objectives. *Healthy People 2030* includes 358 measurable objectives, a significant decrease from the number that were in *Healthy People 2020* (1,000+). Working with fewer objectives will prevent overlap among objectives and help place focus on the most serious issues. Although *Healthy People 2020* began to include specific objectives for the care of older adults, *Healthy People 2030* recognized the growth in this population and the need for more attention to its needs.[7]

New objectives developed for older adults include the following:

- Increase the proportion of older adults with physical or cognitive health problems who get physical activity.
- Reduce the rate of pressure ulcer-related hospital admissions among older adults.
- Reduce the rate of hospital admissions for diabetes among older adults.
- Increase the proportion of older adults with dementia, or their caregivers, who know they have it.
- Reduce the proportion of preventable hospitalizations in older adults with dementia.
- Increase the proportion of adults with subjective cognitive decline who have discussed their symptoms with a provider.
- Reduce infections caused by *Listeria*.
- Reduce the rate of hospital admissions for urinary tract infections among older adults.
- Reduce fall-related deaths among older adults.
- Reduce the proportion of older adults who use inappropriate medications.
- Reduce the rate of emergency department visits due to falls among older adults.
- Reduce the proportion of older adults with untreated root surface tooth decay.
- Reduce the proportion of adults age 45 years and over with moderate and severe periodontitis.
- Reduce hip fractures among older adults.
- Increase the proportion of older adults who get screened for osteoporosis.
- Increase the proportion of older adults who get treated for osteoporosis after a fracture.
- Reduce the rate of hospital admissions for pneumonia among older adults.
- Reduce hospitalizations for asthma in adults age 65 years and over.
- Reduce vision loss from age-related macular degeneration.[7]

There are also recommendations for the following:

- Leading health indicators
- Overall health and well-being measures
- Target-setting methods for objectives
- Stakeholder engagement and communication

Emphasis on health literacy is also included in *Healthy People 2030* as one of its foundational principles and predominant goals. The Health Communication and Health Information Technology (HC-HIT) Workgroup included six objectives that deal with IT and health literacy. *Healthy People 2030* addresses both personal health literacy and organizational health literacy.[7]

Chronic disease affects the older population by decreasing their quality of life, which ultimately leads to higher health-care costs. Chronic conditions cause debilitation and pain. Effective public health strategies currently exist to help older adults remain independent longer, improve their quality of life, and potentially delay the need for long-term care.

Population Growth

The U.S. population has increased between 0.7 and 0.9 percent yearly for the past 10 years due in part to the increase in life span of the population. The country's concerted efforts to expand health insurance coverage, control infectious diseases through immunizations and antibiotics, improve air quality, and provide contaminant-free drinking water and safe food have helped people live longer. In addition, public efforts to address health hazards such as opioid abuse, gun violence, tobacco use, secondhand smoke, the nonuse of seat belts, and unsafe motor vehicles have contributed to longevity.[8] However, the United States ranks only 26 out of the world's 35 wealthiest nations in life expectancy, with men on average living to age 73.1 (2021 data), down from 76 in 2017. In 2021, women's life expectancy dropped to 79.2 years from 81 years in 2017. This drop in life expectancy rates is because of the large number of people who died during the COVID-19 pandemic.

In 1900, people ages 65 and older numbered 3 million, comprising only 3 percent of the U.S. population. In 2000, persons 65 and older numbered 35 million, comprising 12.4 percent of the total population, or 1 in 8 people. In 2021, those over the age of 65 numbered 54 million, or 17 percent of the population. The fastest-growing segment of the population is the age bracket above 65 years.[8]

IMPACT OF COVID-19 ON SENIORS

The COVID-19 pandemic of 2019–2021 illuminated the growing health concerns older adults face in the health-care system. According to the Centers for

Disease Control and Prevention (CDC), the pandemic claimed the lives of nearly 450,000 seniors across the country as of 2021. Of all the COVID-19-related deaths in the United States, approximately 80 percent were citizens 65 years of age and older. Countless others in this age group were affected by the virus but managed to survive. The data also showed that adults ages 65 and older were at a higher risk of hospitalization or death from COVID-19 during the peak of the pandemic.[9]

The CDC 2021 provisional death data report showed a 16 percent increase in the age-adjusted premature death rate for seniors between 2019 and 2020. The estimates placed COVID-19 as the third-leading cause of death in 2020, behind heart disease and cancer. Older adults accounted for the most deaths from COVID-19, with the highest death rates among those ages 85 and older. The COVID-19 vaccination rate for adults 65 or older in 2022 was 67.3 percent, below the *Healthy People 2030* goal. The same population is also experiencing a higher rate of long-COVID syndrome.[9]

As the population of older adults increases, health-care providers must understand the needs and outcomes of care for this population. Current research focuses on the most effective ways of using interventions or programs affecting chronic diseases such as diabetes and arthritis. Many older adults have multiple concurrent chronic or acute diseases. These can be further complicated by poor patient psychological response because of declining mental conditions, limited financial resources, lack of transportation, and the grieving process. Living arrangements become challenging, particularly if older adults live far away from relatives or lack a strong support system. Today's population of older adults has relatively easy access to high-quality health care. However, health care consumes as much as 20 percent of the income of elders, who average $2,000 in out-of-pocket expenses per year. Most health-care expenditures are made in the last 6 months of life.[10]

THE IMPACT OF AN AGING POPULATION

The growing population of older adults in the United States is having major economic consequences for the country, especially for the federal and state programs that help support the health care of this group. The median annual income of older men is only $20,000. And older women fare even worse, with a median annual income of merely $12,500. Eleven percent of older adults live below the poverty level, with another 27 percent categorized as near poor. Women statistically account for 74 percent of poor elders, whose only source of income is Social Security. About half of older women have pensions, and 12 percent subsist on Medicaid[10] used to pay for long-term nursing home care. Many states allow their residents to use Medicaid to cover assisted-living communities or other alternatives, such as in-home care, as well.[10] The demographic shift to a large senior population is not a temporary phenomenon associated only with the baby boomer generation. It is a permanent fixture of American society and will have a long-term impact on the economy. Safety-net programs for older, impoverished adults will likely be cut back as the government looks for ways to pay for recent, huge tax cuts.

> *Older adults accounted for the most deaths due to COVID-19, with the highest death rates among those ages 85 and older.*

Long-Term Effects on Nursing

As more older adults seek health care, the nursing shortage will only become more pronounced. The median age of registered nurses (RNs) in 2022 was 52, up from 46 in 2010, with 19 percent at 65 or older.[11] The average age of RNs entering the workforce is 28 years. It is projected that there will be a shortage of between 200,000 and 800,000 RNs by the year 2025.[11] The nursing education system has made valiant efforts to increase the number of RN graduates from their programs. The number of graduates has increased significantly over the past 10 years and continues to increase but not at a rate fast enough to keep up with the demand.[12] Schools of nursing are not meeting the demand created by older nurses who retire and increase the number of older patients. The Bureau of Labor Statistics (BLS) projects a 7 percent increase in demand for RNs, and a 45 percent increase in demand for advanced practice RNs (APRNs).[12] APRNs are particularly well placed to care for the increasing population of older adults.

Straining the Health-Care System

Most older adults are relatively healthy and able to remain in their homes with minimal assistance. However, as people age, their health-care needs typically increase due to chronic diseases, which strain an already stressed health-care system. As the nursing shortage becomes worse, nurses may need to work back-to-back shifts under highly stressful conditions. These types of working environments have been shown to cause long-term fatigue, accidents and injury, and job dissatisfaction. Research has demonstrated that nurses who work multiple shifts and long hours make more mistakes and have a higher incidence of medication errors.[12] The overall quality of patient care decreases, and nurses who are overstressed begin to leave the profession, which only makes the nursing shortage worse. In 2014, the ANA's position statement on nurse fatigue strongly recommended that nurses not work more than 12 hours in a 24-hour period and not more than 60 hours in a 7-day period. Subsequent documents from the ANA on safe staffing all cite work fatigue as a cause of multiple types of preventable nurse errors.[13]

What Do You Think?

Have you had any direct experiences of the nursing shortage, such as low staffing on a unit? How was the situation handled?

Lack of Geriatric Specialists

With a growing population of older adults comes an increasing need for practitioners who specialize in elder care. The medical community has been slow to respond to this trend, providing nursing with a golden opportunity. Almost all nursing programs today have a course on the care of older patients. Advanced degree programs offer degrees and certification in gerontology for nurse practitioners. With the projected shortage of primary care physicians, nurse practitioners are in a perfect position to fill this need. The reality of the future health-care system is that almost all nurses, except for those working in pediatrics and obstetrics, will be providing care for at least some older patients.

Integrated Care

Increased emphasis on the integration and coordination of patient care is needed across all age ranges, but particularly among older adults. Integrated care requires that chronic diseases are linked with preventive measures such as the involvement of families, screening, counseling, education, and the social determinants of healthy behaviors. True integrated preventive care also involves optimizing cooperation among team members, including community services such as immunization and outreach programs. This type of holistic approach is the foundation of nurse practitioner education.[14]

Many older patients come from other cultures and may not speak English well or at all. To meet the needs of this population, nurses will be required to provide high-quality care in multicultural and multilingual settings (see Chapter 21). In addition, effective treatment of the variety of mental disorders associated with chronic illness in older adults must be part of any care provided. This will also require additional screening and monitoring because these mental disorders are progressive. Mental disorders are the leading cause of compromised self-care and self-management of older adults at home.

> " . . . *effective treatment of the variety of mental disorders associated with chronic illness in the elderly must be part of any care provided.* "

Education Needs of Older Patients

To provide better holistic care, nurses today must educate elders about their health. This education is important in improving the health of the community and the everyday lives of older adults. Because older patients may have limitations such as reduced hearing and visual acuity, poor memory, and disorientation, nurses need to use specialized education techniques to be effective. The goal of all education is to change behavior. The major challenge in teaching older adults is overcoming current behavioral patterns that have developed over their long lifetimes.

One teaching technique that has proven effective is continuous positive reinforcement that can be easily employed in professional practice. Repetition combined with positive reinforcement such as praise, a pleased look, or another type of reward are all positive reinforcements. When the positive reinforcement is linked to a change in behavior, it becomes a motivator. Use of this technique can help build a positive learning environment, add interest and even excitement to the learning sessions, and increase a supportive pattern of trust and communication with all types of patients (see Chapter 11).

In developing an effective teaching plan, it is important to remember that all individuals, but particularly older adults, bring their life experiences to a learning situation. These experiences are based on their religion, gender, ethnicity, economic class, age, sexuality, and mental and physical abilities. Any health teaching must acknowledge and build upon these experiences. Learners also have a set of values that must be identified and incorporated into teaching. In any educational process, a power disparity exists between teachers and students. This disparity may be amplified by a student's cultural background (see Chapter 21). Recognizing this disparity and creating an atmosphere in which the learner does not feel threatened and feels free to ask questions is key to their understanding and remembering the content being taught.[15]

> *In developing an effective teaching plan, it is important to remember that all individuals, but particularly older adults, bring their life experiences to a learning situation.*

Appreciating the Older Population's Spirituality

Older people prefer to remain independent and within their own homes for as long as possible. To an older adult who is either well or ill, this freedom may have a spiritual connection. With aging and changes in health status, many older adults find new meanings for their existence. They prepare for their passage from life to death.[16]

Some nurses have difficulty in their role when managing the needs of old or dying patients due to the nurses' own fear of death. By understanding their own belief systems, nurses may feel more comfortable in addressing the patient's spiritual needs. Nurses can respond to and assist the patient with psychological, physical, spiritual, and emotional support. Nurses must be committed to understanding and be able to assess the importance spirituality plays in patients' daily lives, whether those patients live at home or in a community setting, hospital, or long-term care facility (see Box 22.1).

When nurses provide spiritual support to any patient during a time of illness, the patient develops a sense of inner balance and makes peace with the life they have lived. The same holds true for the older adult. Nurses know how important it is for these patients to be comfortable physically, but nurses also need to take into consideration their patients' spiritual needs. Using spiritual strategies such as empathy and open-ended questions, the nurse can help to improve both the individual's self-esteem and their relationships with other people and with whatever higher power the person may acknowledge. These strategies include asking questions such as "You sound distressed about your condition. What concerns you the most?" Other strategies that can be helpful in reducing pent-up anxiety and frustration are allowing the patient to vent religious or spiritual concerns, supporting the patient's use of prayer and scripture, encouraging family to participate in rituals and prayers, and helping the patient understand the source of spiritual distress as they work through the grieving process. Using these strategies will help older patients find meaning and hope in their lives.[16] (For more information on spiritual strategies, see Chapter 20.)

What Do You Think?

Have you ever had a patient ask you to pray with them? How did you handle the request? If you have not fielded that request yet, how would you handle it?

Spirituality in Nursing Education

Students should be prepared in nursing school not only to understand how spirituality affects older adults and their risks for chronic illness but also to provide spiritual care to this population.[18] Learning spiritual content in nursing school is similar to learning nursing theory or philosophy because it requires

---

Issues in Practice

A Research Investigation in the Spirituality of Older Adults

This study investigated the concept of spirituality in the well older adults who live independently within a community setting in either Southern California or the New York metropolitan area.

The purpose of the study was to investigate the concept of spirituality in this population and their perceived ideas, needs, and concerns. Twenty-six volunteers participated in an unstructured interview. The participants responded to a list of questions pertaining to the role of spirituality in their everyday lives. The data were grouped into respective themes and categories.

Qualitative research methodology explored the meaning of spirituality for older people living within a community setting. The sample size was 26 individuals, ages 65 to 85, who were asked nine open-ended questions used during a face-to-face interview (Box 22.1).

The results indicated that regardless of a person's history, age, gender, work background, or religious upbringing, spirituality played an important role in their daily lives. Participants felt that a powerful spiritual force guides them during periods when they may be lonely or suffering from a feeling of being isolated. Each participant acknowledged the significance of spirituality and the important role it played in his or her life. Participants felt that they had knowledge of the various spiritual modalities and how spirituality plays a significant role in real-life practices. These real-life experiences included prayer and helping others.

Questions for Thought

1. In your care of older adults, have you found that they have a better developed sense of spirituality than younger patients? What do you attribute the difference or lack of difference to?
2. Do you believe that a strong sense of spirituality helps older patients recover more quickly? Give examples of when you have experienced spirituality in this population.
3. Was the sample size of this study adequate to produce reliable results? Does the demographic division of subjects influence the study results?

Sources: *Study conducted in 2012 by Joseph Molinatti, PhD, RN.*[20]

---

the student to analyze situations and use nursing judgment in resolving complex issues.

Just as food and rest are universal needs, so too is spirituality. The more nurses understand about the lived experience of their older patients, the better equipped they will be to provide for the total needs of the individual. Learning about spirituality in nursing school better prepares nurses to assess and respond to the spiritual needs of all their patients, including older adults.

Nurses are beginning to include spirituality in their care and are gaining more knowledge in this arena. The Joint Commission (TJC) has established a standard of patient care that includes spiritual and emotional care for patients. TJC states that the patient's spiritual assessment is to include identification of spiritual practices important to them.[18]

A person does not have to be religious to be spiritual. Spirituality may entail an appreciation of physical experiences such as listening to music, walking along the beach, enjoying art or literature, eating good food, enjoying life, laughing, venting emotional tension, or participating in sexual expression. Often, as a person ages, material things become less significant; however, there is an increased interest in satisfaction of life. Some older adults may even have mystical experiences that may be a response to events in their past or to the many recent changes they have experienced.[18]

Studies have found that as people age, they become more spiritual. These studies found a correlation between age and high spirituality scores. Individuals with high spirituality scores had identified spiritual practices and experiences that they connected to

Box 22.1 Spirituality Questions and Answers

1. "When I say the word *spirituality*, what does the word mean to you?"
   Answered themes: God, faith, religion, one with nature, church
2. "How is spirituality important in your life?"
   Answered themes: Prayer, keeping in touch with self, fascination with other religions, oneness with nature
3. "Are there people, activities, resources that help you meet your spiritual needs?"
   Answered themes: Church, synagogue, family, cultural experiences, friendship
4. "In what way might your definition of spirituality be applied to your life?"
   Answered themes: Respect for life, creation of life
5. "How has spirituality influenced your life?"
   Answered themes: Closer to God, attending mass, a child of a Holocaust survivor
6. "Are you aware of the concept of spirituality?"
   Answered themes: Visiting Israel, church, saints, Ten Commandments
7. "Have you ever had any experience(s) that was particularly spiritually significant to you?"
   Answered themes: Only one responded and spoke of his comrades in a foxhole and God being present. Someone spoke of an out-of-body experience and seeing Jesus Christ and being told to return to her body.
8. "Over time, has the concept of spirituality taken on a different meaning in your life?"
   Answered themes: Sense of spirituality grew over time and relationships, more prayer; simply growing older meant an increased spiritual need and the need to be part of a spiritual community.
9. "What factors influenced your decision to pursue your spiritual needs?"
   Answered themes: Friendship, prayer, religious affiliation, hospice volunteer

Source: Spirituality and health, Familydoctor.org, 2017, https://familydoctor.org/spirituality-and-health.

physical trauma that affected emotions and bodily awareness.[18]

TRANSITION OF CARE

Moving a patient from one setting of care to another, such as from home health to a hospital or assisted-living facility or from the hospital to home health or a rehabilitation setting, is referred to as a **transition of care**, and it presents several challenges to patients and their families. The period following discharge from the hospital is a vulnerable time for all patients, but especially older adults. About half of older patients experience a medical error after hospital discharge, and between 19 and 23 percent undergo an adverse event, with medication errors being the most common. One relatively new challenge for patients and their families as they return home are the increased self-care responsibilities related to shorter hospital stays.[18] Effective planning and coordination of care is essential to increase patient satisfaction, reduce adverse events, and decrease the number of hospital readmissions. Discharge planning needs to begin at the time of admission.[18]

Discharge planning should be undertaken by a multidisciplinary team to better facilitate proper assessments of the needs of patients and their families A team may consist of only a nurse case manager and a social worker, but the team may also include a physical therapist, an occupational therapist, a pharmacist, and other health-care providers.[19] After a comprehensive review of the chart and an in-depth discussion with the patient and the patient's family, the team may suggest a range of discharge options. If they recommend discharge to home, home health services can ensure a smooth transition home and provide supplemental support. The discharge team may recommend discharge to a rehabilitation unit or even a skilled nursing facility.

Keys to Safe and Effective Transitions of Care

Patients who are given an appointment for a follow-up visit prior to discharge are more likely to keep the appointment. Follow-up visits with the provider usually take place within 2 weeks of hospital discharge; however, visits can be scheduled sooner depending on a patient's status. Follow-up appointments can result in lower rates of patient readmission and 30-day mortality, which are key evaluation benchmarks for hospitals.[19] Another effective way of bridging the gap between inpatient and outpatient care is a telephone follow-up conducted a few days after discharge. The person who calls must be fully aware of the patient's recent hospitalization and plan of care at discharge.[19]

Frail older adults and members of other high-risk groups often benefit from home visits by visiting or home health-care nurses. Visiting and home health-care nurses evaluate and assess the home situation for its ability to meet the patient's daily needs. These nurses can also spot potential risks in the home, such as risks for falls, burns, poor nutrition, mismanagement of medications, and even criminal activity.[19]

Nurses should be aware of practice guidelines and recommendations developed by national health organizations as well as their own facility's policies for improving transition care. For example, TJC now requires accredited facilities to "accurately and completely reconcile medications across the continuum of care."[20] The Society of Hospital Medicine has published proposals to reduce the readmission rate after discharge of older patients. The joint Society of Hospital Medicine–Society of General Internal Medicine Continuity of Care Task Force has also developed a systematic review of discharge planning for older adults, with recommendations for improving the transfer of patient information at time of discharge. Research has demonstrated that most errors and adverse events in the transition phase of health care are a result of miscommunication between the hospital team and the patient or the primary care provider.[20]

Better Communication

Ineffective communication at admission and discharge can lead to premature readmissions and increased morbidity. Communication with older patients can be particularly challenging because of the greater likelihood that members of this population will have poor eyesight or hearing, poor

> *Frail older adults and members of other high-risk groups often benefit from home visits by visiting or home health-care nurses.*

comprehension, or failing memories. A full assessment of the older patient's sensory and cognitive abilities needs to be conducted upon admission and noted in the patient's chart so that other providers can use the information. For example, a note on the chart saying, "Make sure the patient's hearing aid is in or he won't be able to hear you," can be valuable for all staff who interact with that patient (see Chapter 11 for more communication tips).

When the older patient is being discharged, instructions should concentrate on the points that are of most importance to the patient's safety and recovery. These key points can include medication changes and expected side effects; the date of the first follow-up appointment; how to care for dressings, drainage tubes, and so forth; activity limitations; signs of developing complications; and who to call if they develop complications.[19] These types of key instructions should be reinforced throughout the hospitalization and not given for the first and only time at discharge. Prerecorded audiovisual instructions can be used when the patient is able to understand them and remain awake during the presentation. They can be used to reinforce verbal instructions by the nurse. When hospital staff cannot communicate fluently in a patient's language, using trained medical interpreters is essential for effective patient teaching and discharge.

Providing patients and family members with clearly written materials in words that are easy to understand (fifth- to sixth-grade reading level) reinforces important self-care instructions when they are at home.[19] Rarely do stressed and worried patients remember all the verbal instructions that are given to them at discharge. Illustrated materials are usually easier to understand than text-only materials, and patients can often remember the illustrations better than a page of typed words. Patients should be provided with a Web address where they can gain access to the same information they received in printed form at discharge. Patients and/or their caregivers should also be asked to demonstrate any new self-care tasks that they will be required to carry out at home, such as changing a colostomy appliance or using eye drops.[20]

Medication Risks

As noted earlier, medication errors are the most numerous types of adverse events during transitions in care.[21] The prescription medications the patient was admitted with are often changed at the transition point, with patients being required to discontinue some medications, switch to a new dosage range of others, or start completely new ones. For more about the three main types of medications errors, see Box 22.2.

Prevention of transition medication errors begins with the admission history. It is important for the admission RN or provider to obtain a comprehensive and accurate medication history at the time of admission. However, the medication list obtained at the time of admission can be affected by the patient's health illiteracy, mental status, language barriers, and pain levels, as well as by the interviewing skills of the provider and time limits.[21]

Those taking a medication history need to consult other important sources of medication information, including family members, prescription lists, pill bottles, and old pharmacy records. By asking the patient an open-ended question or request for information, such as "Tell me about your normal day and what pills you take and when you take them," the history taker can avoid the most common error in the admission medication history, which is omitting a medication taken at home. Reconciling discrepancies in medication histories when they are taken by several different health-care staff will also reduce errors.

A patient's medication regimen can be significantly altered several times during a hospitalization. Acute illness may cause providers to hold certain medications, change long-acting medications to short-acting ones, discontinue others, or change dosages. Most hospitals have closed drug formularies to reduce the cost of medications, and in many cases, hospitals require automatic substitution of a less expensive medication for a more expensive one.[21]

When the older patient is being discharged and referred to their original provider, a comprehensive list of the patient's medications along with a complete file of the patient's recent hospitalization should be given to the provider. Also, at discharge, the patient should receive a list of discharge medications that they are to take at home along with a list of common side effects and instructions for self-administration, written in common words the patient or caregiver can understand. The provider should also point out any changes from the preadmission medications, especially medications that the

---

Box 22.2 How Medication Errors Happen

Errors from the pharmacy: Although pharmacists spend many years in school, they are not perfect. Also, because of the pharmacist shortage, many prescriptions are handled and filled by pharmacy techs who have little education. Sometimes they dispense the wrong dosage, the wrong medication, or the wrong label or information when filling the prescription. Always look carefully at the pill bottles or packaging to make sure it has the right patient's name and right medication name. Open the bottle to confirm that the pills look the same as the ones they are replacing. If they look different, call the pharmacist before administering the medication. It may be that the pharmacy switched suppliers or dispensed a generic form of the medication.

Errors by the physician: Physicians are human, too, and often are very busy. They can fail to thoroughly review the patient's past medical history and may prescribe the wrong medication or the wrong dosage based on outdated information. Physicians are notorious for their poor writing on prescription pads that may cause errors at the pharmacy, although using computers or tablets for writing prescriptions has cut down on these types of errors. Physician assistants and APRNs are also susceptible to these types of errors.

Errors by the nurse (dispensing errors): Errors can also occur if the person giving the medication to the patient is negligent when dispensing it. The nurse must use the five rights (or six rights or 10 rights) for medication administration and double-check the patient's identity. Administering too much or too little or not following the directions for administration are all sources of medication errors.

Source: Medication errors in the elderly, Legal Patriot, 2022, https://legalpatriot.com/medication-errors-and-the-elderly/#:~

patient may still have at home but should no longer be taking.[19]

As the number of older adults continues to rise, hospital admissions for members of this population will also increase. For most admissions, there will also be a discharge, which creates a vulnerable time of transition for the patient. It is important that the transition team prevent this experience from being one of discontinuity and risk but rather create a smooth and secure transfer from one safe environment to another. In today's health-care system, the discharge process can no longer be viewed as the end of health-care providers' commitments to patients but rather the closure of the gap between inpatient and outpatient care through well-planned and effective discharge transition.

Conclusion

The older population is growing and living longer but with increased morbidity because of chronic diseases such as dementia, heart disease, and diabetes. The economic impact of this growing population increased the cost of health care to $4.1 trillion in the United States in 2020.[4] The aging population has an impact on almost all segments of the health-care system. It is straining resources and requiring a shift in paradigm from an illness-oriented system to a prevention-and-maintenance-oriented system. This paradigm shift fits well with the underlying philosophy of professional nursing and the goals of the ACA.

Providing high-quality care for older adults offers a wide range of opportunities for future nurses in all areas of health care. Because most elders are relatively healthy and live independently in the community, community and parish nurses can develop and implement groundbreaking community-based programs. Advanced practice nurses have tremendous opportunities to develop clinics to provide a wide range of services for older adults, ranging from mental health services to screening tests and primary care. RNs who are knowledgeable in the care of older patients will be in great demand in health-care providers' offices and hospital units as well as in nursing education.

CRITICAL-THINKING EXERCISES

- Develop a care plan for an older patient who has a nursing diagnosis of "spiritual distress." What type of assessments would indicate this diagnosis?
- Write a teaching plan for a group of older patients outlining how current changes in the health-care law will affect them in the future.
- How do you think the rapidly increasing aging population will affect your nursing practice?

- Does your nursing program have a class that deals specifically with issues of older patients? Go to the Internet and look up nursing programs that offer a degree in gerontology.
- Use the spirituality questions in Box 22.1 to evaluate one of your older relatives or friends. How did their answers compare to the answered themes?

NCLEX-STYLE QUESTIONS

1. Which of the following statements about the population of older adults in the United States is true?
   1. Most older adults live in some type of assisted-living or nursing home situation.
   2. Older adults as a group are better off financially than their younger counterparts.
   3. Older adults typically seek medical care only for acute illnesses or injuries.
   4. Many older adults live with more than one chronic illness or condition.

2. In which of the following ways do the needs of the older population and the goals of the Affordable Care Act overlap? **Select all that apply.**
   1. Making health insurance premiums more affordable
   2. Focusing on wellness and health maintenance
   3. Switching to electronic health records and user portals
   4. Ensuring coverage of health screenings such as mammograms and colonoscopies
   5. Ensuring coverage of immunizations such as flu shots

3. What is the primary difference between *Healthy People 2020* and *Healthy People 2030*?
   1. *Healthy People 2020* was part of an ongoing federal program to improve the health of the U.S. population that was eliminated by *Healthy People 2030*.
   2. *Healthy People 2030* has fewer objectives than were present in *Healthy People 2020*, making it easier to prioritize the most pressing public health issues.
   3. *Healthy People 2030* provides information on disease prevention and health promotion, whereas *Healthy People 2020* did not include that information.
   4. *Healthy People 2020* has more goals and objectives than *Healthy People 2030* for the health-care of people with COVID-19.

4. The state of having more than one chronic, serious medical condition at the same time is called _____.

5. Which of the following should nurses expect to see in their practice in the future? **Select all that apply.**
   1. An end to the nursing shortage as more RNs graduate from nursing school
   2. More senior patients with complex medical needs
   3. More nurse practitioners who specialize in gerontology
   4. An emphasis on integrated care that stresses prevention through screening, immunization, education, and counseling and that involves patients' families
   5. A decreased need for medical interpreters as older patients learn English

6. Jayden, a nursing student, helped his grandparents make careful disaster preparations before the hurricane season began. This week, a neighbor came to help the couple safely evacuate from their home to a temporary shelter at the local high school. What negative effect are Jayden's grandparents MOST LIKELY to experience related to the disaster?
   1. Disorientation related to the noise, crowding, and unfamiliarity of the shelter
   2. Communication difficulties related to leaving behind the grandfather's hearing aid batteries
   3. Risk of exposure or death related to refusing to leave their home
   4. A hypertensive crisis related to forgetting to bring the grandmother's blood pressure medication

7. Why is learning to provide spiritual care for older patients an important part of nursing education?
   1. To make sure older patients "get right" with God before they die
   2. To help patients feel better about all the mistakes they have made in life
   3. To better assess spiritual distress in older patients and to help ease that distress in accordance with each patient's personal belief system
   4. To enable the nurse to process their own spiritual distress at having a patient who is near the end of life

8. Mr. Hinojosa, age 68, is being discharged home today after a 4-day stay in the hospital for a below-the-knee amputation of his left leg due to complications from diabetes. What is the greatest health risk for Mr. Hinojosa as he transitions from inpatient to outpatient status?
   1. Infection due to impaired healing related to his diabetes
   2. Social isolation due to mobility impairment
   3. Hyperglycemia due to consuming excess "comfort food" made by his wife
   4. Accidental opioid overdose due to misunderstanding the dosing schedule for his pain medication

9. What is a major difference between Medicare and Medicaid for older adults?
   1. Medicare is sponsored by the federal government; Medicaid is administered by each state.
   2. Medicaid is primarily for those over age 65; Medicare is primarily for low-income families and individuals.
   3. Medicare does not cover people with disabilities; Medicaid does.
   4. The ACA increased the number of people who qualify for Medicare, not Medicaid.

10. Eileen, an RN, is admitting Mrs. Jones, age 70, to the medical-surgical unit for treatment of her pneumonia. As part of her new-patient assessment and history taking, Eileen needs to identify and record all the medications Mrs. Jones currently takes. How can Eileen do this? **Select all that apply.**
    1. Ask Mrs. Jones, "Tell me about your normal day and what medications you take and when you take them."
    2. Ask Mrs. Jones's daughter, who helps care for her, about the medications prescribed for Mrs. Jones.
    3. Review the prescription list Mrs. Jones hands her.
    4. Record information from the pill bottles Mrs. Jones brings with her in a plastic bag.
    5. Request records from Mrs. Jones's pharmacy with Mrs. Jones's consent.

References

1. *Navigating the silver tsunami* (August 9, 2019). Advisor Magazine. .https://www.lifehealth.com/navigating-silver-tsunami/
2. Terga. (August 23, 2022). *Common health issues in older age people,* August 23, 2022. https://www.bgpaapd.org/common-health-issues-in-older-age/
3. El Osta A, Webber D, Gnani S, Banarsee R, Mummery D, Mageed A, Smith P. The self-care matrix: A unifying framework for self-care. *SelfCare, 10*(3), 38–56, 2019. https://selfcarejournal.com/wp-content/uploads/2019/07/El-Osta-et-al.-10.3.38-56.pdf
4. NHE fact sheet. CMS.gov, 2023. https://www.cms.gov/Research-Statistics-Data-and-Systems/Statistics-Trends-and-Reports/NationalHealthExpendData/NHE-Fact-Sheet
5. *National Committee to Preserve Social Security Medicare.* Influence Watch, 2021. https://www.influencewatch.org/non-profit/national-committee-to-preserve-social-security-medicare/
6. Taylor N, Meyer T. Inflation Reduction Act of 2022: Key healthcare provisions. *National Law Review,* 2022. https://www.natlawreview.com/article/inflation-reduction-act-2022-key-health-care-provisions
7. Healthy People 2030. *Health.gov,* 2022. https://health.gov/our-work/national-health-initiatives/healthy-people/healthy-people-2030
8. US world and population clock. U.S. Census Bureau, 2022. https://www.census.gov/popclock/
9. 2021 Senior report. America's Health Rankings, 2022. https://www.americashealthrankings.org/learn/reports/2021-senior-report/introduction
10. Eisenberg R. Despite Medicare, health costs are painful for Americans 65+: How high out-of-pocket health costs are causing them financial pain. NextAvenue, October 24, 2021. https://www.nextavenue.org/medicare-costs-americans-65/
11. Registered nurse demographics and statistics in the US. Zippia, 2022. https://www.zippia.com/registered-nurse-jobs/demographics/
12. Hamlin K. Why is there a nursing shortage? *NurseJournal,* March 21, 2022. https://nursejournal.org/articles/why-is-there-a-nursing-shortage
13. Nurse fatigue position statement. American Nurses Association, 2014. https://www.nursingworld.org/~49de63/globalassets/practiceandpolicy/health-and-safety/nurse-fatigue-position-statement-final.pdf#:~
14. Grange K. Treating geriatric patients: 5 tips. EMS1, August 1, 2022. https://www.ems1.com/patient-safety/articles/treating-geriatric-patients-5-tips-for-emts-and-paramedics-feG3rB111kbzJ7T1/
15. 6 Tips on how older adults can prepare for a disaster. National Institute on Aging, 2022. https://www.nia.nih.gov/sites/default/files/disaster-preparedness-infographic-508.pdf
16. Lavretsky H. Spirituality and aging. *Aging Health,* 6(6):749–769, 2010. https://www.medscape.com/viewarticle/740654_
17. Murgia C, Notarnicola I, Rocco G, Stievano A. Spirituality and Religious Diversity in Nursing: A Scoping Review. Systematic Scholar, 2020. https://www.semanticscholar.org/paper/Spirituality-and-Religious-Diversity-in-Nursing%3A-A-Murgia-Notarnicola/f677c193e293fba69f4eb13b9e25b2f279e0f5e2
18. Hoyt J. Senior housing options and retirement guide. SeniorLiving.org, 2022. https://www.seniorliving.org/housing/
19. Blokdyk G. *Discharge planning: A complete guide.* The Art of Service, 2021. https://theartofservice.com
20. Harnett J. The Joint Commission to add health equity standards to accreditation. Modern Healthcare.com, August 12, 2022. https://www.modernhealthcare.com/providers/joint-commission-add-health-equity-standards-accreditations
21. Medication errors in the elderly. Legal Patriot, 2022. https://legalpatriot.com/medication-errors-and-the-elderly/#:~

Patient Education: A Moral Imperative

23

Mary Abadie | Sharon M. Bator | Cynthia Bienemy | Doris Brown | Sandra Brown | Joan Anny Ellis | Betty L. Fomby-White | Anita H. Hansberry | Jacqueline J. Hill | Sharon W. Hutchinson | Karen Mills | Anyadie Onu | Janet S. Rami | Enrica K. Singleton | Wanda Spurlock | Melissa Stewart | Cheryl Taylor | Esperanza Villanueva-Joyce

Learning Objectives

After completing this chapter, the reader will be able to:

- Defend health literacy as a key element in meeting the requirements of today's health-care system
- Appraise the use of self-modeling by nurses as a method of patient education
- Discuss how managed care is interwoven with patient empowerment
- Evaluate the use of the Internet as a source of health-care information
- Analyze how a caring relationship affects the ability of a patient to learn
- Contrast the various communication styles that are used and how educational levels affect communication with a patient

(continued)

INTRODUCTION

Some indicators of the considerable growth of nursing as a profession over the years include the expectation of nurses to provide patient education, the increased emphasis on nursing ethics, and the legal accountability for providing safe and high-quality nursing care. For example, 50 years ago, nurses were prohibited from teaching patients in U.S. hospitals without direct orders from physicians. Many physicians believed that patient teaching in general was not relevant or effective, nor were nurses well enough educated to performing this function.

In the current health-care system, patient teaching is not only an expectation but an ethical and legal requirement. The enactment of the 2010 Affordable Care Act (ACA) provided nurses new opportunities for patient teaching, especially in the area of preventive education. Whether the nurse is teaching health promotion, health maintenance, or health rehabilitation, bringing a patient to a level of personal understanding is morally and ethically the right thing to do; that is, effective patient teaching is a moral imperative.[1] In recent years, several lawsuits have resulted from the failure of nurses to provide adequate patient teaching (Box 23.1).

Providers advise patients to be "smart" and to learn as much as possible about their health-care needs. Expert nurses have modeled ways to incorporate patient education as a priority in care, and nurse theorists provide worldviews and theories imbued with the primacy of patient education. The nation's consumers of health-care services

- Discuss the various collaborative skills a nurse can use
- Relate learner needs to learner characteristics
- Apply the nursing process to the development of a patient teaching plan
- Discuss commonly used teaching strategies and methods appropriate for patients of all ages
- Compare medagogy with pedagogy

Box 23.1 Documenting What You Teach

Always document what you teach patients and their families and include their understanding of what you taught. The classic documentation court case *Kyslinger v. United States* (1975) addressed the nurse's liability for patient teaching. In this case, a Veterans Administration (VA) hospital sent a hemodialysis patient home with an artificial kidney. The patient eventually died (apparently while connected to the hemodialysis machine), and his wife sued, alleging that the hospital and its staff failed to teach her or her husband how to properly use and maintain the home hemodialysis unit.

After examining the evidence, the court ruled against the patient's wife as follows: "During those 10 months that plaintiff's decedent underwent biweekly hemodialysis treatment on the units (at the VA hospital), both plaintiff and decedent were instructed as to the operation, maintenance, and supervision of said treatment as documented by the nurses in the decedent's chart. The Court can find no basis to conclude that the plaintiff or plaintiff's decedent were not properly informed on the use of the hemodialysis unit."

Source: Kyslinger v. United States, 406 F. Supp. 800 (W.D. Pa. 1975).

need their most trusted professionals—nurses—to advance initiatives to address health literacy. **Health literacy** is the ability to find, read, comprehend, and use health-care information in making the correct decisions about health care and the ability to follow directions from providers concerning treatment. Health literacy goes beyond just reading comprehension and includes the ability to understand the terminology used. Problems with health literacy are associated more commonly with ethnic minorities, who have worse outcomes than the majority of the U.S. population. However, even the most educated patients may have difficulty understanding health-care instructions. For example, a well-educated elementary schoolteacher thought the instruction to take pills with food meant wrapping her pills in cheese and then taking them.

The American Nurses Association (ANA) supports the following health-literacy activities:

- Promoting collaborative nursing initiatives to address health-literacy problems
- Using existing research findings to strengthen health-literacy knowledge and skills in nursing school curricula and in registered nurses (RN)'s workplaces
- Advancing nursing research to identify evidence-based practices that promote optimum health literacy[1]

ETHICAL CONSIDERATIONS OF HEALTH SELF-MANAGEMENT

In the United States, nursing students have traditionally been unprepared to educate patients with self-management concerns, particularly chronic illnesses. This lack of nurse preparation creates problems in the long-term wellness goals of patients after they leave an acute care facility, and it increases their risk of harm from pain, infection, medication error, physical disability, and premature death. For people in poverty or those who have little access to health-care, the risk of negative outcomes can be even higher. The unhealthy outcomes produced by nurses' lack of ability to teach patients self-care also causes monetary loss and loss of productivity of health-care institutions.[2] However, nursing schools have begun to remedy the lack of education on how to teach patients, and there is now a certification for nurse patient educators.

ETHICAL CONSIDERATIONS OF "NURSE, HEAL THYSELF"

In an era of increasing health-care costs and increased incidence of chronic disease, providing high-quality preventive care through health education and promotion is critical. By assessing and addressing their own lifestyle behaviors, such as smoking, alcohol use, obesity, and lack of sleep, nurses and nursing students can invest in their future health and that of their present and future patients.

Take the example of obesity. As obesity has reached epidemic proportions, should overweight health-care workers be asked to reduce their weight? A survey of nurses, advanced practice nurses, and nurse educators showed that 54 percent were obese or overweight. But shouldn't nurses serve as role models for healthy diets and lifestyles to positively motivate patients? Put more simply, if experienced health-care providers, who know the health risks of obesity and are informed about intervention techniques, do not follow expert advice, is it realistic to expect the public to do so?[3] One study, in which 93 percent of practicing nurses admitted to being overweight or obese, showed that 76 percent did not even bring up the topics of obesity and weight loss with obese patients.[3] Other studies indicate that limited exercise counseling by nurse practitioners does not match the strong value placed on health promotion by the nursing profession.[4] Do nurse educators avoid the topic of healthy lifestyle choices with their nursing students? If so, what are the health implications for nursing students now and in the future?

> *TJC Standard PC.6.1 requires nursing staff to serve as critical resources by acting as skilled patient educators.*

ACCREDITATION AND REGULATION

Managed care, with its focus on patients taking greater responsibility for their own health and self-care, has contributed to the increased need for patient education. The Institute of Medicine (IOM [now the National Academy of Medicine]) has harshly criticized the disparity in health-care quality and strongly recommends placing patients in control of their own health, making choices based on the best information and knowledge available to them. The IOM established 10 rules for "crossing the quality chasm of care," four of which relate to patient teaching.[5] For many years, nursing theorists and researchers have supported empowering consumers to advocate for their specific health needs, which meshes seamlessly with the goals of managed care.

In addition to the IOM's efforts, The Joint Commission (TJC) has taken steps to regulate patient teaching because it is essential to high-quality care. During their unannounced visits, TJC representatives look for evidence that education standards are being met. TJC Standard PC.6.1 requires nursing staff to serve as critical resources by acting as skilled patient educators. In addition, TJC determines whether learning activities assess the patient's learning needs and adequately address areas in which the patient would like more information. The standard requires all providers to communicate whether the patient's teaching needs are being met (Box 23.2).[6]

IMPLICATIONS OF TECHNOLOGY

Electronic Records

With their capacity to record and store large amounts of data, electronic health records (EHRs) help track when the teaching standards recommended by TJC and the IOM are met. As shown in Table 23.1, the IOM suggests that education should be continuous and customized to each patient and should keep the patient in control with freely shared information.[6]

Other technologies, including telehealth portals and the Internet, can serve as teaching tools for improving patient care. Patients at many facilities can now log on to a website and access their own EHRs. Many providers have patient portals at their offices. Such advances are also good marketing tools for medical facilities. Well-educated learners can use technology successfully in programs such as anticoagulation therapy, suicide

---

Box 23.2 The Joint Committee Standard PC.02.03.01

Standard
Provide patient education and training based on each patient's needs and abilities.

Rationale
- Acute care patients are discharged with instructions for self-care.
- Patient education influences the patient's outcome and promotes healthy behaviors.
- The organization needs to assess the patient's learning needs and use educational methods and instruction that match the patient's level of understanding.

Elements of Performance
- Perform a learning needs assessment that includes the patient's cultural and religious beliefs, emotional barriers, desire and motivation to learn, physical or cognitive limitations, and barriers to communication.
- Provide education and training based on the assessed needs.
- Coordinate patient education and training between all disciplines involved in the patient's care, treatment, and services.
- Based on the patient's condition and assessed needs, the education and training provided to the patient by the hospital include any of the following:
  - An explanation of the plan for care, treatment, and services
  - Basic health practices and safety
  - Information on the safe and effective use of medications (see also MM.06.01.01, EP 9; MM.06.01.03, EPs 3-6)
  - Nutrition interventions (for example, supplements) and modified diets
  - Discussion of pain, the risk for pain, the importance of effective pain management, the pain assessment process, and methods for pain management
  - Information on oral health
  - Information on the safe and effective use of medical equipment or supplies provided by the hospital
  - Habilitation or rehabilitation techniques to help the patient reach maximum independence
  - Fall reduction strategies
- Evaluate the patient's understanding of the education and training.
- Provide education on how to communicate concerns about patient safety issues that occur before, during, and after care is received.

Source: Joint Commission Resources, *2021 Hospital Accreditation Standards Manual*, Oakbrook Terrace, IL: Joint Commission, 2021, pp. 26C–C27. Reprinted with permission.

---

prevention, weight reduction, stress abatement, parenting, and women's health issues.[7]

Working With the Internet
During the time that the COVID-19 pandemic kept people from going out, it made home the center of their lives. Home became many individuals' and families' workspace, workout place, favorite restaurant, and even physician's office. Much of the available health care occurred virtually through technology. The pandemic enhanced pioneering of new methodologies that allowed the population to adjust to a new way of seeking health care that forever transformed patient expectations for how they receive care.

Both patients and health-care personnel quickly learned that if they had the appropriate technology, communication could be interactive, collaborative, in real time, and help everyone involved in giving and receiving care. They learned that patient education could be available on demand. Using printed education materials or educating patients and caregivers in person are now considered outdated modes in

Table 23.1   Building Responsiveness Into Health-Care Systems

Rule	Description
1. Care is based on continuous healing relationships.	Patients should receive care whenever they need it, and in many forms, not just during face-to-face visits. The health-care system must be responsive at all times, and access to care should be provided over the Internet, by telephone, and by other means in addition to in-person visits.
2. Care is customized according to patient needs and values.	The system should be designed to meet the most common types of needs but should have the capability to respond to individual patient choices and preferences.
3. The patient is the source of control.	Patients should be given the necessary information and opportunity to exercise their chosen degree of control over health-care decisions that affect them. The system should be able to accommodate differences in patient preferences and encourage shared decision-making.
4. Knowledge is shared, and information flows freely.	Patients should have unfettered access to their own medical information and to clinical knowledge. Clinicians and patients should communicate effectively and share information.

Source: *Adapted from T. Mirzoev, S. Kane, What is health systems responsiveness? Review of existing knowledge and proposed conceptual framework,* British Medical Journal, *2(4), https://doi.org/10.1136/bmjgh-2017-000486.*

many health-care situations. Using technology-based on-demand education methods empowers people to participate in their own care knowing that they can achieve positive outcomes.[7]

The Internet has been the fastest-growing source of health information for more than a decade. Access to the latest information in virtually any subject is just a click away. In addition, social networking has created a worldwide learning community that patients and health-care providers can tap into. Consequently, patients are better able to increase their own level of responsibility for their health care. This factor has changed nursing practice in that some patients present for care with higher levels of information about their illnesses and possible treatments. Websites such as WebMD, with 16 million users each month, have been a mixed blessing for health-care providers. While patients who use them may have a higher level of health knowledge, providers are also faced with patients who have "diagnosed" themselves online and come in requesting expensive tests or inappropriate medications for themselves or their family members. Note that only a few health-information websites follow privacy policies; it is common for them to share personal health information without the patient's permission or even personal knowledge.[8]

In this information age, demands from patients for sophisticated and better health-care information have increased, and online Web-based classes can impart information as never before. Nursing must keep abreast of these trends and devise accessible, accurate Web-based learning opportunities to improve the quality and outcomes of patient care.

Using Technology in Teaching

Widespread access to the Internet and its huge volume of available information makes it a useful and widely sought tool for both patients and caregivers. The Internet can provide access to medical publications, caregivers, prescription and nonprescription drug information, other patients or family members, and an almost limitless variety of related sources.

Searching for Information

More than half of Americans who have gone online have searched for health or medical information. Daily, far more people seek such information online than actually visit health professionals. These consumers can enhance their own knowledge of health topics through proper use of the Internet.

Many medical professionals are concerned that patients seeking health-care information on the Internet will be misinformed. How can patients know which health-information sites are reliable and which are "fake news"?

Table 23.2 lists some helpful and vetted online health and medical directories. This list is not comprehensive.

Evaluating Results

Part of patient education is teaching patients to evaluate the accuracy and currency of information they find on the Internet. Critical evaluation of a patient's search results is important, and a partnership between caregiver and patient is the best way to undertake it. Both the patient and caregiver should ask these questions:

- Does the site or information have credibility?
- Is it published by a marketing firm or drug manufacturer with a primary focus on sales rather than education?
- Is the content accurate and aligned with the answer being sought? Can the information be checked for accuracy elsewhere?
- Is the information scientifically based or anecdotal? Are disclaimers present; if so, do they state

appropriately that the information is for general use and not diagnostic? (See Chapter 17 for a more detailed discussion.)

To provide the best care, nurses need a thorough understanding of the available Internet learning tools as well as effective techniques for educating patients in person.[8] Of course, nurses must also recognize that not all patients have Internet access or the ability to use a computer. In such cases, the nurse must substitute more traditional methods of sharing information.

To provide appropriate-level reading materials, the nurse must know the patient's literacy level. The Agency of Healthcare Research and Quality has a website (https://www.ahrq.gov/health-literacy/research/tools/index.html#rapid) that helps nurses evaluate literacy levels to tailor the vocabulary and sentence structure of patient-education materials appropriately.

HEALTH PROMOTION FOR OUR TIME

The need for enhanced communication has created a new emphasis on health promotion. One example is the *Healthy People 2030* objectives created by the U.S.

Table 23.2 Online Health and Medical Directories

Name	URL	Description
Hardin Meta Directory (MD)	https://www.lib.uiowa.edu/hardin/md	Health sites listing, selected for connectivity
Everyday Health (A–Z directory)	https://www.everydayhealth.com/conditions/	Consumer health site maintained by health-care professionals
MyHealthfinder	https://health.gov/myhealthfinder	U.S. government–maintained site; uses colloquial language
MedicineNet	https://www.medicinenet.com	Doctor-produced information
Mayo Clinic	https://www.mayoclinic.org	General health information
National Library of Medicine	https://medlineplus.gov/	Current health-care information including videos
Agency for Healthcare Research and Quality	https://www.ahrq.gov/consumer	Primarily aimed at health-care professionals; informative for some patients
CDC Health Topics A–Z	https://www.cdc.gov/az	Information about infectious diseases studied by the Centers for Disease Control and Prevention (CDC)
SafeMedication (American Society of Health System Pharmacists)	https://www.safemedication.com	Information to help patients use medications safely and correctly

Source: *U.S. National Library of Medicine, MedlinePlus, https://medlineplus.gov/.*

Department of Health and Human Services in 2020. The federal government's national prevention agenda for building a healthier nation, *Healthy People 2030* is a statement of national health objectives designed to identify the most significant preventable threats to health and to establish national goals to reduce these threats. Implied throughout this document is the need for high-quality patient education, particularly from nurses.[9]

The vision of *Healthy People 2030* is a society in which all people can achieve their full potential for health and well-being across their lifespan.[9] To achieve its vision, *Healthy People 2030* has established health literacy as a central focus in one of its overarching goals: "Eliminate health disparities, achieve health equity, and attain health literacy to improve the health and well-being of all."[9] *Healthy People 2030* promotes the concept that health literacy is an essential element of communication, patient education, and care. Every person who encounters the health-care system, notwithstanding their level of education, their ability to read, or their ability to understand English, should be able to experience the safest, highest-quality, best-value health-care services in any setting.

Health literacy for *Healthy People 2030* is based on the core principle that all people have the right to health education that aids them in making informed decisions. It addresses the disparities found in minority groups due to the inability to communicate with them. Health information should be presented in ways that are easy to understand and that improve health, longevity, and quality of life for everybody. *Healthy People 2030* is the first Healthy People program to include health literacy as part of its framework. The achievement of health literacy is recognized as a fundamental underpinning of patient education and is why it is included in the *Healthy People 2030* foundational principles and overarching goals.[9]

CARING RELATIONSHIPS MATTER

If patients feel cared for and respected as individuals by nurses and other health-care providers, they will want to learn more about their health and will have more faith in their own ability to learn.[7] Helping patients learn about and develop healthy lifestyles and choices is "one of the most important responsibilities of contemporary nurses."[10]

Now that the ACA has become a part of the health-care landscape and there are fewer uncertainties about health reform, sustaining a caring environment is critical for both the health-care provider and the patient. A non-nurturing interpersonal relationship is profoundly negative to the body, mind, and spirit for both the health-care provider and the patient.

Collaborative Patient Teaching for Healthy Communities

Power is a multifaceted and complex concept that has many definitions (see Chapter 1 for more detail). In the health-care setting, *power* may best be defined as "possession of control, authority, or influence over others or the ability to make others do things they might not otherwise want to do."[11] The perceived power imbalance between patients and nurses is created by the belief that nurses know what is best for the patient because they have "more" medical knowledge than the patient (paternalism). Nurses demonstrate this type of asymmetrical power when they use medical jargon with patients, decide the issues to be discussed, discount the patient's viewpoint, interrupt the patient when they are asking questions, and control the length of the patient–nurse interaction. Other examples may include the nurse giving orders to patients to do something ("take off your clothes and put on this hospital gown") or preventing the patient from doing something ("you can't get out of bed without help").[11]

Shared power underlies successful collaboration. Contemporary nursing practice calls for nurses to work in partnership with patients. Nurses are encouraged to share their power and to empower their patients by providing them information and support. Nurses need to involve patients in their own care by helping them to participate in the health-care decision-making process. In order for nurses and patients to work as partners, nurses must make every effort to equalize the power imbalance. One way to do this is for nurses to share and give information to patients willingly and to be open in their communication with them. Therefore, nursing educators must teach their students the importance of sharing power with patients. When educators mentor shared power, they prepare students to collaborate with one another and with their future patients.[11]

When nurses and patients share power and information, they are engaged in a collaborative relationship to improve the patients' health. The Pew Commission's Final Report stressed that relationship-centered interactions must become central to the education of health professionals. The report emphasized that constructive interpersonal encounters exist when they are culturally sensitive, caring, collaborative, and relationship centered. These types of relationships are critical to the promotion of preventive health care through effective teaching.[11] As noted earlier, effective patient teaching is one way to eliminate the disparities in the access to health care and the quality of health care being provided to various minority groups.

An Evidence-Based Example of a Collaborative Teaching Partnership

For more than 30 years, Dr. David Olds tested a Nurse–Family Partnership (NFP) program in collaboration with nurses and other health-care workers in the fields of medicine, psychology, and public health. This teaching study tracked the effectiveness of home visits by nurses in improving maternal and child health. First-time parents volunteered to take part in the study.

The NFP is committed to enduring improvements in the health and well-being of low-income patients, first-time parents, and their children. Nurses were chosen for this program because of the high public trust of nurses and because nurses can relate to patients in a caring manner.[12]

Box 23.3 summarizes the results of this teaching partnership involving nurses, other health professionals, and first-time parents.[14]

Cultural Aspects of Teaching

Given the vast diversity within the United States, nurses and other health-care providers must be able to adapt teaching to patients whose language, culture, level of education, sexuality, gender identity, and abilities differ from their own. A patient's cultural background and previous experiences with the health-care system strongly influence their attitudes and beliefs about health. Fortunately, the nurse's knowledge of diversity and culturally competent care can facilitate a therapeutic approach to patient teaching (see Chapter 21).

Box 23.3 Improving Care and Saving Money Through Partnership

At an average savings of $13,000 per patient being returned to the government, the following consistent outcomes occurred:

- Reduced emergency department visits
- Fewer hospital readmissions within 30 days
- Increased monitoring of medications for chronic conditions
- Improved coordination among providers
- Increased independence of activity at home
- Reduction in contagious diseases

Source: S. Jaffe, How house calls are saving money for Medicare, *Money,* May 23, 2016, http://money.com/money/4345039/house-calls-medicare; Affordable Care Act model saves more than $25 million in its first performance year [press release], Centers for Medicare and Medicaid Services, June 18, 2015, https://www.cms.gov/newsroom/press-releases/affordable-care-act-payment-model-saves-more-25-million-first-performance-year.

Communication Style

Good communication skills and the ability to establish a caring relationship are essential to an effective educator. These skills also include cultural knowledge and sensitivity. The information provided in Chapters 11 and 12 on communication and dealing with difficult behavior forms the basis for communication in patient education. For example, after surviving a serious illness, surgery, or injury, patients must work their way through the stages of grieving and may even display a type of posttraumatic stress response. Unless the nurse is able to understand what grief stage patients are in and to empathize with them, teaching is likely to be ineffective. With the trend to very short hospital stays and one-day procedures, time for patient education has become extremely short. Assessing what is most important for patients to know when they get home and giving them that information in a succinct and memorable way is key to education success.

Keep in mind that most patients whom nurses teach are adult learners. They bring with them a lifetime of knowledge and information and, sometimes, misinformation. In general, adult learners should not be taught in the same way a child is taught; however, some techniques, such as demonstration and repetition, remain valid.

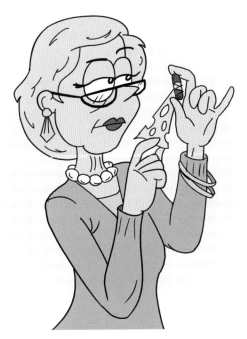

"They said to take it with food."

Language

If the nurse is unable to communicate fluently in the patient's language, then attempting to teach them will be fruitless. In conducting a language assessment, the nurse must determine the patient's fluency in the primary as well as the secondary language.

Brochures in the patient's language may be a teaching option. However, not all patients are able to read, and brochures that have been translated directly from English into another language may not convey the intended message, or the words used may not be familiar to the patient. In that case, a medical interpreter who speaks the patient's language is needed.

A patient may understand elementary English but be unable to translate a lengthy or rapidly spoken technical explanation. Older adult patients may have hearing or vision deficits that can interfere with their ability to take in information. Although television has contributed to wide recognition of terms such as *malignancy* and *cholesterol*, you should not take for granted that a patient understands medical terms and their implications in the same way a nurse does. Nor should you expect the patient to speak up and ask for clarification, particularly if the patient has been hiding a literacy problem for years.

For example, when a patient from an isolated American community was told that her abdominal pain, vaginal bleeding, high blood pressure, and enlarged abdomen were caused by a hydatidiform mole (a type of intrauterine growth that can mimic pregnancy), she became hysterical, believing that a brown, furry animal was living inside her. The patient signed herself out of the hospital and did not return for her scheduled D&C (dilatation and curettage). She was too fearful and ashamed to tell her husband or other family members. Finally, a home-health nurse and a counselor visited the patient at home to assess her condition and determine why she had not returned for the surgical procedure. They quickly determined that the underlying problem was a lack of knowledge—the patient did not understand the meaning of the word "mole" used as a medical term by the physician. The nurse and counselor helped the patient overcome her fear and emotional turmoil by explaining the condition in language she could understand.

Educational Level and Motivation

The higher a person's educational level, the more likely that person is to have received some formal health education and, typically, the higher that person's motivation to learn.

Before attempting to teach a patient, the nurse should ascertain the following information:

- What is the patient's level of motivation to learn?
- What factors will motivate the patient to learn healthy behaviors?

THE CRUX OF PATIENT EDUCATION
Collaborative Skills

The teaching–learning process and the nursing process have more in common than you might think. For example, the need for collaborative skills is implicit in the teaching–learning process, and health-care providers use these skills to empower their patients and help them achieve the best possible quality of life.[11] Collaborative skills include the following:

1. *Consulting:* Consider the nurse as a consultant who helps patients remain in control of their own health choices.
2. *Counseling:* Nurses should be counselors to all patients, reaching out with sensitivity to those who

differ from them in age, education level, gender identity, sexuality, and ethnicity.

3. *Facilitating:* Nurses help the patient understand the relationship between their behaviors and their health.

4. *Assessing:* Nurses need to use their assessment skills to determine patients' barriers to behavior change, including physical limitations, lack of skills, decreased motivation, poor resources, and marginal social support.

5. *Cheerleading:* The ability to encourage patients to commit themselves to change and involve them in the selection of risk factors to eliminate is key to success.

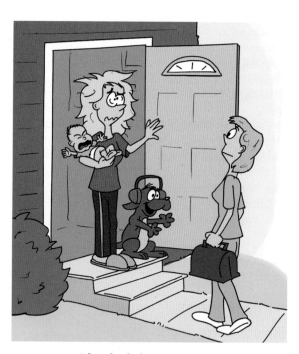

"Am I glad to see you!"

6. *Monitoring:* Evaluating progress through follow-up telephone calls and appointments and activation of the health-care team, including the receptionist and other office staff, will point to areas where additional work is needed.

7. *Role-modeling:* If the nurse is unable to role-model the behaviors they want the patient to display, no amount of teaching will be effective.

8. *Being patient literate:* Every time patients leave an encounter with a health-care professional, they should have more knowledge than when they entered the encounter. If patients do not understand the information nurses and other providers offer or are not given a rationale for lifestyle-change recommendations, they are unlikely to remember the information and may continue making poor choices that may lead to poorer health and even death.

Health-care reform can lead the nation toward a patient-centered, proactive, and preventive model only if consumers understand their providers' instructions.[11]

Steps in a Process

Table 23.3 compares the teaching–learning process and the nursing process. The following discussion examines the teaching–learning process in detail.

I. Assessment

  A. Learner Characteristics

    In assessing learner characteristics and learning readiness, nurses should pay attention to the patient's cultural background, health literacy, education level, age, and gender. For instance, if a woman's religion forbids women from speaking to men outside their family, a male nurse will probably not receive any useful information from this patient.

    Although some patients may be hesitant to talk about their educational level, asking about it is important. For example, a patient who did not finish high school was discharged with a new medication that had complicated instructions concerning how and when to take it. The patient had not been given an educational assessment. Because of the patient's inability to properly understand the directions, he overdosed on the medication with a resulting readmission and adverse event for the hospital.

    On the other hand, do not presume that a highly educated patient understands medical terminology and concepts. The patient may think they understand everything, but in reality, they may misconstrue the entire meaning of a nurse's teaching session.

Table 23.3 Comparison of the Teaching–Learning Process With the Nursing Process

Teaching–Learning Process	Nursing Process

I. Assessment
  A. Learner characteristics
  B. Learner needs
	I. Assessment

II. Development of expected learning outcomes through objectives	II. Diagnosis and planning

III. Development of a teaching plan
  A. Content
  B. Teaching strategies and learning activities
	III. Implementation of the nursing plan

IV. Implementation of the teaching plan	IV. Evaluation

V. Evaluation of expected outcomes
  A. Achievement of learning outcomes
  B. Effectiveness of the teaching process	

Source: *Adapted from C. Edelman, C. Mandel,* Health Promotion Throughout the Life Span *(8th ed., p. 9), Philadelphia, PA: Mosby Elsevier, 2018.*

Finally, be aware that a significant number of patients are unable to read. These patients, along with patients with learning disabilities or developmental delays, require even more attention when explaining new information.

B. Learner Needs

Olds's principles of the Nurse–Family Partnership outlines a step-by-step methodology of working with a patient's learning needs (Box 23.4). A thorough assessment of a patient's learning needs focuses on finding out four basic bits of information. First, finding out what the patient already knows is important because it can help in planning what needs to be taught so that unneeded basic information is not repeated. Second, the nurse needs to find out what the patient wants and needs to learn to help them in dealing with their illness or injury. Third, uncovering what the patient is able to learn involves finding out their comprehension and general intelligence level. The fourth bit of important information to determine is the patient's preferred learning style and the best teaching methods for that style of learning. Most of this information can be obtained by asking questions similar to the following:[14]

- What about your illness or injury most worries or concerns you?
- What would you like to be able to do to take care of yourself when you leave the hospital?
- What do you know about your condition right now?
- What additional information would be most helpful for your recovery and home care?
- Is there anything in your current care that is causing you problems?
- Before you were admitted, what was your primary source of information about your condition?
- Do you ever use a computer to answer your health-care questions?

Box 23.4 Olds's Principles of the Nurse–Family Partnership

1. The patient is an expert on their own life.
2. Follow the patient's heart's desire.
3. Focus on strengths.
4. Focus on solutions.
5. Only a small change is necessary.

Source: D.L. Olds, J. Robinson, R. O'Brien, et al., Home visiting by paraprofessionals and by nurses: A randomized, controlled trial, *Pediatrics,* 110(3):486–496, 2002, https://doi.org/10.1542/peds.110.3.486.

- When you are discharged, what information would be most useful for you to manage your care at home?
- What causes you the most confusion about your disease process (injury) while at the hospital?
- Do you learn best in the morning, afternoon, or evening?
- What is the best way for you to remember new information? Reading it yourself? Having it read to you? The nurse explaining it to you? Watching a video about the topic? A combination of methods?[14]

Interviewing the family is also important in assessing learning ability. Information from the patient's family may present an entirely different perspective on the assessment by filling in missing information, modifying how the nurse understands what the patient said, or reevaluating what the patient's home situation after discharge really is. It is also important to evaluate how involved the family members are in the patient's life and care. Their attendance and participation during scheduled teaching sessions will help to support the patient as they attempt to change health behaviors and to learn new health skills. Table 23.4 outlines a number of teaching strategies and the various types of patients for which they are most useful.

II. Identification of Specific Individualized Learning Needs (Diagnosis)

After collecting as much data as possible through interviewing and other assessment techniques, the nurse needs to analyze the data and organize it to

Table 23.4 Commonly Used Teaching Strategies and Methods

Strategy/Method	Description
Demonstration	Helpful in problem-solving; learner moves from a simple formulation of a problem to a complex understanding of it
Discussion	Verbal communication of ideas; information with participation by both teacher and learner
	Useful in the clinical setting, one-on-one with the patient, or with a small group such as the family
	Allows for assessment of values and knowledge of the topic
	Elicits decision making regarding a situation or a piece of information
Lecture	Formal oral presentation by the teacher
	Useful for larger groups of patients with the same health problem
	Best if oral presentation is accompanied by a handout (e.g., outline, notes) with space for patients to write notes; handouts help learners stay focused
Visual aids, computer instruction, pictures, paintings, posters, PowerPoints, Internet	Useful in the clinical setting for comparison with actual situations
	Useful for increasing motor-skill development, discussing a particular topic, or assessing comprehension of content
	Useful as an adjunct to verbal explanation of concepts and skills
Modeling and teach-back	Teaching by example; learners observe the teacher's behavior and then attempt to repeat the behavior
Trial and error	Learning by experience; used sometimes when the learner has little knowledge of content or of a situation
	Sporadically useful during practice with a computer, engine, or other machine
	Trial-and-error learning is time consuming and frustrating to learners (especially adults) and should be minimized
Role-playing	Acting the part of another person; usually followed by discussion of perceptions or feelings
	Provides a change in perspective

Source: *Adapted from S. Heath, 4 Patient education strategies that drive patient activation, Patient Engagement HIT, April 27, 2017, https://patientengagementhit.com/news/4-patient-education-strategies-that-drive-patient-activation.*

formulate a diagnosis or statement of the patient's learning needs. The diagnosis of learning needs is individualized on the basis of the assessment data collected.[13]

Using clinical judgment skills, the nurse identifies the patient's individual educational and associated physical deficits that may affect learning needs. For example, the needs identification reflects that a 65-year-old male patient has broken both his arms and that this impairment has caused loss of self-care skills, high levels of stress, and a sense of powerlessness, all of which may reduce the patient's ability to learn. Other information that is important to consider is that the patient has type I diabetes, still retains the ability to walk, but has only limited use of his hands, with the casts on both arms. The teaching diagnosis is the basis for the teaching plan.[13]

III. Development of a Teaching Plan Through Goals and Objectives (Planning)

A. **Goals** are generally defined as broad, general statements about what the patient needs and wants to learn. The goals that are formulated collaboratively with the patient will guide their teaching for the duration of the hospitalization and transition back into the community. The goals can be long term or short term. Nurses can better help patients identify their learning goals by working through key questions such as the following: What behaviors do you have that are hindering or harmful to your recovery? What actions or behaviors need to be changed to eliminate this harmful behavior? What actions can I take to help you adopt new, healthy behaviors?[11] For the patient discussed in the previous example, a high-priority goal would be to reduce his high stress levels because stress limits his ability to comprehend and remember new information. This would be a short-term goal because it needs to be achieved before additional learning can take place. The goal might state: The patient will learn techniques to lower his stress levels in two days.

B. *Learning objectives* are derived from the patient's goals and more specifically guide the teaching plan of the patient. Learning objectives are behavioral in their formulation; that is, they emphasize what the learner is

supposed to be able to *do* when learning has occurred. Objectives describe the learning outcomes in clear and understandable language; achievement of the objective, or progress toward it, can be measured. Well-developed behavioral objectives should also specify a time frame in which they are expected to be accomplished.[13]

Key points to keep in mind when developing behavioral objectives include the following:

• Always start the objective with an *action verb* that specifies the behavior that will demonstrate that patient learning has occurred.

• Always focus the objective on how the learner is to perform or complete a behavior. The only way the behavior or action can be observed and measured is if it can be seen, felt, or heard by the nurse.

• Limit each objective to only one specific learning outcome. One of the purposes of assessment, particularly if an outcome is not achieved, is to determine what caused the lack of achievement. Multiple-outcome objectives make that determination very difficult.[13]

The best objectives are created through active collaboration that involves the patient, the health-care team, and the family or community to which the patient returns. Patients are energized by accomplishing simple behaviors conceived collaboratively.

Objectives can fall within three domains, or categories: affective, cognitive, and psychomotor.[14] Different ways of measuring outcomes are used for each domain.

• **Affective domain objectives** center on feelings and emotions, such as interests, values, attitudes, appreciation, and methods of adjustment necessary for a positive effect on the patient's life. Affective skills include positive attitudes, constructive feelings, and values (ethics) that underlie the rapport with the patient.[15] Although affective objectives are more difficult to measure, they are just as important as other categories of objectives. For example, in the patient described earlier, his increased stress may lead to anxiety and interfere with his ability to achieve other objectives, so a goal for him is to lower his stress levels. A possible affective objective may state: Reduce the patient's stress by encouraging him to verbalize his feelings openly; stress reduction is indicated by lower blood pressure and heart rate and reduction in muscle tension, irritability, and expressions of hostility within two days.

- **Cognitive domain objectives** focus on intellectual outcomes, such as knowledge, understanding, and thinking skills the patient needs. Cognitive skills include a patient understanding the management of their injury or illness as well as perceiving self-management care needs after discharge.[15] Many websites offer suggestions for teaching patients about managing chronic illness. The cognitive domain is divided into levels of understanding, from simple to complex. Box 23.5 shows the different levels of learning. An example of a cognitive objective is: Increase the patient's knowledge level concerning the complications of diabetes by the end of the shift. To measure achievement of this cognitive objective, the nurse could ask the patient to list some common complications or could have the patient use a learning module with a posttest.

- **Psychomotor domain objectives** assess learning of motor skills, such as giving self-injections, using mobility assistive devices correctly, using eating utensils after a stroke, or changing a colostomy bag. These objectives can also include changes in diet for weight loss.[15]

Box 23.5 The Cognitive Domain: Levels of Understanding

- Knowledge: Recall of facts and concepts
- Comprehension: Understanding of what concepts mean
- Application: Use of a concept
- Analysis: Ability to examine or explain a concept
- Synthesis: Integration of a concept with other learning
- Evaluation: Judging or comparison of concepts

Source: Adapted from S.B. Bastable, M.F. Alt, Behavioral objectives, Key Nurse, n.d., https://nursekey.com/behavioral-objectives.

For behavioral change to occur, memory from the cognitive domain must be present. Teaching psychomotor skills includes demonstrating and modeling the skills patients will need for self-care.[14] For example, the diabetic patient with two broken arms is going to have a high level of difficulty giving himself insulin injections. After determining that the patient has enough manual dexterity to manipulate a syringe and vial of insulin and is also able to reach the anterior area of both legs, the nurse teaches the patient how to administer his insulin. A psychomotor objective for this patient could be: Demonstrate, by the time of discharge, the ability to use proper technique in self-injecting the appropriate type and amount of insulin, rotating sites on the upper leg.[15]

C. Teaching Content

Nurses can gather the content they need from many resources. Some underused but critical sources are nursing organizations and disease-specific websites, such as that of the American Cancer Society. Good content helps patients make medical decisions; inform themselves about self-care; and understand their condition, their care, or any other area of wellness that needs improvement.[14]

D. Teaching Strategies and Learning Activities

Tables 23.4 and 23.5 summarize this information.[14]

IV. Implementation of the Teaching Plan (Implementation)

It is always important for the nurse to separate what patients *need* to know to improve or maintain their health and what might be *nice* for them to know. Nurses tend to like to tell patients everything about their disease processes. Some patients ask a lot of questions and are very curious about their illness, but the essential element is to teach them what is important to their survival.

The most effective learning occurs when the patient is actively involved in the learning process along with their family. **Passive learning**, wherein the learner is treated like a receptacle for new information, does not change behaviors or attitudes and, therefore, yields poorer outcomes. Although passive learning can be useful when

Table 23.5 Matching Teaching Strategies to Learners

Strategy/Method	Learner
Case study	Adolescents, young adults, adults
Computer	All ages, assuming computer literacy and access to a computer
Demonstration	All ages
Discussion	Preadolescents, adolescents, young adults, adults, older adults
Lecture	Adults, older adults
Media (e-learning)	All ages; especially appropriate for younger learners
Modeling	All ages
Trial and error	Adolescents, young adults
Visual aids	All ages
Role-playing	Children, adolescents, young adults

Source: *Matching teaching strategies with adult learning styles maximizes educational effectiveness*, Strategies for Nurse Managers, *https://ies.ed.gov/ncee/pubs/2021007/pdf/2021007.pdf*

new knowledge must be gained quickly, it is not effective for the long-term success of a patient-education plan.

The implementation of a successful teaching plan will include the following:

A. Visual Aids

Most people, unless they have a visual impairment, are visual learners. High-quality health-care videos are available on almost any subject, from giving self-injections to changing colostomy appliances to managing stress. Use of visual materials is a good way to either introduce or reinforce content that the nurse is attempting to teach. However, it is important to not rely on an electronic presentation as the sole source of educating a patient. The nurse should always review the video content, answer questions, and reinforce the areas they determine are important for the patient's learning.

B. Increasing Motivation

It would seem logical that if a nurse is presenting information about your disease process and how to care for yourself, you would be interested in learning, or motivated to learn. But this is not always the case. Increasing motivation can be a tricky enterprise.

The key to improving patient motivation that produces lasting behavioral changes goes back to establishing a sound nurse–patient relationship through solid communication skills. It is well known that nurses have a caring attitude toward their patients, but patients must be able to recognize and actually *feel* that attitude. One way that nurses can do this is by focusing on clinical care processes that individualize human relationships rather than providing one-size-fits-all care. This change in approach will optimize motivating effects and move patients toward engaging in optimal health behaviors. Patient motivation can be increased by using the following:

• Incentive techniques: Incentives are particularly useful in sparking patient participation in wellness activities ranging from giving themselves insulin injections to walking the length of the hall as an inpatient to climbing a number of steps per day when they are at home. Wellness programs motivate patients to perform wellness activities by offering an incentive or prize at the end. Effective incentive rewards include gift cards to favored stores or eateries, cash prizes, and discounts on bills. An important part of the most effective incentives includes sending regular reminders about the contests and celebratory notes as goals are achieved.

• Apps and social media: Health-related apps and social media provide an opportunity to teach patients and increase their motivation from an external source. There are more than 350,000 health-related apps worldwide. They continue to grow in number and popularity among patients. Some apps are better than others, so the nurse should review an app for quality and content before the patient begins to use it as a component of recovery. The best apps can support patient self-care management.[15] (See Chapters 17 and 24 for methods to evaluate electronic source information.)

Patient education within the app must be targeted and cannot be arbitrary. Increasing the patient's knowledge in ways specifically related to one health behavior can improve compliance and change the behavior. Although health-care motivational apps work best when they convey positive reinforcements, just by using the app, the patient is displaying increased motivation.

- Patient informational materials: Handing patients a pile of photocopied sheets just before they leave the hospital is not the best way to motivate self-care at home. Although information sheets are better than nothing and some patients or their families may actually read the material, they are a one-size-fits-all approach to teaching. Remember that teaching and learning go hand in hand and are intrinsically interrelated. Unless the nurse knows the patient well enough to figure out what type of take-home materials fit their particular learning style, learning will be minimal.

There are two important things to remember when using informational materials. First, do not overwhelm patients with too much information. Too much all at one time will likely crush their motivation to learn or confuse them. Second, while teaching, use the information obtained during the educational assessment to choose teaching methods tailored to an individual patient's preferred learning style. Doing so will improve the patient's retention of important information.[16]

V. Evaluation of Expected Outcomes (Evaluation)
Evaluation is the last and, in some ways, most important phase of the teaching–learning process. It is the review of patients' learning evolution during and after teaching. The purpose of evaluation is to determine whether patients have learned what was taught.

The ability of patients to meet co-created goals and objectives can be easily monitored if follow-up and communication are embedded in the teaching–learning process. Technology- and computer-based learning programs for patients to use at home after discharge can be valuable in reinforcing earlier learning and evaluating self-care. Patients can log on to the facility's website and obtain electronic evaluations that they can do at home. With the provisions in the ACA that call for reimbursement based on meeting patient outcome goals, these types of evaluations become increasingly valuable.

> *Health-related apps and social media provide an opportunity to teach patients and increase their motivation from an external source.*

Evaluating Teaching Effectiveness in Patient Education

Health-care providers must educate patients with the intent of increasing their knowledge and changing their behaviors. The only way to make sure patients understand the information is to ask them to repeat it or to show the nurse how the procedure is done. The question, "Do you understand how to change the tubing on your CAPD system?" can be answered with a yes or a nod of the head, but that response does not ensure the patient can perform the task satisfactorily. A request to "show me how to change the tubing" will provide much more valuable information. This technique, called **teach-back**, or *return demonstration*, has been used in health care for many years. Using teach-back to evaluate patient understanding provides the nurse a concrete measurement of the effectiveness of their teaching.[17]

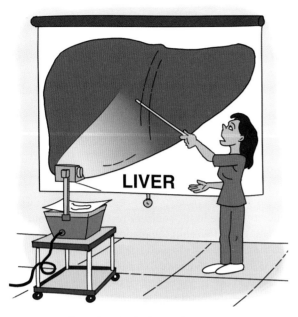

Visual aids help in learning.

Evaluating understanding of content is easily accomplished through testing. True/false, multiple choice, and even essay questions are all viable methods for testing health-care knowledge. Unfortunately, test anxiety is a real phenomenon that can stress a patient already challenged by a health problem. Due to patient anxiety, these types of tests are not likely to produce reliable evaluations of patient learning. Teach-back is a more effective method of evaluating a person's ability to perform a skill. The challenge lies in being able to replicate the behavior as a patient transitions from the inpatient care setting to home.[21]

In documenting patient teaching, it is important to rate how well the patient has learned the information and/or skill that was taught. Here is one rating scale that can be used in evaluating the success of learning:

1. Patient refuses or is unable to learn.
2. Patient is unable to retain fundamental ideas.
3. Patient retains fundamental ideas with help.
4. Patient retains fundamental ideas and replicates skills with help.

5. Patient retains fundamental ideas without help.
6. Patient retains fundamental ideas and replicates skills without help.[17]

Medagogy

Medagogy is a model of patient education that encompasses everything found within the other patient education models; unlike the other models, it focuses the responsibility for health learning on both the teacher (nurse) and the patient.[18] *Medagogy* should not be confused with **pedagogy**, which is the study of the theory and practice of teaching and how these influence student learning. The underlying premise of the medagogy model is the belief in the equal partnership between two experts: the nurse, who is the technical expert, and the patient, who is the expert on themselves. Medagogy then blends in external influences and shows how these lead to a needed change in behavior or no change in behavior if none is required. Although this model was primarily developed to improve patient education, its structure also allows it to be used to evaluate consumer health-information resources. Out of the medagogy model was developed the *integrated conceptual model of health literacy.* Primarily of European origin, medagogy connects hospital-based clinical approaches and public health approaches to health literacy.[18]

Medagogy was one of the first theories focused on patient–nurse information exchange, in which the patient and health-care provider are both learners and educators. Nurse and patient, through knowledge acquired from each other, are able to make informed decisions about health-care choices that are specific to the individual patient.

The goal of medagogy is to move patient education away from the traditional provider-centered model toward a more patient-oriented focus. In the medagogy model, the certified patient educator (CPE), a licensed health-care professional, works to ensure that patients succeed in understanding their health status and the actions or behaviors that can improve their health. In their daily practice, CPEs incorporate various medagogy tools, such as report card teaching plans and evaluation of patient understanding. CPEs empower patients with knowledge so that they can assume a more active role in their personal health care.[18]

Conclusion

With its emphasis on prevention and health maintenance, health-care reform demands that patient education be an essential part of high-quality health care. Since nursing's earliest steps toward a profession, nursing leaders realized that patient education was a moral imperative for nurses. Research shows that a large number of unnecessary readmissions to hospitals and errors in home self-care could have been prevented if patients had received the health-care education they needed before discharge.

It is imperative that nursing schools increase their instruction on patient education. An excellent method to achieve this goal is to have students prepare "teaching sessions" first for their classmates and, later in the program, for groups of patients. Another useful tool is role-play. For example, one student can play the nurse educator, and one student can play the patient. The nurse educator teaches the patient a particular skill, such as changing a colostomy bag and performing stoma care. The volunteers perform their task in front of the class, after which the whole class discusses what was done well (based on their readings and lecture content) and what could be improved. Role-playing is very useful as a teaching tool because it actually uses all three cognitive domains.

Currently, nursing students receive little education on how to teach patients. As a result, they often feel uncomfortable in the educator role and may avoid teaching due to feelings of inadequacy. Practicing teaching skills will aid graduate nurses in developing the skills and confidence to fulfill this key role of the profession. Everyone benefits if patient education is successfully planned and implemented.

CRITICAL-THINKING EXERCISES

- Look back at your own patient teaching and critique what you did well and what could have been improved. Refer to TJC requirements in Box 23.2.
- Review Chapter 6, "Ethics in Nursing," and apply the concepts to the moral imperative for patient teaching.
- Review the legal requirements in charting for patient teaching. Reflect on your own patient teaching charting and describe your strengths and weaknesses in this area.

NCLEX-STYLE QUESTIONS

1. Which of the following is the MAIN difference between medagogy and pedagogy?
   1. *Medagogy* refers to teaching adults; *pedagogy* refers to teaching children.
   2. In *medagogy*, the teacher and the learner share responsibility for health learning; in *pedagogy*, the teacher takes responsibility.
   3. In *medagogy*, the teacher drives the learning process; in *pedagogy*, the learner does.
   4. *Medagogy* refers to the teaching of medical information; *pedagogy* refers to education or learning in general.

2. In a community clinic, Renee, the RN, is preparing to teach LaTisha how to test her blood sugar at home. LaTisha, a 13-year-old honors student, has been recently diagnosed with non-insulin-dependent diabetes mellitus. Which of the following teaching methods would be appropriate for Renee to use with this patient? **Select all that apply.**
   1. Live demonstration
   2. Discussion
   3. Posters
   4. Modeling and teach-back
   5. Trial and error
   6. Role-playing
   7. Video demonstration

3. Mr. Wilson, a 48-year-old white male, is scheduled to have his gallbladder removed laparoscopically. During his pre-op appointment, Mr. Wilson waits until the surgeon has left the examination room and asks the nurse to explain the procedure again. Which of the following is the BEST way for the nurse to begin her response?
   1. "Can you tell me your highest level of education?"
   2. "Is English your native language?"
   3. "Let me call the doctor back to explain it to you again."
   4. "Tell me what you understand so far and what's confusing."

4. Which statement about using the Internet for researching health-care information is TRUE?
   1. All information found on the Internet should be viewed with skepticism.
   2. It easy for well-educated people to identify reliable websites just by reading them.
   3. Tools exist to identify high-quality, reliable websites for health-care information.
   4. Search engines such as Google take you to the most reliable sites for health-care information.

5. Ray, a nurse educator, is teaching a class for patients newly diagnosed with heart disease. The topics the class will cover include quitting use of tobacco products, increasing plant-based foods and limiting animal-based foods in the diet, exercising, and managing stress. Which action by Ray is likely to undermine his teaching plan?
   1. Eating a fast-food hamburger, milkshake, and large fries during lunch with his students.
   2. Driving to the location where the class will be taught.
   3. Telling the class about how he finally succeeded in quitting smoking cigarettes 5 years ago.
   4. Suggesting students try a free yoga class offered by the hospital.

6. Why is health literacy among patients more important now than ever before? **Select all that apply.**
   1. Hospital stays are shorter, so there is less time for patient teaching.
   2. Patients or their families are expected to manage self-care during recovery at home.
   3. Health-care providers are less willing to explain patients' health conditions nowadays.
   4. The managed-care model expects patients to make informed decisions about their own health.
   5. Health literacy allows patients to take steps to prevent or reverse some chronic conditions through nonmedical means, such as diet and exercise.

7. Which of the following BEST describes the relationship between managed care and patient empowerment?
   1. Empowered patients created the need for managed care.
   2. In managed care, the patient, not the provider, is empowered.
   3. Patient education is essential to both managed care and patient empowerment.
   4. Managed care limits patient empowerment but increases the need for patient education.

8. _____ is a collaborative skill that the nurse can use to encourage patients to commit themselves to change and involve them in the selection of risk factors to eliminate.

9. Carol Ann, an RN, is preparing to teach Mrs. Ruiz to care for her surgical wound at home after amputation of her left great toe. In developing her teaching plan, Carol Ann notes that Mrs. Ruiz speaks limited English but that she is interested in learning and asks lots of thoughtful questions through her son, who speaks fluent English. To what step in the nursing process does this part of Carol Ann's teaching plan compare?
   1. Assessment
   2. Diagnosis
   3. Implementation
   4. Evaluation

10. It's a busy day on the unit. Megan has 10 minutes to complete Mr. Jones's discharge teaching before Ms. Richie's blood transfusion is finished and Mrs. Iven's next medication is due. Megan is thinking about her to-do list while she quickly reads aloud the signs of complications from Mr. Jones's information sheet, tells him when his appointment with his primary care physician is, and calls for an aide to wheel Mr. Jones to his daughter's car. How are Megan's actions and attitude most likely to affect Mr. Jones's ability to learn?

1. Because Mr. Jones has a caring relationship with Megan, he will understand that she is busy, and he will be able to learn quickly.

2. Because Megan shows little interest in him or in teaching, Mr. Jones will likely not be able to learn much from this session.

3. Because Megan reviews the most important information with Mr. Jones, he will be able to concentrate on the essentials.

4. Because Mr. Jones has the information sheet to take home, he will be able to learn everything he needs to from that.

References

1. Hendler C. 10 Tactics to improve patient teaching. Wolters Kluwer, August 5, 2022. https://www.wolterskluwer.com/en/expert-insights/ten-tactics-to-improve-patient-teaching

2. Nursing education during times of crisis. National League for Nursing, August 22, 2022. https://www.nln.org/detail-pages/news/2022/08/22/nursing-education-perspectives-publishes-special-themed-edition-for-2022-nln-education-summit-nursing-education-during-times-of-crisis

3. Lee L, Carpenter H. Obesity in nurses. American Nurse, 2023. https://www.myamericannurse.com/obesity-in-nurses/

4. Padden D. The role of the advanced practice nurse in the promotion of exercise and physical activity. *Topics in Advanced Practice Nursing eJournal*, 2(1), 2002. https://www.medscape.com/viewarticle/421475_1

5. Berwick D. A user's manual for the IOM's "Quality Chasm" Report – Medscape. *Health Affairs*, 21(3), 2002. https://www.medscape.com/viewarticle/433216_6

6. The Joint Commission 2021 standards: What's new. Barrins and Associates, February 17, 2021. https://barrins-assoc.com/tjc-cms-blog/hospitals/joint-commission-2021-standards-whats-new/

7. Kozak M. 3 Ways the right technology supports aging in place. CitusHealth, September 1, 2022. https://www.citushealth.com/blog/3-ways-the-right-technology-supports-aging-in-place/

8. Evaluating information: The CRAAP test. McMaster University Health Science Library, 2023. https://hslmcmaster.libguides.com/c.php?g=306752&p=5238186

9. Saukas E. Health People 2030: The significance of health literacy. LinkedIn, September 2, 2022. https://www.linkedin.com/pulse/healthy-people-2030-significance-health-literacy-elizabete-s-/

10. Hirschey R, Tan K, Petermann V, Bryant A. Healthy lifestyle behaviors: Nursing considerations for social determinants of health. *Clinical Journal of Oncology Nursing*, 25(5):42–48, 2021. https://doi.org/10.1188/21.CJON.S1.42-48

11. Loosveld L, Van Gerven P, Vanassche E, Driessen E. Mentors' beliefs about their roles in health care education: A Qualitative study of mentors' personal interpretative framework. *Academic Medicine*, 95(10):1600–1606, 2020. https://doi.org/10.1097/ACM.0000000000003159

12. Nurse-Family Partnership home page. https://www.nursefamilypartnership.org/

13. Morris G. 10 ways nurses and nurse leaders can improve patient education. Nurse Journal, 2022. https://nursejournal.org/articles/tips-to-improve-patient-education/

14. Orr R, Csikari M, Freeman S, Rodriguez M. Writing and using learning objectives. *CBE—Life Sciences Education*, 21(3), 2022. https://doi.org/10.1187/cbe.22-04-0073

15. Number of mHealth apps available in the Apple App Store from 1st quarter 2015 to 3rd quarter 2022. Statista.com, 2022. https://www.statista.com/statistics/779910/health-apps-available-ios-worldwide/

16. Kirk K. Student motivations and attitudes: The role of the affective domain in geoscience learning. *Journal of Geoscience Education*, 2022. https://serc.carleton.edu/NAGTWorkshops/affective/motivation.html

17. Use teach-back method #5. In *Health Literacy Universal Precautions Toolkit*, 2nd ed. Rockville, MD: Agency for Healthcare Research and Quality, 2022. https://www.ahrq.gov/health-literacy/improve/precautions/tool5.html

18. Medagogy - what is that all about? What's brought you here today? The Teaching and Learning Lab, 2020. https://www.whatsbroughtyouheretoday.com/learning/medagogy-what-is-that-all-about/

Nursing Research and Evidence-Based Practice

24

Sharon M. Bator | Cheryl S. Taylor | Joseph T. Catalano | Cindy Krentz | Diane Ream | Karen Webb

Learning Objectives

After completing this chapter, the reader will be able to:

- Discuss the necessity of nursing research as an essential component of comprehensive patient care
- Describe how Magnet status affects evidence-based practice
- Review the history of research ethics and laws that now protect human participants and vulnerable populations
- Describe ways in which nursing research can be used to enhance communication and understanding between cultures
- Discuss the importance of theory, practice, research, and evidence-based practice to quality patient care
- Describe the steps of the quantitative research process to generate further research
- Identify websites that facilitate accomplishing each of the steps of the quantitative research process to generate further research
- Demonstrate the ability to identify the basic similarities and differences related to qualitative and quantitative research designs

(continued)

THE MOST TRUSTED PROFESSION

According to Gallup polls for the past 20 years, the nursing profession is perceived as having the highest level of ethics and honesty.[1] No matter the level of education, nurses are perceived to have the same high values, mission, and ethical standards. What makes a profession ethical? One key element of any highly ethical profession is having a strong knowledge base of practice built on reproducible research. In nursing, practical, evidence-based research contributes to high-quality patient care and outcomes.

This chapter presents an overview of the critical nature of research as scientific support for the nursing profession. The text is directed primarily toward those who are consumers of research to increase their understanding of the research studies they read as well as their ability to distinguish good research from poor research. It also includes frameworks and models to use when performing nursing research as well as common websites helpful for conducting, implementing, and disseminating research.

TAKING THE FIRST STEP

The first, and sometimes most difficult, step in research is finding the gaps in literature and identifying key health-care issues.[2] The National Teaching Institute Evidence-Based Solutions Abstracts (Table 24.1) provide nurses with the categories and classes of past research that deals with improved patient care.[3] In these studies, nurses are the primary investigators.

What Do You Think?

Review the article titles in Table 24.1. Which areas of research do you think are most important in improving patient care and health outcomes?

In addition to the National Teaching Institute, other sources of important topics that may require additional research include the American Nurses Association (ANA), the National League for

- Identify at least four strategies that may help promote implementation of valid research findings in clinical settings
- Describe the barriers to evidence-based practice
- Define and describe the concept and utility of evidence-based practice
- Discuss the research-practice gap as it relates to nursing research and identify some ideas for promoting change

Nursing (NLN), the Association of periOperative Registered Nurses (AORN), the Society of Urologic Nurses and Associates (SUNA), the Emergency Nurses Association (ENA), the Institute of Medicine (IOM, now called the National Academy of Medicine), *Healthy People 2020*, and the Robert Wood Johnson Foundation (RWJF).

Researcher Beware

Nursing research is evolving rapidly because of the technological changes that affect patient care and those that enable more rapid gathering and processing of research data. Digital technology has made dissemination of research faster than ever before. However, proprietary databases can be expensive to use if the researcher does not belong to an organization or institution that subscribes to them. In contrast, **open-access** sources were created with the belief that research information should be available and free to all—patients, consumers, and health-care professionals.[2]

In accessing information, it is important to remember that articles should be valid and reliable, particularly because false and unreliable information has become widespread on social media and the Internet. Validity focuses on the accuracy of a set of research measures, whereas reliability measures the consistency of the research measures.[2] For example, a nurse is not sure whether a newly purchased digital scale used to weigh newborn infants is functioning properly. The nurse takes a large nursing textbook and weighs it on the scale several times. Each time, it measures the same weight; therefore, the scale is reliable. Then the nurse finds a 5-pound traction weight and weighs it. The scale indicates that the weight is 5 pounds; therefore, the scale is valid. The nurse concludes from the results of their research that the scale is accurate and functioning properly.

Researching on the Internet is more complicated because the Internet is strewn with prejudiced, ambiguous, and false information. With the virtually unlimited amount of information available online, it can be difficult to interpret what is true and accurate and what is not. Reliable information comes from dependable sources that are exhaustive, well-thought-out in theory, and based on strong evidence. Some of these sources include the following:

- Scholarly, peer-reviewed articles and books
- Trade or professional articles or books
- Magazine articles, books, and newspaper articles from well-established companies

Other sources, like websites and blog posts, can be reliable but require further evaluation.

Identifying Reliable Sources

Following are some factors that may indicate a source is reliable:

1. *Authority:* Who is the author? What are their credentials? Do they have knowledge and experience in the field they are writing about? What is their academic reputation?

Electronic "bots" can flood the Internet with fake news!

Table 24.1   National Teaching Institute Evidence-Based Solutions Abstracts

Topic	Author(s)
EB1: Veno-Venous Extracorporeal Membrane Oxygenation and Profound Instability: Think Mobility from Cannulation	Jessica Dalton; Lehigh Valley Health Network, Allentown, PA
EB2: Triage of Patients with a Ventricular Assist Device: The Need for Emergent Response to Patient Concerns	Stacy Haverstick, Catherine Johnson; University of Michigan Health System, Ann Arbor, MI
EB3: Measuring True Nursing Competency: How to Improve Your Process	Amy Hiner; Aultman Hospital, Canton, OH
EB4: Increasing Sepsis Awareness in Intensive Care Units	Gabriela Whitener, Michael Thornsberry, Patricia Newcomb; Harris Methodist Hospital, Fort Worth, Arlington, TX
EB5: Peer-to-Peer Accountability as a Method to Increase Delirium Screening	Kimberly Sanchez, Kathrine Winnie, Felisabel Padua; Keck Medicine of USC, Los Angeles, CA
EB6: Preventing Probable Ventilator-Associated Pneumonia	Jessica Schwartz, Matthew Taylor, Timothy Heckman; Christiana Care Health System, Newark, DE
EB7: Central Catheter-Associated Bloodstream Infection Stand-Down Education: Back to Basics	Kelly Papili; Children's Hospital of Philadelphia, Philadelphia, PA
EB8: Increasing PCCN Certification: Strategies for Success	Alexander Nydza, Stephanie Nursey; Cleveland Clinic, Cleveland, OH
EB9: Beat the Bugs: A Campaign Against Hospital Acquired Infection in Critical Care	Leticia Donnelly-Kauffman, Mimi Johnson, Rona Lee; St Joseph Medical Center, Tacoma, WA
EB10: The Interdisciplinary Process of Implementing the ABCDEF Bundle in a Surgical Intensive Care Unit	Taline Marcarian, Katrine Murray; Ronald Reagan UCLA Medical Center, Los Angeles, CA
EB11: Pulmonary Care Unit Chronic Obstructive Pulmonary Disease Initiative	Diana Rose, Kathleen Aidala, Nichelle Lewis; Ellis Hospital, Schenectady, NY
EB12: Breaking the Fall: Creating a Culture of Safety by Implementing a Fall Prevention Bundle in a Heart Failure Unit	Donna Owens, Monette Mabolo; Moses Cone Health System, Greensboro, NC
EB13: Moving X-ray Free for Feeding Tube Placements Using Electromagnetic Technology	Stacy Jepsen, Sharon Wahl; Abbott Northwestern Hospital, Minneapolis, MN
EB14: "I Need HELP!": A Structured Response to Bedside Emergencies in the Intensive Care Unit	Sharon Wahl, Stacy Jepsen, Marina Kern; Abbott Northwestern Hospital, Minneapolis, MN
EB15: Mentoring Nurses to Success in a Cardiothoracic Intensive Care Unit Using a Clinical Ladder Matrix	Barbara Logue; Barnes Jewish Hospital, Saint Louis, MO
EB16: Brain Code: Improving Recognition and Timely Intervention for Intracranial Hypertension and Herniation	Stacy Jepsen, Maximilian Mulder, Matthew Ditmore, Marina Kern; Abbott Northwestern Hospital, Minneapolis, MN
EB17: Daily Line-Necessity Rounds Reduced Hospital-Acquired Infections in a Surgical Transplant Intensive Care Unit	Jose Sala, Ashley Eugene, Michele Ramirez; Methodist Hospital, Houston, TX
EB18: Flash Rounds: Implementing the ABCDEF Bundle in a Surgical Transplant Intensive Care Unit	Jose Sala, Michele Ramirez, Lisa DeGarmo: Methodist Hospital, Houston, TX
EB19: The Rapid Response Nurse: More Than Just a Responder	Elizabeth Avis; Thomas Jefferson University Hospital, Philadelphia, PA
EB20: It Takes a Village to Mobilize a Critically Ill Patient	Mary Beth Leaton, Kristin Ospina; Morristown Medical Center, Morristown, NJ
EB21: Pediatric Intensive Care Unit Medical Supply Waste Reduction	Michelle Chiodini; Children's Hospital Colorado, Aurora, CO

Source: *G. Lobiondo-Wood, J. Haber,* Nursing Research: Methods and Critical Appraisal for Evidence-Based Practice *(9th ed), St. Louis, MO: Elsevier, 2018.*

2. *Precision:* Compare the author's information to that which has already been researched and is known as reliable. Do they match? What are the citations? Does the information seem unfair or biased? If so, does it affect research conclusions?
3. *Handling:* Is the information relevant to the research topic, and does it meet the needs of the research? Does the source have statistics, charts, figures, and graphs that can be used?
4. *Timeliness:* If the research topic is in a constantly developing state, does the source keep pace with latest developments? Although the general rule is to use no references more than 3 to 5 years old, older sources are often appropriate for research on historical topics or past information that has not been updated with more current research.

Although peer-reviewed articles are generally considered the gold standard of research sources, they should still be scrutinized according to the reliability preceding factors. A peer-reviewed article is a manuscript that has been submitted to review by one to as many as five experts in the field of the manuscript's topic before it is published. The reviewers' judgments about the article's validity and reliability determine whether the article will be published.

Bots (short for *robots*) spread false information online by automatically resending the same false information repeatedly. Bots are software programs that run by themselves and share a message much faster than a human could spread it. As much as 42 percent of all Internet traffic is made up of bots.[4]

Like social media, research is susceptible to spreading untrue or invalid information. All researchers should be extremely skeptical of information retrieved from little-known online sources. Researchers must recognize that some sources are densely populated with false stories propagated by bots. It is essential for all researchers to review all their sources for **validity**, credibility, and **reliability**.[2]

A UNIQUE BODY OF KNOWLEDGE

One of the characteristics that defines a profession is the creation and use of a unique body of knowledge and related skills to guide its practitioners. In the nursing profession, the development of a distinct body of nursing knowledge is an ongoing process. Nursing has a long and dignified history as a service and caring profession. It is well established that more

than 150 years ago, Florence Nightingale initiated practice-based health care when working with soldiers in the Crimean War.[5]

Nursing as a scientific discipline continues to evolve, and nurse scientists have been producing research since nursing's earliest days. Nursing research is essential both to the development of the discipline of nursing and to the establishment of an evidence-based foundation for clinical practice. As with every profession, nursing continues to evolve to meet the needs of a changing society and incorporate the rapid development of new technology.

Nursing education, in order to keep pace, had to enhance its teaching of research techniques through ongoing formal development. Nurses at all educational levels are responsible for understanding research and using it to improve patient care.

From Research to Evidence-Based Practice

Using research is essential to improving quality of care for patients. In the 1970s, research became a formal part of nursing education. In the 1990s, evidence-based medicine (EBM) or evidence-based health care (EBHC) became the gold standard for physician care.[6] EBM was the active application of the current best evidence to make the optimal decisions about the treatment of individual patients using statistical data to estimate the risk-benefit ratio that was supported by high-quality research on population samples. To broaden EBM's application from medicine to nursing and to the other health-care professions, the name was changed to evidence-based practice (EBP) and included an increased emphasis on improving the quality of care for both individuals and groups as well as improving health-care outcomes.

Nursing, which had always been involved in conducting research to some degree, shifted its focus from the mere production of research to its use in developing and using EBP in the practice setting. EBP expanded the range of research from strictly quantitative studies to include qualitative studies that were better able to measure and illuminate certain elements of health care that revolved around a patient's personal views of care, such as quality of life, spirituality, and religious and philosophical values. Through the integration of individual clinical expertise, patient preferences and the best available information developed from systematic research, EBP became the gold standard for nursing practice.[7]

Using input from medicine, nursing, and other health-related disciplines, the Agency for Healthcare Research and Quality (AHRQ) in 1999 was given the task of improving the quality of health care and patient safety and improving the efficiency of the health-care system. When the agency exceeded its authority, Congress reacted by changing its name to the National Guideline Clearinghouse (NGC) and scaling back the scope of its authority. The NGC became a database for evidence-based clinical practice guidelines, which was updated weekly and provided the latest information for nurses, physicians, and other health-care team members. Unfortunately, funding for the NGC was cut in 2018, and the database no longer exists. The Alliance for the Implementation of Clinical Practice Guidelines (AiCPG, or the Alliance) is an organization created and operated exclusively for charitable, educational, and scientific purposes. Its primary goal is to freely disseminate evidence-based clinical practice guideline information to the health-care community in order to educate clinicians to improve patient care.[7]

With the current emphasis on EBP, it may be a surprise to learn that only 10 to 15 percent of U.S. health-care providers consistently provide patients with standardized, evidence-based care. The fact that facilities not using EBP experience poorer outcomes as well as a 30 percent increase in cost of operations compared to facilities that do use EBP is a powerful argument for change.[8] However, institutions have found that it may take approximately 20 years to develop a fully functional EBP system of facility-wide patient care.[8]

EBP is foundational in making high-quality clinical decisions, and all nurses need to recognize their responsibility to use it in day-to-day practice.[2] However, barriers remain to be overcome before EBP can be fully used to improve outcomes. The movement toward Magnet status in hospitals has provided an infrastructure for applying evidence-based research to practice, which has helped to overcome most, but not all, barriers to using EBP. (Magnet status is discussed later in this chapter.)

TRIAL AND ERROR

In the past, much of what constituted the practice of nursing was based on the edicts of those in authority. Nursing practice focused on doing exactly what was prescribed by the person in charge, usually the physician. Before the profession started building its own body of knowledge, it made sense to rely on the judgment of those who had more education and were considered by society to be authorities on the issues of health and illness and with whom nurses worked closely.

Experiential learning, also called the *trial-and-error process*, was used for many years in developing the knowledge, skills, and techniques nurses used in the promotion of health and healing. These practices were then passed on from one practitioner to the next. The trial-and-error method was used by humans in a variety of scientific and healing professions before the development of the scientific method and the research process. The experiential method served as the primary source of health-care knowledge for millennia.

> *Nursing as a science depends on valid research evidence to support best practice.*

Today, the trial-and-error process has been replaced by scientific inquiry and the formal research process that not only increase new knowledge but also demonstrate what is best in nursing practice. Research provides the evidence for nursing knowledge that is more reliable and transferable than that afforded by authority, tradition, or past experience. Nursing as a science depends on valid research evidence to support best practice. Research provides the crucial link between theory and practice.

NURSING RESEARCH DEFINED

Nursing research is a systematic process for answering questions through the discovery of new information with the ultimate goal of improving patient care.[2] Another commonly used definition for *research* is that it is a complex process in which knowledge, in this case in the form of discovery, is transformed from the findings of one or more studies into possible nursing interventions, with the ultimate goal of being used in clinical practice.[8]

Research shows which approaches to nursing care are most effective and which do not work. The ability to understand and use research, even if not actually conducting it, is a fundamental competency in nursing; research is also a key element in defining nursing as a profession. As one of a number of health-care professions, nursing discovers and defines its uniqueness through research.

The Goals and Purposes of Inquiry

A major goal of nursing research is to expand and clarify the body of knowledge unique to the discipline of nursing. Scientific inquiry is the tool of choice for achieving the goals of professional clarification, justification, extension, and collaboration (Fig. 24.1). The purpose of nursing research is "to test, refine, and advance the knowledge on which improved education, clinical judgment, and cost-effective, safe, ethical nursing care rests."[2] Nurses are held accountable for their actions and must be able to defend the interventions they use by relying on strong empirical evidence. At the very minimum, nursing care must be safe and effective. In light of contemporary cost-containment issues, nursing interventions are also expected to demonstrate practicality and cost-effectiveness. Nursing will not reach its full status as a profession until scientific inquiry becomes as much a part of daily practice as caring interventions.

Beyond Clinical Practice

Nursing research is not limited to the clinical practice of nursing. In its fullest meaning, nursing research involves a systematic quest for knowledge designed to address any questions and solve any problems relevant to the profession, including issues related to nursing practice, nursing education, and nursing administration.[8]

Redefining the Patient

Nurses know that patients are more than just individuals receiving nursing care within selected clinical settings. Patients are family units, communities, organizations, institutions, corporations, local and state agencies, and populations of a country and the global community. To accurately measure how effectively it meets the needs of an expanding and diverse consumer base, the nursing profession must integrate an expanding and diverse body of scientific knowledge into its daily practice. To do this, nurses must work together to promote better understanding of the research process and encourage their colleagues to seek the evidence needed to explain, modify, and improve nursing practice.

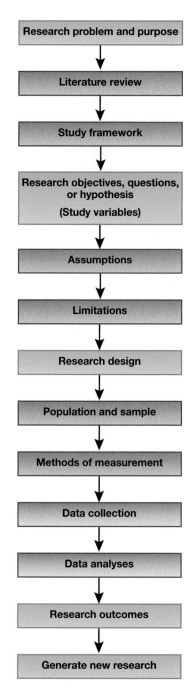

Figure 24.1 Steps in quantitative research.

Setting Priorities and Directions

Clinical decisions and the resulting nursing interventions are justified by scientifically documented findings. Using nursing research, nurse investigators address issues related to cost, safety, quality, and accessibility of health care, and they look ahead to establish priorities and to define the future direction of the nursing profession. Many of the AOS's list of 100 research topics are community oriented and fit well with both the directives of the ACA and nursing's holistic approach to health care.

For many years, the ANA has contributed to setting goals and priorities for the profession. The organization's major expectations for the use of research in nursing can be found on its website. The ANA supports nursing research with a variety of resources, such as the Research Toolkit, and has developed a research agenda to guide the association in identifying priority areas.

Priorities in nursing research can also be set by specific organizations and by local, state, and federal governments.

The Research Problem

Nurses in all areas, including clinical practice, education, health-policy formulation, and research, must be able to identify and state research problems. A clear statement of the research problem, whether it is a completely new area or one that has been the subject of previous research, is the first step in the scientific process and the foundation of the rest of the research study. The research problem can be identified through the problem-solving process, the nursing process, the research process, or the EBP process.

The four major concepts of all nursing theories—patient (person), health, environment, and nursing (see Chapter 3)—should also be considered in identifying areas of research interest. One theory so frequently used that people forget it is a theory is the population, intervention, comparison, and outcome theory (PICO, or sometimes PICOT). (See Box 24.1.) The PICO question flows naturally from nursing's values and focuses primarily on the patient or person.[7] Here is an example: A higher-than-average incidence of infections has been found in infants (the population) in the neonatal intensive care unit (NICU). The PICO question is, What is causing the

Box 24.1 **PICOT Research Methodology**

P	I	C	O	T
Population Patient Problem	Intervention Action Treatment	Comparison	Outcome Measures	Time
Who are the patients? What is the problem? Use general terms.	What do we do to them? What are they exposed to?	With what do we compare the intervention?	What is the outcome? What happened to the patient as a result of the intervention? Can it be measured?	Is the length of time of the study important to the research?
For a patient with a particular disorder, what is their age, gender, ethnicity, race, social group?	What therapy, exposure to a disease, risk behavior, prognostic factor, preventative measure, or diagnostic test is going to be used?	Standard of care? Another intervention? A control group? Absence of disease? Absence of risk factors? A placebo?	Is the disease incidence different? How accurate was the diagnosis? What are the adverse outcomes, survival, or mortality rates?	How long will it take to complete the intervention? How long will the population be observed? When is the outcome going to be measured?

higher-than-average rate of infections in this population? The infants are provided care by registered nurses (RNs) who have artificial fingernails (intervention of interest). The incidence of infections was lower before the RNs started wearing the artificial fingernails (intervention of comparison). After a new policy was implemented that artificial fingernails could no longer be worn by the staff, the number of infections decreased back to the average (positive vs. negative outcome).[9]

Crossing Cultural Boundaries

Culture-related issues (see Chapter 21) provide numerous opportunities for nursing research. Research that seeks to understand and address cultural issues involved in nursing care can improve outcomes, quality of care, and patient satisfaction—and not just for patients of diverse racial, ethnic, or religious groups. Cultural groups that can benefit from nursing research include people who are LGBTQIA+, people with physical or learning disabilities, and people who are homeless. Nursing research can span geographic distances to promote dialogue, investigation, and collaboration with international nursing colleagues.

DEVELOPMENT AND PROGRESSION OF RESEARCH IN NURSING

The Origin of Nursing Research

Florence Nightingale first elevated nursing to the status of a profession. In her first book, *Notes on Nursing*, she introduced the concept of research to the profession and expanded the concept in her subsequent publications. Nightingale believed in the importance of "naming nursing" through the collection and use of objective data. She also used these data to prove that there was a need for wide-ranging health-care reforms, including clinical practices, treatment of injured soldiers, and nursing education. Nightingale recognized the positive impact of combining strong, logical thinking and empirical research in developing a sound scientific base on which to build the practices of the nursing profession.[5]

Methodical Observation

As the first recognized nurse epidemiologist, Nightingale systematically collected objective data and in 1855 described environmental factors that affected health and illness. During the Crimean War, appalled by what she observed in the care of injured soldiers, Nightingale methodically gathered facts, which she eventually used to support her claims that lack of cleanliness, fresh air, proper rest, and adequate nutrition contributed to high levels of disease and death seen in frontline "hospitals" during the war.[5]

Backed by her meticulous research, Nightingale forcefully petitioned the government for more supplies, better food, and cleaner conditions for army hospitals. She also successfully engaged in a media campaign by providing information and statistics to reporters, whose articles garnered public support for her demands. Nightingale's strong advocacy for better care and improved environmental conditions lowered the mortality rate among wounded soldiers from 42 to 2 percent; however, widespread appreciation of her work did not occur until more than a century later.[6]

Even today, the full importance of this one woman's work to the profession of nursing is still being evaluated. Nightingale had few professional role models, relatively little education, a military organization that doubted her value, and meager financial support. In view of these challenges, her accomplishments were phenomenal. It is interesting to speculate about how much more progress would have been

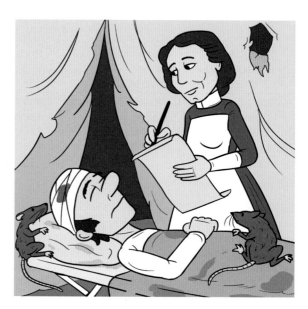

Florence Nightingale's careful observations and statistical analyses formed the early foundation of scientific nursing research.

made in building the unique body of nursing knowledge if other nurses of her time had heeded Nightingale's earliest call for research.

The Development of Research

A Look at Nursing Education

During the 1940s, much research concerning nursing education was done because of the tremendous demand for educated nurses during World War II. For example, nursing education practices were evaluated in a study commissioned by the National Nursing Council for War Service. Findings from this study and others at the time uncovered weaknesses in nursing education.[2] This relatively new wave of research spawned several other studies that looked at nurses' functions, roles, attitudes, acceptance, and interactions with patients.

A Center for Nursing Research

The 1950s saw an increase in the number of nurses with advanced degrees and the formation of a center for nursing research at the Walter Reed Army Institute of Research. The American Nurses Foundation was created during this decade, and the journal *Nursing Research* began publishing nursing research findings. Many of these studies served as the mirror or even the microscope through which nurses studied themselves and their profession. This self-appraisal was an unprecedented research approach for any profession.

New Terminology for Nursing

In the 1960s, phrases such as *conceptual framework, conceptual model*, and *nursing process* made their first appearances in textbooks and other nursing literature (see Chapter 3). Nursing leaders, focused on theoretical support for nursing, continued to lament the relative lack of research.

Many professional nursing organizations set priorities for research during this time. It was also during this time that another visionary nurse heeded the call to logical reasoning and empirical research. According to Virginia Henderson, one of the early nursing theorists, the role of nursing is "to assist individuals (sick or well) with those activities contributing to health, or its recovery or to a peaceful death, that they perform unaided, when they have the necessary strength, will, or knowledge; to help individuals carry out prescribed therapy and to be independent of assistance as soon as possible."[2]

This definition was so conceptually clear that it was accepted by the International Council of Nurses (ICN) in 1960, and Henderson's work went on to identify many relevant research questions for the practice of professional nursing.[2]

A Growth in Research Programs

In the 1970s, the number of graduate nursing programs grew tremendously, and so did the number of nurses who were conducting research. The sheer number of ongoing research studies underscored the need for an improved way to publicize those studies. Three more research journals were developed to meet this need: *Advances in Nursing Science, Research in Nursing and Health*, and the *Western Journal of Nursing Research*. During this time, the research focus began to shift away from the study of nurses toward the study of patient-care needs. Clinical challenges were identified as having the highest priority for nursing research, a trend that continues today.

A Source of National Data

The 1980s witnessed another information explosion when classes of research-trained, graduate-school-educated nurses graduated and computers entered widespread use. Research and writing were both enhanced by electronic databases and the expanding World Wide Web. In 1983, the ANA created the Center for Research for Nursing.

The mission of this center is to serve as a source of national data for the profession. In 1986, the National Center for Nursing Research (NCNR) at the National Institutes of Health was established by congressional mandate. The mission of this organization is to support clinical (applied) and basic research to create a scientific foundation for the care of individuals across the life span. Also during the 1980s, a journal with the specific intention of providing research directed toward the practicing clinical nurse took form in *Applied Nursing Research*.[10]

A New Focus on Practice

In 1993, the NCNR was awarded full institute status, and the National Institute of Nursing Research (NINR) came into being. In 1996, NINR had a reported $55 million budget to promote and support research priorities established during that decade. Since the late 1990s, studies have become more focused on the practice of nursing, the outcomes of nursing and other health-care services, and the building of a stronger knowledge base by replicating previous research using a variety of settings and situations. A significant amount of grant money is still available through NINR's grant application process that can be accessed online.[10]

THE NEXT STEP IN NURSING PRACTICE: CRITICAL DISCERNMENT

Because of the huge volume of literature being published by all health-care professions, including nursing, it is important for researchers to develop critical discernment skills. Critical discernment requires the nurse to understand the research process and to sift through and carefully assess all available and credible research findings. (See Box 24.2.) Once the research has been analyzed and evaluated, recommendations for best-practice techniques can be made on the basis of best evidence.[5]

A Reciprocal Relationship

When theory underlies research, both the validity and reliability of the data produced by the research are increased. In a type of reciprocal relationship, theory helps guide research, and then research helps develop theory. Although a theory is abstract in nature, it can demonstrate the relationship among the variables of the research project. PICO questions are often

---

Box 24.2 Nursing's Top 10 IOM Priorities for Research

1. Preventing and treating overweight and obesity in children and adolescents through school-related interventions such as healthy meal programs, vending machines that sell healthy snacks, and physical activity

2. Developing more effective treatment strategies for atrial fibrillation by comparing treatments such as surgery, catheter ablation, lifestyle changes, and medications

3. Identifying risk factors and preventing falls in older adults through primary prevention methods such as exercise, balance training, and various clinical treatments

4. Evaluating the effectiveness of comprehensive home-care programs for children and adults with severe chronic disease, particularly in minority and ethnic populations that have been identified as having ongoing health disparities

5. Comparing the effectiveness of hearing loss treatments for children and adults in minority groups and ethnic populations; evaluating various methods, including, but not limited to, assistive listening devices, cochlear implants, electric-acoustic devices, rehabilitation methods, sign language, and total communication techniques

6. Preventing obesity, hypertension, diabetes, and heart disease in at-risk groups such as the urban poor, Hispanic, and American Indian populations; comparing the effectiveness of strategies, including, but not limited to, pharmacological interventions, improved community environment, making healthy foods available, or a combination of interventions

7. Reducing or eliminating health-care associated infection (HAI) in adults and children by testing various techniques, particularly where invasive devices such as central lines, ventilators, and surgical procedures are used

8. Determining the best methods for early detection, prevention, treatment, and elimination of antibiotic-resistant organisms (e.g., methicillin-resistant *Staphylococcus aureus* [MRSA]) in both community and institutional settings

9. Determining the best treatments for early detection and management of dementia to be used by caregivers in the community setting

10. Publishing and distributing the findings of CER so that patients, physicians, nurses, and others can use the data to establish best practices

Sources: Institute of Medicine, Committee on Comparative Effectiveness Research Prioritization, *Initial National Priorities for Comparative Effectiveness Research*, Washington, DC: National Academies Press; J. Gray, S. Grove, S. Sutherland, *Burns & Grove's the Practice of Nursing Research: Appraisal, Synthesis, and Generation of Evidence* (8th ed.), St. Louis, MO: Saunders, 2018.

considered a form of conceptual frameworks or conceptual models.[9]

Evidence-Based Practice

Today, the movement to achieve cost-effective, high-quality care based on scientific inquiry generates the drive for EBP, one of today's high-priority nursing issues. Using evidence from the health sciences and other benchmark literature instead of the trial-and-error method of the past is essential for nurses who wish to provide high-quality care to patients, advocate for them, and provide them a safe environment.[11]

Although nurses have been using evidence-based nursing practice in some form since the early days of nursing, it is only recently that the process has become formalized and widespread as a methodology. The current use of EBP in nursing requires a transition from nursing care that is based on opinions, past practices, and tradition to a practice that is based on scientific research and proven evidence. Nurses using EBP obtain the best information available and integrate it into their day-to-day nursing practice with the ultimate goal of improving the quality of care. EBP also accounts for the patient's values and self-determination in providing care and acknowledges the significant role of the patient's family. One important development in EBP is the Magnet Recognition Program, which provides an infrastructure for evidence-based research in hospitals.

Level of Evidence

Data derived from evidence-based research is most helpful when it is classified according to its usefulness, also called its level of evidence (LOE). A responsibility of nurse researchers is to contribute high-quality knowledge to the profession, and this requires being able to evaluate the literature being examined and assess its LOE. Not only does LOE point to the type of research that needs to be conducted, it also assists with the literature search. Several different systems of LOE have been published, but none have been officially adopted by any nursing organizations.

Developing new knowledge requires being able to analyze the literature and data that have already been produced and to identify the level of confidence in their truth and accuracy so that information can be used in the most effective way.

Evidence Reports

Nurses have numerous sources of information to incorporate into their care. Research reported in the literature can be a primary source of high-quality information, but it is not the only one. Other sources include expert opinion, collaborative consensus, published standards, historical data, local quality-assurance studies, and institutional reports, including cost-effectiveness and patient and family preferences and input. The key to using these various sources of information is the ability to grade or rank them so that nursing practice is based on the *best* information available. A list of sites that provide information about research findings in nursing is found in Table 24.2.

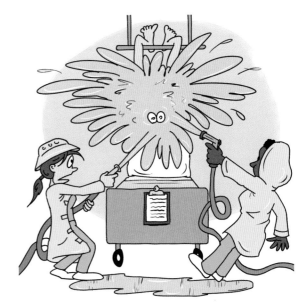

"Are you sure this new bath technique was on the evidence-based practice list?"

Evidence reports located at these sites provide scientific information about a disease or a nursing practice and then integrate those data with actions used in practice. Most reputable sites synthesize previous and current knowledge related to the topic, review the information for quality and documentation, explain how EBP is currently being used, and discuss how useful the EBP is to the clinical practice. The reviews in evidence reports are more detailed than a typical literature review and include broad-based information translated into specific approaches to patient

(text continues on page 669)

Table 24.2 Useful EBP Websites

Resources for EBP Information	Website: Where to Go to Find Information	Information About the Websites
American Nurses Association (United States)	https://www.scribd.com/doc/192569239/American-nurses-association-Nursing-Journal-Toolkit-Quantitative-research-study-critique-guide-to-research-critique	Research Toolkit Helps provide evidence-based care that promotes quality health outcomes: 1. Asking the question 2. Acquiring information 3. Appraising the evidence 4. Essential nursing resources 5. Research glossaries 6. Critique a research article 7. Education about evidence-based practice (EBP) and research 8. Comparative effectiveness research/patient-centered outcomes 9. Subjects protection 10. Research funding 11. Research organizations 12. ANA's research agenda 13. National Database of Nursing Quality Indicators (NDNQI) 14. International Council of Nurses (ICN) EBP resource 15. Research repository [members only—login required]
Joanna Briggs Institute (JBI) (Australia)	https://www.joannabriggs.org/	JBI is the international not-for-profit research and development arm of the School of Translational Science based at the Faculty of Health Sciences, University of Adelaide, South Australia. JBI collaborates internationally with more than 70 entities across the world. Along with its collaborating entities, JBI promotes and supports the synthesis, transfer, and utilization of evidence by identifying feasible, appropriate, meaningful, and effective health-care practices to assist in the improvement of health-care outcomes globally.
Sigma Theta Tau International	https://www.sigmanursing.org	Research library Nursing library Research grants Call for abstracts Research initiatives Research Resources Honor society archives Chapter archivist information **Publications** Books *Reflection on Nursing Leadership* online magazine

Table 24.2   Useful EBP Websites (continued)

Resources for EBP Information	Website: Where to Go to Find Information	Information About the Websites
		Worldviews
		STTIconnect
		STTI Newsletter
		Global Action
		Global initiatives
		STTI and the UN
		Nursing organizations
		Faculty summit
		Global Ambassador Program
Agency for Healthcare Research and Quality (AHRQ) (United States)	https://www.ahrq.gov and https://www.innovations .ahrq.gov	Mission is to produce clinical practice evidence that will increase the safety of health care and produce higher-quality, accessible, unbiased, affordable care. It works within the U.S. Department of Health and Human Services (DHHS) and with other partners to make sure that the evidence is understood and used.
Institute for Healthcare Improvement (IHI) (care bundle information)	http://www.ihi.org	The IHI is a small organization with a very big mission: improvement of patient care. It has many free resources. Learn from experts at IHI conferences and seminars.
		Virtual programs
		Improvement skills training
University of Minnesota, Evidence-Based Healthcare Project	https://www.sph.umn.edu/ research/centers/minnesota -evidence-based-practice -center/	The Minnesota Evidence-based Practice Center (EPC) conducts systematic reviews of health-care topics for federal and state agencies, professional associations, and foundations. Our reviews synthesize the evidence from clinical research studies and assess the quality of that evidence for clinicians, patients, guideline groups, policymakers, purchasers, payors, researchers, and other health-care decision-makers and stakeholders. The mission of the EPC program is to "synthesize scientific evidence to improve quality and effectiveness in health care."
		Excellent tutorial
EBSCOhost	https://www.ebscohost.com	One of the largest privately held and family-owned information services in the United States. For more than 70 years, EBSCO has been partnering with libraries across the country. It offers open access to complete dissertations.
National Library of Medicine	https://www.nlm.nih.gov	Opened in 1879, it has more than 7 million books, journals, technical reports, manuscripts, microfilms, photographs, and other image sources on nursing, medicine, and related sciences, including some of the world's oldest and rarest works.
HIPAA-related issues, U.S. Department of Health and Human Services [HHS]	https://www.hhs.gov/hipaa/ for-professionals/privacy/ laws-regulations/index.html	HIPAA, the Health Insurance Portability and Accountability Act, is a U.S. law designed to provide privacy standards to protect patients' medical records and other health information provided to health plans, doctors, hospitals, and other health-care providers.

(continued)

Table 24.2 Useful EBP Websites (continued)

Resources for EBP Information	Website: Where to Go to Find Information	Information About the Websites
U.S. Office of Human Research Protections (OHRP)	https://www.hhs.gov/ohrp	Provides leadership in the protection of the rights, welfare, and well-being of human subjects involved in research conducted or supported by DHHS. The office's primary duty is the implementation of a set of regulations for IRBs that mirrors the U.S. Food and Drug Administration rules covering clinical research conducted by pharmaceutical companies as well as other regulations under the guidance of the Federal Policy for the Protection of Human Subjects.
Women and minorities in clinical research, NIH policy	https://www.grants.nih.gov/policy/inclusion/women-and-minorities/guidelines.htm	Introduced because of the increasing acknowledgment that the quality and universality of biomedical research in all areas is dependent on inclusion of important biological variables, such as race and gender. Although many research studies still rely heavily on men for research, women now make up approximately one half of all participants in NIH-supported clinical research studies. Under a new policy, researchers are expected to study both male and female vertebrate animals and human subjects (including clinical research) to better improve the understanding of health and disease in men and women.
World Health Organization (WHO), informed consent templates	https://www.who.int/groups/research-ethics-review-committee/guidelines-on-submitting-research-proposals-for-ethics-review/templates-for-informed-consent-forms	Informed consent templates developed by the WHO are to assist the principal investigator in the design of the informed consent forms (ICFs). Principal investigators should adapt the ICF to meet their own requirements of their particular study. The logo of the institution, not the WHO logo, must be used on the ICF.
Internal validity information center	https://conjointly.com/kb/internal-validity/	Includes table of contents; navigating guidelines; foundations; sampling; measurement; design (internal validity); information about establishing cause and effect, single group threats, multiple group threats, social interaction threats Introduction to design Types of design Experimental design **Quasi-experimental design** Relationships among pre-post designs
Random.org research randomizer	https://www.random.org	It is a free resource for researchers and students who may require a quick method to generate random numbers or assign participants to experimental groups. It is useful for most types of research.
Social research methods: Sampling	https://conjointly.com/kb/sampling-in-research/	A free website for researchers involved in applied social research, such as nursing, and evaluation of research. It contains a large database, a research statistics selection program, a concept mapping guide, and a simulation guide.

care. Currently, substantial databases are maintained, and new data are constantly being added to the sites.[11]

What to Look For

Nurses should look for several key elements in evidence reports when attempting to integrate EBP into their care. The first part of the report should include a structured summary statement of the problem, practice, or disease that describes what is in the evidence report. The second part should comprise a lengthy and detailed analysis of the published and unpublished data, including reviews of articles and reports, the populations included in the studies, and the nature of the nursing actions investigated. One of the most important elements in the second part of the evidence report is the ranking or grading of the quality of the evidence.[11]

The level of quality of the evidence, or LOE discussed earlier, is sometimes referred to as the *level of recommendation for use*. Reliable evidence answers yes to the nurse's question, "Is the quality of this information high enough—that is, accurate, valid, and truthful enough—that I can use it in my practice?" Integrative reviews in evidence reports should provide both the type of evidence included and the strengths and consistencies of the information.

How are levels of evidence assessed? One of the most widely used classification systems for evidence is the one developed by Denise F. Polit and Cheryl Tatano Beck.[13] Polit and Beck identify five types, or levels, of evidence that can be present in an evidence report, ranked from I (strongest) to V (weakest):

I. Meta-analysis of multiple well-designed, controlled studies that examines and synthesizes these studies to find similar results
II. At least one well-designed experimental study with a random sample, control group, and intervention
III. Well-designed, quasi-experimental studies, such as nonrandomized controlled, single-group pretest or post-test, cohort studies, or time series studies
IV. Well-designed nonexperimental studies, such as comparative and correlational descriptive studies and controlled case studies
V. Case reports and clinical examples

Further, Polit and Beck rank the strength and consistency of evidence on a five-point scale ranging from A (best) to E (poorest). In general, a B or higher should be present before a nurse integrates the data into EBP. The rankings are as follows:

A. There is type I evidence or consistent findings from multiple studies of types II, III, or IV.
B. There is type II, III, or IV evidence, and the findings are generally consistent.
C. There is type II, III, or IV evidence, but the findings are inconsistent.
D. There is little or no evidence, or there is type V evidence only.
E. Panel consensus: Practice recommendations are based on the opinions of experts in the field.

One potential problem in using a ranking system is that it may not be the best method of analyzing the strength of the evidence. In nursing, much of the research is qualitative or descriptive, or even narrative, because of the difficulty in performing controlled studies with large groups of patients. The nurse needs to check the consistency of the results, even though there may not be any type I, II, or III studies in the evidence report.[14]

The next section of the evidence report focuses on clinical practice and should include practice-focused guidelines or recommendations for specific clinical interventions. Often, this section begins with a statement such as "There is very good evidence that . . ." or "There is no evidence that . . .". The practices outlined should be specific and relevant to the care being given.

The last section of the evidence report is the report source. Reports should be specific and current and should come from high-quality, peer-reviewed (refereed) professional journals.

Evaluating an Evidence Report

Three questions help a nurse evaluate an evidence report. Only if all three questions can be answered in the affirmative should the nurse incorporate the information into his or her practice.

1. *Is this the best available evidence?* Best sources include peer-reviewed journals and reports no more than 3 to 5 years old.
2. *Will the recommendations work for my practice given the patient population and/or medical conditions I routinely see?* If the study population is of young adult white men and the nurse's primary work population is elderly black women, the data generated may not apply.

Issues Now

Magnet recognition is the most prestigious award a health-care organization can receive from the American Nurses Credentialing Center (ANCC). Magnet hospitals are recognized for their commitment to excellence, especially with respect to patient outcomes and the delivery of excellent nursing care. To nurses, a Magnet hospital means a culture in which they can thrive as a professional, increase their knowledge and skills through continuing education, and enjoy professional autonomy and empowerment to make decisions at the bedside.[12]

To maintain Magnet status, health organizations must demonstrate that clinical practice is based on the most up-to-date research. Leaders and organizations such as the National Academy of Medicine (NAM; formerly the Institute of Medicine) also expect continuous improvement of the quality of care and patient outcomes. Because research has demonstrated that EBP leads to improved health and better patient outcomes, the NAM goal for clinical decisions to be evidence based remains at 90 percent. Magnet hospitals integrate EBP into clinical practice by providing nurses the resources, tools, and time needed to learn new information and practice new skills.

The concept of EBP was first introduced to physicians in 1991 and was soon adopted by many other providers, including nurses.[13] The most widely used definition of EBP is "the conscientious, explicit, and judicious use of current best evidence in making decisions about the care of individual patients."[5] The practice of EBHC means integrating individual clinical expertise with the best available external clinical evidence from systematic research. However, the evidence collected to make clinical decisions is just one part of the process. The provider must also consider his or her own clinical expertise as well as patient preferences, values, and beliefs to be able to make clinical decisions that enhance health outcomes and quality care.

The revised definition of EBP specifically for nursing states: "It is the conscientious, explicit, and judicious use of theory-derived, research-based information in making decisions about care delivery to individuals or groups of patients in consideration of their needs and preferences." This definition includes both qualitative and quantitative research and contributes to the utilization of scientific evidence unique to nursing.

Sources: D. Polit, C. Beck, Nursing Research: Generating and Assessing Evidence for Professional Nursing Practice, Philadelphia, PA: Wolters Kluwer, 2021; American Nurses Credentialing Center, ANCC Magnet Recognition Program, https://www.nursingworld.org/organizational-programs/magnet/; B. Melnyk, L. Gallagher-Ford, B. Thomas, M. Troseth, K. Wyngarden, L. Szalacha, A study of chief nurse executives indicates low prioritization of evidence-based practice and shortcomings in hospital performance metrics across the United States, Worldviews on Evidence-Based Nursing, 13(1):6–14; M. Schekel, Nursing education: Past, present, future, in G. Roux, J. Halstead (Eds.), Issues and Trends in Nursing (pp. 27–55), Sudbury, MA: Jones & Bartlett, 2009.

3. *Do the recommendations fit well with the preferences and values of the patients I commonly work with?* If the values of the nurse's patients vary greatly from those of the study group, the recommendations likely will not work well.

Nurses can locate evidence reports from numerous sources, such as the following:

Clinical Journals

Evidence-Based Nursing (https://ebn.bmj.com)
Online Journal of Clinical Innovations (https:// ojin.nursingworld.org/MainMenuCategories/ ANAMarketplace/ANAPeriodicals/OJIN/ TableofContents/Volume62001/No2May01/ ArticlePreviousTopic/ClinicalInnovations.html)

Reformatted STTI *Online Journal for Knowledge Synthesis in Nursing* (https://www.researchgate.net/ publication/14714736_The_Online_Journal_of _Knowledge_Synthesis_for_Nursing) (Must be a member to access)

Other Sources

The Cochrane Collaboration (international): Develops and maintains systematic reviews (http://www.cochrane.org)

Best Practices

Although there is some difference in meaning between the terms *evidence-based practice* and *best practice in nursing*, at the undergraduate level, the difference is probably meaningless. Most of the time, *best practice* is defined as a clinical nursing action that is based on the "best evidence" available from nursing research. The purpose is to achieve patient-care outcomes that exceed the basic standards of care. To be considered a best practice, a practice must be supported by empirical data from multiple institutions that are using the practice, and it must be published in a professional journal. EBP is geared to the goal of improving outcomes and generating high-quality care.[5]

Moving Forward

When nurses integrate EBP and best practices into the care they provide, they raise the level of professionalism in nursing practice. Through the use of EBP and best practices, the quality of patient care improves.

Currently, nurses have the responsibility not only to conduct research but also to evaluate, critique, and apply the research findings of other nurses and health-care professionals in their own practice. Understanding research is more than merely learning simple methods of inquiry. Research skills are expected from nurses at all levels, whether beginning or advanced. For the novice, this means being able to conduct literature searches and select articles to critique. The ability to read, understand, and critique research articles is the first step in improving one's own clinical practice.

THE RESEARCH PROCESS

Long before graduation, nursing students often notice something in the clinical setting that grabs their attention. They may wonder if a different approach would work better, if a technique currently being used can be improved upon, and what evidence exists to support a particular technique or intervention as the "best."

As newcomers to the profession, students may question interventions or solutions that seasoned nurses take for granted. Students may see the experienced nurse's familiar world differently, and their minds may be open to possibilities that those in the field for many years cannot see. Questioning the status quo is a key first step in the research process. Applying critical thinking to a problem often leads to visualizing a research project, developing a plan, implementing that plan, and finally, sharing the findings with others. This process follows a logical progression from abstract ideas to concrete actions.

Research Designs

The word *design* implies both creativity and structure. The design for a research study can be seen as a roadmap or a recipe. It serves as a fairly flexible set of guidelines that will provide the researcher with answers to the questions of inquiry.

What Do You Think?

Have you seen any procedures in your clinical rotations that could be improved? How would you design a research project to test your improved version of the procedure?

To choose a research design, the nurse must first develop a vision of the overall plan for a study, including a general idea of the type of data needed to answer the research question. The design is a critical link that connects the researcher's framework with appropriate types of data. The level of preexisting knowledge in the area of inquiry also helps determine the research design. If little is known about a specific subject, an exploratory study may be the best method for uncovering new information. Exploratory research usually focuses on the qualitative characteristics of data. Hypotheses usually are not required for these studies.

If the researcher is looking at variables that are independent or objective or that demonstrate cause and effect, a quantitative design is most suitable. If the research question invites discovery of meanings, perceptions, and the collection of subjective data, a qualitative design should be used.

Quantitative Versus Qualitative Research

Historically, **quantitative experimental research designs** were the most highly respected; and even today, quantitative research is considered to be the strongest evidence. The gold standard is the randomized clinical trial (RCT).[8] Quantitative designs examine cause-effect with a goal of discerning an underlining time sequence. In searching for the cause that produces a particular effect based on the variables of a study, the researcher must scrutinize causal factors for threats to internal and external validity. Quantitative research data is expressed in numbers.

By contrast, qualitative research looks for meaning and is holistic; it searches for phenomena relevant to human lives. Qualitative research findings are expressed in words. Another method, appropriately called mixed methods, uses elements of both quantitative and **qualitative research design**.

It is important for the nurse researcher to understand the purpose and problem of the research and then select the research design that is most appropriate. In addition, the researcher needs to recognize which level of evidence the research method produces. Although there is a preference for higher levels of evidence, the lower levels are often required to ascertain what questions can be asked at a higher level, such as an RCT.[10]

Qualitative studies were initially developed by social-sciences researchers who view human interactions as complex, highly contextual, and too intricate to be studied using a rigid framework or standard instrument. Another reason for the rise of qualitative studies is that attempting to conduct quantitative research on human subjects often produces serious ethical dilemmas. It is often very difficult to obtain approval for this type of research from the institutional review board (IRB) or the institution's human rights committee, which determines the ethical status and protection of human subjects.

Qualitative Designs

The purpose of qualitative inquiry is to gain an understanding of how individuals construct meaning in their world, visualize a situation, and make sense of that situation. For example, to nurses, the concept of "caring" is very important; yet the nurse will probably perceive caring differently than the patient perceives it. The nurse researcher wishing to measure "caring interventions" might find this concept very difficult to quantify, but a qualitative method could yield much usable information.

Because of the nature of nursing and the usual subject matter (human beings), qualitative designs are best suited to answer questions that interest nurses. The most commonly used of these designs are shown in Box 24.3.

Semistructured interviews using open-ended questions and observations is the most commonly used data-collection method in qualitative studies. Knowledge generated by qualitative research answers questions related to the meaning and understanding of human experiences.[11]

Box 24.3 **Qualitative Research Designs**
Phenomenology
Ethnography
Grounded theory
Historical studies
Case studies

Quantitative Designs

Quantitative designs use approaches that seek to verify data through prescriptive testing, correlation, and sometimes description. These designs imply varying degrees of control over the research material or subjects. Control of the research design can range from very tight to somewhat loose.

The design in quantitative research becomes the means used for hypothesis testing. The design also optimizes control over the variables to be tested and provides the structure and strategy for answering the research question. Highly controlled quantitative designs try to demonstrate causal relationships, whereas flexible designs address relationships between and among variables. Both qualitative and quantitative research follow the basic steps of the research process. For more details on this process, refer to the ANA's Research Toolkit found on its website. It has information for each of the research process steps listed in Figure 24.1.

In quantitative experimental design, a comparison of two or more groups is required. The groups under study must be as similar as possible so that results can be credited to the independent variable and not to differences between the groups. The **independent variable** is the one managed or manipulated by the researcher. The **dependent variable** *depends on*, or is altered as a direct result of, the researcher's manipulation. Table 24.3 summarizes and classifies quantitative research designs.

Neither the quantitative nor the qualitative research design is better than the other. Each research approach is useful in different ways, and both expand understanding of health care and the nursing profession. What *is* important is to choose the methodology that best addresses the questions the researcher is asking and collects whatever data are most useful.

Table 24.3 Quantitative Research Designs	
Experimental Designs	**Nonexperimental Designs**
Pretest/post-test control group	Comparative studies
Post-test only control group	Correlational studies
Solomon four group	Developmental studies
	Evaluation studies
Quasi-experimental designs	Meta-analysis studies
Nonequivalent control group	Methodological studies
Time series	Needs-assessment studies
	Secondary analysis studies
Pre-experimental designs	Survey studies
One group pretest/ post-test	One-shot case study

Comparative Effectiveness Research

Past research often compared two treatments to determine which was more effective, but it seldom took the next step—translating the findings into the practice setting. Comparative effectiveness research (CER) emphasizes the need to use research to establish best-practice standards and to disseminate research that has proven effective. CER also includes studying innovative strategies in health-care delivery, including methods to modify health awareness, lifestyle, diet, or the effect of the environment on health. A CER study must compare health-care actions that lead to a health-related outcome measure. Study methods may include randomized trials with at least two active (non-placebo) intervention groups, database studies, observational studies, model-based studies, and decision analysis. Whereas clinical trials generally use a relatively small collection of patients who meet strict inclusion requirements, CER uses a wide collection of patients who are seen every day in clinical care. For example, a CER study in 2011 investigated the cause of poor compliance with discharge medication for patients who had experienced a myocardial infarction (MI). These

patients had a medication compliance rate in the range of 35 to 49 percent. The hypothesis was that many of the patients who failed to take their medications did so because of the cost and inability to pay for them.

The study compared two groups. The first randomly assigned group was given full prescription coverage with no copay (1,494 insurance plan sponsors with 2,845 patients) for all statins, beta blockers, angiotensin-converting-enzyme inhibitors, and angiotensin-receptor blockers that were prescribed for home use. The second randomly assigned group (1,486 insurance plan sponsors with 3,010 patients) had the usual prescription coverage for the same medications including copays. The researchers' premise was that eliminating out-of-pocket costs might increase medication compliance and produce better outcomes. Although the full-coverage group had a slightly increased compliance rate (40%–55%), the results did not meet the criteria for a statistically significant difference. The cost of medications did not affect compliance. However, the study did yield an unexpected finding. The reduction of incidents of second MIs in the full-coverage group was statistically significant when compared to second MIs in the usual-coverage group.[15]

Systematic Reviews

Systematic reviews present summaries of past research on particular topics that are easy to read and understand. The role of such reviews has become more important as the volume of health-care literature has expanded. Other factors favoring reviews include the inconsistent quality of some research produced, the increased number of treatment approaches resulting from the availability of numerous pharmaceuticals, increasing numbers of health-care products on the market today, and the exponential growth of health-related technology.

Consideration of these factors has prompted the proposal that systematic reviews of existing literature replace primary research as a main source of evidence for clinical decision making. One review of this type could replace many individual studies and free those making clinical decisions from finding, interpreting, and evaluating a collection of published primary research reports and articles.

Some believe that systematic reviews should represent the gold standard in research summaries. But others argue that methods currently used for literature review may not most accurately reflect some of the nursing research being reviewed. The challenge for those who generate systematic reviews is to meet the standards of the "narrowly defined concept of what constitutes good evidence."[16]

Infodemic

Infodemic is a term that may not be familiar to everyone. It is defined as an inundation of online information that contains either false, deceptive, or inaccurate information. Infodemics occur when a need for immediate information in large quantities exists, such as during major crises, elections, disasters, or pandemics. As a result, there is an overproduction of data from multiple sources. The speed at which the new information is created and disseminated affects its quality and ultimately impacts the social and health status of individuals. Although some of the information may be accurate, a large quantity of it is false, inaccurate, deliberately intended to deceive (disinformation), or intentionally biased and manipulated (propaganda). A marked increase in this type of information occurred during the COVID-19 pandemic. Assessing and using information produced during an infodemic period for making health-care decisions requires time and acute discernment. Analyzing the quality of evidence-based infodemic data requires knowledge of the potential harms it can produce.[16]

Primary Research

What about using only primary nursing research studies as a source of information rather than systematic reviews? One recurring criticism of primary nursing research is that much of it is accomplished as single studies, and a single study is rarely adequate for making a decision to incorporate a new procedure or technique in a nurse's clinical practice.[13] Moreover, many excellent qualitative studies are not further validated by more rigorous quantitative studies. One solution to that problem would be to make replication studies a high research priority, particularly for research addressing clinical nursing issues.

NARROWING THE RESEARCH–PRACTICE GAP

Increasingly, nurses are becoming academically astute in the area of research. Unfortunately, education alone does not ensure transfer of what is learned in the classroom into the daily practice of nursing. Like the basic but critical skill of sterile technique, research will become a part of each nurse's practice only when it is used regularly.

Two Different Cultures

Academic and clinical nursing are two entirely different cultures. The critical and creative thinking so valued and promoted in the academic environment may fall victim to time and budget constraints in the clinical setting. To support what is best for patients, clinical practice areas such as hospitals must find ways to ensure that research finds its way into the culture of practice. The implementation of research in practice will depend on inquisitiveness, development of cognitive skills, the ability to question one's own practice, and professional discipline. Nurses also must understand that sometimes research findings will conflict with practices rooted in tradition.[5]

There has been an emphasis on nursing research for more than two decades, and nurses on the front lines of clinical practice are beginning to actively use research as a way to improve their practice.

Barriers to Adopting Research Findings in Practice

The research–practice gap remains a challenge to the nursing profession. Research is more widely available than in the past, which is a good thing. Yet the availability of research leads some to ask, "Why generate new research when the findings already generated have not been fully adopted in practice?" Following are a few of the challenges nurses encounter in trying to apply research findings to their practice.

An Isolated Skill

One challenge to the use of research in practice is that research skills are often taught to nursing students in isolation from other nursing subjects. Learning about research in this way reinforces the division between research and practice by separating the two elements early in the nurse's professional development and education. Recommendations set forth in the NAM report on the future of nursing, in addition to recommendations by major professional nursing organizations, point to the need to focus inquiry on and link research findings to clinical practice early in the education process. If these EBPs are adopted by and incorporated into nursing education, the research–practice gap should shrink and eventually be eliminated.

Lack of Understanding

Another challenge to the implementation of research in the health-care setting is that some researchers do not understand practice issues from the bedside nurse's viewpoint. As a result, these researchers' solutions may not be practical for bedside care. Nurses who attempt to use such research studies to answer their practice questions will feel frustrated and may doubt the usefulness of research.

Conversely, some nurses skilled in clinical practice may lack the knowledge to understand or interpret the language of research. Published research can often be abstract and complicated. Researchers must find ways to communicate their conclusions so that practicing nurses can easily understand and apply evidence-based solutions to the care issues they are facing.

What Do You Think?

Have you read a research report that you did not understand or could not apply to clinical practice? Was the problem overly complicated language in the report or a lack of knowledge on your part? What did you do to resolve the problem?

Entrenched Practices

Entrenched nursing practices present yet another challenge to the adoption of research findings in the clinical setting. In the not-too-distant past, nursing practices were handed down from expert nurses to novice nurses and accepted without question. A few nursing traditions remain so deeply entrenched as fact that they are hardly ever questioned and therefore evade the scrutiny of testing. However, best practices may never be identified without testing all approaches, even those that have been accepted "forever."

For example, the Homans sign test was devised by Dr. John Homans in 1941 as a physical examination technique for the assessment of lower extremity vascular compliance. It was taught in nursing and other health-care professions' assessment classes for many years. Homans, a vascular surgeon, noted that many patients with redness and irritation of the posterior calf muscle seemed to be developing early deep vein thrombosis (DVT), or a blood clot in the lower leg. One problem with the use of the Homans sign test was that calf pain with ankle dorsiflexion can signal a number of medical conditions—herniated vertebral discs, cellulitis, muscle spasms, muscle tears, muscle strains, or neurologic disorders—not just DVTs. Moreover, the test was also often misinterpreted or not conducted correctly.

Research in the 1960s and in later years demonstrated that the Homans sign test was accurate only about 8 percent to 15 percent of the time for detecting a positive DVT; however, it was taught in nursing schools long after that date. Even more troubling, later studies found that performing the test might dislodge clots if they were present, precipitating a cerebrovascular incident (stroke). Current thinking is that the Homans sign is unreliable as a clinical sign of DVT in most cases and should not be used in assessing for DVT.[17]

Lack of Incentive

Historically, due to budget limitations, few hospitals or other agencies had offered encouragement or rewards to nurses who were willing to seek out and use research findings in an effort to improve practice. One survey, conducted to identify barriers to implementation of research from clinicians' perspectives, revealed "insufficient authority and insufficient time" as the two obstacles most often cited.[10] However, these roadblocks have crumbled because of accreditation requirements by The Joint Commission and recommendations from the NAM.

Resistance From Managers

A final obstacle to implementing research findings in nursing practice may be frontline managers. Some research suggests that unit managers may view an environment of updates and change as unfavorable to maintaining a committed and cohesive staff. Some managers describe change as a threat to the constancy necessary for safe and expeditious patient care.[8] Nurses willing to incorporate best-practice evidence into clinical protocols must have confidence in their own professional judgment. They must be prepared to respectfully and diplomatically persuade reluctant managers to at least try implementing new best practices.

Incorporating Best Practices Into Nursing Practice

One strategy that can help nurses use research for the improvement of nursing care is attending conferences in which clinical research findings and ideas for practice are presented. Other strategies include

1. Incorporating research findings in textbooks, basic and continuing nursing education programs, and clinical policy and procedure manuals.
2. Explicitly connecting research use to institutional goals and objectives.
3. Developing joint committees between colleges of nursing and hospital nursing departments.
4. Inviting staff nurses to find and present summaries and abstracts during unit meetings and clinical case conferences, in an effort to increase the interest of colleagues working on their units.[11]

Almost all of the most widely read, clinically focused nursing journals have added research or EBP sections or routinely include research articles. The presence of these articles increases access to research, ensures a wider distribution of current clinical research findings, and promotes the incorporation into clinical settings of best practices based on credible evidence. Often, these articles are more accessible than the original studies because they simplify or explain some of the abstract language of research. Such articles also underscore the importance and practical nature of clinical research.

Evidence-Based Practice

The time of unquestioned nursing practice traditions is over. Nowadays, nurses must be able and willing to use evidence to inform their practice. Health-care administrators are interested in EBP because of its potential to increase quality of care and decrease the cost of health-care delivery. In addition, standards of nursing practice, clinical guidelines, and routine performance audits promote the use of research findings.

How Useful Is It?

Successful implementation of EBP depends on how practical and useful the research information is to the practicing nurse. To assess usefulness, the nurse must evaluate several factors, including potential benefits versus possible harm, cost effectiveness, availability of ongoing support resources, and willingness of the health-care staff and patients to accept change.

The challenge of implementing EBP demands critical and creative thinking for the following reasons:

• Nurses must access, understand, evaluate, and disseminate a rapidly expanding body of nursing and other health-related information.
• Nurses must be able to recognize commonalities and uncover inconsistencies regarding the values of the profession, the values of the organization that employs them, the needs of patients for whom they advocate, and even the popular culture that exerts pressure on the public's ability to make safe choices.
• Nurses must support research into complex health-care issues and promote successful implementation of changes in professional practice.

> *Successful implementation of EBP depends on how practical and useful the research information is to the practicing nurse.*

EBP and COVID-19

When the COVID-19 pandemic confronted the health-care system, it created great challenges for nurses and other health-care professionals. Nurses found themselves in uncharted waters in attempting to provide care in response to the SARS-CoV-2 virus. EBP is based on an existing body of research evidence that has accumulated over years of medical and nursing practice. Professional nurses had only minimal time to investigate evidence about the novel coronavirus when the first cases arrived in the state of Washington. It took at least 6 months before epidemiologists and the health-care system began to have a realistic understanding of COVID-19, how it spread, and what could be done to treat it. While thousands of people died, misinformation or conjecture about the virus was broadcast on both mainstream media and social media.[12]

Because of the lack of both old and new knowledge, existing evidence, and valid research, nurses entered a period of great uncertainty as they cared for increasing numbers of patients in the pandemic. The Centers for Disease Control and Prevention (CDC) and the World Health Organization (WHO) had previously published protocols and guidelines for dealing with novel acute respiratory infections to prevent and control pandemics, but these mostly applied to foreign countries. Because the mode of transmission is often unknown in novel diseases, best practice sanctioned by the CDC and WHO early in the pandemic specified the use of the highest level of infection control measures.[12] This included the use of the N95 respirator-mask for all health-care providers caring for patients who were infected. The N95 mask was not an item generally stocked in most hospitals, and their supply was soon depleted. Manufacturing companies were unable to meet the demand because many of them had been shut down due to fear of the virus. During the early weeks and months of the pandemic, the CDC changed its recommendations rapidly and frequently, increasing the confusion among health-care providers. At times, the recommendations from the CDC and WHO and other officials conflicted with each other. At one point, the CDC recommended that health-care providers use scarves and bandanas if there were no N95 masks available.[12] This recommendation does not seem to have been based on EBP.

After the pandemic, critical appraisals of EBP were undertaken. Through this evaluation process, several key questions about the use of EBP became apparent:

1. What if there is no evidence to review?
2. What if the known best-practice interventions are not available?
3. What if the trustworthy authorities' guidelines and recommendations contraindicate each other and/or the best evidence?[12]

What did nurses do when faced with an onslaught of sick and dying patients without any EBP to fall back on? They gathered whatever research evidence they could find and used their clinical knowledge, including evidence from patient assessment, internal evidence, available health-care resources, and their clinical decision-making skills, to develop treatment methodologies to meet the needs of their patients. They even fell back on trial-and-error methodologies to solve difficult care problems.[2]

Essential Features of EBP

The goals of EBP include cost-effective practice based on the data produced by research, the dissemination of data, and the implementation of best-practice interventions into the nurse's practice. But what are the essential features of EBP? EBP

- Is problem based and within the scope of the practitioner's experience.
- Narrows the research–practice gap by combining research with existing knowledge.
- Facilitates application of research into practice by including both primary and secondary research findings.
- Is concerned with quality of service and is therefore a quality-assurance activity.
- Requires team support and collaborative action.
- Supports research projects and outcomes that are cost effective.[11]

Evidence-based researchers conduct systematic reviews of existing literature. These reviews are necessary because of the large quantity of health-care literature already in existence that has not yet been assimilated into practice. The mission of EBP researchers is to evaluate and present the available evidence on a specific topic in a clear and unbiased way. Clinical recommendations evolving from this process present nurses with sound decisions based on evidence of best practice. Consequently, researchers not only will know what questions have been satisfactorily answered but also will be better able to identify where gaps in the knowledge still exist.

Networking: Where to Begin

As more evidence becomes available to guide practice, agencies and organizations are developing EBP guidelines. Guideline Central (GC) has been working closely with a variety of medical and nursing specialty organizations for two decades to develop and distribute summaries of evidence-based clinical practice guidelines. While most of GC's data sources are free, it offers a number of published products that can be purchased.[18] Other clinical resources are available through GC's mobile app and website.

Another searchable database that provides access to the best evidence from recent research is Evidence-Alerts. It supports evidence-based clinical decisions, and it offers open access to the public and health-care providers, although registration is required.

Most nursing students and many practicing nurses are familiar with PubMed as a source of articles about nursing and a multitude of biomedical topics. Although its more than 28 million documents can be difficult to search for sources of EBP, when used appropriately, it can be a rich source for finding clinical guidelines. Rather than going to the PubMed main page to search for information, the trick is to use the advanced search builder tool to find EBP-related information.

The American Pain Society, the Oncology Nursing Society, and the Gerontological Nursing Interventions Research Center provide EBP materials, and the Evidence-Based Practice Network synthesizes information from a number of sources.

RESEARCH ROLES BY EDUCATIONAL LEVEL

Leaders and educators within nursing agree that there is a role for every nurse in research, regardless of education level. A minimum requirement for all 21st-century nurses is the ability to develop *and use* basic research skills. The goal is to educate students at all levels of nursing education to understand research strategies.[3] Nurses striving to improve their individual practice are increasingly committed to building a body of knowledge specific to nursing. Findings from scientific inquiry define the unique and valuable roles and the challenges of nursing. The NLN's Research Priorities in Nursing Education tasks nurse educators with cultivating the next generation of nurse scientists. To attain this objective, nursing programs at every level must prepare nurses to capably utilize research in their practice and, with higher education, be able to produce original knowledge for nursing practice.

Areas of Competency

In its classic document *Commission on Nursing Research: Education for Preparation in Nursing Research*, the ANA identified research competencies for each classification of the nursing education program. The ANA presumes that professional nurses committed to lifelong learning will cultivate their research expertise throughout their careers. The following are the ANA's expectations and proficiencies of nursing research roles at different educational levels.

Associate Degree Nursing Graduate

1. Demonstrates awareness of the value or relevance of research in nursing

> *The ANA presumes that professional nurses committed to lifelong learning will cultivate their research expertise throughout their careers.*

2. Assists in identifying problem areas encountered in nursing practice or identifies potential research problems
3. Assists in collection of data within an established structured format

Associate degree nurses are expected to demonstrate an awareness of the value of research in nursing by becoming knowledgeable consumers of research information and by helping identify problems within their scope of nursing practice that may warrant exploration.

Baccalaureate Degree Nursing Graduate

1. Reads, interprets, and evaluates research for applicability to nursing practice
2. Identifies nursing problems that need to be investigated and participates in the implementation of scientific studies
3. Uses nursing practice as a means of gathering data for refining and extending practice
4. Applies established findings of nursing and other health-related research to practice
5. Shares research findings with colleagues

Nurses with a baccalaureate education are expected to be intelligent consumers of research by having a basic understanding of the research process. Baccalaureate-prepared nurses can interpret, evaluate, and determine the credibility of research findings. They understand the basic elements of EBP and can actively participate in research projects. These nurses must be alert to and uphold the ethical principles of any research involving human participants and oversee the protection of individual rights as specified in the ANA Code of Ethics.[19]

Master's Degree in Nursing

1. Analyzes and identifies nursing-practice problems so that scientific knowledge and scientific methods can be used to find solutions
2. Enhances quality and clinical relevance of nursing research by providing expertise in clinical problems and providing knowledge about the way in which these clinical services are delivered

3. Facilitates exploration of problems in clinical settings by contributing to a climate supportive of investigative activities, collaborating with others in investigations, and enhancing nurses' access to patients and data

4. Investigates for the purpose of monitoring the quality of nursing practice in a clinical setting

5. Develops and directs teams and assists others in applying scientific knowledge in nursing practice

Doctorate Degree in Practice-Focused Nursing or a Related Discipline

1. Provides leadership for the integration of scientific knowledge with other types of knowledge for the advancement of practice-specific knowledge into complex clinical interventions

2. Uses advanced leadership knowledge to appraise the translation of studies into practice and works together with investigators on original health-policy research opportunities

3. Translates scientific knowledge into complex clinical interventions

4. Conducts investigations to evaluate the contributions of nursing activities to the well-being of patients

5. Develops methods to monitor the quality of nursing practice in a clinical setting and to evaluate contributions of nursing activities to the well-being of patients

Graduates of a practice-focused doctoral program may have the degree of doctor of nursing (ND), doctor of nursing practice (DNP), or doctor of nursing science (DNSc). Graduates are prepared to concentrate on the evaluation and utilization of research rather than on the conduct of the research.

Graduate of a Research-Oriented Doctoral Program

1. Develops theoretical explanation of phenomena relevant to nursing by empirical research and analytic processes

2. Uses analytical and empirical methods to discover ways to modify or extend existing scientific knowledge so that it is relevant to nursing

3. Develops methods for scientific inquiry of phenomena relevant to nursing[8]

Research-focused doctoral programs grant the degree of doctor of philosophy (PhD). Graduates are expected to plan and carry out an independent program of research before receiving the degree.

ETHICAL ISSUES IN RESEARCH

Although guidelines that govern human behavior have always been a part of recorded history, the need for ethical standards in research became apparent after World War II, when evidence of the Nazis' brutal medical experimentation was revealed.

The Nuremberg Code

During the trials of German war criminals in Nuremberg, Germany, Nazi physicians tried to justify the atrocities they committed by calling them "medical research." As a result, the American Medical Association was asked to develop a code of ethics for research that would serve as a standard for judging the Nazi war crimes. This standard still exists and is known as the *Nuremberg Code* (Box 24.4).

National Research Act

Researchers from all disciplines are bound by ethical principles that protect the rights of the public. One set of these principles comes from the 1974 National Research Act. This act established the National Commission for Protection of Human Subjects in Biomedical and Behavioral Research.[20]

Part of the act mandated the establishment of IRBs, whose primary responsibility is to safeguard, in every way, the rights of any individual participating in a research study. IRBs are panels that review research proposals in detail to ensure that ethical standards are met in the protection of human rights. The mission of IRBs is to ensure that researchers do not engage in unethical behavior or conduct poorly designed research studies.

Every university, hospital, and agency that receives federal monies must submit assurances that they have established an IRB composed of at least five members. These members should reflect a variety of professional backgrounds, occupations, ethnic groups, and cultures in an effort to uphold complete and unbiased project reviews.[20]

Code of Ethics for Nurses

The profession of nursing has its own code of ethics to which all nurses are legally and ethically bound. The development of this code was initiated by the ANA board of directors and the Congress on Nursing Practice in 1995. In June 2015, the ANA House

Box 24.4 Articles Adapted From the Nuremberg Code

1. The voluntary consent of human subjects is absolutely necessary.
2. The experiment should yield fruitful results for the good of society.
3. The experiment should be so designed and based on results of animal experimentation and knowledge of . . . the disease or problem under study that the anticipated results will justify performance of the experiment.
4. The experiment should be conducted so as to avoid all unnecessary physical and mental suffering and harm.
5. No experiment should be conducted where there is an a priori reason to believe that death or . . . injury will occur.
6. The degree of risk . . . should never exceed that determined . . . by the importance of the problem to be solved by the experiment.
7. Proper preparations should be made . . . to protect the experimental subject against even remote possibilities of injury, disability, or death.
8. Only scientifically qualified people must conduct the experiment. The highest degree of skill and care should be required through all stages of the experiment.
9. During the course of the experiment, the subject should be at liberty to bring the experiment to an end.
10. During the course of the experiment, the scientist . . . must be prepared to terminate the experiment at any stage.

Source: Adapted from International Military Tribunal, *Trials of War Criminals Before the Nuremberg Military Tribunals Under Control Council Law No. 10; Nuremberg, October 1946–April 1949* (vol. 2, pp 181–182), Washington, DC: U.S. Government Printing Office, 1949.

of Delegates voted to accept a revised code of ethics, and in July 2015, the Congress on Nursing Practice and Economics voted to accept the new language, resulting in a fully approved document called *Code of Ethics for Nurses With Interpretive Statements* (see Chapter 6).

Embedded in nurses' professional code of ethics is the charge to protect every person from harm. This responsibility extends beyond nursing *research* to include any patient-related issue, any type of behavioral or biomedical research, and any questionable procedure.[2]

Informed Consent

One protection of human research subjects is the requirement that they have the information they need to make informed decisions. Patients have the right to be fully informed, not only about the care they receive but also about any research in which they participate. Informed consent is both an ethical and a legal requirement in the research process. The ethical principle of self-determination is central to the concept of informed consent.

Certain groups of individuals are considered particularly vulnerable to coercion and thus unable to give informed consent. These groups include children, people with developmental disabilities, elderly individuals, those with terminal diseases, homeless people, prisoners, and those who may have altered levels of consciousness as the result of a disease, medication, or sedation.

Nurses are well aware of the need for informed consent and the provision of information before procedures. This knowledge can serve nurses well in their obligation to obtain informed consent before conducting research.

The language of the consent form must be clear and understandable, written in the primary language of the patient, and designed for those with no more than an eighth-grade reading level. Technical language should never be used. The Code of Federal Regulations states that subjects must never be asked to waive their rights or to release the investigation from liability or negligence. Twelve key elements of informed consent are listed in Box 24.5, but various institutions and researchers, in an effort to protect

Box 24.5 Key Elements of Informed Consent

1. Researcher is identified and credentials presented.
2. Subject selection process is explained.
3. Purpose of the research is described.
4. Study procedures are discussed.
5. Potential risks are identified.
6. Potential benefits are described.
7. Compensation, if any, is discussed.
8. Alternative procedures, if any, are disclosed.
9. Assurances regarding anonymity or confidentiality are explained.
10. The right to refuse participation or withdraw from the study at any time is assured.
11. An offer to answer all questions honestly is made.
12. The means of obtaining the study results is described.

Source: R.M. Nieswiadomy, *Foundations of Nursing Research* (7th ed.), Upper Saddle River, NJ: Pearson/Prentice Hall, 2018.

research participants even further, include more than these 12 criteria.

Process Consent

In qualitative research, an important concept is *process consent*, which requires that the researcher renegotiate a subject's consent if any unanticipated events occur during the interview or observation.[2] An example of this might be a situation in which two parents with a small child in the hospital have given consent for the taping and study of "a day in the life of a hospitalized toddler."

During taping, the parents are informed by the physician that their child must undergo an unexpected lumbar puncture. The parents may become visibly upset by this turn of events. In such a case, the researcher should find a way of reconfirming the couple's ongoing interest in being part of the research study. When this family is given the opportunity to renegotiate the original agreement, it confirms the nurse researcher's role of advocate and proceeding in the best interest of all participants.

Detecting the Ethical Components of Written Research

It can be difficult to critique the ethical features of written research reports. If there is evidence that permission to conduct the study was granted by an IRB, it is highly likely that the participants' rights were protected. Box 24.6 provides the guidelines for critiquing ethics in research.

IMPLEMENTING RESEARCH IN THE PRACTICE SETTING

Knowledge that is generated by research and then translated into policy and procedure becomes the ultimate guide to the scientific practice of nursing. A primary responsibility of every nurse conducting research is the distribution of the findings (evidence) that have application in the patient-care setting. Conversely, the professional responsibility of every nurse caring for patients is that all nursing interventions be planned on the basis of reliable research findings.

Nursing research is of no value to the profession or to the patient if the practice supported by the research is not used in the clinical setting. Unlimited opportunities for the generation and dissemination of new knowledge exist in nursing, but the truly daunting task is transforming that knowledge into practice.

Box 24.6 Guidelines for Critiquing the Ethical Features of Research

1. Was the study approved by an IRB?
2. Was informed consent obtained from every subject?
3. Is there information regarding anonymity or confidentiality?
4. Were vulnerable subjects used?
5. Does it appear that any coercion may have been used?
6. Is it evident that potential benefits of participation outweigh the possible risks?
7. Were participants invited to ask questions about the study and told how to contact the researcher, should the need arise?
8. Were participants informed how to obtain results of the study?

Source: R.M. Nieswiadomy, *Foundations of Nursing Research* (7th ed.), Upper Saddle River, NJ: Pearson/Prentice Hall, 2018.

The Call for Implementing Research

Research is critical to the professional practice of nursing. For example, The Joint Commission's accreditation guidelines specify that patient-care intervention must be based on information from scientifically valid and timely sources.

The mandate of the modern health-care system is that nurses make practice decisions based on the best scientific information available. Standard VII of the ANA Standards of Clinical Nursing Practice states that "the nurse uses research findings in practice." Nurses may participate in research activities in a number of ways. They can conduct reviews of literature, critique research studies for the possibility of application to practice, or "[use] research findings in the development of policies, procedures and guidelines for patient care."[21]

Approaches to Using Research

Nursing is not the only profession that is transforming research into practice. Almost every health-care discipline is trying to close the research–practice gap. Currently, there are several models that nurses can use to apply research findings that support EBP. One model that appears both practical and relatively uncomplicated is presented in Box 24.7.[12]

Promoting Change

Nurses must promote an environment conducive to change. In many hospitals, maintaining the status quo is seen as a priority. The professional nurse committed

---

Box 24.7 Model for Application of Nursing Research

Assess the need for practice changes:
(a) Involve all nurses who have a stake in the intervention or change.
(b) Identify problems associated with the current practice.
(c) Compare available information.

Link the problem intervention and outcomes:
(a) Identify possible interventions.
(b) Develop outcome indicators.

Produce best evidence for consideration:
(a) Conduct a review of existing literature.
(b) Compare and contrast the evidence found.
(c) Determine feasibility (including cost in dollars and time).
(d) Consider benefits and risks.

Design a proposed practice change:
(a) Define the anticipated change.
(b) Identify necessary resources.
(c) Develop a plan based on desired outcomes.

Implement and evaluate the proposed change:
(a) Conduct a pilot study.
(b) Assess the process and the outcomes.
(c) Make a decision to alter, accept, or reject the proposed change.

Support the change with ongoing evaluations of the outcomes:
(a) Communicate the desired change to those involved.
(b) Conduct in-service education sessions.
(c) Revise standards of practice (policy/procedures) reflecting the change.
(d) Monitor the ongoing process and results.

Source: M. Smith, P. Liehr, *Middle Range Theory for Nursing*, New York, NY: Springer, 2018.

to using "best evidence" to provide the best patient care needs to find simple approaches that create an environment receptive to new research findings. Following are some helpful tactics:

- Read clinical journals regularly but also critically. Nursing professionals are well informed and believe in the concept of lifelong learning.
- Attend clinically focused nursing conferences where the latest patient-care interventions are presented and discussed.
- Learn to look for evidence that clearly supports the effectiveness and feasibility of updating nursing interventions.

- Seek work environments that promote the use of research findings and evidence-based care.
- Collaborate with a nurse researcher. Apprenticeship to one who has mastered a skill is an old but venerated means of learning that skill.
- Learn to critically scrutinize the status quo. Many worthwhile ideas for change come from students and nurses who are "in the trenches" and at the bedside.
- Pursue the possibility of proposing and implementing a project. If the nurse finds a research idea for clinical care interesting, then taking the steps to research it can be productive.

Conclusion

Modern health care has become so complex and demanding that simple trial-and-error approaches to practice do not provide the quality required for the safe, effective, and economical care demanded by well-informed consumers. The nursing profession is quickly moving away from the "I do it because it's always been done this way" method of care to scientifically rooted care practices based on research. As a result, nurses are gaining increased recognition as key members of the health-care team.

Nurses are now required to be able to analyze and evaluate research findings to determine which studies are of high quality and can be used as a guide for nursing practice. Similarly, nurses are required

to contribute to the body of nursing knowledge by participating in nursing research studies conducted at their facilities. It is presumed that nurses with advanced degrees will initiate and conduct high-quality research.

The ability of nurses to make thoughtful use of research is an important first step in the development of EBP. Society's call for cost containment, high-quality care, and documented outcomes of health-care services will continue to fuel the engine of positive health-care developments. As nursing looks to its future, research and EBP will become increasingly more important factors that guide and inform the day-to-day practice of nurses.

CRITICAL-THINKING EXERCISES

- Obtain and read both a qualitative and a quantitative research study. What are the main differences between the two studies? What are the similarities? Which produced the more reliable data?
- Identify the problem statement in each research article. Are they clearly stated? Do they contain more than one idea? How do they form the foundation for the research?
- Look up the topics of the two articles on one of the EBP websites given in this chapter. Was either article listed as a high-quality resource?

- Select a procedure you have observed or some problem you have encountered in your clinical rotations. Write a research problem statement for the issue. What type of research would be most appropriate for studying this issue?
- Reread the two articles you selected earlier. What, if any, ethical issues were involved in the studies? How did the researcher deal with them?
- Read about the Nuremburg Trials. How do the results of these trials affect nursing research today? What were the primary violations the defendants were accused of?

NCLEX-STYLE QUESTIONS

1. Which elements do qualitative and quantitative research designs have in common? **Select all that apply.**
   1. Dependent and independent variables
   2. A research question
   3. Structured interviews
   4. A comparison of two or more groups
   5. A plan for the study that identifies the type of data needed to answer the question
2. A nurse in an assisted-living facility wants to study the effects of room temperature on patients' osteoarthritis pain. Which of the following is potentially an ethical concern of this proposed research?
   1. The fact that the research subjects are in an assisted-living facility
   2. The lack of process consent in case an unanticipated event occurs
   3. The age of the research subjects
   4. The possibility that manipulation of a variable (temperature) might increase some subjects' discomfort
3. What prompted the development of laws related to the treatment of human research subjects?
   1. In the 1960s, experiments by psychologist Stanley Milgram found that most people were willing to torture others because someone in authority told them to.
   2. After World War II, Nazi physicians tried to justify atrocities they committed by calling them "medical research."
   3. The Geneva Convention formed the basis for laws related to the treatment of human research subjects.
   4. Military commanders were alarmed by Florence Nightingale's research on human subjects during the Crimean War.
4. Which scenario is most likely to encourage nurses to incorporate evidence-based practice into their patient care?
   1. Research skills are taught in their own class, not as a part of other nursing topics, in nursing school.
   2. New nurses at a facility are expected to accept and adopt the nursing practices of their nurse-mentors.
   3. The unit is consistently short staffed, and nurses lack time to read the nursing literature.
   4. The nurse manager devotes time during each staff meeting for one nurse to share an EBP idea and for the group to discuss how the unit might implement it.
5. The unit manager in a hospital's intensive care unit (ICU) wants to promote implementation of valid research findings in the unit's patient care. Which strategy would be effective for the manager to use? **Select all that apply.**
   1. Reimburse conference fees and travel costs for nurses who attend and report back on conferences in which clinical research findings and ideas for practice are presented.
   2. Develop a research committee consisting of ICU nurses and members of nursing faculty at a nearby university.
   3. Update the ICU's new-nurse training and the clinical policy and procedure manuals using the latest research findings.
   4. Hand out copies of research articles and require ICU nurses to read the article, write a summary, and submit it to the manager.
   5. Tell nurses that pay raises are now tied to evidence that they have conducted original research.
6. _____ is the conscientious, explicit, and judicious use of current best evidence in making decisions about the care of individual patients.
7. Place the following steps of the research process in the order they should occur.
   _____1. Develop a research plan.
   _____2. Question the status quo.
   _____3. Implement the plan.
   _____4. Apply critical thinking to the problem.
   _____5. Share research findings with others.
8. Which statement BEST describes the relationship between nursing research and patient care?
   1. Nursing research answers questions through discovery of new information with the goal of improving patient care.
   2. Nursing research conducted by academics yields practices that are unsuited for clinical use with patients.

3. Nursing research confirms scientifically what nurses previously learned through trial and error in patient care.

4. Nursing research is most concerned with defining the profession of nursing and less concerned with patient care.

9. A hospital is working toward gaining Magnet status. Which of the following existing conditions at the facility will need to change in order for it to qualify for this status?

1. The hospital has experienced no sentinel events this year.

2. The hospital's robust continuing-education program is free to nurses.

3. Nurses are generally encouraged to use EBP, but the EHR system has no mechanism for noting or recording this information.

4. Nurses report that they have more autonomy and empowerment here than at hospitals where they worked previously.

10. A professor asks the class to suggest ways in which nursing research could be used to enhance communication and understanding between cultures. Which answer requires correction from the professor?

1. "Researchers could investigate the comparative effectiveness of in-house medical interpreters and interpreter tele-help services in patient teaching for patients whose primary language is not English."

2. "Researchers could study how LGBTQ patients interact with nursing staff who are also LGBTQ."

3. "Research on traditional herbal remedies of different cultures could be used to improve the quality of history-taking and medication reconciliation during an initial nursing assessment."

4. "Research on Muslim women's experiences in the U.S. health-care system could be used to improve patient satisfaction for a Somali woman in active labor and her family."

References

1. Gallup: Nurse are the most trusted profession for 20th straight year. Yale School of Nursing, February 7, 2022. https://nursing.yale.edu/news/gallup-nurses-are-most-trusted-profession-20th-straight-year

2. Fain J. *Reading, Understanding and Applying Nursing Research* (6th ed). Philadelphia, PA: F.A. Davis, 2021.

3. 2022 National Teaching Institute evidence based-solutions abstract. *Critical Care Nurse*, 42 (2):e10–e36, 2022. https://doi.org/10.4037/ccn2022820

4. Chinnasamy V. 42% of Internet traffic is from bots. What is your cybersecurity gameplan? Light Reading, August 22, 2022. https://www.lightreading.com/42-of-internet-traffic-is-from-bots---what-is-your-cybersecurity-gameplan-/a/d-id/779854

5. Nightingale F. *Notes on Nursing*. Haverhill, MA: D. Appleton & Company, 1860.

6. Evidenced based nursing. University of Massachusetts Boston, 2022. https://umb.libguides.com/EBN

7. Alliance for the Implementation of Clinical Practice Guidelines [home page]. https://aicpg.org/

8. Tappen R. *Advanced Nursing Research: From Theory to Practice* (3rd ed.). Burlington, MA: Jones & Bartlett Learning, 2023.

9. What is PICOT? Centennial Libraries, 2023. https://libguides.cedarville.edu/picoquestion/what_is_picot

10. National Institute of Nursing Research [home page]. https://www.ninr.nih.gov/

11. EBP checklists. University of Glasgow, n.d. https://www.gla.ac.uk/schools/healthwellbeing/research/generalpractice/ebp/checklists/

12. Yingling J. Rationing evidence-based nursing practice: Considering a resource-based approach. *OJIN: The Online Journal of Issues in Nursing*, 26(1), October 29, 2020. https://doi.org/10.3912/OJIN.Vol26No01PPT62

13. Polit D, Beck C. *Essentials of Nursing Research*. New York, NY: Wolters Kluwer, 2021.

14. AACN levels of evidence. American Association of Critical-Care Nurses, n.d. https://www.aacn.org/clinical-resources/practice-alerts/aacn-levels-of-evidence

15. Choudhry N, Avorn J, Glynn R, et al. Full coverage for preventive medications after myocardial infarction. *New England Journal of Medicine*, 365(22):2088–2097, 2011. https://doi.org/10.1056/NEJMsa1107913

16. Borges do Nascimento I, Pizarro A, Almeida J, Azzopardi-Muscat N, Goncalves M, Bjorklund M, Novillo-Ortiz D. Infodemics and health misinformation: A systematic review of reviews. *Bulletin of the World Health Organization*, 100(9):544–561. https://doi.org/10.2471%2FBLT.21.287654

17. Deep vein thrombosis. Family Practice Notebook, n.d. https://fpnotebook.com/HemeOnc/CV/DpVnThrmbs.htm

18. About Guideline Central. Guideline Central, n.d. https://www
.guidelinecentral.com/about/

19. Brand S, Menzies J, Vijayakumaran N, Bijou-Rowe C. Engaging
student nurses in research 1: Research-delivery placements.
Nursing Times, August 8, 2022. https://www.nursingtimes.net/
roles/nurse-educators/engaging-student-nurses-in-research-1
-research-delivery-placements-08-08-2022/

20. 1974: National Research Act. Alliance for Human Research
Protection, 2022. https://ahrp.org/1974-national-research-act/

21. Nursing Scope and Standards Workgroup. ANA standards of
nursing practice. January 5, 2016. https://westafricaneducated
nursesdotorg.files.wordpress.com/2016/01/ana-standards-of
-nursing-practice-table.pdf

Integrative Health Practices

25

Lydia DeSantis | Joseph T. Catalano

Learning Objectives

After completing this chapter, the reader will be able to:

- Describe the interrelationship between integrative health practices and complementary and alternative practices

- Compare the philosophy and objectives of alternative and complementary healing (ACH) modalities with those of conventional Western medicine

- List major reasons why a growing number of people use ACH modalities

- Describe major types of ACH modalities

- Summarize methods by which nurses and patients can obtain information about ACH modalities

- Evaluate a patient for use of ACH modalities

- Identify the strengths and weaknesses of ACH modalities

A DIFFERENT KIND OF HEALING

Complementary and alternative health-care practices, now called *integrative practices*, have been widely used by a large percentage of the world's population. Their popularity continues to increase dramatically with patients of all ages and backgrounds. Integrative practices include a range of traditional therapies and treatments that are not usually used or taught in conventional Western health care. Although some people use the terms *alternative health care* and *integrative health care* synonymously, integrative care is more inclusive. It attempts to integrate the best of Western scientific medicine with a broader understanding of the nature of illness, healing, and wellness. It also includes ACH but goes beyond to include the care of the whole person, focusing on health rather than illness. A complementary health-care practice is a non-mainstream practice that is used *together with* conventional medicine, whereas an alternative health-care practice is used *in place of* conventional medical practices. Very few people use only alternative medicine but often combine these practices with conventional treatments. There are many definitions of "integrative" health care, but all the definitions involve combining conventional and complementary approaches in a coordinated way.

Based on evidence from research, integrative practice, also sometimes called *functional health care*, involves the individual in their own care to achieve the highest level of health and well-being. Integrative health practice is highly inclusive, "integrating approaches to treatment from the allopathic, complementary, alternative, psychological, spiritual, environmental, nutritional, and self-help arenas."[1] With integrative health practices, patients are aided in using their illness crises as the starting point to making positive changes in their lives and reaching their full potential in wellness. It is important for nurses to have a solid understanding of this type of health care to ensure their patients' safety and well-being and to be supportive of their practices.

According to the World Health Organization (WHO), 80 percent of the world's population uses what Americans call "alternative" practices as their primary source of health care. Because of the widely accepted use of these practices, WHO has officially sanctioned the incorporation of "safe and effective [alternative] remedies and practices for use in public and private health services." Currently, between 34 and 42 percent of Americans (60 to 83 million people) use ACH practices, as do 20 to 75 percent of people in western Europe, 33 percent in Finland, and 49 percent in Australia.[2]

Issues Now

The Federal Government Supports Integrative Medicine

The U.S. Health Resources and Services Administration (HRSA) has approximately $35 million available for research into complementary and alternative modalities. These are competitive grants. To qualify, programs must demonstrate how evidence-based integrative medicine is being used in existing preventive medical residencies.[3]

The 2010 Affordable Care Act (ACA) included several provisions that benefit integrative medicine and complementary and alternative medicine (CAM). With its emphasis on preventing insurance companies from denying coverage, the ACA includes a provision that patients who are participating in clinical trials of alternative health-care methods cannot lose their coverage. Under the law, insurance companies are required to cover all routine costs of medications and treatments used during the trial. The goal of the law is to make trials available to patients who otherwise might not be able to participate and to make it easier for researchers to conduct successful trials that will improve health care and treatments for others.

However, certain criteria must be met. First, the patient must be categorized as "qualified." This means that the patient must be authorized by their health-care provider for participation. The provider must also provide "medical and scientific information establishing that the individual's participation in such trial would be appropriate."

Second, the clinical trial must be "approved." An approved clinical trial, ranging from phase I to phase IV, is conducted to advance the prevention, detection, or treatment of cancer or another life-threatening disease or condition. The trial must meet at least one of three conditions: it must be federally funded or approved, approved by the Food and Drug Administration (FDA), or conducted by the federal government.

The bill also includes provisions to prevent insurance companies from discriminating against CAM practitioners. Practitioner coverage now includes acupuncturists, chiropractors, and naturopathic doctors who may prescribe dietary supplements. Some CAM practitioners believe the new provisions open the door for future growth of alternative health-care practices.

One overarching goal of the ACA is to educate the public about methods to prevent illness and improve health-care status. To achieve this goal, the law supports the development of wellness plans to be implemented through community health centers, particularly in lower-income and underserved areas. These centers provide wellness assessments, health education, and a selection of dietary supplements that have FDA-approved health claims. Some supplements that are available are folic acid, calcium, vitamin D, omega-3 fatty acids, and multivitamins. Supplements are targeted for at-risk groups; for example, calcium and vitamin D are targeted for older patients.

Another section of the ACA promotes increased participation for CAM practitioners in the development of health-care policy. The National Healthcare Workforce Commission was created in 2010 as part of the ACA, but it was never completely funded. As of June 2019, most of its key elements remain in effect, and the commission works with the U.S. Department of Health and Human Services. One of its main projects created community health teams, which must include licensed CAM practitioners.

Sources: *CAM, supplements included in healthcare reform bill, Natural Products Insider,* March 24, 2010, https://www.naturalproductsinsider.com/legal -compliance/cam-supplements-included-health-care-reform-bill; *Grants and funding, National Center for Complementary and Integrative Health,* 2022, https://www.nccih.nih.gov/about/offices/od/director.

The trend toward alternative practices has grown in the United States since the 1990s. Studies show that 40 percent of people have developed an increasingly positive attitude toward alternative practices, whereas only 2 percent had more negative opinions. Both the general public (72 percent) and health maintenance organizations (HMOs; 73 percent) expect consumer demand for this area of health care to remain moderate to strong. Approximately 25 percent of the medicines used in modern therapy are derived from herbal plant sources used in traditional healing practices. Although there has been rapid growth in biomedical knowledge and technology during this time period, the demand for alternative therapies continues to increase.[2]

DEFINING INTEGRATIVE HEALTH PRACTICE

Integrative health practice finds its origins in the definition of health presented by the WHO: health is "a state of complete physical, mental and social well-being and not merely the absence of disease or infirmity."[2] It is patient focused. The integrative approach to health is based on the belief that patients, after an illness or injury, have the capability to regain their overall health and maintain wellness during their life spans. The work of the practitioner using integrative health practices is to become familiar with each patient's particular health needs and then personalize their care using the full range of elements that affect health, including physical, mental, spiritual, social, and environmental factors. Taking into consideration the complex relationship between mind, body, and spirit, integrative health care addresses both the short-term care needs and long-term issues of the patient.[3]

Integrative health care has the potential to affect the health status of patients across the spectrum of the health-care system. For nursing practice, it includes the ability to incorporate conventional health-care diagnoses and treatments with evidence-based practice (EBP), nonconventional complementary and alternative treatments, environmental factors, and nutritional therapies into their nursing skills set. Nurses must be able to bring to patients an awareness of how emotional, spiritual, cultural, and environmental factors in their lives affect their health and long-term well-being. On the patients' part, they need to develop a personal understanding of the causes and meanings of their illnesses and be willing to make a commitment to the healing process. Only then will they achieve the best outcomes from their treatments.[1]

Integrative health-care practices differ from ACH in that integrative health care looks past the mere treatment of symptoms and attempts to identify and treat the underlying cause of the illness. However, complementary and alternative modalities are an essential element in achieving the goal of integrative health. Integrative health care is moving toward becoming a specialty of its own. A number of postgraduate programs on integrative health are available, such as the Arizona Center for Integrative Medicine (United States), the British College of Integrative Medicine (United Kingdom), the European University Viadrina (Germany), and the National Institute of Integrative Medicine (Australia). This chapter focuses primarily on complementary and alternative treatment modalities, keeping in mind that they are one element in an integrative approach to wellness.

DEFINING ACH

Several definitions are used for complementary and alternative health-care practices. They are sometimes defined as practices outside of conventional, science-based Western medicine and not sanctioned by the official health-care system. A considerable range of practices and concepts is included in ACH. These practices are generally used in place of conventional practices or used to enhance the effectiveness of standard medical treatments.

An Outdated Definition

There is no universally accepted definition of complementary and alternative health-care practices. Many of these practices originated long ago within cultural belief systems and healing traditions. A commonly used definition in the United States for complementary and alternative modalities comes from the National Center for Complementary and Integrative Health (NCCIH), an agency of the National Institutes of Health. The NCCIH definition is "those treatments and healthcare practices not taught widely in medical schools, not generally used in hospitals, and not usually reimbursed by medical insurance companies."[4]

However, this definition is quickly becoming outdated. Several medical and nursing schools now include courses on complementary and alternative health-care practices. Also, the practice of alternative medicine is gradually becoming part of conventional health care. Health-care providers, nurses, and other health-care professionals are responding to the growing public use of these practices by incorporating selected modalities into their own patient care. Physicians and other providers have begun referring patients to a variety of alternative healers and using alternative therapies for their own health.

A Holistic Basis

For the purposes of this discussion, CAM is defined as the understanding and use of healing therapies not commonly considered part of Western biomedicine. The focus here is mainly on methods of self-care, wellness, self-healing, health promotion, and illness prevention. Therapies and practices are called *alternative* when used alone or with other alternative therapies and called *complementary* when used with conventional therapies.

The use of the terms *healing, modalities,* and *therapies* to refer to ACH is preferred to *medicine.* Integrative health care and complementary and alternative modalities typically are based in holistic philosophies, which go beyond treatment or cure of the physiological and psychological dimensions of care commonly associated with modern, scientific biomedicine. *Holism* refers to treatment of the whole person (body–mind–spirit) in that person's environmental context (i.e., physical, biological, social, cultural, and spiritual).

> *" Integrative health-care and complementary and alternative modalities typically are based in holistic philosophies, which go beyond treatment or cure of the physiological and psychological dimensions of care commonly associated with modern, scientific biomedicine. "*

What Do You Think?

Do you use any alternative health-care practices? What are they? Why do you use them? How do they help you?

USE OF INTEGRATIVE THERAPIES

Although forms of integrative therapies have been used for many years in the United States, the passage of the ACA has the potential to increase their use even more. Section 2706 of the ACA makes it illegal for insurance companies to discriminate against patients who use integrative therapies. Providers of integrative therapies must be reimbursed by the insurance companies at the same rates as providers of traditional procedures. There are other references to integrative therapies in the wellness and prevention sections of the ACA. As of the time of publication, this regulation was still in effect. The one sticking point is that the individual states can write their own language concerning which practitioners receive how much reimbursement for integrative practices.

What Are They Used For?

Complementary and alternative therapies are used to treat a wide variety of health problems as well as to maintain and promote a healthy body and mind. The most common diseases treated by alternative therapies include pain in any part of the body, mild to severe depression, high blood pressure in older adults, cancer treatment side effects, memory loss, and a variety of chronic diseases.[5] During the initial surge of the COVID-19 pandemic, there were no effective prevention therapies or treatments, particularly vaccines. People who had never used complementary and alternative therapies before turned to them as preventive measures and treatments. According to a 2022 study, almost 84 percent of participants reported that they used one or more complementary and/or alternative medicines during the COVID-19 pandemic.[5] Use of at-home yoga and meditation increased sharply during the pandemic because of closed fitness centers, gyms, and pools due to lockdown regulations.

Many individuals who survived a severe episode of COVID-19 have been diagnosed with long-COVID, or long-haul-COVID, which produces a variety of symptoms, including brain fog, respiratory distress, severe fatigue, pins-and-needles sensations in the arms and legs, headaches (from mild to severe), faintness and dizziness (from low blood pressure), body aches (mild to moderate), joint pain, and anxiety.[6] Chiropractic treatment is being used by some patients with long-COVID to support the heart and lungs and to restore healthy breathing. Chiropractors are using their hands and touch modalities to improve circulation and movement of lymph to help clear toxins and carbon dioxide from the body.[7] Rest and relaxation help reduce stress and anxiety, as do certain herbal medications, meditation, and rhythmic breathing. Two clinical studies suggested that Chinese herbal medications were effective in relieving symptoms of pulmonary dysfunction found in patients with long-COVID.[3]

Who Uses Them?

In most national studies of alternative therapy users, ethnic and racial minorities are underrepresented, particularly among persons who do not speak English. Such exclusions raise questions about whether the use rate of alternative therapies in the United States may exceed 62 percent, up from 42 percent 10 years ago.[2] The use of alternative therapies among immigrant populations and those with lower incomes tends to be high. Many such populations have grown up with these therapies as "folk" medicine, and their worldviews encompass different concepts of health, illness, and healing. Conversely, alternative health-care practices are most popular among women, people ages 35 to 49 years, people with higher educational levels (some graduate education), and those with annual incomes of more than $50,000.

Why Their Use Has Increased

Three general theories have been advanced to explain the growing use of integrative healing: (1) dissatisfaction with conventional health care, (2) a desire for greater control over one's health, and (3) a desire for cultural and philosophical congruence with personal beliefs about health and illness. Many other patient-specific reasons have also been postulated, such as belief in the effectiveness of integrative therapies and the individual's health status (Box 25.1). The rising cost of conventional medications and health care may play a role as well.

Box 25.1 Reasons for Use of Integrative, Alternative, and Complementary Modalities

People use integrative and alternative therapies alone or together with conventional health care for a variety of reasons. There is no single predictor of use, and the reasons for use may vary from situation to situation. Persons who seem to benefit most from the alternative approach are those who

- Prefer a personal relationship with healers.
- Refuse to give up hope and hopefulness, regardless of illness or life state.
- Desire to focus on wellness, health promotion and maintenance, and illness prevention.
- Are concerned with gentle alleviation and management of suffering and illness rather than aggressive management of the end-stage of life through technology, medications, surgery, and other invasive procedures.
- Wish to participate actively in decision making about their health care.
- Believe in the holistic aspects of existence rather than in the primacy of biological and physiological aspects.
- Are "culture creatives"—persons at the leading edge of innovation and culture change who have been exposed to alternative lifestyles and worldviews compatible with those from which complementary and alternative modalities and theories have arisen.
- Share cultural and philosophical views similar to those from which complementary and alternative modalities have developed.

Source: J.A. Austin, Why patients use alternative medicine, *Journal of the American Medical Association*, 279:1548, 1998; from Aspen Reference Group, *Holistic Health Promotion & Complementary Therapies Manual*, Clifton Park, NY: Thomson Delmar Learning, 1998. Reprinted with permission from Delmar Learning.

Dissatisfaction

The increasing use of integrative therapies is due in part to the feeling that conventional health care is unable to deal with major health problems or improve a person's general health. People who have a high degree of distrust in conventional health care often rely primarily on integrative therapies. This lack of trust has increased recently for several reasons, including the following:

- Conflicting information from health-care-related studies and clinical trials about risk prevention and health promotion. For example, patients no longer know what to believe about salt intake, normal cholesterol levels, alcohol use, or hormone replacement therapy.
- Continuing emphasis of conventional health care on curative rather than preventive aspects of care. The lack of emphasis on illness prevention limits the ability of individuals to live long lives relatively free of disability from major chronic illnesses, such as arthritis, diabetes, cancer, and cardiovascular disease.
- Growing concern about costs, safety, and access to conventional health care. Many people are concerned about the increased incidence of hospital-acquired diseases, deadly medication errors, invasive procedures, antibiotic-resistant bacteria, and reliance on impersonal technology.

Desire for Control

Some people who use integrative therapies believe conventional care is too intolerant, authoritarian, and impersonal. They feel that some conventional health-care professionals lack sensitivity to the wishes of patients and their families when developing treatment plans. Patients believe they should be partners in decision making about their care rather than just having decisions handed down to them.

In the United States, the majority of people report being reluctant to tell conventional health-care professionals that they use integrative therapies. Although almost all (89 percent) who use integrative therapies do so under the supervision of an integrative healer, about half of this same group do not consult a conventional health-care professional before they begin. Fourteen percent of persons see both conventional health-care professionals and integrative healers. Similar patterns of self-care and nondisclosure to conventional health-care professionals are found throughout the industrialized world.[4]

Holistic Philosophy

Conventional health care is often faulted for its limited focus on the physiological dimension of health and curing to the exclusion of the unity of mind–body–spirit healing. Another negative characteristic of conventional health care is its excessive dependence on medicine, surgery, and technology rather than on natural and noninvasive alternative approaches that focus on self-care and self-healing.

What Do You Think?

If you use integrative therapies, do you tell your physician or primary health-care provider? What is their response?

Belief in Effectiveness

Patients who use alternative therapies do so because they believe those therapies will work, either alone or when combined with conventional treatments. Persons who consider their health to be poor or who have chronic illnesses report greater benefits from alternative than conventional health care and are more likely to try both at the same time. Referral from conventional health-care professionals, friends, or other users of integrative therapies is also a prominent reason for the simultaneous use of both systems. For many patients, integrative therapies simply make them feel better than conventional health care does.

> *Patients who use alternative therapies do so because they believe those therapies will work, either alone or when combined with conventional treatments.*

Cost of Alternative Care

Estimated costs of alternative medicines (herbs and nutritional supplements), diet products, equipment, and books and courses totaled $102 billion in 2021, up from $32 billion in 2017. Sixty-seven percent of HMOs cover one or more ACH modalities, but coverage is uneven and varies regionally. Chiropractic is the most common covered service (65 percent), followed by acupuncture (31 percent), massage therapy (11 percent), and vitamin therapy (6 percent). HMOs expect to increase coverage for acupuncture to 36 percent, acupressure to 31 percent, massage therapy to 30 percent, and vitamin therapy to 27 percent. The most important reasons for adding coverage for these services are public demand, legislative mandate, and demonstrated clinical effectiveness.[5]

CLASSIFYING INTEGRATIVE METHODS

The underlying goals of any type of health care include preventing illness, promoting and maintaining health, and caring for people while alleviating the suffering caused by illness. However, despite these common elements, health-care practices vary profoundly in their modalities (technologies), practitioner education and monitoring, underlying concepts (models) of health and illness, modes of care delivery, and social and legal mandates to provide care. Because of the large number of variables, a confusing array of health-care systems, practitioners, and healing modalities has developed. A system that can be used to help define and classify complementary and alternative therapies is the NCCIH classification.[4]

The NCCIH Classification

In 1992, Congress mandated the establishment of an Office of Alternative Medicine in the National Institutes of Health to enhance the study of ACH. In 1998, the Office became the National Center for Complementary and Alternative Medicine (NCCAM). Its mission was to conduct and support basic and applied research and training and to disseminate ACH information to conventional health-care professionals, alternative healers, and the public. In 2014, the NCCAM was renamed the NCCIH.

Five major categories identified by the NCCIH are defined and subdivided into practices that (1) fall under CAM, (2) are found in conventional health care but reclassified as behavioral medicine, and (3) are overlapping—that is, they can fall in the domain of either CAM or behavioral medicine. Table 25.1 summarizes the NCCIH classifications.

Category I: Integrative Medical Systems

Category I includes alternative systems of theory and practice developed outside Western biomedicine. For example, acupuncture is grounded in **traditional Chinese medicine**. Also in this category are traditional indigenous systems, comprising all medical systems other than traditional Chinese medicine that developed outside of Western biomedicine. This category also includes unconventional Western systems not classified elsewhere that were developed in the West but are not considered part of biomedicine, such as **homeopathy**.

Finally, category I includes **naturopathy**, an unconventional medical system that has recently gained attention in the United States. This eclectic approach consists of various natural systems, such as herbalism, lifestyle therapies, and diet as therapy.

Category II: Mind–Body Interventions

Category II includes mind–body practices, religion and spirituality, and social and contextual areas.

Mind–body medicine involves a variety of approaches to health care. Mind–body systems are seldom practiced alone but are usually combined with lifestyle interventions.

Mind–body methods may be used as a supplement to a traditional medical system. They are sometimes used in conventional health-care practices; however, they are characterized as CAM when used for conditions for which they are not normally prescribed. Religion and spirituality include treatments directed toward biological functions or clinical conditions. Social and contextual areas include treatment methods that are not included in other categories, such as cultural and symbolic interventions.

Category III: Biologically Based Therapies

Biologically based therapies include products, interventions, and practices that are natural in origin and biologically based. They may or may not overlap with conventional medicine and its use of dietary supplements.

Phytotherapy, or herbalism, is the use of plant-derived products for purposes of prevention and

> *Biologically based therapies include products, interventions, and practices that are natural in origin and biologically based.*

(text continues on page 696)

Table 25.1 Categories of Alternative Practice

I. Integrative Medical Systems

Traditional Chinese Medicine

Acupuncture	Herbal formulas
Diet	Massage and manipulation (tui na)
External and internal qigong	Tai chi

Traditional Indigenous Systems

Ayurvedic medicine	Traditional African medicine
Curanderismo	Traditional Aboriginal medicine
Central and South American	Unani-tibbi
Kampo medicine	Siddhi
Native American medicine	

CAM   **Overlapping**

Alternative Western Systems

Homeopathy	Anthroposophically extended medicine
Naturopathy	
Orthomolecular medicine	

II. Mind–Body Interventions

CAM   **Behavioral Medicine**   **Overlapping**

Mind–Body Methods

Yoga	Hypnosis	Art, music, and dance therapies
Tai chi	Meditation	Humor
Internal qigong	Biofeedback	Journaling

CAM

Religion and Spirituality

Confession	Nontemporality	"Special" healers
Nonlocality	Soul retrieval	Spiritual healing

CAM   **Overlapping**

Social and Contextual Areas

Caring-based approaches (e.g., holistic nursing, pastoral care)	Community-based approaches (e.g., Native American "sweat" rituals)
Intuitive diagnosis	Explanatory models
	Placebo

III. Biologically Based Therapies

Phytotherapy or Herbalism

Aloe vera	Echinacea	Ginseng	Mistletoe
Bee pollen	Evening primrose	Green tea	Peppermint oil
Biloba	Garlic	Hawthorne	Saw palmetto

Table 25.1   Categories of Alternative Practice (continued)

Cat's claw	Ginger	Kava	Witch hazel
Dong quai	Ginkgo	Licorice root	Valerian

Special Diet Therapies

Atkins	McDougall	Fasting	Paleolithic
Diamond	Ornish	High fiber	Vegetarian
Kelly-Gonzalez	Pritikin	Macrobiotic	
Gerson therapy	Wigmore	Mediterranean	
Livingston-Wheeler	Asian	Natural hygiene	

Orthomolecular Therapies

Single Nutrients (Partial Listing)

Amino acids	Folic acid	Lysine	Potassium	Thiamine
Ascorbic acid	Glutamine	Manganese	Selenium	Tyrosine
Boron	Glucosamine sulfate	Magnesium	Silicon	Vanadium
Calcium triglycerides	Iodine	Medium-chain	Glandular products	Vitamin A
Carotenes	Inositol	Melatonin	Riboflavin	Vitamin D
Choline	Iron	Niacin	Taurine	Vitamin K
Fatty acids	Lipoic acid	Niacinamide	Taurine	

III. Biologically Based Therapies

Pharmacological, Biological, and Instrumental Interventions

Products

Antineoplastons	Cone therapy	Hyperbaric oxygen
Bee pollen therapy	Enderlin products	Induced remission
Cartilage	Enzyme therapies	Ozone
Cell therapy	Gallo immunotherapy	Revici system
Coley's toxins	H_2O_2	

Procedures/Devices

Apitherapy	Electrodiagnostics	Neural therapy
Bioresonance	Iridology	
Chirography	MORA device	

IV. Manipulative and Body-Based Methods

Chiropractic Medicine

Massage and Bodywork

Acupressure	Feldenkrais technique	Reflexology
Alexander technique	Osteopathic manipulative therapy (OMT)	**Rolfing**
Applied kinesiology	Pilates method	Swedish massage
Chinese tui na massage	Polarity	Trager bodywork
Craniosacral OMT		

(continued)

Table 25.1 **Categories of Alternative Practice** (continued)		
Unconventional Physical Therapies		
Colonics	Heat and electrotherapies	Light and color therapies
Diathermy	Hydrotherapy	
	V. Energy Therapies	
Biofield Therapies		
External qigong	Healing touch	Reiki
Healing science	Huna	Therapeutic touch
Bioelectromagnetically Based Therapies*		
Alternating and direct current fields	Magnetic fields	Pulsed fields

*Unconventional use of electromagnetic fields.

Sources: *National Center for Complementary and Integrative Health, https://nccih.nih.gov; C.J. Fries, Classification of complementary and alternative medical practices, Canada Family Physician, 54(11):1570–1571.e7, 2008.*

treatment. Diet therapies use special diets to reduce risk factors or treat chronic diseases. **Orthomolecular medicine** is the use of nutritional products and food supplements that are not included in other categories for prevention and treatment of disease. Pharmacological, biological, and instrumental interventions are those not covered in other categories and administered in an unconventional manner.

Category IV: Manipulative and Body-Based Methods

Manipulative and body-based methods include body manipulation, body movement, or both. **Chiropractic** care specializes in adjustments and manipulation of the spine, returning the body to its optimal alignment. This type of care is most often used when people have pain in their lower back, shoulders, and neck. However, chiropractic is often considered to be holistic, and these manipulations may also improve the overall state of wellness.

The ancient healing art of acupressure was first recognized in Asia approximately 5,000 years ago. The acupressure practitioner uses their fingers to gradually press key points throughout the body. It is believed that this pressure stimulates the body's own healing mechanisms. It can also be self-performed to relieve stress and tension, boost the immune system, reduce some types of pain, and improve health.

However, just because something is traditional or "natural" or effective does not mean it is always safe for everyone. For example, the acupressure point used to relieve headaches—the meaty V between the thumb and forefinger—is widely known and used. What is less well known is that the same pressure point promotes uterine contractions and can cause spontaneous abortion in someone who is pregnant. This pressure point should never be used on a pregnant person unless the goal is to actually induce labor.

Category V: Energy Therapies

Energy therapies are based on manipulation of biofields with bioelectromagnetically based therapies. Biofields include energy systems and energy fields internal and external to the body that are used for medical purposes. Bioelectromagnetics is the use of electromagnetic fields in an unconventional manner for medical reasons.[4] Although it is called **therapeutic touch** (TT), in this treatment modality there is no actual contact with the body or only very light touch. The use of TT is believed to redirect energy flow and treat pain and disease. Research shows that in some individuals, TT is effective on wound healing, pain, and anxiety, but the reports of results have been mixed.

COMPARING CONVENTIONAL, ALTERNATIVE, AND INTEGRATIVE PRACTICES

Many similarities exist among integrative, alternative, and conventional health care. As they attempt to achieve similar goals, they overlap in methodology, even though the methods are derived from different concepts of healing and different theoretical models. Table 25.2 summarizes characteristics often cited as

Table 25.2   Contrasts Between Conventional and Integrative Health Care

Conventional	Integrative
Chemotherapy	Plants and other natural products
Curing/treating	Healing/ministering care
Disease category	Unique individual
End-stage	Hope/hopefulness
Focus is on disease and illness	Focus is on health and wellness
Illness treatment	Health promotion and illness prevention
Individual is viewed as disease category	Individual is viewed as unique being
Nutrition is adjunct and supportive to treatment	Nutrition is the basis of health, wellness, and treatment
Objectivism: person is separate from disease	Subjectivism: person is integral to the illness
Patient/client	Person
Practitioner as authority	Practitioner as facilitator
Practitioner paternalism/patient dependency	Practitioner as partner/person empowerment
Positivism/materialism: data are physically measurable	Metaphysical: entity is energy system or vital force
Reductionist	Holistic
Specialist care	Self-care
Symptom relief	Alleviation of causative factors
Somatic (body biologic and physiologic) model	Behavioral–psychosocial–spiritual model
Science is most reliable source of knowledge and truth	Multiple sources of knowledge and truth
Technological/invasive	Natural/noninvasive

common to alternative healing and contrasts them with those usually associated with conventional health care.

Consider a patient who suffers from migraine headaches. What alternatives does this patient have to treat their pain and other migraine symptoms when conventional treatments are ineffective? **Therapeutic massage** may help. By pressing or rubbing on different pressure points on the body, a trained massage therapist can reduce a patient's migraine pain. Significant pain reduction occurs in about 50 percent of patients who use massage therapy three times a week.[3] However, massage therapy is not for everyone. People with an active case of flu or cold, an acute injury, bleeding disorders, contagious skin problems, or recent surgery or fractures in the upper part of the body should avoid massage. As with most treatments, pregnant women should get their provider's approval before starting massage therapy. Side effects are rare and are usually associated with the application of too much pressure, such as bruising or soreness.

Another alternative treatment for migraine headaches is the use of essential oils. The oils are typically inhaled (**aromatherapy**) or applied in a diluted form in small amounts to the skin. Essential oils should not be applied at full strength or in large amounts or be ingested. Lavender is the oil of choice for migraine headaches and often helps reduce the pain and other symptoms. Treatment usually consists of inhaling the lavender oil every 15 minutes for 2 hours. There have been no reported side effects.

The patient with migraine headaches may seek chiropractic treatment but may not experience much relief from it. Spinal adjustments or manipulations are the central focus of the therapy. A number of side effects are associated with chiropractic treatment, including headaches, dizziness, tiredness, and general body soreness. It is important to find a chiropractor who has the proper licensing and education and has a reputation for being a high-quality practitioner.

A number of over-the-counter supplements claim to be the ultimate treatment for relieving migraine pain.

Many of these supplements even cite data from small clinical trials to support their claims. However, none of these products are FDA approved or controlled by any organization. Patients who choose to use them do so at their own risk. No serious side effects have been reported so far, and some of these products can be expensive.

A Reductionist Philosophy

In general, conventional medicine focuses on the physical or material part of the person, the body. It is concerned with the structure, function, and connections or communication between material elements that comprise the body, such as bones, muscles, and nerves. Conventional medicine generally views all humans as being very similar biologically. Disease is seen as a deviation from what is generally considered to be a normal biological or somatic state.

Conventional medicine is sometimes considered reductionist because it tends to reduce very complex entities (humans) to seemingly equal and more simple beings who are all anatomically and physiologically similar. From this perspective, it is believed that all individuals will respond in more or less the same ways to causative agents, such as bacteria and viruses, and respond similarly to common treatments, such as medicines and surgery. In other words, a person with measles, cirrhosis of the liver, or breast cancer will have the same course of illness as other persons with those illnesses and will respond to treatments in basically the same manner. The opposite of reductionism is holism.

Diagnosis by Category

Conventional medicine has developed extensive disease categories, and great emphasis is placed on diagnosis and cure based on the assessment of physical signs and symptoms. Most newly developed medications, when they are in the human-testing phase, are tested on White men between the ages of 25 and 35 years, with the presumption that the drugs will work similarly in women, older adults, children, and people of color. That presumption is not always accurate, and there is a growing trend at pharmaceutical companies to test medications on groups of persons for whom they are more likely to be used.

Integration of Nonmaterial Factors

The physical body is the primary focus of conventional medicine. Because of its almost exclusive focus on the physical body, conventional medicine often does not consider or include the nonmaterialistic aspects of health and illness in diagnosis and treatment decisions. Consequently, spiritual, psychological, sociocultural, behavioral, and energy system aspects play little or no role in conventional medical treatment.

Although there has been some movement to a more holistic approach to patient care in medical schools that train doctors of medicine (MDs), overall conventional medical practice does not generally view the patient as an integrated person-body that is affected simultaneously by both material and nonmaterial factors during everyday life. The integration of these elements is often not viewed as significant to the person's state of wellness or illness; therefore, therapies based on the concept of holism are not deemed to be essential in treatment. However, schools of osteopathic medicine that train doctors of osteopathy (DOs) have been producing physicians with a holistic view of patient care for many years. One major difference between the medical education of MDs and DOs is that DO programs require 300 to 500 hours of study and practice of integrative practices, including hands-on manipulation of the human body.

The Holistic Approach

In contrast to reductionist conventional medicine, the integrative and alternative approaches view the person-body as consisting of multiple, integrated elements that incorporate both the materialistic and nonmaterialistic aspects of existence. These elements include the physical (material), spiritual, energetic, and social bodies. This view allows for various interpretations of how the different components of the person-body interact and

> *In contrast to conventional medicine, the integrative and alternative approaches view the person-body as consisting of multiple, integrated elements that incorporate both the materialistic and nonmaterialistic aspects of existence.*

function to affect health and illness and respond to different therapeutic interventions.

The Multiple-Body View

The integration of multiple aspects into a unified but distinctly individual person-body results in the belief that the person-body responds as a whole to factors that affect its state of well-being. Although the signs and symptoms of illness for one person are similar to those for another person, they may indicate different underlying causes depending on variable risk factors. From this viewpoint, diagnostic measures and interventions cannot be based on only one aspect of the person's being but must be tailored to the person-body of each individual.

A Capacity for Self-Healing

A variety of integrative modalities are often needed to diagnose and treat each individual holistically. It often is not obvious when the health problems of the physical body correspond to the dynamics of the energetic body or when the energetic body merges with the spiritual body, nor is it always obvious how the physical, energetic, and spiritual bodies are eventually integrated into the psychosocial body. The mediating role of the psychosocial body in the integrative approach emphasizes each person's capacity for self-healing. The importance of the mind–body interaction to elicit the placebo response and the need for patients to participate actively in the monitoring and maintenance of their health and well-being are positive factors in the diagnosis and treatment of their illness.

The multiple-body view found in some alternative health-care practices requires an eclectic approach to health promotion and maintenance. The diagnosis and treatment of illness from a multiple-body view require more than dependence on a single healing tradition centered on a one-body concept or on a fixed set of diagnostic criteria. The integrative approach requires active participation of both well and ill persons to better promote health or diagnose and treat disorders, rather than passive acceptance of a diagnosis and treatment plan from conventional health-care professionals. The goal is lifelong wellness.

Combining Modalities

The integrative philosophy includes both the material and nonmaterial aspects of the individual, stimulation of the self-healing forces, and the determination of a person's unique needs. It uses the concepts and treatment modalities of both alternative and conventional healing traditions simultaneously. These modalities are based on different worldviews or concepts of reality and address the individual healing needs of each person.

For example, acupuncturists may also use massage and other types of bodywork and energy-system methods; chiropractors may incorporate diet, herbs, and other kinds of naturopathic methodologies into chiropractic spinal manipulations; and massage therapists may include mind–body techniques such as meditation, imagery, and visualization. These alternative modalities are used to treat various patient symptoms, whereas integrative practices attempt to select the best of both conventional and alternative treatments and combine them to produce a long-term state of health[8] (Box 25.2).

Box 25.2 The Principles of Integrative Medicine

1. A partnership between patient and practitioner in the healing process
2. Appropriate use of conventional and alternative methods to facilitate the body's innate healing response
3. Consideration of all factors that influence health, wellness, and disease, including mind, spirit, and community as well as body
4. A philosophy that neither rejects conventional medicine nor accepts alternative therapies uncritically
5. Recognition that good medicine should be based in good science, be inquiry driven, and be open to new paradigms
6. Use of natural, effective, less-invasive interventions whenever possible
7. Use of the broader concepts of promotion of health and the prevention of illness as well as the treatment of disease
8. Training of practitioners to be models of health and healing, committed to the process of self-exploration and self-development

Source: Integrative medicine defined, American Board of Physician Specialties, 2018, https://www.abpsus.org/integrative-medicine -defined; What is integrative medicine? Dr. Weil, 2013, https:// www.drweil.com/health-wellness/balanced-living/meet-dr-weil/ what-is-integrative-medicine.

What Do You Think?

Name someone you know or know of who recovered from an illness they were not expected to recover from. Why do you think this happened?

The concept of a multiple-body individual is central to integrative healing. Healers function as facilitators in the promotion of health and healing (Box 25.3). In contrast, conventional therapy relies primarily on the concept of the physical-body individual, and conventional health-care providers function as experts in determining the meaning of physical signs and symptoms of health or illness and prescribing interventions to promote health or cure illness. The concepts of wellness and holism, self-healing, energy systems, nutrition, and plant-based medicine can be used to compare and contrast integrative and conventional methods of healing.

Box 25.3 Defining Integrative Healers

Integrative healers are conventional health-care professionals who incorporate hands-on complementary and alternative modalities into their conventional patient care and are sometimes called *integrative practitioners*. They should undergo the same educational, certification, and licensing processes as both conventional and alternative healers for the modalities they use.

Creating a universally applicable definition of integrative healers is extremely difficult because of the wide variety of healing traditions in use and the number of specialized healing techniques they encompass. The difficulty is compounded by the fact that many alternative healers incorporate various modalities from different healing traditions into their practices. For example, chiropractors commonly use therapeutic touch, acupuncture, acupressure, massage therapy, and naturopathic or homeopathic therapies. Massage therapists may combine multiple types of massage (e.g., Alexander, Swedish, Trager, and sports) with therapeutic touch, aromatherapy, reflexology, nutritional supplements, and electromagnetic therapies. The growing use of alternative practices by conventional health-care professionals is demonstrating the trend toward alternative healing practice.

Wellness and Holism

The term *wellness* is often used interchangeably with *good health*, generally meaning an absence of disease or illness; however, in the context of this chapter, it includes much more. The term *holism*, first used in discussion of systems theory, is often defined as the totality or entirety of a system that is more than the sum of its parts. The system being looked at in health care is the human person.

Therapy From Outside

Wellness, from the perspective of traditional medicine, tends to focus on individuals who are seen as being at risk for illness. Prevention often begins when signs or symptoms arise and is directed at alleviating them rather than treating or removing their underlying cause. Because of the strong belief in the ethical principal of autonomy or self-determination, at-risk individuals are often permitted to engage in risky behaviors as long as conventional health care can find treatments or palliative measures for the symptoms of diseases it cannot prevent. For example, a patient who smokes develops a chronic cough but does not yet have any of the smoking-related diseases (i.e., emphysema, bronchitis, lung cancer). This person would likely receive from a non-holistic physician a strong warning about smoking, but the major focus of care would be to provide the patient with medication to eliminate the cough. From this perspective, the absence of an active specific disease is considered synonymous with wellness.

Because the focus of traditional medicine is on individual body systems or organs, it is considered to be reductionist (breaking apart) rather than holistic. It emphasizes the biological–physiological (body) dimension of the patient and treats only the disease process for which signs and symptoms are already evident. The cause of illness is usually attributed to external forces or risk factors that "invade" the body from the surrounding physical, social, or biological environments.

From the biomedical view, treatment usually centers on identifying potentially dangerous or invading agents and then destroying, immobilizing, or extracting them from the person's body. Interventions consist mainly of chemotherapeutic agents (medications), surgery, or other externally imposed treatments to prevent a person considered at risk from becoming ill or to prevent signs and symptoms from becoming full-blown diseases.

Therapy From Within

In contrast to traditional medical care, the integrative model views wellness as a state in which individuals are in harmony or balance with their internal and external worlds.[8] A holistic understanding of wellness is much broader than the traditional concept of health. It implies that the patient is aware of their present and future state of health in all its aspects (physical, mental, emotional, spiritual, environmental, social, and occupational). To be able to achieve a true state of wellness requires the patients to maintain, alter, balance, and evaluate their health in each one of the health aspects.

This approach to wellness forms a common thread in many nursing models or theories of health (see Chapter 3). Integrative modalities hold that wellness can rarely be imposed on a person by an outside entity or agent. Rather, wellness is achieved mainly by individuals through the process of self-care. The individual assumes responsibility for maintaining their own state of health or wellness. The individual, when ill, works to return to a state of wellness by restoring both the internal and external (environmental) states of balance and harmony.

For example, in the case of the smoker who does not yet have an active disease process, the integrative health-care provider would also treat the cough but would spend much more time with the patient to attempt to determine which stressors in their life trigger the urge to smoke. The integrative provider would likely offer the patient methods either to reduce or eliminate these stressful situations. The provider would discuss with the patient ways to stop smoking, including use of stop-smoking aids, hypnotherapy, and smoking-cessation groups to help the patient gain control over the addiction and return to a healthy, balanced state of life.

External Disruptions

External disruptions—such as work stress, personal tragedy, a troublesome interpersonal relationship, or illness of a parent, spouse, or child—are seen as capable of affecting internal harmony and producing signs and symptoms of physical, emotional, or spiritual illness. This provides a holistic view of individuals in which they are one with their internal and external environments, thereby requiring holistic care. Treatment must address the whole individual (body–mind–spirit) in an environmental (physical, biological, social, cultural, and spiritual) context.

Spirituality is an essential part of holistic treatment (see Chapter 20). The human spirit incorporates the values, perception of meaning, and purpose in life that can positively or negatively affect the ability to heal and achieve wellness. From this perspective, health (balance or harmony), or the absence of illness, is but one aspect of wellness.

Self-Care

In the integrative model, first-level measures involve self-care aimed at wellness and can generally be performed independently. Some examples include exercising, eating a well-balanced diet, nurturing the spirit, getting enough sleep, cleaning the house, using defensive driving measures, doing monthly breast self-examinations, applying sunscreen when outside, eliminating destructive habits, and practicing good hygiene.

> *Integrative, alternative, and conventional health care all include the belief that the body has the capacity to heal itself.*

The next level of self-care requires seeking the assistance of others to achieve balance in self and the environment. This level includes getting help to find satisfying employment, seeking prenatal care, taking parenting classes when pregnant, going to community meetings to address environmental safety and citizen quality-of-life issues, seeking conventional health screening examinations (e.g., mammography and dental check-ups), obtaining glasses or contact lenses to correct vision problems, and getting vaccinations and keeping them up to date. Alternative measures, such as acupuncture and energy therapies, can also be used in this level of care.

The third level of self-care requires a high degree of specialist assistance from integrative and alternative healers to deal with major disruptions in internal or external well-being. Measures from this level focus on the spiritual dimension and include searching for personal awakening, enlightenment, and self-actualization. Effective modalities to achieve this goal are often rooted in other systems of health care such as traditional

Chinese medicine and spiritualism. In some cases, individuals may require the use of both alternative modalities and conventional health care when a single treatment modality is no longer effective.[7]

Self-Healing

Integrative, alternative, and conventional health care all include the belief that the body has the capacity to heal itself. The integrative and alternative systems place self-healing as the central principle of their models and see it as the basis of all healing. Thus, integrative and alternative healers focus on helping people determine why the cells of their body are sick and search for imbalances from a holistic perspective. Conventional health care views the ability of the body to self-heal primarily through the normal process of replacing cells; examples include the physiological and biological processes involved in wound healing. Conventional care approaches the concept of body self-healing by questioning why the cells are not replacing themselves and attempts to facilitate healing through external means, which are potentially invasive, such as surgery or medications.

The Placebo Response

Conventional health practitioners tend to dismiss the effects of healing after integrative and alternative modalities have been used by attributing them to the placebo response. They feel that healing takes place only because the individual believes the treatment is effective. In conventional medicine, the term *placebo* has come to signify a type of sham treatment instituted to please difficult or anxious patients, or a sugar pill given when health-care professionals have nothing more to offer the patient. In biomedical clinical research, a placebo is an inactive or nontreatment given to the control group under the assumption that it will not change any physiological responses and will therefore prove the effectiveness of the active treatments.[9]

What Do You Think?

What are the ethical issues involved in using placebos? If you were being given a placebo and you found out, how would you feel? What if you improved with the placebo? Would you still feel the same way?

> *Relaxation therapies and other types of stress-reducing and stress-controlling techniques are believed to promote the release of endorphins that relieve pain.*

The placebo response plays an important part in the testing of new drugs. The commonly used double-blind study requires that neither researchers nor study participants know which group is receiving the study drug and which group is receiving an inert substance (placebo). At the conclusion of the study, researchers compare results and decide whether a higher percentage of the experimental group experienced the hoped-for results from the active medication than the control group received from the placebo. However, clinical studies have shown that some participants respond positively to placebo medications between 30 and 70 percent of the time.[9] The patients with the highest positive results from placebos include those with

- Pain from chronic disease, such as cancer, arthritis, back pain, angina pectoris, and gastrointestinal tract discomfort.
- Autonomic nervous system disorders, such as phobias, psychoneuroses, depression, and nausea.
- Neurohormonal disorders, such as asthma, other bronchial airflow conditions, and hypertension.

How Does It Work?

Researchers do not have a good understanding of the mechanism by which the placebo response produces positive results. Some believe that the placebo effect is at work in all therapeutic interventions regardless of whether the intervention is an alternative or a conventional treatment. Five possible factors have been examined:

1. An endorphin-mediated response
2. Belief of the patient
3. Belief of the healer
4. The patient–healer relationship
5. Remembered wellness[9]

Endorphin-Mediated Response

Endorphins are the body's natural painkillers; they are released primarily when a person experiences fear, stress, or pain. Endorphins work by binding with opioid receptor sites in order to reduce pain as well as cause a change in mental status, such as a degree of euphoria. There are more than 20 types of endorphins; however, the beta-endorphins are the most powerful with an effect stronger than morphine. Relaxation therapies and other types of stress-reducing and stress-controlling techniques are believed to promote the release of endorphins that relieve pain. When experimental groups were given medications that block the release of beta-endorphins, patients with postoperative dental pain reported an increase in pain.[9]

Belief of the Patient

A person's belief in the effectiveness of the therapy is an important factor in its success and may be just as important as the therapy itself. Studies of patient compliance in taking prescribed beta-blocker heart medications, conducted in the first year after myocardial infarction, showed that mortality rates were almost equal for those failing to take either the beta blocker or the placebo. Mortality rates for both these groups were higher than the rates for those who faithfully took their prescribed medications or placebos.[10]

Belief of the Healer

Healers who believe in the therapeutic effectiveness of interventions and are able to convey that belief to their patients achieve more positive responses than healers who remain skeptical about the interventions they are prescribing. An attitude of caring and being in control tends to alleviate patients' anxieties and fears while increasing their hope and positive expectations.

Patient–Healer Relationship

A trusting and close relationship between the patient and healer has a positive psychological effect on patients and can become the mental catalyst they need for recovery. This relationship is essential for the success of the integrative approach. The ability of healers to communicate in an empathic manner increases patient satisfaction with care; increases compliance with mutually set goals; increases feelings of empowerment, self-confidence, and self-worth; and decreases depression and anxiety.

Although conventional health care considers many of these approaches as speculative, incomplete, or insufficient to explain the placebo response, integrative healers see the placebo response as measurable and reproducible evidence that the mind and body are intertwined. The placebo response is viewed as proof that feelings, thoughts, and beliefs can change the physiological and structural functioning of individuals.

Remembered Wellness

The term *remembered wellness* is the physiological response that occurs after positive therapeutic interventions. Remembered wellness includes the person's prior learning, experiences, environment, beliefs, and perceptions. It can also include biological and genetic factors.

Remembered wellness is triggered by memories of past events or times when good health and feelings of confidence, strength, hope, and peace were part of the person's life. Alternative therapies access these memories by stimulating relaxation, such as the quieting of the body and mind to promote healing. Clinical research has demonstrated relaxation to be effective in treating anxiety, pain, high blood pressure, and tachycardia and in managing stress. Research studies have confirmed a close relationship between the central nervous system and immune system and have shown that interaction occurs between the two mind–body pathways: the autonomic and neuroendocrine systems.

> *Remembered wellness is triggered by memories of past events or times when good health and feelings of confidence, strength, hope, and peace were part of the person's life.*

Much more research is required for a full scientific explanation of how the mind and body interact to produce the placebo response and why remembered wellness produces the positive responses it often does. The placebo response remains an enigma to conventional health care and implies an element of deceitfulness when used deliberately in patient treatments. For integrative healing, the placebo response and remembered wellness are forces that can be harnessed to bring about healing.

Energy Systems

It has long been known scientifically that the human body is regulated by its own internal biochemical electrical energy system called the *neurological system*. Human beings cannot survive without the low levels of electricity that sustain and regulate life at the cellular and molecular levels. Electrochemical reactions are produced in the nervous system and help regulate other body systems, electrical impulses trigger heartbeats, and minute electrical currents regulate the production of hormones. The blood is composed largely of iron; therefore, magnetic forces exist in all parts of the body.[11]

Conventional Uses of Energy

Conventional health care has long used various types of energy systems (e.g., electrical, magnetic, microwave, and infrared) for screening, diagnosis, and some types of treatment. Commonly used modalities include electrocardiograms (ECGs), magnetic resonance imaging (MRI), electroencephalograms (EEGs), electromyograms, x-rays, radiation treatments for cancer, low-frequency electric current to stimulate growth of bone cells (osteoblasts) to accelerate healing of fractures, types of electric shock therapy for cardiac arrest, cardioversions for cardiac arrhythmia, pacemakers, and electroconvulsive therapy (ECT) for a number of severe mental health disorders.

Conventional health care also uses bioenergy (body energy) to determine the degree of injury and estimate recovery times through the study of cells as they decompose, die, reproduce, and respond to pathogens and traumas. The majority of conventional treatments for many diseases are chemical (medications) or surgical or involve immobilizing or manipulating the affected body part. They are used primarily *after* the disease has been diagnosed.

Energy in Alternative Healing

Conventional medicine has long been cynical about integrative practices and, as a result, has been slow to recognize how the energy of the body can be used for health promotion and healing. Alternative therapies refer to energy systems as fields, vital essences, balance, and flow that patients can use to prevent illness, promote health, and heal themselves. The basic concept is that external forces are not able to cause harm if the person is in the well state. Alternative healers may be needed to help individuals manipulate the energy system primarily for self-protection or healing. Major complementary and alternative modalities using bioenergy and other energy fields include **energy medicine**, vital essences and balance, and external energy forces.[11]

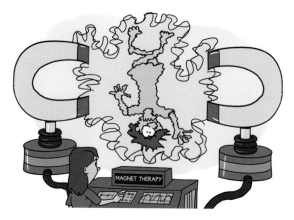

Energy field manipulation with magnets is believed to promote healing and wellness.

Energy Medicine

This therapy includes a number of techniques that use external energy sources to stimulate tissue regeneration or improve the immune system response. Relaxation of muscles through electrical stimulation is thought to promote general body relaxation, increase circulation, enhance waste removal, improve nutrition and oxygenation, and restore energy balance. Examples of energy medicine include biofeedback, magnet therapy, and sound and light therapy.

Vital Essences and Balance

In the integrative models, illness reflects blockage, loss, or imbalance of body energy or vital essence. Disturbance of internal body energy can result from external or internal factors. Treatment may be directed at removing the blockage of energy flow through such measures as acupuncture, acupressure, chiropractic adjustment, craniosacral therapy, or reflexology.[11] It may also be directed at increasing the amount of energy and vital essence to restore balance in the body.

Ways of inducing these changes include diet, herbs, exercises, and spiritual techniques, such as **yoga, meditation, qigong,** and **tai chi.** Therapies related to the creative arts, such as music, drawing, singing, chanting, and dancing, are also used to restore balance and vital essences.

External Energy Forces

It is believed that external energy forces have the capacity for healing. Some of these external forces involve treatments with actual external energy sources, such as whole-body vibration (WBV) therapy (WBVT) and electroacupuncture.

Scientists have long known that everything in the universe vibrates at its own particular frequency, whether it is an iron bar or a human being. WBV involves stimulating the patient's body with low-frequency vibration in the range of 0.5 to 80 Hz.[12] To be most effective, the vibration should be administered over a wide contact area, using a platform to stimulate the feet when standing, a special chair to stimulate the buttocks when sitting, or a vibrating surface to stimulate the whole back when lying down. For maximal effect, the patient should experience some fatigue or low-level stress after the treatment.[12]

It is believed that the vibration causes the body to learn how to adapt to external stress, which produces increased circulation, improved muscle tone, better joint motion, and activation of osteoblasts that increase bone density.[12] By connecting wires to two acupuncture needles at a time and passing a low-voltage pulsating current of electricity between them, it is believed that electroacupuncture augments the acupuncture experience and is especially effective in the treatment of pain. Several pairs of needles can be electrified at the same time, and the procedure should not last more than half an hour.

Other energy-force treatments include mobilizing the healing energy of faith, spirituality, prayer, shamanism, crystals, and hand-mediated energetic healing techniques, such as TT and healing touch (Box 25.4).

Nutrition

Nutrition and diet have long been recognized by both integrative and conventional healing systems as important in health promotion and illness treatment. They can also be risk factors for or can even cause disease. In conventional health care, nutrition and diet are usually considered as adjuncts to treatment with medication. In integrative systems, nutrition is commonly seen as a way of life and as a method of preventing illness.

Benefits of Organic Foods

Currently in the United States, there is a trend to use the terms *natural foods, all-natural foods*, and *organic foods* interchangeably; however, there are significant differences among these terms. The definitions for

---

Box 25.4 Therapeutic Touch

Therapeutic touch (TT) and healing touch (HT) are two forms of hand-mediated energetic healing. TT refers to the Krieger-Kunz method and HT to the techniques taught to health-care professionals and certified by the American Holistic Nurses Association. HT relies on the ability of practitioners to choose appropriate energy healing techniques through their interpretation of the patient's energy flow, whereas TT follows a set of rules and protocols based in traditional or ancient healing concepts of energy, such as aura (electromagnetic field), chakras, and prana (life force or vital essence in ayurvedic medicine).

No physical contact takes place between practitioner and patient in either technique. The practitioner's hands are held, palms down, 2 to 6 inches away from the patient. Slow, rhythmic motions are made over the patient from head to toe to detect blockage in the normal energy flow in the body. When energy blockages or imbalances are detected or sensed, they are rectified by transference of energy from the practitioner's hands to the patient's energy field, replenishing the patient's energy flow, removing energy obstructions, and releasing energy congestion. The transference of energy stimulates the healing powers of the body through reduction of stress and anxiety, promotion of relaxation, and relief of pain. TT is also believed to relax crying babies; relieve asthmatic breathing; increase wound healing; and reduce fever, inflammation, headache, and postoperative pain.

---

natural and *all-natural* foods have little meaning because of the lack of established quality standards for them. The implication in labeling a product as natural is that the food is unprocessed or only minimally processed, suggesting that it does not contain "unnatural" or manufactured substances. However, these products may contain natural substances such as salt, and they may be grown with the use of pesticides and chemical fertilizers and may be irradiated after harvesting and still be called *natural*.[13]

In contrast, the term *organic* has been legally defined and has agreed-upon international standards. Foods can be labeled organic only if they are grown using organic farming methods, which eliminate the use of all synthetic products, such as chemical pesticides and synthetic fertilizers, during their growth cycles. In addition, organic foods are not irradiated or chemically cleaned and do not contain any synthetic food additives after harvesting. Producers must obtain a special certificate from the U.S. government to market their products as organic.[13]

Conventional health care commonly focuses on the need for food and a well-balanced diet without close regard to food production or processing. The safety of food sources in the contemporary diet has been called into question by both alternative healers and conventional health-care professionals because of increasing evidence of toxins in the food chain. These include

- Pesticides used in agricultural production, lawn care, and pest control.
- Industrial pollutants discharged into the air and water in which plants and animals live and obtain nutrients.
- Chemicals added to food for preservation, to increase shelf life, or to make food more aesthetically appealing and pleasing in texture and taste.
- Irradiation used to kill organisms, retard sprouting, and preserve shelf life.
- Antibiotics, hormones, and other drugs given to animals to improve their health and increase their size, weight, and speed of growth.
- Alteration of nutrients during food processing.
- Genetic alteration of foods for improved production rates and drought resistance.[13]

Integrative modalities recommend only foods produced in a natural manner and in their natural environment. Emphasis on organic products can be attributed to four primary factors:

1. Concerns about food production and processing
2. The belief that the person-body, as both an energy system and a physical entity, is designed to live in a natural environment
3. The belief that what is eaten directly affects an individual's health
4. Concerns about increased consumption of nutrient-poor and energy-rich foods

Scientific evidence indicates that the more sedentary lifestyle and greater affluence experienced by many have resulted in excessive and unhealthy eating. The end result is a nation that has high rates of obesity, coronary artery disease, micronutrient deficiencies, congenital abnormalities, and cancer. Most integrative health practitioners advocate consumption of plant-based, whole foods and complex carbohydrates. Increasing the amounts of food lower on the food chain helps decrease the amounts of meat, saturated fats, and processed foods that dominate many diets. Examples of natural food diets include macrobiotic, vegetarian, and vegan diets.

Dietary Supplements

The FDA defines dietary supplements as a product intended for ingestion that contains a "dietary ingredient" intended to add further nutritional value to (supplement) the diet. A "dietary ingredient" may be one, or any combination, of the following substances:

- A vitamin
- A mineral
- An herb or other botanical
- An amino acid
- A dietary substance for use by people to supplement the diet by increasing the total dietary intake
- A concentrate, metabolite, constituent, or extract

> *Some dietary supplements can help ensure an adequate dietary intake of essential nutrients; others may help to reduce the risk of disease.*

Dietary supplements may be found in many forms, such as tablets, capsules, softgels, gelcaps, liquids, or powders. Some dietary supplements can help ensure an adequate dietary intake of essential nutrients; others may help to reduce the risk of disease.[14]

However, buyer beware! Some substances that are sold or promoted as supplements are useless scams; others are potentially harmful—for example, supplements containing licorice root to relieve gastrointestinal symptoms should not be taken by people with hypertension. Licorice is useful in alleviating an upset stomach, but it also raises blood pressure. Fake cure-all products have a long history harkening back to the "snake oil" salesmen who sold their elixirs from the back of a horse-drawn wagon.

Supplements as Prevention

Conventional health-care professionals typically view nutritional supplements (vitamins and minerals) as replacement or preventive therapy for nutrition-deficient conditions. For example, adequate vitamin D and calcium intake are essential to prevent rickets and osteoporosis; adequate ascorbic acid (vitamin C) intake prevents scurvy; and the majority of neural tube defects in newborns can be prevented by sufficient maternal intake of folic acid (vitamin B_9) during the prenatal period. Niacin has been shown to lower cholesterol levels. On the basis of research by the National Academy of Sciences, the FDA has established maximum recommended daily allowances (RDAs) for vitamin and mineral intake. These levels are usually well above the amount at which deficiency diseases occur but below the level at which the patient would experience toxic side effects.

Rethinking RDA Levels

Studies indicate that approximately two-thirds of adults fail to consume the RDAs of fruits and vegetables.[15] Also, some studies suggest that RDA levels may be too low for certain vitamins, minerals, and micronutrients to prevent the onset of chronic diseases in persons whose diets do not meet the recommended daily nutrient requirements. Especially susceptible are growing children; alcoholics; people with conditions preventing normal nutrient absorption; and pregnant, lactating, and postmenopausal women. Conventional health-care professionals consider general daily supplements, such as vitamin pills, sufficient to prevent deficiency diseases in persons with special dietary needs.

Alternative systems, like conventional health care, regard nutritional supplements as useful to ensure adequate dietary intake and as replacement therapy for conditions caused by nutrition deficiency. Alternative systems also consider orthomolecular therapy or megavitamin therapy (the administration of "megadoses" far in excess of RDAs for vitamins and minerals) as being effective in curing diseases, increasing vitality, and enhancing overall well-being.

Regulation of Supplements

Concern about nutritional supplements also exists because, unlike drugs and most food additives, they are not regulated by the FDA. If manufacturers make no claims that supplements are effective against a disease, the supplements do not need to be tested for safety and effectiveness before they are sold to the public. However, there has been a gradual increase in the regulation of these products over the past 25 years. The 1994 Dietary Supplement Health and Education Act (DSHEA) created a special category of 20,000 protected substances previously sold as supplements.[15] The DSHEA defined supplements as including vitamins, minerals, amino acids, herbs, botanicals, and other plant-derived products and the extracts, metabolites, constituents, and concentrates of supplements. The DSHEA is updated every year.

What Do You Think?

Should dietary supplements be considered medications? What are the advantages and disadvantages of classifying supplements as medications? Do you take any supplements?

The FDA can remove supplements from the market if it receives reports of their adverse effects and then proves that they are dangerous to consumers' health. The FDA issues public warnings when supplements are linked to safety concerns. The DSHEA also gave the FDA authority to improve and enforce product labeling, package inserts, and accompanying literature. To enhance product comparison, guidelines instituted in 1999 require labels to carry a panel of "supplemental facts" or a "nutrition facts box," which includes ingredients.

The U.S. Postal Inspection Service and the Federal Trade Commission (FTC) also regulate nutritional supplements and herbal products. The U.S. Postal Inspection Service monitors products purchased by mail and may intercept supplements shipped through the mail for false claims, such as the statement that they can cure AIDS or cancer.

The FTC has issued guidelines to ensure that advertising claims are substantiated by reliable

> *If manufacturers make no claims that supplements are effective against a disease, the supplements do not need to be tested for safety and effectiveness before they are sold to the public.*

scientific evidence. Claims of effectiveness and safety based on testimonials and other anecdotal evidence are no longer acceptable. Also outlawed are vague disclaimers, such as "results may vary." The term *traditional use* (e.g., folk remedy), which implies that the product is effective even without scientific evidence, has also been banned. The risks or qualifying information of any product must be prominently displayed and easily understood.

Plants as Medicine

Both alternative and conventional health care use plants as medicine. Herbalism, or **botanical medicine**, also known as **phytotherapy** or **phytomedicine** in England and other parts of Europe, is the study and use of herbs or crude-based plant products for food, medicine, or prophylaxis. Herbs can also be used to heal, treat, or prevent illness and improve the spiritual and physical quality of life[16] (Box 25.5).

Herbs may be angiosperms (flowering plants, trees, or shrubs), algae, moss, fungus, seaweed, lichen, or ferns. Herbs used as medicines come from some part of the plant (leaf, root, flower, fruit, stem, bark, or seed), its syrup-like exudates, or some combination of these. In some herbal traditions, nonplant products are used alone or in combination, with or without plants. They may include animal secretions and parts (e.g., bones, organs, or tissues), stones and gemstones, minerals and metals, shells, and insects and insect products.[16]

Box 25.5 Top 10 Phytotherapy (Herbal) Supplements

Medicinal Herb	Healing Properties
Raw garlic	Anti-inflammatory, boosts immune system, lowers blood pressure, relieves allergies, helps with heart disease, fights fungal and viral infections, reverses alopecia, lowers blood sugar
Ginger root	Antioxidant, anti-inflammatory
Turmeric root	Antimutagenic, antimicrobial, fights cancer, anti-inflammatory, potent antioxidant
Ginseng root	Stress reducer, weight loss agent, bronchodilator, reduces blood sugar, anti-inflammatory, boosts immune system, treats sexual dysfunction
Milk thistle	Increases gastrointestinal function, anti-inflammatory, helps with skin health and aging, lowers cholesterol, general body detoxification
Feverfew (flower)	Reduces fever; reduces pain; helps with infertility, menstrual irregularities, and labor
St. John's wort	Antidepressant, improves mood during menopause, anti-inflammatory, reduces skin irritations, treats obsessive-compulsive disorder, relieves premenstrual syndrome symptoms
Ginkgo biloba	Improves mental activity including memory and concentration; reduces risk for dementia, Alzheimer's, anxiety, and depression, vision problems; reduces attention deficit-hyperactivity disorder symptoms, increases libido
Saw palmetto	Anti-inflammatory, boosts immune system, bronchodilator, antianxiety effect,
Aloe vera	Constipation aid, reduces skin inflammation, colic treatment, antifungal agent, antihelminth

Source: Understanding the benefits and risks of using herbal medications, *Midland Daily News*, August 14, 2022, https://www.ourmidland.com/news/article/Understanding-benefits-risks-of-using-herbal-17372737.php; Hassan G, Belete G, Carrera K, et al., Clinical implications of herbal supplements in conventional medical practice: A US perspective, *Cureus*, 14(7), 2022, https://doi.org/10.7759%2Fcureus.26893.

Botanical healing in the form of herbal medicines was widely used in the United States until the early 19th century, when it was gradually displaced by the increasing prominence of the scientific method and was labeled quackery. Phytomedicine continues to be a prominent branch of conventional health care in Europe. Botanicals are used by 40 percent of German and French physicians in their daily practices.

Scientists have yet to determine the pharmaceutical qualities of most plants, and little is known about what toxicities they can produce. The world supports an estimated 390,900 flowering plant species, but only 5,000 have been researched for their pharmacological effects.[16]

Herbal Traditions

The use of herbal therapies varies according to culture and tradition. The three major groups of herbal therapies recognized throughout the world are from Western medicine, traditional Chinese medicine, and ayurvedic medicine.

Western Pharmacology

The Western herbal tradition relies primarily on the pharmacological action of herbs. Approximately 123 plant-derived pharmaceutical medicines are in use today. Almost all food supplements and herbal over-the-counter products, except for minerals, are plant based.[16] The compounds and chemicals found in plants constitute about 25 percent of prescriptions by conventional health-care professionals.

Traditional Chinese Medicine

Herbology is used in traditional Chinese medicine to enhance the flow and amount of **chi**, restore the harmonious balance of the complementary forces of **yin and yang**, and balance the five elements (fire, earth, metal, water, and wood). In the Chinese system, plants are prescribed according to their effects on the five elements and their corresponding body processes, including organs, tissues, emotions, and temperatures (climates).[17]

According to traditional Chinese medicine, the five elements give rise to the five tastes that produce particular medicinal actions. Bitter-tasting herbs (fire) dry and drain. Sweet-tasting herbs (earth) reduce pain and increase tone. Acrid herbs (metal) rid the body of toxins. Salty herbs (water) nourish the kidney. Sour herbs (wood) clean, helping preserve chi and nourishing yin. Herbs are also symbolically classified according to temperature changes they are thought to produce in the body: cold, cool, neutral, warm, and hot.[17] The temperatures correspond to the symbolic climate qualities of the organs and the five elements.

Ayurvedic Medicine

Ayurvedic medicine is the traditional medical system that has been used in India for over 3,000 thousand years and is considered to be the oldest medical system.[18] It focuses on producing health by balancing the three key substances of the body. A body out of balance is considered to be in a state of illness, and plant-based substances are used to achieve a balance in the body and restore a state of health. The ayurvedic system also considers the taste, or "essence," of the herb as an integral element in herbology. Ayurveda recognizes six essences (sweet, sour, salty, pungent, bitter, and astringent) and five elements (ether, water, fire, air, and earth). The elements are manifested as three doshas, or humors (*vata, pitta,* and *kapha*), that govern body functioning and that must be kept in balance to maintain or restore a healthy state.[18]

Vata, the principle of air, wind, or movement, is decreased by herbs that are sweet, sour, and salty, which exert a symbolic heating effect on the body. *Vata* is increased by herbs that are pungent, bitter, astringent, and cooling. *Pitta,* the principle of fire, is decreased by herbs that are sweet, bitter, astringent, and cooling and is increased by those that are pungent, sour, salty, and heating. *Kapha,* the principle of water, is decreased by herbs that are pungent, bitter, and astringent; and heating and is increased by those that are sweet, sour, salty, and cooling.[18]

Concerns About Herbal Therapies

There is growing concern in the United States about the use of herbal preparations by the general public without consultation with either conventional

> " *. . . the FDA has found that as many as 20 percent of herbal preparations imported from India and China contain higher-than-allowed levels of heavy metals such as lead, arsenic, and mercury.* "

health-care professionals or alternative healers. Sales of herbal preparations have been growing tremendously, and the safety of the products is a concern. For example, the FDA has found that as many as 20 percent of herbal preparations imported from India and China contain higher-than-allowed levels of heavy metals such as lead, arsenic, and mercury. Some imported herbs have been banned from entry into the United States. Another concern is the lack of licensing and standards for herbalists. Except for naturopaths, most herbalists have no foundation in phytochemistry or botanical medicine.[14]

In some cultural traditions, herbs are not prescribed for the biological effects of their chemical ingredients. Instead, they are prescribed according to the "doctrine of signatures," or their physical and taste characteristics. For example, herbs with heart-shaped leaves may be used to treat heart problems, those with red flowers or leaves may be used to control bleeding or blood disorders, and those with a sour taste may be given to decrease swelling or counteract the effects of "sugar" on the body (diabetes mellitus).

Additional problems with herbal remedies may arise because the public views them as natural products and therefore considers them to be pure, safe, relatively harmless, and more healthy than manufactured medicines. Recent problems with some natural products indicate that there is no guarantee of safety.

Street Drug or Medicine?

Marijuana

Using the strict definitions just discussed, marijuana is a natural product, and if grown without using fertilizer, insecticides, or other chemicals, it can be classified as organic. When it is mixed in with foods or liquids to drink, it can be classified as an herb. Unfortunately, marijuana produces effects that caused the federal government to classify it as a Schedule 1 controlled substance so that its use or possession is punishable by fines or jail time. The use of the word *is* in the preceding sentence is correct. Marijuana use or possession is still a federal crime, although the Department of Justice has chosen to ignore the law for many years.

In the summer of 2022, Senator Chuck Schumer (D-New York) introduced a bill in the Senate called the Cannabis Administration and Opportunity Act (CAOA). This bill or ones similar to it have passed the House of Representatives seven times, but they keep being blocked in the Senate. The bill also contains language that would protect cannabis industry workers' rights, establish impaired driving standards, allow access to banks by marijuana sellers, and establish penalties for possessing or distributing large quantities of marijuana without a federal permit.[19]

According to a Gallup poll in 2022, more Americans were smoking marijuana than smoked cigarettes. The percentage of Americans who said they smoke marijuana was 16 percent, the highest percentage ever recorded. Also, about 14 percent said they consumed edible marijuana products; however, there is a significant overlap between the two groups.[20] Some of the increase in marijuana use can be traced to patients attempting to treat COVID-19 or especially long-COVID.[6] U.S. adults who admitted to smoking tobacco during the same time period was 11 percent, a drop from a whopping 43 percent in 1972.[20]

The number of states legalizing the medical use of cannabis at the time of publication is 38. Each state has its own criteria regarding what medical or psychiatric conditions cannabis can be prescribed for, how much can be used, and what the process is for issuing medical marijuana licenses to qualified residents.[20] According to the National Conference of State Legislatures, 19 states have legalized the adult use of marijuana for recreational purposes. As with medical marijuana, the laws vary from state to state on how much can be purchased at one time, how much an individual may carry on their person, and where and when its use is restricted[20] (Boxes 25.6 and 25.7).

Some states are more restrictive than others. Proponents of medical cannabis cite numerous studies that show the value of the plant in treating ailments such as pain, cancer, multiple sclerosis, rheumatoid arthritis, and inflammatory bowel disease; there is even newer research into the usefulness of cannabis in treating neurological disorders such as Alzheimer's disease.[19] Proponents also point to the American Medical Association's call to conduct clinical research to develop new cannabinoid-based medicines that do not need to be smoked. Large pharmaceutical companies have also seen the potential for profits in developing non-smokable cannabis-based medications and are beginning to accelerate research into these substances. Cannabis oil can be mixed with lotions and used on the skin or made into a paste-like

Box 25.6 U.S. States and Territories That Have Legalized Medical Marijuana

Alaska	Hawaii	Missouri	Oklahoma	West Virginia
Alabama	Illinois	Montana	Oregon	District of Columbia
Arizona	Louisiana	Nevada	Pennsylvania	Puerto Rico
Arkansas	Maine	New Hampshire	Rhode Island	Guam Northern Mariana Islands
California	Maryland	New Jersey	South Dakota	US Virgin Islands
Colorado	Massachusetts	New Mexico	Utah	
Connecticut	Michigan	New York	Vermont	
Delaware	Minnesota	North Dakota	Virginia	
Florida	Mississippi	Ohio	Washington	

Box 25.7 U.S. States and Territories That Have Legalized Recreational Marijuana

Alaska	Illinois	Nevada	Rhode Island	Guam
Arizona	Maine	New Jersey	Vermont	Northern Mariana Islands
California	Massachusetts	New Mexico	Virginia	
Colorado	Michigan	New York	Washington	
Connecticut	Montana	Oregon	District of Columbia	

substance and used like dip or put in food. Cannabis can also be turned into a traditional-looking tablet to be taken orally.

Opponents of the legalization of medical cannabis point to the fact that federal statutes still consider cannabis a Schedule I controlled substance, and possession of large quantities is a felony. Federal law always supersedes state law, although states can choose to ignore and not enforce a federal law. States that are considering allowing the use of medical marijuana face a confusing array of legal and legislative regulations. Any facility that receives federal funds, including most drug stores that take Medicare insurance, banks that are Federal Deposit Insurance Corporation (FDIC) insured, Indian health-care dispensaries, or any of the military drug stores, are controlled by federal laws and are unable to dispense cannabis-based medications. As a result, the states have to establish their own regulations for standalone cannabis dispensaries that are not able to sell any other type of medical substance.[19]

Opponents note that testing has shown that "medical-grade" cannabis is the same as cannabis bought off the street and that cannabis contains more than 400 potentially dangerous chemical compounds if it is smoked. Medical-grade plants have also tested positive for fungi, bacteria, pesticides, and other dangerous substances that are aerosolized and inhaled when smoked.[19] However, oils produced from the plants do not contain the chemicals that make a person "high" and have many fewer contaminants. The long-term effects of their use have yet to be determined.

Opponents also highlight the dangerous effects on the lungs of smoking any substance and the demonstrated neurological effects, such as paranoia and psychosis, sometimes seen in long-time cannabis smokers. The effects of secondhand cannabis smoke on infants and children in houses or cars where cannabis is being used have not been investigated, but from experiences with secondhand cigarette smoke, the effects would probably be similar.

Overall, opponents feel that taking shortcuts to get around the scientific and testing processes used for FDA approval of other medications for the purpose of hastening the use of medical cannabis is a mistake and will have long-term negative consequences on the health of many patients.

Where Did Cannabis Laws Come From?

It is a common belief that cannabis was made illegal in the United States because of its abuse potential and its role as a gateway drug to more addictive substances. However, these arguments were first made long *after* the original laws outlawing cannabis were passed. A major shift in many Americans' positive or neutral attitudes toward cannabis occurred early in the 1900s. This shift was at least partly the result of prejudice against the large number of Mexicans who immigrated to the United States around the time of the 1910 Mexican Revolution. Police officers in Texas fueled public fears about these new immigrants and the marijuana some of them used with claims that the drug incited people to commit violent crimes and aroused blood lust.[19]

The fact is, research has shown that alcohol is a more dangerous drug than marijuana. In addition, cannabis use does not really incite people to violence and may have the exact opposite effect. Even the U.S. Drug Enforcement Administration's own fact sheet on the drug says that "no death from overdose of marijuana has been reported." Despite the lack of evidence to support the dramatic and negative claims that were made about cannabis, many states began to restrict its sale around 1906, and by the mid-1930s, cannabis was regulated as a drug in every state. The Marihuana Tax Act of 1937 was the first national regulation of cannabis, and it was passed despite objections from the American Medical Association related to medical usage.[19] The Controlled Substances Act of 1970 finally outlawed cannabis for any use, including medical use.

THE PARADOX OF INTEGRATIVE HEALING PRACTICES

Nurses often feel uncomfortable with the use of herbal products and unconventional therapies. Their discomfort is due to unclear definitions of various integrative practices along with the widespread, yet often unregulated, use of alternative products and healers.

This paradox arises because most nursing knowledge comes from the biomedical sciences, but most integrative modalities (1) have not yet been scientifically validated or proven safe by the scientific method and (2) are based in concepts of holism, self-care, and theoretical constructs that emanate from worldviews different from that of biomedicine and the scientific perspective.

A Lack of Validation

Put simply, for many integrative treatment modalities, there is little scientific research about whether or how they work, their side effects, or their interactions with conventional or other integrative treatments. Although scientific research is increasing in this area, claims regarding the effectiveness of these treatments still come largely from testimonials of users or integrative healers rather than from evidence in scientific studies. Equally limited is valid knowledge about the effectiveness of the various integrative modalities in specific conditions and about their short- and long-term effects.

The nursing profession has worked for many years to build its decision-making skills on knowledge derived from the scientific method and on the use of critical thinking and cultural competence. The push toward EBP reinforces this belief that the scientific method is the most reliable source of knowledge. Nurses promote self-care in patients by teaching them to make informed choices about their health-care options. Many of the integrative health-care practices in use today conflict with the nursing profession's movement toward EBP.

Few Regulatory Standards

The technical competence and knowledge of integrative healers are of considerable importance to nurses caring for patients who pursue integrative practices. Nurses and the general public are accustomed to determining the qualifications, assumed competency, and scope of practice of conventional health-care practitioners through external regulation. These external regulations include graduation from an accredited school, state-regulated licenses, credentialing, and attainment of specialty certifications from professional organizations or institutions of higher education. No such external processes or criteria exist to validate the competence and knowledge of most integrative practitioners.

The relative lack of regulatory standards makes selection of competent integrative practitioners exceedingly difficult. It is a major concern of conventional health-care practitioners, insurers, and the general public because patients may be subject to financial exploitation, ineffective therapies, and even psychological or physical abuse.

A Challenge to Nurses

The challenge presented to nurses by integrative healing modalities relates to professional accountability. Nurses must learn about integrative modalities, their general safety and efficacy, and their use in specific health and illness conditions.

Human caring and cultural competence require that nurses be able to develop therapeutic partnerships with culturally diverse patients and empower them to take charge of their lives and health care. Nurses need to preserve the patient's right to self-determination and to incorporate whenever possible the patient's cultural health practices, as well as to pursue a variety of conventional or integrative therapies, with or without consulting alternative healers or conventional health-care professionals. Nurses must keep an open mind while relying on sound evidence for recommendations about alternative practices and practitioners.

> " *Nurses must learn about integrative modalities, their general safety and efficacy, and their use in specific health and illness conditions.* "

Ask Questions

Box 25.8 lists some questions nurses need to ask when determining the quality and validity of information about an integrative modality. It is important to teach patients to ask similar questions so that they can decide about integrative therapy and sort out conflicting advice from family, friends, conventional health-care professionals, integrative healers, and the media.

Many patients use integrative healing modalities without ever talking to a conventional health professional about them. Some patients may fear a negative reaction; others are not aware of potential harm that may occur, especially when they combine integrative therapies or alternative and conventional therapies.

Some patients may consider the scientific evidence and mistakenly conclude that noninvasive and non-drug alternative therapies are harmless. Others may wrongly assume that integrative therapies are regulated by the government and would not be available if they were dangerous.

Find Information

Lack of scientific information about integrative healing modalities is of concern to integrative healers, conventional health-care professionals, and patients. For nurses and their patients, the need to know where and how to find up-to-date, reliable information on integrative therapies is a must.

Information Resources

- International College of Integrative Medicine (ICIM): https://www.faim.org/international-college -of-integrative-medicine.
- MedlinePlus is one of several authoritative sources on herbal medicines available for practitioners and patients: https:// medlineplus.gov/herbal medicine.html.
- The FDA maintains a site for reporting and obtaining information about adverse effects and interactions of herbals through MedWatch (800-FDA-1088): https:// www.fda.gov/safety/medwatch-fda-safety -information-and-adverse-event-reporting -program.
- Davis's DrugGuide.com (https://www.drugguide.com/) and the U.S. Pharmacopeia (https://www.usp.org/) include searchable sections on herbal medicines.
- The American Botanical Society (800-313-7105) has a website (http://abc.herbalgram.org/site/ PageServer) and publishes *Herbalgram*, a newsletter on herbal medications.
- Tyler's *The Honest Herbal* is one of the most reputable guides for the use of herbs.[6]
- *The Physicians' Desk Reference for Herbal Medicine* contains scientific findings on the efficacy, potential interactions, clinical trials, and case reports of herbs, as well as indexes on Asian, ayurvedic, and homeopathic herbs.[7]

Box 25.8 Questions to Ask About Integrative Modalities

1. What evidence exists that the therapy is effective or harmful?
   - Is there experimental evidence? How effective is the alternative modality when examined experimentally?
   - Is there clinical-practice evidence? How effective is the alternative modality when applied clinically?
   - Is there comparative evidence? How effective is the modality when compared with other treatments?
   - Is there summary evidence? Has the modality been evaluated and a consensus reached regarding its use and effectiveness for various health conditions?
   - Is there evidence of demand? Is the modality wanted by patients, practitioners, or both?
   - Is there evidence of satisfaction? Does the alternative modality meet the expectations of patients and practitioners?
   - Is there cost evidence? Is the modality covered by health insurance? Is it cost effective?
   - Is the meaning evident? Is the modality the best and right one for the patient?
2. How strong is the evidence? Is it based on testimonials, clinical observations, or scientific research?
3. Can the results be attributed to the placebo effect? Is the benefit from the placebo effect adequate to the patient's needs?
4. Does evidence exist that the benefits of the therapy outweigh the risks?
   - Is the alternative modality potentially useful?
   - Is the modality essentially without value except for the potential placebo effect?
   - Is the modality potentially harmful?
5. Is there another way to obtain the same hoped-for results?
6. Who else has tried this alternative modality, and what was their experience?
7. Are there reputable (licensed and certified) alternative healers available? What has been their experience with this alternative modality?
8. What information do regulatory agencies have about the modality or the alternative healers?
9. What information is available in the popular media about the modality or alternative healers? Has it been or can it be verified by clinical observations or research studies?

Sources: Complementary, alternative or integrative. What's in a name? National Center for Complementary and Integrative Health, 2021, https://www.nccih.nih.gov/health/complementary-alternative-or-integrative-health-whats-in-a-name; Integrative medicine: Alternative becomes mainstream, Mayo Clinic, 2022, https://www.mayoclinichealthsystem.org/services-and-treatments/complementary-medicine.

- Quackwatch (https://www.quackwatch.org) offers fact sheets and reviews of specific alternative modalities, as well as those associated with certain illnesses. It also has sections on how to determine whether a website devoted to alternative modalities is trustworthy.

Ask the Patient

It is important to ask patients about their use of integrative therapies. Not doing so may place them at risk for adverse health outcomes. When and how to assess for the use of ACH during the patient assessment process is a matter of judgment and should be guided by the nurse's knowledge of individual patients. An appropriate time is often after the chief complaint has been documented because this is when questions are asked about the patients' reasons for seeking

health care and what they have already done for their problem.

The following dialog demonstrates how the nurse might obtain information about a patient's use of over-the-counter medications, herbal preparations, home remedies, vitamins, other supplements, and other health practices.

RN: Thank you for going over all your prescribed medications with me. Now, can you tell me if you take any over-the-counter medications, the kind anyone can just buy at the drug store?

Patient: Oh, sure. I take ibuprofen when I have a headache or muscle pain and a stool softener when I have constipation problems.

RN: How about any home remedies or herbal preparations that you take?

Patient: I take two turmeric with black pepper capsules each day for my arthritis. I use tulsi powder to help with my digestion and Boswellia extract capsules to help with inflammation.

RN: Do you take any vitamins or minerals regularly?

Patient: I take a multivitamin tablet each morning with breakfast.

RN: Can you tell me about any activities or practices you do for your health?

Patient: I meditate daily and use deep breathing exercises at least three times a day. I try to get a massage followed by a steam sauna once a week, and I drink warm water and ginger tea throughout the day.

RN: And do these practices help?

Patient: Yes, I believe they help detoxify my body and improve my mind, spirit, and body connection.

RN: Are there any other practices or substances you use for health reasons that we have not discussed already?

What Do You Think?

Does the facility where you do your clinical practice ask about integrative therapies during the admission assessment? Are there checkboxes for this information on the admission sheet? Are you taught to assess for this information in your nursing program?

Using good communication techniques, such as open-ended questions and encouraging statements, will help elicit information that patients might not otherwise discuss. In some cultures, herbs and other therapies may not be considered medicinal, so the nurse may need to use somewhat different vocabulary to ask about these topics. Discuss the patient's use of integrative therapies tactfully and supportively. Keep complete and accurate documentation of all interactions with patients about integrative therapies and healers. And as much as possible, help direct patients toward the safest therapies and the most qualified practitioners.

Conclusion

Integrative, alternative, and nontraditional health-care practices are a growing part of health care in the United States. It is essential that nurses become aware of what these practices entail and how they may affect or interact with conventional therapies that the patient is already receiving. When patients enter the health-care system for whatever reason, admission assessments for these practices should become a routine part of patient evaluation. Nurses traditionally have approached health care from a holistic viewpoint that addresses all the patient's needs—mind, body, and spirit. As health care moves more toward integrative practices, nurses are the logical choice to coordinate a comprehensive approach to health care that includes both traditional and alternative practices.

CRITICAL-THINKING EXERCISES

- Contact three of the websites on alternative practices listed in this chapter. Evaluate them according to their quality, content, and usefulness to your practice.
- Identify a nurse practitioner, physician, or other health-care provider in your area who uses integrative practices. Interview that person and arrange for a presentation to the class about alternative health-care practices.
- Select a patient from your clinical experiences who is having pain. How might alternative practices help this patient? Develop a care plan using both traditional and alternative methods for pain control.
- Identify and discuss three advantages of and three problems with integrative health-care practices.
- Select three nursing theories from Chapter 3 that use a holistic approach to nursing. Identify how and what alternative practices would work well with each one of these theories.
- Have a class debate about the pros and cons of the use of medical cannabis.

NCLEX-STYLE QUESTIONS

1. Which of the following best describes the relationship between integrative medicine and complementary and alternative health practices?
   1. Integrative medicine is another name for complementary and alternative health practices.
   2. Integrative medicine has more in common with complementary health practices than it does with alternative health practices.
   3. Integrative medicine combines appropriate complementary and alternative health practices with conventional Western scientific practices.
   4. Integrative medicine is primarily conventional Western medicine that includes a few complementary and alternative health practices.

2. The focus of complementary and alternative health practices differs from the focus of conventional Western medicine. On which of the following topics do complementary and alternative health practices focus? **Select all that apply.**
   1. Specific diseases
   2. Illness prevention
   3. Healing
   4. Practitioner care
   5. Symptom relief
   6. Self-care
   7. Health and wellness

3. Yolanda is having unpleasant side effects from her chemotherapy for breast cancer. She tells the oncology nurse that she is seeking treatment for her nausea, insomnia, and neuropathy from a practitioner of traditional Chinese medicine. Which of the following responses indicates that the nurse practices an integrative approach to health care?
   1. "You should have asked the oncologist for help with these side effects."
   2. "Traditional Chinese medicine can be very effective. What treatments is your practitioner using? Are they relieving your symptoms?"
   3. "Tell me why you are dissatisfied with the current treatment plan or medication."
   4. "Between you and me, I'd use traditional Chinese medicine instead of chemotherapy if I had cancer."

4. _____ therapies, including therapeutic touch, are based on manipulation of biofields, energy systems internal and external to the body that are used for medical purposes.

5. Which of the following is a unique characteristic of biologically based therapies?
   1. The application or ingestion of naturally occurring substances
   2. The direction of spiritual treatments toward biological functions
   3. The use of body manipulation and/or movement to return the body to optimal alignment
   4. The manipulation of energy fields internal or external to the body for medical purposes

6. Which of the following are reliable sources for information about complementary and alternative health practices? **Select all that apply.**
   1. *The Physicians' Desk Reference for Herbal Medicine*
   2. https://goop.com, a lifestyle website developed by actress Gwyneth Paltrow
   3. International College of Integrative Medicine
   4. *Paleo Magazine*, a guide to "modern day primal living"
   5. National Center for Complementary and Alternative Medicine (NCCAM)

7. The conventional Western practice of pharmacology is most similar to which alternative health practice?
   1. Acupuncture
   2. Homeopathy
   3. Therapeutic touch
   4. Phytotherapy

8. Marcus, an RN, is conducting an admission assessment of Mr. Reza. In addition to documenting any prescription medications Mr. Reza regularly takes, Marcus needs to know about any other herbs, supplements, or other substances he uses for his health. Which question is most likely to elicit a complete answer from the patient?
   1. "You don't take any vitamin supplements or herbal preparations, do you?"
   2. "Can you tell me about any vitamins and minerals, over-the-counter medications, and herbal or home remedies you take on a regular basis?"

3. "What complementary or alternative therapies do you regularly use?"

4. "Can you tell me about any supplements you take?"

9. Practitioners of conventional Western medicine typically have reservations about ACH practices. Which of the following may be seen by Western practitioners as a weakness of CAM? **Select all that apply.**

1. Little or no scientific validation for many health claims

2. Few regulatory standards for CAM practitioners

3. Reliance on the placebo effect

4. Conventional providers' lack of knowledge about CAM treatment modalities

5. Reliance of some ethnic minorities on familiar CAM treatment modalities

10. Which of the following statements about integrative medicine is true?

1. Integrative medicine is more similar to holistic theories of nursing practice than it is to conventional Western medicine.

2. Integrative medicine has more in common with complementary and alternative therapies than it does with conventional Western medicine.

3. Integrative medicine focuses on the practitioner's role in curing or treating illness through surgical or chemotherapeutic means.

4. Integrative medicine does not rely on the diagnoses and treatments that research in conventional Western medicine supports.

References

1. Complementary, alternative or integrative. What's in a name? National Center for Complementary and Integrative Health, 2021. https://www.nccih.nih.gov/health/complementary-alternative-or-integrative-health-whats-in-a-name

2. World Health Organization. *WHO traditional medicine strategy: 2014–2023.* Geneva, Switzerland: World Health Organization, 2013.

3. Kamei S. What benefits can alternative healthcare provide? The Joint Chiropractic, n.d. https://www.thejoint.com/georgia/augusta/washington-crossing-04015/192946-what-benefits-can-alternative-healthcare-provide

4. Statistics on CAM use. Healthy Place, 2016. https://www.healthyplace.com/alternative-mental-health/treatments/statistics-on-cam-use

5. Complementary and alternative medicine market. PR Newswire, August 25, 2022. https://finance.yahoo.com/news/complementary-alternative-medicine-market-reach-233000654.html?fr=yhssrp_catchall

6. Tucker J. Treatment for long COVID: supplementation, oxygenation, and suggested treatment modalities. Chiropractic Economics, August 12, 2022. https://www.chiroeco.com/treatment-for-long-covid/

7. The advantages of an integrative approach in the primary healthcare of post-COVID-19 and ME/CFS patients. American Myalgic Chronic Fatigue Syndrome Society, 2022. https://ammes.org/tag/alternative-health-care/

8. What is integrative therapy? BetterHelp.com, 2022. https://www.betterhelp.com/advice/therapy/some-of-the-benefits-of-integrative-therapy/

9. Wong E, Dulai P, Marshall J, Jairath V, Reinisch S, Narula N. Predictors of placebo induction response and remission in ulcerative colitis. *Clinical Gastroenterology and Hepatology*, 21(4):1050–1060, 2022. https://doi.org/10.1016/j.cgh.2022.08.015

10. Saling J. What is the placebo effect? WebMD, February 8, 2022. https://www.webmd.com/pain-management/what-is-the-placebo-effect

11. Cronkleton E. Energy therapy: What to know? Medical News Today, 2022. https://www.medicalnewstoday.com/articles/energy-therapy

12. Laskowski E. Is whole-body vibration a good way to lose weight and improve fitness? Mayo Clinic, April 12, 2022. https://www.mayoclinic.org/healthy-lifestyle/fitness/expert-answers/whole-body-vibration/faq-20057958

13. Robinson L, Segal J. Organic foods: What you need to know. Help Guide.org, 2022. https://www.helpguide.org/articles/healthy-eating/organic-foods.htm

14. Deboest A. What you need to know about dietary supplements. North Kansas City Hospital, August 23, 2022. https://www.nkch.org/blog/what-you-need-to-know-about-dietary-supplements

15. Dietary guidelines for Americans. Health.gov, 2022. https://health.gov/our-work/nutrition-physical-activity/dietary-guidelines

16. Understanding the benefits and risks of using herbal medications. *Midland Daily News*, August 14, 2022. https://www.ourmidland.com/news/article/Understanding-benefits-risks-of-using-herbal-17372737.php

17. Traditional Chinese medicine (TCM). Natural Healing Hawaii, 2022. https://www.naturalhealinghawaii.com/chinese-medicine/

18. Yadav P. Difference between ayurveda and siddha medicine. Ask Any Difference, 2022. https://askanydifference.com/difference-between-ayurveda-and-siddha-medicine/

19. Jaeger K. Senate bill to federally legalize marijuana and promote social equity finally filed by Schumer, Booker and Wyden. Marijuana Moment, July 21, 2022. https://www.marijuanamoment.net/senate-bill-to-federally-legalize-marijuana-and-promote-social-equity-finally-filed-by-schumer-booker-and-wyden/

20. Avery D. Marijuana laws in every state: Where is weed legal? CNET, March 8, 2022. https://www.cnet.com/news/politics/marijuana-laws-in-every-state/

Preparing for and Responding to Disasters

26

Joseph T. Catalano

DISASTERS ON THE INCREASE

According to the Center for Disease Control (CDC), the world has witnessed an unprecedented increase in natural and human-made calamities during the past decade. These include weather-related catastrophes, such as tornadoes, hurricanes, droughts, forest fires, crop failures, and floods; devastating biological disasters such as the COVID-19 and monkeypox pandemics; and horrendous human-generated events, particularly mass shootings.[1]

Most credible scientists believe that because of climate change, natural disasters will become more frequent and more destructive for decades to come. In addition, scientists also recognize that biological catastrophes will also increase. The Centers for Disease Control and Prevention (CDC) currently has a top 10 list of potential pandemic-producing diseases that they are watching. The combination of climate-change-induced population migration and potent disease-producing viruses and bacteria increases the risk for another, even more deadly, pandemic.[1]

By 2020, scientists noted that the planet as a whole had warmed 2.2°F since the beginning of the Industrial Revolution in 1880. Satellite imagery from NASA and the German Aerospace Center's twin Gravity Recovery and Climate Experiment (GRACE) shows that between 2002 and 2022, Greenland's ice mass melted approximately 300 gigatons, or almost 3.3 percent per year, and the rate is increasing as global warming continues.[2] Similar melting of other large ice masses, such as Antarctica's "Doomsday Glacier," will raise the sea level by as much as 10 feet during the next decade. Between 1992 and 2022, the world's oceans rose by 3.3 inches, a rate of 0.15 inches per year. At this rate, the oceans will be 6 to 10 inches deeper in 10 years, submerging as many as 50,000 ocean-front properties.[3] The carbon dioxide level, which is the primary driver of global warming, has increased globally by 24 percent in recent years; however, U.S. carbon dioxide levels decreased slightly between 2019 and 2022. The other primary greenhouse gas, methane, increased in the United States during the same time period.[1]

- Discuss the nurse's role in a bioterrorism attack and the plan of care for exposure to the different biological agents
- Explain the differences in the mechanisms of action of the three types of chemical weapons
- Name and explain the three key factors for effective treatment of chemical injuries
- Define *decontamination* and identify the steps in the process for both chemicals and biological agents
- Distinguish between the different classes of protective wear for chemical or biological contamination
- Discuss current issues in disaster preparedness, including intruder safety
- Identify the methods to respond to intruders and active shooter incidents

Scientists also point to hurricanes and superstorms such as Hurricane Ian (2022) that tore apart the western coast of Florida; Hurricane Zeta (2020) that blasted Louisiana; Hurricane Sally (2020) that devastated Gulf Shore, Alabama; Hurricane Florence (2018) that submerged much of North and South Carolina; Hurricane Harvey (2017) that inundated Houston, Texas, and surrounding areas under feet of water; and Hurricane Maria (2017) that shocked Puerto Rico and wiped out its power grid for almost a year. Hurricanes Ian, Harvey, and Maria were all category 4 (out of 5) storms with winds in excess of 155 miles per hour. Florence and Sally were "only" category 2 storms, but they produced rainfall measured in feet, not inches. More than 5 years after the storms made landfall, many of these areas were still recovering.

Weather scientists also study the tornadic events that took place in 2011 in Joplin, Missouri, and in 2013 in Moore and El Reno, Oklahoma, all of which were rated as EF5 tornadoes. An EF5 tornado is the most powerful windstorm on earth, with winds in the range of 200 to 300 miles per hour or more and the ability to uproot large trees, vacuum up pavement, and completely demolish a well-built house, remove it from its foundation, and then remove the foundation also.

Tornadoes in the United States and Canada are rated on a scale from 0 to 5, based on the amount of damage they produce. This scale was initially developed by Dr. Tetsuya Fujita in 1971 (the Fujita scale) and revised in 2007 to be able to classify the more powerful tornadoes being seen; it is now named the Enhanced Fujita (EF) scale. A portable Doppler radar truck monitoring the May 5, 2003, Oklahoma City

tornado clocked the EF5 with the fastest winds ever recorded on earth at 319 miles per hour. In the past, EF5 tornadoes were very rare, with one occurring only once a year; that's about one out of every 1,000 tornadoes that occur every year in the United States. The Moore and El Reno tornadoes occurred within weeks of each other. Moreover, the El Reno tornado was the largest tornado on record so far, measuring almost 3 miles wide. Just 4 months later, an EF4 tornado struck Washington, Illinois, killing eight people and removing the town from the map. Fortunately, there have not been any more EF5 tornadoes in the United States since the Moore and El Reno tornadoes, although there has been a large number of F3 and F4 storms that can produce large tracts of total destruction.

> ❝ *A portable Doppler radar truck monitoring the May 5, 2003, Oklahoma City tornado clocked the EF5 with the fastest winds ever recorded on earth at 319 miles per hour.* ❞

Disaster Defined

Simply defined, a disaster is a catastrophic event that leads to major property damage, a large number of injuries, displaced individuals, and/or major loss of life. The International Federation of the Red Cross defines a disaster as "a sudden, calamitous event that seriously disrupts the functioning of a community or society and causes human, material, and economic or environmental losses that exceed the community's or society's ability to cope using its own resources. Though often caused by nature, disasters can have human origins."[5] Natural disasters include hurricanes, tornados, storms, floods, tidal waves, earthquakes, volcanic eruptions, droughts, blizzards, pestilence, famines, and wildfires. Human-made disasters include explosions, building collapses, commercial transportation wrecks, leakage and spills of toxic chemicals, radiation contamination, building fires, and other situations.[5]

Personal and Family Preparation for a Disaster

It is virtually impossible to make preparations to *avoid* disasters caused by acts of terrorism and catastrophic human engineering failures. Most natural disasters have a warning period ranging from a few minutes to several hours. However, the aftermath of all disasters is very similar, and preparations can be made to deal with those circumstances. Relief and rescue workers generally arrive quickly after a disaster, but they cannot take care of all the injured or trapped at the same time. During the time between the occurrence of the disaster and the rescue, individuals must rely on themselves to survive.

Extreme disaster preparedness is carried out by *doomsday preppers* or just *preppers*. Some of these individuals may build large, elaborate underground structures costing anywhere from a few hundred thousand dollars to several million dollars. Preppers typically make sure to have enough food, water, and other supplies to last up to 6 months without any contact with the outside world. They may have electrical generators and special air-filtration devices to keep out unwanted viruses and toxins. Preppers also generally arm themselves with a variety of powerful weapons to keep out individuals or groups who might seek shelter in the preppers' subterranean enclaves. However, even these strongly built structures can be destroyed by natural events such as earthquakes and floods or man-made devices such as large bombs.

Most U.S. residents cannot afford, nor would they even want, this type of extreme disaster preparation. What can the rest of us do when faced with an impending disaster? There are a number of relatively straightforward measures that can be taken when coping with a disaster and its aftermath. These can be modified to some degree to accommodate the most common types of disasters that are likely to be encountered in a given area. For example, an underground storm shelter is great protection in an area that experiences tornadoes regularly, but it would not be appropriate in a coastal area, where hurricanes usually cause flooding.

As health-care providers, nurses need to make the same basic emergency preparations as the general public to ensure their safety during the emergency so that they can effectively aid those injured during the disaster. An injured health-care provider is just another victim who needs care.

The Federal Emergency Management Agency (FEMA), in conjunction with the Red Cross, recommends the following four steps in preparing for a disaster:

1. Get informed.
2. Make a plan.
3. Assemble a kit.
4. Update the plan and the kit.[6]

What Do You Think?

What was the last disaster that affected you or your community? What type of response was available after the disaster? Do you have a disaster preparation kit? Why or why not?

Get Informed

Knowledge is the best preparation for any kind of disaster. Before a plan can be formulated, a sufficient amount of information must be gathered about potential dangers and ways to deal with them. The local emergency management office or local American Red Cross chapter is a good place to start the search for information. Some areas are more likely than others to experience certain types of disasters. Find out what disasters the community has experienced in the past. Is it on a fault line and likely to have earthquakes? Is it located in "tornado alley"? Is it in the shadow of a dormant volcano? Is it along the sea coast where coastal flooding and hurricanes occur? When was the last time a wildfire broke out? There may be some potential human-made hazards associated with the community. Does it have large fertilizer or fireworks plants that may explode? Does a large oil or natural gas pipeline run under the town? How old is the freshwater dam that is located upstream from the community?

All communities should have a written disaster plan that provides information such as how local first responders are to organize rescue efforts, where community emergency shelters are located, and which roads are designated as evacuation routes. These plans will probably be located at the local Red Cross office or at firehouses. Ask for a copy of it. Other valuable information includes mass transportation plans. In the event that personal transportation is unavailable or has been destroyed, are other means of transportation available to evacuate people? Also find out what types of internal disaster plans schools, businesses, and hospitals have to protect the children, employees, and patients.[6]

Disaster Warning Signals

All communities should have some type of early warning signals. These are usually sirens or horns, but it is important to learn before a disaster event what these signals sound like and know how much time there is between when the signals sound and when the disaster hits. Most community disaster plans have some provision for how local authorities and rescuers will provide information to the public before, during, and after a disaster has occurred.

A commonly used method of notification is the National Oceanic and Atmospheric Administration (NOAA) weather radio system and the Emergency Alert System (EAS). Although emergency warnings can be broadcast over the network television system, purchasing an inexpensive NOAA alert radio can provide warnings 24 hours a day. The automatic alert system sends a signal that triggers the radio to turn on. The speakers and audiovisual alert screen automatically turn on to provide instant alerts of conditions that may affect life and property. These radios have Specific Area Message Encoding (SAME) technology, allowing the radio to be programmed to receive only information specific to a particular geographic area. Most cellular phones and tablets can access apps that announce warnings and provide instantaneous, location-specific weather-alert information from the National Weather Service, local TV stations, or The Weather Channel.

The Wireless Emergency Alerts (WEA) system has become an indispensable part of preparing America

> *All communities should have a written disaster plan that provides information such as how local first responders are to organize rescue efforts, where community emergency shelters are located, and which roads are designated as evacuation routes.*

for disasters and emergencies. Since it was started 2012, the WEA system has been used more than 70,000 times to warn the public about dangerous weather, missing children, and other life-threatening situations by placing alerts on cell phones and other mobile devices. WEA is a national public safety system that permits individuals who own compatible mobile devices to receive geographically targeted text messages alerting them of imminent threats to safety in their area, such as tornado alerts for Oklahoma City and its environs.[7]

Make a Plan

After gathering sufficient information, sit down with all family members and develop a plan for possible disasters. The following sections discuss some key elements to be included in all emergency disaster plans.

An out-of-town contact person. A contact person should be a friend or relative who lives a considerable distance from the community and is therefore unlikely to be caught in the disaster. The person's phone number needs to be programmed into all family members' cell phones or memorized by everyone. After a disaster has struck, family members should call to inform this person where they are and what their condition is. Because of damage to the cell phone system or overload of the system by high call volume after a disaster, it is often easier to reach someone by a long-distance call than to reach a family member who may be only a few blocks away.[7] Also, the phone's texting feature uses a different system than the voice phone, and it is often less problematic to send and receive text messages than to make voice calls.

A preselected meeting place. Most of the time, disasters do not occur when everyone is together in one place. They are more likely to occur when family members are widely dispersed, such as at school and work, and family members may be unable to return home because of public transportation shutdowns, road closings due to damage and debris, and so on. Therefore, a disaster plan should include a preselected, centrally located meeting place that is likely to survive the disaster.[6]

A family communication plan. All contact information for all family members at all times should be easily accessible. This includes work and school phone numbers. Other useful numbers can include the National Poison Control Center (1-800-222-1222), local hospitals, and close relatives. These numbers can be programmed into phones or, in case of damage or loss of the phone, listed on a card or a form that should be carried at all times by all family members. A sample of this type of form can be found at https://www.ready.gov. This website also provides blank wallet cards on which contact information can be recorded and carried in a wallet, purse, backpack, and so on, for quick reference.[9] It is a good idea to get the cards laminated to make them more durable and able to survive if they get wet. You might want to obtain several so that they can be available in different locations. Children must be taught how to call the emergency phone numbers and in what situation it is appropriate to do so. Also, post a copy of the communication plan near each landline house phone, if these are present.

Escape routes and safe places. Draw a floorplan of the home that shows all the rooms and the location of stairways, doors, and windows that lead outside. The locations of the utility shutoff points, particularly gas and electricity, should also be shown. There should be at least two ways to exit each room, such as a door and a window or two doors.[7] Everyone in the family should know the best escape routes out of the house and where the safe places are in the house for each possible type of disaster (e.g., if a tornado approaches, go to the storm shelter or basement or the lowest floor of the home or to an interior room or closet with no windows). It is recommended that emergency evacuation drills be conducted at least two times a year and whenever any changes are made in the escape plan or the building's structure.

> *It is recommended that emergency evacuation drills be conducted at least two times a year and whenever any changes are made in the escape plan or the building's structure.*

Disaster Preparation for Older Adults and Disabled Family Members

Recent natural disasters have pointed out the special needs of older adults in a disaster situation. Disaster planning often does not include any special preparation for elders, who are more likely to have mobility limitations and chronic diseases that decrease their ability to cope with major disasters. It may be difficult even to convince older adults to leave their homes. If they do evacuate, they may leave behind life-sustaining medications and assistive devices that they need for their normal daily activities. For bed-bound individuals who have caregivers, the caregivers need an alternative plan if no one else is at home. Power companies should be notified if the disabled person is dependent on life-support technology such as a ventilator.[9] Most of these devices have some type of battery backup system for short-term power outages, but there should be a plan for an alternative power source for long-term outages. The plan may require moving the person to another location.

Although the ability to move elders quickly to a rescue center may save their lives, it can have a profound negative effect on their level of orientation and quality of life. Often, shelters consist of large rooms with rows of cots and have little ability to meet the health needs of older adults. Disaster planning for older adults and those with disabilities should include the following measures:

- Assembling a team of relatives or neighbors who can aid in moving immobile individuals safely. The team should include at least one individual who can move or carry heavy objects, such as mobility devices and life-support equipment.
- Providing one or more of the team members with a key to the older person's house.
- Naming one or more of the team members as a legal health-care decision-maker in case the primary decision-maker is injured in the disaster.
- Assembling a "to-go" emergency kit in a sturdy toolbox or small suitcase that, in addition to the supplies listed for the emergency kit, also include at least 7 days'

worth of items the person routinely uses, such as all medications, adult diapers, ostomy supplies, sanitizing supplies, syringes and alcohol pads for people with diabetes, dressings for those with wounds, and sterile water. Keep the kit near the door that is commonly used for exiting the residence.

- Keeping commonly used mobility devices such as wheelchairs, crutches, and canes near the door of exit.
- Knowing how to get to the nearest special-needs shelter.
- Having a written list of the person's everyday routine, including times of medicines, treatments, and dressing changes, along with the supplies, in case caregivers become separated.[16]

A plan for pets. Pets can create considerable problems for rescue workers. Some people refuse to leave their pets when they are asked to evacuate; other times, pets, especially large dogs, become protective of their injured owners and will not allow rescue workers to approach them. If forced to evacuate, take the pet along if at all possible. Some individuals have many pets and taking all of them may not be possible. In the past, emergency shelters did not allow any animals other than service animals because of hygiene issues.[8] However, with the many disasters that have occurred in recent years, these rules have been relaxed to some degree. Some shelters are divided into no-pet and pet sections. Identify boarding facilities, veterinarians, and pet-friendly hotels that would be willing to accept pets when a disaster occurs.

Actions to Take Before a Disaster
Check key utilities locations. Learn how to turn off water, gas, and electricity at the main switches or valves. Show all family members where these are located and how to shut them off. If a special wrench or tool is required, buy a spare one and keep it near the valve or shutoff.[8]

Check insurance coverage. Most people tend to automatically renew their homeowner insurance coverage each year when they receive the renewal notification. It is a good idea to sit down with an insurance agent every 1 to 2 years and discuss what is actually covered in the policy. The worst time to find out that an insurance policy does not cover roof or siding damage is after a wind or hailstorm. Homeowner insurance does not cover flood damage. Special flood insurance is

available from the U.S. government.[11] Most home insurance does not routinely cover earthquakes either. Special additional coverage must be purchased.

Take a first aid/cardiopulmonary resuscitation (CPR) and automated external defibrillation (AED) class. Contact the local American Red Cross chapter to find out when classes are offered. The American Heart Association also provides CPR classes and can be contacted for locations and times of classes. Most hospitals hold classes also, generally for their employees, but they often allow community members to attend.

Take an inventory of all home possessions. In the past, this type of inventory required several written pages of information.[8] With the advent of cell phones and other digital devices with built-in cameras, it now is easy to inventory your belongings. Make a movie of the house inside and out, with particular focus on high-dollar items such as the 70-inch LED smart TV and computer equipment. Because the device also records audio, comments such as when it was purchased and particular additional features, such as 3D capability, are helpful in establishing its value.

Some policies have a total replacement value clause that will replace the item with a new one just like it no matter how old it is. These policies are more expensive, obviously. Most homeowner policies prorate the value of the item on its age. For example, if a computer cost $3,000 five years ago, it may be worth only $1,500 today. The $1,500 is all that the insurance company will reimburse the homeowner for this item. Also, make a video recording of outbuildings, cars, boats, and recreational vehicles. Obtain professional appraisals of jewelry, collectibles, artwork, and other items that may be difficult to evaluate. Make copies of receipts and canceled checks showing the cost for valuable items. Store this information in a place safe from flood, fire, and other disasters. Paper documents can be safely stored in a safe-deposit box at a local bank. Electronic data can be stored on a flash drive that also can be kept at the bank. In addition, electronic data can be stored at off-site electronic data storage facilities or even in the cloud.

Protect important records and documents. Important documents include photocopies of all credit cards, home titles, birth and marriage certificates, Social Security cards, passports, wills, deeds, and financial information such as checking account numbers, insurance policies, and immunizations records. Ideally, these should be kept in a safe-deposit box, but fire- and waterproof home safes and strongboxes can provide adequate protection and are more convenient to access.

Assemble a Kit

A disaster-supplies kit is a collection of basic items a family would probably need to stay safe and be more comfortable during and after a disaster.[3] Store these items in plastic or metal portable containers kept as close as possible to the exit door or in a secure place such as a storm shelter. At least once a year, the kit should be opened and all items checked. Family members' needs may have changed, and certain items will have exceeded their expiration date. Smaller emergency kits can be kept in each vehicle and at work.

A well-stocked disaster supply kit should include the following:

- Three-day supply of boxed and canned ready-to-eat nonperishable food
- A manual can opener, knives, and other eating utensils (can be plastic)
- Three-day supply of water (1 gallon of water per person, per day)
- Portable, battery-powered radio, citizen band (CB) radio, or small television with extra batteries
- Flashlight, portable LED lantern with many extra batteries
- Well-stocked first aid kit with sufficient supplies to stop major bleeding injuries
- Sanitation and hygiene items (hand sanitizer, moist towelettes, feminine hygiene items [pads and/or tampons], and toilet paper)
- Matches or a lighter in waterproof containers
- Whistle, horn, or some other type of device that can be used for signaling if trapped
- Extra sturdy clothing and warm blankets
- Photocopies of identification and credit cards
- Cash (several hundred dollars if possible) and coins
- Special-needs items such as prescription medications, eyeglasses, contact lens solution, and hearing aid batteries

- If applicable, items for infants, such as formula, diapers, bottles, and pacifiers
- Basic tools (hammer, large pliers, screwdrivers, small pry bar) and, if applicable, pet supplies
- Jacket or coat
- Long pants and long-sleeve shirt
- Sturdy shoes and socks
- Sleeping bag or warm blanket[2]

Update the Plan and the Kit

Ideally, the plan should be reevaluated every 6 months. Ask family members about it and get their input. Check expiration dates on food and medical supplies and replace items that have expired; replace drinking water every 6 months.[7]

Even with every precaution and preparation in place, when a disaster strikes, it is going to be both physically and emotionally traumatic to the whole family. Keeping a cool head and knowing what to do enables all involved to make the best of a bad situation.

It is important to follow the instructions of the professional first responders who have trained and planned for a variety of disasters. If a radio or television is available, valuable information can be obtained concerning the location of emergency shelters, the estimated time for rescuers to respond, and the general condition of the surrounding community.

It is important to wear sturdy clothing such as jeans and particularly important to protect feet by wearing sturdy shoes or boots.[7] If attempting to evacuate an area, it is best to use only the travel routes specified by local authorities. Emergency routes are generally the first ones cleared after a disaster, while alternate routes and shortcuts may be blocked by debris or water and be impassable or dangerous. If at home after a disaster, only use flashlights if it is dark. There may be undetectable gas leaks or other dangerous fumes that can be ignited by matches or candles. Also, keep at least one general-purpose fire extinguisher in an easily accessible location.[8]

Downed high-voltage power lines pose a particularly lethal threat to those who are near them.

> ❝ *It is important to wear sturdy clothing such as jeans and particularly important to protect feet by wearing sturdy shoes or boots.* ❞

Even if a downed power line is not sparking, it may still be live, and stepping on it or driving over it is a potentially deadly mistake. If water is present near the power line, it too can become electrified and cause a fatal shock several feet from the actual power line.

Many people have purchased portable generators in recent years as a backup source of power after a disaster. These pose their own set of dangers. The biggest one is carbon monoxide poisoning.[11] Some people think that running the generator in an attached garage is safe because the fumes go out the big open door. This is false! Generators should be run only outside in a well-ventilated area. In addition, refueling a generator while it is still hot or while it is running can cause a serious fire. Electricity is dangerous, and there is always the potential for electrical shock or fire if the wiring is not connected correctly.

There are many resources for dealing with all types of disasters. FEMA's Community and Family Preparedness Program and American Red Cross Community Disaster Education are available online. Almost every agency that deals with disasters has written information that is available.[8]

HEALTH-CARE PROFESSIONAL AND FIRST RESPONDER PREPARATION FOR A DISASTER

The preceding information is general guidance that all citizens, including health-care providers and first responders, should know in preparing for a variety of disasters. However, by the very nature of their work, health-care providers and first responders require additional knowledge and preparation in dealing with disasters. People look to them for help during their time of need. Although some of the knowledge overlaps, a higher level of preparation is expected of professionals. The information that follows focuses on this specialized knowledge.

Disaster Phases

Although there is a considerable amount of overlap, all disasters can be divided into three basic phases: the preimpact phase, the impact phase, and the postimpact phase. Nurses should learn what they need to do to provide care in all of the disaster phases.

The Preimpact Phase

Certain types of natural disasters are preceded by a warning period. For a tornado, this may range from

---

Issues in Practice

The 10 Commandments of Disaster Preparedness

Nurses and the general public should take the following preparation steps well before a disaster strikes:

1. Discuss the type of hazards that could affect your family. Know your home's vulnerability to storm surge, flooding, and high winds.
2. Locate a safe room or the safest areas in your home for high wind hazard. In certain circumstances, the safest areas may not be in your home but in your community.
3. Determine escape routes from your home and places to meet.
4. Designate an out-of-state friend or relative as a single point of contact for all your family members.
5. Make a plan now for what to do with your pets if you need to evacuate.
6. Post emergency telephone numbers by your phones and make sure your children know how and when to call 911.
7. Check your insurance coverage—flood damage usually is not covered by homeowner insurance.
8. Stock nonperishable emergency supplies and a disaster supply kit.
9. Purchase and know how to use an NOAA weather radio. Remember to replace its battery every 6 months.
10. Take first aid, CPR, and disaster preparedness classes.

Source: *Disaster preparedness plan. SafetyCulture, 2022. https://safetyculture.com/topics/disaster-preparedness-plan.*

a few minutes to as much as an hour; for hurricanes, it may be as long as several days. During the warning stage, also called the *preimpact phase*, the focus is on preparation for the aftereffects of the event. This preparation is primarily at the local community level.[12]

Even before a catastrophic event is predicted, first responders and health-care professionals in disaster-prone regions practice with disaster drills. These drills provide valuable training in a low-stress environment and identify the types of resources that may be needed during a disaster. This type of preparation helps identify unique risk situations for the community and builds the skills and knowledge disaster responders must have to meet the needs of the population.

Mitigation is a type of preparation that includes efforts to diminish susceptibility to disaster impacts such as physical harm, loss of life, and damage to property. These efforts may be long term, such as improving building codes to reinforce buildings against wind, updating zoning and land use management to remove homes and businesses from flood-prone areas, and solidifying infrastructure such as public utilities. Or they may be short-term efforts, such as taping or boarding windows to make individual homes more resilient to a catastrophic event.

> **❝ *During the warning stage, also called the* preimpact phase, *the focus is on preparation for the aftereffects of the event.* ❞**

When the disaster becomes imminent and a warning is issued, preparations such as evacuations are put into operation by the local emergency response unit. Since Hurricane Katrina, FEMA, the Red Cross, and other government agencies have begun the practice of stockpiling essential supplies to be used after the disaster somewhere close to the disaster target area where they can be reached quickly and easily for distribution.

Preimpact for a Pandemic

Preparing for the next new pandemic is almost impossible. As far back as 2009, the federal government had developed a plan for pandemics; however, it did not seem to work well for the COVID-19 outbreak.[13] During the initial outbreak of the pandemic, scientists and researchers scrambled to collect blood and sputum samples from people who had inexplicably developed high fevers, persistent coughs with congestion, and shortness of breath. In a short period of time, it became evident that the disease-causing offender was an animal virus that was completely new to humans. These types of viruses are particularly dangerous because people do not have any time to develop even low levels of immunity to them.[14]

The World Health Organization (WHO) has a system to track developing public-health threats across the planet through its Global Outbreak and Alert Response Network (GOARN). GOARN also provides emergency assistance to countries confronting any type of infectious disease outbreaks.[15] However, a large portion of GOARN's funding comes from the United States, and the Trump administration had cut funding to the point where U.S. scientists and researchers in foreign countries were recalled, and their research eliminated. GOARN is now refunded under the Biden administration and can continue to fulfill its responsibilities that extend beyond contagious disease outbreaks to include crises in food safety, natural and human-made disasters, and the release of chemical toxins.[15]

The CDC also has a parallel worldwide surveillance for emerging pathogens, funding for which was similarly cut by the Trump administration, leaving the United States vulnerable to dangerous organisms. Now that its funding is back, the CDC can keep teams abroad as well as mobile infectious disease investigators ready to fly anywhere around the world to provide assistance if countries ask for it.[14] Finding and treating infectious diseases in other counties can prevent pandemics in the United States. The emergence and re-emergence of infectious diseases in other countries continues to threaten the health of Americans.[13]

Unlike natural disasters or terrorist events, which are localized, viral pandemics are widespread, affecting multiple areas of the United States and other countries at the same time. A pandemic is an extended event with multiple waves of outbreaks; each outbreak wave can last from weeks to months. Waves of outbreaks may occur for a year or more and may re-cluster in the same geographic locations as the organism mutates. Supporting research and development preparedness efforts are new epidemiology and surveillance programs, extended capacity for vaccine production, and strong and coordinated communication structure. The degree of preparedness governs the speed and effectiveness of the response.[13] Preparedness research efforts provide the biological components needed for vaccine production and evaluation of effectiveness, the laboratory infrastructure for production, and the study requirements needed for a vigorous research response to a future pandemic.[14]

Pandemic preparedness plans focus chiefly on viruses and other organisms that could cause epidemics or pandemics. They prioritize research on prototype-pathogens, typical pathogens from viral families already known to infect humans, and high-priority animal pathogens most likely to threaten large numbers of humans. Important early research and development assesses how people respond to medical countermeasures, such as vaccines, therapeutics, and monoclonal antibodies.[15]

Communication Is Critical

One key improvement in recent disaster response is the ability of the various agencies involved to communicate with each other. The lack of efficient communication between agencies became painfully evident after the terrorist attacks on September 11, 2001. Fire and rescue, law enforcement, and other first responders; public health and government agencies; and health-care services were using radios set to different frequencies and were unable to exchange essential information. President George W. Bush's administration authorized the government to spend large sums of money to correct this problem so that victims could receive the best possible care in a timely manner. Efficient communication leads to a well-coordinated response. All agencies must have

agreements in place and understand the role that each agency is to serve in the disaster. This preparation helps to eliminate the arguments sometimes seen among agencies.[7] In rural areas, agreements with nearby communities also become important for obtaining mutual aid.

The news media plays a large part in disaster reporting; however, planning for the news media and the flow of information is often overlooked in disaster preparations. Nurses are likely to hear about a disaster from breaking news reports before they learn about it through official channels. During the beginning of the COVID-19 pandemic, official agencies were slow in providing information about the disease-causing organism, how it was transmitted, and what safety measures should be taken. Health-care workers received false, incomplete, and conflicting information from social and public media. One fear that can become a reality because of this type of unregulated information is group panic. Generally, all information released from a health-care facility should go through the facility's public relations representative or designated spokesperson. Before any information is released, it should be determined how the news will affect particular populations. Families of victims often cling to every word and may misinterpret what is being said. Social media sources may not provide reliable information. Avoid using these sources as your primary basis for action.

> *Persons designated to speak for the health-care facility should have experience with public speaking and be able to convey the information clearly and in terms that the general public can understand.*

Persons designated to speak for the health-care facility should have experience with public speaking and be able to convey the information clearly and in terms that the general public can understand. They should also be able to think on their feet when responding to questions. However, question-and-answer sessions should be limited, especially when national media are involved. Reporters ask the same questions repeatedly, even when there is no new information about the subject.

When people are under stress or have high levels of anxiety, communication must be direct, honest, and to the point. Long, technical explanations will only confuse the facts. The public should also be calmed by reassurances that everything possible is being done. Regular updates every 30 to 60 minutes, even if there is little new information, are helpful in reducing anxiety levels.

Who to Contact
The following agencies can help with planning during the preimpact phase:

- *Disaster Medical Assistance Team (DMAT).* A group of frontline medical personnel, including nurses, who provide health-care after a disaster. These may include terrorist, natural, or environmental disasters.
- *Medical Reserve Corps.* Part of the USA Freedom Corps, which was developed in 2002 in response to Americans' desire to volunteer and serve their communities in the wake of the 9/11 terrorist attacks.
- *American Red Cross.* Registered nurses (RNs) can join their local Red Cross and receive specialized training in disaster and bioterrorism preparedness.
- *Commission Corps Readiness Force.* Deploys teams to respond to public health emergencies.[6]
- *National Disaster Medical System (NDMS).* Mobilizes comprehensive disaster relief and works closely with local fire, police, and emergency medical services. NDMS also uses volunteer disaster response teams called International Medical/Surgical Response Teams (IMSuRTs), of which nurses are an essential component. IMSuRTs provide emergency medical services at any place in the world where there is a lack of resources.
- *Centers for Disease Control and Prevention (CDC).* Headquarters at 1600 Clifton Road, Atlanta, GA 30329 USA. 800-CDC-INFO | (800-232-4636) | TTY: (888) 232-6348. https://wwwn.cdc.gov/DCS/ContactUs/Form
- *World Health Organization (WHO).* Headquarters at Avenue Appia 20, 1211 Geneva, Switzerland. Telephone: +41 22 791 21 11. America contact: 525 23rd Street NW, Washington, DC 20037. Telephone: +1-202-974-3000, fax: +1-202-974-3663, website: https://www.paho.org/

The Impact Phase
When the actual disaster strikes, the impact phase begins. The goal during the impact phase is to respond to the disaster, activate the emergency response, and reduce the long-term effects of the disaster as much as possible.[7] Activation of the emergency response plans developed during the preimpact phase mobilizes all agencies involved. Because fire, rescue, and police are usually the first on the scene, they provide and establish the command post from which all other efforts will be coordinated. Their goal is to identify and remove victims from dangerous situations, deal with unstable structures, and provide first aid to those who have been injured.

Because of concern about terrorism, law enforcement, particularly the Federal Bureau of Investigation (FBI) or Homeland Security, may initially take control of the disaster scene until it can be determined that the cause was not a criminal act such as a bombing or arson. Even with natural disasters such as tornadoes or floods, law enforcement is often first on the scene and, because of their training, tend to take control. Nurses working in the early stages of disasters sometimes feel frustrated by law enforcement officers, who may limit nurses' ability to provide care. It is important to remember that law enforcement is concerned with identifying a crime, catching criminals, and preserving evidence that may be used later in criminal prosecutions. The whole disaster area is considered a crime scene until released by law enforcement, and everyone there is considered a potential witness who may be questioned.

The incident management system (IMS) is an effective tool in bringing some order to the confusion that always surrounds any disaster event. Based on a military model, IMS is a hierarchy with a well-defined chain of command. At the top is the incident commander or manager, who is responsible for coordinating all rescue efforts. A *job sheet*, really a vertical organizational chart, lists all the key people from all the essential agencies involved. It also outlines the responsibilities of each person and agency and must be followed throughout the disaster event for the best coordination of emergency services.[8] Most IMS plans now include hospitals within the service area. Information flows freely from the commander down to paramedics and from the street level back to the top.

Medical assistance is provided in hospitals, in local clinics, or at the disaster site itself. Deployable Rapid Assembly Shelters (DRASHs) are mobile shelters that can be used by the IMSuRT as a small, independent hospital. The DRASH is designed with triage emergency care, intensive care units, and surgical rooms.

During the peak of the pandemic, when the number of patients was overwhelming the capacity of many hospitals, DRASH structures were set up outside hospitals to be used as prehospital diagnosis and treatment areas. The DRASH units were supplied and set up by local National Guard units whose soldiers often remained to help with staffing. In some places, the DRASH units were used as shelter hospitals and played an important role in improving the ability to treat COVID-19 and prevent its spread. Patients who were crowded into emergency rooms (ERs) due to the lack of hospital beds were transferred to the DRASH shelter hospitals, which helped control the source of the infection and reduced its transmission. Only those with low to moderate COVID-19 infections were placed in the shelter hospitals, leaving more hospital beds available for severe and critically ill patients.[16]

Protection for First Responders

Nurses and other first responders must always be aware of the potential dangers of any disaster. If the health-care providers become injured during rescue attempts, they can no longer provide care to the victims and instead become another victim who needs care. As a result, protecting the lives and health of the first responders takes priority over rescue efforts. Because of the wide range of potential hazards, including chemicals such as nerve gas, biological substances, radioactive agents, and explosive devices, care providers must wear appropriate protective equipment.[7] Images of rescue personnel wearing bulky yellow or blue biohazard suits have become ingrained in the public consciousness. Biohazard suits, otherwise known as *personal protective equipment (PPE)*, come in different types and have a range of protective abilities against many types of substances[17] (Box 26.1 and Fig. 26.1).

What's a Nurse to Wear?

It wasn't until March 2020, several months into the pandemic, that the Food and Drug Administration (FDA) first issued an enforcement policy for gowns and other protective equipment to be worn during the COVID-19 pandemic in health-care settings. At this time, the transmissibility of COVID-19 was still not fully understood; however, the FDA recommended

Box 26.1 Protective Levels of Biohazard (Hazmat) Suits

Level A: Resistant to all types of chemicals and biological and radioactive substances and is used in situations in which splashing or exposure to unknown agents is possible. Totally encapsulates personnel and has its own internal air supply.

Level B: Has a hood but does not totally encapsulate personnel. Is splash resistant to most chemicals. Has its own internal air supply.

Level C: Has a hood but does not totally encapsulate personnel. Is less resistant to chemical penetration than previous levels. Equipped with a respirator that can filter out most chemical contaminants and biological and radioactive substances.

Level D: Used when there are no chemicals or agents that can affect the respiratory system or penetrate through the skin. Generally consists of a jumpsuit or scrub suit.

that the choice of gown should be made based on the level of risk of contamination:

- Level 1: *Minimal risk*, to be used, for example, during basic care, standard isolation, visitor precautions (e.g., cover gowns), or in a standard medical unit
- Level 2: *Low risk*, to be used, for example, during blood draw, suturing, in the intensive care unit (ICU), or in a pathology laboratory
- Level 3: *Moderate risk*, to be used, for example, during arterial blood draw, when inserting an IV line, in the emergency department (ED), or for trauma cases
- Level 4: *High risk*, to be used, for example, during long, fluid intense procedures; during surgery; when pathogen resistance is needed or infectious diseases are suspected (both airborne and non-airborne)[18]

Gowns are intended to provide broad barrier protection. Certain areas of surgical and isolation gowns are defined as "critical zones" where direct contact with blood, body fluids, and/or other potentially infectious materials is most likely to occur. These critical zones include the front of the body from top of shoulders to knees and the arms from the wrist cuff to above

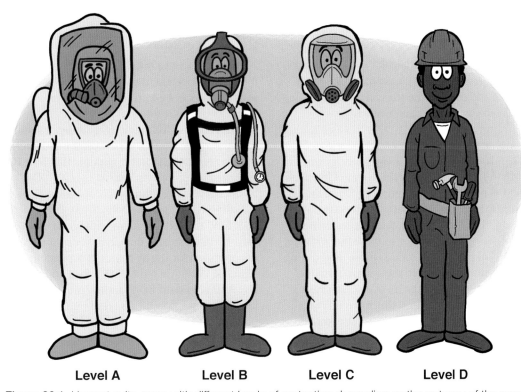

Level A   Level B   Level C   Level D

Figure 26.1 Hazmat suits come with different levels of protection depending on the potency of the agent.

the elbow. Level 3 and Level 4 gowns provide this type of protection. When wearing gowns for protection against infective organisms, it is important that they have sufficient overlap of the fabric so that the gown wraps around the body to cover the back (ensuring that if the wearer squats or sits down, the gown still protects the back area of the body).[18]

By the time scientists determined that the COVID-19 virus was primarily transmitted by respiratory droplets and physical contact with the virus, most hospitals, using their own protection protocols, were already requiring their personnel to wear full Level A or Level B hazmat-type PPE, some with the self-contained breathing aparatus.[19] Although this type of PPE was not necessary, it did provide extra layers of protection and large profits for the companies that manufactured the equipment. The CDC actually recommended against the full-body-type coveralls because of the ease of self-contamination when removing them. As research continued, it became known that low-level virus transmission could occur

via conjunctival secretions, asymptomatic carriers, fecal-oral routes, vertical transmission (mothers to newborns), as well as sexual transmission.[19]

The FDA recommended that nonsterile disposable patient examination gloves, which are used for routine patient care in health-care settings, be worn for the care of patients with suspected or confirmed COVID-19. Double-gloving and heavy protective gloves were not necessary and were a waste of precious PPE. The FDA also recommended the use of face shields or goggles and hair covers if there was a risk of splashing or aerosolization of secretions containing the virus.[18]

Prior to the COVID-19 pandemic, most nurses had not received training in donning, wearing, or performing procedures in Level A or Level B biohazard suits. If nurses find themselves in situations in which they may be required to wear such protection, it is important to recognize some of the limitations. The heavy gloves significantly reduce manual dexterity, and even routine procedures, such as starting IV lines or dressing wounds, become extremely difficult if not impossible.

The hood restricts peripheral vision, and the plastic view plate may distort the visual field. Even cursory physical examination, including the ability to use a stethoscope, becomes more difficult. Nurses may also find that the suit itself causes claustrophobia. The unusual taste and smell of the self-contained breathing equipment can sometimes cause nausea.

Wearing Masks or Respirators

Masks are made to stop droplets and particles when a person exhales, coughs, or sneezes. They are intended to protect the patient from the nurse's potentially harmful organisms. A wide variety of masks are available ranging from those that have little effectiveness such as the neck pull-up masks, to those that provide a higher level of protection, such as those used during surgical procedures. However, these masks provide little protection for the inhalation of disease-causing organisms, particularly viruses, which are very small in size. On the other hand, **respirators**, also known as facepiece filtering respirators or respirator masks, are devices that are designed to protect the individual wearing it by fitting closely on the face and containing materials that filter out very small particles, including the virus that causes COVID-19. They also act as masks by blocking droplets and particles exhaled by

the person wearing them. The N95 is considered a respirator and provides much higher protection than an ordinary mask.[20]

When wearing a mask or respirator, such as N95, it is most important to choose one that fits appropriately and can be worn correctly. The mask needs to fit closely to the face and to completely cover the mouth and nose Although tight-fitting, it should still be comfortable enough to be worn for long periods of time (Fig 26.2). Other respirators that have been approved for protection against the COVID-19 virus by the National Institute of Occupational Safety and Health (NIOSH) include N99, N100, P95, P99, P100, R95, R99, and R100 (with or without an exhalation valve).[20] Interestingly, these types of respirators were not approved for use by health-care personnel until March 2, 2020, when the FDA issued an Emergency Use Authorization (EUA) authorizing their use in health-care settings.[20] These respirators were previously only used by industries that had a possibility of exposure to toxic materials.

After exposure to any type of chemical, biological, or radioactive agent, personnel must go through a decontamination procedure. These procedures vary widely, depending on the type of agent and the equipment the personnel are wearing. They range from

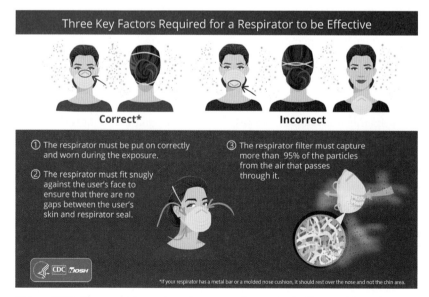

Figure 26.2 The correct way to put on a respirator mask. *Source:* Three key factors required for a respirator to be effective. Centers for Disease Control and Prevention, National Institute for Occupational Safety and Health, 2021. https://www.cdc.gov/niosh/npptl/pdfs/KeyFactorsRequiedResp01042018-508.pdf

simply removing clothes and showering with water to extensive treatment with various neutralizing agents. Most emergency response teams have a decontamination tent that provides some privacy (however, personal privacy is low on the list of priorities) and contains the equipment necessary for thorough decontamination, such as disinfectants and a shower.

Decontamination procedures for personnel wearing hospital-type PPE are different from the procedures for firefighters or individuals wearing Level A or Level B equipment that can be sprayed with sanitizing or disinfecting agents, then hosed-down with water. Unless the health-care facility or DRASH units have an ultraviolet light–C (UVC) room or tent where personnel can walk in after covering their eyes and exposed skin, the only way to decontaminate after being exposed to COVID-19 is to carefully remove and dispose of garments and protective items.[21] Sanitization reduces the number of live microorganisms such as bacteria and viruses to a level at which they can no longer cause disease, generally defined by the U.S. Environmental Protection Agency (EPA) as 99.9 percent. Disinfection kills or inactivates *all* microorganisms at or above 99.9999 percent. Research showed that the live COVID-19 virus was detectable in aerosols for up to 3 hours, on copper surfaces for up to 4 hours, on cardboard for up to 24 hours, and on plastic and stainless steel for up to 3 days.[19]

Although inhalation is the primary mode of viral spread, it is possible for a person to get COVID-19 by touching a contaminated surface or object and then touching their own mouth, nose, or eyes. Cross-contamination, which is the unintentional transfer of a virus or bacterium from one person to another or from a surface to a person, needs to be monitored closely. Phones and other personal items should not be taken into rooms that are contaminated, and personnel should not use each other's phones or other work items and equipment such as stethoscopes or clamps. All items should be cleaned and sanitized *before* and *after* use by other nurses.[18] Careful removal and proper disposal of virus-exposed, single-use PPE, which includes almost all of what is worn by the nurse, needs to take place. Respirators should never be removed while the person is still in a contaminated area. The respirator should be the next-to-last item removed after all other PPE has been taken off except for the gloves. Thorough hand washing and use of hand sanitizer should follow the removal of any PPE

that has been used in a contaminated area. A hot shower with an antimicrobial soap and washing of the hair should also take place before leaving the facility if at all possible. If any of the PPE is contaminated with blood or other potentially infectious liquids or secretions, it should be disposed of in a biohazardous container.[19]

The Postimpact Phase

The postimpact phase begins as soon as the disaster ends and may continue for hours to months.[6] With some disasters, it may continue for years, as in the aftermath of Hurricane Harvey in Texas, Hurricane Katrina in New Orleans, the attacks on the World Trade Center in New York, and the COVID-19 pandemic. Postimpact activities focus on recovery, rehabilitation, and rebuilding. One vital step during the postimpact phase is the evaluation of the disaster preparations and of how rescue and recovery efforts could be improved.

Many Roles for the Nurse

Every disaster poses its own unique challenges. The role of the nurse in a specific disaster depends on its nature and on the type and numbers of injuries. Although most nurses have some familiarity with the role of nurses when they provide aid in a disaster, they may assume many other roles and function outside their usual practice setting in meeting the needs of the disaster victims.[6] Nurses must be able to perform under stressful and sometimes physically dangerous conditions.

After the hurricanes in Florida, large numbers of disabled and elderly patients who had been living in nursing homes and extended care facilities were displaced to schools and shelters. Nurses assumed the primary responsibility for caring for these individuals who, because they could not care for themselves and lacked essential medications, needed care at a level above what rescue workers could provide.

Triage Nurse

When the number of injured is very high, more than 1,000, the incident is classified as a mass casualty, and multiple agencies, from local to federal, become involved. Nurses can provide direct treatment, which may be brief, or they may be involved in more complex roles, such as providing care in mobile surgical units (Box 26.2).

Box 26.2 Responsibilities of the Disaster Nurse

Short Term

1. Performs triage at the scene or in the emergency department.
2. Provides emergency medical assistance at the scene or in the emergency department. Special attention is given to vulnerable groups, such as people with disabilities, children, and elderly persons.
3. Provides assistance in the mobilization of necessary resources such as food, shelter, medication, and water.
4. Works in collaboration with existing disaster organizations and uses available resources.

Long Term

1. Provides assistance with resettlement programs and psychological, economic, and legal needs.
2. Partners with independent, objective media; local and national branches of government; international agencies; and nongovernmental organizations.
3. Warns patients to be aware that many scam artists are present after any disaster and advises patients of factors to consider in detecting a scam.

However, in the early stages of many disasters, nurses may find a lack of essential resources in the field, in the hospital, and in the ED, as was seen with the pandemic. Nurses have a long history of being able to improvise and get by with what is available, and disasters certainly challenge their creativity. When there are large numbers of victims in major disasters, nurses are often responsible for triage (from the French word meaning "to sort"), assessing victims and prioritizing care for the best use of resources. Mass casualty situations require a different type of thinking than is usually used in everyday health care. The traditional classification of victims into low-risk, intermediate care, and immediate care is reordered. The overriding goal in a disaster is to provide the best care possible for the greatest number of victims. Often, this involves providing only palliative care to those with critical injuries, allowing more resources

to be used for those with a better chance of surviving the disaster.[5]

Triage is performed either in the field or in the ED. In the field, few medical resources are typically available, quick evacuation is not possible, and no one knows how soon higher-level medical care will arrive. Standard triage systems were developed for fewer numbers of victims who could be moved quickly to a health-care facility; however, they fall short when there are many victims who must remain in the disaster zone for a longer period of time.

The medical disaster response (MDR) system is designed to quickly evaluate and classify victims, immediately after a disaster, who cannot be evacuated for a substantial period of time. It requires the specialized training of local health-care providers, particularly nurses and first responders. It relies on a dynamic triage methodology that allows for ongoing triage that may last for hours or even days. The goal is to maximize victim survival and make the best use of existing resources.

Classification Systems

The MDR system is based on the traditional simple triage and rapid treatment (START) method but is modified to use palpation of the radial pulse in place of the more difficult capillary refill assessment along with respiratory rate and basic neurological assessment (i.e., Can the victim respond to commands?). MDR can also be combined with the secondary assessment of victim endpoint (SAVE) system of triage that was developed to better use limited resources for victims who were most likely to survive and recover. Trauma statistics serve as the basis for the SAVE system, which attempts to determine which victims will best survive with the various types of injuries they have suffered.[22] The formula used is

Probability of survival (%) = benefit ÷ available resources

If it is determined that a victim has a 50 percent or greater chance of surviving, they receive treatment. Basically, the person conducting the triage makes a cost-benefit analysis in deciding which victims will benefit most from the limited resources on hand. The system places all victims into one of three categories:

Category 1: Those who will die anyway, no matter what resources are used to help them

Category 2: Those who will survive whether or not they are treated

Category 3: Those who can be helped and will gain long-term benefit from intervention and use of resources

The key to the success of the system is to identify and treat those who fall into Category 3 as quickly as possible. The first and second category victims will receive only palliative care. Colored tags are also affixed to the victims according to their physical condition and injuries:

Green (Category 2): Victims who are able to get up and walk around and require minimal or no treatment to save life or limb.

Red (Category 3): Victims who require help breathing or assistance with their airways or whose respiratory rate is greater than 30 breaths per minute. Also included in this group are patients who are breathing but have no pulse at the wrist (radial pulse) and victims who are unable to respond to commands. Some of these victims can be saved and require immediate intervention, but they require the use of a large quantity of already scarce resources.

Yellow (Category 3—nonurgent): Victims who do not meet the criteria for the red category but are not able to walk. These individuals require intervention but usually can tolerate some delay in treatment.

Black (Category 1): Victims who are so severely injured that they have no chance for survival—fatalities.

Other factors that enter into the decision-making process include the victim's age and severity of any preexisting conditions. For example, an elderly victim with a head injury and a Glasgow Coma Scale score of 5 (out of a possible 15—unresponsive to all stimuli) who is wearing a MedicAlert bracelet that says they are on anticoagulant medications would require the use of significant medical resources and would still not likely survive the injury. This person would receive a black tag and be placed in the "expectant" area. However, a middle-aged adult with 20 percent second-degree burns of the legs that require minimal treatment with dressings and pain medications and who has an excellent chance of surviving with full recovery would receive a yellow tag and be moved to a "treatment" area. Victims need to be reassessed frequently because conditions change, and they may need to be moved to another area. The MDR-SAVE methodology is a systematic approach to use triage as a tool to maximize victims' survival in the immediate aftermath of a catastrophic disaster.

COVID-19 Triage

The triage system used during the pandemic is radically different from the MDR-SAVE system. A pandemic triage system is, in its intent and purposes, closer to the way organ transplant donation decisions are made than to field triage decisions. The first step is to ascertain knowledge of the patient's health condition before they became infected with the virus, at the time of presentation at the hospital, and their prognosis, all before recommending treatment.[23] Pandemic triage decisions should be based on a protocol, considering the need for medical measures and therapy benefits. Next, exclusion of treatment criteria should be considered, such as being in a state of irreversible shock or total organ failure and the overall risk of death, to decide who is a candidate for mechanical ventilation.[23]

Prior to beginning mechanical ventilation, the patient and their family should be informed about how closely the patient's physiological responses to the treatment will be monitored and the possibility that, at some point, the patient may be disconnected from the ventilator. The patient then should be evaluated frequently to determine the progression of their health status. If the patient's condition continues to deteriorate and oxygenation declines despite the use of ventilation therapy, ventilator weaning should be considered, particularly if there is a shortage of ventilators.[23] This is one of the most difficult decisions that

> *All triage and decision-making systems are faced with fundamental ethical issues such as the right to self-determination, distributive justice, obligations and duties of health-care personnel, and the right to life.*

health-care providers have to make, and they often receive strong pushback from the family. To avoid situations in which a longer ventilation time may have resulted in a patient's survival, sufficient time should be allowed before evaluating their response to intensive treatment. Other elements to consider in the allocation of scarce equipment in making a pandemic triage decision include first come, first served and who has the most severe condition.

Triage Ethics

All triage and decision-making systems are faced with fundamental ethical issues such as the right to self-determination, distributive justice, obligations and duties of health-care personnel, and the right to life. Some facilities attempted to use pandemic decision-making systems that absolutely excluded patients from ventilation because of the patient's age, certain underlying diseases such as cardiac disease, end-stage renal disease, moderate to advanced cancer, severe genetic disorders, and so forth. Other facilities used a system that automatically classified all COVID-19 patients as DNR/AND.[23] These types of systems were soon dropped by most facilities. Although not ethically bullet-proof, the type of triage system described earlier is based on a public health model that focuses primarily on population-level health outcomes in which the interests and rights of individuals are secondary to the common good.[23] Some hospitals did not have any type of triage system for pandemic patients but simply attempted to treat everyone who entered their doors until they ran out of PPE and ventilators.

BIOTERRORISM

Biological weapons include any organism (e.g., bacteria, viruses, or fungi) or toxin found in nature that can be used to kill or injure people. Toxins, such as the botulism toxin, are poisonous compounds produced by organisms. **Bioterrorism** is defined as the intentional weaponization and dissemination of a biological agent or its toxins for the purpose of killing or incapacitating targets including individuals or populations to achieve military or political goals. It is the use of a disease-causing microbe or its components as an instrument of terror.[24]

An Acute Health Issue

Biological weapons are one category of weapons of mass destruction because of their ability to disable or kill large numbers of people at one time. Unfortunately, biological weapons are relatively easy and inexpensive to produce. Biological agents can be spread through the air, through water, or in food. It is also possible to use robotic delivery of agents by remote-control devices such as drones. Biological agents can also be spread by "suicide coughers" who have purposely been given the disease and who spread it from person to person in a crowded space such as a subway or an airport. After being released, microorganisms can go undetected for an extended period because their effects are not immediate and the initial symptoms are often nonspecific or flu-like. Person-to-person transmission may continue for days or even weeks before the source is detected and a specific disease-causing organism is identified.[24]

Although the COVID-19 virus was not a bioterrorism weapon, it revealed the vulnerability of the United States to the effects of a biological attack. In addition, the biological weapons programs of the former Soviet Union produced some deadly weaponized biological agents that cannot be located; this knowledge has increased national anxiety concerning bioterrorism in the United States. Since 1998, the American Nurses Association (ANA) has worked in conjunction with the American College of Emergency Physicians (ACEP) to develop strategies for health-care providers to use in responding to nuclear, biological, and chemical incidents.

Early Recognition

For nurses and other clinicians, the key to an effective response is early recognition of a bioterrorist attack.[25] Some biological agents can be detected in the environment using high-tech detection devices (sniffers). Portable sniffer models include the

> *Although the COVID-19 virus was not a bioterrorism weapon, it revealed the vulnerability of the United States to the effects of a biological attack.*

Biological Aerosol Warning System (BAWS), which was first used widely in the Iraq War in 2003, and the portable biofluorosensor (PBS). Newer technology, such as the handheld monoclonal antibody biological detection unit, is even more sensitive and can detect a wider range of substances. These devices include the fiberoptic bio-sniffer, which may also be used in the future as a breath analyzer to detect respiratory and other infections, and metal–organic frameworks, which are thin, film-coated optical-fiber sensors that can detect everything from biotoxins to nerve gas.[25] Even newer technology is in the development phase and can play a key part in the future of early detection of biological agents. The latest research is focused on developing tiny electronic chips containing living nerve cells that could be worn like a radiation-detection badge. They would warn of the presence of a wide range of bacterial and viral organisms. Another experimental device that would help identify specific pathogens such as botulism and smallpox consists of fiberoptic tubes coated with antibodies. Light-emitting molecules would shine through the antibodies, and the different colors produced would indicate which organism is present.[25]

However, biological agents are most often identified by specific blood tests and cultures or the report by a health-care provider of a particular set of symptoms indicative of a particular disease. Another early warning sign is an unusually large number of ill or dead animals, particularly birds, found throughout the community. They are often the first to catch lethal illnesses. Health-care providers must be able to identify victims early and recognize the patterns of the disease. If there are a large number of people with the same unusual symptoms, reports of dead animals, or other consistent findings, a biological warfare attack should be suspected. Early detection of a biological agent in the environment allows for early and specific treatment and enough time to treat others who were exposed. Currently, the U.S. Department of Defense is evaluating devices to detect clouds of biological warfare agents in the air at higher altitudes.

Are Nurses Ready?

Studies conducted as recently as 2022 indicate that nurses are still not as well prepared as they should be to respond to biological warfare agents.[26] Although much was learned by dealing with the COVID-19 pandemic, biological attacks require a different mindset and orientation. Nurses have been and will remain among the frontline first responders to all emergency situations, including a biological attack. Nurse preparedness can increase only through improved education and training in early recognition, detection, and treatment of infected persons. To help achieve this goal, several computerized education programs have been developed to raise the knowledge level of nurses and other first responders.

To educate nurses about bioterrorism, the CDC has produced online teaching and learning modules. A more comprehensive education program has been developed by the University of California–Los Angeles in conjunction with content experts. It consists of six interactive case studies that require participants to use their knowledge to identify each biological agent. Pretest and post-test results indicate a marked increase in participant knowledge and ability to detect and distinguish among various biological agents.[26]

In 1999, the CDC and the Association for Professionals in Infection Control and Epidemiology have developed a Bioterrorism Readiness Plan: A Template for Healthcare Facilities, which is available on the CDC's website at https://emergency.cdc.gov/bioterrorism/prep.asp.

Recognizing and treating outbreaks as early as possible is critical for rapid implementation of measures to prevent the spread of disease. Response to bioterrorist attacks is similar to the traditional public health response when communicable disease outbreaks occur naturally, but the focus is on early detection. However, early recognition is challenging because terrorists may use weaponized biological agents that have extremely short incubation periods or produce unusual initial symptoms or symptoms that are ignored until they become debilitating.

Clinical Presentation

Nurses and other clinicians must be familiar with the specific symptoms and clinical syndromes caused by bioterrorism agents (Box 26.3). One of the first indications of a biological attack is an increase in the number of individuals seeking care from public health agencies, primary care providers, and EDs. Because many of these agents are viruses, the early symptoms often look like a case of the flu. Hospitals, health-care providers, nurses, and public health professionals

Box 26.3 Epidemiological Clues to a Biological Attack

- Many patients with the same disease, indicating the sudden development of a large epidemic
- Multiple patients with unusually severe symptoms or diseases with unusual routes of exposure
- Diseases occurring where they normally do not, or during the wrong season, or at a time when the normal vector is absent (e.g., West Nile virus in the winter—no mosquitoes)
- Multiple simultaneous epidemics of different diseases
- Outbreak of zoonotic disease (diseases transferred from animals to humans)
- Larger than normal numbers of sick, dying, or dead animals in the community
- Unusual strains of contagious organisms or large numbers of antibiotic-resistant organisms
- Higher rates of disease than would normally be seen in persons exposed to the organism
- Reports of a credible threat of a biological attack by official authorities
- Direct evidence of biological attack

will be on the front lines of any attack. A heightened level of suspicion, plus knowledge of the relevant epidemiological clues, should help in the recognition of changes in illness patterns.[26]

Biological Agents

The CDC has developed a list of biological agents that are considered most likely to be used in a bioterrorist attack (Table 26.1). Infective agents were included for their ability to produce widely disseminated infections, high mortality rates, potential for major public health impact, and ability to cause panic and social disruption. Those that require special action for public health preparedness were also included. Category A agents possess the highest immediate risk for use as biological weapons; category B agents pose the next highest risk. Category C agents have a potential for use but are not considered an immediate risk as biological weapons.

Effective Response

In the event of a widespread bioterrorism attack, nurses in all levels and types of health-care settings will likely become involved. To develop a prompt and effective response, nurses and other health-care providers must know the modes of transmission, incubation periods, symptoms, and communicable periods of these diseases, as outlined by the CDC.[26]

Identification and Management

Once a potential outbreak is detected, it must be brought to the attention of the appropriate health-care agencies or specialists in infective diseases. The CDC is always called in and may commandeer the hospital to prevent further spread of the biological agent. In cases of suspected bioterrorism, the CDC is given the authority of federal law enforcement personnel.

All nurses should have accurate around-the-clock information on the resources available for their geographic area. Once appropriate notifications have been made, nurses use their skills of clinical evaluation and history taking to identify the infective organism, mode of transmission, and source of exposure. In addition, nurses have a critical role in managing postexposure prophylaxis and its complications, as well as psychological and mental health problems brought on by the event.

What Do You Think?

Have you received any specialized training in disaster or bioterrorism preparedness? If you did, did it help you in the care of COVID-19 patients? If you do not eventually receive this training, is it something that you think is important enough to seek out on your own? Do you feel prepared to care for these victims?

Response Training

The ACEP, in alliance with the ANA, submitted a list of recommendations to the U.S. Department of Health and Human Services (DHHS) Office of Emergency Preparedness in April 2001. One of the recommendations is that all basic nurse education programs include information on how to respond to mass casualty events. The task force also recommended that self-study modules and other types of specialty programs be developed for ED nurses to provide more in-depth

Table 26.1	**Critical Biological Agent Categories for Public Health Preparedness**	
Category	**Biological Agent**	**Disease**
A: Highest immediate risk	*Variola major*	Smallpox
	Bacillus anthracis	Anthrax
	Yersinia pestis	Plague
	Clostridium botulinum (botulinum toxins)	Botulism
	Francisella tularensis	Tularemia
	Filoviruses and arenaviruses (Ebola and Lassa viruses)	Viral hemorrhagic fevers
B: Next-highest risk	*Coxiella burnetii*	Q fever
	Brucella species	Brucellosis
	Burkholderia mallei	Glanders
	Burkholderia pseudomallei	Melioidosis
	Alphaviruses	Encephalitis (VEE, EEE, WEE)
	Rickettsia prowazekii	Typhus fever
	Toxins (e.g., ricin, staphylococcal enterotoxin B)	Toxic syndromes
	Chlamydia psittaci	Psittacosis
	Food-safety threats (e.g., *Salmonella* species, *Escherichia coli* O157:H7)	Salmonellosis, diarrheal illness, sepsis, HUS
	Water-safety threats (e.g., *Vibrio cholerae*, *Cryptosporidium parvum*)	Cholera, cryptosporidiosis
C: Potential, but not an immediate risk	Emerging-threat agents (e.g., Nipah virus, hantavirus)	

EEE = eastern equine encephalitis; HUS = hemolytic uremic syndrome; VEE = Venezuelan equine encephalitis; WEE = western equine encephalitis.

information on the detection and management of bioterrorism.

The ANA is actively involved in developing ways to better prepare nurses to respond to bioterrorist events. In collaboration with the DHHS, it established the **National Nurses Response Team (NNRT)**. This joint effort was unveiled at the ANA's 2002 biennial convention. These teams have been deployed to numerous disaster sites over the past decade.[27]

Activation and Deployment

In the event that the president declares a bioterrorism state of disaster, the NNRT will be activated to respond by providing mass immunization or chemoprophylaxis to a population at risk. The NNRT, under the auspices of the DHHS, will be quickly deployed in response to a major national event.

The goal of the ANA and federal officials is to recruit 10 regional teams of 200 nurses. The ANA is working to recruit these nurse teams and will provide ongoing education to the NNRT in disaster response. The DHHS is responsible for the screening and processing of potential nurse team members after they have been recruited by the ANA.

When the NNRT is deployed, the members become "federalized," and the federal government pays their salaries, reimburses them for travel, and covers their housing costs during the duty period. In case of a terrorism disaster, the deployment is limited to 2 weeks to minimize the impact on the nurses' employers.[27]

The public depends on nurses to be the frontline responders and to protect them from the effects of bioterrorism. Nurses must be able to communicate medical information and educate the public quickly after a crisis. It is imperative that the nursing profession train nurses in appropriate, effective responses to ensure the best outcome in a frightening, unfamiliar event.[13]

MEDICAL RESERVE CORPS

Nurses interested in working with disaster victims might want to consider joining the **Medical Reserve Corps (MRC)**, sponsored by the office of the Surgeon General of the United States. The MRC is a national network of local response units of volunteers committed to improving the health, safety, and resiliency of their communities, and anyone can join. The largest single group of volunteers in the MRC is nurses. Each MRC unit is organized and trained to address a wide range of challenges, from public health education to disaster response. The training is specific for the types of disasters that are seen in the units' communities and range from setting up aid stations and administering immunizations to the aftercare of displaced elderly victims. Nurse volunteers who are trained and certified can respond to a variety of different types of disasters, including those that are out of state. Normally, nurses are not allowed to practice nursing in states in which they are not licensed, but because MRC certification is national, states have agreed to allow certified nurses who are unlicensed in a state to practice within their boundaries during disaster events. State boards of nursing also have the power to allow nurses not licensed in their states to practice in case of disasters, and the State Compact Law allows nurses to practice in other states if they belong to the agreement.

CHEMICAL WEAPONS

Although the Chemical Weapons Convention (CWC) of 1993 banned, under the legal threat of punishment, the worldwide production, stockpiling, and use of chemical weapons, a number of countries, including the United States, maintain large, aging stockpiles of these horrific weapons. Their storage and use are generally rationalized as a means of defending the country against attack from a hostile aggressor.

Definition

Chemical weapons (CW) are generally defined as devices that use any one of a number of chemicals mixed in such a way as to inflict death or harm to human beings. CWs, along with biological and nuclear devices, are generally known as *weapons of mass destruction* (WMDs). CWs, also called the poor man's WMD, take many forms, including gases, liquids, and solids, that often kill or destroy targets other than the one intended.[28]

Toxins are poisonous chemicals usually produced by living organisms and as such might be considered biological. However, toxins are addressed by the CWC because they act and are treated like chemicals and because they can be and have been used as chemical weapons. Two toxins, ricin and saxitoxin, are in fact explicitly listed in Schedule 1 and are among the deadliest CW agents available. In addition, a large number of toxins can be synthesized in laboratories without resorting to the organisms or plants that produce them in nature. A number of toxins are also synthetic dual-use chemicals, meaning that under the CWC, amounts needed for legitimate activities are permitted.[28]

There are two general classes of CWs—unitary and binary agents. Unitary chemical agents are effective by themselves and do not require any other substances to be mixed with them to make them lethal. These agents are highly volatile (unstable and return to a gas state quickly) and are the types of agents most commonly stockpiled by nations in their weapons arsenals and preferred by terrorists. Chemical agents developed after World War II are more deadly than those produced before or during that conflict. They require less saturation (i.e., smaller quantities), are colorless and odorless, have the ability to incapacitate their targets in mere seconds, and can kill within a minute.[28]

Binary CWs become lethal only when two relatively nondangerous chemicals are mixed together

> *In the event that the president declares a bioterrorism state of disaster, the NNRT will be activated to respond by providing mass immunization or chemoprophylaxis to a population at risk.*

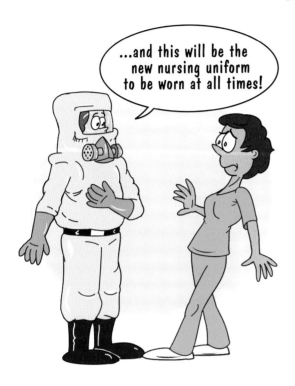

...and this will be the new nursing uniform to be worn at all times!

to create a third dangerous chemical. These are more difficult to manufacture and more complicated to activate. Binary CWs were developed primarily by the Soviet Union during the Cold War but are now available to most countries on the black market. These chemical agents often have Russian names such as Novichok or letters and numbers such as M687, GB2, or A234. These CWs are almost always potent nerve agents, some five times more potent than the nerve agent VX. Although difficult to weaponize to produce mass casualties, this type of CW has been used in recent years to assassinate North Korean leader Kim Jong-un's half-brother Kim Jong-nam in 2017 and to almost kill Sergei Skripal and his daughter Yulia Skripal in England in 2018. Quick treatment saved the Skripals' lives; however, they had a long recovery period and have residual neurological damage. A234 is so toxic that two hotel workers became sick from its residue months after the Skripals were initially poisoned.[28]

The reason airline passengers must limit the liquids they carry on board to 3-ounce increments is also related to CWs. Terrorists in Great Britain in 2006 plotted to use binary agents poured into shampoo bottles and then mixed when they were on the plane with the intention of bringing down international flights.[28]

Horrific Results

The first widespread military use of CWs was in Europe during World War I. The injuries caused by them were so horrific that, although most major countries now have stockpiles of these weapons, they have been very reluctant to use them. The Japanese used CWs against the Chinese at the beginning of World War II, but after seeing the effects, they decided to discontinue their use. The Aum Shinrikyo cult used sarin, a deadly colorless, odorless nerve gas, on a Tokyo subway in 1995, killing 12 people and injuring more than 5,500.[13] In addition, Saddam Hussein used CWs against the Kurds in the northern part of Iraq, killing thousands of people. Parts of the country became a chemical desert because CWs annihilated all living things and made the area uninhabitable for decades due to contamination of water and food supplies. The half-life of certain CWs is decades.[28]

In 1997, the U.S. Senate ratified the United Nation's CWC, a global chemical-weapons ban treaty signed by more than 80 nations. However, terrorist groups do not abide by treaties and, because of the horrific effects and great fear generated by CWs, may wish to obtain and use them.

Letters sent to the U.S. president and several high-ranking government officials in the spring of 2013 were laced with ground castor beans, the key ingredient in the deadly poison ricin; however, they were intercepted before they could cause any harm. More recently, a joint inquiry of the UN and the Organization for the Prohibition of Chemical Weapons found that the Syrian government used the nerve agent sarin in an April 2017 attack on rebel sites.[29]

Since the September 11, 2001, terrorist attacks on America, the threat of CWs has become a concern for both citizens and the government. The government has made preparations to protect the population against CWs and has created a plan for action in response to a CW attack. However, the technology used to produce CWs is widely available, and key chemicals are available at tens of thousands of chemical-manufacturing plants throughout the world.

Types of Chemical Weapons

The three major groups of CWs are nerve agents, blister agents, and choking agents. They are generally dispensed as aerosols, liquids, or vapors that enter the body through the eyes, lungs, or skin. There are also blood agents, which are inhaled. The overall effectiveness of any CW depends on how old the agent is, its purity, weather conditions such as temperature and humidity, the strength and direction of the wind, the size of the environment where they are released, and how they are introduced into the environment.[28]

Many of the newer CWs kill in a matter of minutes; others can take hours or even days, providing victims with a chance of survival if they are quickly decontaminated and treated with the appropriate antidote if one is available. Although symptoms vary depending on the class of agent, some general symptoms to look for include immediate failure of the respiratory or nervous system (paralysis), seizures, severe skin irritations and blisters, headaches, irregular heartbeat or palpitations, vomiting, and convulsions (Table 26.2).

Nerve Agents

Nerve agents are among the most toxic of all CWs. They are particularly deadly when released in an enclosed area such as a subway train or an airplane. These agents were initially developed just before World War II for the purpose of controlling insect infestations on farms. Chemically related to the organophosphorus insecticides that are in wide use today, they work by inhibiting the production of acetylcholinesterase throughout the nervous system and causing paralysis of smooth muscles. German scientists of the 1930s soon recognized the lethal potential of these chemicals and began producing concentrated, weaponized forms that could be used on the battlefield and in the gas chambers of the concentration camps.[28]

Causing an excessive accumulation of acetylcholine in the nerve endings of the parasympathetic system, nerve agents inhibit the smooth muscles all along the vagus nerve (cranial nerve X), including the iris of the eye, ciliary bodies in the bronchial tree and gastrointestinal tract, bladder, and blood vessels. They also paralyze the salivary glands and secretory glands of the gastrointestinal tract, the respiratory tract, and eventually the cardiac muscle tissue. Although respiratory symptoms are generally the first to appear after inhalation of nerve-agent vapors, gastrointestinal symptoms are usually the first to appear if the agent is ingested. The early symptoms often mimic a heart attack, manifesting with tightness in the chest, shortness of breath, elevated blood pressure, and abnormal heart rhythms. As the effect of the toxin becomes more systemic, the victim experiences increased fatigue and generalized weakness, which increases with activity. Soon after, involuntary muscular twitching, scattered involuntary muscle contractions, and intermittent muscle cramps develop. The skin may be pale due to vasoconstriction. Left untreated or treated too late, nerve agents lead to organ failure, complete shutdown of the nervous system, and death.[28]

The primary treatment is immediate decontamination and the administration of atropine sulfate IV as soon as possible. Atropine blocks the effects of

Table 26.2 Classes of Chemical Agents		
Nerve Agents	**Blister Agents**	**Respiratory Agents**
Tabun (GA)	Sulfur mustard (Yperite) (HD)	Phosgene (CG)
Sarin (GB)	Nitrogen mustard (HN)	Diphosgene (DP)
Soman (GD)	Lewisite (L)	Chlorine (Cl)
Cyclosarin (GF)	Phosgene oxime (CX)	Chloropicrin (PS)
Methylphosphonothioic acid (VX)		

"G" or "G Series" stands for gases developed by Germany during World War I and World War II. The second letter seems to be associated with the relative order of development (A before B). "V" or "V Series" stands for gases in the "venomous" category (no relation to snakes). The "X" has no particular significance. The "V" gases were developed in Great Britain. "H" in the H Series gases most likely stands for "Hun Stuff" (Hun as a slang term for German). "C" or "C Series" stands for chlorobenzalmalonitrate, which is one of the cyanocarbon or cyanide related poisons. The second letter does not seem to have any significance. "P" in PL is just a military designation for the substance.

the parasympathetic system and helps breathing by drying secretions and dilating the airways. Atropine also suppresses other symptoms of nerve agents, including nausea, vomiting, abdominal cramping, low heart rate, and sweating. Atropine, however, does not prevent or reverse paralysis. Another medication, pralidoxime chloride, may also be given. It belongs to a family of compounds called *oximes* that bind to organophosphate-inactivated acetylcholinesterase, thereby "regenerating" or "reactivating" acetylcholinesterase and allowing the synapses to function again.[14] Unfortunately, if it is not given soon after exposure, it may not be able to break the molecular bonds in the synapse, and it will be ineffective. The combination injection DuoDote (administered via an antidote treatment nerve agent, auto-injector [ATNAA]) includes both atropine and pralidoxime chloride. If treated early, the serious signs and symptoms of nerve-agent toxicity rarely last more than a couple of hours.

Generally, if the victim survives the initial exposure and peak toxic effects, the symptoms disappear within 1 day, and the survival rate is excellent. Victims who were exposed but show no symptoms are usually observed for at least 18 hours because some signs and symptoms can present later.

Blister Agents

Blister agents, sometimes called *vesicants*, burn and blister the exposed skin on any part of the body they contact. With enough exposure or if inhaled in large quantities, they can kill people, but they are more often used to produce large numbers of serious casualties that need extensive care, thus diverting resources needed for fighting. These agents also force the enemy to wear full protective equipment, making their ability to fight more cumbersome and less effective. When thickened and applied to land, ship decks, or the surfaces of aircraft or vehicles, blister agents become a persistent hazard that makes it challenging to defeat enemies.[30]

Although exposed skin is usually the first area of the body affected, blister agents also can cause major damage to the eyes, mucous membranes, linings of the lungs, and blood-forming organs (thymus, bone marrow, spleen, lymph nodes). In addition, when ingested, they cause vomiting and diarrhea. The most feared and oldest of the blister agents is mustard gas. It is easily made, very stable chemically, and remains dangerous on surfaces almost indefinitely; there is no effective treatment for it even today, making it hard to decontaminate.[30] Mustard gas was first used in World War I, and the gruesome burns it produced frightened even the soldiers who released it.[30]

Exposure to mustard gas is not always immediately evident because of the latent and symptom-free period that may occur after skin exposure. This may result in delayed decontamination or failure to decontaminate at all. However, this agent must be removed from the skin quickly and efficiently. After even as little as a 2-minute exposure, a drop of mustard gas on the skin can cause serious blisters and burns.

Initial treatment, as with all chemical agents, is immediate decontamination. Chemical chlorination has proven somewhat effective in disabling mustard gas and several other of the blister agents. There is no practical drug treatment available for preventing the internal effects of mustard gas. Infection is the most serious complication after exposure to blister agents. Although there is little agreement on the best way to treat exposure to blister agents, most mustard gas victims survive but have protracted and painful recovery periods with the need for multiple skin grafts.[30]

> *Mustard gas was first used in World War I, and the gruesome burns it produced frightened even the soldiers who released it.*

Choking Agents

Choking or respiratory agents work by attacking the tissues of the lungs and produce massive pulmonary edema. The most dangerous of this group of toxins, phosgene, is the one that terrorists are most likely to use. Phosgene was used for the first time in 1915, and it accounted for 80 percent of all the deaths attributed to CWs during World War I. Initial symptoms include coughing, choking, a feeling of tightness in the chest, nausea and occasionally vomiting, headache, and excessive tear production.[31]

When phosgene is delivered in very high concentrations, a painful and agonizing death can occur

Issues Now

Disaster Preparedness for . . . Scams?

After disasters, scam artists show up like flies at a picnic, and there are as many different scams as there are flies. The Better Business Bureau has dubbed these scam artists "storm chasers" because they show up after every major storm or disaster. (By the way, scammers like to use business cards that say "Approved by the BBB." Although BBB *can* stand for Better Business Bureau, unless the name is spelled out, the letters probably stand for something else—Big Blue Buttons, Big Best Barbeque, or maybe Bob's Best Bikes).

There were so many scams after Hurricane Katrina in 2005 that the Department of Justice created a new agency, the National Center for Disaster Fraud, a central information clearinghouse for more than 20 federal agencies where people can report suspected fraudulent activities tied to disasters of all types. If you are the victim of a disaster, here are some things to keep in mind to avoid being scammed:

- There are *never* fees to apply for FEMA or Small Business Administration (SBA) assistance or to receive property damage inspections. If someone is asking for money, it is a scam.
- Utilities do not charge for turning *off* services. Some charge a small fee for turning them back on, although in disaster situations, they often waive the fees.
- If someone claims to be from the government, always ask to see a government-issued photo ID and take a picture of it with your cell phone. In fact, they should volunteer to show you an ID.
- Business cards *are not* official IDs. With all the online, do-it-yourself business card companies these days, it is very easy to make professional-looking business cards that say just about anything.
- Government workers or people associated with government agencies will *never* ask for payment to perform their duties or offer to increase your assistance grant for a fee.
- If private insurance adjusters and local building code inspectors visit your property, they too should provide identification on demand. They do not charge fees.
- *Never* hire a laborer or contractor on the spot; good ones do not need to solicit work door to door. Also, check with your neighbors to see if they suffered damage similar to what is being cited at your place.
- For major repairs, get at least three estimates based on the same specifications and materials. Check the references, licensing, and registration information of all contractors with the National Association of State Contractors Licensing Agencies (NASCLA), and read reviews posted by the Better Business Bureau.
- Require written contracts that specify work to be done, materials to be used, start and end dates, responsibility for hauling away debris, and costs broken down by labor and materials. Verify that the contractor's name, address, phone number, and license number are included, as well as any verbal promises and warranties.
- *Never* sign a contract that contains blank spaces. Unscrupulous contractors sometimes enter unacceptable terms after the contract is signed.
- *Never* give out Social Security numbers, credit card numbers, bank account numbers, or personal information about your finances. Employees of legitimate organizations will never ask for them.
- Read the fine print. Some shady contracts include clauses allowing substantial cancellation fees if you choose not to use the contractor after your insurance company has approved the claim. Others require you to pay the full price if you cancel after the cancellation period has expired.
- Ask your contractor to provide proof of their company's current insurance that covers workers' compensation benefits, property damage, and personal liability. Depending on the size of the job, you may want a performance bond, which protects you if work is not done according to the contract. Contractors do not like to get these.

> ## Issues Now (continued)
>
> - You will probably be asked to pay an upfront deposit to cover initial materials—one-quarter to one-third is reasonable upon delivery of materials to your home and once work begins. Get a signed receipt for the money you paid.
> - Never pay in full in advance, and do not pay cash. Have the contract specify a schedule for releasing payments, and before making the final payment, ask the contractor to provide proof that all subcontractors have been paid—if they have not been paid, you could be liable for their fees.
> - If you suspect anyone—whether an inspector, contractor, disaster survivor, or someone posing as one—of fraudulent activities in relation to a natural or human-made disaster, call FEMA's toll-free Disaster Fraud Hotline at 866-720-5721 or local law enforcement officials.
> - If it sounds too good to be true, it probably is.
> - If someone uses high-pressure sales tactics, requires full payment up front, asks you to get necessary permits, or offers to shave costs by using leftover materials from another job, it is a scam.
>
> We generally think of older people as being most susceptible to scam artists, but these crooks are so slick that anyone can fall for their sales pitches. They know that people who are under stress are much more vulnerable to scams than those who feel secure. Many post-disaster victims have a mild form of posttraumatic stress disorder (PTSD) that may last for many months or even years after the disaster. Making people aware of scams, although not usually thought of as a nursing function, certainly falls into the category of caring.
>
> Sources: *How to avoid fraud and scams after a disaster, Internal Revenue Service, September 27, 2021, https://www.irs.gov/newsroom/how-to-avoid-fraud-and-scams-after-a-disaster; Be alert to fraud after a disaster, FEMA, July 31, 2022, https://www.fema.gov/press-release/20220731/be-alert-fraud-after-disaster.*

within several hours. With lower concentrations, death usually occurs in 12 to 24 hours. There is no specific antidote or treatment. Respiratory support by ventilation with positive end-expiratory pressure (PEEP) can usually maintain adequate oxygenation of the body. Use of osmotic diuretics can reduce the fluid load in the lungs. Other supportive measures commonly used for persons in pulmonary edema may be helpful. If the victim survives the initial exposure, they will usually begin to recover within 48 hours, although there may be permanent lung damage. Respiratory infection is the major complication. If victims survive longer than 48 hours, they usually make a full recovery.[31]

General Principles of CW Preparation

In reality, many of the measures used by nurses and first responders for preparation and protection for bioterrorism are also effective with CWs. It is imperative that nurses and emergency personnel wear Level A or Level B personal protective suits when dealing with chemical contamination due to the persistent nature of some of the agents. Decontamination of the victims as soon as possible is essential to reducing their exposure to the toxins, as is providing appropriate medical treatment, such as specific antidotes, that will increase their chances for survival.[27]

Personal Protective Equipment

First responders and ED personnel are at serious risk for exposure to chemically contaminated areas (known as *hot zones*). The victims themselves automatically become hot zones, and the hot zones can move if the victim is not completely decontaminated. If first responders are unprotected, direct contact with the CW or inhalation of vapors automatically makes them victims as well. If a liquid chemical agent was used, handling the skin and clothing of victims exposes rescue personnel to the same chemical.[28]

Full level A hazardous material (hazmat) suits should be worn until the source of contamination has been completely eliminated. A hazmat suit is an impermeable whole-body garment that is worn as protection against a variety of hazardous materials. To protect against chemical exposures, these suits are made of barrier materials such as Teflon, heavy PVC plastic, corrosive-resistant synthetic rubber, or Tyvek (a brand name for cloth made from flash-spun high-density polyethylene fibers). These suits can cost anywhere from $150 to $1,500 each and are almost always destroyed after use.[27]

High-level suits have self-contained, filtered breathing systems to eliminate any exposure to airborne toxins. These are similar to the suits used for bioterrorism, except that they are more resistant to the corrosive effects of some chemical agents. Also, biological protective suits must have fully sealed systems and positive-pressure breathing systems to prevent entry of the biological agent, even if the suit is punctured or torn. Although hazmat suits are used primarily by firefighters, researchers, personnel responding to toxic spills, specialists cleaning up contaminated facilities, and workers in toxic environments, most health-care facilities have them available for personnel who are likely to come into contact with hazardous chemicals.[28]

Decontamination

Decontamination is the physical and chemical removal of toxic agents from people's skin, clothing, equipment, and any environmental surfaces where the agents were disseminated. Hazardous chemicals remaining on clothing, skin surfaces, and even in the respiratory system can be a source of exposure to others.[16] This is called *secondary exposure* and is the most common type of exposure experienced by first responders and ED personnel. Immediate decontamination is a major treatment priority for those with CW exposure. It should include the following:

- Removing all contaminated clothes and jewelry from the victim and washing the unclothed body thoroughly with warm water and soap.
- Avoiding the use of very hot water and vigorous scrubbing because these may actually force more of the chemical into the skin.
- Decontaminating all victims who have been exposed, even if it is unknown whether the agent was a vapor or liquid. Vapor exposure alone may not require decontamination; however, some vapors cling to

clothing and skin and can be inhaled from these surfaces.
- Decontaminating victims as close as possible to the site of exposure. This minimizes the time of exposure and prevents moving the hot zone to another area. Most hospitals that are certified to treat chemical exposures have policies and procedures about where victims may be decontaminated. Usually, it is an area outside the ED, where a tent is erected to perform initial decontamination before people and equipment are allowed entry into the hospital. Portable decontamination equipment with showers and runoff water collection systems are commercially available. Some larger facilities have in-house decontamination areas with showers, special ventilation, and various decontamination rooms. All hospitals should have the capacity to safely decontaminate at least one person at a time.[16]

Supportive and Specific Therapy

Health-care providers should follow the ABCs of emergency care: airway, breathing, and circulation. Keeping the airway open and making sure victims are able to breathe or are well oxygenated is always the first priority. Intubation and oxygen delivery equipment must be available. Until the specific agent is identified, health-care providers should treat the most serious and life-threatening symptoms first. However, laboratory tests used to identify specific chemical agents are not available in all hospitals. Confirmation of the chemical agent may take several hours or even days. Once the agent has been identified, specific antidotes known to be effective should be used.

The CDC is the authority on chemical weapons and their treatments. It has information on treatment options and a decision tree that can be used for determining what treatments are most likely to be successful.

The Odds Are Good

Realistically, the chances of being exposed to CWs or chemical agents in the United States are miniscule. Although some terrorist organizations have been successful in obtaining and releasing chemical agents, the reality is that making effective delivery systems is extremely difficult. It is more likely that an individual would be exposed to a chemical agent from an

(text continues on page 751)

Issues Now

Intruder Safety

It is a sad commentary on the status of our society that we even have to have this topic in a nursing text. However, the reality of today's life is that unstable and extremely dangerous individuals have relatively easy access to a wide range of deadly weapons. What can you do to help keep yourself and others safe?

Be Aware of Suspicious Activity or Persons

Situational awareness involves, *at all times*, looking around you where you are, being observant, and noticing any unusual or suspicious objects, people, or behavior. What might make someone or something suspicious includes, but is not limited to, the following:

- Unusual items or situations:
  - A strange vehicle parked in an unusual location
  - A package left unattended in a strange place
  - An open window or door that is usually closed
  - Other out-of-the-ordinary situations
- Eliciting information:
  - A person unknown to you asks questions at a level beyond normal curiosity about a building's purpose, operations, security procedures, and/or personnel.
- Observation or surveillance:
  - A stranger paying unusual attention to facilities or buildings beyond a normal interest
  - A person loitering for a lengthy period of time without explanation (particularly in concealed locations)
  - Unusual, repeated, and/or prolonged observation of a building or personnel (e.g., with binoculars or video camera)
  - Someone taking notes or measurements, counting paces, sketching floor plans, and so on

Types of Intruders

There are several different types of intruder situations, and each one requires a somewhat different response on your part. These include the unarmed intruder outside a building, the unarmed intruder inside a building, the armed intruder inside a building who wants to commit robbery only, and the active shooter either inside or outside a building.

Unarmed Suspicious Person Outside a Building

This is a person who is just walking around the property, maybe trying doors to see if they are open or looking in or pushing on windows.

- Evaluate the situation:
  - How big is the person?
  - How big are you? (Size really does matter here!)
  - How threatening do they look?
  - How comfortable are you with approaching them and asking questions?
- If you feel uncomfortable at all approaching the person:
  - Call security or 911 right away.
  - Tell security or 911 who or what you saw, providing as much detail as possible:
    - Description of the person (approximate height, weight, and age; clothing; hat; facial hair; distinguishing marks)

(continued)

Issues Now (continued)

- The time when you saw them
- Where the suspicious person was
- What they were doing/why the person seemed suspicious to you
- Whether the person is still there
- If not, in what direction they went
- If you feel comfortable approaching the person:
- Approach them slowly.
- Keep a safe distance (at least the person's arm's length) away
- Ask nicely, "Is there something I can help you with?"
- Do not be confrontational.
- If the person says something such as "I need to talk to . . ." or "My car is out of gas," direct them to the person they are looking for or to the nearest gas station.
- Do **not** give the person money.
- If you can approach the person from inside your car, it is much safer.
- If the person runs away as you approach, call security or 911.
- If they are threatening, hostile, or aggressive, back away and call 911.
- If they are still hanging around after a period of time, call security or 911 and report a suspicious person. The police will come and investigate.

Unarmed Intruder Inside a Building

- Your response will depend somewhat on what building you are in, the time of day, and whether any other people are with you.
- If you are by yourself and it is after the usual hours for the building to be open, call security or 911 immediately. The intruder should not be in there.
- Provide the information listed previously.
- Seek a safe place or room that can be locked from the inside and barricaded.
- Wait quietly until police arrive.
- Do not argue with, try to talk to, or chase the intruder. They are trespassing, and that is a crime.
- If you find a suspicious stranger in a building during normal operating hours, use the process outlined under Unarmed Suspicious Person Outside a Building.
- If the person has a legitimate reason for being there, direct them to the appropriate location for help.
- If you encounter any type of resistance or hostile response, leave the area immediately and call security or 911.
- Because colleges can be open at unusual hours for night and weekend classes and other events and because we actually want people to attend these, it may be more difficult to identify an unwanted intruder on campus.
- *Security personnel:* If there are security guards, they are the frontline responders in identifying suspicious individuals, but it is everyone's responsibility to be vigilant.
- Look for any unusual behavior that might indicate the person has issues, including pacing, shaking, twitching, uneven or unsteady gate, crying, angry or loud outbursts, temper tantrums, swearing, or emotional language. If you are by yourself:
- Stop the person near the doors if possible and ask if they need help.
- If the person responds aggressively, call security or 911 immediately.
- Do not argue with the person.

Issues Now (continued)

- Do not attempt to restrain or force the person out of the building.
- If the person is walking around in the building, follow them at a safe distance until the police arrive.
- Remain calm and in control—confrontation always increases anxiety.

Armed Intruder Inside a Building Who Wants to Commit Robbery Only
- In general, these intruders do **not** want to hurt anybody. They want to get money or loot and then get out.
- They will use their weapons if they encounter resistance or if any attempt is made to overtake them.
- The goals in dealing with these people are to prevent the injury or death of anyone and to get the intruders out of the building as quickly as possible.
  - Remain calm. These people are already anxious because of what they are doing. Your nervousness will only escalate their feelings.
  - Follow their directions.
  - Do not talk to them at all.
  - Do not stare at them or look them directly in the eyes—these actions can be interpreted as acts of aggression.
  - Do not argue, threaten, or try to reason with them.
  - Give them what they want. Are the contents of your wallet worth your life?
  - Try to memorize what they look like, what they are wearing, and other details.
  - Call security or 911 when they are gone—calling when they are still present may cause them to discharge a weapon or may produce a hostage situation if law enforcement arrives before they leave.
  - Try to observe what the vehicle they are driving looks like and which direction it goes when they leave.
  - If you have your own weapon, *leave it where it is!* Nothing precipitates gun violence more than another gun.

Active Shooter
- This is a relatively new phenomenon in society and one of the most lethal ever.
- An average of 16.4 active shooter incidents occur each year in the United States.
- These intruders seek to kill as many people as possible.
- They will likely keep shooting until they are out of ammunition or are stopped.
- Many are suicidal and want to die themselves, often committing "suicide by cop."
- Active-shooter incidents are unpredictable and can occur at any time or place, although they are more common when a group of people is gathered together in one place, such as a church service, a lecture hall, or a movie theater.
- Dealing with active-shooter incidents requires a radical shift in thinking and acting that may seem counterintuitive at first.
- The reality is that people are going to die, and the goal is to reduce that number as much as possible.
- The one and only goal is your personal survival.
- The goal of law enforcement is to neutralize (disarm or kill) the shooter as quickly as possible.

How to Respond to an Active Shooter Incident
- An active-shooter incident at college is most likely to occur in an area where a large number of people are congregated (cafeteria, meeting room, etc.).
- Active-shooter incidents are often over within 10 to 15 minutes, which may mean they are over before law enforcement arrives on the scene.
- All individuals must be prepared both mentally and physically to deal with an active-shooter incident and do whatever it takes to survive.

(continued)

Issues Now (continued)

Actions for Responding to an Active Shooter Situation

- Be aware of your environment and any possible dangers.
- Note where the two nearest exits are located in any facility you visit.
- When an active-shooter event begins, you will hear gunshots (people describe it sometimes as the sound of firecrackers going off or of a car backfiring). You may hear the shooter yelling and the screams of the victims.
- If someone has already been shot, do **not** listen to or follow the shooter's commands. This person is there only to kill people. If they tell you to freeze and you do, you become an easy target.
- Try to determine as quickly as possible the shooter's location and run in the opposite direction toward an exit.
- **GET OUT OF THE BUILDING** is the golden rule for survival of an active-shooter event. When you are out, do not stop—just keep going.
  - If law enforcement is present when you are coming out, raise your hands over your head and spread out your fingers.
  - Leave your belongings behind. The shooter does not want them.
  - Do **not** try to drag wounded persons out of the building. You both become slow-moving targets.
- The first person out the door should call security or 911. Tell them your location and use the term "active shooter." All police agencies have had some type of training in active-shooter situations, and the term will trigger a rapid response.
  - Never go back in the building while the shooter is still active.
  - Hiding in-place has been shown to be the *least effective* action for survival. You just become a stationary target if you are under a desk or behind a table. You are much harder to hit if you are running.
  - Do not try to hide in a closet or bathroom unless the door can be securely locked and barricaded with something besides a person's body.
  - Stay away from the door. An AR-15, the weapon of choice for active shooters, can easily shoot through a 2-inch-thick solid wood door. It can also shoot the lock off with little difficulty. A 9mm semiautomatic handgun, the second-most favored weapon of active shooters, may or may not be able to shoot through a solid wood door depending on the type of ammunition being used. Hollow-core doors barely stop the pellets from BB guns.
- Make noise, scream, and create as much confusion as possible while running out of the building. This is exactly the opposite of what you do in the other intruder situations. The noise and motion may help disorient or distract the shooter.
- Fight back if you are relatively close to the shooter and cannot get away. Throw any objects you can get your hands on at the shooter's head. Hard or sharp items are best, such as textbooks, phones, and purse items. It is hard to shoot when you are dodging objects coming at your head.
- Run away from the shooter while throwing things.
- **If you are armed AND**
  - have a clear shot without risk of hitting other people,
  - are proficient with the weapon,
  - are close enough for a sure shot,
  shoot to kill.

Issues Now (continued)

- Keep shooting until the intruder is down and not moving or you are out of ammunition.
- Remember that if you miss, you will automatically become the shooter's primary target.
- The weapon the shooter is using must be reloaded periodically with a new magazine. This process takes a few seconds, but that is the best time to attack.
- As a *last resort*, attempt to physically take the active shooter down.
  - When the shooter is at close range and you *cannot* flee, your chance of survival is much greater if you attack and try to knock down and incapacitate the shooter.
  - Attack the shooter from behind—hit the back of the legs at the knee level. The shooter is focused on what is in front of them.
  - Swarm the shooter with one or two or more people, grabbing each of the intruder's arms and legs. Numbers increase the chance of success.
  - At least one person should grab the weapon with both hands, push the muzzle toward the floor, and yank it will all their strength.
  - Act as aggressively as possible against the shooter. Yell, scream, and growl—try to instill fear.
  - Be fully committed in body, mind, and soul to this action, or it will not work.
- If you do manage to incapacitate the shooter,
  - Remove the weapon and put it in a place out of reach and out of sight. **Do not hold it.**
  - Do whatever it takes to keep the shooter down until the police arrive—tie or tape the shooter's hands or legs, sit on the shooter, or render them unconscious.
- **When the police arrive, NEVER, NEVER, NEVER be holding a weapon!**
  - In an active-shooter incident, police are trained to shoot the person who is holding the gun.
  - Put your hands up, spread your fingers, and keep them visible at all times. Do not make any quick or sudden moves.
  - Follow the instructions of any police officers. Do not ask them questions, just follow directions.
- After the police have the shooter restrained and in custody and have finished their initial questioning of the bystanders, try to help the wounded.
- Nurses, health-care providers, and other emergency personnel can lead the way and direct others on what to do.
- By the mere fact that you were in the building at the time of the shooting, you are a witness. Law enforcement will want to question you and obtain your name and address. This may be completed later.
- Do not leave the site until the police say you can leave.

Sources: *Active shooter preparedness*, AlertMedia, April 12, 2022, https://www.alertmedia.com/blog/active-shooter-preparedness; Intruder preparedness and response, Georgia Center for School Safety, n.d., https://www.gacss.org/resources-category/intruder-preparedness-and-response.

industrial or vehicular accident. Numerous chemical factories across the nation are creating chemical toxins that are more deadly than any ever used in weapons. Because of the volatile nature of the chemicals they make, these chemical factories can explode from time to time and spread the toxins over wide areas. In addition, toxic chemicals are regularly shipped by trains and tractor-trailers to all parts of the country. It is not unusual to see a train accident where the large black tank cars lie broken on their sides near a populated area. The chemicals these cars contain are often highly toxic.

Dangerous Aging Weapons

More concerning are the aging stockpiles of CWs owned by the U.S. military. Many of these weapons were manufactured more than 80 years ago and put into containers made to last only a few years. Binary weapons become even more dangerous with age because the barrier separating the two chemicals is designed to rupture either on impact or as a result of a detonator. Because of the corrosive nature of these chemicals, many of the containers are developing leaks, exposing personnel to the toxic agents. The only sure way to dispose of these toxins is to burn them at extremely high temperatures, 2,500°F to 3,000°F, reducing them to their basic elements and rendering them harmless. Unfortunately, only a few disposal plants for chemical weapons exist in this country. Disposal of the many aging chemical warheads would require shipping them cross-country by rail or truck to the disposal sites. The dangers of accidents and widespread contamination make this method of eliminating them very dangerous. Some companies have developed large "indestructible" stainless steel tanks located in stable underground salt caves that can theoretically keep these weapons in safe storage for centuries. Unfortunately, no one knows for certain how safe these tanks and salt caves really are.

Nurses must be prepared to deal with all types of disaster. Education for disaster preparedness needs to start in nursing school and continue throughout each nurse's career. It is highly unlikely that a nurse would not experience some type of disaster during his or her career. Knowledge and skills development are the best preparation.

Conclusion

Nurses need to be prepared for all types of disasters, including bioterrorism, natural disasters, and chemical weapon exposure. The COVID-19 pandemic revealed how poorly prepared the United States was to deal with disasters. In response, legislation was enacted at federal and state levels that began to address the many issues associated with terrorist acts. Large sums of money were expended to purchase equipment and train health-care workers to be better able to deal with a variety of potential disasters.

Collaboration between emergency-response groups has improved dramatically since the beginning of the pandemic. DHHS and the ANA have worked closely together to educate nurses in disaster and bioterrorism responses, and their efforts have been rewarded. Better preparation was demonstrated in the aftermath of the EF5 Oklahoma tornadoes of 2013 than was evident after the EF5 tornado of 2005, and the post-disaster phase of Hurricane Harvey in 2017 was managed significantly better than the aftermath of Hurricane Katrina in 2005. However, there is still room for improvement, as the delayed, fragmented, and insufficient response to 2017's Hurricane Maria in Puerto Rico showed.[26] Nurses have dealt with disasters for many years in EDs and as first responders in the field. Most of their knowledge was accumulated on the job after years of experience. Nowadays, it is essential that the principles of disaster preparation and emergency aftercare be taught to nurses before they graduate from nursing school.

CRITICAL-THINKING EXERCISES

- Obtain the policy and procedure manuals from your nursing school and your primary clinical location. Try to find the procedures for disaster preparedness (note that they are sometimes separate documents). Compare the school's and the facility's policies with each other and with the plan in this chapter. How do they compare? Where are the areas that need improvement?
- If you do not yet have a disaster plan or kit for your family, start putting one together. Involve your family in this activity so that everyone knows the plan and is aware of what is in the kit.
- Volunteer to work with your local Red Cross chapter. Write a report about what it does and how it is funded.
- Look up the word *acetylcholinesterase*. Prepare a short presentation to the class about how nerve agents affect the sympathetic and parasympathetic nervous systems. Explain why atropine is an effective antidote.
- Interview someone who had severe COVID-19 and was hospitalized for a lengthy period of time. Ask them about the nursing care they experienced and how it might have been improved.

NCLEX-STYLE QUESTIONS

1. After an explosion at a chemical plant, the local emergency department is preparing to receive eight victims with chemical injuries. No other details are available at this time. Which of the following should the nursing staff do immediately to prepare for patients with chemical injuries? **Select all that apply**.
   1. Set up a decontamination area.
   2. Gather necessary equipment for drawing blood samples.
   3. Ensure that everyone who will be in contact with patients dons personal protective equipment.
   4. Gather intubation and oxygen-delivery equipment.
   5. Locate the CDC decision tree on chemical exposures and their treatments.

2. Natural disasters related to the weather appear to be increasing in frequency and intensity. What do scientists think is the major reason for these increases?
   1. The migration of population centers from central regions to the coasts
   2. Climate change as evidenced by the warming of the planet, the rise of sea levels, and the rising level of CO_2
   3. The faster rotation of the earth on its axis that has occurred over the last millennium
   4. It is part of the natural cycle of weather events that increase and then decrease in severity over thousands of years

3. The physical and chemical removal of toxic agents from people's skin, clothing, equipment, and any environmental surfaces where they were disseminated is called _____.

4. A terrorist organization threatened to release a biological weapon in the city today. At 9:00 a.m., EMTs are called to a subway station. There, they find an otherwise healthy, 25-year-old man in severe respiratory distress. Witnesses report that the man's symptoms began suddenly after he exited the train. What action should the EMTs take first?
   1. Assess the man's ABCs—airway, breathing, and circulation.
   2. Quarantine the subway station, allowing no one to leave.
   3. Don personal protective equipment.
   4. Call for backup and report a possible bioterrorism incident.

5. Which statement about the postimpact phase of a disaster is true? **Select all that apply.**
   1. It is the longest of the three disaster phases.
   2. It involves activating the emergency response procedures.
   3. It is when scam artists prey on victims of a disaster.
   4. It involves identifying and removing victims from dangerous situations.
   5. It is a time for evaluating the effectiveness of disaster preparations.

6. Professor Velázquez has asked for volunteers to list ways people can protect themselves from post-disaster scams. Which answer indicates a need for clarification?
   1. "Verify that the contractor or agent has a business card that indicates that they are approved by the BBB."
   2. "Be suspicious of high-pressure sales tactics or 'limited time only' offers."
   3. "Never sign a contract that contains blank spaces."
   4. "Don't pay for work in full in advance."

7. Brittany, a nursing student in Oklahoma, decides that her family needs a disaster-preparedness plan. Which of the following elements should her plan include? **Select all that apply.**
   1. A disaster supply kit that includes nonperishable food, water, clothing, and medications, among other things
   2. Flotation devices in case of storm surge or flooding
   3. Verification that everyone in the family who is old enough takes first aid and CPR classes
   4. An evacuation plan that includes their cat, Penny
   5. Locating escape routes from the home and agreeing on a place to meet

8. Which of the following is the best definition of *disaster*?
   1. A catastrophic event that leads to major property damage, a large number of injuries, displaced individuals, and/or major loss of life
   2. An event caused by weather, volcanoes, or earthquakes that causes human suffering
   3. An event caused by human error or deliberate actions that leads to property damage and loss of life
   4. A catastrophic event that occurs without warning, inflicts major property damage, and results in injury or loss of life

9. After a devastating hurricane in a neighboring state, Cedric, an RN, wants to help. How can Cedric legally practice nursing in a state in which he is not licensed? **Select all that apply.**
   1. Join the Medical Reserve Corps (MRC).
   2. Get a waiver from the neighboring state's board of nursing.
   3. Fully disclose to the coworkers and patients he is helping that he is not licensed in that state.
   4. Use his State Compact license because both states belong to the agreement.
   5. Look for victims to help on his own, away from other first responders.

10. A group of nursing students is having a study session on the second floor of the library when they hear gunshots erupt from the first-floor lobby. What action should the members of the study group take immediately?
    1. Gather their belongings and prepare to exit the building.
    2. Prepare to look for gunshot victims and try to help them.
    3. Call campus security to report the shooting.
    4. Get out of the building as quickly as possible.

References

1. Constable H, Kushner J. Stopping the next one: What could the next pandemic be? BBC, 2022. https://www.bbc.com/future/article/20210111-what-could-the-next-pandemic-be
2. Hubbard A. Greenland ice sheet is shrinking faster than forecast, locking in sea level rise: Study. Talking Points Memo, August 29, 2022. https://talkingpointsmemo.com/cafe/greenland-ice-sheet-sea-level-rise-study
3. Jacobo J. Antarctica's melting "Doomsday glacier" could raise sea levels by 10 feet, scientists say. ABC News, September 6, 2022. https://abcnews.go.com/International/antarcticas-melting-doomsday-glacier-raise-sea-levels-10/story?id=89415405
4. Ritchie H, Roser M. United States: CO_2 country profile. Our World in Data, 2022. https://ourworldindata.org/co2/country/united-states#year-on-year-change-what-is-the-percentage-change-in-co2-emissions
5. Disaster. *Britannica*, 2022. https://www.britannica.com/science/disaster
6. Disaster preparedness plan. SafetyCulture, 2022. https://safetyculture.com/topics/disaster-preparedness-plan/
7. Wireless emergency alerts. Federal Communications Commission, 2022. https://www.fcc.gov/consumers/guides/wireless-emergency-alerts-wea
8. Make a plan. Ready.gov, 2022. https://www.ready.gov/
9. People with disabilities. Ready.gov, 2022. https://www.ready.gov/disability
10. Sinnock B. Rising disaster coverage costs could be coming to a head for housing. *National Mortgage News*, August 16, 2022. https://www.nationalmortgagenews.com/news/rising-disaster-coverage-costs-could-be-coming-to-a-head-for-housing
11. Clinical guidance for carbon monoxide (CO) poisoning after a disaster. Centers for Disease Control and Prevention, 2022. https://www.cdc.gov/disasters/co_guidance.html
12. Phases of a disaster. Restore Your Economy, 2020. https://restoreyoureconomy.org/main/phases-of-disaster/
13. Pandemic preparedness plan. Child and Family Services Agency, 2009. https://cfsa.dc.gov/sites/default/files/dc/sites/cfsa/publication/attachments/cfsa%25202009%2520pandemic%2520preparedness%2520plan_0.pdf
14. Park A. How virus hunters are preparing for the next pandemic. *Time*, August 1, 2022. https://time.com/6202044/preparing-for-next-pandemic-virus-hunters/
15. NIAID pandemic preparedness plan. National Institute of Allergies and Infectious Diseases, 2021. https://www.niaid.nih.gov/sites/default/files/pandemic-preparedness-plan.pdf
16. Zhou F, Gao X, Li M, Zhang Y. Shelter hospital: Glimmers of hope in treating coronavirus 2019. *Disaster Medicine and Public Health Preparedness*, 14(5):e3–e4, 2020. https://doi.org/10.1017/dmp.2020.105
17. Hazmat suits level of protection. Hazwoper-OSHA.com, n.d. https://hazwoper-osha.com/blog-post/hazmat-suits-levels-of-protection/
18. Personal protective equipment: Questions and answers. Centers for Disease Control and Prevention, 2019. https://www.cdc.gov/coronavirus/2019-ncov/hcp/respirator-use-faq.html
19. Mukhra R, Krishan K, Kanchan T. Possible modes of transmission of Novel Coronavirus SARS-CoV-2: A review. *Acta Biomedica*, 91(3), 2020. https://doi.org/10.23750%2Fabm.v91i3.10039
20. How to use the N95 respirator mask. Centers for Disease Control and Prevention, March 16, 2022. https://www.cdc.gov/coronavirus/2019-ncov/prevent-getting-sick/use-n95-respirator.html#:~

21. Biosafety Manual. *West Virginia University: Environmental Health and Safety*, 2023. https://www.ehs.wvu.edu/

22. Disaster response and recovery. Department of Homeland Security, 2022. https://www.dhs.gov/disaster-response-and-recovery

23. Kucewicz-Czech E, Damps M. Triage during the COVID-19 pandemic. *Anesthesiology Intensive Therapy*, 52(4):312–315, 2020. https://doi.org/10.5114/ait.2020.100564

24. Johnson A. What is bioterrorism in biotechnology? ScienceOxygen, 2022. https://scienceoxygen.com/what-is-bioterrorism-in-biotechnology/

25. Pampaplakis G, Kostoudi S. Chemical, Physical, and Toxicological Properties of V-Agents. *Multidisciplinary Digital Publishing Institute*, 2023. https://www.mdpi.com/1422-0067/24/10/8600

26. The lack of preparation for bioterrorism puts health workers at risk. *Hospital Employee Health*, December 1, 2000. https://www.reliasmedia.com/articles/47330-lack-of-preparation-for-bioterrorism-puts-health-workers-at-risk

27. National Response Team (NRT) member roles and responsibilities. Environmental Protection Agency, 2022. https://www.epa.gov/emergency-response/national-response-team-nrt-member-roles-and-responsibilities

28. Arnold J. Chemical Warfare. Emedicine Health, 2023. https://www.emedicinehealth.com/chemical_warfare/article_em.htm#risk_of_exposure_to_chemical_weapons

29. Deutsch A. Chemical weapons watchdog blames Syrian air force for Douma attack. *Reuters*, 2023. https://www.reuters.com/world/middle-east/chemical-weapons-watchdog-blames-syrian-air force-douma-attack-2023-01-27/

30. Blister agents. Virginia Department of Health, n.d. https://www.vdh.virginia.gov/emergency-preparedness/public-preparedness-guidance/chemical-agents/blister-agents/

31. Choking agent poisoning. Drugs.com, 2022. https://www.drugs.com/cg/choking-agent-poisoning.html

Developments in Current Nursing Practice

27

Joseph T. Catalano

Learning Objectives

After completing this chapter, the reader will be able to:

- Discuss the requirements for becoming and the roles of a forensic nurse, sexual assault nurse examiner, legal nurse consultant, forensic death investigator, forensic psychiatric nurse, correctional nurse, nurse entrepreneur, nurse navigator, nurse coder, patient safety officer, and telehealth nurse

- Discuss ways in which to develop a nurse-run business

NEW ROLES FOR THE RN

The profession of nursing is dynamic. Nursing roles evolve and develop in response to the needs of society. Many nursing professionals hoped that the Patient Protection and Affordable Care Act 2010 (ACA) would open even more doors for professional nurses and provide opportunities for expanded practice, allowing nurses to practice to the full extent of their education and licensure, as identified by the Institute of Medicine (IOM). This chapter discusses the new and exciting practice roles in nursing. Included are discussions of forensic nursing, nurse entrepreneurs, nurse case managers, legal nurse consultants, and telehealth nurses.

FORENSIC NURSING

Forensic nursing forms an alliance among nursing, law enforcement, and the **forensic sciences**. The term *forensic* means anything belonging to or pertaining to the law.

Continuum of Care

Forensic nursing, as defined by the International Association of Forensic Nurses (IAFN), is "the application of nursing science to public or legal proceedings; the application of the forensic aspects of health care combined with the biopsychosocial education of the registered nurse (RN) in the scientific investigation and treatment of trauma and/or death of victims and perpetrators of abuse, violence, criminal activity and traumatic accidents."[1] **Forensic nurses** provide a continuum of care to victims and their families, beginning in the emergency department (ED) or at the crime scene and leading to participation in the criminal investigation and the courts of law.[1]

Nurses, particularly ED nurses, have long provided care to victims of domestic violence, sexual assault, gunshot wounds, stabbings, and other injuries resulting from criminal acts. These nurses have collected, preserved, and documented legal evidence, often without formal training. It was not until 1992 that the term *forensic nursing* was coined.

What Do You Think?

Do you know any nurses who are involved in forensic nursing? Is this a role that you might be interested in pursuing after graduation?

The IAFN was founded in the summer of 1992. Seventy-four nurses, primarily sexual assault nurse examiners, came together in Minneapolis, Minnesota, to develop an organization of nurses who practice within the arena of the law. This very diverse group includes, but is not limited to, legal nurse consultants, forensic nurse death investigators, **forensic psychiatric nurses**, and forensic correctional nurses.

The organization's membership tripled within its first year. By 1999, the IAFN had more than 1,800 members. The American Nurses Association (ANA) recognized forensic nursing as a subspecialty in 1995, and the Scope and Standards of Forensic Practice was established in 1997. Although this area of practice has existed for more than 30 years, new technology and types of criminal activity, such as terrorism and active shooters, make the forensic nurse role continue to expand and evolve. With the formation of the IAFN and the designation of the forensic specialty, nurses were given an identity and recognition for a role they have long been performing.

Forensic nurses specialize in several diverse roles and find employment in a variety of settings, such as the following:

• SANE (Sexual Assault Nurse Examiner)
• Medical examiner's office
• Medical legal nurse consultant
• ED nursing
• Medicolegal death investigator
• Evidence collection trainer
• Expert medical witness
• Law enforcement teams
• Forensic nurse death investigator
• Forensic psychiatric nurse
• Forensic correctional nurse[2]

Sexual Assault Nurse Examiner

A SANE is an RN trained in the forensic examination of sexual assault victims. This person has an advanced education and clinical preparation to specialize in this area.

Patients who have been sexually assaulted have unique medical, legal, and psychological needs. As crime victims, they require a competent collection of evidence that assists in both investigation and prosecution of the incident. The victim's body and clothing become a key part of the crime scene and are essential for collection of evidence. The SANE offers the type of compassionate care that is often lacking among law enforcement personnel. The care provided by SANEs is designed to preserve the victim's dignity and reduce psychological trauma. Research data collected in recent years indicate that the SANE's comprehensive forensic evidence collection leads to more effective investigations and more successful prosecutions.[2]

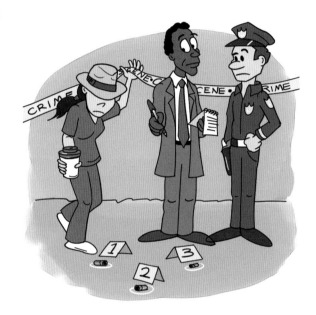

Forensic nurses' care can begin at the crime scene.

Usually, SANEs work in a hospital or ED with other members of a sexual assault response team (SART). The other team members may include health-care providers, law enforcement personnel, social workers, child and adult protective service workers, and therapists.

In their training, SANEs learn all aspects of the care of sexually assaulted patients. Their responsibilities include interviewing the victim, completing the physical examination, collecting specimens for forensic evidence, and documenting the findings. They also provide emotional support for victims and family members. When the case goes to court, the SANE testifies as an expert legal witness about how evidence was collected and the physical and psychological condition of the patient. The SANE may offer an opinion as to whether a crime occurred.

To become a SANE, an RN must complete an adult/adolescent SANE education program. These programs are available either through a traditional university setting or online. The training includes a minimum of 40 contact hours of instruction or three semester units of classroom instruction by an accredited school of nursing. Trainees also must have clinical supervision until they demonstrate competency in SANE practice. After successful completion of the program, the candidate is able to take the certification examination.[3]

Legal Nurse Consultant

The legal nurse consultant is a licensed RN who has a minimum of 5 years' experience as a practicing nurse and who passes the Legal Nurse Certification examination. This role includes critically evaluating and analyzing health-care issues in medically related lawsuits; being a liaison between health-care providers, attorneys, and patients; and being bold and confident in sharing decisions and opinions. Because the legal system is involved, nurses acting as consultants are considered to be practicing forensics. Whether they are self-employed or employees of a law firm, legal nurse consultants uniquely combine their medical expertise with legal knowledge to assess compliance with accepted standards of health-care practice.

Legal nurse consultants work in collaboration with attorneys and other legal and health-care professionals. They may have independent practices, work in the hospital setting in risk management, or be employed by law firms or health insurance companies.

The following activities performed by legal nurse consultants distinguish their specialty practice:

1. Drafting legal documents under the supervision of an attorney
2. Interviewing witnesses
3. Educating attorneys and other involved parties on health-care issues and standards
4. Researching nursing literature, standards, and guidelines as they relate to issues within a particular case

5. Reviewing, analyzing, and summarizing medical records
6. Identifying and conferring with expert witnesses
7. Assessing causation and issues of damages as they relate to the case
8. Developing a case strategy in collaboration with other members of the legal team
9. Providing support during the legal proceedings
10. Educating and mentoring other RNs in the practice of legal nurse consulting[4]

Forensic Nurse Death Investigator

The role of the forensic nurse death investigator (FNDI) is to advocate for the deceased. In general, a death investigator is a professional with experiential and scientific knowledge who can accurately determine the cause of death. The FNDI is an RN with specialized education who is functioning in the death investigator's role. FDNIs are called upon when law enforcement suspects a death resulted from natural causes, such as a heart attack at home. Because uniformed officers are usually the first to respond to these types of calls, they often also are the only representatives of the legal establishment present when the FNDI arrives and pronounces the victim dead. The victims are then typically removed by funeral home personnel, and no additional investigation is required. FNDIs may also be called for deaths that are suspicious and not clearly from natural causes. In these cases, many more representatives from the law enforcement community are present, including detectives, forensic evidence technicians, and even MD **coroners**. In these situations, the FNDI takes on the role of assisting where required.

> *FNDIs may also be called for deaths that are suspicious and not clearly from natural causes.*

The FNDI's role has several different titles, such as forensic nurse investigator, death investigator, and deputy coroner. In some areas of the country, nurses actually practice as coroners. In the United States, there are currently no standard definitions of *nurse death investigator* or any national credentialing or education requirements. Each region of the country specifies the requirements in its own jurisdiction.

A complete death investigation must have three key elements: (1) history of the victim, including psychological, medical, and social history; (2) a detailed and thorough examination of the victim's body; and (3) a search for evidence in the immediate and extended death area.[5] Nurses who have been trained and certified in forensic investigation and crime techniques are ideal for these types of investigations. To qualify for forensic training, the nurse should have 2 to 5 years of work experience in a critical care setting such as an ED or critical care unit, a high level of critical-thinking ability, and well-developed assessment skills. The nurse must also be able to cope with often violent and gruesome crime scenes.

The basic knowledge and skills in which all nurses are educated, such as physical assessment, pharmacology, anatomy, physiology, growth, and development, are minimum requirements for the death investigator role. This nursing knowledge allows the investigator to sort out factors involved in a death. Nurses also learn advanced communication skills and knowledge of the grief process during their education. These skills are required for notifying the victim's survivors and interviewing witnesses.[5] (For a more complete list of skill requirements for nurse death examiners, see Box 27.1.)

Box 27.1 Required Skills for a Forensic Nurse Death Investigator

The ability to

- Collaborate with other disciplines and agencies
- Use basic nursing knowledge such as anatomy, physiology, pharmacology, and communication techniques during investigations
- Formulate insightful questions using an evidence-based practice knowledge base
- Help families and survivors work through the grieving process
- Know and follow state codes about obtaining evidence and submitting death reports
- Conduct postmortem sexual assault and abuse examinations
- Work with organ and tissue procurement agencies to identify appropriate donors
- Act as a liaison between medical personnel and police investigative staff

FNDIs can use their skills in a variety of ways and at a number of locations. Work settings range from a coroner's or **medical examiner's** laboratory to accident sites or sites where a suspicious death has occurred to police precincts with homicide detectives. FNDIs have many responsibilities. They respond to scenes of death or accidents and work in collaboration with law enforcement. At the scene, they examine the body, pronounce death, and take tissue and blood samples. They take pictures of the body and evidence at the scene. FNDIs must be able to recognize and integrate other evidence collected during the investigation, such as patterns of injury, types of wounds, and estimated time of death. They are responsible for record-keeping and arranging for the transport of the body to the morgue or to the coroner's office to undergo **autopsy** for further examination. FNDIs work with the forensic pathologist to collect additional evidence in the laboratory during the autopsy. There still remain a number of states that require physicians or coroners to pronounce a person dead.

What Do You Think?

Have you ever been involved in a court case or lawsuit? What was your role? How would being a nurse trained in legal issues have changed what you did or said?

Forensic Psychiatric Nurse

Forensic psychiatric nurses work with individuals who have mental health needs and who have entered the legal system. These nurses generally practice in state psychiatric institutions, jails, and prisons.[6]

Nurses in this role perform physical and psychiatric assessments and develop care plans for the patients entrusted to their care. At the most basic level, forensic psychiatric nurses assist patients with self-care, administer medical care and treatment, and monitor the effectiveness of the treatment. Psychiatric interventions are developed to promote coping skills and improve mental health in a therapeutic environment.[6]

Forensic psychiatric nurses may also have advanced practice certification. RNs who have master's degrees in psychiatric–mental health nursing practice work as clinical nurse specialists or nurse practitioners (NPs). Nurses in this role are able to diagnose and treat individuals with psychiatric disorders and often are

Issues in Practice

If You Were the Nurse on Duty, What Would You Do?

The following scenarios exemplify typical situations for the nurse in general practice. Identify your probable response. Critically analyze each situation in terms of what you know and do not know. What types of facts or skills are not part of your current knowledge base?

You are working on a maternity unit when an inmate from a correctional institution is admitted in an advanced stage of labor. A correctional officer is in attendance; the woman is shackled at the feet and hands. As she is wheeled to the labor room, you note that the patient has had 10 previous pregnancies and four live births.

Questions for Thought

1. What factors make the care of this woman different from that of other pregnant women?
2. Is she dangerous?
3. How do you maintain confidentiality with this patient?
4. As an offender in custody, does she surrender any rights?

You work in a hospital setting that is experiencing an increase in workplace violence. Perpetrators of street, child, and domestic violence often follow their victims to the hospital and continue to pose a significant threat to the whole hospital community. It is important to assess the potential for violence.

Questions for Thought

1. How will you contribute to the reduction of risk in the workplace?
2. Identify risk factors and cues for violence.
3. How would you implement strategies to assist violence management in the acute care setting?

A halfway house for paroled offenders is due to be constructed in your community. Residents are angry and afraid to have ex-convicts living in their neighborhood. A town meeting is scheduled in which the issue will be discussed. Does nursing have anything to contribute to the discussion?

Questions for Thought

1. What do we know about mentally ill offenders, sex offenders, perpetrators of domestic violence, and others?
2. What is the therapeutic outcome for those mentally ill offenders who have completed rehabilitation programs?
3. What is the risk to the community?
4. What stress management strategies are helpful to a community?

You work at a junior high school, providing sex education and health promotion programs for young teenagers. You notice that increasing numbers of young people are wearing gang colors and using gang-related language and hand signals.

Questions for Thought

1. How does this situation affect your work?
2. Does it change your priorities?
3. Are there referrals or strategies that should be initiated because of the gang affiliations of your students?

allowed to prescribe medications. They may function as primary care medical and mental health providers, psychotherapists, and consultants. Advanced practice forensic psychiatric nurses may practice independently or in mental health centers, state facilities, and health maintenance organizations (HMOs).

Forensic Correctional Nurse

Correctional facilities reflect the demographics of the general population, with an increasingly aging incarcerated population who have age-related health problems. Forensic **correctional nurses** provide health care for inmates in correctional facilities such as juvenile centers, jails, and prisons. They manage acute and chronic illness, develop health-care plans, dispense medications, and perform health screenings and health education. Forensic correctional nurses conduct psychiatric assessments and respond to emergency situations. The role of the forensic correctional nurse offers a high level of autonomy compared with other nursing roles.

Evolving Requirements

Nurses can obtain certification as a forensic nurse specialist or SANE. Many nurses working in forensic roles believe certification requirements will develop as the specialty of forensic nursing continues to evolve and becomes better defined. Nursing education is beginning to develop classes that teach forensic nursing as a part of their curriculum.

NURSE ENTREPRENEUR

An entrepreneur is someone who establishes and runs their own business. A nurse entrepreneur starts a business by combining nursing experience and knowledge with business knowledge.[7]

Should You Be Your Own Boss?

Starting a business can be risky financially and certainly is far different from the nurse's traditional role as an employee in an institution. However, nurses are educated to think independently and are sometimes willing to take risks for the benefit of their patients. As professionals who can translate their expertise and confidence into new arenas, nurses are capable of achieving personal and financial success running their own businesses.[6]

Historically, nurse-run businesses have included temporary staffing agencies, nurse managers, nurse educators, FNDIs, nurse midwives, nurse paralegals, psychiatric nurses, legal nurse consultants, SANEs, and nurse consultants in education and leadership. NPs in some rural areas set up their own primary care clinics and provide care for populations that do not have access to any other type of primary care. However, not all states give NPs full practice authority to fulfill these roles independently; some states require collaborative agreements between NPs and physicians.

> *Key qualities needed for success are a high degree of self-motivation and a passion for the business to succeed. Nurse entrepreneurs are limited only by their creativity and desire to succeed.*

Here are the top 10 nurse entrepreneur ideas:

1. Start an in-home senior care service
2. Become a nutritionist
3. Start a private nurse service
4. Start a health-care training business
5. Become a hospice caregiver
6. Become a freelance writer
7. Build a medical app
8. Start a doula service
9. Create an online course
10. Start a fertility business[7]

Assess Your Nursing Skills

In making the decision to start a business, nurses need to first assess their nursing experience to determine what type of business would be appropriate for their skill set and knowledge levels. For example, a SANE may contract services to EDs or law enforcement agencies. A critical care nurse may start a home care agency offering high-tech services. Nurses may develop self-defense courses they can market to high-risk professions, such as forensic psychiatric and forensic correctional nurses.

After nurses determine what skills and knowledge they possess, they need to develop a plan on how to establish the business. A basic knowledge about finances and the business start-up process is essential for success. The hopeful entrepreneur needs to consider the customers who will be seeking the services, what customers need and desire, what start-up costs will be, and who the competition may be. Answering these questions helps the nurse to assess the potential risks and rewards of the business.[7]

Any nurse can start a business. Generally, no advanced degrees are required unless the business involves diagnosis and treatment. Key qualities needed for success are a high degree of self-motivation and a passion for the business to succeed. Nurse entrepreneurs are limited only by their creativity and desire to succeed.

CASE MANAGEMENT

Other titles for this position are care coordinator, care manager, transitional care coordinator, transitional care nurse, nurse care coordinator, wellness nurse, and patient care coordinator. The Case Management Society of America (CMSA) defines case management as "a collaborative process of assessment, planning, facilitation and advocacy for options and services to meet an individual's health needs through communication and available resources to promote quality, cost-effective outcomes."[8] Effective collaboration among all members of the health-care team is essential to meet the needs of patients in today's complex health-care system.

Case Managers in a Pandemic

COVID-19 had an extraordinary impact on nurse case managers' professional and personal lives. They were dealing with a pandemic that not only could infect patients but also could infect and debilitate the very system tasked with halting the outbreak. In addition to physicians and nurses being on the front lines

> *The goal of the nurse case manager is to help the patient obtain high-quality, cost-effective care while preventing the duplication and fragmentation of care.*

of the pandemic, case managers also had to face incredible risks and make difficult choices every day without a triage system in place.[9]

Although many case managers worked from home during the acute stage of the pandemic, they faced an increased caseload of patients, greater complexity of systems, and increased responsibilities. With the advent of social distancing, case managers could no longer walk down the hall to confer with a physician or nurse about a patient's needs or condition. Attempting to coordinate people and services without the benefit of human connections amplifies the loss of work–life balance. For example, a case manager was unable to arrange critical follow-up appointments for cancer patients because oncology offices were closed. A 2-year-old unstable asthma patient was suddenly discharged to home without discharge instructions or medications because his pulmonologist was needed in the ICU to monitor patients connected to ventilators. Other patients were discharged from the hospital after being tested for the COVID-19 virus and were instructed to self-quarantine but then were unable to get their test results.[9]

Finding placement for critically ill patients was a major challenge, and many patients became stranded in EDs or tents outside the hospital. A primary role for case managers was to improve those conditions from a remote location with little support and in the middle of a system plagued by glitches and breakdowns.

Case managers battled this disaster from behind the scenes by planning for patients' care for the next six months. Their work world revolved around making frantic phone calls at all times of the day and night, staying focused on the needs of patients, and making decisions about when people need the approval for surgery or where the patient was going next.[9] They worked hard to ensure the best outcome for patients and families.

A Care Coordinator

In the era of health-care reform, nurse case managers are serving a larger role than previously experienced. The ACA includes the Hospital Consumer Assessment of Healthcare Providers and Systems (HCAHPS) survey among the methods used to calculate value-based incentive payments. The HCAHPS survey asks discharged patients 27 questions that help evaluate their stay in the facility. It is administered randomly between 48 hours and 6 weeks after discharge. Hospitals must submit the results of the HCAHPS survey to receive their full inpatient prospective payment system (IPPS) annual increases in funding. This evaluation system has broad implications for case managers in controlling the resources used in patient diagnosis and treatment. Case managers play a key role in ensuring that preadmission tests and results are communicated throughout the health-care system so that tests are not unnecessarily repeated.[8]

Nurse case managers act as advocates for patients and their families by coordinating care and linking the patient with the health-care provider, other members of the health-care team, resources, and the payer. The goal of the nurse case manager is to help the patient obtain high-quality, cost-effective care while preventing the duplication and fragmentation of care. One of the important goals of the ACA was to reduce the rate of readmissions occurring within 30 days of discharge. Early readmissions currently cost Medicare in excess of $26 billion per year. The nurse care coordinator is in the perfect position to help reduce readmissions by coordinating the quality of care and support between the hospital and outpatient post-care entities. Hospitals with relatively high rates of readmissions receive a reduction in Medicare payments. Research data indicate that active participation by a nurse case manager in the care of a patient positively affects the patient's outcomes.[9]

What Do You Think?

Do you know any nurses with the title "case manager"? Interview them and note what duties they perform as part of their roles.

Nurses are uniquely prepared by their education and professional experiences to fulfill the role of case manager. The holistic health-care approach has been an underlying principle of nursing care since the time of Florence Nightingale. Nurses have experience in arranging referrals, providing patient education, and acting as a liaison between health-care providers and specialty care.

Any patient who may face challenges regarding care and recovery can benefit from case management. Included are hospitalized patients, those with complex medical conditions, those requiring specialty care, and those who have personal or psychological circumstances that may interfere with recovery. Factors that indicate the need for a nurse case manager include

1. A complex treatment plan that requires coordination or a plan that is unclear.
2. An injury or illness that may permanently prevent the patient from returning to their previous level of health.
3. A preexisting medical condition that may complicate or prolong recovery.
4. A need for assistance in accessing health-care resources.
5. Environmental stressors that may interfere with recovery.

A Guide for Health-Care Providers

The CMSA Standards of Practice for Case Management cite health-care provider and case manager collaboration as essential for successful case management.[8] Recent research shows that patients benefit from case management; however, some health-care providers are hesitant to use it. A consensus paper was developed between health-care providers and case managers to better integrate the use of case management into medical practice. This paper serves as the guiding document to identify both barriers and ways to promote effective, collaborative use of case management by health-care providers (Box 27.2).

The research that attributes improved patient outcomes directly to case management is compelling. It appears that nurse case managers will continue to expand their role in the health-care system of the future.

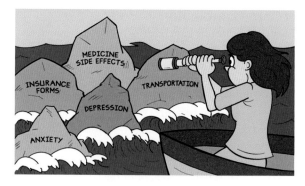

Nurse navigators look out for barriers to care.

NURSE NAVIGATOR/CARE NAVIGATOR

Although the nurse navigator (also called a *care navigator*) role is similar to that of the case manager, it tends to be more focused on only one specialty area, such as cancer patients. The role revolves around patients and families to help them deal with complex care issues. The nurse navigator attempts to eliminate barriers and serves as an advocate for the patient to make moving through the treatment maze easier. Some of the obstacles that patients face include lack of transportation; a myriad of confusing insurance forms; change in financial status; and lack of knowledge about the disease, its treatment options, and the side effects of powerful medications. The nurse navigator also works with the patient's family, caregivers, and employers to help reduce the patient's anxiety and/or depression.[10]

After receiving a referral from a health-care provider, the nurse navigator contacts the patient, and together they develop an individual plan of care that addresses the patient's particular needs. This referral can even be made before the patient undergoes surgery or first treatments. The nurse navigator takes into consideration the patient's perceptions and beliefs about the disease process and the modalities of treatment. It is important that the patient maintains a sense of empowerment while undergoing treatment. Regular contact is maintained with the patient throughout the treatment regime by personal contact, phone, or e-mail. The patient is reassured that the nurse navigator is available to answer any questions or concerns at any time.

Office appointments often can trigger anxiety and can be confusing for a patient. In such cases, the nurse navigator will accompany the patient to the office or clinic to reduce the patient's apprehension and help them understand the treatments or instructions the patient receives. The nurse navigator also may write up a summary of the interaction with the care provider so that the patient can better remember the instructions given and the date and time for the next appointment.[10] An interprofessional approach to care is used by involving other members of the health-care team, such as a social worker, financial counselor, dietitian, chaplain, and, if needed, a mental health professional. Subsequently, the patient is encouraged to participate in rehabilitation programs and other support services.

Some facilities focusing on women's health now have a full-time nurse navigator to serve as a patient advocate and liaison between women of all ages and their health-care providers. The nurse navigator guides women and their families through the health-care process by assisting with coordinating multiple appointments, explaining complicated health concerns, and providing education about various health topics. The nurse navigator can connect patients to support networks and community services. Some of the care women's nurse navigators can perform includes explaining in detail how a particular medication works, providing guidance in finding and making an appointment with a specialist, and answering personal health-care questions. Women's health nurse navigators offer personalized care depending on the patient's stage of life and unique circumstances.

Nurses who choose this role find it very rewarding. They observe patients go from the depths of treatment and illness to a new state of wellness. Average salaries for nurse navigators depend on the region, but they generally range between $74,000 and $113,985 annually.[11] Many facilities are seeking nurse navigators post-pandemic, and the job market is wide open, especially for nurses with several years of floor experience.[10]

NURSE CODER

Most of the time, nurses do not think much about the process that allows them to be paid. They get their money direct-deposited into their bank accounts periodically, and as long as it shows up, they do not ask questions. However, the process is much more complicated. The reimbursement systems used to pay facilities for individual patients from insurance companies and the government are dependent on a coding system for diseases and injuries. Each patient is assigned a code or several codes when they are treated. The 10th revision of the International Classification of Diseases (ICD-10) coding system has more than 72,748 codes; the previous revision had only 14,000. These codes are not static but are revised on a yearly basis. In 2022, for example, 159 new codes were added, 32 previous codes were removed, and 20 codes were revised.[12] These revisions in codes provide for more precise identification of illness and meet the demands of a changing health-care system. For 2022, a number of new codes were added for COVID-19- and cannabis-related conditions.[12]

The switch in coding systems was challenging for hospitals and other health-care providers to master,

but it opened the door for new nursing roles—certified RN-coders and certified RN-auditors. Because coding is now much more complicated, the knowledge and expertise of nurses will be a remarkable asset.[13]

The origins of the American Association of Clinical Coders and Auditors (AACCA) can be traced back to 2003 when a group of RNs who held master's and doctorate degrees, in conjunction with several physicians and a physician's assistant, met to discuss how to improve the quality of coding. Mistakes in coding were costing health-care facilities huge sums of money from third-party payers. The group came up with the idea of certifying individuals who were doing coding by providing a valid test of their coding knowledge and skills. The test would also determine if coders were in compliance with the coding rules and documentation, which would help to reduce fraud and abuse of the system. The group established a bank of questions and tested them for validity and reliability. Currently, the AACCA has more than 4,000 members and has tested/credentialed 3,682 members, 99 percent of whom are RNs. Certification testing is completed online, and results are provided immediately after test completion.[14]

There are training courses for coders online and in person. These courses vary in length from a few weeks of full-time classes to as much as 15 weeks taking classes one day a week.[13] The cost is rather high,

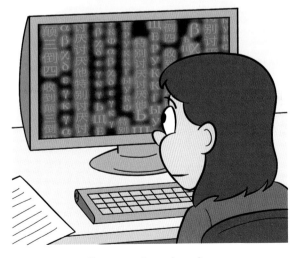

Nurse coders decode confusing health information.

ranging from around $1,000 on the low end to $4,000 on the high end. Most high-end courses include the cost of the certification examination, which is around $400 for members of the AACCA and $1,200 for nonmembers. Some colleges and universities offer a bachelor's degree in coding.[13]

Job responsibilities include the following:

• Confirm accurate diagnostic data following the international classification standards.
• Evaluate patient records to detect any missing or possibly inaccurate coding.
• Change coding on patient records to increase accuracy.
• Train physicians, staff, and secretaries on how to code accurately.
• Maintain currency in certification and knowledge of annual changes in coding.

Nurse coding positions analyzed by the U.S. Bureau of Labor Statistics (BLS) are predicted to have a faster-than-average job growth rate, about 9 percent per year, between 2025 and 2030. Job growth is due in part to an aging population and the transition to the ICD-10 program. Use of more advanced electronic technology also contributes to the growth in the market for professional coders. The BLS reported that nurse coders' annual wages were $74,180 per year.[14]

> *Insurance companies and law firms may also hire certified patient safety nurses to use their expertise in reducing costly lawsuits and injury settlements.*

PATIENT SAFETY OFFICER

Also known as a *patient safety nurse* or *patient safety specialist*, RNs in this position work to lower the risk factors that cause poor or adverse patient outcomes. Unlike traditional quality-assurance programs that focus primarily on satisfying The Joint Commission and the requirements of other regulatory bodies, patient safety officers plan and implement protocols and procedures to eliminate health-care errors. Under the auspices of the National Patient Safety Foundation (NPSF), these nurses provide a more comprehensive approach to safety, including reporting and analyzing adverse events, looking for trends, implementing risk-reduction activities, and developing medication error reduction strategies. They also monitor the effectiveness of the protocols and maintain systems that increase patient safety.[15]

One of the most difficult elements of the role is attempting to change the traditional health-care culture that attributes errors in patient care to carelessness and incompetence. The patient safety officer attempts to establish a new culture of safety in which both individual health-care providers and the organization as a whole see safety in all elements of care. The institution collectively must have an awareness of patient safety and make it a part of its mission. An important part of the patient safety officer's role is to educate other nurses on the causes of errors and how to eliminate them using evidence-based safety strategies. Although the position can be filled by a relatively new graduate RN, nurses with experience in risk management and quality assurance are frequently recruited for the role.

The IOM initial report in 2000 revealed an excess of 90,000 patient deaths per year caused by medical errors. Current estimates of deaths caused by medical errors are around 250,000 per year.[15] Although quality of care and patient safety are related, they are not the same thing. Patient safety is a subset of quality of care; however, without safety, there is no quality of care. The patient safety officer role evolved from the IOM's goals for high-quality care, including safe, effective, patient-centered, timely, efficient, and equitable care.

Traditionally, nursing students were taught the bare minimum about patient safety in their classes (see Chapter 14). Although this trend is beginning to wane, most nurses in practice today learned about safety and its application to health care while on the job. In many of the larger health-care facilities, nurse safety officers are required to have a master's or higher degree in nursing. They also need to take and pass the patient safety examination to become certified.[16]

In smaller facilities, the patient safety officer often fills one or more roles at the same time, such as infection control or nurse educator. In larger facilities, the patient safety officer position may be the only job the nurse has. In extremely large facilities, several patient safety officers may be assigned to individual units that tend to have high error rates with poor outcomes, such as the ED, intensive care unit, or obstetrical unit. Insurance companies and law firms may also hire certified patient safety nurses to use their expertise in reducing costly lawsuits and injury settlements.[16]

Most nurses in the safety officer role have a high degree of satisfaction with their position. They get to observe the decrease in errors and the overall increase in safety and quality of care. Because they are usually classified as administration, salaries for patient safety officers range from around $50,000 to more than $100,000 per year.[15]

TELEHEALTH NURSING

Have you ever seen a medical TV show or movie with a nurse answering an emergency phone call and providing information that helps deliver a baby or stop the bleeding from a gunshot wound? Telehealth nursing is similar to this but different because it incorporates the nursing process to provide care for individual patients over the phone or other electronic communication media. *Telehealth nursing, telehealth,* and *nursing telepractice* are all interchangeable terms. According to the American Telehealth Association, telehealth nursing is a tool for delivering nursing care remotely to improve efficiency and patient access to health care.

Some of the current places in which nurses practice telehealth include

- Physician offices
- Hospitals
- Trauma centers
- Crisis hotlines
- Outpatient care facilities
- Poison control centers

Patient care responsibilities for telehealth nurses include the following:

- Scheduling appointments and referring patients to specialists
- Assisting and consulting with patients over the phone or via video chat services
- Educating patients on different ways to manage their symptoms
- Monitoring patient's oxygen levels, health rate, respiration, and blood glucose
- Providing presurgical and postsurgical care
- Assisting doctors in reducing patient load

- Providing medical advice for patients with minor health issues
- Supporting medical response teams in bringing patients into the hospital
- Telephone triage
- Health information and education
- Disease management
- Interactive two-way video technology (i.e., home care)
- Robotic examinations

Telehealth nursing, or *telenursing,* is usually defined as the use of distant technology to provide nursing care and carry out nursing practice. The Health Resources and Services Administration defines *telehealth* as "the use of electronic information and telecommunications technologies to support long-distance clinical health care, patient and professional health-related education, public health and health administration."[17] The ANA has defined *telenursing* as a subset of telehealth in which the focus is on the specific profession's practice (i.e., nursing).[8]

Who can work as a telehealth nurse (TN)? The requirements vary somewhat from state to state. However, because the TN's role is to present health care at a provider level, TNs are usually advanced practice registered nurses (APRN) with at least 5 years of practice experience. Many are family nurse practitioners who are well prepared to work in the home-care setting where much of the telehealth care takes place, although other settings may require different skills, such as a certified nurse midwife for an obstetrical setting or a psychiatric nurse practitioner for a psychiatric setting. Because TNs provide nursing care to patients who are primarily in ambulatory care settings such as their homes, they should have the knowledge, skills, and competencies to provide care to these patients. For this reason, it is recommended that they obtain the Ambulatory Care Nursing Certification (RN-Board Certified) for their telehealth practice through the American Nurses Credentialing Center. At this time, there is not a specific certification for telehealth nursing.[17] The TN must have an active license in good standing at their practice level where they live and a license for each state in which they practice telenursing.

The recent APRN Compact, initiated by the National Council of State Boards of Nursing (NCSBN), allows an APRN in one compact state to hold a multistate license with privileges to practice in other compact states. This compact is also known as the Enhanced Nurse

Licensure Compact (eNLC). The goal of the multistate license plan is to make requirements more consistent and licenses more portable from state to state, allowing APRNs to practice at the highest level of their education and training. According to NCBSN officials, eNLC states have aligned their licensing standards so that applicants for a multistate license need to meet only one set of standards, which include federal and state fingerprint-based criminal background checks.

The COVID-19 pandemic brought unparalleled disruption to the normal functioning of the health-care system across the world. Telehealth played an essential role in balancing the care demands between social distancing and providing everyday care services to the public. Telehealth was used for triage and management of COVID-19 patients. Patients who may have had early symptoms of COVID-19 were initially contacted remotely via telephone or video to reduce the risks of virus spreading. Nurse practitioners made remote consultations, such as taking a history, performing remote physical examination, making decisions for management, and providing advice on whether to have further in-person assessment at a clinic or ED.[18]

During the peak of the pandemic, Congress passed a bill to allow critical telehealth flexibilities, including provisions to waive provider and patient location limitations, remove in-person requirements for tele-mental health, ensure continued access to clinically appropriate controlled substances without in-person requirements, and increase access to telehealth services in the commercial market, including for those with a high-deductible health plan coupled with a health savings account. The bill also allowed adults ages 65 and older Medicare coverage for telehealth visits, including some audio-only visits, regardless of where the patient lived relative to the health-care provider rather than limiting the service to rural areas. Under the pandemic's telehealth flexibilities bill, all Medicare-enrolled providers could bill for telehealth services. Also, Medicare covered telehealth visits that took place from the patient's home as well as from medical facilities. The flexibilities provisions applied only to Medicare reimbursement for telehealth, but private insurers are likely to follow suit.[19]

During the lockdown, virtual teaching and learning gained popularity and became the only way for nursing schools to keep courses running. Virtual teaching involved both theoretical content and skills presentations.[20] On April 6, 2021, the American Association of Colleges of Nursing (AACN) released an updated core competencies for nursing education. Technology competency is identified as one of the most critical abilities for nursing students to master. These competencies include distinguishing and describing various information communication technology (ICT) tools used in clinical care; using ICT tools to gather data, create information, and generate knowledge; using ICT tools to deliver safe care to diverse populations in a variety of settings; documenting care and communicating among providers, patients, and all system levels; and using ICT in accordance with ethical, legal, professional, and regular standards and workplace policies.[18]

Although the use of distant technology changes the way nursing care is delivered and requires additional technical skills, the skills of assessment, clinical judgment, and analysis by means of the nursing process remain the same. APRNs must still practice within their designated scope of practice. Nurses practicing through telenursing are required to assess, plan, intervene, and evaluate the outcomes of nursing care, but they do so using technologies such as the Internet, computers, telephones, digital assessment tools, and telemonitoring equipment. Teletechnology continues to expand the number and type of health-care services provided (see Chapter 17).

The delivery of telehealth care is not limited to health-care providers and nurses; it includes other health disciplines, such as radiology, pharmacy, and psychology. A wide range of services can be offered over telehealth systems, depending on the needs of patients and the resources that are available. One of the newer technologies, infrared scanning and sensor devices, has markedly increased the remote monitoring capabilities of nurses. Falls, traumatic injuries, or sudden illness are easier to detect using these systems that offer almost immediate care to patients. However, the continuous monitoring nature of these devices may prove to be an infringement of patients' rights to privacy and therefore an ethical issue for health-care providers to consider.

As with all electronic technology, confidentiality in telehealth remains one of the top concerns.

Issues Now

The Green Wave: A New Role for Nurses

As of 2022, the U.S. Food and Drug Administration (FDA) had approved 12 cannabinoid-based medicines:

Ado-trastuzumab emtansine (Kadcyla)

Brentuximab vedotin (Adcetris)

Inotuzumab ozogamicin (Besponsa)

Gemtuzumab ozogamicin (Mylotarg)

Moxetumomab pasudotox-tdfk (Lumoxiti)

Polatuzumab vedotin-piiq (Polivy)

Enfortumab vedotin-ejfv (Padcev)

Sacituzumab govitecan-hziy (Trodelvy)

Trastuzumab deruxtecan-nxki (Enhertu)

Belantamab mafodotin-blmf (Blenrep)

Loncastuximab tesirine-lpyl (Zynlonta)

Tisotumab vedotin-tftv (Tivdak)

Support for medical marijuana, also called the Green Wave, continues to push its way across the country. By the end of 2022, 37 states plus Washington, DC, Guam, and Puerto Rico had approved the use of medical marijuana. Several other states are considering legalizing medical marijuana or have laws pending in their legislatures. These states have chosen to ignore and not enforce the federal law that still considers any use of marijuana illegal.* Unlikely as it may seem, marijuana is now creating a new category of medications with a wide range of uses.

Although the laws vary widely from state to state, the approval of cannabis for medical use has opened the door for a whole new role in nursing: the cannabis nurse. The American Cannabis Nurses Association (ACNA) defines cannabis nursing as care that incorporates the knowledge of

- The endocannabinoid system, which includes the group of cannabinoid receptors located in the brain and throughout the central and peripheral nervous systems.
- The safe use of herbal cannabis products.
- The legal complexities associated with the use of herbal cannabis products.**

The cannabis nurse's role also requires a wide range of knowledge of all medications and their interactions with cannabis substances. There is no standardization of most cannabis products, so close monitoring of the effects is essential. Also, because the routes to administer cannabis include inhaling, vaporizing, smoking, eating infused gummies or brownies, massaging with creams or balms, absorbing transdermally by a patch, and even dissolving sublingual strips, the cannabis nurse must select the method that is most appropriate for each patient. Educating patients about possible side effects and drug interactions and helping patients titrate doses and evaluate which strains are most effective are keys to being a successful cannabis nurse.

(continued)

Issues Now (continued)

As of 2022, there were neither specific education requirements for a cannabis nurse nor any certification available. However, it is obvious that cannabis nursing requires a nurse who is educated in multiple disciplines, such as pharmacology and counseling, that go above and beyond basic RN education. Nurses can earn a certificate that shows completion of cannabis education courses. Earning this certificate demonstrates professionalism, continued education, and a goal to meet industry standards.

The ACNA is in the process of developing the first Scope of Practice and Standards for Cannabis Nurses, and an APRN certification will likely be the minimum requirement. According to nurses who already practice in this role, those considering it as a career should have thick skins. Because there is still a stigma attached to the drug, some medical personnel and many laypeople think that the role involves getting patients high.*

In reality, the active ingredient that causes a "high" has been removed in approved cannabis medications, and only the substances that directly affect the pain centers are left. Cannabis nurses help treat a wide range of patients, including those with cancer, opioid addiction, nausea, anxiety disorders, insomnia, cachexia, depression, and chronic pain. As medical cannabis continues to be more accepted across the country, the need for nurses educated in the use of these substances will continue to increase. Wherever there are people with cancer, chronic pain, seizure disorders, and other illnesses, nurses educated and skilled at medical cannabis administration can bring hope and quality to their patients' lives.

Sources: *K. Hayes, Marijuana laws by state in 2022, Fox9, September 12, 2022, https://www.fox9.com/news/marijuana-laws-by-us-state-2022.

**J.Y. Jean, What is cannabis nursing? NurseJournal, 2022. https://nursejournal.org/articles/what-is-cannabis-nursing.

With recent events such as electronic interference in the 2016 U.S. election and loss of vast amounts of customer data by various companies, the security of telehealth becomes paramount. Telehealth sessions should retain the confidentiality of an office visit between a provider and a patient. Enclosed rooms without traffic or others present on both ends of the telehealth session are imperative to maintain privacy. Health-care providers need to be conscious of who is in attendance for the session and respect privacy and confidentiality of the patient. Patient information should be transmitted over secure lines. New wireless technologies, increased use of e-mail by providers for gathering information, and the continual threat of hackers and computer viruses increase the need for security and confidentiality of patient data.[17]

In addition to confidentiality, other issues need to be settled as well. The APRN's scope of practice varies quite a bit from one state's nurse practice act to another. Should the eAPRN know what each state's scope of practice includes? Some states still do not allow full independence of practice for APRNs. If a

TN is providing care for a patient in one of those states, do they need a supervising physician? Also, if errors that harm a patient are committed by an eAPRN, who should discipline the provider: the state board where the eAPRN lives and practices or the state where the error occurred and the patient lives? What about providing telenursing to a patient on a cruise ship in the open ocean or in a foreign country? What practice guidelines should be followed?

The critical telehealth flexibilities just discussed were due to expire in April 2023; however, more than 370 organizations sent a joint letter to bipartisan leaders of the U.S. Senate to pass a two-year extension of important telehealth policies enacted at the start of the COVID-19 pandemic. The bill has already passed the House but is being held up in the Senate.[20]

The average salary for a telehealth nurse with a BSN ranges between $74,017 and $85,095. Salaries for advanced practice telehealth nurses are in the $100,000+ range, depending on years of practice and certification.[18] Since the end of the pandemic, there has been great demand for telehealth nurses.[19]

Conclusion

Florence Nightingale wrote in 1859 that "no man, not even a doctor, ever gives any other definition of what a nurse should be than this—'devoted and obedient.' This definition would do just as well for a porter. It might even do for a horse!"[21] The profession of nursing has come a long way since Nightingale made the first efforts to move nursing out of its position of servitude to physicians.

Nursing is constantly evolving and defining itself as it strives to include expanded roles of practice. Many new and exciting roles for nurses—forensic, legal consultant, entrepreneur, case management, nurse navigator, nurse coder, and nurse safety officer—have developed in response to the needs of society.

Although nurses have practiced in these areas for many years, they are only now beginning to be recognized for the unique skills and qualities they bring to these roles. For example, the job description of an ED nurse has long included interviews with and assessments of crime victims, collection and proper handling of evidence, and accurate and complete documentation of injuries and information provided by crime victims. In the role of patient advocate, nurses have always been case managers through assessment of patient needs, coordination of referrals for specialized or long-term care, and coordination of non-nursing services such as diet teaching and social services.

All nurses have the knowledge of anatomy, physiology, growth, and development that is required for the death examiner position. As more nurses seek the specialized training now available for many of these roles and obtain nationally recognized certification as a demonstration of their knowledge, they will gain acceptance as highly qualified and valuable members of these specialized health-care teams.

ASSOCIATIONS AND WEBSITES

American Academy of Forensic Sciences: https://www.aafs.org

American Association of Legal Nurse Consultants: https://www.aalnc.org

American College of Forensic Examiners Institute: https://www.omicsonline.org/universities/American_College_of_Forensic_Examiners_Institute/

American Forensic Nurses: www.amrn.com

American Psychiatric Nurses Association: https://www.apna.org

International Association of Forensic Nurses: https://www.iafn.org

Journal of Forensic Nursing: https://journals.lww.com/forensicnursing/pages/default.aspx

Legal Nurse Consultant: How to become one in 2023. Career Employer, 2023. https://careeremployer.com/nursing/rn/legal-nurse-consultant/

National Alliance of Sexual Assault Coalitions: https://www.endsexualviolence.org/who-we-are/about-naesv

National Commission on Correctional Health Care: https://www.ncchc.org

National Nurse Practitioner Entrepreneur Network (NNPEN): https://www.nnpen.org/

National Nurses in Business Association: https://nnbanow.com

Office for Victims of Crime: https://www.ovc.gov/news/index.html

Office for Victims of Crime Resource Center: http://www.ncjrs.org

Rape, Abuse, and Incest National Network (RAINN): https://www.rainn.org

Sexual Assault Resource Service (SARS): https://www.sane-sart.com

Violence Against Women Office: https://www.gallaudet.edu/title-ix/violence-against-women-act

CRITICAL-THINKING EXERCISES

SHERLOCK RN

For each of the following scenarios, answer these questions:

1. What additional information would help you make a decision about guilt or innocence?
2. What are the victim's legal rights?
3. What are the accused's legal rights?
4. What is the forensic nurse investigator's role in defining and protecting the rights of everyone involved?

- A married father of two, an upstanding member of the community with no previous allegations of wrongdoing, is accused of child molestation. The stress of the allegations causes a mental breakdown, and he is admitted to the unit for psychiatric evaluation. A judge orders him to submit samples for blood type and DNA analysis.

- An inmate becomes pregnant in prison. Although the primary suspect is a guard, the inmate does not want anyone to know who the father is. All the guards are required to submit saliva samples for DNA analysis.
- A young man with a history of substance abuse and severe bipolar disorder steals a car. He refuses to take the medication that controls his psychotic behavior and is confined in a forensic psychiatric facility. He claims that he is incompetent to stand trial for the car theft.
- A mother of an infant is being interviewed in a suspected child abuse case. She admits that she was sexually and physically abused as a child and throughout her marriage. The priority is to establish her role in the current charges involving injury of her 3-month-old infant.

NCLEX-STYLE QUESTIONS

1. Which of the following is true of nurse entrepreneurs?
   1. They are required to have advanced degrees or certification.
   2. They practice under the supervision of a physician.
   3. They need business skills in addition to nursing skills.
   4. There are very few options for nurses who want to be entrepreneurs.
2. Tobias, an RN in a busy medical-surgical unit, wants to change his work situation so that he can be at home with his infant daughter. Tobias is extremely detail oriented and has excellent computer skills. Which nursing role best suits Tobias's abilities and his desire to be at home with his daughter?
   1. Nurse navigator
   2. Nurse coder

   3. Patient safety officer
   4. Case manager
3. Mrs. Jones is a 78-year-old African American woman with diabetes whose kidney function has decreased significantly over the past year. After seeing the nephrologist, Mrs. Jones is scheduled for surgery to create an A-V fistula. She will begin dialysis 6 weeks later. Mrs. Jones lives with her daughter, who travels often for her job, and grandchildren, whom Mrs. Jones helps care for. Which factors in the scenario indicate the need for case management for Mrs. Jones? **Select all that apply.**
   1. She is 78 years old.
   2. She has diabetes.
   3. She is getting an A-V fistula.
   4. She is a caregiver for her grandchildren.
   5. She lives with her daughter.
   6. Her daughter travels for work.

4. Jenny is giving a presentation to her nursing class on the role of the sexual assault nurse examiner (SANE). Which of the following statements should her classmates question?
   1. "The SANE interviews victims of sexual assault."
   2. "An important task of the SANE is to complete a physical examination and collect specimens for forensic evidence."
   3. "The SANE provides ongoing counseling to survivors of sexual assault."
   4. "The SANE testifies in court about how evidence was collected and the physical and psychological condition of the victim."

5. What is the main difference between a nurse case manager and a nurse navigator?
   1. Case managers help patients with a variety of health issues; nurse navigators focus on one specialty area.
   2. A case manager advocates for patients, but a nurse navigator does not.
   3. A nurse navigator helps the patient obtain high-quality, cost-effective care; the case manager's focus is on reducing readmissions.
   4. Nurse case managers work for the facility; nurse navigators work for the patient.

6. In the United States, what trend in the incarcerated population mirrors the general population?
   1. The rates of HIV and tuberculosis are increasing.
   2. Obesity-related illnesses are increasing rapidly.
   3. Correctional nurses focus on wellness rather than illness.
   4. The population is aging and requires care for age-related health-care problems.

7. A _____ works to lower the risk factors that cause poor or adverse patient outcomes by eliminating health-care errors.

8. Telehealth is a growing field in nursing. Which of the following is of special concern in telehealth?
   1. The qualification of nurses and other providers
   2. The confidentiality of patient information
   3. Nurses practicing outside their scope of practice
   4. The inability of technology to accommodate the nursing process

9. Technology allows telehealth nurses to remotely monitor patients for falls, sleep apnea, and a variety of other concerns. What principle of nursing ethics could potentially be violated by the use of these technologies?
   1. Autonomy
   2. Beneficence
   3. Justice
   4. Fidelity

10. Ernesto Vazquez, RN, was an ICU nurse for several years and is now a legal nurse consultant. In which of the following facilities is he most likely to work?
    1. A cardiology group practice
    2. A law firm
    3. An outpatient clinic
    4. A small rural hospital

References

1. What is a forensic nurse? *NurseJournal*, 2022. https://nursejournal.org/careers/forensic-nurse/
2. International Association of Forensic Nursing. TheForensicNurse.com, 2022. https://www.theforensicnurse.com/IAFN.cfm
3. Pass the SANE exam. TheForensicNurse.com, 2022. http://www.theforensicnurse.com/Pass_SANE_exam.cfm
4. What is a legal nurse consultant? Coursera, September 15, 2022. https://www.coursera.org/articles/what-is-a-legal-nurse-consultant
5. Schindell J. The forensic nurse as a death investigator. International Association of Forensic Nurses, n.d. https://www.forensicnurses.org/page/DeathInvest
6. Franjic S. Role of the nurse in forensic psychiatry. *Scientific Journal of Research and Reviews*, 1(1), 2018. http://dx.doi.org/%2010.33552/SJRR.2018.01.000504
7. Walls Pat. 38 Nurse entrepreneur ideas in 2022 [nursing business ideas]. Starter Story, September 9, 2022. https://www.starterstory.com/nurse-business-ideas
8. CMSA Standards of practice for case management. Case Management Society of America, 2022. https://cmsa.org/sop22/

9. Shelton W. Case managers on the frontline of COVID-19. LinkedIn, March 31, 2020. https://www.linkedin.com/pulse/case-managers-other-frontline-covid-19-wil-shelton

10. What is a nurse navigator and what do they do (with skills)? Indeed, 2021. https://www.indeed.com/career-advice/finding-a-job/what-is-nurse-navigator#:~

11. Care navigator salaries in the United States. Indeed, 2022. https://www.indeed.com/career/care-navigator/salaries

12. 2022 New ICD-10 codes changes: What you need to know to get paid. DocCharge, February 13, 2022. https://doccharge.com/blog/2022-new-icd-10-codes-changes-what-you-need-to-know-to-get-paid/

13. Feeney A. RN coder. *Nurse Journal*, November 18, 2022. https://nursejournal.org/registered-nursing/rn-coder

14. American Association of Certified Medical Coders and Auditors [home page]. AACMCA, 2022. https://aacmca.org/

15. Knapp C. How many deaths are cause by medical errors? Knapp & Roberts, December 14, 2021. https://www.knappandroberts.com/how-many-deaths-are-caused-by-medical-errors/

16. VanGeest J, Cummins D. *An Educational Needs Assessment for Improving Patient Safety Results of a National Study of Physicians and Nurses*. Boston, MA: National Patient Safety Foundation, 2003. https://cdn.ymaws.com/www.npsf.org/resource/collection/ABAB3CA8-4E0A-41C5-A480-6DE8B793536C/Educational_Needs_Assessment.pdf

17. Telehealth: Healthcare from the safety of your own home. Telehealth.HHS.gov, 2022. https://telehealth.hhs.gov/

18. Wu Y. Utilization of telehealth and the advancement of nursing informatics during COVID-19 pandemic. *International Journal of Nursing Sciences*, 8(4):367–369, 2021. https://doi.org/10.1016%2Fj.ijnss.2021.09.004

19. Gaines K. Career guide series: Telehealth nurse. Nurse.org, September 16, 2022. https://nurse.org/resources/telehealth-nurse/

20. Landi H. Amazon, Walmart and hundreds of providers lobby the Senate for the extension of telehealth policies. Fierce Healthcare, September 14, 2022. https://www.fiercehealthcare.com/health-tech/amazon-walmart-and-hundreds-providers-lobby-senate-extension-telehealth-policies

21. Nightingale F. *Notes on Nursing*. Oxford, UK: Dover, 1860.

Next Generation NCLEX®: What You Need to Know

28

Joseph T. Catalano

Learning Objectives

After completing this chapter, the reader will be able to:

- Describe the NGN-RN test plan
- Discuss the NGN-RN test format
- Analyze and identify the different types of questions used on the NGN-RN
- Select the most appropriate means for preparing for the NGN-RN

I DON'T WANT TO TAKE THIS EXAM!

The primary purpose of licensure examinations is to protect the public from unsafe or uneducated practitioners of a profession. When you pass the National Council Licensure Examination (NCLEX), now called the Next Generation NCLEX (NGN) or Next Gen NCLEX,[1] it indicates that you have the minimal level of knowledge or competency deemed necessary by the state to practice nursing without injury to clients. Licensure is a legal requirement for all professions that deal with public health, welfare, or safety.

Most people have varying levels of anxiety before taking an examination. The more important the examination, the higher the anxiety level. Anxiety is sometimes defined as fear of the unknown. This chapter presents key information about the NGN test plan to help you better understand and anticipate what you will encounter when you take the examination. The more familiar you become with the design of the test, how it is scored, and how the questions are asked, the better chance you have of answering correctly.

The chapter also includes some suggestions for studying for the NGN and *dos* and *don't*s for the examination. This information should help lower your anxiety about the NGN. Sample practice questions throughout the chapter give you an idea of how the NGN asks about different types of nursing information. This chapter should be used in conjunction with Bonus Chapter 29 on the Fadavis.com site. Try to answer these questions as you read. The answers and rationales are found at the end of the chapter.

NGN TEST PLAN

You will take the NGN on a personal computer at a Pearson Professional Center. The NGN is a computerized, **criterion-referenced examination** that you take after you graduate from nursing school. Unlike a **norm-referenced examination**, which bases a passing score on the scores of others who took the examination, criterion-referenced examinations compare your knowledge to a preestablished standard. If you meet or exceed the standard, you pass. The NGN measures nursing knowledge of a wide range of subject matter, but it primarily measures your ability to think critically and make sound judgments about nursing care. With computerized adaptive tests such as the NGN, the computer selects questions in accordance with the test plan and how you answered previous questions. After you answer a question and move to the next question, you cannot go back to a previous question.

How Changes in the Test Plan Are Made

Every 3 years, the National Council of State Boards of Nursing (NCSBN) undertakes an analysis of current nursing practice, with the most recent changes beginning April 1, 2023. An expert panel of nine nurses conducts a survey that asks approximately 12,000 newly licensed nurses about the frequency and importance of performing the 15 NGN test-plan nursing care activities.[2] These activities are then analyzed in relation to the frequency of performance, impact on maintaining client safety, and client care settings where the activities are performed.

THINGS THAT ARE STAYING THE SAME

Questions Distributed by Category

Although there was little information at the time of publication about the distribution of questions by category for the NGN, it appears that the distribution of questions will be similar to what was presented on the examination in 2022.[3] Questions dealing with management and management issues comprise 17 to 23 percent of the examination, the highest percentage of any single type of question. Pharmacology-related questions will remain around 12 to 18 percent of the examination.

The NGN for Registered Nurses (NGN-RN) test plan is organized into three primary components: (1) client needs, (2) level of cognitive ability, and (3) integrated concepts and processes. The third component includes nursing process, caring, communication, cultural awareness, documentation, self-care, and teaching and learning. A number of new format questions (see later in chapter) are now being used; however, the time to complete the test remains at 5 hours.[4]

Client Health Needs

The NGN asks questions about four general groups of material called *client health needs*:

- Safe and effective care environment
- Physiological integrity
- Psychosocial integrity
- Health promotion and maintenance needs

Safe and Effective Care Environment (25 to 38 percent)

A. Management of care: 17 to 23 percent of NGN questions
B. Safety and infection control: 9 to 15 percent of NGN questions

The questions in this category make up between 25 and 38 percent of the total questions on the NGN. These questions deal with overt safety issues in client care (e.g., use of restraints), medication administration, safety measures to prevent injuries (e.g., putting up side rails), prevention of infections, isolation precautions, safety measures with pediatric clients, and special safety needs of clients with psychiatric problems.

This needs category also includes questions about laboratory tests, their results, and any special nursing measures associated with them; legal and ethical issues in nursing; a small amount of nursing management; and quality assurance issues. Questions on these issues are interspersed with other questions throughout the examination.

Physiological Integrity (38 to 62 percent)

A. Basic care and comfort: 6 to 12 percent of NGN questions
B. Pharmacological and parenteral therapies: 12 to 18 percent of NGN questions
C. Reduction of risk potential: 9 to 15 percent of NGN questions
D. Physiological adaptation: 11 to 17 percent of NGN questions

The physiological integrity needs are concerned with adult medical and surgical nursing care, pediatrics, and **gerontology**. This category comprises the largest groups of questions, with about 38 to 62 percent of the total number of questions on the NGN. The more common health-care problems, both acute and chronic conditions, that nurses deal with on a daily basis include the following:

- Diabetes
- Cardiovascular disorders
- Neurological disorders
- Renal diseases
- Respiratory diseases
- Traumatic injuries
- Immunological disorders
- Skin and infective diseases

This component also asks questions about nursing care of the pediatric client, such as these topics:

- Growth and development
- Congenital abnormalities
- Child abuse
- Burn injury
- Fractures and cast and traction care
- Common infective diseases in children
- Common childhood trauma such as eye injuries

Psychosocial Integrity (6 to 12 percent)

Psychosocial integrity needs are health-care issues that revolve around the client with psychiatric problems. This material also deals with coping mechanisms for high-stress situations, such as acute illness and life-threatening diseases or trauma. These clients do not necessarily have any psychiatric disorders. This category constitutes, at most, 12 percent of the examination and includes questions about the care of clients with eating disorders, personality disorders, anxiety disorders, depression, schizophrenia, and organic mental disease. Also included in the psychosocial needs section are questions about therapeutic communication, crisis intervention, and substance abuse.

Health Promotion and Maintenance (6 to 12 percent)

Health promotion and maintenance needs deal with birth control measures, pregnancy, labor and delivery, care of the newborn infant, growth and development, and contagious diseases, particularly sexually transmitted diseases. This section constitutes approximately 12 percent of the total examination. Teaching and counseling are important parts of the nurse's client care during pregnancy, and knowledge of diet, signs and symptoms of complications, fetal development, and testing used during pregnancy is necessary.

Also, there are questions about alternative therapies and how they interact with traditional treatments and medications.

Integrated Concepts and Processes

The integrated concepts and processes component includes the following:

- Nursing process
- Concepts of caring
- Therapeutic communication
- Cultural awareness
- Documentation
- Self-care
- Teaching and learning

These concepts are integrated throughout the examination and are included as elements in the four needs categories. You will also find that pharmacology questions tend to be integrated in other areas even though they are a separate category.

NGN FORMAT

The Clinical Judgment Measurement Model

Based on the data obtained from research over a number of years, the NCSBN came to the decision that new graduate nurses, who are responsible for a large percentage of medical errors, had difficulty using clinical judgement (CJ) in caring for patients (see Fig. 28.1). The NCSBN defines clinical judgment as "the observed outcome of critical thinking and decision-making."[6] It is similar to critical thinking in that it uses the nurse's nursing knowledge to observe and assess care situations, prioritize a patient's problem, and produce the best possible evidenced-based resolution to the problem using safe patient care. The model for CJ proposed by the NCSBN consists of what they refer to as "layers," which are like conceptual building blocks in which one layer leads to the next one based on the critical decision made by the nurse. The goal of using the layers is to build a cognitive construct that is measurable in a higher order thought process.[5]

The end result of the research and cognitive development by the NCSBN was the production that became known as the Clinical Judgment Measurement Model (CJMM). The model is designed to measure your capability to use sound clinical judgment and decision

The NCSBN Clinical Judgment Measurement Model

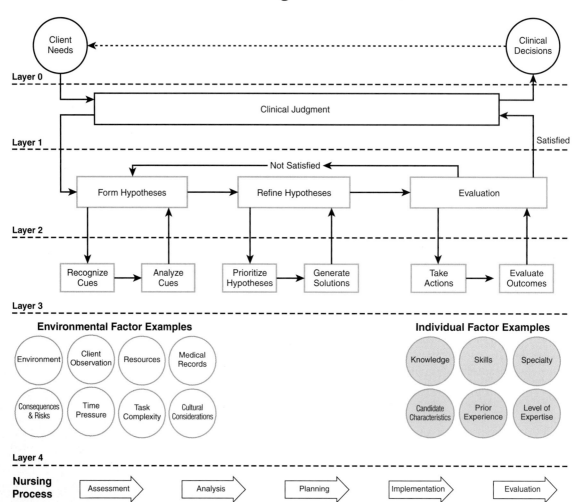

Figure 28.1 The NCSBN Clinical Judgment Measurement Model. The model provides a method for measuring and making valid decisions about how well new graduate nurses use their clinical judgment and decision-making skills. *Source:* Copyright 2019, NCSBN. All Rights Reserved.

making on the NGN and then later in your actual nursing practice. The test questions that use this model are more applicable to the real-world nursing practice seen in current health-care settings, particularly because of the increase in acuity of hospitalized patients. These questions are also more difficult than questions on past examinations.[3]

The CJMM was designed to be used with case studies or case scenario questions (see later in chapter) where your thought processes and actions

are built in layers as the six interrelated items or questions require you to use your best clinical judgment. Although the layers are numbered, they are not necessarily meant to be taken in order. Rather, they can be thought of as a circular construct wherein the layers denote a type of repetitive system of emerging answers built on each other. The layers do not stand alone but rather network with one another, moving you from the level of assessment to the level of CJ and finally to a solution to a clinical problem.[6]

The layers of the CJMM include:

Layer 0—Responding to Layer 2. Determining the patient's needs. What are their problems? Why are they seeking care?

Layer 1—Responding to Layer 0. Using clinical judgment. What is the response to the problem? What is the outcome for the patient? Can the outcome be evaluated?

Layer 2—Responding to Layer 1. Is the solution to the problem satisfactory? Then move on. Is the solution to the problem unsatisfactory, and does it fail to solve the problem? Go back to Layer 0 and repeat the cycle of layers until you produce the right outcome. Layer 2 interacts with Layer 3, which will break down the process into greater detail. In Layer 2, the nurse takes three steps: (1) form a hypothesis, (2) refine the hypothesis, and (3) evaluate the hypothesis. For each one of these steps, there are two steps in Layer 3 that make up each of the steps in Layer 2.

Layer 3—Responding to Layer 2. Contains six steps (two steps for each of the three in Layer 2) that work along with Layer 2 to use all available data, knowledge, and resources to solve a clinical problem.

Layer 4—Responding to Layers 2 and 3. Provides the context for the clinical judgment steps in Layers 2 and 3. Context items refer to information in the case scenario's presentation that may affect the outcome. These might include cultural elements, negative habits of the patient, or the nurse's knowledge and skill. External factors that might affect the outcome include available resources for care or family influence.[5]

The CJMM may seem very complicated, and that is because it is. But if you relate it to the nursing process, which is a similar type of problem-solving method that uses critical thinking, it may be easier to understand. Actually, the layers of the CJMM are designed to work with the nursing process, but the layers fill in detail and add specificity to the critical thinking that goes into it. Remember that the nursing process is a systematic way to plan and provide nursing care.[5] The steps of the nursing process are as follows:

- Assessment (Layers 0 & 1)—Observe objective and subjective signs and symptoms that are used to identify and define the patient's need or problems.

- Diagnosis (Layers 0 & 1)—Define the problem (nursing diagnosis).
- Planning (Layers 3 & 4)—Establish outcome goals that are used in the implementation of nursing interventions.
- Implementation (Layers 3 & 4)—Carry out the nursing interventions.
- Evaluation (Layers 2 & 4)—Did the interventions resolve the problem? If not, start over.[2]

Nursing Process

The nursing process has traditionally been a very important part of the NGN. The NGN uses the five-step nursing process: assessment, analysis, planning, intervention and implementation, and evaluation, which is integrated with the CJMM.[5] Each of the questions you will be asked on the NGN falls into one of the five nursing process categories.

It is important that you keep in mind the steps of the nursing process when answering questions. Often, questions that ask, "What should the nurse do first?" are looking for an assessment-type answer because that is the first step in the nursing process. Questions on the nursing process are no longer equally divided on the examination.

Assessment

The assessment phase primarily establishes the database on which the rest of the nursing process is built. Some components of the assessment phase include both subjective and objective data about the client, significant history, history of the present illness, signs and symptoms, environmental elements, laboratory values, and vital signs. Often, the examination will ask you to distinguish between appropriate and inappropriate assessment factors. An example of an assessment phase question follows:

1. What would be the most important information for the nurse to obtain when a client is admitted for evaluation of recurrent episodes of Stokes-Adams syndrome?
   1. Ability to perform aerobic exercises for 15 minutes
   2. Bradycardia and increases in blood pressure
   3. Changes in level of consciousness
   4. Ability to discuss fat and sodium diet restrictions

Analysis

The analysis phase of the nursing process involves developing and using a nursing diagnosis for the care of the client. The NGN uses the NANDA International (NANDA-I) nursing diagnosis system. Questions concerning nursing diagnosis often ask you to prioritize the diagnoses. (See online Bonus Chapter 29 for detailed information about prioritization.) The basic rules for prioritization are to use Maslow's hierarchy of needs and the ABCs you learned in CPR (airway, breathing, and circulation). Following is an example of an analysis phase question:

2. A client is admitted to the unit with a diagnosis of bronchitis, congestive heart failure, and a fever. The nurse assesses him as having a temperature of 101.8°F, peripheral edema, dyspnea, and rhonchi. The following nursing diagnoses are all appropriate, but which one has the highest priority?
   1. Anxiety related to fear of hospitalization
   2. Ineffective airway clearance related to retained secretions
   3. Fluid volume excess related to third spacing of fluid (edema)
   4. Ineffective thermoregulation related to fever

Planning

The planning phase of the nursing process primarily involves setting goals for the client. Included in the planning phase are such factors as determining expected outcomes, setting priorities for goals, and anticipating client needs based on the assessment. These questions may ask you to identify the most appropriate goal or may ask you to identify the highest-priority goal from several appropriate goals. You can prioritize goals the same way you did the nursing diagnosis. Remember that a good goal is measurable, client centered, time limited, and realistic. Here is an example of a planning phase question:

3. A client is found to be in respiratory failure and is placed on oxygen. Which goal has the highest priority for this client?
   1. Walk the length of the hall twice during a nurse's shift.
   2. Complete his bath and morning care before breakfast.
   3. Maintain an oxygen saturation of 90% throughout the shift.
   4. Keep the head of the bed elevated to promote proper ventilation.

Intervention and Implementation

The intervention and implementation phase of the nursing process involves identifying nursing actions that are required to meet the goals stated in the planning phase. Following are some of the material in the intervention and implementation phase:

- Providing nursing care based on the client's goals.
- Preventing injury or spread of disease
- Providing therapy with medications and their administration
- Giving treatments
- Carrying out procedures
- Charting and record-keeping
- Teaching about health care
- Monitoring changes in condition

An example of an intervention and implementation phase question follows:

4. When the nurse ambulates a client who has been on bedrest for 3 days, he suddenly becomes very restless, displays extreme dyspnea, and complains of chest pain. Select the most appropriate nursing action.
   1. Call a code blue.
   2. Continue to help the client walk but at a slower pace.
   3. Give the client an injection of his ordered pain medication.
   4. Return the client to bed and evaluate his vital signs and lung sounds.

Evaluation

The **evaluation** phase of the nursing process determines whether the goals stated in the planning phase have been met through the interventions. The evaluation phase also ties the nursing process together and makes it cyclic. If the goals have been achieved, it is an indication that the plan and implementation were effective, and new goals need to be established. If the goals were not met, then you have to go back and find the difficulty. Were the assessment data inadequate? Were the goals defective? Was there a deficiency in the implementation?

Evaluation is a continuous process. Material in the evaluation phase includes comparison of actual outcomes with expected outcomes, verification of assessment data, evaluation of nursing actions and client responses, and evaluation of the client's level of knowledge and understanding. Evaluation questions are often worded very similarly and are relatively easy to identify after you have experienced a few of them. Here is an example of an evaluation question:

5. A client is being prepared for discharge. He is to take theophylline by mouth at home for his lung disease. Which statement by the client indicates to the nurse that her teaching concerning theophylline medications has been effective?
   1. "I can stop taking this medication when I feel better."
   2. "If I have difficulty swallowing the time-released capsules, I can crush them or chew them."
   3. "If I have a lot of nausea and vomiting or become restless and can't sleep, I need to call my physician."
   4. "I need to drink more coffee and cola while I am on these medications."

A Thinking Process

As with the nursing process, the goal of the CJMM is simply to help you learn to progress through a very specific set of steps in your thinking when you are using your clinical judgment to resolve a patient's problem. Later in this chapter, you will see a sample of an evolving case scenario with questions that use the steps or levels of the CJMM (Fig. 28.15). Apply the information about the CJMM to the scenario and see if it is easier to understand.

Almost all the questions on the NGN are at Level 3 or 4 with very few basic knowledge questions.[1] Also, no longer do all questions on the NGN stand alone. "Standing alone" means that the question does not have any association with another question even though a similar situation may be repeated. Case study or scenario type questions on the NGN have multiple layers of answers that are based on the information in the case study. The scenario is created by the writers based on a situation that could happen in the real world of nursing care. It assesses the graduate's ability to work through a realistic nursing situation. The scenario provides the graduate with information about a patient including their history, medical diagnosis, current assessment findings, medications they are taking, recent and past laboratory results, and a presenting problem. Based on this information, the graduate must then make decisions on what they judge to be the best care.[3]

TYPES OF QUESTIONS

Up to 80 percent of the new NGN contains the same type of questions that have been on the previous NCLEXs. These are the questions found in Figures 28.2 to 28.7. All of these questions are stand-alone questions and are graded as either correct or incorrect or without partial credit. The NGN may have between 52 and 117 standalone items with up to 3 evolving case studies worth 18 points.[5]

Multiple Choice Questions

Questions that are in a multiple-choice format are constructed similarly. They include a client situation, a question stem, and four answer choices, like the sample questions you have seen so far in this chapter. Three answer choices are distractors, or incorrect answers, and one choice is the correct answer.

For the multiple-choice questions, you are asked to select the best answer from among the four possible choices. No partial credit is given for a "close" answer; there is only one correct answer for any particular question. The questions are totally integrated from the content areas that were previously discussed along with the approximate percentages that were identified. Each question carries an equal weight or value toward the final score.

When the question appears on the screen, read the question and answers using the process described in online Bonus Chapter 29. When you decide what the correct answer is, place the cursor in the circle in front of the answer and click to select the answer (see Fig. 28.2). If you decide to change the answer (seldom a good idea), place the cursor on the answer you selected and click again. It will remove the indicator, and you can move the cursor to another answer. Or change the answer by placing the cursor in a new circle and clicking. When you are sure you have selected the correct answer, click the NEXT button at the bottom of the screen or strike the "n" key on the keyboard. That question will disappear, and a new one will appear. You cannot go back and change an answer after you click the NEXT button.

Alternative Format Questions

In 2004, alternative format questions (AFQs) were first added to the NCLEX examination; in 2010, three new types of AFQs were added. The NGN now uses AFQs on all examinations.

There are several types of AFQs. They are given a difficulty rating based on the same criteria as the multiple-choice questions. NGN review books contain

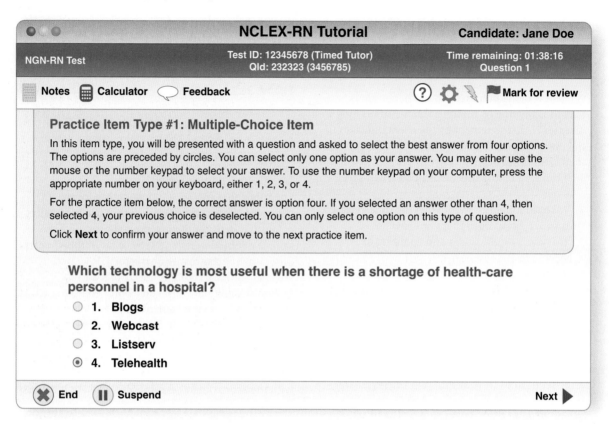

Figure 28.2 Sample multiple-choice question. Select the answer by placing the cursor in the circle and click or type in the answer number. If you decide to change the answer (never a good idea), place the cursor on the answer you selected and click again. It will remove the indicator, and you can move the cursor to another answer. Or, change the answer by placing the cursor in a new circle and clicking. Move to the next question by clicking the NEXT button at the bottom of the screen.

practice AFQs; however, they are difficult to reproduce just on paper. Most review books come with either disks or access to a website where AFQs can be taken. The important thing to remember about these types of questions is to read and follow all directions carefully.

Fill in the Blank

These AFQs may ask for a range of information. They may be calculation questions or may ask for knowledge. After you read the question, you need to type the answer in the box provided. If it is a calculation question, you may use the pop-up calculator, accessible by clicking on the Calculator symbol on the question screen or the "C" on the keyboard (Fig. 28.3). After you have typed in your answer, you can go back and change it. Once you have decided that it is correct, click the NEXT button, and a new question will appear.

Multiple Response

With multiple-response questions, you are given a list of options or answers and must select all that are correct. It is possible that only one option is correct or that all of them are correct; however, in practice, there are almost always at least two correct options. These types of questions can be difficult, but if you think about the options individually as being either true or false, the questions become easier. Read the question, then read the first answer. Is it true or false? If true, click on it. Do the same for the rest of the answers. To select the answers you think are correct, place the cursor in the circle or box before the option and click (Fig. 28.4). If you decide that one of the options is not really the one you want, you can click on the circle again to deselect it. When you decide you have the options you want, click the

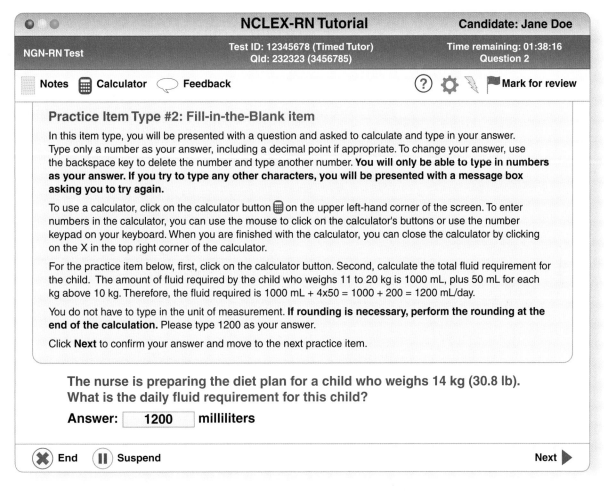

NCLEX-RN Tutorial   Candidate: Jane Doe

NGN-RN Test

Test ID: 12345678 (Timed Tutor)
Qld: 232323 (3456785)

Time remaining: 01:38:16
Question 2

Notes   Calculator   Feedback   (?)   ⚙   ⚡   🚩 Mark for review

Practice Item Type #2: Fill-in-the-Blank item

In this item type, you will be presented with a question and asked to calculate and type in your answer. Type only a number as your answer, including a decimal point if appropriate. To change your answer, use the backspace key to delete the number and type another number. **You will only be able to type in numbers as your answer. If you try to type any other characters, you will be presented with a message box asking you to try again.**

To use a calculator, click on the calculator button 🖩 on the upper left-hand corner of the screen. To enter numbers in the calculator, you can use the mouse to click on the calculator's buttons or use the number keypad on your keyboard. When you are finished with the calculator, you can close the calculator by clicking on the X in the top right corner of the calculator.

For the practice item below, first, click on the calculator button. Second, calculate the total fluid requirement for the child. The amount of fluid required by the child who weighs 11 to 20 kg is 1000 mL, plus 50 mL for each kg above 10 kg. Therefore, the fluid required is 1000 mL + 4x50 = 1000 + 200 = 1200 mL/day.

You do not have to type in the unit of measurement. **If rounding is necessary, perform the rounding at the end of the calculation.** Please type 1200 as your answer.

Click **Next** to confirm your answer and move to the next practice item.

The nurse is preparing the diet plan for a child who weighs 14 kg (30.8 lb). What is the daily fluid requirement for this child?

Answer: 1200   milliliters

(✖) End   (❚❚) Suspend   Next ▶

Figure 28.3 Alternative format question—fill in the blank. Fill in the blank by clicking on the answer box at the lower left corner. To use the calculator, click on the calculator button on the upper left-hand corner of the screen. Do not use spaces or commas in the answer. Close the calculator by clicking on the X button on the calculator screen.

NEXT button, and the next question will appear on the screen.

Sequencing Items (Ordered Response)
Sequencing questions provide you with a question and four or more options (items) that are related to the question. Your task with this type of question is to place them in the proper sequence (Fig. 28.5). Sequencing questions use a drag-and-drop answer system whereby you can click and hold on the answer you think is number 1, then drag it and drop it in the number 1 box. This design presents a series of items in a box on the left side of the screen and a set of empty boxes on the right. The same method works

for the rest of the answers. If you want to change an answer, click and hold and then drag it to another box. When you have the options sequenced the way you think they should be, click the NEXT button, and a new question will appear on the screen.

Identify the Area (or Hot Spot)
Hot spot questions provide you with a picture, graph, or diagram and ask you to identify an area of or a specific element on the picture (Fig. 28.6). You place the cursor on the area that you think is correct and click. An X appears. If you decide that is not where you really want the X, you can click the X again to remove it and then place the cursor in a new spot and

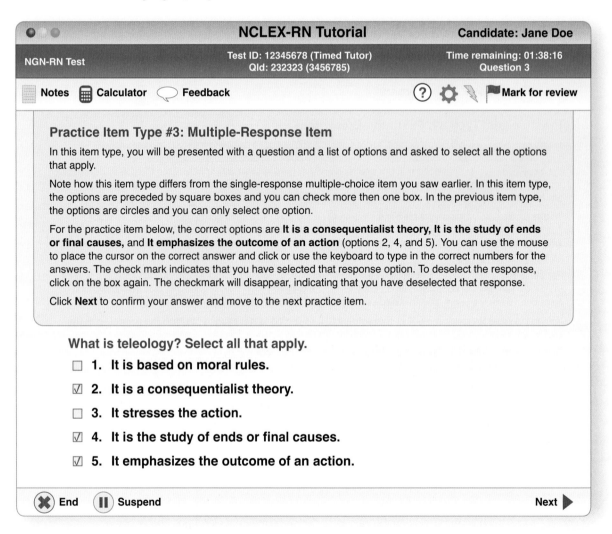

Figure 28.4 Alternative format question—multiple response.

click again. The X does not have to be on the exact right spot because there is a "zone" of correctness around it. Once you have it where you want it, click the NEXT button, and the next question will appear on the screen.

Chart/Exhibit Items (Type 1)

A chart or exhibit item presents you with a chart, graph, or some other picture or graphic item or with a series of charts, graphs, or other pictures. You need to be able to read the chart, graph, or picture to obtain the information to answer the question. Then you will be asked to select the correct answer from four or more options by using the information you gleaned from the chart, graph, or picture.

Exhibit Items (Type 2)

With this type of question, you are presented with either a question or a problem. To answer the question or solve the problem, you must click an Exhibit button. Each exhibit contains three tabs with dropdowns; you must click each tab and read the information (Fig. 28.7). The question will ask you to find some data provided by one of the tabs. Once you determine which chart or graph (tab) has the correct information, you must select the one corresponding

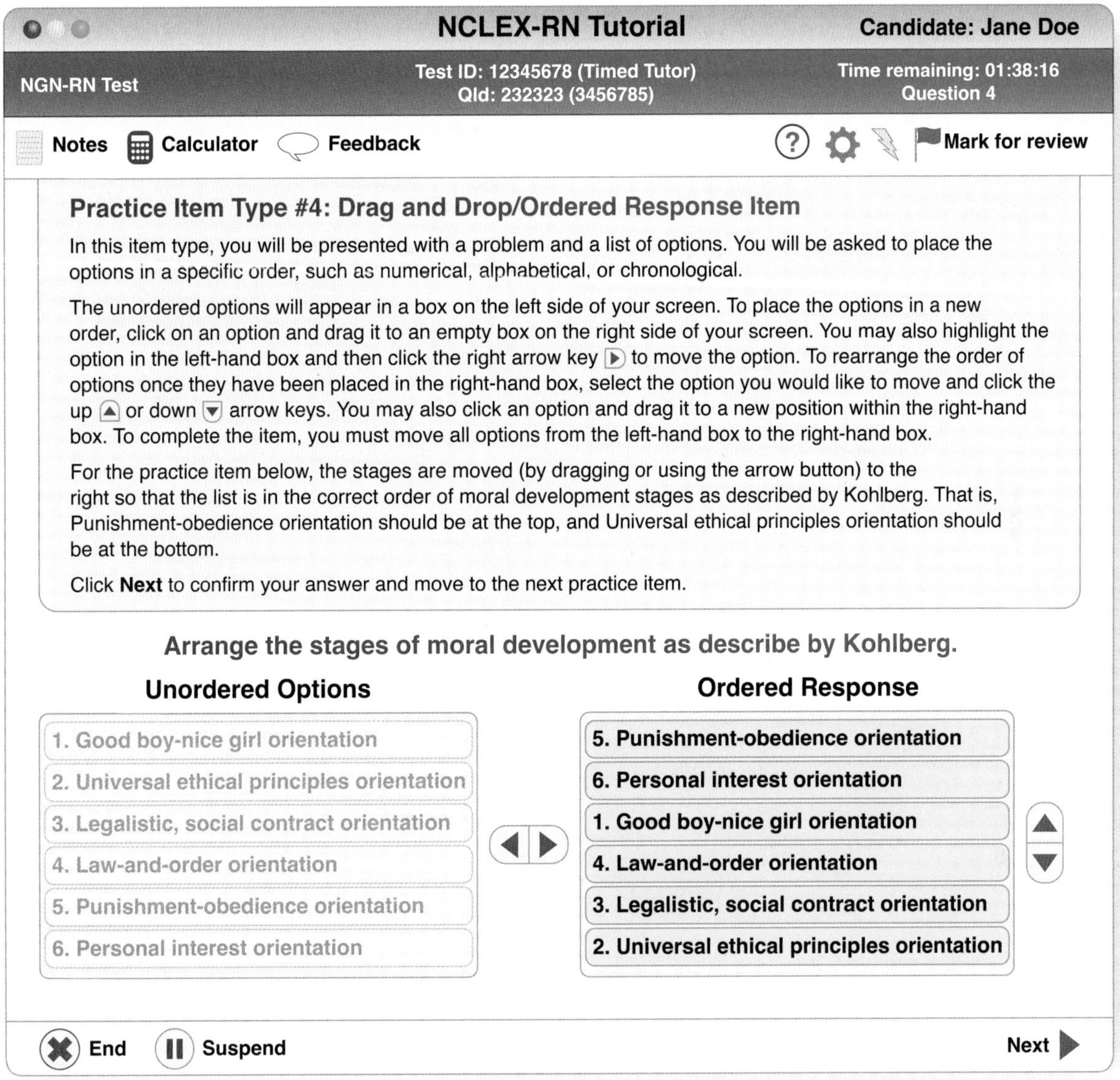

NCLEX-RN Tutorial   Candidate: Jane Doe

NGN-RN Test

Test ID: 12345678 (Timed Tutor)   Time remaining: 01:38:16
Qld: 232323 (3456785)   Question 4

▦ Notes   🖩 Calculator   ⬭ Feedback   ⑦ ⚙ ⚡   🚩 Mark for review

Practice Item Type #4: Drag and Drop/Ordered Response Item

In this item type, you will be presented with a problem and a list of options. You will be asked to place the options in a specific order, such as numerical, alphabetical, or chronological.

The unordered options will appear in a box on the left side of your screen. To place the options in a new order, click on an option and drag it to an empty box on the right side of your screen. You may also highlight the option in the left-hand box and then click the right arrow key ▶ to move the option. To rearrange the order of options once they have been placed in the right-hand box, select the option you would like to move and click the up ▲ or down ▼ arrow keys. You may also click an option and drag it to a new position within the right-hand box. To complete the item, you must move all options from the left-hand box to the right-hand box.

For the practice item below, the stages are moved (by dragging or using the arrow button) to the right so that the list is in the correct order of moral development stages as described by Kohlberg. That is, Punishment-obedience orientation should be at the top, and Universal ethical principles orientation should be at the bottom.

Click **Next** to confirm your answer and move to the next practice item.

Arrange the stages of moral development as describe by Kohlberg.

Unordered Options   **Ordered Response**

1. Good boy-nice girl orientation   5. Punishment-obedience orientation

2. Universal ethical principles orientation 6. Personal interest orientation

3. Legalistic, social contract orientation   1. Good boy-nice girl orientation

4. Law-and-order orientation   ◀ ▶   4. Law-and-order orientation   ▲ ▼

5. Punishment-obedience orientation   3. Legalistic, social contract orientation

6. Personal interest orientation   2. Universal ethical principles orientation

✖ End   ⏸ Suspend   Next ▶

Figure 28.5 Alternative format question—ordered response.

correct item from the four options provided. Then you click the NEXT button and move on to the next question.

Exhibit item questions test your ability to use information correctly. This type of question responds to the increase in the use of evidence-based practice in the health-care setting. If a nurse cannot understand and interpret research findings correctly, the safety of clients becomes an issue.

Audio Items

This type of question requires the use of a headset. When the question comes up, you will initially see what looks like the audio bar from a DVD with the usual symbols for play, pause, forward, stop, and reverse.

Four options (answer choices) will be displayed underneath the bar. You must put on the headset and click the arrow-shaped play button to listen to the audio clip. The volume can be adjusted using the

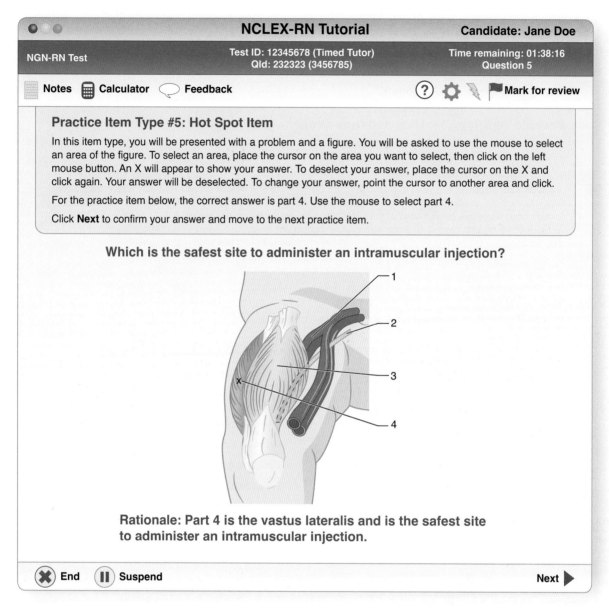

NCLEX-RN Tutorial **Candidate: Jane Doe**

NGN-RN Test | Test ID: 12345678 (Timed Tutor)
Qld: 232323 (3456785) | Time remaining: 01:38:16
Question 5

▦ Notes 🖩 Calculator ⬭ Feedback   (?) ⚙ ✎ ⚑ Mark for review

Practice Item Type #5: Hot Spot Item

In this item type, you will be presented with a problem and a figure. You will be asked to use the mouse to select an area of the figure. To select an area, place the cursor on the area you want to select, then click on the left mouse button. An X will appear to show your answer. To deselect your answer, place the cursor on the X and click again. Your answer will be deselected. To change your answer, point the cursor to another area and click.

For the practice item below, the correct answer is part 4. Use the mouse to select part 4.

Click **Next** to confirm your answer and move to the next practice item.

Which is the safest site to administer an intramuscular injection?

— 1
— 2
— 3
— 4

Rationale: Part 4 is the vastus lateralis and is the safest site to administer an intramuscular injection.

(✖) End (❚❚) Suspend   Next ▶

Figure 28.6 Alternative format question—hot spot. With this type of question, you are given a diagram or picture and asked to locate a structure or area. Place the cursor on the area you think is correct and click. An X will appear in that area. To deselect the answer, click the X and move the cursor to the new area. When finished, click Next on the question screen or "N" on the keyboard.

volume slide bar. After listening to the clip, you must select the one correct option related to it. You can repeat the clip as often as you want, stop it, or pause it by clicking the appropriate audio bar symbols. After selecting your answer, click the NEXT button to move on to the next question.

The NCSBN has not indicated what you might find on these audio clips. Logically, it would seem that anything a nurse usually "hears" in the course of a day's work could be included: heart sounds, breath sounds, bruits, and even client statements (e.g., based on which you might be asked, Is this client depressed,

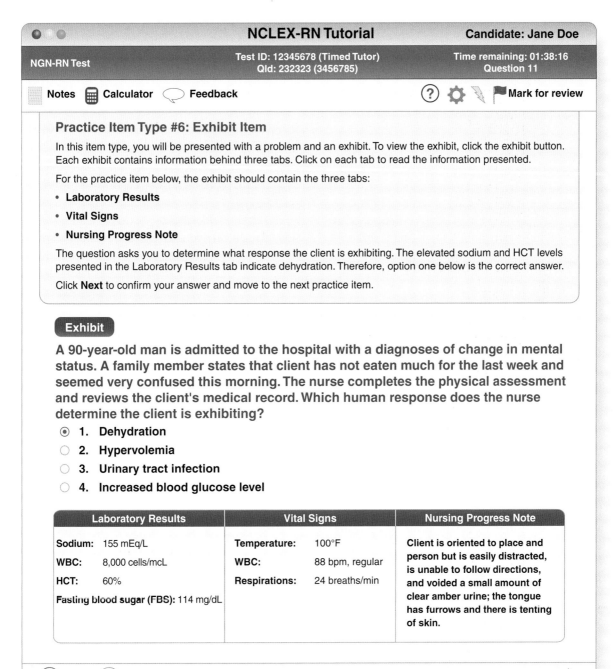

Notes   Calculator   Feedback   (?) ⚙ 🗲 ⚑ Mark for review

Practice Item Type #6: Exhibit Item

In this item type, you will be presented with a problem and an exhibit. To view the exhibit, click the exhibit button. Each exhibit contains information behind three tabs. Click on each tab to read the information presented.

For the practice item below, the exhibit should contain the three tabs:

- **Laboratory Results**
- **Vital Signs**
- **Nursing Progress Note**

The question asks you to determine what response the client is exhibiting. The elevated sodium and HCT levels presented in the Laboratory Results tab indicate dehydration. Therefore, option one below is the correct answer.

Click **Next** to confirm your answer and move to the next practice item.

Exhibit

A 90-year-old man is admitted to the hospital with a diagnoses of change in mental status. A family member states that client has not eaten much for the last week and seemed very confused this morning. The nurse completes the physical assessment and reviews the client's medical record. Which human response does the nurse determine the client is exhibiting?

- ◉ 1. **Dehydration**
- ○ 2. **Hypervolemia**
- ○ 3. **Urinary tract infection**
- ○ 4. **Increased blood glucose level**

Laboratory Results	Vital Signs	Nursing Progress Note
Sodium: 155 mEq/L	**Temperature:** 100°F	Client is oriented to place and person but is easily distracted, is unable to follow directions, and voided a small amount of clear amber urine; the tongue has furrows and there is tenting of skin.
WBC: 8,000 cells/mcL	**WBC:** 88 bpm, regular	
HCT: 60%	**Respirations:** 24 breaths/min	
Fasting blood sugar (FBS): 114 mg/dL		

(✖) **End**   (❚❚) **Suspend**   **Next** ▶

Figure 28.7 Alternative format question—exhibit item.

angry, anxious, or expressing echolalia?). These audio items might be difficult.

Graphic Items

These questions are similar to the traditional multiple-choice questions in that there is a written question. However, the question presents four pictures or graphics, not written options, as answer selections. As with the audio items, the NCSBN has not provided any indication of the types of graphics you might encounter. They could be charts of disease frequencies, pictures of rashes or wounds, ECG strips, types of syringes, medication labels on bottles, or just about anything a nurse might see during a work shift.

THINGS THAT WILL BE DIFFERENT

How Many Questions?

On the NGN, you may take a minimum of 85 and a maximum of 150 questions, of which a minimum of 70 to a maximum of 135 count as scored items. Of the first 85 questions, only 70 count. The other 15 are "trial" or "pretest" questions that will be used on future examinations; however, they are completely integrated with the other questions, and there is no way to know which ones do not count, so do your best on all of them.[1] The NCSBN is attempting to establish reliability and validity data on the new trial questions.

If you get a lot of questions in a particular category—for example, pediatrics—it may mean one of two things. The NCSBN may be testing pediatric questions on your examination, so you are receiving a lot of them, and some do not count; or you may be having some problems answering pediatric questions correctly. The computer will continue to give you questions in a particular content area until you meet the requirements of the test plan. The computer randomly draws the questions you are seeing from a pool of more than 4,000 questions. It creates your test as you go along and gives you new questions depending on how you answered previous questions.[4]

A short, 30-minute questionnaire called the Special Research Section (SRS) will be offered to some candidates, as part of their examination, immediately after finishing the NGN. When you register for the NGN (NCLEX), you can check the box stating you are willing to participate in the study. If you do and if you are selected, you will get a short 30-minute questionnaire immediately after you complete the NGN. These additional questions, like the pretest questions that everybody takes, are not graded, and the NCSBN assures participants that the SRS questionnaire does not affect their chances of passing the NGN. The SRS is used to test the new question formats. This helps the NCSBN ensure that the new question layouts are understandable, appropriately coded, and representative of the latest standards of care.[6]

If the computer determines that there is not enough time left for you to take the SRS, it will not appear on your screen. Also, if you did check the box for the SRS and then decide not to take it, or if you stop taking it after you have started, your NGN score will not be affected in any way.[3]

The NGN is given by computerized adaptive testing (CAT); therefore, increases in the passing standard do not necessarily require you to answer more questions correctly. However, a new passing standard does require that you answer questions correctly at a slightly higher difficulty level than the previous year's graduates (i.e., the examination is going to be a little more difficult to pass). Questions are assigned a difficulty value on a seven-unit scale called the NGN *logit scale*, ranging from the easiest (minus 3 logits), which all graduates should answer correctly, to the most difficult (plus 3 logits), which almost all graduates would be expected to miss (Fig. 28.8).

New Questions—Based on the Old Format

The NGN has several new types of questions that are somewhat similar to questions using a format found in previous examinations. All questions are presented on a split-screen with a case study on the left side and the question items on the right. Also, partial credit, or what is called *polytomous scoring*, will be given for one or more correct answers. This type of scoring allows graduates to earn credit for partial understanding of a subject; however, they can lose points for an incorrect answer.

These questions include the following:

• Extended multiple response
• Select all that apply
• Select *N*
• Extended drag and drop
• Cloze
• Drop-down

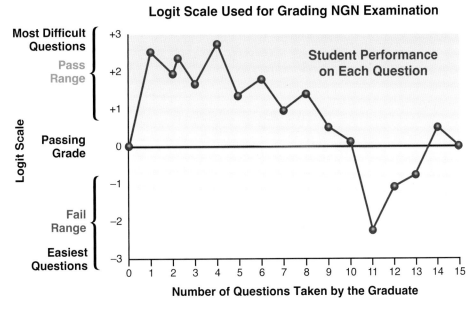

Figure 28.8 Logit scale used for grading examinations.

• Highlight (enhanced hot spot)
• In text
• In table [5]

Extended Multiple Response

These questions are similar to Figure 28.3 except that the list of possible options is longer. These questions better mimic real-world situations. When your patient takes a turn for the worse, you do not have just four or five options to choose from in their care; you may have as many as 10!

These items are scored the same as the basic multiple-choice questions. You earn a point for each correct option selected, and one point is deducted when you select an incorrect option. The points are then added together for a total question score.

Extended Drag and Drop

These questions are similar to the drag and drop (ordered response) type questions found in previous examinations (Fig. 28.9) except that they include more information and can better assess the graduate's ability to make sound clinical judgments. They require you to drag and drop items into the correct order or select all that apply. The main difference is that you are dragging the answer over rather than

clicking a button. In some cases, there might be more boxes available than there are correct answers, which means that not all response options are required or correct, so you must select which ones actually apply to the patient in the case study. This is scored per item as either correct or incorrect. The sum of the scores is across all the answer choices, and the maximum score is the same as the number of answer choices.

Cloze (Drop-Down)

This is a short-answer type question. The question requires you to choose from possible options in a drop-down menu or list that appears in a sentence, chart, or table (Fig. 28.10). There can be up to six responses for each option. It is very similar to fill-in-the-blank questions, but instead of keying in an answer, you select a response from the drop-down. For example, you are given a sentence about how the nurse evaluates a patient with a disease process. The sentence contains a blank box that you must fill in. You point the curser on the box, a menu drops down with several options in it, and you select your answer. Some sentences may contain more than one box. This type of question is scored per item, either correct or incorrect. The sum of the correct items is the score for the question.

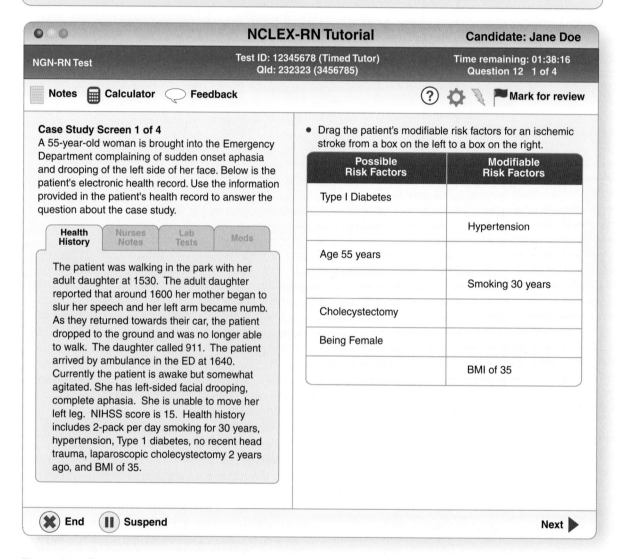

Extended Drag and Drop

These questions require that you choose the correct answer and then drag and drop the answer items into the correct order or to select all that apply and drag and drop them into the next column. In some cases, there might be more boxes available than there are correct answers. These questions are scored per item as either correct or incorrect.

NCLEX-RN Tutorial   **Candidate: Jane Doe**

| NGN-RN Test | Test ID: 12345678 (Timed Tutor) Qld: 232323 (3456785) | Time remaining: 01:38:16 Question 12 1 of 4 |

Notes   Calculator   Feedback   (?) ⚙ ✎ 🚩 Mark for review

Case Study Screen 1 of 4

A 55-year-old woman is brought into the Emergency Department complaining of sudden onset aphasia and drooping of the left side of her face. Below is the patient's electronic health record. Use the information provided in the patient's health record to answer the question about the case study.

Health History | Nurses Notes | Lab Tests | Meds

The patient was walking in the park with her adult daughter at 1530. The adult daughter reported that around 1600 her mother began to slur her speech and her left arm became numb. As they returned towards their car, the patient dropped to the ground and was no longer able to walk. The daughter called 911. The patient arrived by ambulance in the ED at 1640. Currently the patient is awake but somewhat agitated. She has left-sided facial drooping, complete aphasia. She is unable to move her left leg. NIHSS score is 15. Health history includes 2-pack per day smoking for 30 years, hypertension, Type 1 diabetes, no recent head trauma, laparoscopic cholecystectomy 2 years ago, and BMI of 35.

- Drag the patient's modifiable risk factors for an ischemic stroke from a box on the left to a box on the right.

Possible Risk Factors	Modifiable Risk Factors
Type I Diabetes	
	Hypertension
Age 55 years	
	Smoking 30 years
Cholecystectomy	
Being Female	
	BMI of 35

(X) End   (II) Suspend   Next ▶

Figure 28.9 Extended drag and drop. Move or place response options into answer spaces. This question type is similar to ordered response items, but not all response options may be required to answer the question—that is, there may be more response options than answer spaces.

Enhanced Hot Spots (EHS)

Similar to hot spot questions found in previous examinations (Fig. 28.5) that asked you to click on specific information to show you know which information is important to your clinical decision making, these questions may ask you to highlight, by dragging your cursor across certain information, information in case studies, illustrations, charts, or diagrams (Fig. 28.11). EHS items are similar to receiving a written report from a nurse going off shift, and inside

Cloze (Drop-Down)

These questions are similar to fill-in-the-blank questions, but instead of filling in the blanks without any idea about the answer, the candidate has a choice of answers from a drop-down box in the blank. Click on the blank and select the correct answer from the drop-down box that appears. There may be more than one blank to fill in.

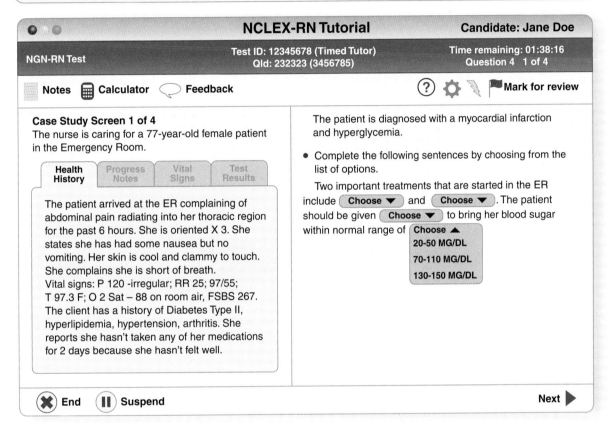

Figure 28.10 Cloze (drop-down). Similar to fill-in-the-blank questions, but instead of filling in a blank, you select one answer from a drop-down list. Drop-down lists can be used as words or phrases within a sentence or within tables and charts.

that report there are several bits of information that you have to identify as important for the care of the patients on your shift or things that require your immediate action. While less common, hot spot questions will have you select a particular area in a graphic that answers the question. Partial credit can be earned for these questions. You earn 1 point for selecting a correct option and lose 1 point for selecting an incorrect option, with a minimum score no lower than 0 and a maximum score of the number of correct options.

BRAND NEW FORMAT NGN QUESTION

Because the NCSBN's last survey found that nurses in today's health-care system are more often caring for patients who are critically ill than has been true even in the recent past, they decided that the NGN questions need to be more difficult, with increased focus on caring for more critically ill patients. These questions require a high degree of critical thinking, analysis, and decision-making skills. The new format questions discussed next are substantially different from what nursing graduates have been used to seeing as students.

Enhanced Hot Spot (Highlighting)

With these types of questions, the candidate is to place the cursor and click on the highlighted section of the nurses' notes that answers the question asked in the question part of the screen.

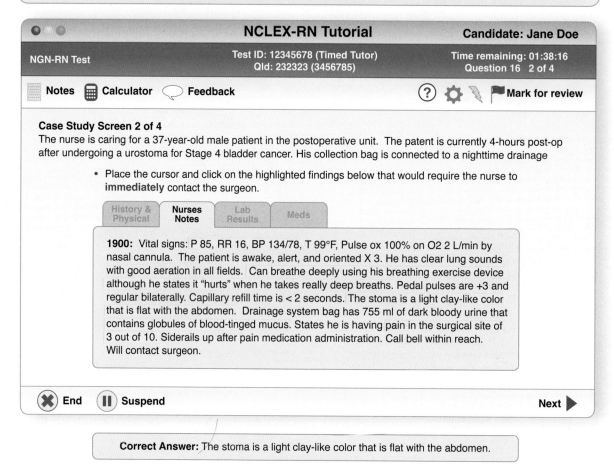

Figure 28.11 Highlighting (also referred to as enhanced hot spot). This is a type of hot spot question but requires identifying critical information in a scenario. Test takers read the patient's medical record and then select and click on the highlighted section that answers the question correctly.

Traditionally, most test questions have been stand-alone questions, meaning that each question has no relationship to any other question. These questions are much easier to write and score. In the new NGN, each case study will have six questions related to and derived from it. When you see these case studies, they will provide you with a patient record with several tabs at the top and a split screen. The patient record will be on one side, usually the left, and questions will appear on the other. Selecting a tab with the cursor will bring down information that can be used to answer a question. Tabs on the right side of the screen will bring down new questions. Partial credit will be given for these questions.[1] These questions will include the following:

- Matrix/grid
- Multiple response
- Multiple choice
- Bowtie
- Trend
- Unfolding case studies[5]

Matrix/Grid (Matrix and Grid)

If you have ever filled out a satisfaction survey on the computer, maybe after having your car worked on or visiting a hotel, you have completed a matrix/grid questionnaire. On the NGN, matrix/grid questions test your ability to choose one or more options in rows and columns that ask you to categorize the options as

- Essential/nonessential
- Contraindicated/effective/ineffective/unrelated
- Risk factor/not a risk factor
- Anticipated/not anticipated for the patient (Fig. 28.12)

You may be asked to select a single answer (matrix/grid multiple choice), or you may be asked to choose from multiple answers (matrix/grid multiple response). A matrix/grid question works like a case study that unfolds as you answer questions. It can allow the graduate to select multiple answers and

---

Matrix/Grid

Matrix/Grid questions require the candidate to choose one or more answers from a row of answers by placing the cursor and clicking on a radio button under the appropriate heading. There must be one response for each row.

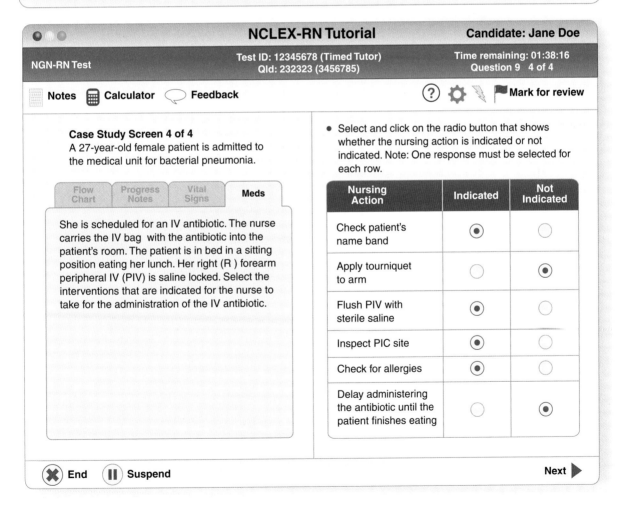

Figure 28.12 Matrix/grid. In this multiple-answer question, test-takers select one or more answer options for each row and/or column. It is useful in measuring multiple aspects of the clinical scenario with a single item.

different options on each row, usually indicated by radio buttons. These buttons can be round or square. You can select only one radio button on each row. Square buttons indicate more than one correct answer per row in a different column. This is all part of the CJMM, which assesses your ability to make safe client care decisions.

There are two types of matrix/grid questions, and each one is scored differently. The matrix/grid multiple response gives you 1 point for a correct answer and −1 point for an incorrect answer. The matrix/grid multiple choice just gives you 1 point for a correct answer but does not take any points away for an incorrect answer.

Bowtie

The bowtie question is one of the most complicated of all the questions on the NGN. However, you have to answer it to be able to move on in the examination. It is given the name "bowtie" because of the shape in which the answer boxes are arranged and has nothing to do with bows or ties. The bowtie item requires you to use all six functions of clinical judgment in answering the question: recognizing cues, analyzing cues, generating solutions, prioritizing hypotheses, taking action, and evaluating outcomes. You are first presented with a case scenario; then you have to work your way through the clinical judgment functions.

To answer this question, first figure out the primary problem the patient is suffering from (diagnosis) based on the information provided in the case scenario (Fig. 28.13). Then, under the heading "Potential Condition," select what you think is wrong with the patient and drag it up to the appropriately labeled box. Next, you have to figure out which two items under the "Actions to Take" would be the best for this patient's condition. Keep in mind that more than two may be appropriate, but you have to select the two that are "best" or are the ones that will keep your patient alive. Once you decide, drag them into their appropriate spaces. Finally, you must figure out what you should be looking for after you have taken your action (evaluation). Under the "Parameters to Monitor" heading, choose the two best items and drag them into their spaces.

The tabs or boxes in a bowtie question may be labeled differently, such as Nurses' Notes, History and Physical, Laboratory Results, Vital Signs, Admission Notes, Intake and Output, Progress Notes,

Medications, Diagnostic Results, and Flow Sheet. You can move the items around after you first select them by dragging them back to where they came from and then dragging the new answers into the answer boxes or tabs. This is *not* a good strategy because your first selections are usually the best ones.

Bowtie items are standalone questions. You can receive partial credit for the item. Because there are two possible options for the left two boxes, two possible options for the right two boxes, and one possible option for the middle box, the maximum number of possible points is 5. You earn 1 point for each correct response, but no points for any incorrect response. Therefore, you can earn between 0 and 5 points for this type of question.

Trend Items

A trend item gives you a case scenario that looks like a medical record divided up into progressive time intervals ranging from minutes to hours to days or longer. You must review and analyze the information in the medical record and see how it trends over the given time interval. The case scenarios (tabs) for trend items can vary and include nurses' notes, history and physical, laboratory results, vital signs, admission notes, intake and output, progress notes, diagnostic results from x-rays or other tests, and other flow sheets. After you analyze the case scenario and decide on a diagnosis for the client (in Fig. 28.14, based on the child's age and symptoms, it probably is pyloric stenosis), you need to make a decision about what to do next. In this case, think about the types of diagnostic tests that are needed to make a definitive diagnosis for pyloric stenosis.

Trend items are standalone questions and can be scored as correct or incorrect or as partial credit, depending on the type of responses listed. The sample question, Figure 28.14, probably uses a partial credit format due to the multiple correct responses.

Unfolding (Evolving) Case Study

The unfolding, or evolving, case study and case scenario is one of the new types of questions on the NGN designed to measure your clinical judgment. These case studies are made up of sets of six items presented in an unfolding sequence (hence the name). The unfolding case scenario starts by presenting a real-world clinical situation and patient information in one or two sentences or paragraphs, which are

Bowtie

Bowtie questions combine all six steps of the Clinical Judgment Measurement Model (CJMM) into the question. A bowtie question usually presents a patient case study along with patient information that is either normal or abnormal. Nursing actions options must be chosen from the list of **Actions to Take** cues to complete the left side of the bowtie. Place the cursor and click on the appropriate action, then drag it up to one of the two **Action to Take** boxes of the bowtie graphic and drop it. After selecting the two actions to perform (from the list of **Action to Take** cues), and filling in the left-side bowtie boxes, choose the **parameters to monitor** on the right side of the bowtie (using the **Parameters to Monitor** cues) and slide them up to the right-side bowtie **Parameters to Monitor** boxes. Finally, using the same process as for the right- and left-side boxes for Potential Conditions, slide the one correct answer from the Potential Conditions list of cues up to the **Potential Condition** box in the center of the bowtie. These are stand-alone questions.

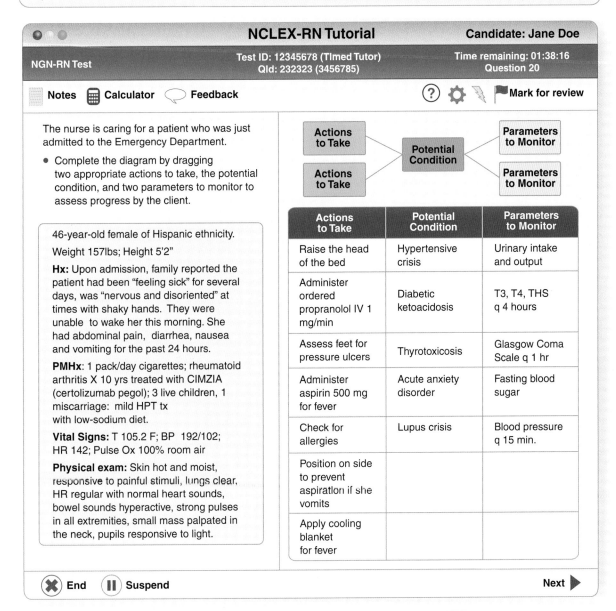

The nurse is caring for a patient who was just admitted to the Emergency Department.

- Complete the diagram by dragging two appropriate actions to take, the potential condition, and two parameters to monitor to assess progress by the client.

46-year-old female of Hispanic ethnicity.

Weight 157lbs; Height 5'2"

Hx: Upon admission, family reported the patient had been "feeling sick" for several days, was "nervous and disoriented" at times with shaky hands. They were unable to wake her this morning. She had abdominal pain, diarrhea, nausea and vomiting for the past 24 hours.

PMHx: 1 pack/day cigarettes; rheumatoid arthritis X 10 yrs treated with CIMZIA (certolizumab pegol); 3 live children, 1 miscarriage: mild HPT tx with low-sodium diet.

Vital Signs: T 105.2 F; BP 192/102; HR 142; Pulse Ox 100% room air

Physical exam: Skin hot and moist, responsive to painful stimuli, lungs clear, HR regular with normal heart sounds, bowel sounds hyperactive, strong pulses in all extremities, small mass palpated in the neck, pupils responsive to light.

Actions to Take	Potential Condition	Parameters to Monitor
Raise the head of the bed	Hypertensive crisis	Urinary intake and output
Administer ordered propranolol IV 1 mg/min	Diabetic ketoacidosis	T3, T4, THS q 4 hours
Assess feet for pressure ulcers	Thyrotoxicosis	Glasgow Coma Scale q 1 hr
Administer aspirin 500 mg for fever	Acute anxiety disorder	Fasting blood sugar
Check for allergies	Lupus crisis	Blood pressure q 15 min.
Position on side to prevent aspiration if she vomits		
Apply cooling blanket for fever		

End   Suspend   Next ▶

Answers to the question:
Actions to take: Check for allergies; Apply cooling blanket for fever.
Potential Condition: Thyrotoxicosis.
Parameters to Monitor: T3, T4, THS q 4 hours; BP q 15 minutes

Figure 28.13 Bowtie. This standalone item is set up as an advanced drag and drop and looks like a bowtie.

Trend

Trend questions have a patient case study with vital signs, condition, and other findings that change over a designated period of time. There is a question, usually one or more multiple choice questions or a multiple response question about the information in the case study. Trend questions could ask about client needs, nursing interventions, or anticipated health-care provider orders, among other things. These questions can be stand-alone or part of an Unfolding Case Study question

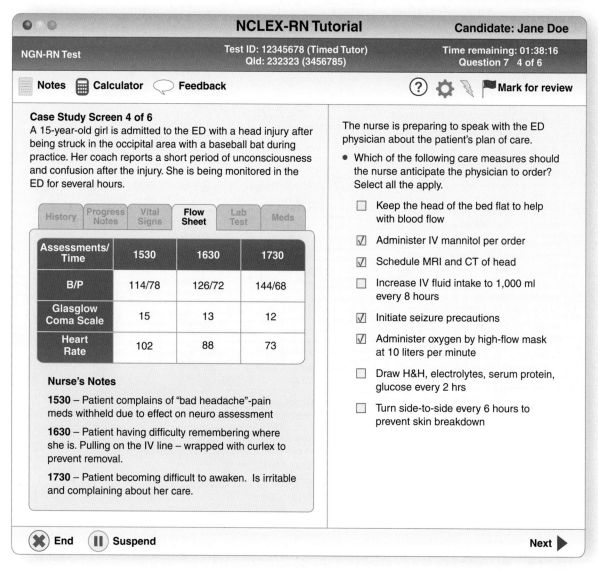

Figure 28.14 Trend. This question type addresses multiple steps of the Clinical Judgment Measurement Model by having the candidate review the patient's condition over time. A standalone item, it can feature any of the item response types.

generally in a medical record format. The patient scenarios place you into the patient situation and measure your ability to recognize key data and make the appropriate care-planning decisions. An unfolding scenario includes more than one phase of care for one client. It may include up to four phases, depending on the complexity of the case scenario. The initial clinical scenario changes over time as the patient's condition evolves.

On the left-hand side of the first computer screen of the scenario, a "card" with the initial patient information will appear. The card has tabs at the top with identifiers such as Health History, Nurse's Notes, Physician's Orders, and Laboratory Profile. By clicking on the tabs, you will move to the next screen, which will show a card with the same basic patient information with new data added to the scenario that has evolved over a period of time (minutes, hours, days, and so forth). As you read through the patient information, you must pick out the most important data to be able to answer the questions for that particular screen. To help you keep track of where you are, the upper left-hand corner of each card is numbered, such as "1 of 6," "2 of 6," and so forth.

The computer screen is divided down the middle (like the other questions you have already seen), and on the right-hand side are the questions you need to answer about the scenario. Rather than assessing your knowledge and understanding of information, as some of the standalone questions do, these questions act as prods for you to use your clinical judgment. The questions might focus on your ability to identify cues in the scenario or on how you determine additional data that needs to be collected, interpret patient problems and concerns, and analyze laboratory values. Some of the questions may ask you to take specific actions in a situation, both immediate and long term, or to identify outcomes for improvement in a patient's condition. Unfolding case studies may present questions in any of the standalone formats already discussed, such as select the best answer, select all that apply, matrix/grid selection, highlight the answer, or fill in the blank. Figure 28.15 shows a select-all-that-apply question, which is likely one of the most common formats you will see.

As you click on each tab sequentially, one question for each tab will appear, for a total of six questions based on the *same* case scenario

(i.e., all six questions refer to the same scenario and do not stand alone). Make sure you select the tabs sequentially because you *cannot* go back. There are three unfolding case scenarios on each examination; each case scenario has six items, for a total of 18 items. The three unfolding cases are distributed in the test so that graduates who need to take only the minimum 85 questions will have a chance to answer this type of question. There is one unfolding scenario within the first 70 questions, another one near the 100th question, and a final one before the 150th question. NGN case studies are delivered according to the CAT model, which is based on the increasing difficulty of each question.

Scoring on the unfolding case scenarios is complex. Even though all six questions are related to the scenario, each question within the group of six for a particular case scenario is independent of the others and is scored according to the type of answers presented. For example, if the question says, "Select the one best option," then there is only one correct answer, and it is scored as correct or incorrect. If instead the question says, "Select all that apply," it is likely graded on a partial basis. As with the rest of the items on the NGN, on the case scenarios, you will not be able to go back to view previous questions. A composite score will be computed from your responses to each item in the six-question case study, and the score for the entire case study determines which item you will see next.

Who Is Responsible?

The NCSBN, which is responsible for designing the NGN, publicly states that no graduates are randomly selected by the computer to take all 150 questions. You can pass or fail the test with 85 or 150 questions or any number in between.

The passing standard for 2023 to 2026 is 0.00 logits, the same as it has been since 2020. In past years when substantial changes were made in the examination, the national pass rate was usually lowered. The NGN is designed to focus on evaluating how nursing graduates make clinical judgments and decisions about patient care and how they use their critical-thinking skills. It does not explicitly test for clinical knowledge. Rather, graduates must have nursing knowledge about clinical skills and disease processes to be successful and obtain the correct answer. Although the majority

> ## Unfolding (Evolving) Case Study — Question 1 (Extended Multiple Choice)
>
> This question type assesses your ability to work through a realistic patient situation. Note the highlighted tab at the top of the left-side question box. The highlighted tab indicates that this is an unfolding case study, NOT a stand-alone question. The case study has six layers of questions based on the information provided in ONE unfolding case study. Questions can be any of the question types found in the Question Tutorial. Clicking on each tab to the right of the highlighted tab allows you to access more information related to the case. Make sure you view ALL tabs and answer the associated questions on each tab because *you can NOT go back and click on a previous tab to the left.* Each tab's question is based on the totality of information provided by previous tabs up to the current tab.

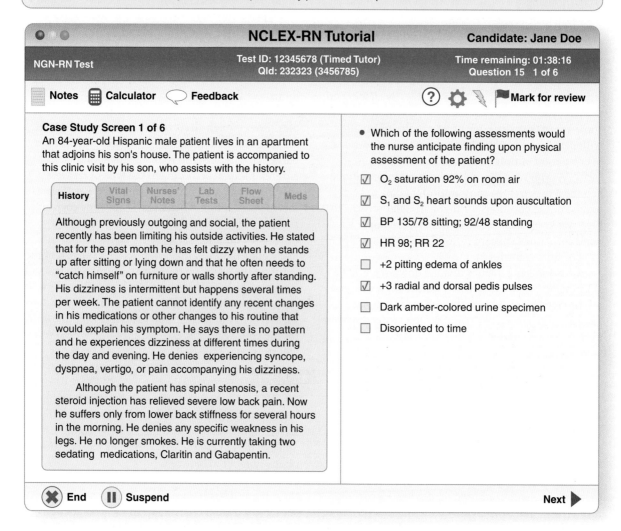

Figure 28.15 Unfolding, or evolving, case study questions and answers are dependent on the case scenario as it unfolds over time.

of the content will remain unchanged, the graduate can expect more questions on virtual and remote patient-teaching environments, greater emphasis on community health, and more questions on patient communication.[2]

How Long Do I Have?

There is a maximum time limit of 5 hours for the entire examination, although there is no minimum time limit. You can take breaks at any time during the examination, but remember that you will lose this time from your total time for the examination.[1]

The examination is not really timed except for the overall time limit. Theoretically, you could sit at the computer for the full 5 hours with question number 1 on the screen. The computer does not make you take questions at any particular rate. Most people can answer a multiple-choice question in about 45 seconds. As a rule of thumb, if you are spending more than 3 minutes on any single question, put an answer down and move on to the next question.

If you calculate that you could take as many as 150 questions in 5 hours, it comes out to a little less than 2 minutes per question. Some of the alternative-format questions, such as the evolving case studies and bowtie questions, may take a little longer to answer, although some may take less time than the multiple-choice questions. Take a watch along, but *not* a smartwatch (the proctor will take it away). Keep an eye on the Time Remaining box at the top of the screen. Again, if you are spending more than 3 minutes on any one question, select the best answer you can and move on to the next question. Wasting a lot of time on one question that you do not know the answer to is not productive.

What Grade Do I Need to Get to Pass?

The NGN is graded on a statistical model that compares your responses with a pre-established standard. If you can demonstrate a knowledge level consistently above the standard, you will pass the examination.

Because the findings of previous NCSBN surveys indicate an increase in the complexity of care in the health-care industry, the difficulty level required to pass has been gradually increased over the years. The need for a new examination was initially identified in 2017, following a massive nationwide RN Nursing Knowledge Survey. During this survey, it became evident that a nurse's scope of practice is now broader than it has ever been before. Meanwhile, patients are sicker on average, and caring for them requires deeper knowledge and more complex decisions. Based on these results, the NCSBN believed that it was essential for even recent graduates to think critically when providing care. This finding was consistent with previous research showing that clinical judgment is essential to the safe practice of nursing at the entry level.

The aim of the new type of test questions is to more closely simulate a hospital's work setting to produce better patient outcomes. The focus is on evaluating nursing graduates' judgment, decision making, and critical-thinking skills.[6]

You may have heard someone ask, "Do I need a 50 percent or 60 percent or 70 percent on the NGN to pass it?" It does not really matter—percentages are meaningless on this examination. Your answer from the question you just answered is analyzed by the computer as either correct or incorrect; however, you may earn partial credit on some of the new items! The computer then decides the difficulty level of the next question, which will probably be at a slightly higher difficulty level if you answered the previous question correctly. If you seem to be getting a lot of hard questions, that is a good sign! You need to demonstrate to the computer that you can, with a 95 percent confidence interval, answer medium-difficulty-level questions correctly at least 50 percent of the time. Why such a high confidence level (95 percent)? The state board of nursing wants to be confident that as a new RN you are not going to hurt or kill someone on your first day on the floor!

You must answer enough questions ranked above the pass criteria to demonstrate that you can practice nursing safely. If you do that, you pass the NGN. Even if you answer many questions correctly that are below the passing standard, they do not help you pass the examination, and you will fail.

Level of Difficulty

The difficulty level of the questions is determined by the writers and question reviewers. It is based on such factors as when the material is usually presented in nursing programs (material presented earlier is considered less difficult), the complexity of the material, and how you use your critical-thinking skills to make sound clinical judgments. To you, the test-taker, difficulty level is somewhat relative. If you know the answer to a question, then it will seem relatively easy to you even if it is classified by the test writers as being of a higher difficulty level. Similarly, if you do not know the answer, that question will be difficult for you even if it is determined to be at a relatively low difficulty level.

No Happy Questions

Keep in mind also that there are no "happy" questions on the NGN. There is always something wrong, and if there is a problem in the question, you need to worry about it. Also, as a general guiding principle, anything you know really well from your classes will *not* be on the NGN, so anticipate difficult questions.

Your Zone of Knowledge

After you finish the mandatory tutorial on the use of the computer, the first real question you get will be at a medium difficulty level, probably a little above or a little below the pass criteria. If you answer it correctly, the next question will be a little more difficult. If you answer that one correctly, the next question will also increase in difficulty, and so forth, until you start missing questions. Then the computer will give you slightly less difficult questions until you start answering them correctly again. The space between when you start missing questions and then start getting them correct again is your "zone of knowledge." If that zone is above the pass standard, then you will pass the examination (see Figure 28.8).

If the computer can determine with a 95 percent accuracy that your zone of knowledge is above the pass criteria within the first 85 questions, it will stop the test and ask you to complete the SRS if you signed up for it and have enough time. The reason many graduates take more than 85 questions is that the computer is having difficulty establishing a clear zone of knowledge above or below the pass standard. The computer will keep giving questions until a 95 percent accurate determination of your knowledge level is made. Graduates who take all 150 questions have answered questions above and below the pass standard throughout the whole examination but not enough to establish a clear 95 percent passing zone. If you do have to take all 150 questions, it does not necessarily mean you failed, but your examination will be graded using a different method.

Remember that it is probably a good sign that you are getting difficult questions. It means that you are answering questions above the pass standard. You do not want a lot of easy questions on the NGN. Also keep in mind that the NGN is designed so that no one can answer all the questions correctly. Even your most knowledgeable nursing instructor would not be able to answer some of the questions on the examination. Do not look for exceptions: think horses, not zebras, when answering a question. The examination writers do not intentionally write questions with the goal of tricking you. Each examination is different

and unique to the person taking it because future questions depend on how you answered previous questions.

NGN BACKGROUND INFORMATION

After you graduate from your nursing program, you must apply to the state board of nursing for permission to take the NGN. Once you have been approved by the state board, that information is sent to the NGN, which sends you an authorization to test card or document. You will receive your authorization document more quickly if you select the e-mail option on the application form for the examination.

You make an appointment at the center that is most conveniently located for you to take the test. Appointments are made on a first-come, first-served basis. The centers are required to schedule the examination within 30 days from the time you apply. Each state establishes its own maximum time interval for the graduate to take the examination after graduation, usually 1 year.

There are both morning and afternoon sessions of 6 hours' duration. Depending on the size of the center, between 8 and 15 graduates may be taking the test at the same time. In addition, there may be other people at the center taking examinations in other disciplines at the same time as the nursing graduates.

Test Vendor and Logistics

The test vendor for the NGN is Virtual University Enterprises (VUE), a subsidiary of National Communication Systems (NCS). The tests are given at Pearson Professional Centers. The test items and the format of the examination always stay the same, even if vendors change, because the examination is owned by the NCSBN, which contracts with vendors to administer it.

Testing by Computer

The computer skills required are minimal. The mouse is used for most of the examination, with minimal typing required. A digital picture, palm print scan, and your signature are taken at the time you enter the examination room, and that picture, along with your personal information, appears on one of the computer screens in the room.

You sit at the computer with your picture on it and complete a tutorial with the use of the mouse and computer. You have two attempts at completing the tutorial successfully. If you are unable to do so after the second try, a person who is working at the testing center will come and help you. After the examination is completed, you will be asked to complete a short computerized personal data questionnaire and an evaluation of the examination site.

Questions appear one at a time on the computer screen, with a button bar on the bottom of the screen and a "time remaining" box in the upper corner. After you select an answer, the question is replaced with another question and answer options. No question is ever repeated, nor are you able to change the answer once you have clicked the NEXT button.

An on-screen pop-up calculator is available for answering dosage and other questions that require calculations; you can access it by clicking the Calculator button on the screen. Because of the increased emphasis on pharmacology and concern about medication errors, it is probably safe to assume that the difficulty level of future calculation questions will increase markedly.

Security

Security is very tight at the examination sites. Lockers are provided, and you must place all your personal belongings, including your phone and all electronic devices, in a locker, so do not bring a lot of things with you. If you refuse to secure your phone, you will not be allowed to take the examination and will forfeit your examination fee.

All examination sessions are videotaped, and there is a proctor in the room monitoring all the test-takers. Although cheating on the NGN is virtually impossible—each test-taker has a different examination—it is important to not even look as if you are attempting to cheat. Do not talk to the person next to you. Keep your eyes on your own computer. Do not take out any papers or electronic devices during the examination. Magic slates are generally provided for use as "scrap paper," so you will not need any paper or pens during the test.

How the Test Is Graded

The NGN is graded on a pass/fail basis. The results are checked twice for accuracy. If the graduate fails, they must take the entire examination again. The NCSBN requires a 45-day waiting period before repeating the test, and first-time test takers are given preference over those who are repeating the examination. Several states have restricted the number of times the

graduate can retake the test (usually up to three) or have placed a time limit of 1 or 2 years on retaking it. Check with your state board of nursing for the particular regulations.

When the computer shuts off, it knows whether you passed or failed, but it will not give you that information at that time. At the end of the day, after the last testing session, results are downloaded electronically to NCSBN in Chicago, Illinois. The next business day, NCSBN notifies the state board of nursing electronically and sends a hard copy; then it is up to the state board of nursing to notify you.

The official examination results may be sent to you by mail, usually within 7 to 10 days after the examination has been completed, although this time frame varies from state to state. Most states now offer official online results within 72 hours after the test. Check with your state board of nursing to make sure it offers this service and to find out how to access the site. The NCSBN offers a "quick results" service that allows you to obtain unofficial results 2 business days after you take the examination. The cost is about $10. Not all states participate in the service, and your employment agency may or may not accept the results, since they are unofficial.

Some graduates have found a very quick way to get unofficial results in as little as 2 or 3 hours, but more commonly by the next day. After you take the NGN and return home, log on to the Pearson VUE site. Attempt to register for the NGN again under your original login. Register for the exact same test, just as you did when you originally registered. Continue through the registration process until you find the message asking you to pay for the examination. If the site allows you to put in your credit card information, it is an indication that you might have failed the examination. It is best not to do anything else until you get the official results from your state board of nursing. If you get a message saying that you are unable to schedule the NGN because one is already on record, you most likely passed the examination. To double check, try the registration process again later to see if you get the same message.

NGN STUDY STRATEGIES

There are several ways to prepare for examinations, including the NGN. To attempt to take the examination with an attitude of "If I don't know it by now, I never will" is to court failure. Carefully directed study and preparation will considerably increase the chances of passing the test. Review online Bonus Chapter 29 for general tips on how to study for and take examinations. Following is some specific information on preparing for the NGN.

The NCSBN and Pearson VUE Websites

The NCBSN website (https://www.ncsbn.org) can provide significant help as you prepare to take the NGN. It offers the most recent information on any changes in the test and simply lays out the steps to register for the examination. The Pearson VUE site (www.vue.com/nclex) also has a wealth of information, including free sample examination questions. The more you learn about the examination before you take it, the lower your anxiety will be and the better you will do.

Review Books

The material covered by review books is the key material found on the NGN. These books usually follow the NGN test plan very closely. However, a review book is just that: it reviews the material that you should already know. Reviewing is important to reinforce learning and recall of information you may not have used in a year or more.

What Do You Think?

When was the last time you sat in on a group study session? List three of the problems you encountered at the session. How could they be solved?

Review books are not really designed to present any new information about key material. If you are totally unfamiliar with the material in a particular section of the review book, reading a more comprehensive textbook on that particular subject area will be necessary.

An important function of a review book is to point out areas of weakness. If you find a section that seems to contain "new" material, it is important to investigate that section in more detail. If you find most of the material familiar and easy to grasp, you are probably well on your way to passing the NGN.

Group Study

Group study can be an effective method of preparation for an examination such as the NGN. Study groups generally meet once or twice a week.

To optimize the results of group study sessions, several rules should be followed:

Rule 1: Be very selective when choosing the members of the study group. They should have a similar frame of mind and orientation toward studying. They should be graduates who are also going to be taking the NGN. The ideal size for a study group is between four and six people. Groups larger than six become difficult to organize and handle. After the group has been formed and has begun its study sessions, it may be necessary to ask an individual to leave the group for not participating or for being disruptive to the study process or displaying negative attitudes about the examination.

Rule 2: Have each individual prepare a particular section for each group study session. For example, if next week the group is going to study the endocrine system, assign group member 1 the anatomy and physiology of the system, member 2 the pathological conditions, member 3 the medications used for treatment, and member 4 the key elements of nursing care. When the group comes together, have each individual present their prepared section. This type of preparation prevents the "What are we going to study tonight?" syndrome that often plagues group study sessions.

Following this process organizes the study group and allows for more in-depth coverage of the topic. It also permits the members of the group to ask questions of the other members, thereby reinforcing the information being discussed.

Rule 3: Limit the length of the study session. No single study session should be longer than 60 to 90 minutes. Sessions that go longer tend to get off the topic and foster a negative attitude about the examination. Try to avoid making group study sessions into party time. A few snacks and refreshments may be helpful to maintain the group's energy level, but a real party atmosphere will detract significantly from the effectiveness of the study session.

Rule 4: Use role-playing to reinforce information. The more senses you can involve in the learning process, the better the learning.

Rule 5: Remain positive. Although group study times should not be party times, relax and have some fun with the study.

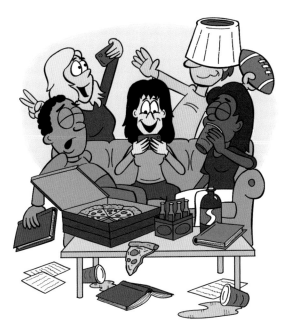

Group study time is not party time!

Individual Study Tips

No matter what other study and preparation methods are used, individual preparation for the NGN is a necessity. This preparation can take several forms:

Tip 1: Use a review book. As previously discussed, use of a review book is valuable to indicate areas of deficient knowledge. Reading and studying the appropriate textbooks and study guides can be helpful when approached correctly. It is important that the graduate mentally organize the information being read into a format similar to that found in the NGN. After reading each page of a textbook or study guide, the graduate should be able to ask three or four multiple-choice questions about that information. These questions can be asked silently or written out and should answer the question, "How might the NGN test my knowledge of this material?"

Tip 2: Take practice examinations on the computer and learn the NGN format. Practice answering questions similar to those found on the examination you are going to take. Most of the review books come with a CD or a link to a website that has practice questions on it. It is almost impossible to replicate the new NGN questions on paper. The disk or electronic access will give you a more realistic sample of what you will see on the actual examination.

The practice questions will help alleviate some of the unknowns, particularly if you have not had a lot of experience with computer-based examinations. Experts recommend that you take between 3,000 and 5,000 practice questions before you take the NGN. Try to take at least 1,000 questions using a computerized format and AFQs. Obviously, starting early in this process (6 months) is important, as are planning and time management. Do not try to take 1,000 questions at a time! For maximum learning, take 50 to 100 at a sitting and review the answers to understand why you missed the ones you missed.

When you answer practice questions, the following important mental processes occur:

Getting comfortable. First, you are becoming more familiar with and therefore more comfortable with the format of the examination. In research, this process is termed the *practice effect*; it must be accounted for when analyzing the results from pretest/post-test types of research projects. Individuals will have better results after a test, even without any type of intervention, because of having practiced answering questions on the pretest. Similarly, your score on the NGN may increase by as much as 10 percent through answering practice questions.

Reinforcing information. A second result of answering practice questions is that it reinforces the information already studied. Although it is unlikely that a question on the NGN examination will be identical to a practice question, there are many similarities. Realistically, only a limited number of questions can be asked about any given subject. After a while, the questions will begin to sound very similar.

Identifying weak spots. A third advantage of answering practice questions is that it quickly reveals subject areas that you need to study. It is relatively easy to say, "I understand the renal system pretty well." It is quite another to answer correctly 10 or 15 questions about that system. If you answer the questions correctly, you can move on to the next topic. If you miss the majority of the questions, however, further review is required.

After you have answered the questions, you need to review them and compare your answers with the answers provided in the study book. You should also look at the rationales and the categories into which the questions fall. Try to understand why you missed the questions you did. Was it lack of knowledge? Did you not read the question carefully? Did you not use critical thinking?

Tip 3: Complete a 150-item test in one sitting in 5 hours. Many websites provide testing materials and sample examinations that will allow you to do this.

Tip 4: Take the NGN as soon as possible after graduation. The NCSBN has done some studies that show the following:

- The NGN taken less than 26 days after graduation has a 91 percent average pass rate.
- The NGN taken between 27 and 39 days after graduation has an 80 percent average pass rate.
- The NGN taken between 40 and 62 days after graduation has a 72 percent average pass rate.
- The NGN taken more than 62 days after graduation has a 45 percent average pass rate.

Formal NGN Reviews

The NCSBN does not endorse or sponsor any review courses for the NGN directly, but many companies offer reviews shortly after graduation. An online comprehensive review course for the NGN examination on the NCSBN website is offered by an independent company. Many of the companies used by nursing schools to provide testing throughout their programs also offer a concentrated NGN review program or course toward the end of the program or just after the student graduates. These review courses range from 2 to 5 days and basically cover the information found in review books. These standalone courses are rather expensive, and the quality of NGN reviews varies. In general, they are only as good as the people who are presenting the material. Also, look at the reported pass rate of the graduates after they take the review. Courses with higher pass rates are probably better. Take the NGN as soon as possible after you finish the review course.

PREPARING FOR THE BIG DAY

Several Months to One Week Before the Examination

1. Get mentally and physically prepared. Eat a good healthy diet; emphasize foods with protein, vitamin K, and calcium. These foods have been shown to help control long-term stress. Exercise regularly. Drink lots of water (64 ounces per day) to rid your body of accumulated toxins. Avoid alcohol, street drugs, and even over-the-counter medications such as antihistamines that can affect your ability to concentrate and think. Ease off on the caffeine, and stop smoking. Start taking a memory-enhancing supplement.
2. Practice doing NGN-type questions—lots of them!
3. Avoid major life-altering activities, such as buying a car or planning a wedding, major vacation, or baby shower!

The Day Before the Examination

1. Do not work. Most employers understand that the NGN produces anxiety and are willing to let you have the day off. If your stress levels are high, it may be difficult for you to concentrate on your work, possibly compromising the health and well-being of your clients.
2. Do something fun and relaxing, but do not overdo it. Activities that involve some moderate exercise will help with anxiety levels. Avoid alcohol and recreational drugs!
3. Eat citrus fruits or drink liquids with vitamin C. Vitamin C has been shown to decrease short-term stress.
4. If you are unfamiliar with the area where the test center is located, drive to the test site. Note parking facilities and places where you can get a meal. This preparation will save you from getting lost the next day and help you be on time.

The Night Before the Examination

1. Make sure you have all the materials you will need for the examination, including two forms of photo ID, authorization to test card, and Social Security card.
2. Review formulas, common medications, and information that can be summarized in tables or on cards and lists. It is probably not a good time to pull out all your old textbooks and notes and try to read them. Concentrate on things that are visual and may have caused you some problems in the past—for example, the list of cranial nerves or the glands and hormones in the endocrine system. Do not try to study everything. The "if I don't know it now, I never will" attitude is a negative thought process. You can always learn something.

3. Avoid strange or exotic foods that you have never eaten before. This can be a real temptation if you have to travel away from home and stay in a hotel the night before the examination. Stick to your usual diet. New or unusual foods may cause some gastrointestinal consequences that can be very distracting during the test.

4. Go to bed at a reasonable hour. It is probably best to stick to your normal schedule. Staying up all night trying to study is counterproductive. You will be nervous and may have some problems sleeping, but stay away from sleep aids. They will interfere with your decision-making ability on the examination. Even if you are not sound asleep, the fact that you are resting will be helpful. Use a relaxation technique involving deep breathing and thought focus.

The Day of the Examination

1. Stick to your regular schedule and routine as much as possible. Avoid drinking excessive amounts of caffeine or sugary beverages to try to stay awake. They will only make you nervous and may increase the amount of time you need to spend on breaks in the restroom.

2. Eat breakfast, especially if you are scheduled for the morning session. Eat something with some glucose for a quick start (bread with jelly) and something with protein to get you through the morning (cereal and milk; eggs and bacon). Drink some cinnamon tea, eat some lemon drop candies, or chew some peppermint gum. These flavors have been reported to enhance learning and sharpen thought processes. If you are taking the examination in the afternoon, eat lunch, but avoid a large meal with a lot of greasy food. It will make you sleepy and sit in your stomach like a lump.

3. Do not let the security at the site fluster you. Security personnel will take a digital picture, palmprint, and signature. They will make you leave all your belongings in lockers at the door. Someone will be walking around the room during the examination, watching the test-takers. Just concentrate on your computer and answer the questions, and you will do fine.

4. Wear comfortable clothes. You do not get extra points on the NGN for looking like a fashion model. Dress appropriately for the season, but keep in mind that some buildings are cool in the summer because of air conditioning and hot in the winter because of heating. Wear something you have worn before. Gym clothes (washed) are a good choice, particularly because you can dress in layers.

5. Think positively! If you truly believe you will do well, you will do well. If you go into the examination with an "I'm never going to pass this—I'm too dumb" attitude, you probably are not going to do as well.

Conclusion

Taking and passing the NGN is a necessary step in the process of becoming a professional registered nurse. Like all licensure examinations, its purpose is to protect the public from undereducated or unsafe practitioners. The examination is comprehensive and includes material from all areas of the graduate's nursing education. Although most graduates have some anxiety about taking this test, knowledge about its format and content and strategies for taking it can lower anxiety.

CRITICAL-THINKING EXERCISES

- Obtain an NGN-RN, CAT review book. Analyze the questions in the practice examination for type, cognitive level, and level of difficulty.
- Identify three to five other students in your class with whom you would feel comfortable working in a study group. Organize a study group session before the next major course examination.
- When you get the results of your next course examination, identify why you missed the questions you missed and what strategies might have been used to answer those questions correctly.

ANSWERS TO QUESTIONS IN CHAPTER 28

1. **Correct answer: 3.** Stokes-Adams syndrome is a suddenly occurring episode of asystole. The client becomes unconscious quickly.
2. **Correct answer: 2.** Nursing diagnoses that deal with the airway always have highest priority.
3. **Correct answer: 3.** Choice 1 is unrealistic for this client; choice 2 is not client-centered; choice 4 is a nursing intervention, not a goal. Maintaining an oxygen saturation of 90 percent is realistic, measurable, and within normal limits.
4. **Correct answer: 4.** These are symptoms of a pulmonary embolism, which is a common complication of prolonged bed rest.
5. **Correct answer: 3.** Answer 3 lists some side effects of theophylline medications that may indicate the onset of toxicity. The physician needs to know about these toxic side effects so that the medication can be stopped and the dosage of the medication reduced when it is restarted.

NCLEX-STYLE QUESTIONS

1. Which activity associated with the American Nurses Association (ANA) has the greatest impact on the quality of care provided by a nurse at a patient's bedside?
   1. Accrediting nursing education programs
   2. Publishing standards of professional nursing practice
   3. Lobbying economic issues impacting the profession of nursing
   4. Mentoring the professional development of future registered nurses
2. A nurse in a health clinic is assessing a preschool-age child. Which behaviors that may indicate a developmental delay should the nurse bring to the attention of the health-care provider? **Select all that apply.**
   1. Goes up and down stairs using both feet on each step
   2. Is unable to dress self without assistance
   3. Has imprecise fine motor skills
   4. Uses magical thinking
   5. Falls frequently
3. An upper-level nurse manager is assessing the qualities of several nurses who demonstrate leadership abilities for a promotion to a first-level management position. Which ability is required of a nurse manager that is not a necessity for a leader?
   1. Thinks critically
   2. Understands budgets
   3. Collaborates effectively
   4. Demonstrates competence
4. Which activity is appropriate for an unlicensed assistive personnel (UAP) to implement?
   1. Collecting urine for a 24-hour creatinine clearance test
   2. Giving an obese client a brochure on an 1,800-calorie diet
   3. Placing a tube feeding pump on hold while bathing a client
   4. Helping with the insertion of a nasogastric (NG) tube by a health-care provider
5. Which documentation regarding the administration of a medication is recorded accurately according to The Joint Commission?
   1. Coumadin 5 mg QOD for 7 days
   2. Heparin 5,000 units Sub-Q daily
   3. $MgSO_4$ 1.0 g for hypertension
   4. Calcium 600 mg po qd
6. A nurse is planning care for a client who is a Jehovah's Witness. What action is most appropriate?
   1. Ensure that a kosher menu is provided for meal selection.
   2. Verify with certainty that the client does not want a blood transfusion.
   3. Assign a female UAP to help the client with activities of daily living.
   4. Consult with the dietitian regarding the avoidance of meat and milk during the same meal.

7. A health-care provider orders a dose of a medication for a child at 2 mg/kg of body weight. The child weighs 64 pounds. How much medication should be given to the child? Round to the nearest whole number.

_____

8. A nurse is caring for an older adult and suspects that the client may be experiencing hypovolemia. Which clinical indicator supports the nurse's suspicion?
   1. Distended neck veins
   2. Bradycardia
   3. Dilute urine
   4. Weak pulse

9. A nurse must obtain a sputum specimen from a client with an endotracheal tube. Place the following steps in the order in which they should be performed.
   _____ 1. Verify the order and wash the hands.
   _____ 2. Don a protective eye shield and sterile gloves.
   _____ 3. Apply suction when the patient coughs or when meeting resistance.
   _____ 4. Lubricate the catheter tip with normal saline and advance it into the endotracheal tube.
   _____ 5. Remove the catheter and attach the tubing on the specimen container to the attached adapter.

10. A nurse is preparing to teach a client about the medication atorvastatin (Lipitor). Which information is important to emphasize in the teaching?
   1. Replace monosaturated oils in the diet with polyunsaturated fatty acids.
   2. Notify the health-care provider of muscle pain, weakness, or fever.
   3. Avoid crushing and mixing the medication with applesauce.
   4. Take this medication during a meal or with food.

References

1. Morris G. What you need to know about NCLEX changes. *NurseJournal*, 2022. https://nursejournal.org/articles/what-you-need-to-know-about-nclex-changes/
2. Seidu Y. What is changing on the NextGen NCLEX? Nurse-Pective, 2022. https://nursepective.com/next-gen-nclex-2023/
3. The Next Generation NCLEX. RegisteredNurseRN.com, 2022. https://www.registerednursern.com/next-generation-nclex/
4. The Next Generation NCLEX (NGN). NurseAchieve, 2022. https://www.nurseachieve.com/ngn
5. Betts J, Muntean W, Kim D, Kao S. The Next Generation NCLEX®: Test plan. *Next Generation NCLEX News*, Winter 2022. https://ncsbn.org/public-files/NGN_Winter22_English_Final.pdf
6. NGN FAQs for candidates. National Council of State Boards of Nursing, 2022. https://ncsbn.org/exams/next-generation-nclex/NGN+FAQS/ngn-faqs-for-candidates.page

Glossary

Inclusion of particular ideas or practices in this glossary does not imply endorsement of them. Healthcare practitioners and their clients must carefully evaluate the claims and qualifications of integrative healing practices and practitioners before coming to conclusions about them.

3D bioprinting A process, still experimental, whereby 3D printers are able to reproduce a variety of medical implants and even implantable organs.

abandonment Leaving a client without the client's permission; terminating the professional relationship without providing for appropriate continued or follow-up care by another equally qualified professional.

accountability Concept that each individual is responsible for their own actions and the consequence of those actions; professional accountability implies a responsibility to perform the activities and duties of the profession according to established standards.

accreditation Approval of a program or institution by a voluntary professional organization to provide specific education or service programs.

acculturation The altering of a person's own cultural practices in an attempt to become more like members of the new culture or major culture.

act Legislation that has become law.

active euthanasia Acts performed to help end a sick person's life.

active shooter An individual who uses a firearm with the intention of wounding or killing people in a confined or populated area.

act utilitarianism A theory of ethics based on consequentialism that states that a person's act is morally right if (and only if) it produces the best possible results or the greatest good in that specific situation.

acute-severe condition Health problem of sudden onset; a serious illness or condition.

adaptation Process of exchange between a person and the environment to maintain or regain personal integrity; the key principle in the Roy model of nursing.

administration The act or process of running an organization. As a noun, one of the three main branches of government that approves and enforces legislation.

administrative rule or regulation An operating procedure that describes how a government agency implements the intent of a statute; state boards of nursing implement the nurse practice act.

advanced nursing education Master's- or doctoral-level education that provides knowledge and skills in areas such as research, education, administration, and clinical specialties.

advanced placement A process by which a student is given credit for a required course through transfer or examination rather than by enrolling in and completing the course.

advanced practice Extended role; increased responsibilities and actions undertaken by an individual because of additional education and experience; nurse practitioners, nurse midwives, and nurse anesthetists are all advanced practice nurses.

advocate One who pleads for a cause or proposal; one who acts on behalf of another.

affective domain objectives Goals established in conjunction with the client that are directed toward changing feelings, values, and attitudes necessary for a positive effect on the client's health.

affidavit Written, sworn statement.

affiliation agreement A formal agreement between an educational institution and another agency that agrees to provide clinical areas for student practice.

aggressiveness Harsh behavior that may result in physical or emotional harm to others.

Alexander technique A technique developed by Frederick Matthias Alexander that realigns body posture through imaging and relaxation. Decreases muscle tension and fatigue, stress, and back and neck pain. Based on the belief that poor posture during daily activities contributes to physical and emotional problems.

allopathic medicine A synonym for conventional Western medicine. Practitioner uses medicines to counteract symptoms or heal by producing different effects or a second condition different from the one being treated. From the Greek words *allos* (other) and *pathos* (suffering).

ambulatory care center Type of primary care facility that provides treatment on an outpatient basis.

anesthesia A loss of sensitivity to pain; commonly artificially induced before or during surgical procedures by administering gases or injecting medications.

anesthetics Medications that cause loss of sensitivity to pain; can be local or general; include medications such as narcotics, analgesics, sedatives, opiates, and others.

answer Document filed in the court by the defendant in response to the complaint.

anticipatory grief A deep feeling of anguish, sadness, emotional pain, and suffering that an individual experiences before an imminent loss, such as the death of a loved one or loss of a body part such as a limb.

anxiety Uneasiness or apprehension caused by an impending threat or fear of the unknown.

apathy Lack of interest.

appeal Request to a higher court to review a decision in the hope of changing the ruling of a lower court.

appellant Person who seeks an appeal.

applied ethics One of the three divisions of the philosophy of ethics that attempts to develop a framework by which decisions can be judged as ethical or unethical. Applied ethics combines normative ethics and metaethics to help determine the morality of specific actions.

applied kinesiology Study of muscle activity, strength, and health effects through the muscle–gland–organ link. Muscle dysfunction may be counteracted by nutrition, manual procedures (e.g., massage), pressure over muscle attachment points, and realignment.

arbitrator Neutral third party who assesses facts independently of the judicial system.

aromatherapy A type of herbal therapy that uses the odors of essential oils extracted from plants to treat various conditions, such as headaches, tension, and anxiety. Chemical composition of the oils produces pharmacological effects that include antibacterial, antiviral, antispasmodic, diuretic, vasodilative, and mood-harmonizing actions. The oils may be applied by massage, inhaled, placed in baths, and other forms of hydrotherapy, or taken internally.

art therapy Use of artistic self-expression through drawing, sculpture, and painting to diagnose and treat behavioral or emotional problems.

articulation Type of education program that allows easy entry from one level to another; for example, many BSN programs have articulation for nurses with associate degrees.

artificial insemination Insertion of sperm into the uterus with a syringe.

artificial intelligence An electronic device or system that can accurately interpret input data, modify its internal systems from the data, and use the modified data to achieve specific goals or tasks through the application of flexible adaptation.

assault An overt threat to violate a person's right to self-determination or an overt threat of bodily harm coupled with an apparent, present ability to cause the harm. The actual production of harm is *battery*.

assertiveness Ability to express thoughts, feelings, and ideas openly and directly without fear.

assessment Process of collecting information about a client to help plan care.

assignment Designating tasks for ancillary personnel that fall under their *own level of practice* according to facility policies, position descriptions, and, if applicable, state practice act.

assisted suicide Also known as "aid-in-dying," is a decision made by a person to end their life with the help of another person. The other person may be a medical professional, relative or friend who agrees to participate in the act. It is illegal in most states.

associate degree nursing program Type of nursing education program that leads to an associate degree with a major in nursing; usually located in a community or junior college, these programs normally last 2 years.

asymmetrical information The use of multiple data sources in economics and business that produces a better understanding of day-to-day economic activity.

audit Close review of records or documents to detect the presence or absence of specific information.

aura Magnetic field thought to surround every person, plant, and animal. Adjustment of the field is believed to affect health, emotions, spirit, and mind.

auriculotherapy A method developed in France in which points on the external ear are stimulated with acupuncture needles, massage, electronics, or infrared treatment. These points are believed to have neurological connections to other body areas. Also called *ear acupuncture.*

auscultation Assessment technique that requires listening with a stethoscope to various parts of the body to detect sounds produced by organs.

authoritarian Type of leadership style in which the leader gives orders, makes decisions for the group as a whole, and bears most of the responsibility for the outcomes. Also called *autocratic, directive,* or *controlling.*

automated external defibrillator (AED) A defibrillator that performs all the functions by computer (analyses rhythm, selects an energy level, charges the machine, and shocks the patient). The operator applies adhesive paddles and turns the machine on, then makes certain that no one is in contact with the patient.

autonomy State of being self-directed or independent; the ability to make decisions about one's future.

autopsy Examination of a body after passing to determine the cause of death.

ayurvedic medicine A personalistic, holistic, and naturalistic approach to health maintenance and treatment of illness, originating in India. Maintains balance of the three doshas (bioenergies) of the body through diet and herbs, meditation, breathing exercises (pranayama), massage with medicated oils, yoga and other forms of vigorous exercise, and exposure to the sun for higher consciousness.

baccalaureate degree nursing program Type of nursing education program that leads to the bachelor's degree with a major in nursing; usually located in a college or university, the length of the program is 4 years.

Bach flower essences Homeopathic preparations of oil concentrates extracted from flowers. Originated by Edward Bach, an English physician, this method is aimed at emotional states rather than the signs and symptoms of physical illness. Specific concentrates or combinations of concentrates are associated with various emotional states. Each client is diagnosed individually because there is no corresponding psychological equivalent for every physical state.

bargaining agent Organization certified by a governmental agency to represent a group of employees for the purpose of collective bargaining.

baseline data Initial information obtained about a client that establishes the norms for comparison as the client's condition changes.

basic human rights Those considerations society deems reasonably expected for all people: right to self-determination, protection from discomfort and harm, dignity, fair treatment, and privacy.

battery Nonconsensual touching of another person that does not necessarily cause harm or injury.

behavior modification Method to change behavior through rewards for positive behavior.

behaviorism Psychological theory based on the belief that all behavior is learned over time through conditioning.

belief Expectations or judgments based on attitude verified by experiences.

benchmarking Written outcome standards used to classify acceptable levels of performance to maintain high-quality care.

beneficence Ethical principle based on the beliefs that the health-care provider should do no harm, prevent harm, remove existing harm, and promote the good and well-being of the client.

bereavement State of sadness brought on by the loss or death of a loved one.

best practices Clinical nursing actions that are based on the "best evidence" available from nursing research.

bias An influence that produces a distortion in the results of a research study.

bill Proposed law that is moving through the legislative process.

bill of rights List of statements that outline the claims and privileges of a particular group, such as the Client's Bill of Rights.

bioethical issues Issues that deal with the health, safety, life, and death of human beings, often arising from advances in medical science and technology.

bioethics The study of ethical situations and questions that relate to the spectrum of human health-related life sciences such as biology, psychology, medical experimentation, biotechnology, scarce resources, genomics, and more.

biofeedback Ability to control autonomic responses in the body through conscious effort.

Biological Aerosol Warning System (BAWS) A high-tech biological agent detection device that is capable of detecting biological agents in the environment.

bioterrorism The use of microorganisms with the deliberate intent of causing infection to achieve military or political goals.

black belts Individuals certified as Six Sigma consultants through the Institute of Industrial and Systems Engineers or the American Society for Quality who are trained employees of Six Sigma working as well-paid consultants for hospitals and other institutions.

blameless reporting The ability of an employee to recount a negative incident to a superior in the work environment without the fear of chastisement or retribution.

body substance isolation (BSI) Universal precautions; guidelines established by the Centers for Disease Control and Prevention (CDC) and the Occupational Safety and Health Administration (OSHA) to protect health-care professionals and the client from diseases carried in the blood and body fluids, such as HIV and hepatitis B; involves the use of gloves whenever one is in contact with blood or body fluids and the use of masks, gowns, and eye covers if a chance exists of aerosol contact with fluids.

bodywork General term used to describe various forms of massage therapy, energy balancing, deep-tissue manipulation, and movement awareness.

bot Short for *robot*, a repetitive software program that is inserted into the Internet or social media to present false or misleading information to large groups of people.

botanical medicine The use of plant-based medications or treatments, such as algae, fungi, leaves, roots, and liquid substances produced by various plants, for illness or a disease process or for the maintenance of a healthy state.

brain death Irreversible destruction of the cerebral cortex and brain stem manifested by absence of all reflexes; absence of brain waves on an electroencephalogram.

breach of contract Failure by one of the parties in a contract to fulfill all the terms of the agreement.

bullying A type of uncivil behavior that could reasonably be considered humiliating, intimidating, threatening, or demeaning to an individual or group of individuals. It can occur anywhere and at times becomes habitual, being repeated over and over.

burden of proof Requirement that the plaintiff submit sufficient evidence to prove a defendant's guilt.

burnout syndrome A state of emotional exhaustion that results from the accumulative stress of an individual's life, including work, personal, and family responsibilities.

cadaver donor Clinically dead or brain-dead individual who previously agreed to allow organs to be taken for transplantation.

capitated payment system System of reimbursement in which a flat fee is paid for health-care services for a prescribed period of time. Expenses incurred in excess of this fee are provider losses.

capricious Unpredictable; arbitrary.

career ladder Articulation of educational programs that permit advancement from a lower level to a higher level without loss of credit or repetition of coursework.

career mobility Opportunity for individuals in one occupational area to move to another without restrictions.

care pathways Standardized sets of processes or management guidelines that guide the health care for patients with specific conditions; used to improve the quality of care by guiding the plan of care from first contact with a health-care provider to attainment of specified health outcomes.

case management Health-care delivery in which a client advocate or health-care coordinator helps the client through the hospitalization to obtain the most appropriate care.

case manager Health-care provider who coordinates cost-effective quality care for individuals who are generally at high risk and require long-term complex services.

case study An in-depth qualitative study of a selected phenomenon involving a person, a group of people, or an institution.

causal relationship A relationship between variables in which the presence or absence of one variable (known as the "cause") will determine the presence or absence of the other variable (known as the "effect").

certification Official recognition of a degree of education and skills in a profession by a national specialty organization; recognition that an institution has met standards that allow it to deliver certain services.

chain of command The order in which authority and power in an organization are wielded and delegated from top management to every employee at every level of the organization. It is usually outlined in the organization's administrative flow chart.

chakras Ancient Sanskrit term for energetic circles found along the midline of the body, in alignment with the spinal cord, that distribute energy throughout the body. If they are blocked, energy flow is inhibited.

challenge examination Examination that assesses levels of knowledge or skill to grant credit for previous learning and experience; passing a challenge examination gives the individual credit for a course not actually taken.

chart Legal document that contains all the pertinent information about a client who is in a hospital or clinic; usually includes medical and nursing history, medical and nursing diagnosis, laboratory test results, notes about the client's progress, physician's orders, and personal data.

charting Process of recording (written or computer-generated) specific information about the client in the chart or medical record.

chelation therapy Use of minerals combined with amino acids, given intravenously or orally, to help cleanse the body of unnecessary or toxic minerals that block blood circulation. From the Greek word *chele* (to bind or to claw).

chemotherapy (also chemo, CTX, or CTx) The treatment of disease by the use of chemical substances ranging from low-toxicity chemical agents such as antibiotics to agents with a high level of toxicity such as those used to treat cancer.

chi (qi, shi) From traditional Chinese medicine. Chi is the invisible life force that circulates through the body along meridians, or channels. Maintaining or restoring the flow of chi restores and promotes health.

chiropractic A Western medical system postulating that partial joint dislocations (subluxations) cause the body to be misaligned. Removal or adjustment of subluxations balances the spinal–nervous system and restores and maintains health.

civil law Law concerned with the violation of the rights of one individual by another; it includes contract law, treaty law, tax law, and tort law.

claims-made policy Type of malpractice insurance that protects only against claims made during the time the policy is in effect.

client More modern term for *patient;* an individual seeking or receiving health-related services.

client goal Statement about a desired change, outcome, or activity that a client should achieve by a specific time.

clinical component The portion of a student's nursing education program that involves applying knowledge learned in the classroom to the actual treatment and care of patients in a health-care setting.

clinical education Hands-on part of a nursing program that allows the student to practice skills on actual clients under the supervision of a nursing instructor.

clinical forensic nurse Professional nurse who specializes in management of crime victims from trauma to trial through collection of evidence, assessment of victims, or making judgments related to client treatment associated with court-related issues.

Clinical Judgment Measurement Model (CJMM) A model developed by the National Council of State Boards of Nursing that measures the graduate's ability to make valid decisions using their clinical judgment and decision-making skills. This model serves as the basis for Next Generation NCLEX.

clinical ladder Type of performance evaluation and career advancement in which nursing positions for direct client care have two or more progressive levels of required skill leading to advancement in salary and responsibility; it allows nurses to remain in direct client care while making career advancements rather than having to move into administration.

clinical nurse specialist (CNS) An advanced practice nurse who specializes in one or more areas of nursing practice; works in a wide variety of health-care settings; and provides diagnosis, treatment, and ongoing management of patients. The CNS also provides expertise and support to nurses caring for patients at the bedside, helps drive practice changes throughout the organization, and ensures the use of best practices and evidence-based care to achieve the best possible patient outcomes.

clinical pathways Case-management protocols used to enhance quality of care, encourage cost-effectiveness, and promote efficiency.

closed system System that does not exchange energy, matter, or information with the environment or with other systems.

code of ethics Written values of a profession that act as guidelines for professional behavior.

coping skills (coping strategies or coping mechanisms) Tools and techniques that can be used to deal with difficult emotions, such as anger, anxiety, sadness, or stress, and establish or maintain a sense of internal order. Coping skills can be either healthy or unhealthy.

clustered regularly interspaced short palindromic repeat (CRISPR) A family of DNA sequences found in the genomes of prokaryotic (without a nucleus or internal membrane) organisms such as bacteria and archaea (single-celled organisms without nuclei). CRISPR technology is used by research scientists to selectively modify the DNA of living organisms; it plays a key role in the antiviral defense system, providing a form of acquired immunity.

cognitive domain objectives Most basic type of objectives for client learning that merely outline the knowledge that will be taught to the client.

collaboration A cooperative venture among those with a common goal.

collective bargaining Negotiations for wages, hours, benefits, and working conditions for a group of employees.

collective bargaining unit Group of employees recognized as representatives of the majority, with the right to bargain collectively with their employer and to reach an agreement on the terms of a contract.

committee Group of legislators, in the House or Senate, assigned to analyze bills on a particular subject.

common law Law based on past judicial judgments made in similar cases.

community rating A method of calculating health insurance premium costs that is based on the risk factors attributed to all people in a particular region or the nation as a whole. It requires health insurance companies to charge everyone in the group the same rates and prevents them from changing rates based on the history of claims or the health status of any one or small group of individuals. It is rarely used in the private insurance market but widely used by the government.

comparable worth Method for determining employees' salaries within an organization so that the same salary is paid for all jobs that have equivalent educational requirements, responsibilities, and complexity regardless of external market factors.

comparative effectiveness research (CER) A method to determine the priority of research topics developed by the Institute of Medicine, based on client outcomes both in and outside the institutional setting.

compensatory damages Awards that cover the actual cost of injuries and economic losses caused by the injury in a lawsuit including all medical expenses related to the injury and any lost wages or income that resulted from extended hospitalization or recovery period. Also called *actual damages*.

competencies Behaviors, skills, attitudes, and knowledge that an individual or professional has or is expected to have.

Competency Outcomes and Performance Assessment (COPA) model An assessment tool used by medical schools and some schools of nursing to validate the skills and knowledge of their graduates and promote competency for clinical practice at all levels.

competency-based education Courses or programs based on anticipated student outcomes.

complaint Legal document filed by a plaintiff to initiate a lawsuit, claiming that the plaintiff's legal rights have been violated.

compliance Voluntary following of a prescribed plan of care or treatment regimen.

computer technology Use of highly advanced technological equipment to store, process, and access a vast amount of information.

concept Abstract idea or image.

conceptual framework Concept, theory, or basic idea around which an educational program is organized and developed.

conceptual model Group of concepts, ideas, or theories that are interrelated but in which the relationship is not clearly defined.

confidentiality Right of the client to expect the communication with a professional to remain unshared with any other person unless a medical reason exists or unless the safety of the public is threatened.

conflict management The use of interpersonal communication skills and reason to reduce the tension and disagreement between employees who hold strong opinions and views about a particular project or idea with the goal of achieving conflict resolution.

conflict resolution Using conflict management skills to bring together individuals or groups who disagree so that conflicts are resolved fairly and closure is achieved on the disagreement, moving the group toward achievement of the ultimate goal.

consensus General agreement between two or more individuals or groups regarding beliefs or positions on an issue or finding.

consent Voluntary permission given by a competent person.

consortium Two or more agencies that share sponsorship of a program or an institution.

constitutional law Law contained within a federal or state constitution.

continuing care Nursing care generally provided in geriatric day-care centers or in the homes of elderly clients.

continuing education Formal education programs and informal learning experiences that maintain and increase the nurse's knowledge and skills in specific areas.

continuing education unit (CEU) Specific unit of credit earned by participating in an approved continuing education program.

continuous positive airway pressure (CPAP) A type of noninvasive ventilation (NIV) similar to PEEP, but the pressure applied is maintained throughout the respiratory cycle (during both inspiration and expiration), preventing the collapse of the alveoli at the end of the respiratory cycle.

continuous quality improvement (CQI) Type of total quality management whose primary goal is the improvement of the quality of health care.

contract Legally binding agreement between two or more parties.

contractual obligation Duty to perform a service identified by a contract.

copayment Percentage of the cost of a medical expense that is not covered by insurance and must be paid by the client.

core curriculum Curriculum design that enables a student to leave a career program at various levels, with a career attained and with the option to continue at another higher level or career; it is organized around a central or core body of knowledge common to the profession.

coroner Elected public official, usually a physician, who investigates deaths from unnatural causes, including homicide, violence, suicide, and other suspicious circumstances.

correctional/institutional nurse Registered nurse who specializes in the health care of those in custody in secure settings such as jails or prisons.

correlation The degree of association between two variables.

cost sharing (cost matching) Medication or health-care costs that are not paid by an insuring agency but are covered by other entities, including cash from the patient, awards, or coverage from other insurers such as the federal government.

craniosacral therapy Manipulation of the bones of the skull to treat craniosacral dysfunctions caused by restriction in the flow of cerebrospinal fluid and misalignment of bones. *Cranio* refers to the cranium and *sacral* to the sacrum.

credentialing Process whereby individuals, programs, or institutions are designated as having met minimal standards for the safety and welfare of the public.

crime Violation of criminal law.

criminal action Process by which a person charged with a crime is accused, tried, and punished.

criminal law Law concerned with violation of criminal statutes or laws.

criterion-referenced examination Test that compares an individual's knowledge to a predetermined standard rather than to the performance of others who take the same test.

critical discernment The ability to sift through and carefully assess all available and credible research findings by analysis and judgment so that recommendations for using the best practice techniques can be made on the basis of best evidence.

critical incident An occurrence, mistake, accident, or event that is unusual, sudden, and unexpected that may produce physical harm, emotional stress, or a threat to life.

critical incident stress debriefing (CISD) A process to help health-care providers deal with major acts of violence and trauma. The process is performed by teams of mental health professionals specially trained in crisis intervention, stress management, and treating posttraumatic stress disorder with the goal of encouraging the participants to verbalize their feelings and thoughts, identify and develop their coping skills, and generally lower overall grief and anxiety levels.

critical pathways Plans that organize and demonstrate health-care goals for patients and develop the sequence and timing of actions necessary to achieve these goals; are a method to standardize care, increase efficiency in the use of resources, and improve health care quality; also known as *critical paths, clinical pathways,* or *care paths.*

critical thinking The intellectual process of rationally examining ideas, inferences, assumptions, principles, arguments, conclusions, issues, statements, beliefs, and actions for which all the relevant information may not be available. This process involves the ability to use the five types of reasoning (scientific, deductive, inductive, informal, practical) in application of the nursing process, decision making, and resolution of ambiguous issues.

crystal therapy Use of quartz and other gemstones, believed to emit electromagnetic energy. Frequently used with light and color therapy. Also called *gem therapy.*

cultural competence The provision of effective care for clients who belong to diverse cultures, based on the nurse's knowledge and understanding of the values, customs, beliefs, and practices of the culture.

cultural synergy The commitment that health-care providers make not only to learn about other cultures but also to immerse themselves in those cultures. Nurses achieve cultural synergy when they begin to selectively include values, customs, and beliefs of other cultures in their own world views.

cupping From traditional Chinese medicine and ayurvedic practice. Method using a heated cup placed over the skin to draw out impurities, decrease blood pressure, increase circulation, and relieve muscle pain.

curanderismo Healing tradition, found in Mexican American communities, based in concepts of supernaturalism, balance, and holism. From the Spanish verb *to heal.*

curriculum Group of courses that prepare an individual for a specific degree or profession.

customary, prevailing, and reasonable charges The typical rate in a specific locale that payers traditionally reimburse physicians.

damages Money awarded to a plaintiff by a court in a lawsuit that covers the actual costs incurred by the plaintiff.

dance therapy Use of dance movement to enhance wellness and aid healing. Sharpens levels of awareness, enhances self-confidence, helps with motor coordination and physical skills, and assists with communication, especially with severely disturbed psychiatric clients.

dashboards Electronic tools that act as a scorecard providing retrospective or real-time data to assess the quality of client care and assisting the process of quality improvement.

data cleaning The process of detecting and correcting (or removing) corrupt or inaccurate data points, including identifying incomplete, incorrect, inaccurate, or irrelevant parts of the data set and then replacing them with accurate information after data has been entered into the system.

database Information collected by a computer program on a specific topic in a specified format.

death panels A political term coined to falsely suggest that the Affordable Care Act allowed bureaucrats to decide which persons should live and which should die as a cost-saving measure.

decoding In human communication, it is the process of receiving a message, both verbal and nonverbal, from a sender, then analyzing and interpreting the message so that the receiver can understand the meaning of the sender's message. In electronic data management, it is the process of converting electronic characters into the original sequence of letters, numbers, or other symbols.

defamation of character Communication of information that is false or detrimental to a person's reputation.

defendant Person accused of criminal or civil wrongdoing. A party to a lawsuit against whom the complaint is served.

defibrillator A device that delivers an electrical shock that completely depolarizes the myocardium, producing a brief period of asystole. The goal of defibrillation is to let the sinoatrial node recover control of the heart's electrical activity and terminate potentially fatal heart rhythms, such as ventricular tachycardia and ventricular fibrillation.

delegation Assignment of specific duties by one individual to another individual.

democratic Type of leadership style in which the leader shares the planning, decision making, and responsibilities for outcomes with the other members of the group. Also called *participative leadership.*

deontology Ethical system based on the principle that the right action is guided by a set of unchanging rules.

dependent practitioner Provider of care who delivers health care under the supervision of another health-care practitioner; for example, a physician's assistant is supervised by a physician, and an LPN is supervised by an RN.

dependent variable *Depends on,* or is altered as a direct result of, the researcher's manipulation.

deposition Sworn statement by a witness that is made outside the courtroom; sworn depositions may be admitted as evidence in court when the individual is unable to be present.

diagnosis Statement that describes or identifies a client problem and is based on a thorough assessment.

diagnosis-related groups (DRGs) The classification system as the basis of the prospective payment method used by the U.S. government and many insurance companies that pay a flat fee for treatment of a person with a particular diagnosis.

differentiated practice Organizational process of defining nursing roles based on education, experience, and training.

dilemma Predicament in which a choice must be made between two or more equally balanced alternatives; it often occurs when attempting to make ethical decisions.

directed services Health-care activities that require contact between a health-care professional and a client.

discharge planning Assessment of anticipated client needs after discharge from the hospital and development of a plan to meet those needs before the client is discharged.

disease Illness; a functional disturbance resulting from an individual organism's inability to adapt to certain stressors; an abnormal physiologic state caused by microorganisms, cancer, or other conditions.

distributive justice Ethical principle based on the belief that the right action is determined by that which will provide an outcome equal for all persons and will also benefit the least fortunate.

donut hole A gap in prescription drug coverage during which a person may pay more for prescription drugs. A person enters the donut hole when the Medicare Part D plan has paid a certain amount toward prescription drugs during a coverage year, making the individual pay more out of pocket for the cost of prescriptions until a yearly limit is reached. After exiting the donut hole, a person will receive *catastrophic coverage,* meaning that they will pay 5 percent of a drug's cost or a small copay.

doshas Three basic metabolic types (*vata, pitta,* and *kapha*), life forces, or bioenergies in ayurvedic medicine. Each has certain characteristics and tendencies that combine to determine a person's constitution. When they are in balance, mind and body are coordinated, resulting in vibrant health and energy. When they are out of balance, the body is susceptible to outside stressors, such as microorganisms, poor nutrition, and work overload.

due process Right to have specific procedures or processes followed before the deprivation of life, liberty, or property; the guarantee of privileges under the 5th and 14th Amendments to the U.S. Constitution.

duty Obligation to act created by a statute, contract, or voluntary agreement.

electronic signature (or e-signature) A type of signature on a totally electronic record or document that has the same legal standing as a handwritten signature as long as it adheres to the requirements of the National Institute of Standards and Technology–Digital Signature Standard (NIST-DSS) regulations in the United States.

emerging health occupations Health-care occupations that are not yet officially recognized by government or professional organizations.

empirical evidence Objective data gathered through use of the human senses.

employee Individual hired for pay by another.

Employee Retirement Income Security Act (ERISA) Federal law that grants incentives to employers to offer self-funded health insurance plans to their employees.

employer Individual or organization that hires other individuals for pay to carry out specific duties during certain hours of employment.

empowerment Process in which the individual assumes increased autonomy and responsibility for their actions.

encoding In human communication, it is the process of a sender transforming an abstract idea by using words, symbols, pictures, sounds, or other communication techniques, into a message that the reader can understand. In electronic data management, it is the process of converting a sequence of characters (letters, numbers, punctuation, symbols, and even human language) into a specialized format or code that a computer or electronic device can read for transmission or storage.

end product Output of a system not reusable as input.

endorsement Reciprocity; a state's acceptance of a license issued by another state.

energy Capacity to do work.

energy medicine Measurement of electromagnetic frequencies emitted by the body. The object is to diagnose energy imbalances that may cause or contribute to present or future illnesses and to use electromagnetic forces to counteract imbalances and restore the body's energy balance.

entry into practice Minimal educational requirements to obtain a license for a profession.

environment Internal and external physical and social boundaries of humans; all those things that are outside a system.

environmental medicine Method that explores the role of environmental and dietary allergens in health and illness.

epidemiologist One who studies the distribution and determinants of health and illness and the application of findings as a means of promoting health and preventing illness.

essentials for accreditation Minimal standards that a program must meet to be accredited.

ethical dilemma Ethical situation that requires an individual to make a choice between two equally unfavorable alternatives.

ethical rights (moral rights) Rights that are based on moral or ethical principles but have no legal mechanism of enforcement.

ethical standards Standards determined by principles of moral values and moral conduct.

ethical system System of moral judgments based on the beliefs and values of a profession.

ethics Principles or standards of conduct that govern an individual or group.

ethnic group Individuals who share similar physical characteristics, religion, language, or customs.

ethnography A qualitative research approach involving the study of cultural groups.

euthanasia A word that is derived from Greek, '*Eu*' meaning 'good' and '*thanatos*' meaning 'death.' Together, euthanasia simply means 'a good death'. It is divided into two types: Active Euthanasia and Passive Euthanasia.

evaluation Fifth step in the nursing process; used to determine whether goals set for a client have been attained.

evaluation criteria Outcome criteria; desired behaviors or standards.

evidence reports Documents that provide a scientific basis for a disease or a nursing practice and then integrate research data into actions used in practice. They synthesize previous and current knowledge related to the topic, review the information for quality and documentation, explain how evidence-based practice (EBP) is currently being used, and discuss how useful the EBP is to the clinical practice.

evidence-based practice (EBP) The selective and practical use of the best evidence, as demonstrated by research, to guide health-care implementation and decisions.

expanded role Extended role; increased responsibilities and actions undertaken by an individual because of additional education and experience.

experience rating Similar in concept to risk rating, experience rating establishes insurance premiums based on the history of the individual. Often used in calculating lost work days due to illness or injury in workman's compensation cases, it compares the lost days of the individual to what would normally be expected for individuals in the same class.

experimental research design A quantitative research design that meets all of the following criteria: an experimental variable that is manipulated, at least one experimental and one comparison group, and random assignments of participants to either the experimental or the comparison group.

expert witness Individual with knowledge beyond the ordinary person, resulting from special education or training, who testifies during a trial.

exploratory study The descriptive examination of available data to become as familiar as possible with the information.

external degree Academic degree granted when all the requirements have been met by the student; a type of outcomes-based education in which credit is given when the individual demonstrates a certain level of knowledge and skill, regardless of how or when these skills are attained; challenge examinations are often used.

false imprisonment Intentional tort committed by illegally confining or restricting a client against his or her will.

family Two or more related individuals living together.

Federal Tort Claims Act Statute that allows the government to be sued for negligence of its employees in the performance of their duties; many states have similar laws.

fee for service Payment is expected each time a service is rendered. Includes physicians' office visits, diagnostic procedures (laboratory tests, x-rays), and minor surgical procedures.

feedback Reentry of output into a system as input that helps maintain the internal balance of the system.

feedback loop As used in systems theory or nursing care models, it is the continuous provision of information about the effectiveness of treatments back to the health-care provider that allows them to adjust the treatments for optimal effectiveness.

Feldenkrais method A type of bodywork or physical movement developed by Moshe Feldenkrais that stresses awareness through movement and helps the body work with gravity. Incorporates imaging, active moving, and forms of directed attention designed to reeducate the nervous system, teach subjects how to learn from their own kinesic feedback, and avoid movements that strain joints and muscles.

fellowship Scholarship or grant that provides money to individuals who are highly qualified or highly intelligent.

felony Serious crime that may be punished by a fine of more than $1,000, more than 1 year in jail or prison, death, or a combination thereof.

fidelity The obligation of an individual to be faithful to commitments made to self and others.

foreign graduate nurse Individual graduated from a school of nursing outside the United States. This individual is required to pass the U.S. NCLEX-RN CAT to become a registered nurse in the United States.

forensic nurse Registered nurse who specializes in the integration of forensic science and nursing science to apply the nursing process to individual clients, their families, and the community, bridging the gap between the health-care system and the criminal justice system.

forensic psychiatric nurse Registered nurse who specializes in application of psychosocial nursing knowledge linking offending behavior to client characteristics; nurse specializing in forensic psychological evaluation and care of offender populations with mental disorders.

forensic science Body of empirical knowledge used for legal investigation and evidence-based judgment in police or criminal cases.

for-profit Health-care agencies in which profits can be used to raise capital to pay stockholders dividends on their investments. Also called *proprietary agencies.*

fraud Deliberate deception in provision of goods or services; lying.

functional nursing Nursing care in which each nurse provides a different aspect of care; nurses are assigned a set of specific tasks to perform for all clients, such as passing medications.

garbage in, garbage out (GIGO) Inaccurate data entry results in inaccurate data output, which can produce wrong decisions, incorrect solutions, and medical errors.

general damages Monetary awards in a lawsuit for injuries for which an exact dollar amount cannot be calculated including pain and suffering, loss of companionship, shortened life span, loss of reputation, and wrongful death.

general systems theory Set of interrelated concepts, definitions, and propositions that describe a system.

genetics Scientific study of heredity and related variations.

gerontology Study of the process of aging and of the effects of aging on individuals.

Gerson therapy Metabolic therapy developed by Max Gerson, a German physician. It is based on the belief that cancer results from metabolic dysfunctions in cells that can be countered by detoxification, a vegetarian diet, coffee enemas to stimulate excretion of liver bile, the exclusion of sodium, and an abundance of potassium.

Global Outbreak and Alert Response Network (GOARN) A system to track developing public-health threats such as new viruses across the planet through its strategically placed laboratories. It also provides emergency assistance to countries confronting any type of infectious disease outbreaks.

goal Desired outcome.

Good Samaritan Act Law that protects health-care providers from being charged with contributory negligence when they provide emergency care to persons in need of immediate treatment.

grievance Complaint or dispute about the terms or conditions of employment.

grounded theory An inductive approach to research using a systematic set of procedures to develop a theory that is then supported by, or "grounded in," the data.

group practice Three or more physicians or nurse practitioners in business together to provide health care.

guided imagery A facilitated flow of thoughts that helps a person see, feel, taste, smell, hear, or touch something in the imagination. The power of the mind or imagination is used to stimulate positive physical responses and provide insight into health and an understanding of emotions as a cause of ill health.

healing touch Healing tradition based on the belief in a universal energy system. Humans are seen as interpenetrating layers of energy systems just above and outside the body that are integrated with energy fields in the environment. Manipulation of such energy fields through touch can help restore a person's energy balance and health.

health Complete physical, mental, and social well-being; a relative state along a continuum ranging from severe illness to ideal state of being; the ability to adapt to illness and to reach the highest level of functioning.

health insurance purchasing cooperative (HIPC) Large groups of people or employers who band together to buy insurance at reduced costs. HIPCs may be organized by private groups or the government.

health literacy A client's ability to read, comprehend, and act on health-care instructions provided by a nurse or other health-care worker.

health maintenance organization (HMO) Prototype of the managed health-care system; method of payment for a full range of primary, secondary, and tertiary health-care services; members pay a fixed annual fee for services and a small deductible when care is given.

health policy Goals and directions that guide activities to safeguard and promote the health of citizens.

health practitioner Individual, usually licensed, who provides health-care services to individuals with health-care needs.

health promotion Interventions and behaviors that increase and maintain the level of well-being of persons, families, groups, communities, and society.

health systems agency (HSA) Local voluntary organization of providers and consumers that plans for the health-care services of its geographic region.

health-care consumer Client or patient; an individual who uses health-care services or products.

health-care team Group of individuals of different levels of education who work together to provide help to clients.

hearsay Evidence not based on personal knowledge of the witness and usually not allowed in courts.

Hellerwork A type of bodywork developed by Joseph Heller as an outgrowth of rolfing. It combines dialogue, body movement education, and deep touch to achieve greater mind–body awareness and structural body alignment with gravitational forces. Therapy is individualized to different body types.

herbal medicine Use of the chemical makeup of herbs in much the same way as conventional medicine uses pharmaceuticals. The most ancient known form of health care, herbal medicine is basic to traditional Chinese, ayurvedic, and Native American medical systems. Also called *botanical medicine, phytotherapy,* and *phytomedicine.*

higher-quality care Health care that is being provided at a level that is above an accepted standard that is issued by an official health-care rating entity. For example, the Netherlands has a much higher quality of care as measured by the Health Care Access and Quality (HAQ) index than the United States.

historical study Qualitative research involving the systematic collection and synthesis of data regarding people and events of the past.

holistic Treatment of the total individual, including physical, psychological, sociological, and spiritual elements, with emphasis on the interrelatedness of parts and wholes.

home health care Health-care services provided in the client's home.

home-automation system (Smart Home) A method of connecting many or all home electrical devices into one central computer–controlled network in which everything is assigned its own Internet Protocol (IP) address, and can be programmed, monitored, and accessed remotely.

homeopathy A Western medical system based on the principle that "like cures like." Natural substances are prescribed in minute dilutions to cause the symptoms of the disease they are intended to cure, helping the body cure itself.

honesty, integrity, respect, responsibility, and ethics (HIRRE) Type of honor code in which students and faculty sign a pledge not to cheat or plagiarize.

horizontal violence Type of peer-to-peer incivility or negative interaction.

hospice care Alternative way of providing care to terminally ill clients in which palliative care is used; the major goals of hospice care are control of pain, provision of emotional support, promotion of social interaction, and preparation for death; family support measures and anticipatory grief counseling are also used if appropriate.

hospital privileges   Authority granted by a hospital, usually through its medical board, for a health-care practitioner to admit and supervise the treatment of clients within that hospital.

huddle   In health care, they are brief staff meetings that are used to alert all health-care staff on the unit to staffing shortages, upcoming events, important policy updates, critical changes in patients' condition, and other unexpected events on the unit.

human factor   The interaction of a human being with a technology such as an electronic device or automated process, often to the detriment of either the human or the technology.

humor therapy   Deliberate use of laughter to improve quality of life by encouraging relaxation and stress reduction, distracting individuals from awareness of constant pain, and providing symptom relief.

humor-me approach   A communication method used with clients in the denial stage of grief to help them comply with the treatment regimen.

hydrotherapy   Use of hot, cold, or contrasting water temperatures to maintain or restore health. Water, steam, or ice may be used in combination with baths, compresses, hot and cold packs, showers, and enemas or colonic irrigations. Minerals, herbs, and oils may be added to enhance the therapeutic effects. Also known as *water cure.*

hypnotherapy   Use of hypnosis, power of suggestion, and trancelike states to access the deepest levels of the mind. Used to bring about changes in behavior, treat health conditions, and manage medical and psychological problems.

hypothesis   Prediction or proposition related to a problem, usually found in research.

ideal role image   Projection of society's expectations for nurses that clearly delineates the obligations and responsibilities, as well as the rights and privileges those in the role can lay claim to. Is often unrealistic.

illness   Disease; a functional disturbance resulting from an individual organism's inability to adapt to certain stressors; an abnormal physiologic state caused by microorganisms, cancer, or other conditions.

implementation   Fourth step in the nursing process, in which the plan of care is carried out.

incidence   Number of occurrences of a specific condition or event.

incident report   Document that describes an accident or error involving a client or family member that may or may not have resulted in injury; the purpose of the incident report is to track incidents and to make changes in the situations that caused them; the incident report is not part of the chart.

incivility   Failure to be civil; any speech or behavior that disrupts the harmony of the work or educational environment.

incompetency   Inability of an individual to manage personal affairs because of mental or physical conditions; the inability of a professional to carry out professional activities at the expected level of functioning because of lack of knowledge or skill or because of drug or alcohol abuse.

indemnity insurance   Health insurance in which the contractual agreement is between the consumer and the insurance company. Providers are not involved in these arrangements, and rates are not preestablished.

independent   Being free from outside control or another's authority; acting with autonomy as to one's own opinion, actions, and care.

independent nurse practitioner   Nurse who has a private practice in one of the expanded roles of nursing.

independent practice association (IPA)   Type of HMO usually organized by physicians that requires fee-for-service payment.

independent practice organization (IPO)   Type of IPA in which a group of providers deals with more than one insurer at a time.

independent practitioner   Health-care provider who delivers health care independently with or without supervision by another health-care practitioner.

independent variable   The one managed or manipulated by the researcher.

indirect services   Health-care actions that do not require direct client contact but that still facilitate care, such as the supply and distribution department of a hospital.

individual mandate The requirement that all U.S. citizens must purchase some type of health insurance with the goal of spreading the costs across a large population and lowering premiums.

infodemic A word that blends *information* and *epidemic;* refers to an excessive amount of information, often obtained from the Internet or social media, about a problem, disease, or some event that is typically unreliable, spreads rapidly, and makes a solution more difficult to achieve.

informed consent Permission granted by a person based on full knowledge of the risks and benefits of participation in a procedure or surgery for which the consent has been given.

injunction Court order specifying actions that must or must not be taken.

input Matter, energy, or information entering a system from the environment.

inquest Formal inquiry about the course or manner of death.

institutional licensure Authority for an individual health-care provider to practice that is granted by the individual's employing institution; the institution determines the educational preparation, training, and functions of each category of provider it employs; no longer legally permitted, unlicensed assistive personnel (UAPs) act under a form of de facto institutional licensure.

institutional review board (IRB) A panel established at an agency, such as a hospital or university, to review all proposed research studies and to set standards for research involving human subjects.

integration One or more electronic devices sharing data with another device, regardless of whether or not this was the original goal of the device.

integrative medicine The practice of conventional health-care professionals who prescribe a combination of therapies from both systems.

integrative review A method of data analysis that summarizes past empirical or theoretical literature to provide a more comprehensive understanding of a particular health-care problem. It allows for the inclusion of diverse methodologies and informs research, practice, and policy initiatives to make a judgment about the quality of the data.

intentional tort A willful act that violates another person's rights or property and may or may not cause physical injury.

interoperability The ability to use, or share, data among any number of devices regardless of the type or brand of device.

interprofessional education Two or more students from different professions learning about, from, and with each other to enable effective collaboration and improve health outcomes.

interrogatories Written questions directed to a party in a lawsuit by the opposing side as part of the discovery process.

intervention Nursing action taken to meet specific client goals.

invasion of privacy Type of quasi-intentional tort that involves (1) an act that intrudes into the seclusion of the client, (2) intrusion that is objectionable to a reasonable person, (3) an act that intrudes into private facts or published as facts or pictures of a private nature, and (4) public disclosure of private information.

iridology Iris diagnosis. In this belief system, each area of the body has a corresponding point on the iris of the eye. Thus, the state of health (balance) or disease (imbalance) can be diagnosed from the color, texture, or location of pigments in the eye.

Jin Shin Jyutsu A Japanese form of massage in which combinations of healing points on the body are held for a minute or more with the fingertips. The purpose is to enhance or restore the flow of chi.

Joint Commission, The Formerly the Joint Commission on Accreditation of Healthcare Organizations (JCAHO), an organization that performs accreditation reviews for health-care agencies.

judgment Decision of the court regarding a case.

junk policies Low-cost health insurance policies that sound good when advertised but include riders that severely limit what is covered. They are marketed to people who tend not to read the fine print such as young adults and the elderly.

jurisdiction Authority of a court to hear and decide lawsuits.

just culture The establishment of a positive work environment that has a commitment to safety and quality, transparency, using errors as learning opportunities, and allowing employees to report errors and near misses voluntarily and anonymously. Also called a *blame-free culture.*

justice Fairness; giving people their due.

Kardex Portable card file that contains important client information and a care plan.

laissez-faire Type of leadership style in which the leader does little planning, sets few goals, avoids decision making, and fails to encourage group members to participate. Also called permissive or nondirective leadership.

lateral violence Also known as *horizontal violence,* lateral violence is found in the workplace and can include name calling; threatening body language; physical hazing; bickering; fault finding; negative criticism; intimidation; gossip; shouting; blaming; put-downs; raised eyebrows; rolling of the eyes; verbally abusive sarcasm with rude tones; physical acts such as pounding on a table, throwing objects or shoving a chair against a wall; unfair assignments; marginalizing a person; refusing to help someone; ignoring; making faces behind someone's back; refusing to work with certain people; whining; sabotage; exclusion; and fabrication.

law Formal statement of a society's beliefs about interactions among and between its citizens; a formal rule enforced by society.

Leapfrog Group Launched in 2000 by the Robert Wood Johnson Foundation, the Leapfrog Group's mission is to promote giant leaps forward in the safety, quality, and affordability of health care by using incentives and rewards.

legal complaint Document filed by a plaintiff against a defendant claiming infringement of the plaintiff's legal rights.

legal obligations Obligations that have become formal statements of law and are enforceable under the law.

legal rights (welfare rights) Rights that are based on a legal entitlement to some good or benefits and are enforceable under the legal system with punishment for violations.

legislator Elected member of either the House of Representatives or the Senate.

legislature Body of elected individuals invested with constitutional power to make, alter, or repeal laws.

liable Obligated or held accountable by law.

libel Written defamation of character.

license Permission to practice granted to an individual by the state after the individual has met the requirements for that particular position; licensing protects the safety of the public.

licensed practical nurse (LPN) Licensed vocational nurse; technical nurse licensed by any state, after completing a practical nursing program, to provide technical bedside care to clients.

licensing board Government agency that implements the statutes of a particular profession in accordance with the Professions Practice Act.

licensure Process by which an agency or government grants an individual permission to practice; it establishes a minimal level of competency for practice.

licensure, accreditation, certification, and education (LACE) A model developed in 2008 by the APRN Consensus Work Group and the National Council of State Boards of Nursing (NCSBN) APRN Advisory Committee addressing the lack of common definitions regarding APRN practice, the ever-increasing numbers of specializations, the inconsistency in credentials and scope of practice, and the wide variations in education for advanced practice registered nurses.

licensure by endorsement Method of obtaining a license to practice by having a state acknowledge the individual's existing comparable license in another state.

licensure examination Method of obtaining a license to practice by successfully passing a state-board examination.

light therapy A method by which light is converted into electrical impulses, travels along the optic nerve to the brain, and stimulates the hypothalamus to send neurotransmitters to regulate the autonomic nervous system. Various colors of light are believed to stimulate different parts of the body.

literature review An exploration of available information to determine what is known and what remains unknown about a subject.

living will Signed legal document in which individuals make known their wishes about the care they are to receive if they should become incompetent at a future date; it usually specifies what types of treatments are permitted and what types are to be withheld.

lobbyist Person who attempts to influence political decisions as an official representative of an organization, group, or institution.

locality rule standard of care Legal process that holds an individual nurse accountable both to what is an acceptable standard within their local community and to national standards as developed by nurses throughout the nation through the American Nurses Association, national practice groups, and health-care agencies.

logit The unit of measurement of difficulty for each question on the Next Generation NCLEX® ranging from a −3 to a +3 on a 7-point scale.

magnet hospital A medical facility considered to have reached the gold standard for nursing practice and health care innovation that is certified by the American Nurses' Credentialing Center (ANCC) as institutions where nurses are empowered to not only take the lead on patient care but to be the drivers of institutional health care change and innovation.

magnet therapy A type of electromagnetic therapy or energy medicine in which magnets are used to stimulate circulation, increase oxygen to cells, and facilitate healing by correcting disturbed or malfunctioning electromagnetic frequencies that the body emits.

malfeasance Performance of an illegal act.

malpractice Negligent acts by a licensed professional based on either omission of an expected action or commission of an inappropriate action resulting in damages to another party; not doing what a reasonable and prudent professional of the same rank would have done in the same situation.

managed care System of organized health-care delivery systems linked by provider networks; health maintenance organizations are the primary example of managed care.

mandatory licensure Law that requires all who practice a particular profession to have and to maintain a license in that profession.

manslaughter Killing of an individual without premeditated intent; different degrees of manslaughter exist, and most are felonies.

mantra A type of sound therapy used in ayurvedic medicine to reach a higher level of spiritual and mental functioning. It changes the "vibratory patterns of the mind" to release unconscious negative thoughts, psychological stress, and emotional distress. Often achieved by uttering a mystical word or phrase and associated with meditation.

medagogy A model of client education that encompasses everything found within the other client education models and focuses the responsibility for health learning on both the teacher (nurse) and the client.

mediation Legal process that allows each party to present their case to a mediator, who is an independent third party trained in dispute resolution.

Medicaid State health-care insurance program, supported in part by federal funds, for health-care services for certain groups unable to pay for their own health care; amount and type of coverage vary from state to state.

medical examiner Coroner; a physician who investigates deaths that appear to be from other than natural causes.

Medical Reserve Core (MRC) A nationwide network of community-based response units sponsored by the Office of the Surgeon General of the United States who are committed to improving the health, safety, and resiliency of their communities.

medically indigent Individuals who cannot personally pay for health-care services without incurring financial hardship.

Medicare Federally run program that is financed primarily through employee payroll taxes and covers any individual who is 65 years of age or older as well as blind and disabled individuals of any age.

Medicare Utilization and Quality Peer Review Organization (PRO) Organization that reviews the quality and cost of Medicare services.

medication formulary A list of medications that a health insurer agrees to pay (at least partially) for a predefined or specified health condition or disease.

Medigap policies Health insurance policies that are purchased to cover expenses not paid by Medicare.

meditation Use of contemplation to exercise the mind. A form of mental cleansing that enhances self-awareness and awareness of one's environment. Also called *mind-cure,* this is an unseen force of healing. Thoughts and deep feelings are considered the primary arbiters of health through relaxation.

megavitamin therapy A type of orthomolecular medicine in which diseases are prevented and cured by large doses of vitamins and other supplements. Dosages exceed the normal or recommended amounts needed for general good health or prevention of deficiencies. The disease to be treated or prevented determines the type, dosage, and mode of administration of vitamins, minerals, and nutrient supplements.

meridians Invisible channels by which chi flows through the body. Blockage along a meridian causes illness. From traditional Chinese medicine.

messenger RNA (mRNA) (ribonucleic acid) A single strand of genetic material that consists of nucleotides copied from a segment of DNA that carries the genetic code from the DNA (or another strand of RNA) for a particular protein out of the nucleus to the site of protein synthesis in the cytoplasm to be reproduced or translated into a new identical protein.

metaparadigm The broadest perspective of a discipline giving an overview of the key theoretical models.

middle-range descriptive theories Nursing theories that are created and tested using descriptive research methodology; are either qualitative or quantitative in design.

middle-range explanatory theories Nursing theories that describe why a relationship exists between two concepts and the degree to which one concept is related to another concept or how it affects the other concept. These theories are produced and tested using correlational research that is usually quantitative in design.

middle-range predictive theories Nursing theories that attempt to predict relations between concepts (rather than just explaining them) through the process of identifying how changes in one element affects other elements. Testing of this type of theory uses experimental research models and quantitative designs.

middle-range theory A set of relatively concrete concepts or propositions that lie between a minor working hypothesis found in everyday nursing research and a well-developed major nursing theory. They are less comprehensive and more focused than the major nursing theories but not as specific or concrete as situation-specific practice theories, and they generally contain only a few basic ideas or concepts that the researcher is attempting to prove or illustrate.

midwife Individual experienced in assisting women during labor and delivery; the individual may be a lay midwife, who has no official education, or a certified nurse midwife, who is an RN in an expanded role, having received additional education and passed a national certification examination.

mind–body medicine Healing based on the interconnectedness of the mind and body, individual responsibility for self-care, and the self-healing capabilities of the body. Uses a wide range of modalities, such as imaging, massage, hypnotherapy, meditation, yoga, concepts of balance, herbs, and diet.

misdemeanor Less serious crime than a felony; punishable by a fine of less than $1,000 or a jail term of less than 1 year.

mixed-method (triangulation) A research method that uses both quantitative and qualitative research in the same study.

model Hypothetical representation of something that exists in reality. The purpose of a model is to attempt to explain a complex reality in a systematic and organized manner.

Modular Synthetic Research Evaluation and Extrapolation Tool (mSTREET) A learning game developed by the Community Health Nursing Serious Game designed to deliver computerized virtual training. In the game, students can investigate and respond to a variety of settings as they "walk" through the streets of a virtual city.

moral injury A trauma to an individual's ethical conscience that arises when faced with situations that deeply violate their integrity or threaten their core values, resulting in an internal struggle with guilt and anger and an overwhelming feeling of being unable to forgive themselves or others.

moral obligations Obligations based on moral or ethical principles but not enforceable under the law.

moral rights *See* ethical rights.

morality Concept of right and wrong.

moral imperative Something that must be done because it is extremely important and considered the right thing to do; a principle that compels an individual to act ethically.

morals Fundamental standards of right and wrong that an individual learns and internalizes during the early stages of childhood development, based primarily on religious beliefs and societal norms.

mores Values and customs of a society.

mortality Property or capacity to die; death.

motivation Internal drive that causes individuals to seek achievement of higher goals; desire.

multicompetency technician Allied health-care provider who has skills in two or more areas of practice through the process of cross-training.

multiculturalism A process whereby individuals who migrate into a new culture from other cultures maintain many of their traditional cultural practices and languages while slowly learning aspects of the new culture.

multiskilled practitioner Health-care professional who has skills in more than one area of health care, such as an RN who has training in physical therapy.

music therapy Use of music to enhance well-being and promote healing. Helps improve physical and mental functioning, alleviate pain, ease the psychological discomfort of illness, and improve quality of life, especially for terminally ill persons. Aids ability of the mentally handicapped, autistic persons, and elderly persons with dementia to interact with others, learn, and relate to their environments.

national health insurance Proposed system of payment for health-care services whereby the government pays for the costs of the health care.

National Nurses Response Teams (NNRT) Teams of nurses under the auspices of the U.S. Department of Health and Human Services; the teams can be quickly deployed in response to major national bioterrorism events to provide mass immunization or chemoprophylaxis to high-risk populations.

naturopathy A Western healing system that uses safe, natural therapies. Promotes holism and use of natural substances, treats cause rather than effect (symptoms), empowers and motivates individuals to take responsibility for their own health, prevents disease through lifestyle and education, and does no harm.

negative entropy Also known as *negentropy*. Tendency toward increased order in a system.

negligence Failure to perform at an expected level of functioning or the performance of an inappropriate function resulting in damages to another party; not doing what a reasonable and prudent person would do in a similar situation.

neurolinguistic programming A system that focuses on how individuals learn, communicate, and change. *Neuro* refers to the way the brain works and the consistent and observable patterns that emanate from human thinking. *Linguistic* refers to the expression (verbal and nonverbal) of those patterns of thinking. *Programming* refers to the ways such patterns of thinking are interpreted and how they can be changed. Changing the patterns gives people the ability to make better choices for healthy behavior.

never events A list of reasonably preventable medical errors that occur in hospitals that will no longer be paid for by Medicare in an attempt to control costs.

Next Generation NCLEX® (NGN) The new National Council Licensure Examination launched in 2023 with new question types based on the Clinical Judgment Measurement Model (CJMM).

no-code order Do not resuscitate (DNR) order; an order by a physician to withhold cardiopulmonary resuscitation and other resuscitative efforts from a client.

nonfeasance Failure to perform a legally required duty.

nonmaleficence Ethical principle that requires the professional to do no harm to the client.

nonprobability sampling A sampling process in which a sample is selected from elements of a population through methods that are not random. Convenience, quota, and purposive sampling are examples.

nonsummativity The degree of connection among the system's parts. The higher the degree of nonsummativity, the greater the interdependence of parts.

nontraditional education Methods of education that do not follow the traditional lecture and clinical practice methods of learning; may include computer-simulated learning, self-education techniques, or other creative methods.

nonverbal A type of communication that uses any methods except written and spoken messages and constitutes 93 percent of the communication between individuals. It includes body language, gestures, facial expression, tone, pace, personal space, and so on.

normal damages Money awarded when the law requires a judge and jury to find a defendant guilty but no real harm happened to the plaintiff. The award is usually very small, generally in the sum of $10.00.

normative ethics Questions and dilemmas requiring a choice of actions whereby there is a conflict of rights or obligations between the nurse and the client, the nurse and the client's family, or the nurse and the physician.

norm-referenced examination Examination scored by comparison with standards established on the performance of all others who took the same examination during a specific time; the National League for Nursing achievement examinations are norm referenced.

not-for-profit (nonprofit) organizations Agencies in which all profits must be used in the operation of the organization.

nucleotide The basic unit of genetic material for all living things that exists in chains that encode the information necessary to copy and replicate RNA and DNA (protein synthesis) and also function in cell signaling, metabolism, and enzyme reactions.

Nuremberg Code A code of conduct that serves as one of the recognized guides in the ethical conduct of research.

nurse clinician Registered nurse with advanced skills in a particular area of nursing practice; if certified by a professional organization, a nurse clinician may also be a nurse practitioner, but more often this designation refers to nurses in advanced practice roles such as nurse specialists.

nurse practice act Part of state law that establishes the scope of practice for professional nurses, as well as educational levels and standards, professional conduct, and reasons for revocation of licensure.

nurse practitioner Nurse specialist with advanced education in a primary care specialty, such as community health, pediatrics, or mental health, who is prepared independently to manage health promotion and maintenance and illness prevention of a specific group of clients.

nurse specialist (clinical nurse specialist) Nurse who is an expert in providing care focused on a specialized field drawn from the range of general practice, such as cardiac nurse specialist.

nurse theorist Nurse who analyzes and attempts to describe what the profession of nursing is and what nurses do through nursing models or nursing theories.

nursing assessment Systematic collection and recording of client data, both objective and subjective, from primary and secondary sources using the nursing history, physical examination, and laboratory data, for example.

nursing diagnosis Statements of a client's actual or potential health-care problems or deficits.

nursing informatics (NI) The use of nursing skills in tandem with information and technology to improve health-care outcomes.

nursing order Statement of a nursing action selected by a nurse to achieve a client's goal; may be stated as either the nurse's or the client's expected behavior.

nursing process Systematic, comprehensive decision-making process used by nurses to identify and treat actual and potential health problems.

nursing research Formal study of problems of nursing practice, the role of the nurse in health care, and the value of nursing.

nursing standards Desired nursing behaviors established by the profession and used to evaluate nurses' performances.

obligations Demands made on individuals, professions, society, or government to fulfill and honor the rights of others. Obligations are often divided into two categories—moral and legal (welfare).

occurrence policy A type of malpractice insurance that protects against all claims that occurred during the policy period regardless of when the claim is made.

omission Failure to fulfill a duty or carry out a procedure recognized as a standard of care; often forms the basis for claims of malpractice.

oncology Area of health care that deals with the treatment of cancer.

open access A free source of electronic data that can be used by any person.

open curriculum Educational system that allows a student to enter and leave the system freely; often uses past education and experiences.

open system System that can exchange energy, matter, and information with the environment and with other systems.

option rights Rights that are based on a fundamental belief in the dignity and freedom of humans.

ordinance Local or municipal law.

orthodox medicine A synonym for conventional, Western, scientific, biomedicine, or official health-care system.

orthomolecular medicine A system that treats physiological and psychological disorders by reestablishing, normalizing, or creating the optimal nutritional balance in the body. Vitamins, minerals, amino acids, and other types of nutritional substances are administered. (*Ortho-* means "normal" or "correct.")

osteopathy A Western system of medicine that considers the structural integrity of the body the most important factor in maintaining and restoring the person to health. The structural integrity or balance of the musculoskeletal system is maintained through physical therapy, joint manipulation, and postural reeducation.

outcome criteria Standards that measure changes or improvements in clients' conditions.

out-of-pocket expenses Amount the client is responsible for paying for a health-care service.

output Matter, energy, or information released from a system into the environment or transmitted to another system.

oxygen therapy Use of various forms of oxygen to destroy pathogens and promote body healing. Includes hyperbaric, ozone, and hydrogen peroxide therapies.

palliative Type of treatment directed toward minimizing the severity of a disease or illness rather than curing it; for example, for a client with terminal cancer, relief of pain (palliative care), rather than cure, is the main goal.

pandemic A widespread occurrence of an infectious disease over an entire country or the world during a particular time period.

panel of approved providers A list of physicians, nurse practitioners, pharmacies, and other health-care providers that are approved by an insurance plan and to whom reimbursement will be made by the insurer.

paraverbal The tone, pitch, volume, and diction used when delivering a verbal message that comprises approximately 38 percent of the nonverbal communication and is often considered part of nonverbal communication.

passive euthanasia The withholding or withdrawing treatment which is necessary for maintaining life. Do not resuscitate (DNR) orders are a type of passive euthanasia commonly practiced in most acute care facilities and has almost no legal implications.

passive learning A type of client education in which the material is merely presented to the client without their involvement. Least-effective type of learning because it usually does not change attitudes or behaviors.

patient Client; an individual seeking or receiving health-care services.

patient day Client day; the 24-hour period during which hospital services are provided that forms the basis for charging the patient, usually from midnight to midnight.

patient goals Also known as *patient-centered goals*. Diagnosis-specific treatment outcomes or results that are specific to the patient and help align the patient's wishes with those of the health-care provider's treatment plan.

pedagogy The study of the theory and practice of teaching and how these influence student learning.

pediatrics Study and care of problems and diseases of children younger than the age of 18.

peer review Evaluation against professional standards of the performance of individuals with the same basic education and qualifications; formal process of review or evaluation by coworkers of an equal rank.

perceived role image The individual's own definition of the role, which is usually more realistic than the ideal role, involving rejection or modification of some of the norms and expectations of society.

percussion Physical examination involving the tapping of various parts of the body to determine density by eliciting different sounds.

performed role image The duties performed by the practitioner of a role. Often produces reality shock in new graduate nurses.

perjury Crime committed by giving false testimony while under oath.

permissive licensure Law that allows individuals to practice a profession as long as they do not use the title of the profession; no states now have permissive licensure.

personal protective equipment (PPE) Protective clothing, helmets, gloves, face shields, goggles, facemasks and/or respirators, or other equipment designed to protect the wearer from injury or the spread of infection or illness. Commonly used in health-care settings such as hospitals, doctor's offices, and clinical laboratories, PPE acts as a barrier between infectious materials such as viral and bacterial contaminants from contact with skin, mouth, nose, and eyes or other mucous membranes.

personal space The distance from others that individuals maintain around themselves in most casual social situations. Is often culturally based.

pharmacognosy Scientific study of the chemical properties of plants and natural products. A goal is to standardize herbal products to make sure they are free of harmful components and contain the identical amount of active ingredients.

phenomenology Philosophical approach that holds that consciousness determines reality in space and time.

physician-assisted suicide (PAS) The voluntary termination of a patient's own life by administration of a lethal medication or substance by the patient with the help of a physician. It is different from active euthanasia in that the physician only provides the necessary means to end the patient's life and the patient performs the act rather than the physician performing the act.

phytomedicine/phytotherapy A branch of botanical medicine, especially prominent in Europe, that includes the pharmaceutical study and therapeutic use of herbs, herbal derivatives, and herbal synthetics. Merges ancient herbal traditions with contemporary scientific investigation to standardize the active ingredients of herbal products.

PICO question A question in which *P* represents "population" or "patient"; *I* stands for "phenomenon of interest"; *C* stands for "comparative," and *O* stands for "outcome."

plaintiff Individual who charges another individual in a court of law with a violation of the individual's rights; the party who files the complaint in a lawsuit.

point-of-service plans Insurance plans in which consumers can select providers outside of a prescribed provider panel if they are willing to pay an additional fee.

polarity therapy A combination of bodywork and other hands-on techniques to restore the natural flow of energy through the body. Other therapies may include reflexology, hydrotherapy, and breathing techniques.

political action Activities on the part of individuals that influence the actions of government officials in establishing policy.

political capital The goodwill or favorable sentiment that a politician gains after winning an election, initiating a successful program, passing other politicians' bills, or making a public appearance after a natural disaster that accentuates their leadership abilities. It is sometimes called the "honeymoon" period of a presidency and, like money, must be spent soon or it will evaporate.

political involvement Group of activities that, individually or collectively, increase the voice of nursing in the political or health-care policy process.

politics Process of influencing the decisions of others and exerting control over situations or events; includes influencing the allocation of scarce resources.

polytomous scoring A type of scoring on the Next Generation NCLEX® that allows graduates to earn credit for partial understanding of a subject; however, they can lose credit for an incorrect answer.

positive end expiratory pressure The maintenance of positive pressure (above atmospheric pressure) in a patient's airway at the end of expiration to distend distal alveoli, assuming there is no airway obstruction. PEEP is provided by mechanical ventilation or noninvasive ventilation (NIV), CPAP (continuous positive airway pressure).

practical nursing program Vocational nursing program; a program of study leading to a certificate in practical nursing, usually 12 to 18 months in length; these programs are located in a vocational or technical school or in a community or junior college; after passing the NCLEX-LPN CAT examination, students become licensed practical nurses (LPNs).

prana Vital energy or life force that runs through the body. From ayurvedic medicine.

pre-authorization requirements A formal request by a provider or supplier to the insuring entity to receive authorization or approval that the requested treatments or procedures may be rendered to the patient. Similar to a pre-claim review.

precedent Decision previously issued by a court that is used as the basis for a decision in another case with similar circumstances.

preceptor Educated or skilled practitioner who agrees to work with a less-educated or less-trained individual to increase the individual's knowledge and skills; often a staff nurse who works with student nurses during their senior year.

precertification Approval for reimbursement of services before their being rendered.

predictive analytics The analysis and use of cleaned data to make predictions or recommendations for improvements in care using the principles of cognitive science and artificial intelligence.

preferred provider organization (PPO) Method of payment for employee health-care benefits in which employers contract with a specific group of health-care providers for a lower cost for their employees' health-care services but require the employee to use the providers listed.

premium Amount paid on a periodic basis for health insurance or HMO membership.

prescriptive authority Legal right to write prescriptions for medications, granted to physicians, veterinarians, dentists, and advanced practice nurses.

presumed consent law A law that presumes that all reasonable and prudent persons would normally wish to donate their organs upon their death. It is often associated with the issuance of a new driver's license; however, those not wishing to be organ donors are able to opt out of the process, which is a reversal of the current process of asking for consent to donate.

preventive care Well care; nursing care provided for the purpose of maintaining health and preventing disease or injury, often through community health clinics, school nursing services, and storefront clinics.

primary care Type of health care for individuals and families in which maintenance of health is emphasized; first-line health care in hospitals, physicians' offices, or community health clinics that deal with acute conditions.

primary care nurse Hospital staff RN assigned to a primary care unit to provide nursing care to a limited number of clients who are followed by the same nurse from admission to discharge.

primary intervention Health promotion, illness prevention, early diagnosis, and treatment of common health problems.

primary research source A report or account of a research study written by the researcher(s) conducting the study. In historical research, a primary source might be an original letter, diary, or other authenticated document.

private-duty nurse Nurse in private practice; nurse self-employed for providing direct client care services either in the home or the hospital setting.

privileged communication Information imparted by a client to a physician, lawyer, or clergyman that is protected from disclosure in a court of law. Communication between a client and a nurse is not legally protected, but nurses can participate in privileged communication when they overhear information imparted by the client to the physician.

process consent A requirement that the researcher renegotiate the consent if any unanticipated events occur during the process of gathering data.

profession Nursing; an occupation that meets the criteria for a profession, including education, altruism, code of ethics, public service, and dedication.

professional performance standards A list of requirements or goals for patient treatment and care that are developed by members of a professional organization; used to guide practice and performance and maintain safety and high-level quality of care.

professional review organization Multilevel program to oversee the quality and cost of federally funded medical care programs.

professional standards of care Evidence-based guidelines developed by a collaboration of nursing professionals that specify the level of appropriate treatment or care. They determine how a reasonable and prudent professional should act in similar situations under similar conditions and can be used to determine the level of negligence and liability for malpractice lawsuits.

Professional Standards Review Organization (PSRO) An organization established to monitor health-care services paid for through Medicare, Medicaid, and Maternal and Child Health programs to ensure that services provided are medically necessary, meet professional standards, and are provided in the most economic, medically appropriate health-care agency or institution.

professionalism Behaviors and attitudes exhibited by an individual that are recognized by others as the traits of a professional.

prospective payment system (PPS) System of reimbursement for health-care services that establishes the payment rates before hospitalization based on certain criteria, such as diagnosis-related groups (DRGs).

protocol Written plan of action based on previously identified situations; standing orders are a type of protocol often used in specialty units that have clients with similar problems.

provider Person or organization who delivers health care, including health promotion and maintenance and illness prevention and treatment.

provider panel Health-care providers selected to render services to a group of consumers within a managed-care plan.

proximate cause Nearest cause; the element in a direct cause-and-effect relationship between what is done by the professional and what happens to the client. For example, when a nurse fails to raise the side rails on the bed of a client who has received a narcotic medication, and the client falls out of bed and breaks a hip as a result.

psychomotor domain objectives Goals established with input from the client that deal with changes in behavior or learned skills.

public policy Decision made by a society or its elected representatives that has a material effect on citizens other than the decision-makers.

punitive damages Money awarded in a lawsuit in addition to compensatory and general damages when the actions that caused the injury to the client were judged to be willful, malicious, or to have demonstrated an extreme measure of incompetence and gross negligence. The primary purpose of punitive damages is to "punish" the defendant and deter them from ever acting in the same way again. Also called *exemplary damages.*

qigong (chi kung, chi gong) Technique from traditional Chinese medicine that combines movement, meditation and deep relaxation, and regulation of breathing. Enhanced flow of chi throughout the body nourishes vital organs.

qualitative research design Investigates the why and how of decision making and not just what, where, and when it happened with the goal of gathering an in-depth understanding of human behavior and the reasons that govern such behavior.

quality Level of excellence based on preestablished criteria.

Quality and Safety Education for Nurses (QSEN) Nursing education curriculum designed to prepare future nurses with the knowledge, skills, and attitudes (KSAs) necessary to continuously improve the quality and safety of the health-care system in which they work.

quality assurance Activity conducted in health-care facilities that evaluates the quality of care provided to ensure that it meets preestablished quality standards.

quality indicators Measures of health-care quality from easily accessible inpatient hospital administrative data that includes prevention, inpatient, patient, and pediatric safety and are used to focus efforts on potential quality concerns so they may be addressed by further investigation as well as tracking changes over time.

quality metrics (QM) Data collection tools ranging from questionnaires to electronic patient check lists that help quantify health-care processes, outcomes, patient perceptions, and organizational structure and/or systems and are used to provide high-quality health care and/or care that relate to one or more quality goals for health care.

quantitative experimental research designs Research that is guided by a somewhat rigid set of rules that gives the most importance to the *process* of inquiry and is highly respected by researchers.

quasi-experimental design A type of experimental design in which there is either no comparison group or no random assignment of participants.

quasi-intentional tort A violation of a person's reputation or personal privacy.

random sample A selection process that ensures that each member of a population has an equal probability of being selected.

rapid response team (RRT) Team of individuals from various disciplines who can rescue clients whose conditions are deteriorating to prevent codes and in-hospital deaths using specific communication models to make interdisciplinary communication clearer, a workspace that promotes efficiency and waste reduction, professional support programs, and liberalized diet plans and meal times.

rapid task switching (multitasking) A mental and/or motor ability that some individuals develop that allows them to seemingly perform more than one task at a time; in reality, they are switching from one task to the next in quick succession. Performance on multiple tasks causes a disruption in performance when there is a switch from one task to another that decreases quality of performance and accuracy and is known as the *switch cost.*

reality shock (transition shock) A sudden and sometimes traumatic realization on the part of the new graduate that the ideal or perceived roles do not match the actual performed role.

recertification Periodic renewal of certification by examination, continuing education, or other criteria established by the accrediting agency.

reciprocity Endorsement; a state's acceptance of a license issued by another state.

reflexology Pressure applied to the hands or feet to unblock nerve impulses. In this belief system, every part of the body has a corresponding area on the hands and feet. Thus, body parts can be stimulated by pressure applied to the appropriate sites. Reflexology is used to relieve tension, improve circulation, promote relaxation, and restore energy balance.

registration Listing of a license with a state for a fee.

registry Published list of those who are registered; the agency that publishes the list of individuals who are registered.

regulations Rules or orders issued by various regulatory agencies, such as a state board of nursing, which have the force of law.

rehabilitation Restoration to the highest possible level of performance or health of an individual who has suffered an injury or illness.

reiki An ancient Buddhist version of healing touch practiced in Tibet and Japan. The word also means *universal life force*. Energy is transferred to the person through the hands of the healer to restore energy balance in the body.

relative intensity measure (RIM) Method for calculating nursing resources needed to provide nursing care for various types of clients; helps determine the number and type of staff required based on client acuity and needs.

relaxation response Physiological mechanism described by Herbert Benson in which body stress is reduced through regulation of internal activity, such as reduced metabolism and slowing of other physiological reactions.

relaxation therapy Use of the relaxation response to reduce stress through release of physical and emotional tension. Various therapies are commonly included in other types of therapeutic programs. Examples are mind–body therapies such as biofeedback, hydrotherapy, imaging and visualization, meditation, qigong, tai chi, and yoga.

reliability The dependability or degree of consistency with which an instrument measures what it is intended to measure.

replication study A research study designed to repeat or duplicate earlier research. A different sample or setting may be used while the essential elements of the original study are kept intact.

rescission The practice of health insurance companies to cut or cancel health-care plans already in place usually because of the high costs associated with the client's illness.

research design A blueprint for conducting a research study.

research process A process that requires the comprehension of a unique language and involves the ability to apply a variety of research processes.

respirator An apparatus worn over the mouth and nose or the entire face to prevent the inhalation of dust, smoke, or other noxious substances.

respondeat superior (Latin) Legal doctrine that holds the employer or supervisor responsible for the actions of the employees or of those supervised; for example, under this doctrine, RNs are held responsible for the actions of unlicensed assistive personnel under their supervision.

responsibility Accountability; the concept that all individuals are accountable for their own actions and for the consequences of those actions.

restorative care Curative care; nursing care that has as its goal cure and recovery from disease.

restrictive provider network A health insurance or benefit plan that limits the payment of medication and other health-care benefits, in whole or in part, to the use of the providers that have entered into a contractual arrangement with the insurer to provide health-care services to covered individuals.

résumé Curriculum vitae; a summary of an individual's education, work experience, and qualifications.

retrospective payment system Payment system for health care in which reimbursement is based on the actual care rendered rather than on preset rates.

right Just claim or expectation that may or may not be protected by law; legal rights are protected by law, whereas moral rights are not.

risk management Evaluating the risk of clients and staff for injuries and for potential liabilities and implementing corrective and preventive measures.

risk rating A method of calculating the rate for health insurance premiums based on various characteristics of an individual or small group of individuals, such as previous history of claims filed, characteristics of the individual's or group's health practices, or changes in the individual's or group's overall health status that might increase the risk for claims. It is the most commonly used method of calculating health insurance premiums and allows companies to change their rates at will.

rolfing Technique of deep massage developed by Ida Rolf. Use of the knuckles is meant to counteract the effects of gravity on body balance. Fascia, connective tissue, and muscle are loosened and lengthened to help them return to their correct positions.

root-cause analysis A type of assessment that tracks events leading to error, identifies faulty systems, and processes and develops a plan to prevent further errors.

Rosen technique A type of bodywork in which muscle tension is seen as repressed emotional conflicts. Deep and gentle pressure is applied as persons are questioned about what they are experiencing.

rushed labor insertion The use of senior-level nursing students to work as staff during the COVID-19 pandemic.

sample A subset of a population selected to participate in a study as representative of that population.

scientific inquiry A logical, orderly means of collecting data for the generation and testing of ideas.

secondary care Nursing care usually provided in short-term and long-term care facilities to clients with commonly occurring conditions.

secondary intervention Acute care designed to prevent complications or resolve health problems.

secured settings Any institutional setting imposing restriction of movement, confinement, and limitations to activity and access; jails, locked units or locked mental institutions, prisons.

sentinel event Unexpected occurrence involving death or serious physical or psychological injury, or the risk thereof, including loss of limb or function. Relatively infrequent, occurring independently of a client's condition, that commonly reflects hospital system and process deficiencies and results in negative outcomes for clients. Sentinel events are not the same as medical errors.

sequential compression device (SCD) Also called intermittent pneumatic compression (IPC) device. Inflatable sleeves, jackets, or boots used to surround a limb that requires treatment to prevent deep vein thrombosis (DVT) or pulmonary embolism (PE). Usually, the device has multiple internal chambers that work together to inflate in a series to squeeze the limb in a "milking action."

service insurance Health insurance in which services are provided for a prescribed fee that is established between the providers and the insurance company.

sexual assault nurse examiner (SANE) A registered nurse specializing in care of victims of sexual assault, performing physical and psychosocial examination, collection of physical evidence, and therapeutic interventions to minimize trauma.

shamanism Ancient healing approach found in most cultural systems. Shamans communicate with the spirit world through trances and other altered states of consciousness. They attempt to control spirits and effect change in the physical world. The belief is that the soul of the shaman separates from the body and explores the cosmos in search of cures for ill clients.

shared governance A type of management system or process that promotes inclusive and collective decision making that is designed to empower all members of the workforce and encourage them to express their individual ideas and opinions.

shiatsu Japanese form of massage, literally meaning *finger pressure*. Consists of firm pressure in a sequential and rhythmic manner. Pressure is exerted for 3 to 10 seconds on points along the body that correspond to acupuncture meridians. It is designed to "awaken the meridian."

significant other Individual who is not a family member but is emotionally or symbolically important to an individual.

Situation, Background, Assessment, Recommendation (SBAR) Communication technique used between members of the health-care team when a client's condition requires immediate attention and action; an easy-to-remember, concrete mechanism frames the conversation efficiently.

Six Sigma Business management strategy that has been adapted to the health-care industry to identify wasteful practices and lower costs while improving the overall quality of care.

slander Oral defamation of character.

sliding-scale fees Fees for services that are based on the client's ability to pay.

slow-code order Physician's order that the efforts for resuscitation of a client who is terminally ill should be initiated and conducted at a leisurely pace; the goal of a slow-code order is to allow the client to die during an apparent resuscitation. Slow-code orders are not acceptable practice and do not meet standards of care.

sound therapy Use of sound to affect different parts of the brain, regulate corticosteroid hormone levels, and affect the body's own rhythmic patterns.

special damages Money awarded to the plaintiff for out-of-pocket expenses related to the trial. It would cover the expenses of taking a taxi back and forth to the courthouse, use of special assistive equipment and home health-care providers, and other expenses that are not covered under actual damages.

spiritual healing Cosmic healing energy transferred or channeled from practitioner to client through laying on of the hands.

staff nurse Nurse generalist who works as an employee of a hospital, nursing home, community health agency, or some other organization providing primary and direct nursing care to clients.

standard of best interest A type of decision made about an individual's health care when they are unable to make the informed decision for their own care; based on what the health-care providers and/or the family decide is best for that individual.

standards Norms; criteria for expected behaviors or conduct.

standards of care Written or established criteria for nursing care that all nurses are expected to meet.

standards of nursing practice A set of guidelines and principles developed by the American Nurses Association to help elevate the nursing profession by defining the values and priorities for registered nurses across the nation. The guidelines provide direction to all nurses, influence legislation, and implement a framework to objectively evaluate nursing excellence.

standards of practice Written or established criteria for nursing practice that all professional nurses are expected to meet.

standing order Written order by physician for certain actions or medication administration to be initiated or given in certain expected circumstances; similar to protocols.

statute Law passed by a government's legislature and signed by its chief executive.

statute of limitations Specific time period in which a lawsuit must be filed or a crime must be prosecuted; most nursing or medical lawsuits have a 2-year statute of limitations from the time of discovery of the incident.

statutory law Law passed by a legislature.

stem cell A cell that has yet to develop into a particular cell variation (undifferentiated) that can divide to produce offspring cells that are the same as the original cells or to produce cells that are different from the original cell (differentiated or specialized).

step therapy for prescription medications An attempt to lower health insurance costs by first prescribing the least-expensive medication to treat a disease and, if that medication is proven ineffective, moving to the next more expensive medication, and so forth, until the most expensive medication is reached. Also called *fail-first medication therapy.*

stereotype Fixed or predetermined image of or attitude toward an individual or group.

stress Crisis situation that causes increased anxiety and initiation of the flight-or-fight mechanism.

stress debriefing A highly specific, structured crisis intervention to aid individuals in coping with the physical and/or psychological symptoms that are the result of stress due to traumatic events. Debriefing allows individuals experiencing traumatic incidents to process the event and develop coping skills.

stressor Internal or external force to which a person responds.

structure criteria Physical environmental framework for client care.

subpoena Court document that requires an individual to appear in court and provide testimony; individuals who do not honor the subpoena can be held in contempt of court and jailed or fined.

subsystem Smaller system within a large system.

summary judgment Decision by a judge in cases in which no facts are in dispute.

sunset law Law that automatically terminates a program after a preestablished period of time unless that program can justify its need for existence.

supervision A set of activities carried out by a person to make certain that tasks or actions performed by another person are appropriate, safe, high quality, and meet preestablished standards.

support system Environmental factors and individuals who can help an individual in a crisis cope with the situation.

Swedish massage The most common form of massage, focusing on superficial muscle layers. Practitioner uses kneading, friction, and long, gliding strokes to relieve muscle tension and promote relaxation.

systems theory Theory that stresses the interrelatedness of parts in any system in which a change in one part affects all other parts; often, the system is greater than the sum of its parts.

tai chi From traditional Chinese medicine. Derived from qigong but practiced at a much slower pace. Also one of the body–mind therapies. Combines contemplation (meditation) with movement or "moving meditation" and coordinated breathing.

taxonomy Classification system.

teach-back A method of teaching a client that requires that the client perform the task being demonstrated to better evaluate the client's understanding and provide the nurse a concrete measurement of the effectiveness of their teaching and the client's learning.

team nursing Method of organizing nursing care in which each client is assigned a team consisting of RNs, LPNs, and nursing assistants to deliver nursing care.

technician Individual who carries out technical tasks.

technology Use of science and the application of scientific principles to any situation; often involves the use of complicated machines and computers.

telehealth The use of electronic information and communications technologies to provide and support health care when distance separates the health-care provider and the client; telehealth can be provided using "plain old telephone service" (POTS), highly sophisticated digitized cameras, telemetry, voice systems, and even interactive robots that can be controlled by the practitioner to assess clients and administer treatments.

telemedicine One of the services provided by the overall telehealth system that primarily involve consultation with a physician.

teleology Utilitarianism; an ethical system that identifies the right action by determining what will provide the greatest good for the greatest number of persons. This system has no set, unchanging rules; rather, it varies as the situation changes.

tertiary care Nursing care usually provided in long-term care and rehabilitation facilities for chronic diseases or injuries requiring long recovery.

tertiary intervention Provision of advanced and long-term health-care services to acutely ill clients, including the use of advanced technology, complicated surgical procedures, rehabilitation services, and care of the terminally ill.

testimony Oral statement of a witness under oath.

theoretical framework A framework based on propositional statements derived from one theory or interrelated theories.

theory Set of interrelated constructs (concepts, definitions, or propositions) that presents a systematic view of phenomena by specifying relations among variables with the purpose of explaining and predicting phenomena.

therapeutic massage Manipulation of soft tissues through a variety of techniques to affect the circulatory, lymphatic, and nervous systems.

therapeutic touch A healing touch modality that does not involve actual touching of the client's body. The therapist's hands are used to sense and interact with the client's energy field to redirect it, alleviate energy blockage, and restore balance.

third-party payment Payment for health-care services by an insurance company or a government agency rather than directly by the client.

third-party reimburser Organization other than the client, such as an employer, insurance company, or governmental agency, that assumes responsibility for payment of health-care charges for services rendered to the client.

throughput Matter, energy, or information as it passes through a system.

tort Violation of the civil law that violates a person's rights and causes injury or harm to the individual. Civil wrong independent of an action in contract that results from a breach of a legal duty; a tort can be classified as unintentional, intentional, or quasi-intentional.

tortfeasor Person who commits a tort.

total quality management (TQM) Method for monitoring and maintaining the quality of health care being delivered by a particular institution or health-care industry.

trackable medications Tablets or capsules with tiny sensors, about the size of a grain of sand, embedded in them that contain copper, magnesium, and silicon (safe ingredients found in foods) and generate an electrical signal when they come in contact with stomach acid (a process similar to generating a current with a potato battery).

traditional Chinese medicine A complete system of healing based on the concept of the uninterrupted flow of chi, or vital essence, and the concept of balance (yin and yang), representing corresponding and interrelated elements in the internal world of the body and the external world. All illness is attributed ultimately to a disturbance of chi.

Trager therapy A method of bodywork, developed by Milton Trager, meant to develop the ability to move more effortlessly. Use of gentle, rhythmic touch and movement exercises to assist in the release of accumulated tensions. Uses sensory-motor feedback or mental gymnastics (mentastics) to learn how the body moves.

transactional relationship A relationship in which the involved partners stay together because they receive benefits or support from it, such as money, status, education, or a future outcome. It does not depend on love, affection, or compatibility.

transition of care The movement of patients between health-care providers, health-care facilities, nursing homes, and other settings based on changes in their conditions and needs. It is a potentially risky time for patients because ineffective care transition usually caused by poor communication between providers and facilities often leads to adverse events and higher hospital readmission rates.

treble damages A provision in the laws of some states that allows the judge, in certain instances, to triple the actual damage award amount as an additional form of punitive damages in a lawsuit.

trial Legal proceedings during which all relevant facts are presented to a jury or judge for legal decision.

Tri-Council Nursing group composed of the American Nurses Association (ANA), National League for Nursing (NLN), American Association of Colleges of Nursing (AACN), and American Organization of Nurse Executives (AONE).

two plus two (2 + 2) program Nursing education program that starts with an associate (2-year) degree and then moves the individual to a baccalaureate degree with an additional 2 years of education.

Uniform Anatomical Gift Act Legislation providing for a legal document signed by an individual indicating the desire to donate specific body organs or the entire body after death.

unintentional tort A wrong occurring to a person or that person's property even though it was not intended; negligence.

universal health-care coverage Health-care reimbursement benefits for all U.S. citizens and legal residents.

universal precautions Body substance isolation; guidelines established by the Centers for Disease

Control and Prevention (CDC) and the Occupational Safety and Health Administration (OSHA) to protect health-care professionals and clients from diseases carried in the blood and body fluids, such as HIV and hepatitis B; involves the use of gloves whenever in contact with blood or body fluids, and masks, gowns, and eye covers if a chance exists of contact with aerosol fluids.

upward mobility Movement toward increased status and power in an organization through promotion.

utilitarianism Teleology; an ethical system that identifies the right action by determining what will provide the greatest good for the greatest number of persons. This system has no set, unchanging rules; rather, it varies as the situation changes.

utilization guidelines Guidelines that stipulate the amount of services that can be delivered by a health-care provider.

validity The ability of an instrument to measure the variables that it is intended to measure.

value Judgment of worth, quality, or desirability based on attitude formed from need or experience; a strong belief held by individuals about something important to them.

values clarification Process by which individuals list and prioritize the values they hold most important.

variable Any trait of an individual, object, or situation that is susceptible to change and that may be manipulated or measured in quantitative research.

veracity The principle of truthfulness. It requires the health-care provider to tell the truth and not intentionally deceive or mislead clients.

verbal A type of communication based on written or spoken messages that constitute approximately 7 percent of the total communication between individuals.

vertical violence The use of inappropriate coercive power by a superior to harass and bully subordinates.

veto Signed refusal by the president or a governor to enact a bill into law. If the president vetoes a bill, the veto may be overridden by a two-thirds vote of the membership of both the House and Senate.

vibration medicine Healing systems that treat the body on an energy level. Cure is effected by ingestion of substances that adjust energy or rate of energy field vibration. Homeopathy is an example.

vicarious liability Imputation of blame on a person for the actions of the other.

victimization Experience of physical, emotional, or psychological trauma in which the individual suffers injury, fear, self-blame, and/or other dysfunction.

visualization Also called *guided imagery, centering, focusing, meditation,* or *distraction.* Use of the imagination or power of the mind to get in touch with one's inner self. Involves all, several, or one of the senses to bridge the mind, body, and spirit.

vocational nursing program Licensed practical nursing program in Texas and California; a program of study leading to a certificate in vocational nursing, usually 12 to 18 months in length; these programs are located in vocational and technical schools and community and junior colleges; after passing the NCLEX-LPN CAT examination, students become licensed vocational nurses (LVNs).

welfare rights *See* legal rights.

workaround The result of the human factor interacting with a difficult technology in which the human finds a way to modify the technology or completely bypasses it to achieve the goal.

yin/yang Complementary but opposing phenomena or correspondents in Taoist philosophical thought that form the underpinning of traditional Chinese medicine. Yin and yang represent the interdependence of all elements of nature and body and mind. Yin represents the female force and passive, still, reflective aspects. Yang represents the male force and active, warm, moving aspects. For health to be maintained and wellness achieved, yin and yang must be in balance.

yoga Literally meaning *union,* or the integration of mental, physical, and spiritual energies. Part of ayurvedic medicine. The integration is accomplished through exercise in the form of assuming different body postures, meditating, and breathing.

INDEX

Note: *b* indicates box; *f*, figure; and *t*, table

A

abandonment, 189–190
abortion, 149–151
 use of fetal tissue from, 152–153
absolute statements, 307
abuse
 child, 171–173
 elder, 175–177
Academic Progression in Nursing (APIN)
 program, 76
acceptance stage of grief, 353
accountability, 426
 defined, 429
 in delegating, 428–433
 professionalism and, 15
 responsibility and, 4
accreditation, 76, 100, 637
Accreditation Commission for Education in
 Nursing (ACEN), 76–77, 105
acculturative stress, 592
accusations, 306
achievement behavioral subsystem, 53
acknowledging what was said, 304
active listening, 260*b*, 261, 300
active shooters, 749–751
activities of daily living (ADLs), 48
actual damages, 194
act utilitarianism, 128–129
acupuncture, 19
administrators and incivility, 452
advance directives, 162–165, 162*b*, 166*f*, 199*b*
 nurse's role in, 201
advanced practice registered nurses
 (APRNs), 10–11
 certification of, 100–101
 definitions and roles of, 101, 103
 doctoral-level education and, 86–87
 education for, 84–87, 103–104
 health-care reform and, 102
 LACE model, 101
 need for, 560
 political issues and, 511
 scope of, 85–86
 specializations for, 11
 in telehealth, 767–768, 770
 titles for, 103
Advanced Research Projects Agency
 (ARPA), 480
Advances in Nursing Science, 663
advocacy, patient, 763

affidavit, 193
Affordable Care Act (ACA), 73, 101, 143,
 147, 219, 371–372, 496, 507, 543
 concerns about, 374
 COOPS and, 390
 cost-effectiveness of, 557–558
 debate over, 556, 558
 goals of, 372–373
 Hospital Consumer Assessment of
 Healthcare Providers and Systems
 (HCAHPS), 763
 new roles for RNs and, 756
 nursing and, 374–375
 nursing informatics and, 496
 older adults and, 622–623
 passage of, 547, 559
 patient teaching and, 635
 quality care and, 417
ageism, 620
Agency for Healthcare Research and Quality
 (AHRQ), 406, 417, 659
aggressive communication, 296–297
aging in place, 621
aging population. *See* older adults
aging weapons, 751–752
Akron Children's Hospital, 480
alliances, political, 532–533
allow-natural-death (AND) orders,
 201–202
alternative and complementary healing
 (ACH)
 compared to conventional and integrative
 practices, 696–712, 697*t*
 defining, 689–690
 holistic approach in, 698–699
 plants as medicine in, 708–709, 708*b*
 self-care in, 701–702
 self-healing and, 702–704
 use of, 690–693, 691*b*
 See also integrative practices
alternative format questions, 781–788,
 783–787*f*
alternative health care. *See* integrative
 practices
altruism, 5, 7–8
always events, 418
ambulatory care centers, 63
American Academy of Nursing (AAN), 421
American Association of Clinical Coders
 and Auditors (AACCA), 765

American Association of Colleges and
 Nursing (AACN), 10, 66, 66*t*, 88
 on the nursing shortage, 508
 on professional standards, 461
 on quality care, 415–416
 transcultural nursing and, 593–594
American Association of Retired Persons
 (AARP), 557
American Bar Association (ABA), 8
American Botanical Society, 713
American College of Healthcare Executives
 (ACHE), 267
American Holistic Nurses Association
 (AHNA), 577
American Hospital Association (AHA), 8
 Blue Cross insurance plans established
 by, 547
American Journal of Nursing, 29, 133, 533
American Medical Association (AMA), 8,
 102, 546, 679
American Medical Informatics Association
 (AMIA), 496
American Nurse, 533
American Nurses Association (ANA), 8,
 10, 29, 64
 on bioterrorism, 738–739
 on bullying, 447
 Code of Ethics, 8, 133, 134, 437–438, 458,
 460, 679–680
 on delegation, 425–426
 entry into practice and, 106
 on health-care reform, 556–557
 on health literacy, 636
 on incivility, 446
 legislation and, 106
 membership, 105–106
 on multicultural content in nursing
 curricula, 606
 on nursing research, 655–656
 political action by, 506–507, 533
 position paper on education for
 nurses, 74
 purposes, 105
 on QSEN-structured curricula, 417
 recognition of forensic nursing, 757
 recognition of nursing informatics, 486
 on staffing, 270, 273
 standards of practice, 106
 on supervision, 427
 on wisdom, 477